NATURAL STANDARD HERBAL PHARMACOTHERAPY

An Evidence-Based Approach

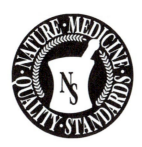

NATURAL STANDARD HERBAL PHARMACOTHERAPY

An Evidence-Based Approach

Natural Standard Research Collaboration
www.naturalstandard.com

CHIEF EDITOR
Catherine Ulbricht, PharmD
Natural Standard Research Collaboration
Somerville, Massachusetts
Department of Pharmacy
Massachusetts General Hospital
Boston, Massachusetts

ASSOCIATE EDITOR
Erica Seamon, PharmD
Natural Standard Research Collaboration
Somerville, Massachusetts

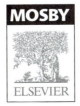

11830 Westline Industrial Drive
St. Louis, Missouri 63146

NATURAL STANDARD HERBAL PHARMACOTHERAPY: AN EVIDENCE-BASED APPROACH 978-0-323-05184-2
Copyright © 2010 by Mosby, Inc., an affiliate of Elsevier Inc.

All rights reserved. No part of this publication may be reproduced or transmitted in any form or by any means, electronic or mechanical, including photocopying, recording, or any information storage and retrieval system, without permission in writing from the publisher. Permissions may be sought directly from Elsevier's Rights Department: phone: (+1) 215 239 3804 (US) or (+44) 1865 843830 (UK); fax: (+44) 1865 853333; e-mail: healthpermissions@elsevier.com. You may also complete your request on-line via the Elsevier website at http://www.elsevier.com/permissions.

Notice

Knowledge and best practice in this field are constantly changing. As new research and experience broaden our knowledge, changes in practice, treatment and drug therapy may become necessary or appropriate. Readers are advised to check the most current information provided (i) on procedures featured or (ii) by the manufacturer of each product to be administered, to verify the recommended dose or formula, the method and duration of administration, and contraindications. It is the responsibility of the practitioner, relying on their own experience and knowledge of the patient, to make diagnoses, to determine dosages and the best treatment for each individual patient, and to take all appropriate safety precautions. To the fullest extent of the law, neither the Publisher nor the Author assumes any liability for any injury and/or damage to persons or property arising out of or related to any use of the material contained in this book.

The Publisher

Natural Standard herbal pharmacotherapy : an evidence-based approach / Natural Standard Research Collaboration; chief editor, Catherine (Kate) Ulbricht ; associate editor, Erica Seamon. — 1st ed.
    p. ; cm.
  Includes bibliographical references and index.
  ISBN 978-0-323-05184-2 (hardcover: alk. paper) 1. Herbs–Therapeutic use. I. Ulbricht, Catherine E. II. Seamon, Erica. III. Natural Standard (Firm)
  [DNLM: 1. Phytotherapy–methods. 2. Evidence-Based Medicine–methods. 3. Herbal Medicine–methods. 4. Plant Preparations–therapeutic use. 5. Plants, Medicinal. WB 925 N2854 2010]
  RM666.H33N387 2010
  615'.321–dc22

2009008616

Vice President and Publisher: Linda Duncan
Senior Editor: Kellie White
Senior Developmental Editor: Jennifer Watrous
Editorial Assistant: April Falast
Publishing Services Manager: Patricia Tannian
Senior Project Manager: Sarah Wunderly
Design Direction: Amy Buxton

Printed in Canada

Last digit is the print number: 9 8 7 6 5 4 3 2 1

Natural Standard Contributors

EDITORS

Glen F. Aukerman, MD
Jason Barker, ND
Ernie-Paul Barrette, MD, FACP
Ethan Basch, MD, MSc, MPhil
Brent A. Bauer, MD
William Benda, MD, FACEP, FAAEM
Deena Beneda-Khosh, ND
Samuel D. Benjamin, MD, MD (H)
Stephen Bent, MD
Lee S. Berk, DrPH, MPH, FACSM, CHES, CLS
Timothy C. Birdsall, ND
Reid B. Blackwelder, MD
Heather Boon, BScPhm, PhD
Thomas Brendler
Stefan Bughi, MD
Mark S. Chambers, DMD, MS
Theresa Charrois, BScPharm, MSc
Richard Philip Cohan, DDS, MS, MBA
William Collinge, MPH, PhD
Julie Conquer, BSc, MSc, PhD
B.H. Cook, MD, PhD
Cathi Dennehy, PharmD
J. Donald Dishman, DC, MSc
John Douillard, PhD
Sarah Elsabagh, BSc, PhD
Joan Engebretson, DrPH, RN
Edzard Ernst, MD, PhD, FRCP
Mitchell A. Fleisher, MD, DHt, FAAFP, DcABCT
Harley Goldberg, DO
Joerg Gruenwald, PhD
Ruoling Guo, BSc MSc PhD
William R. Hamilton, PharmD
Paul Hammerness, MD
Donna Hebbeler, MPH, DrPH
Evelyn Hermes-DeSantis, PharmD, BCPS
Kevin Hoehn, BS, PharmD, MBA, CGP
Charles Holmes, MD, MPH
Karen Hopenwasser, MD
Ioncla O. Hubbard, LAc, MAOM, QME
Paul Ingraham, RMT
Courtney Jarvis, PharmD
Joseph K. Jordan, PharmD, BCPS
Karta Purkh Singh Khalsa, CDN, RH (AHG)
Catherine DeFranco Kirkwood, MPH, CCCJS-MAC
Benjamin Kligler, MD, MPH
David J. Kroll, PhD
Vasant Lad, MASc
Dana J. Lawrence, DC
Zhongxing Liao, MD
Richard Liebowitz, MD
Yanze Liu, PhD
Ann M. Lynch, RPh, AE-C
John S. Markowitz, PharmD
Sonia Elisa Masocco
Jörg Melzer, MD
Jennifer Minigh, PhD
Shri Kant Mishra, ABMS (BHU), MD, MS, FAAN, FIAA
Wadie Najm, MD, MSEd
Carolyn Williams Orlando, MA, PhD candidate
Steven G. Ottariano, BS Pharm, RPh
Todd D. Porter, PhD
Pamela Hemrajani Ramer, DC, PhD[c]
John Redwanski, PharmD
Adrianne Rogers, MD
Aviva Romm, BSc, RH (AHG), CPM
Michael Rotblatt, MD, PharmD
Andrew L. Rubman, ND
Nancy C. Russell, DrPH
Kenneth Sancier, PhD
Elad Schiff, MD
Robb Scholten, MSLIS
David Shannahoff-Khalsa

Hari Sharma, MD, FRCPC
Amy Heck Sheehan, PharmD
Judith Smith, PharmD, FCCP, BCOP
Michael Smith, MRPharmS, ND
Ivan Solà, Bs C
David Sollars, MAc, HMC
Philippe Szapary, MD
Candy Tsourounis, PharmD
René Vega, MD
Andrew Weil, MD
Wynn Werner
Roger Wood, LMT, Dipl. ABT (NCCAOM)
Jay Woosaree, MAg, PAg
Steven H. Yale MD, FACP
Youko Yeracaris, MD
Mario M. Zeolla, PharmD, CPS
Robert Zori, MD

AUTHORS

Clement Abedamowo, MD: Harvard School of Public Health
Lena Abraham, PharmD: Massachusetts College of Pharmacy
Winnie Abrahamson, ND: Private Practice
Tracee Abrams, PharmD: University of Rhode Island
James David Adams, Jr., PhD: University of Southern California School of Pharmacy
Imtiaz Ahmad, MD: Harvard School of Public Health
Qlaitan Akinade, PharmD: Massachusetts College of Pharmacy
Aceele Al-Saleh, PharmD: MCPHS—Worcester
Catherine Armato, BA: Northeastern University
Nicole Armbruester, PhD: analyze & realize ag
Jennifer Armstrong, PharmD: University of Rhode Island
Johanna Assies, MD, PhD: Academic Medical Center, Amsterdam
Rawan Barakat, PharmD: Massachusetts College of Pharmacy
James P. Barassi, DC, DACBSP: Harvard Medical School
Steve Bediakoh, PharmD: Northeastern University
Karl Berger, ABT, LMT: Hvd. Vanguard Altern. Paths to Health
Anja Bevens, PharmD: Northeastern University
Michael Bodock, RPh: Massachusetts General Hospital
Jay Bradner, MD: Brigham and Women's Hospital
Rebecca Bramwell, PharmD: Northeastern University
Ashley Brigham, PharmD: Northeastern University
Larry Callanan, MD: Beth Israel Deaconess Healthcare
Elizabeth Camacho, PharmD: University of Rhode Island
Carolyn Carley, PharmD: Northeastern University
Danielle Carter, PharmD: Massachusetts College of Pharmacy
Franco Casagrande Jr, PharmD: Northeastern University
James Ceurvels, PharmD: Northeastern University
David Chantal, PharmD: Massachusetts College of Pharmacy

Cristina Cho, PharmD: Massachusetts College of Pharmacy
Alice Chung, PharmD: Northeastern University
John Clark, PharmD: Massachusetts General Hospital
Jessica Clubb, PharmD: Northeastern University
Craig Coffenberg, PharmD: University of Rhode Island
Christopher Coleman, RN, ACRN: University of Pennsylvania
Colleen Collins, PharmD: Massachusetts General Hospital
Jeffrey Collins, MD, PhD: Brigham and Women's Hospital
Julie Conquer, PhD: RGB Consulting
Michelle Corrado, PharmD: Harvard Vanguard Medical Associates
Mary Couillard, PhD, RN, FNP: North County Children's Clinic
Renn Crichlow, MD: Harvard Medical School
Michael A. Czerniewski, PharmD: Massachusetts College of Pharmacy
Cynthia Dacey, PharmD: Natural Standard Research
Alicia Dalton, PhD: Harvard University
Sean Dalton, MD, MPH, PhD: University of Cambridge (UK)
Chi Dam, PharmD: Northeastern University
Theresa Davies-Heerema, PhD: Boston School of Medicine
Molly Davis, PharmD: University of Rhode Island
Kamal Dhanota, PharmD: Northeastern University
Diana Do, MD: Johns Hopkins University Medical School
Mary Dulay, PharmD: Northeastern University
Samantha Duong, PharmD: Massachusetts General Hospital
Benjamin Ebert MD, PhD: Harvard Medical School
Antoinette Edmondson, PharmD: Massachusetts College of Pharmacy
Sarah Elshama, PharmD: Massachusetts College of Pharmacy
Edzard Ernst, MD, PhD: Peninsula Medical School, Universities of Exeter & Plymouth
Carla Falkson, MD: University of Alabama
Jennifer Fass, PharmD: Nova Southeastern University
Phillip Fong, PharmD: Natural Standard Research Collaboration
Ivo Foppa, MD, PhD: University of South Carolina
Steve Gabardi, PharmD: Brigham and Women's Hospital
Levi Garraway, MD, PhD: Harvard Medical School
Anait Gasparyan, PharmD: Northeastern University
Cristina Gavriel, PharmD: Massachusetts College of Pharmacy
Gerald Gianutsos, PhD, JD: University of Connecticut
Mary Giles, PharmD: University of Rhode Island
Peter Glickman, MD: Harvard Medical School
Darrick Glidden, PharmD: Massachusetts College of Pharmacy
Michael Goble, PharmD: Massachusetts College of Pharmacy
Juliann Goodfriend, PharmD: Northeastern University
Matthew Greene, PhD: North Carolina State University
Penelope Greene, PhD: Harvard School of Public Health
Jaspal Gujral, MBBS: Medical College of Georgia

Rita Guldbrandsen, PharmD: Northeastern University
Adarsh Gupta, RPh: Children's Hospital
Shlomit Halachmi, MD
Michelle Harrison, PharmD: University of Rhode Island
Sadaf Hashmi, MD, MPh: Johns Hopkins School of Hygiene and Public Health
Ernest B. Hawkins, MS, BSPharm, RPh: Health Education Resources, Inc.
Jamie Hegarty, PharmD: Massachusetts College of Pharmacy
Jo Hermanns, PhD: Naresuan University, Thailand
Quyen Hoang, PharmD: Massachusetts College of Pharmacy
Charissa Hodgeboom, PhD, Lac
Taras Hollyer, ND: Canadian College of Natural Medicine
Kathy Iglesias, PharmD: Northeastern University
Amy Ingargiola, PharmD: Massachusetts College of Pharmacy
Petra Jancar, PharmD: University of Ljubljana
Jason Jang, Bs.C., DC: Palmer Chiropractic West
Sooyoun Kang, PharmD: Massachusetts College of Pharmacy
Sun Kang, PharmD: Northeastern University
Kelly Karpa, BSPharm, PhD: Penn State University College of Medicine
Beth Kerbel PharmD: New England Medical Center
David Kiefer MD, University of Arizona
Helena Kim: PharmD: Northeastern University
Jenny Kim, PharmD: Massachusetts College of Pharmacy
John Kim, PharmD: Massachusetts College of Pharmacy
Eileen Kingsbury, PharmD: University of Rhode Island
Mitchell Knutson, MPH: Harvard School of Public Health
Paul Kraus, PharmD: Northeastern University
Brad Kuo, MD: Massachusetts General Hospital
Grace Kuo, PharmD: Baylor College of Medicine
Ellen Kurek, ELS: Kurek Communications
Emily Kyomitmaitee, PharmD: University of Rhode Island
James Lake, MD: Pacific Grove
Rebecca Lawrence, ND: Lawrence Natural Medicine
Anh Le, PhD: Emory University
Son Le, PharmD: Massachusetts College of Pharmacy
Thuy-Duong Le, PharmD: Oregon State University
Melissa Leck, PharmD: Massachusetts College of Pharmacy
David Lee, PharmD: Massachusetts College of Pharmacy
James Lee, PharmD: Northeastern University
Erik Letko, MD: Massachusetts Eye and Ear Infirmary
Yue-Chiao Liang, PharmD: Massachusetts College of Pharmacy
Nikos Linardakis, MD
Anita Lipke, PharmD: Natural Standard Research Collaboration
Anthony Lisi, DC: Palmer College of Chiropractic West
Garth MacDonald, PharmD: University of Rhode Island
Kerri MacWhorter, PharmD: University of Rhode Island
Martha Maguire, PharmD: Massachusetts College of Pharmacy
Nicole Maisch, PharmD: St. John's University
Keri Marshall, MS, ND: Makai Naturopathic Center
Timothy McCall, MD: Author, *Examining Your Doctor*
Meaghan McGrath, PharmD: University of Rhode Island
Adam McLean, MPharm: University of Nottingham, United Kingdom
Tarek Mehanna, PharmD: Massachusetts College of Pharmacy
Michelle Mele, PharmD: Northeastern University
Victor Mendoza, MD: Washington University Medical Center
Tamara Milkin, PharmD: Northeastern University
Lucy Miller, PharmD: Massachusetts College of Pharmacy
Jennifer Minigh, PhD: Medical Communication Consultants
Arielle Mizrahi-Arnaud, MD: Children's Hospital Boston
Julie Montalbano, PharmD: Massachusetts College of Pharmacy
Timothy Morris, ND: Bastyr University
Audrey Nealon, PharmD: Northeastern University
Jamie Nelsen, PharmD: University of Rhode Island
Ly Nguyen, PharmD: Northeastern University
Phuong Nguyen, PharmD: Massachusetts College of Pharmacy
William Nguyen, PharmD: Massachusetts College of Pharmacy
Katie Nummy, BS: Northeastern University
David Olson, MD: Boston Medical Center
Elizabeth O'Neill, L.Ac.: First Health of Andover
Kimberly Pacitto, PharmD: Massachusetts College of Pharmacy
Regina Pacor, ND, MW: Private Practice
Stephen Papadoulias, PharmD: MCPHS—Worcester
George Papaliodis, MD: Massachusetts Eye and Ear Infirmary
Christine Park, PharmD: Northeastern University
Vrutika Patel, PharmD: Massachusetts College of Pharmacy
Jeff Peppercorn, MD: Harvard Medical School
An T Pham, PharmD: Northeastern University
Cam Pham, PharmD: Massachusetts College of Pharmacy
Linda Poon, PharmD: Massachusetts College of Pharmacy
Jesse Potash, PhD: Massachusetts Institute of Technology
Karen Powell, PharmD
Venessa Price, PharmD: Harvard Vanguard Medical Associates
Swee-Peck Quek, PhD: Harvard University School of Public Health
Victoria Rand, MD: University of California San Francisco
Carol Rainville, ND: Private Practice
Cathleen Rapp, ND
Michael Rashti, PharmD: Northeastern University
Swathi Reddy, PharmD: Massachusetts College of Pharmacy
Celtina K. Reinert, PharmD: UMKC School of Pharmacy
April Reynolds, MS, ELS
J. Daniel Robinson, PharmD: University of Florida
Andrew Ross, MD: Harvard Medical School
Idalia Rychlik, PharmD: Massachusetts College of Pharmacy

Haleh Sadig, PharmD: Massachusetts College of Pharmacy
Ana Sanchez, PharmD: Massachusetts College of Pharmacy
Anabela Santos, PharmD: Northeastern University
Toni Schaeffer, PhD, PharmD: Albany College of Pharmacy
Jana Schipper, PharmD: Massachusetts College of Pharmacy
Lisa Scully, PharmD: Massachusetts College of Pharmacy
Payal Shah, PharmD: Massachusetts College of Pharmacy
Huaihai Shan, Qigong Master, MD: Shanghai University, China
Natalia Shcherbak, PhD: St. Petersburg State Medical University
Elizabeth Sheehan, PharmD: Northeastern University
Scott Shurmur, MD: Nebraska Medical Center
Tina Sindwani, MD: University of Arizona
Charlene So, PharmD: University of Michigan
Carolyn Soo, PharmD: Northeastern University
Anne Spencer, PharmD, BCPS: Medical University of South Carolina
Tera Stock, PharmD: Massachusetts College of Pharmacy
Rebecca Strauss, PharmD: Northeastern University
Kristopher Swinney, PharmD: Massachusetts College of Pharmacy
Isabell Syelsky, PharmD: Northeastern University
Brian Szczechowski, PharmD: Massachusetts College of Pharmacy
Nancy Tannous, PharmD: Northeastern University
Kellie Taylor, PharmD: Northeastern University
Sarah Taylor, PharmD: University of Pittsburgh
Vera Terry, PhD, LLB: Children's Hospital, Westmead, Australia
Amanda Thomas, PharmD: Massachusetts College of Pharmacy
Thu Tieu, PharmD: Massachusetts College of Pharmacy
Natasha Tiffany, MD: Massachusetts General Hospital
Huy N Tran, PharmD: Northeastern University
Nicole Trelour, ND: Symbion Health
Kenneth Triptow, PharmD: Drake University
My Le Truong, PharmD: Northeastern University
Verda Tunaligil, MD, MPh: Harvard School of Public Health
Minney Varghese, BS: Northeastern University
Ruslan Voloshin, PharmD: Massachusetts College of Pharmacy
Dietrich von Stechow, MD: Harvard Medical School
Mamta Vora, PharmD: Natural Standard Research
Kirstin Wadewitz, PharmD: Massachusetts General Hospital
Shannon Welch, PharmD: Northeastern University
Lisa Wendt, PharmD: University of Albany
Deborah Wexler, MD: Harvard Medical School
Peter Wolsko, MD: Harvard Medical School
Denise Wong, PharmD: Northeastern University
Jerod Work, PharmD, MBA: University of Minnesota
Jack Wylie, MD: Harvard Medical School
Xiaoyan Sherry Xie, PharmD: Massachusetts College of Pharmacy
Kui Xu, PhD: Northeastern University
Meng Yeng, PharmD: ACS-Consultec, Inc.
Heeja Yoon, PharmD: Drake University
Monica Zangwill, MD, MPH: Beth Israel Deaconess Medical Center
Robert Zakroff, PhD: University of Rhode Island

RESEARCH TEAM

Kimberly Blozie
Robert Brandon
J. Kathryn Bryan
Dilys Burke
Wendy Chao, PhD*
Candice Clarke
Dawn Costa*
William Gienepp
Nicole Giese
Simon Gorelikov
Regina Gorenshteyn
Dana A. Hackman
Nicole Halpenny
Whitney Hancock
Gabriel Hayes
Elizabeth Helig
Jenna Hollenstein
Kelly Laprade
Emily Marsters
Brian McCarthy
Michelle Nhuch
Nam Nguyen
Michael Richardson
Leigh Taginski
Shaina Tanguay-Colucci
Chris Tonelli
Christine Ulbricht
Melissa Vandawalker
Gabriel Volpicelli
Anja Wallace
Wendy Weissner*
Jen Woods*

*Special Acknowledgment

We are sincerely grateful for the ongoing contributions of Natural Standard's authors, peer reviewers, and editors since the founding of our international research collaboration *(see About Us on www.naturalstandard.com)*. The hard work and dedication of the following content team members deserve special recognition for helping make this particular book available: Wendy Chao, Dawn Costa, Wendy Weissner, and Jen Woods. Additionally, we thank our operational, outreach, member services, and technical support teams, along with our Board of Directors for their ongoing support of evidence-based integrative medicine research.

Preface

Natural Standard Herbal Pharmacotherapy educates readers on the proposed mechanisms of action of herbal products, as well as the safety and efficacy of these products in humans. Natural Standard uses an evidence-based teaching approach that helps students and clinicians practice safe and effective herbal pharmacotherapy to accomplish integrative care—considering all preventative and therapeutic health care options. The text capitalizes on knowledge gained from over a decade of cumulative academic research completed by over 500 contributors to the prestigious Natural Standard Research Collaboration (www.naturalstandard.com). Authors have aggregated, analyzed, and applied evidence-based information to real-life patient care scenarios to facilitate the learning process and practical application in the field.

DISTINCTIVE FEATURES

Natural Standard Herbal Pharmacotherapy was authored by health care professionals and subjected to blinded peer review by multidisciplinary research and clinical faculty at major academic centers to assure quality and eliminate bias.

Unique to this book is The Natural Standard Evidence-Based **Grading Scale** that categorizes the level of effectiveness for each herbal therapy presented based on the available scientific research. Efficacy is graded as strong (A), good (B), or unclear or conflicting evidence (C). Herbs with fair negative evidence (D) or strong negative evidence (F) are also included. This validated and reproducible grading scale consolidates treatment options and the supporting evidence, or comparative effectiveness, which practitioners can use to guide therapeutic recommendations.

The **Integrative Care Plan** provides information on how to assess patients, and includes prevention, diet exercise, and conventional therapies along with evidence-based information surrounding possible herbal therapy treatment options. Health care professionals and students can refer to this section to learn how to counsel patients on herbal therapies with more reliability and confidence than with other commercially available references. Natural Standard is a trustworthy source.

The rigorous **Safety appendix** describes adverse effects and clinically significant interactions between herbs and other botanicals (including plants, fungi, algae, and common constituents), nutrient depletion, prescription and over-the-counter drugs, as well as pharmacokinetics. An additional **Pregnancy and Lactation appendix** contains scientific evidence regarding the safety and efficacy of herbal products in mothers' pregnancy and lactation.

A full-color photo insert, organized by plant species, is included to help identify botanical therapies in the field.

BENEFITS OF USING THIS BOOK

The popularity of herbal products has increased significantly over the last decade. Because of high utilization rates and consumer self-treating, it is critical for all health care providers to have access to exceptional decision support tools. This comprehensive reference provides the standard in evidence-based integrative patient care.

Herbal therapies may be beneficial for many conditions; infact, some herbs are sources of established pharmaceuticals. However, because many herbs contain pharmacologically active constituents, they may also pose health risks similar to conventional therapies. Furthermore, they may interact or potentiate the effects of drugs or other herbs and supplements and cause nutrient depletion. Many software programs used in pharmacies do not yet recognize these interactions (although a growing number of pharmacies are integrating such information thanks to Natural Standard research). This up-to-date teaching text aggregates the available safety data and concisely states the contraindications of each therapy so that users can apply their new-found knowledge to patient care in real time.

This trusted decision-support tool allows practitioners to communicate with their colleagues and patients with confidence about important topics in this emerging area of medicine.

HOW TO USE THIS BOOK

The text is organized by medical condition. Each chapter is divided into the following sections:
- **Learning Objectives**—Help identify goals related to study of the material using a condition-based approach.
- **Overview**—Topics covered include pathophysiology, clinical presentation, and diagnosis.
- **Selected Herbal Therapies**
  - Natural Standard Grade captures the scientific evidence for effectiveness based on available research
  - Mechanism of action
  - Discussion
  - Doses

- **Herbal Therapies with Limited Evidence**—Includes popularly and traditionally used herbs, herbs that have exerted effects but lack high-quality clinical trials supporting use, and herbs studied in combination with other agents, making it difficult to determine which ingredient may offer a beneficial effect.
- **Adjunct Therapies**—Provides herbal, botanical, and supplemental treatments that may assist primary treatments, prevent or treat the side effects of such treatments, or aid potential comorbidities.
- **Integrative Therapy Plan**—Trains students and practitioners in patient assessment and provision of well-rounded, evidence-based medical treatment, including conventional and herbal treatment options plus diet and exercise or lifestyle management techniques.
- **Case Studies**—Illustrate practical application of new-found knowledge to real-life patient cases, using well-designed simulated clinical situations.
- **Herb Tables by Class**—Summarize key information by therapeutic class to help search for treatment options and screen for interactions.
- **Review Questions**—More than 200 review questions with answers incorporated into the text to assess understanding of the information presented in each chapter and the practical application to patient care.

BONUS ONLINE RESOURCES AVAILABLE VIA EVOLVE

Log on to the accompanying Evolve website for these additional resources: References for all chapters and appendices; Traditional Chinese Medicine chapter; Herb Effectiveness by Grade Charts; and scientific animations that show concepts from the book in detail.

ABOUT NATURAL STANDARD

Natural Standard (www.naturalstandard.com) is an international research collaboration that aggregates and synthesizes data on complementary and alternative therapies. Using a comprehensive methodology and reproducible grading scale, information is created that is evidence-based, consensus-based, and peer-reviewed, tapping into the collective expertise of a multidisciplinary Editorial Board. The mission of this collaboration is to provide objective, reliable information that aids clinicians, patients, and health care institutions to make more informed and safer therapeutic decisions. Natural Standard is widely recognized as one of the world's premier sources of information in this area. Additional trusted resources from Natural Standard include: *Natural Standard Medical Conditions Reference: An Integrative Approach* (Elsevier, 2009); *Natural Standard Herb and Supplement Reference: Evidence-Based Clinical Reviews* (Elsevier, 2005); and *Natural Standard Herb and Supplement Handbook: The Clinical Bottom Line* (Elsevier, 2005).

Contents

1 Introduction to Herbal Pharmacotherapy, 1
2 Evidence-Based Integrative Care, 8
3 Psychiatric Disorders, 11
4 Anxiety and Insomnia, 17
5 Depressive Disorders, 29
6 Physical and Cognitive Enhancement, 39
7 Parkinson's Disease, 53
8 Seizure Disorders, 61
9 Pain, 69
10 Alzheimer's Disease and Related Disorders, 86
11 Hypertension, 102
12 Congestive Heart Failure and Diuresis, 114
13 Angina, 127
14 Ischemic Disease and Heart Rhythm Disorders, 134
15 Coagulation Disorders, 155
16 Lipid Disorders, 170
17 Respiratory Disorders, 196
18 Diabetes Mellitus, 216
19 Pituitary and Thyroid Disorders, 241
20 Obesity, 252
21 Menopause, 266
22 Osteoporosis, 281
23 Arthritis, 291
24 Gastrointestinal Disorders, 315
25 Liver Disorders, 343
26 Genitourinary Disorders, 359
27 Bacterial Infections, 380
28 Parasitic and Fungal Infections, 408
29 Viral Infections, 427
30 Cancer, 444

APPENDICES

A Safety: Adverse Effects, Interactions, Pharmacokinetics, 486
B Pregnancy and Lactation, 570

Answers to Review Questions, 593

1 Introduction to Herbal Pharmacotherapy

Outline

TEXT OVERVIEW
COMPLEMENTARY AND ALTERNATIVE MEDICINE
   Background
   Prevalence
DIETARY SUPPLEMENTS
   Herbs
      Forms of Herbs
   Supplements
   Combination Products
   Safety and Purity
   Active Ingredients
   Interactions

REGULATION OF HERBS AND SUPPLEMENTS
   Labeling
   Nutrient Content Claims
   Structure and Function Claims
   Health Claims
STANDARDIZATION OF HERBS AND SUPPLEMENTS
   Third-Party Testing
DOSAGES OF HERBS AND SUPPLEMENTS
EVIDENCE-BASED INTEGRATIVE CARE
PATIENT COUNSELING

TEXT OVERVIEW

Natural Standard Herbal Pharmacotherapy helps educate readers on the important field of herbal pharmacology plus practical application of evidence-based medical care. Healthcare providers and patients can now make rational decisions in this area, considering all therapeutic options beyond just conventional drugs, leading to a whole body integrative health care plan.

The robust chapters are organized by medical condition. Along with disease state information and conventional treatment protocols, potential herbal therapies are investigated. Scientific research on clinical effectiveness, mechanism of action, pharmacokinetics and dynamics, adverse effects, and interactions of herbals are detailed throughout the book. Evidence-based application of these principles occurs through integrative care plans and case-based methods, along with review questions and answers. Additional instructor materials, including a large test question bank and audio/visual slide presentations, are available online, along with reference lists and a teaching curriculum that should be adopted as the standard for university courses on herbal pharmacotherapy.

COMPLEMENTARY AND ALTERNATIVE MEDICINE

Background

The term *complementary and alternative medicine* (CAM) has been variably defined but is generally regarded as encompassing a broad group of healing philosophies, diagnostic approaches, and therapeutic interventions that do not belong to the politically dominant (conventional) Western health system.[1,2] Some authors separately define *alternative* therapies as those used in place of conventional practices, whereas *complementary* or *integrative* medicine can be combined with mainstream approaches.[2,3] Other terms used to refer to CAM include *folkloric, holistic, irregular, nonconventional, non-Western, traditional, unconventional, unorthodox,* and *unproven* medicine.

In the United States, CAM is defined by the National Center for Complementary and Alternative Medicine (NCCAM) as a group of diverse medical and health care systems, practices, and products that are not normally considered to be conventional or *allopathic* medicine.[1] NCCAM classifies CAM therapies into five categories, or domains: *alternative medical systems* (e.g., homeopathic medicine, traditional Chinese medicine), *mind-body interventions* (e.g., meditation, prayer), *biologically based therapies* (e.g., dietary supplements, herbal products), *manipulative and body-based methods* (e.g., chiropractic manipulation, massage), and *energy therapies* (e.g., Qi gong, Reiki).[4]

The term *integrative medicine* is currently becoming more popular and is preferred by innovative academics and practitioners. Perpetuating a multidisciplinary approach to healthcare based on educated safe decisions in this area is a goal of Natural Standard. *Integrative medicine* has been defined by the Consortium of Academic Health Centers for Integrative Medicine as "the practice of medicine that reaffirms the importance of the relationship between practitioner and patient, focuses on the whole person, is informed by evidence, and makes use of all appropriate therapeutic approaches, providers, and disciplines to achieve optimal health and healing."[5] This definition has been adopted by dozens of medical schools in the United States. Integrative medicine calls on conventional, complementary, and alternative medical knowledge to make well-informed, rounded healthcare decisions.

Use of CAM appears to be more common among those with a higher educational level, those with higher income, women, younger persons, those undergoing chemotherapy or surgery, and those with a history of CAM use before diagnosis. Surveys vary in their definitions of CAM and in the specific types of therapy included in questionnaires, complicating the assessment of overall prevalence.

The safety and efficacy of many CAM approaches are not well studied, although the body of research is growing. In 1992 the U.S. Congress established the Office of Alternative Medicine within the National Institutes of Health (NIH) with a budget of $2 million to "investigate and evaluate promising unconventional medical practices." In 1998, Congress elevated the status of the Office of Alternative Medicine to an NIH center, renaming it the National Center for Complementary and Alternative Medicine (NCCAM). The NCCAM budget has progressively increased, from $50 million in fiscal year 1999 to more than $122 million in 2006, advancing its mission to "support rigorous research on CAM, to train researchers in CAM, and to disseminate information to the public and professionals on which CAM modalities work, which do not, and why."

In addition to NCCAM, the National Cancer Institute (NCI) established the Office of Cancer Complementary and Alternative Medicine (OCCAM) in October 1998 to coordinate and enhance the activities of NCI, and to increase the amount of high-quality cancer research and information on the use of complementary and alternative modalities. In 2005, NCI supported approximately $121 million in CAM-related research. This represents more than 400 projects in the form of grants, cooperative agreements, and supplements or contracts.[6] Other NIH institutes also contribute funds to CAM research, with estimates of almost $500 million for all institutes and centers combined.

Prevalence

According to the National Toxicology Program, headquartered at the National Institute of Environmental Health Sciences, over 1,500 herbal products and dietary supplements are currently on the market.[7] Approximately $17.8 billion was spent on dietary supplements in the United States in 2001, of which $4.2 billion was for herbs and botanical preparations. An estimated 44% of the U.S. population used at least one CAM therapy in 1997.[8-11] Findings on Americans' use of CAM were released in May 2004 by NCCAM and the National Center for Health Statistics (NCHS), part of the Centers for Disease Control and Prevention (CDC). The 2002 edition included detailed questions on CAM and was completed by 31,044 adults age 18 years or older from the U.S. civilian noninstitutionalized population. The report found that 36% of adults use some form of CAM. When the definition of CAM is expanded to include megavitamin therapy and prayer used specifically for health reasons, the number rises to 62%.[12]

DIETARY SUPPLEMENTS

The U.S. Congress defined the term "dietary supplement" in the Dietary Supplement Health and Education Act (DSHEA) of 1994 as a product (other than tobacco) taken by mouth that contains a "dietary ingredient" intended to supplement the diet.[13] Dietary ingredients may include vitamins, minerals, herbs or other botanicals, amino acids, and substances such as enzymes, organ tissues, and metabolites. Dietary supplements come in many forms, including extracts, concentrates, tablets, capsules, gelcaps, liquids, and powders. These products often appear on store shelves alongside over-the-counter (OTC) medications, such as aspirin and antihistamines, which are closely regulated by the U.S. Food and Drug Administration (FDA). However, dietary supplements are largely unregulated. DSHEA places dietary supplements in a special category under the general umbrella of "foods," which excludes drugs. It is required that every supplement be labeled a "dietary" supplement.

DSHEA states that "dietary supplements may be legally marketed with truthful and non-misleading claims to affect the structure or function of the body (structure/function claims), if certain conditions are met." Claims may not intend "to prevent, diagnose, mitigate, treat, or cure disease"—lest they be considered as drug claims. Exceptions to this rule are specific health claims for certain foods and supplements that are authorized by the FDA.

Any therapeutic claims (e.g., to treat or cure a disease or condition) will be regarded as a drug claim by the FDA. Drugs cannot be sold in the United States unless rigorous clinical trials have demonstrated sufficient efficacy and safety for FDA approval. If manufacturers of functional foods and dietary supplements make unfounded health claims on labeling or in advertising, they may be disciplined not only by the FDA but also by the Federal Trade Commission (FTC). In 2007, the FTC fined the manufacturers of four weight-loss supplements $25 million for making spurious health claims in advertising.

One problem that complicates and inhibits the regulation of dietary supplements is that it is often difficult to know the active ingredient or mechanism of action of many products. For example, herbal products come from plants, but plants contain many different substances, any of which could be the active constituent. For many substances, researchers have done laboratory and animal tests in an attempt to isolate the active ingredient(s).

The Office of Dietary Supplements (ODS) at the NIH was designed to strengthen the knowledge and understanding of dietary supplements by evaluating scientific information, stimulating and supporting research, disseminating research results, and educating the public to foster an enhanced quality of life and health for the U.S. population.[14] The ODS provides information on more than 2000 brands of dietary supplements, including their ingredients, uses, and manufacturers, so that users can determine the ingredients in specific brands and compare the ingredients in different brands.

The U.S. Department of Agriculture (USDA) provides leadership on food, agriculture, natural resources, and related issues based on sound public policy, the best available science, and efficient management. The USDA has developed the Dietary Supplement Ingredient Database (DSID) that helps monitor the levels of ingredients in dietary supplement products.[15] Natural Standard aggregates data found in all of these and multiple other resources to provide a clearinghouse of integrative medicine information,[16] a subset of which is included in this teaching text.

Herbs

For over 5000 years, since the dawn of Ayurvedic and traditional Chinese medicine, herbs and other natural products have been principal sources of pharmacologically active compounds; in fact, many conventional drugs used today come from natural sources.[16] Aspirin, one of the most widely used drugs in the world,[17] is derived from salicylic acid, a constituent found in the bark of the willow tree (*Salix* spp.) and some other plant species.[16] The narcotic alkaloids found in the latex sap of the opium poppy *(Papaver somniferum)* are used to make drugs in the class known as *opiates,* such as morphine, codeine, and heroin.[7] Metformin, a popular antidiabetic drug and the 11th most commonly prescribed generic drug in the country,[18] is a biguanide derivative of the guanidines found in galega *(Galega officinalis)* and considered to be an "essential medicine" by the World Health Organization (WHO).[19] Other notable herb-based drugs include digoxin (extracted from the foxglove plant *Digitalis purpurea*), paclitaxel (isolated from the bark of the Pacific yew tree *Taxus brevifolia*), and yohimbine (a constituent of the bark of the yohimbe tree *Pausinystalia yohimbe*).[16]

An herb is a plant that may be used for food flavoring or medicinal purposes. The botanical definition of "herb" excludes woody plants, trees, and shrubs; however, some texts may classify woody plant products (such as yohimbe bark extract) as herbs. Non-plants such as algae (e.g., spirulina) and fungi (e.g., shiitake mushroom and red yeast rice) may also be classified as herbs. Regardless of their origin, herbs may be sold in many different forms, including capsules, tablets, tinctures, teas, dried herbs, powders, and creams. Herbs are widely used for health maintenance, disease prevention, and even disease treatment. Herbal supplements have become increasingly popular in recent years, and currently constitute a multibillion dollar industry. Some of the most popular herbs in the United States include echinacea, St. John's wort, *Ginkgo biloba,* garlic, saw palmetto, ginseng (and the unrelated Siberian ginseng), goldenseal, aloe, and valerian.

Forms of Herbs

Tea

A tea is an aromatic beverage of leaves, seeds, or roots prepared by infusion in boiling water.

Decoction

A decoction is the act or process of boiling, usually in water, so as to extract the flavor or "active principle" (the resultant extract). This process is different than making a tea because the fluid is boiled (usually for about 5-10 minutes). Decoctions are taken orally.

Infusion

An infusion refers to an herbal product or tea made by soaking or steeping herbs in hot water to extract the potentially therapeutic properties. Teas are examples of infusions. Delicate parts of the plant, such as flowers or leaves, are most often used.

Homeopathy

Homeopathy is a method of healing in which minute amounts of a substance that causes symptoms in a healthy person are given to a sick person to cure the same symptoms. Homeopathic remedies are thought to stimulate the body's ability to heal itself. Homeopathy also refers to a system of medicine founded by Dr. Samuel Christian Friedrich Hahnemann (1755-1843), based on the theory that large doses of drugs that cause the symptoms of a disease will cure the symptoms when administered in small doses (i.e., "like cures like"). For example, in homeopathy, a substance that causes vomiting when used full strength is thought to cure nausea when used in a very low concentration.

Extracts

Extracts are pills, powders, liquids, or other forms of herbs that contain a concentrated and usually standard amount of therapeutic ingredients. The most common extracts are fluid or liquid extracts, solid extracts, powdered extracts, tinctures, and native extracts.

FLUID EXTRACTS. A fluid extract is a concentrated solution of the soluble constituents of plant drugs, containing alcohol as both a solvent and a preservative, in which 1 milliliter (mL) is equivalent to 1 gram (g) of the original plant material. Fluid extracts are typically hydroalcoholic solutions with strength of 1 part solvent to 1 part herb. However, the alcohol content varies with each product.

SOLID EXTRACTS. A solid extract is a highly concentrated herbal product with a thick, syrup-like consistency.

POWDERED EXTRACTS. A powdered extract is prepared from a native extract by diluting to the specified strength with starch, lactose, or other diluents or with anticaking agents, such as magnesium carbonate, followed by drying, usually under vacuum, to yield dry solids. It is ground into powder to yield powdered extracts or granulated to produce *granular extract*.

TINCTURES. A tincture is a therapeutic solution made by soaking an herb in a mixture of water and alcohol to extract the pharmacologically active constituents of an herbal product. The strength is then noted as a ratio of the percent of herbal product used to the amount of alcohol/water.

NATIVE EXTRACTS. A native extract is a viscous, semisolid botanical extract prepared by removing the solvent from a liquid extract.

Poultices

A poultice is a thick paste of hot, moist herb or a soft mush, prepared by wetting powders or other absorbent substances with oils or water. Poultices are applied directly to the skin to alleviate pain, reduce inflammation, or promote healing.

Essential Oils

An essential oil is a highly volatile, aromatic, concentrated oil extracted from plants. Also known as *volatile oils, ethereal oils*, or *essences*, they can be highly toxic. Therefore, essential oils are usually complex mixtures of a wide variety of organic compounds, mostly volatile terpene derivatives that evaporate when exposed to air. These diluted mixtures may be applied to the skin, sprayed in the air, or inhaled. Massage is a common means of delivering oils into the body through the skin, and is considered the most effective method of delivery of essential oils by aromatherapists. Essential oils can be highly toxic, and should not be taken internally or applied full strength directly on the skin.

Supplements

A supplement can be a vitamin, mineral, or other nutritional ingredient taken in addition to a person's normal dietary intake. Commonly used supplements include multivitamins, chondroitin sulfate, and glucosamine. Supplements are available in many dosage forms, including tablets, capsules, liquids, and teas.

Combination Products

Many OTC products contain multiple ingredients. Sometimes these products are labeled according to the condition they are marketed to treat rather than by their constituents (e.g., Memory Booster, Fat Burner, Immune Support, MenoSupport). Combining ingredients can make it challenging to determine the constituent(s) that may cause positive effects or adverse reactions. Standardization is not always reliable to ensure that constituent amounts and formulations are consistent across (or even within) batches. Nonetheless, it is important to recognize the long tradition of combining herbs in multiple-medicinal systems; therefore this model may require reconciliation with the current Western paradigm of developing and scientifically evaluating agents based on a single active ingredient.

Safety and Purity

The FDA does not function to guarantee the strength, purity, or safety of dietary supplements in the United States. Such responsibilities lie with the manufacturers. As a result, the contents of products may vary from one brand or even one batch to the next. Consumers should review product labels carefully, realizing that inconsistencies have been reported in the scientific literature and by organizations that systematically test the contents of commercially available products. There have been proposals to require that manufacturers regularly evaluate the purity, quality, strength, and composition of their supplements (but not to demonstrate that products are safe or effective).

Active Ingredients

Many herbs and other supplements contain biologically active ingredients. In the same way that prescription and nonprescription drugs act on the body, many herbs and supplements cause side effects and adverse reactions; they may also interact with other medications, herbs, supplements, or foods. The idea that an herb is "natural" does not mean it has no harmful effects on the body. In fact, some common drugs were derived from naturally occurring constituents, such as aspirin from salicylic acid (found in willow bark).

Interactions

Most herbs and supplements have not been thoroughly tested for interactions with other herbs, supplements, drugs, or foods, nor with laboratory and diagnostic tests. Manufacturers of herbs and supplements are not required to do specific testing to discover the adverse effects or interactions of their products. In a survey of the leading 44 pharmaceutical herbal companies published in 2003 in the *Archives of Internal Medicine*, only 15 of these companies responded to a questionnaire about herb-drug interactions. Only three of the 44 companies reported that they conduct studies on herb-drug interactions, and only two stated they allocate funds to such research.[3]

Though many herbs have known pharmacological effects, the fact that they are "natural" has led to a widespread and somewhat ironic notion that all herbs are safe. Rather, adverse and toxic effects have been documented for many herbal products — sometimes due to contaminants, but often due to the constituents of the herbs themselves.[16] Potential interactions between herbs and conventional drugs are also possible,[20] but are often overlooked despite the fact that many herbs not only possess known pharmacological effects but also serve as sources for conventional drugs.[16,21] The classification of herbs as "dietary supplements" rather than as drugs,[22] even when taken for health reasons, has indeed complicated the regulation of herbal products.

REGULATION OF HERBS AND SUPPLEMENTS

Before DSHEA was signed into law in October 1994,[22] dietary supplements were subject to the same regulatory requirements as other foods. Herbal products and other dietary supplements are not regulated as drugs and cosmetics, for safety, purity, or efficacy, under the Federal Food, Drug and Cosmetic Act. Instead, these products are governed by the DSHEA regulations, which are generally less stringent. For example, if a manufacturer of prescription or OTC drugs wants to make a claim about a product's safety or effectiveness, the company must prove the claim to the satisfaction of the FDA before marketing the product. This is not the case with dietary supplements covered by the DSHEA regulations. Topics discussed in DSHEA include product labeling and content, structure/function, and health claims.

Labeling

Dietary supplements have special requirements for labeling. Labels must contain a descriptive name of the product stating that it is a "supplement." Labels must also contain the name and location of the manufacturer, packer, or distributor; a complete list of ingredients; and the net contents of the product. Additionally, each dietary supplement must have nutrition labeling in the form of a "supplement facts" panel and must identify each dietary ingredient contained in the product (Figure 1-1).

Nutrient Content Claims

Nutrient content claims characterize the level of a nutrient or dietary substance in a food product, using such terms as *free, high,* and *low,* or compare the nutrient content to that of another food, using terms such as *more, reduced,* and *light* (or *lite*). For example, a product containing 500 mg of calcium may claim "high in calcium."

Structure and Function Claims

Structure/function claims explain the role of a nutrient or dietary ingredient intended to affect normal structure or function in humans; for example, "calcium builds strong bones." These claims also may characterize the means by which a nutrient or dietary ingredient acts to maintain such structure or function (e.g., "fiber maintains bowel regularity") or may describe general well-being from consumption of a nutrient or dietary ingredient (such as calcium).

Structure/function claims may also describe a benefit related to a nutrient deficiency disease (e.g., vitamin C and scurvy), as long as the statement includes the extent of the disease in the United States. The manufacturer is responsible

Supplement Facts
Serving Size 1 Capsule

Amount Per Capsule	% Daily Value
Calories 20	
Calories from Fat 20	
Total Fat 2 g	3%*
Saturated Fat 0.5 g	3%*
Polyunsaturated Fat 1 g	†
Monounsaturated Fat 0.5 g	†
Vitamin A 4250 IU	85%
Vitamin D 425 IU	106%
Omega-3 fatty acids 0.5 g	†

* Percent Daily Values are based on a 2,000 calorie diet.
† Daily Value not established.

Ingredients: Cod liver oil, gelatin, water, and glycerin.

Figure 1-1 "Supplement facts" panel identifies each dietary ingredient contained in the product. (Available at http://www.cfsan.fda.gov.) (Courtesy U.S. Food and Drug Administration.)

for ensuring the accuracy and truthfulness of these claims; these are not preapproved by the FDA and must be truthful and not misleading. If a dietary supplement label includes such a claim, the following statement must appear on labels:

THESE STATEMENTS HAVE NOT BEEN EVALUATED BY THE FDA. THIS PRODUCT IS NOT INTENDED TO DIAGNOSE, TREAT, CURE, OR PREVENT ANY DISEASE.

Health Claims

Health claims describe a relationship between a food, food component, or dietary supplement ingredient and a health-related condition. Health claims are not about treating, mitigating, or curing diseases. The FDA exercises its oversight in determining the health claims that may be used on a label, or in labeling for a food or dietary supplement, in the following three ways:

1. The 1990 Nutrition Labeling and Education Act (NLEA) provides for the FDA to issue regulations authorizing health claims for foods and dietary supplements, after the FDA's careful review of the scientific evidence submitted in health claim petitions.
2. The 1997 Food and Drug Administration Modernization Act (FDAMA) provides for health claims based on an authoritative statement of a scientific body of the U.S. government or the National Academy of Sciences; such claims may be used after submission of a health claim notification to the FDA.
3. The 2003 FDA Consumer Health Information for Better Nutrition Initiative provides for qualified health claims when the quality and strength of the scientific evidence

fall below that required for the FDA to issue an authorizing regulation.

Such health claims must be qualified to ensure accuracy and non-misleading presentation to consumers. Examples of health claims approved by the FDA include calcium for osteoporosis; dietary fats and cancer; dietary saturated fat and cholesterol and risk of coronary heart disease (CHD); folate and neural tube defects (in pregnancy); fiber-containing grain products, fruits, and vegetables and CHD risk; fruits and vegetables and cancer; sodium and hypertension; dietary sugar alcohol and dental caries; soy protein and CHD risk; plant sterol/stanol esters and CHD risk; whole-grain foods and risk of heart disease and certain cancers; and potassium and risk of high blood pressure and stroke.

According to the DSHEA, the manufacturer of an herbal preparation is responsible for the truthfulness of claims made on the label and must have evidence that the claims are supported by clinical studies. However, no set standard for the evidence is required, and evidence does not need to be submitted to the FDA as does information for drugs.

STANDARDIZATION OF HERBS AND SUPPLEMENTS

The government does not regulate the purity of dietary supplements as it does OTC medications (e.g., pain relievers, antihistamines). Instead, the consumer must rely on manufacturers to ensure the quality and strength of their own products.

Currently, lack of regulation makes it difficult to know whether the consumer is assured of receiving the labeled dosage of a particular product. Clinicians may suggest doses of herbs and supplements based on those most often used in human trials and based on clinical experience. With natural products, however, the optimal doses to balance effectiveness and safety are often unclear because scientific data are lacking, and different products may contain varying amounts of active ingredients in the same reported dose.

Preparation and purity may vary from manufacturer to manufacturer and from batch to batch with the same manufacturer. The effects and side effects of different brands may not be the same because the exact ingredients and manufacturing process may not be the same.

Third-Party Testing

Although many manufacturers of herbs and supplements test the chemical ingredients of their own products, wide variations in quality have been detected when independent laboratories test products. Testing has frequently shown that the ingredients in herbs and dietary supplements often do not match the labels.

Third-party testers include Consumer Labs, Consumer Reports, Natural Products Association, NSF International, and U.S. Pharmacopeia (USP). Consumer Reports, for example, has tested multiple brands of *Ginkgo biloba* and reported that the active ingredients claimed on the label were not always present.

A 2006 test of 10 brands of ginger found substantial brand-to-brand variation in the amount of ginger present in pills.[23] Consumer Reports has tested *Echinacea*, saw palmetto, glucosamine, and chondroitin with similar conclusions. Consumer Labs has also tested numerous herbs, supplements, vitamins, and minerals, reporting variable presence of proposed ingredients.[24] This company provides the names of products that performed better or worse in their testing. However, some third-party testers are paid by some manufacturers for testing, a potential source of bias that has led to some criticisms of possible conflict of interest.

Complicating matters further, herbs have many constituents, and the active ingredients are not always clear. This makes it difficult to determine a standard formula or dose. Given these limitations and that even advertised "standardized" products do not always contain the claimed ingredients when tested, one strategy is to purchase the brand that has been used in positive scientific studies.

The doses provided in this text are based on the best available scientific evidence or on practitioner opinion when research is not available. As the body of scientific data in this area grows and impartial third parties evaluate more products "off the shelf," it may become easier to find reliable brands.

DOSAGES OF HERBS AND SUPPLEMENTS

Healthcare providers are encouraged to suggest doses of herbs and supplements based on those most frequently used in positive human trials substantiated by multiple third-party testers and clinical experience. Again, however, with natural products the optimal dose in balancing effectiveness and safety is often unclear because of a lack of scientific data. Further research is warranted.

EVIDENCE-BASED INTEGRATIVE CARE

Evidence-based integrative care is the application of the best available evidence in combination with clinical expertise in considering *all* preventative and therapeutic options (conventional *and* CAM) to render optimal patient care (Figure 1-2). The practice of *evidence-based medicine* (EBM) has five components: assess the patient, ask clinical questions, acquire the best evidence, appraise the evidence, and apply evidence to patient care.

As the consumer demand for complementary therapy increases, so must the knowledge of the health care professional. Clinicians should apply EBM standards to CAM, leading to a fully integrated whole-body approach. Providers and patients should know how and where to seek reliable CAM information as the processes for locating reliable CAM information often differ from routine strategies. There is abundant misinformation on the Internet, in texts, and anecdotes, and anti-advocacy CAM groups also exist.

An evidence-based approach to CAM includes literature searching and study evaluation. Databases such as Medline may be useful starting points, but are incomplete. Many

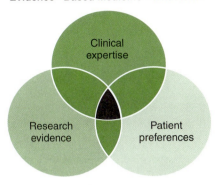

Figure 1-2 Evidence-based medicine. (Modified from Kleinbart J et al: *Introduction to evidence-based medicine.* Available at http://www.slideshare.net/maxedmond/evidence-based-medicine-intro.)

secondary databases have important limitations. A combination approach to searching the literature is often required for CAM and involves the use of specialized databases. The evidence-based integration of CAM also requires strong evaluation techniques. Because of variable study quality, lack of randomized controlled trials, and safety data not systematically evaluated, validated scales are imperative (e.g., *JAMA* guidelines, Jadad scores). Furthermore, there is often conflicting evidence and lack of expert consensus about CAM therapies, so reproducible/validated scales (e.g., U.S. Preventive Services Task Force, ACP-ASIM, McMaster, Natural Standard) should be used as well as multidisciplinary peer review to help eliminate bias.

Thus, a clinical practitioner who wants to integrate evidence-based care must be skillful in information retrieval and evaluation. A basic understanding of research design and statistics, anatomy and pathophysiology, drug and herbal pharmacology, and pharmacotherapy is essential. Natural Standard combines all of this work to save user time and provides trustworthy decision support tools in user-friendly print resources such as this book, online, and for handheld systems.

PATIENT COUNSELING

Studies suggest that many patients do not reveal their use of herbal remedies because of concern about being judged or criticized. Asking patients respectfully about herb and supplement use should therefore be routine when taking a medication history. Clinicians can provide information about recommended doses, frequencies, and specific brand-name products used in clinical trials while helping to avoid adverse effects or interactions, and successfully monitor patient results.

Herbs contain pharmacologically active constituents and may interact with or potentiate the effects of drugs. Clinicians may advise against initiating the administration of multiple herbal preparations simultaneously, or adding such therapies at the same time as starting prescription or other OTC drugs, because this can make it more difficult to determine which specific therapy is effective or harmful.

Many software programs used in pharmacies do not recognize these herb-drug interactions, although a growing number are integrating such crucial information with the help of Natural Standard. Healthcare providers should become familiar with this data to gain the skills and comfort needed to counsel patients and colleagues confidently about the overall safety and effectiveness of herbal pharmacotherapy within an integrative care plan.[25-27]

References for Chapter 1 can be found on the Evolve website at http://evolve.elsevier.com/Ulbricht/herbalpharmacotherapy/

2 Evidence-Based Integrative Care

Outline

NATURAL STANDARD RESEARCH COLLABORATION
   The Authority on Integrative Medicine
   Search Strategy
   Selection Criteria
   Data Analysis
   Review Process
   Update Process
NATURAL STANDARD GRADING SCALE
TEXT CHAPTER OUTLINE

NATURAL STANDARD RESEARCH COLLABORATION

The Authority on Integrative Medicine

Natural Standard is an international research collaboration that aggregates and synthesizes data on complementary and alternative medicine (CAM) therapies.[1] Using a comprehensive methodology and reproducible grading scales, Natural Standard creates systematic reviews that are evidence based, consensus based, and peer reviewed, tapping into the collective expertise of a multidisciplinary editorial board. The mission of this collaboration is to provide objective, reliable information that aids clinicians, patients, and healthcare institutions to make more informed and safer therapeutic decisions. Natural Standard is widely recognized as one of the world's premier sources of information in this area. For further information, see www.naturalstandard.com.

As CAM safety concerns and scientific research volume increases, clinicians and patients are faced with progressively complex therapeutic decisions. These issues, coupled with a growing consciousness among practitioners that many patients use CAM therapies, have created a need for high-quality information services and decision support utilities.

However, rigorous, peer-reviewed, evidence-based resources in this area are scarce. Sources of CAM information often are outdated, rely on anecdotal evidence rather than an evidence-based approach, are not rooted in academic health centers, are not scientifically rigorous, and do not encompass a multidisciplinary approach. In response to this need, the Natural Standard Research Collaboration was formed as a multidisciplinary, multi-institution initiative in 1999. Natural Standard's content and rigorous research methodology are designed to address issues of safety and efficacy that directly pertain to the questions raised by clinicians, patients, and health care institutions, thereby perpetuating open communication and integrative healthcare.

Complementary and alternative medicine is one part of a larger health care context that is becoming progressively integrated. Natural Standard aspires to raise the standards for CAM information, toward improving the quality of health care delivery overall.

Search Strategy

To prepare each Natural Standard systematic review, electronic searches are conducted in several databases, including AMED, CANCERLIT, CINAHL, CISCOM, Cochrane Library, EMBASE, HerbMed, International Pharmaceutical Abstracts, Medline, and NAPRALERT among multiple other resources. Search terms include the common name(s), scientific name(s), and all listed synonyms for each topic. Hand searches are conducted of over 20 additional journals (not indexed in common databases) and of bibliographies from more than 50 selected secondary references. No restrictions are placed on language or quality of the publications. Researchers in the CAM field are consulted for access to additional references or ongoing research.

Selection Criteria

All herbal literature is collected pertaining to efficacy in humans (regardless of study design, quality, or language), dosages, precautions, adverse effects, use in pregnancy/lactation, interactions, alteration of laboratory assays, and mechanism of action (in vitro, animal research, human data). Standardized inclusion/exclusion criteria are used for selection.

Data Analysis

Data extraction and analysis are performed by health care professionals conducting clinical work and research at academic centers, using standardized instruments that pertain to each systematic review section (defining inclusion/exclusion criteria and analytical techniques, including validated measures of study quality). Data are verified by a second reviewer.

Review Process

Blinded review of systematic reviews is conducted by multidisciplinary research-clinical faculty at major academic centers with expertise in epidemiology and biostatistics, pharmacology, toxicology, CAM research, and clinical practice. In cases of editorial disagreement, a three-member panel of the Editorial Board addresses conflicts and consults experts when applicable. Authors of studies are contacted when clarification is required.

Update Process

Natural Standard regularly monitors scientific literature and industry warnings. When new, clinically relevant data emerge, best efforts are made to update content in a timely manner. In addition, regular updates with renewed searches occur every 3 to 18 months, variable by topic.

NATURAL STANDARD GRADING SCALE

Natural Standard evidence-based grades reflect the level of available scientific evidence in support of the efficacy of a given therapy for a specific indication. Evidence of harm is considered separately. The criteria on which each grade is based are specified in the table below.

Natural Standard Evidence-Based Grading Scale™

LEVEL OF EVIDENCE	CRITERIA
Grade A Strong scientific evidence	Statistically significant evidence of benefit from more than two properly conducted randomized controlled trials (RCTs), *or* evidence from one properly conducted RCT *and* one properly conducted meta-analysis, *or* evidence from multiple RCTs with a clear majority of the properly conducted trials showing statistically significant evidence of benefit *and* with supporting evidence in basic science, animal studies, or theory.
Grade B Good scientific evidence	Statistically significant evidence of benefit from one or two properly conducted RCTs, *or* evidence of benefit from one or more properly conducted meta-analyses *or* evidence of benefit from more than one cohort/case-control/nonrandomized trial *and* with supporting evidence in basic science, animal studies, or theory.
	This grade applies to situations in which a well-designed RCT reports negative results but stands in contrast to the positive efficacy results of multiple other, less well-designed trials or a well-designed meta-analysis, while awaiting confirmatory evidence from an additional well-designed RCT.
Grade C Unclear or conflicting scientific evidence	Evidence of benefit from one or more small RCTs without adequate size, power, statistical significance, or quality of design by objective criteria* *or* conflicting evidence from multiple RCTs without a clear majority of the properly conducted trials showing evidence of benefit or ineffectiveness; *or* evidence of benefit from one or more cohort/case-control/nonrandomized trials *and* without supporting evidence in basic science, animal studies, or theory; *or* evidence of efficacy only from basic science, animal studies, or theory.
Grade D Fair negative scientific evidence	Statistically significant negative evidence (i.e., lack of evidence of benefit) from cohort/case-control/nonrandomized trials, *and* evidence in basic science, animal studies, or theory suggesting a lack of benefit.
	This grade also applies to situations in which more than one well-designed RCT reports negative results, notwithstanding the existence of positive efficacy results reported from other, less well-designed trials or a meta-analysis. (*Note:* If one or more negative RCTs are well designed and highly compelling, this will result in a grade of F, notwithstanding positive results from other, less well-designed studies.)
Grade F Strong negative scientific evidence	Statistically significant negative evidence (i.e., lack of evidence of benefit) from one or more properly randomized, adequately powered trials of high-quality design by objective criteria.*
Lack of evidence†	Unable to evaluate efficacy due to a lack of adequate available human data.

*Objective criteria are derived from validated instruments for evaluating study quality, including the 5-point scale developed by Jadad et al.,[2] in which a score below 4 is considered to indicate lesser quality methodologically.
†Listed separately in the Herbs with Limited Evidence section.

TEXT CHAPTER OUTLINE

Most chapters in this textbook include the following sections:
- **Learning Objectives:** These objectives help identify goals related to study of the material.
- **Overview:** Topics covered in this section include signs and symptoms, pathophysiology, and diagnosis.
- **Selected Herbal Therapies:**
  — Natural Standard evidence grade, based on level of available scientific evidence for effectiveness
  — Mechanism of action
  — Pharmacokinetics (see Appendix A)
  — Scientific evidence of effectiveness
  — Dose
  — Adverse effects (see Appendix A)
  — Interactions (see Appendix A)
    - Drug
    - Herb/supplement
    - Food
    - Laboratory (includes nutrient depletion)
- **Other Herbal Therapies:** The herbs in this section include traditionally used herbs, herbs that may have demonstrated proposed effects but lack statistically significant clinical trials supporting efficacy, popularly used herbs that lack scientific evidence, and combination products.
- **Herb Tables by Class:** Tables list herbs by therapeutic class based on proposed mechanism of action, therapeutic, or adverse effects.
- **Adjunct Therapies:** Additional herbal treatments that may be used to assist primary treatments, prevent or treat side effects, or help comorbidities are discussed.
- **Integrative Care Plan:** Patient assessment techniques, lifestyle changes including diet and exercise, and conventional therapies plus evidence-based herbal therapy treatment options are discussed (see sample in box).
- **Case Studies:** Practical application of newfound knowledge to patient cases using real-life clinical situations.
- **Review Questions:** Provided at the end of each chapter to assess learning progress.

References for Chapter 2 can be found on the Evolve website at http://evolve.elsevier.com/Ulbricht/herbalpharmacotherapy/

Integrative Care Plan

- Understand patient's goals.
- Determine concomitant disorders.
- Establish length of symptom presentation.
- Obtain thorough medication history including prescriptions, over-the-counter (OTC) drugs, herbs, and supplements.
- Confirm allergy profile.
- Verify proper dosing.
- Question females to determine if pregnant or breastfeeding or trying to become pregnant.
- Agree to a therapeutic, monitoring, and follow-up plan.
- Advise the patient to take the dosage and frequency that have been studied in clinical trials, tested by third-party testers, and not exceed qualified dosing regimens.
- Counsel the patient, when possible, to use the same brand name product administered in positive clinical trials.
- Recommend standardized preparations that have the name and address of the manufacturer, a lot number, the date of manufacture, and an expiration date.
- Warn against administering herbal preparations to pregnant women, nursing mothers, infants, and children.
- Advise patients who are anticipating surgical procedures to discontinue use of herbs before surgery because of increased bleeding risk associated with many herbs.
- Recommend against the administration of several herbal preparations simultaneously.
- Encourage consulting with a qualified healthcare provider prior to taking herbs with prescriptions or OTC drugs.
- Notify the patient that many interactions and adverse effects of herbal products are not known.
- Urge the patient to communicate his or her therapeutic plan with all of his or her healthcare providers.
- Determine if the condition to be treated requires further professional medical care and make appropriate referrals. Be alert to patients self-treating serious diseases.
- Discuss costs of interventions and insurance coverage.

3 Psychiatric Disorders

Outline

OVERVIEW
    Psychiatric Disorders
        Psychotic Disorders
SELECTED HERBAL THERAPIES
    Betel Nut *(Areca catechu)*
    Coleus *(Coleus forskohlii)*
    Evening Primrose *(Oenothera biennis)*

HERBAL THERAPIES WITH LIMITED EVIDENCE
HALLUCINOGENIC HERBS
ADJUNCT THERAPIES
INTEGRATIVE THERAPY PLAN
CASE STUDIES
REVIEW QUESTIONS

Learning Objectives

- Recognize the signs and symptoms of psychiatric disorders.
- Describe the efficacy of herbal neuroleptics.
- Understand the side effects of herbal neuroleptics.
- Identify potential interactions with herbal neuroleptics.
- Counsel a patient on appropriate and inappropriate herbal treatments for psychiatric disorders.

OVERVIEW

Psychiatric Disorders[1-4]

Psychiatric disorders, also called *psychological disorders,* are conditions that disrupt thinking, feelings, moods, and ability to relate to others (Figure 3-1). The various types of psychiatric conditions may be classified as anxiety disorders, mood or thought disorders, adjustment disorders, developmental disorders, somatoform disorders, dissociative disorders, personality disorders, and psychotic disorders. Psychiatric disorders can occur in anyone, regardless of gender, age, race, ethnic background, or medical history.

Researchers believe a combination of factors, including genetics, brain chemistry, and environmental stimuli (e.g., traumatic events), may lead to the development of mental illnesses. These factors may also determine how the disorders are treated, and how successful a treatment is. Various therapies, including psychotherapy and medications, may help manage symptoms and prevent relapses.

Family, friends, and caregivers may also benefit from *psychoeducation* to help them learn how to cope with the patient's illness. Support groups are also available for both patients and their loved ones.

Neuroleptics are used to treat mental illnesses such as schizophrenia and mood disorders. Mental illnesses are thought to be primarily an imbalance in the brain involving a number of neurotransmitters; thus, many neuroleptics act on the neurotransmitters or their receptors. Traditional neuroleptics mostly have inhibitory effects on dopamine and serotonin receptors.

To maximize the effectiveness of medications, patients with psychiatric illnesses are advised to take medications exactly as prescribed, and to not change or discontinue drug regimens without first consulting their health care providers. Patient noncompliance is a continuing problem in psychiatric illnesses, often because of the inherent nature of these diseases; furthermore, patients may not believe that they are ill.

Psychotic Disorders

Psychotic disorders, also called *psychosis* (pl. *psychoses*), occur when patients are unable to differentiate between what is real and unreal. Psychotic symptoms may include hallucinations, irrational thoughts and fears, disorganized thoughts, and bizarre or inappropriate behavior. Different types of psychotic disorders include schizophrenia, schizoaffective disorder, schizophreniform disorder, and brief psychotic disorder.

The underlying causes of psychotic disorders are not well understood. Schizophrenia affects about 1% of the general population, compared to 10% of those with family histories of schizophrenia. Thus, it is very likely there is a genetic component of schizophrenia and perhaps other psychotic disorders. Chemical abnormalities in the brain may also contribute to the development of psychotic disorders.

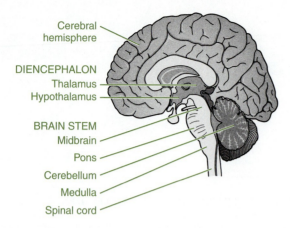

Figure 3-1 Brain and spinal cord (lateral sagittal view). The brain and spinal cord together form the central nervous system. (Modified from Fehrenbach MJ, editor: *Dental anatomy coloring book*, St Louis, 2008, Saunders-Elsevier.)

Signs and Symptoms

Schizophrenia causes patients to suffer from delusions and hallucinations for more than 6 months. *Delusions* occur when patients lose touch with reality. Other common symptoms of schizophrenia include social withdrawal, intense anxiety, feelings of altered reality, loss of appetite, poor hygiene, difficulty processing information, poor memory, depressed mood, and sense of being controlled by outside forces. The behavior of schizophrenic patients varies widely. Men usually develop symptoms of schizophrenia while in their teens or 20s. Women usually develop the disorder between 20 and 30 years of age.

Patients with *schizoaffective disorder* have symptoms of schizophrenia in addition to serious mood or affective disorders (e.g., depression bipolar disorder, or mania). Patients with *schizophreniform disorder* have symptoms of schizophrenia, but unlike schizophrenia, symptoms last 6 months or less. *Brief psychotic disorders* occur when patients have short periods of psychotic behavior, usually in response to stressful events (such as death in the family). Patients usually recover within a month.

Diagnosis

Clinical testing is generally not used to diagnose psychotic disorders. However, patients usually first undergo physical examinations to rule out conditions that may lead to similar symptoms, such as seizure disorders, metabolic disorders, brain tumors, or thyroid dysfunction. A psychological evaluation is then recommended. A mental health professional diagnoses the specific psychotic disorder after reviewing the patient's symptoms and personal and medical history. The *Diagnostic and Statistical Manual of Mental Disorders* (DSM), published by the American Psychiatric Association, contains guidelines used by mental health professionals to diagnosis mental health disorders, including schizophrenia.[4]

SELECTED HERBAL THERAPIES

 Note

To help make this educational resource more interactive, all pharmacokinetics, adverse effects, and interactions data have been compiled in Appendix A. Safety data specifically related to pregnancy and lactation are listed in Appendix B. Please refer to these appendices when working through the case studies and answering the review questions.

Psychiatric disorders are serious illnesses, and an individual should be evaluated by a physician or mental health professional before using any herbal therapy.

Betel Nut *(Areca catechu)*

Grade C: *Unclear or conflicting scientific evidence*

Note: Despite widespread recreational use, betel nut cannot be considered safe for human use, particularly when used chronically or in high doses, because of the documented toxicity associated with acute or chronic chewing and oral consumption.[5, 8-17] See Appendix A.

Mechanism of Action

Arecoline, a constituent of betel nut, has been found to be a potent muscarinic agonist that rapidly crosses the blood-brain barrier and induces parasympathetic effects.[6,7] Such cholinergic effects provide a promising pharmacological explanation and understanding of arecoline's benefits in patients with schizophrenia.

Scientific Evidence of Effectiveness

Two clinical trials reported improvements in betel nut chewers with schizophrenia. Patients scored significantly lower on the positive and negative subscales of the *Positive and Negative Syndrome Scale* (PANSS).[8,9] However, it is not clear from these trials if betel nut chewing was the cause of improved symptoms, or if the patients may have had higher baseline scores on the PANSS.

Dose. Insufficient available evidence.

Adverse Effects, Interactions, Pharmacokinetics. See Appendix A.

Coleus *(Coleus forskohlii)*

Grade C: *Unclear or conflicting scientific evidence*

Mechanism of Action

Schizophrenic patients may have reduced cyclic adenosine monophosphate (cAMP). Forskolin, the major active constituent found in *Coleus forskohlii*, may act as an activator of adenylate cyclase, which directly raises levels of the second-messenger cAMP.[18,19]

Scientific Evidence of Effectiveness
One preliminary study involving five schizophrenic patients found that intravenous forskolin, given in a 75-minute infusion, improved mood.[20]

Dose
The exact dose of coleus for schizophrenia has not been determined.

Adverse Effects, Interactions, Pharmacokinetics. See Appendix A.

Evening Primrose (Oenothera biennis)

Grade D: *Fair negative scientific evidence*
It is believed that the omega-6 essential fatty acid *gamma-linolenic acid* (GLA) is the active ingredient of evening primrose oil (EPO). Membrane phospholipid metabolism may be abnormal in schizophrenic patients; it has been shown that essential fatty acids (particularly arachidonic acid and docosahexanoic acid) in red blood cell membranes are lower in schizophrenic patients relative to healthy control subjects.[21] Thus, it was surmised that boosting the levels of essential fatty acids may help reduce the symptoms of schizophrenia.

Changes in diet, which modify membrane levels of fatty acids, can have significant effects on symptoms of schizophrenia and tardive dyskinesia (involuntary movements). Schizophrenic patients who eat more (n-3) fatty acids in their normal diet may have less severe symptoms. However, clinical evidence thus far does not support the hypothesis that essential fatty acid supplementation, including EPO and fish oil, may benefit schizophrenia. One trial reported no difference in mental status score (PANSS) between EPO and placebo subjects.[21] A double-blind, crossover study found no significant therapeutic effect in 13 schizophrenic patients who received EPO for 2 to 4 months.[22]

HERBAL THERAPIES WITH LIMITED EVIDENCE

Bacopa (Bacopa monnieri)
Bacopa is claimed to be a neuroleptic and psychotropic herb. However, there is a lack of evidence to support the use of bacopa for psychiatric disorders. Beneficial effects may be due to increased cholinergic activity and antioxidant effects.

Chaparral (Larrea tridentata, Larrea divaricata)
Chaparral tea was once used for its purported effects of removing lysergic acid diethylamide (LSD) residue, thereby preventing recurrent hallucinations. The chaparral component nordihydroguaiaretic acid (NDGA) has been evaluated as a treatment for various conditions, including psychiatric and neurological disorders.[1] However, due to risk of renal and hepatic toxicity it is considered unsafe and not recommended for use.

Oleander (Nerium oleander, Thevetia peruviana)
In South China, oleander is used to treat a variety of neurological and psychiatric illnesses. However, oleander ingestion is considered unsafe, and has led to fatal poisonings.[23]

HALLUCINOGENIC HERBS

Note
Not recommended (contraindicated in psychiatric conditions).

Agaric (Amanita muscarina)
Agaric, or fly amanita, has been used traditionally as a hallucinogen. Case reports of hallucinations and delirium exist with agaric use. In near fatal doses, it causes swollen features, high rage and madness, characterized by bouts of mania followed by periods of quiet hallucination.

Angel's Trumpet (Brugmansia and Datura spp.)
Angel's trumpet has been traditionally used for hallucinogenic purposes,[24] and it is increasingly being used by young people as a substitute for the hallucinogen LSD.[25-27] Ingestion of angel's trumpet flowers or tea may result in an alkaloid-induced central nervous system (CNS) anticholinergic syndrome characterized by such symptoms as fever, delirium, hallucinations, agitation, and persistent memory disturbances.[25]

Calamus (Acorus calamus)
Calamus has appeal in the psychedelic realm, stemming from its traditional use among Native Americans as an ingredient of ritual snuff. In 2005, a study reported that calamus was an ingredient of some commercially available products for recreational use as a hallucinogen and/or stimulant.[28]

Damiana (Turnera diffusa)
Turnera diffusa, also known as *Turnera aphrodisiaca*, is commonly marketed on the internet for recreational hallucinogenic effects and purported aphrodisiac effects.[28]

False Pennyroyal (Hedeoma spp.)
American pennyroyal is considered a toxic herb and may cause injury to the brain, kidneys, and liver. Ingestion of pennyroyal oil has led to hallucinations, psychosis, and delirium.[29-31]

Guarana (Paullinia cupana)
The active ingredient in guarana was formerly called guaranine (tetramethylxanthine), but was later found to be caffeine. Guarana has the same stimulatory effect as caffeine and is often used for energy, weight loss, and as an additive to

soft drinks. Guarana is an ingredient in products advertised on the internet for recreational hallucinogenic use.[28]

Kava *(Piper methysticum)*

Kava beverages, made from dried roots of the shrub *Piper methysticum*, have been used ceremonially and socially in the South Pacific for hundreds of years and in Europe since the 1700s. The drink is reported to have pleasant mild psychoactive effects, similar to alcoholic beverages. Recreational use of kava has spread over the last 20 years to Aboriginal communities in Australia, where it is often consumed in combination with alcohol. In 2005, a survey of products sold for recreational use included products containing kava.[28]

Peyote *(Lophophora williamsii)*

Peyote is classified as a hallucinogen and has been reported to induce psychosis.[32,33] The hallucinogen *mescaline* is found in peyote and may have activity similar to LSD.

Salvia *(Salvia divinorum)*

Salvia is a hallucinogenic plant traditionally used by the Mazatec culture in central Mexico.[34] Salvia is grown in California and other parts of the United States, where it is used as a legal hallucinogen and is becoming popular with teenagers and young adults. Laws in Finland, Denmark, and Australia prohibit cultivating, consuming, or dealing with salvia.[35] *Salvia divinorum* has several known constituents, but salvinorin A is usually known as the active component[36] and is selective for kappa(1)-opioid receptors[34,37] Salvinorin A, a neoclerodane diterpene, is a naturally occurring hallucinogen and has been compared to the synthetic hallucinogen LSD in potency.

Yohimbe *(Pausinystalia yohimbe)*

Traditionally, yohimbe bark was used as an aphrodisiac and mild hallucinogen. However, much of the information related to its efficacy is folkloric, anecdotal, or extrapolated from studies of yohimbine hydrochloride.

ADJUNCT THERAPIES

1. Patients with psychiatric disorders such as schizophrenia also experience anxiety and agitation. *Valerian* and *lemon balm* may be used for such symptoms.
2. Psychiatric disorders may also be accompanied by depression. *St. John's wort* is used for depressive disorders and may also provide benefit in anxiety symptom reduction. However, St. John's wort appears to be an inducer of cytochrome P450, and extreme caution is advised with concurrent use of many drugs.
3. Memory impairment has also been reported in patients with psychiatric disorders such as schizophrenia and bipolar disorder. *Ginkgo* may provide benefit for memory enhancement.
4. Dehydroepiandrosterone is an *endogenous* hormone (made in the human body) secreted by the adrenal gland. DHEA serves as a precursor to male and female sex hormones (androgens and estrogens). Initial research reports that DHEA supplementation may help manage the negative, depressive, and anxiety symptoms of schizophrenia.[38] In addition, DHEA may help reduce some side effects of prescription drugs used to treat the disorder.
5. In a double-blind trial of schizophrenic patients, *Ginkgo biloba* was added to the antipsychotic haloperidol (Haldol) and was found to reduce side effects and enhance the drug's effectiveness.[39] More research is warranted to determine *Ginkgo biloba's* role in schizophrenia.

Herbs with Antipsychotic Properties*

HERB	SPECIFIC THERAPEUTIC USE(S)†	HERB	SPECIFIC THERAPEUTIC USE(S)†
Apricot	Psychiatric disorders (neuropsychometric symptoms in AIDS patients)	Ginseng	Psychotic disorders, psychoasthenia
		Gotu kola	Psychiatric disorders
Ayurveda herbs	Psychiatric disorders	Ground ivy	Psychiatric disorders (monomania)
Bael fruit	Psychiatric disorders	Lavender	Psychotic disorders
Bitter almond	Psychiatric disorders (neuropsychometric symptoms in AIDS patients)	Organic food	Psychiatric disorders
		Perilla	Schizophrenia
Chinese medicine	Schizophrenia	Podophyllum	Psychiatric disorders
Devil's club	Psychiatric disorders	Pygeum	Psychotic disorders
Germanium	Psychiatric disorders, schizophrenia	Raspberry	Psychiatric disorders, psychotic disorders
Ginkgo	Schizophrenia	Rhodiola	Schizophrenia

*This is not an all-inclusive or comprehensive list of herbs with antipsychotic properties; other herbs and supplements may possess these qualities. A qualified health care provider should be consulted with specific questions or concerns regarding potential antipsychotic effects or interactions.
†Based on expert opinion, anecdote, case reports, and/or preliminary trial evidence.
AIDS, Acquired immunodeficiency syndrome; *LSD*, lysergic acid diethylamide.

INTEGRATIVE THERAPY PLAN

- Determine if the patient with a psychiatric disorder has had a thorough physical and mental evaluation as well as laboratory workup.
- Identify any potential comorbidities, including substance abuse.
- The pharmacotherapeutic plan should include monitoring for potential side effects.
- Combination treatment strategies may be of value in treatment-resistant patients.
- Strong supportive evidence is lacking for the use of herbs in psychiatric disorders. Adding EPO or making changes in diet to include essential fatty acids may help improve symptoms of schizophrenia and tardive dyskinesia (involuntary movements). However, EPO may lower the seizure threshold and precipitate seizures in patients taking certain drugs (e.g., phenothiazines). Patients should seek medical advice before starting any dietary supplement.
- The patient and the family should be provided psychoeducation, including education about the illness, symptoms, long-term treatment, and methods to improve adaptive functioning.

Case Studies

CASE STUDY 3-1

GT is a 40-year-old man who was recently diagnosed with schizophrenia. His physician calls to tell you that GT does not want to take prescription medication. He asks you if there is an herbal agent that GT can try. How do you respond?

Answer: Theoretically, coleus may be beneficial in schizophrenic patients and may be an herbal treatment option for GT. Explain to GT's physician that forskolin, the major active constituent found in coleus, may act as an activator of denylate cyclase that directly raises levels of second-messenger cAMP. Intravenous forskolin in a 75-minute infusion improved mood in five schizophrenic patients. However, evidence is lacking on the oral use of coleus.

CASE STUDY 3-2

TV is a 35-year-old woman who has a 4-year history of bipolar disorder. Her symptoms are somewhat controlled by lithium carbonate, but she feels very depressed and sometimes anxious. She asks you if there is an herbal therapy she can use. How do you counsel?

Answer: St. John's wort (SJW) is used for depressive disorders and may also provide benefit in anxiety symptom reduction. However, SJW is an inducer of cytochrome P450, and extreme caution is advised with concurrent use of many drugs. The interaction between SJW and lithium is not well understood. If TV is interested in trying SJW, her physician should be notified so that TV's symptoms and lithium levels can be properly monitored.

References for Chapter 3 can be found on the Evolve website at http://evolve.elsevier.com/Ulbricht/herbalpharmacotherapy/

Review Questions

1. There have been case reports of _____ associated with the use of evening primrose oil.
   a. hepatotoxicity
   b. kidney failure
   c. arrhythmia
   d. seizures

2. Which constituent of betel nut has been found to possess cholinergic properties and extrapyramidal side effects?
   a. Arecoline
   b. Tannins
   c. Chavicol
   d. Guvacine

3. True or false: Studies have reported improvements in only negative symptoms of schizophrenia in betel nut chewers.

4. Evening primrose oil has been well tolerated at what dose?
   a. 3 g twice daily for up to 1 year
   b. 3 mg daily for up to 1 year
   c. 3 g daily for up to 1 year
   d. None of the above

5. All the following statements are true *except:*
   a. Patients being treated with drugs such as phenothiazines, which may lower the seizure threshold, should avoid using evening primrose oil.
   b. Based on studies demonstrating abnormal membrane phospholipid metabolism in patients with schizophrenia, it has been theorized that betel nut may play a role in the treatment of schizophrenia.
   c. Betel nut is not considered safe for recreational or medicinal use.
   d. Changes in diet, which modify membrane levels of fatty acids, can have significant effects on symptoms of schizophrenia and tardive dyskinesia.

Answers are found in the Answers to Review Questions section in the back of the text.

4 Anxiety and Insomnia

Outline

OVERVIEW
    Anxiety Disorders
        Signs and Symptoms
        Generalized Anxiety Disorder
        Panic Disorder
        Social Anxiety Disorder
        Posttraumatic Stress Disorder
        Obsessive-Compulsive Disorder
        Phobias
        Diagnosis
    Insomnia
        Signs and Symptoms
SELECTED HERBAL THERAPIES
    Bacopa (*Bacopa monnieri*)
    Borage (*Borago officinalis*)
    Chamomile (*Matricaria recutita*, syn. *Matricaria suaveolens*, *Matricaria chamomilla*, *Anthemis nobilis*, *Chamaemelum nobile*, *Chamomilla chamomilla*, *Chamomilla recutita*)
    Gotu Kola (*Centella asiatica*)
    Hop (*Humulus lupulus*)
    Kava (*Piper methysticum*)
    Lavender (*Lavandula angustifolia*)
    Lemon Balm (*Melissa officinalis*)
    Passion Flower (*Passiflora incarnata*)
    Rosemary (*Rosmarinus officinalis*)
    St. John's Wort (*Hypericum perforatum*)
    Sandalwood (*Santalum album*)
    Valerian (*Valeriana officinalis*)
HERBAL THERAPIES WITH NEGATIVE EVIDENCE
HERBAL THERAPIES WITH LIMITED EVIDENCE
ADJUNCT THERAPIES
    Anxiety
    Insomnia
INTEGRATIVE THERAPY PLAN
    Anxiety
    Insomnia
CASE STUDIES
REVIEW QUESTIONS

Learning Objectives

- Define characteristics of anxiety.
- Discuss herbs that possess antianxiety and hypnotic properties.
- Review data currently available to support herbal treatment selection for anxiety and insomnia.
- Explain mechanism of action, adverse effects, and interactions associated with herbs used for anxiety and insomnia.
- Educate patients regarding an integrative pharmacotherapy plan.

OVERVIEW

Anxiety Disorders[1-3]

Anxiety is a complex and unpleasant feeling of nervousness, fear, and worry; it is often accompanied by physical sensations such as heart palpitations, nausea, angina, shortness of breath, and tension headaches.

Anxiety disorders affect about 40 million Americans over the age of 18 each year. Only about one third of persons with anxiety disorders receive treatment, yet they are reported to account for annual treatment costs of more than $42 billion in the United States. Unlike the relatively mild, brief anxiety that is normal in stressful events (e.g., testing, job interview, death of a loved one, public performance/speaking), anxiety disorders last at least 6 months and can worsen if untreated.

Anxiety disorders often occur in conjunction with other mental or physical illnesses (e.g., alcohol/substance abuse, depression, bipolar illness), which may mask or worsen anxiety symptoms.

Types of anxiety disorders include generalized anxiety disorder, obsessive-compulsive disorder, panic attack/panic disorder, posttraumatic stress disorder, phobias, separation anxiety, and social anxiety/social phobia. Individuals with anxiety disorders are three to five times more likely to seek medical treatment and six times more likely to be hospitalized for psychiatric disorders than those without anxiety disorders.

Sympathetic nervous system activation occurs with anxiety, resulting in increased neuron firing and release of neurotransmitters (e.g., epinephrine, norepinephrine). The sympathetic nervous system is primarily responsible for "fight or flight" responses as well as the symptoms typically seen in anxiety

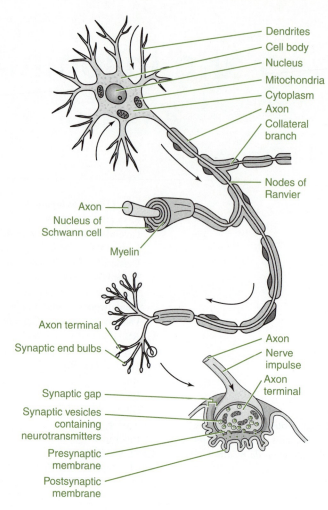

Figure 4-1 A typical neuron. (Modified from Salvo S: *Massage therapy: principles and practice*, ed 2, St Louis, 2003, Saunders-Elsevier.)

disorders. *Gamma-aminobutyric acid* (GABA) and *glutamate* play major roles in the control of neuron signal conduction (Figure 4-1). GABA is an inhibitory neurotransmitter, and glutamate is an excitatory neurotransmitter; an increase or decrease in either will result in a complementary response based on the action of GABA or glutamate. Anxiolytic (antianxiety) and hypnotic drugs and herbs are central nervous system (CNS) depressants, and reduce neuronal firing to exert sedative and tranquilizing effects.

Signs and Symptoms

The primary symptoms of anxiety disorders are driven by cognitive and emotional components that produce fear, apprehension, and worry. However, anxiety disorders are also characterized by other emotional and physical symptoms.

Physical Symptoms

Many physical symptoms of anxiety disorders are cardiopulmonary, including heart palpitations, angina, and shortness of breath. These may lead to hot flashes or chills, cold and clammy hands, and sweating. Gastrointestinal symptoms of anxiety may include stomach upset, nausea or queasiness, diarrhea, or constipation. Other common symptoms include frequent urination, vertigo, tremors, muscle tension or aches, fatigue, and insomnia.

Emotional or Psychological Symptoms

Emotional or psychological symptoms of anxiety disorders can include feelings related to nervousness, such as uneasiness, restlessness, and jumpiness. Feelings of anxiety may also be related to fear—such as apprehension, avoidance, dread, nightmares, fear of dying or "going crazy," self-consciousness, insecurity, and a strong desire to escape. Concentration may be impaired, and anxiety patients may have confusion or selective attention. Behavioral problems are common, especially in children and adolescents.

Generalized Anxiety Disorder

Specific symptoms for generalized anxiety disorder (GAD) include chronic exaggerated worry, tension, and irritability; these appear to have no cause or are more intense than warranted by various situations. Physical signs (e.g., restlessness, trouble falling or staying asleep, headaches, trembling, twitching, muscle tension, sweating) often accompany these psychological symptoms.

Panic Disorder
Panic disorders are characterized by recurrent severe panic attacks. Physical symptoms include heart palpitations, angina, shortness of breath, lightheadedness or dizziness, nausea, hot flashes or chills, sweating, shaking or trembling, choking, numbness, or tingling. Emotions include feelings of imminent danger, fear of dying, feelings of unreality, and feelings of going crazy. Because many of the symptoms of panic disorder mimic those found in other conditions (such as heart disease, thyroid problems, and breathing disorders), people with panic disorder frequently seek medical attention, convinced they have life-threatening illnesses.

Social Anxiety Disorder
Specific symptoms of social anxiety disorder (SAD) include blushing, sweating, trembling, nausea, rapid heartbeat, dizziness, and headaches. Some people with SAD may have intense fears of a specific social or performance situation (e.g., giving speeches, talking to salespersons, making phone calls) but may be perfectly comfortable in other social settings. Others may have a more generalized form of SAD, manifesting as anxiety in a variety of routines, clinging behavior, and throwing tantrums.

Posttraumatic Stress Disorder
Posttraumatic stress disorder (PTSD) is a type of anxiety that occurs after a physically or emotionally traumatic event. Situations reminiscent of the traumatic event may provoke intense distress or even panic attacks. PTSD is characterized by three major types of symptoms: (1) re-experiencing the trauma through intrusive and distressing recollections of the event (flashbacks) and nightmares; (2) emotional numbness and avoidance of anything (places, people, or activities) reminiscent of the trauma; and (3) increased irritability (e.g., difficulty sleeping and concentrating, feeling jumpy, and easily becoming angered).

Obsessive-Compulsive Disorder
Obsessive-compulsive disorder (OCD) manifests as recurrent and persistent thoughts, impulses, or images that are intrusive and cause significant distress and anxiety. A common obsession of OCD patients is a constant, irrational worry about dirt, germs, or contamination. Other common emotions are feelings that something bad will happen if certain items are not in an exact place, position, or order. OCD patients may fear that their negative or blasphemous thoughts or images will cause personal harm or harm to loved ones; they may also ruminate about accidentally or purposely injuring other people. In OCD, it is also common to be preoccupied with losing objects with little or no value. Persons with OCD usually recognize that their obsessions are not based in reality and are indeed irrational.

To decrease the anxiety that results during these irrational thoughts and images, people with OCD typically perform repetitive behaviors or mental acts called *compulsions*. Some common compulsions, which typically are linked to particular obsessions, include repeatedly bathing, washing the hands, or cleaning household items for hours at a time. Compulsions may manifest in constantly checking and rechecking (several to hundreds of times per day) to make sure doors are locked, stoves are turned off, and appliances are unplugged. OCD patients may seem unable to stop repeating names, phrases, or tunes. They often exhibit excessive, methodical, and painstakingly slow approaches to daily activities. Hoarding is another common OCD behavior, and involves saving common or useless items (e.g., old newspapers or magazines, bottle caps, rubber bands).

Because they may consume many hours of each day, obsessions and rituals can substantially interfere with normal routines, schoolwork, jobs, families, or social activities. Children can also have OCD, but unlike adults, they often do not realize that their obsessions and compulsions are excessive and ritualistic.

Phobias
Specific phobias are characterized by strong, irrational, and involuntary reactions to particular objects, places, or situations. These phobias lead people with phobias to dread confronting common, everyday situations; alternatively, they may avoid certain situations altogether, even though there may be no logical or conscious threat of danger. Some typical phobias include fear of heights, flying in airplanes, public transportation, confined spaces, or elevators. Other common phobias include fear of certain animals (such as insects, spiders, or snakes), fear of dental procedures, and fear of thunder. People with phobias generally acknowledge that their fears are unfounded; however, they will continue to avoid the objects of their phobias at all costs. When confronted with feared situations or objects, people with phobias may even have panic attacks.

Diagnosis
The *Diagnostic and Statistical Manual of Mental Disorders*, (DSM) published by the American Psychiatric Association, contains guidelines used to diagnose mental health disorders (including anxiety) in both children and adults.

Insomnia
Insomnia may involve difficulty falling asleep, difficulty staying asleep, or waking up too early in the morning. It is a common health problem that can cause excessive daytime sleepiness and lack of energy.[4-10] Up to 25% of Americans report occasional sleeping problems, and insomnia is chronic in about 10% of people.[11] According to the pharmaceutical consulting company IMS Health, consumers spent $3.6 billion on prescription sleep medications in 2006.[12] Those suffering from insomnia may feel tired, depressed, or irritable. They may also have trouble paying attention, learning, and remembering; they may not be able to perform fully on the job or at school. Severe insomnia can result in neurochemical changes, which may cause further problems such as depression and anxiety. Insomnia may be

classified as *transient* (occasional), *mild,* or *severe,* depending on how often and for how long it occurs. Insomnia that lasts for less than a month is known as short-term (or *acute*) insomnia. *Chronic* insomnia is defined as having symptoms at least three nights per week for more than a month.

Insomnia is a component of most common psychological problems, including anxiety, stress, and depression. In fact, insomnia may be an indicator of depression. Many people will have insomnia during the more severe phases of a mental illness, such as in mania of bipolar disorder.

Medical conditions can also cause insomnia. These include chronic pain (e.g., arthritis, fibromyalgia, cancer), sleep apnea, enlarged prostate, cystitis (common in women), overactive thyroid, congestive heart failure (CHF), gastroesophageal reflux disease (GERD, heartburn), chronic obstructive pulmonary disease (COPD), gastrointestinal disorders (e.g., diarrhea, ulcers, irritable bowel syndrome), and neurological disorders (e.g., Alzheimer's, Parkinson's).

Certain prescription and nonprescription medications may also cause acute or chronic insomnia. If the insomnia is related to a medication side effect, a normal sleep/wake pattern should be achieved shortly after discontinuing the medication. A variety of drugs with stimulant properties can cause insomnia, including pseudoephedrine, beta-2 agonists (bronchodilators), decongestants, theophylline, antidepressants, and thyroid medications. Caffeine, alcohol, and nicotine may also contribute to insomnia by altering brain chemistry, thereby disrupting the normal sleep/wake cycle. The abrupt discontinuation of alcohol in chronic users can also contribute to insomnia. Similarily, abrupt cessation of some medications (e.g., sleeping pills, hypnotics, antianxiety drugs, antidepressants) can also cause acute insomnia.

Signs and Symptoms

The main signs and symptoms of insomnia revolve around difficulty sleeping. This may involve having trouble falling asleep, or waking up often or too early. Insomnia is typically, followed by a distinct feeling of fatigue (tiredness) the following day. Most often, daytime symptoms will bring people to seek medical attention. Daytime problems caused by insomnia include anxiousness, irritability, fatigue, poor concentration and focus, impaired memory or motor coordination and impaired social interaction. Motor vehicle accidents have been attributed to fatigued, sleep-deprived drivers.

SELECTED HERBAL THERAPIES

Note

To help make this educational resource more interactive, all pharmacokinetics, adverse effects, and interactions data have been compiled in Appendix A. Safety data specifically related to pregnancy and lactation are listed in Appendix B. Please refer to these appendices when working through the case studies and answering the review questions.

Bacopa *(Bacopa monnieri)*

Grade C: *Unclear or conflicting scientific evidence*

Mechanism of Action

The exact mechanism by which bacopa reduces anxiety is not well understood.

Scientific Evidence of Effectiveness

Bacopa is commonly called "brahmi" and is used in the Ayurvedic system of medicine in India. One study reported a significant improvement in 35 patients with anxiety who took bacopa syrup for 1 month.[13] Anxiety symptoms were evaluated 2 and 4 weeks after the start of bacopa treatment, and observation of clinical relief was based on improvement of symptoms such as nervousness, palpitation, insomnia, headache, lack of concentration, fatigue/exhaustion, anorexia, tremors, dyspepsia/flatulence, and irritability. Physiological changes associated with bacopa treatment included decreased anxiety, adjustment, disability levels, and mental fatigue rate. Physiological changes associated with treatment involved the pulse rate, blood pressure, body weight, rate of respiration, and breath-holding time.

Dose

A dose of 30 milliliters (mL) of bacopa syrup daily, representing 12 grams (g) of dry crude extract, has been used for 1 month in patients with anxiety.[13]

Adverse Effects, Interactions, Pharmacokinetics. See Appendix A.

Borage *(Borago officinalis)*

Grade C: *Unclear or conflicting scientific evidence*

Mechanism of Action. Insufficient available evidence.

Scientific Evidence of Effectiveness

Borage *(Borago officinalis)* is an herb native to Syria that has spread throughout the Middle East and Mediterranean. Borage seeds are often pressed to produce oil very high in gamma-linolenic acid (GLA). Clinical evidence suggests that borage oil decreases cardiovascular reactivity to acute stress.[14]

Dose. Insufficient available evidence.

Adverse Effects, Interactions, Pharmacokinetics. See Appendix A.

Chamomile *(Matricaria recutita,* syn. *Matricaria suaveolens, Matricaria chamomilla, Anthemis nobilis, Chamaemelum nobile, Chamomilla chamomilla, Chamomilla recutita)*

Grade C: *Unclear or conflicting scientific evidence*

Mechanism of Action

The sedative action of chamomile remains unclear. In one mouse model it was suggested that the apigenin flavonoid component of chamomile is a ligand for benzodiazepine receptors, and thus exerts slight sedative effects.[15]

Scientific Evidence of Effectiveness

In the United States, chamomile is most widely found in herbal tea preparations, and used as a mild sedative. Many practitioners believe that chamomile possesses calming properties, and it is frequently consumed with this intention. However, limited evidence supports the use of chamomile for sedation. In a case series examining the cardiac effects of chamomile, 10 of 12 patients undergoing cardiac catheterization fell asleep shortly after drinking chamomile tea.[16]

Dose

Most American chamomile products are not standardized to any particular constituent. Many German chamomile products, such as Kamillosan (20 mg of chamomile essential oil per 100 g of cream), are standardized to minimum values of the constituents chamazulene and alpha-bisobolol. Tablets and capsules of chamomile may be standardized to contain 1.2% apigenin and 0.5% essential oil per dose. For sedation, doses (based on herbal and folkloric medicine) have included 3 cups of tea daily, or 1 to 4 mL of tincture three times daily. One to 4 cups of tea daily (or as needed) may also be used.

Adverse Effects, Interactions, Pharmacokinetics. See Appendix A.

Gotu Kola (Centella asiatica)

Grade C: *Unclear or conflicting scientific evidence*

Mechanism of Action

The exact mechanism by which gotu kola may reduce anxiety is unclear. Intraperitoneal administration in rodents has been shown to produce CNS depression and increased sleeping time after giving hexobarbital, a barbiturate with sedative-hypnotic properties, possibly through a cholinergic mechanism.[17]

Scientific Evidence of Effectiveness

In the traditional Indian system of Ayurvedic medicine, gotu kola is believed to develop the *crown chakra,* or the energy center at the top of the head, and to balance the right and left hemispheres of the brain. It has traditionally been used by yogis as a food for meditation. Animal research has demonstrated anxiolytic properties of gotu kola.[18,19] In one randomized controlled trial (RCT), subjects received a single 12-g dose of gotu kola, mixed with 300 mL of grape juice, or placebo.[20] At 30 and 60 minutes after ingestion, the group who received gotu kola experienced a significant decrease in the acoustic startle response compared to the placebo group.

Dose

A dose of 12 g of gotu kola in grape juice was used in one clinical study to relieve anxiety[20]; however, doses of 120 milligrams (mg) daily have also been used.[21]

Adverse Effects, Interactions, Pharmacokinetics. See Appendix A.

Hop (Humulus lupulus)

Grade C: *Unclear or conflicting scientific evidence*

Mechanism of Action

Mouse models have found hop to have sedative, hypnotic, hypothermic, antinociceptive, and anticonvulsant properties.[22] In vivo, the 2-methyl-3-butene-2-ol in the volatile fraction has been identified as a principal sedative-hypnotic constituent of hop.[23] In fresh hop there are only traces of this constituent, but the concentration of 2-methyl-3-butene-2-ol has been shown to increase continuously after drying, reaching maximum levels (~0.15%) within 2 years of storing at room temperature (18°-24° C or 64.4°-75.2° F).

Scientific Evidence of Effectiveness

Plants in the Cannabacea family, including hop, have been traditionally used for relaxation, sedation, and to treat insomnia. A number of methodologically weak human trials have investigated hop in combination with valerian *(Valeriana officinalis)* for the treatment of sleep disturbances, and several animal studies have examined the sedative properties of hop monotherapy.[22] Improved subjective sleep parameters and quality of life have been noted in studies examining hop in combination with valerian.[24,25]

Dose

Two tablets of standardized extracts of a valerian (187 mg) and hop (41.9 mg) combination for 28 days improved subjective sleep parameters.[24,25]

Adverse Effects, Interactions, Pharmacokinetics. See Appendix A.

Kava (Piper methysticum)

Grade A: *Strong scientific evidence*

Kava is a shrub from the South Pacific islands that has been used for centuries to produce calming effects in humans. Currently, pharmaceutical preparations of the herb are widely used in Europe and the United States as anxiolytics; however, kava has been withdrawn from markets in several countries because of safety concerns about liver toxicity.[26-32]

Mechanism of Action

Kavapyrones, the active substances found in kava, have been indicated in depression of the limbic system, a set of brain structures implicated in the control of emotional processes. As a result, the kavapyrones in kava may cause the suppression of various moods and emotional states.[33] Kavapyrones may potentiate the binding of GABA-A receptors and increase the number of GABA binding sites.[34] Additionally, the blockade of voltage-gated cation channels may depress neuronal function and cause sedation.[35]

Scientific Evidence of Effectiveness

Short-term use (<1-2 months) of kava may be beneficial in patients with mild to moderate anxiety disorders; it may also provide relief to patients with sleep disorders associated with anxiety.[36] The effects of kava for generalized anxiety disorders and chronic anxiety is equivocal.[37] Kava may offer similar symptom relief as observed with prescribed benzodiazepine drugs, such as diazepam (Valium).[38,39] In one clinical trial, kava's effects were reported to be similar to buspirone (Buspar), which is used for generalized anxiety disorder.[40] Kava extracts standardized to 70% kavalactones appear to be superior to placebo for the treatment of anxiety.[38,41-44]

Dose

For anxiety disorders, most clinical trials have used 105 to 210 milligrams (mg) of kavalactones (standardized to 70% kavalactones) for less than 4 weeks.[38,41-44] Most clinical trials have used the German kava extract WS 1490. Manufacturers typically recommend 150 to 300 mg, once to three times daily as needed for anxiety.

Adverse Effects, Interactions, Pharmacokinetics. See Appendix A.

Lavender (*Lavandula angustifolia*)

Grade B: *Good scientific evidence*

Mechanism of Action

Linalool, a constituent of lavender, has been shown to reduce motor activity in mice because of a dose-related binding to glutamate, a primary excitatory neurotransmitter of the central nervous system. The hypnotic effects of lavender may be caused by the potentiation of the neurotransmitter GABA.[45]

Scientific Evidence of Effectiveness

In general, the evidence supporting lavender aromatherapy and topically applied lavender as an anxiolytic is weak; however some research suggests a small positive effect in relieving anxiety.[46-50] In one study, intensive care unit patients massaged with lavender reported less anxiety after the session.[48] Lavender aromatherapy was also noted to decrease anxiety as measured by the *Hamilton Anxiety Scale* (HAM-A), which quantifies the severity of anxiety symptoms, in chronic renal failure patients receiving hemodialysis.[49] However, the inherent difficulties in designing blinded or placebo-controlled studies of an olfactory therapy must be overcome before compelling results can be generated. Additionally, many experts and patients believe that lavender aromatherapy is an effective hypnotic. When aromatherapeutic lavender was compared as an alternative to conventional hypnotics (temazepam, promazine, chlormethiazole), geriatric patients reported similar sleep times with the lavender aromatherapy treatment compared to conventional oral hypnotics.[39]

Dose

Lavender products are not standardized in the United States; each species of lavender has unique chemical constituents and activity. The flowers are the part of lavender most often used medicinally. The exact dose of lavender for anxiety has not been determined. Lavender oil has been used for massage or in hot baths.[47,49,50,52,53] For massage, 1 to 4 drops per tablespoon of base oil may be used. Aromatherapy typically involves adding 2 to 4 drops into 2 to 3 cups of boiling water, followed by inhalation of the vapors. Aromatherapy can be administered intermittently or daily as needed.

Adverse Effects, Interactions, Pharmacokinetics. See Appendix A.

Lemon Balm (*Melissa officinalis*)

Grade C: *Unclear or conflicting scientific evidence*

Mechanism of Action

In animal studies, lemon balm extract was reported to have calming effects;[54] however, the exact mechanism by which lemon balm exerts its calming effects is not known. An ethanolic extract of lemon balm was tested for affinity to the GABA-A–benzodiazepine site, and moderate activity was reported.[55]

Scientific Evidence of Effectiveness

In a randomized, placebo-controlled trial, subjects were given a combination product (27 mg lemon balm, 36 mg orange peel, 16 mg cinnamon, and 4 mg myristica in 5 mL) at a dose of 0.23 mL per kilogram (kg) body weight three times daily for 8 weeks, resulting in relief of symptoms associated with anxiety.[56] Significant differences between the treatment group and the placebo group were reported for the dimensions of nervousness and excitability; however, because this study used a combination product, the exact role of lemon balm in reducing anxiety remains unclear. A combination product of lemon balm (80 mg) and valerian (160 mg) was found to be superior to placebo in relieving insomnia in a double-blind trial.[57] Although these results appear promising, studies evaluating lemon balm monotherapy are warranted.

Dose

The amount of essential oil that can be obtained from lemon balm leaves can range from 0.08 to 0.25 mL/100 g, and from the herb, 0.06 to 0.167 mL/100 g.[58] The content and quality of essential oils from lemon balm may also differ, depending on the height and location of the harvest cut of a particular plant, the vegetation period of the plant, and between different populations of the plant. For example, the oil content in lemon balm appears to be highest in the top third of the plant, and the percentage of the constituents may be highest when the plant is cut in the basipetal direction (from top to base).[58-65] Clinical trial data suggest that different preparations of lemon balm may result in products that exhibit different properties depending on the process used for the sample preparation.[66]

Adverse Effects, Interactions, Pharmacokinetics. See Appendix A.

Passion Flower *(Passiflora incarnata)*

Grade C: Unclear or conflicting scientific evidence

Mechanism of Action

Chrysin, a flavonoid found in passion flower, has demonstrated antianxiety effects and altered benzodiazepine receptor binding.[67-60]

Scientific Evidence of Effectiveness

Passion flower has traditionally been used by Native South Americans as a mild sedative. In a small pilot study of 36 patients, passion flower was shown to be as effective as oxazepam in treating generalized anxiety disorder.[70] Other studies have evaluated passion flower in combination with other agents, which makes it difficult to extrapolate to its use as monotherapy.[71,72]

Adverse Effects, Interactions, Pharmacokinetics. See Appendix A.

Rosemary *(Rosmarinus officinalis)*

Grade C: Unclear or conflicting scientific evidence

Mechanism of Action

The exact mechanism by which rosemary reduces anxiety and improves alertness has not been completely elucidated; however, one study investigated the effects of rosemary aromatherapy on alertness and electroencephalogram (EEG) activity and found that patients showed decreased frontal alpha and beta power that suggested increased alertness.[73] Patients also had lower state anxiety scores, reported feeling more relaxed and alert, and they were faster (but not more accurate) at completing the math computations after the aromatherapy session.

Scientific Evidence of Effectiveness

Rosemary extract is frequently used in aromatherapy for treatment of a variety of conditions, including anxiety, mood enhancement, and alteration of pain perception, as well as to increase alertness. In two aromatherapy studies, rosemary alone and in combination with lavender and peppermint was reported to decrease stress levels and increase alertness.[74,75] Rosemary extract was reported to be more beneficial in reducing "confusion and bewilderment" than lavender.

Dose

There is no standardization widely used for extract of rosemary. The active ingredients are thought to be caffeic acid and its derivatives, including rosmarinic acid. Rosemary aromatherapy has been studied for its effects on anxiety; however, no effective standard dose has been determined.

Adverse Effects, Interactions, Pharmacokinetics. See Appendix A.

St. John's Wort *(Hypericum perforatum)*

Grade C: Unclear or conflicting scientific evidence

Mechanism of Action

Evidence from animal research suggests that the total extract of *Hypericum perforatum* affects exploratory behavior and exerts anxiolytic effects in rats.[76] In this study the anxiolytic activity of total *H. perforatum* extract was blocked before treatment with the benzodiazepine antagonist flumazenil, suggesting that the anxiolytic effects of St. John's wort may be caused by benzodiazepine receptor activation. Hypericin, the main constituent of *H. perforatum*, reduced the GABA-activated chloride currents, whereas administration of pseudohypericin (another constituent of *H. perforatum*) resulted in an opposite effect, and GABA-activated chloride currents were increased. Furthermore, both hypericin and pseudohypericin were shown to inhibit the activation of *N*-methyl-D-aspartate (NMDA) receptors.[76]

Scientific Evidence of Effectiveness

Extracts of St. John's wort have been traditionally used for a wide range of medical conditions. The most common modern-day application of St. John's wort is the treatment of depressive disorders. Some studies of depression have reported benefit in anxiety symptom reduction.[77,78] Case reports have shown St. John's wort to improve DSM-defined generalized anxiety disorder.[79]

Dose

A dose of 900 mg of St. John's wort (standardized to 0.3% hypericin) once or twice daily for 2 to 4 weeks has been used in patients with DSM-defined generalized anxiety disorder.[79]

Adverse Effects, Interactions, Pharmacokinetics. See Appendix A.

Sandalwood (Santalum album)

Grade C: *Unclear or conflicting scientific evidence*

Mechanism of Action

The main compound of sandalwood, alpha-santalol, is likely responsible for its distinctive scent;[80] however, the exact mechanism by which sandalwood reduces anxiety is not well understood.

Scientific Evidence of Effectiveness

One clinical trial evaluating 1% sandalwood oil aromatherapy massage reported positive results in reducing anxiety.[81] Another study evaluating the topical effects of sandalwood oil found physiological changes in blood oxygen saturation, blood pressure, breathing rate, eye-blink rate, pulse rate, skin conductance, skin temperature, and surface electromyogram, which were interpreted in terms of a relaxing/sedative effect.[82] However, sandalwood has also caused alertness.[80] More research is needed to clarify these results.

Dose

The dose of sandalwood for anxiety has not been determined.

Adverse Effects, Interactions, Pharmacokinetics. See Appendix A.

Valerian (Valeriana officinalis)

Grade C: Unclear or conflicting scientific evidence (anxiety)

Grade B: *Good scientific evidence (insomnia)*

Mechanism of Action

The flavonoid glycoside linarin, the flavone 6-methylapigenin, and the flavanone glycoside 2S(–) hesperidin have been suggested to possess anxiolytic or sedative properties.[83] A combination of these compounds may impart clinical activity to valerian.[84-86] Valerian may cause sedation by increasing the amount of GABA in the synaptic cleft. Extracts have been reported to increase synaptosomal GABA concentrations, possibly by enhancing GABA release and inhibiting GABA uptake.[84,87-89] Valerenic acid has also been shown to inhibit an enzyme that breaks down GABA. It is not known if the GABA found in valerian extracts can cross the blood-brain barrier and contribute to its sedative effects.

Scientific Evidence of Effectiveness

Valerian has been proposed as a treatment for anxiety and panic disorder. One clinical study showed that valerian improved scores on HAM-A and *state-trait anxiety inventory* (STAI-trait) after 4 weeks of use.[90] Valerian is more frequently used as a treatment for insomnia. Preliminary data from several human trials suggest that valerian improves subjective measures of sleep quality and sleep latency for up to 4 to 6 weeks, and greater effects have been noted in poor sleepers than in those who do not typically have insomnia. Preliminary evidence suggests that ongoing use may be more effective than acute (single-dose) use, with progressive effects over 4 weeks.[91-92] However, most available studies have been methodologically weak, and in most cases, results have not been confirmed using objective sleep pattern data in a sleep laboratory or validated measurement scales. Preliminary studies of combination products containing valerian and hop (*Flores humuli*)[24,25] are promising, but again, these results have been obtained using insufficient study methodology.

Dose

Extracts are often standardized to contain 0.3% valerenic acid, although other chemical constituents may be responsible for the pharmacological activity. Some products are standardized to contain 0.8% valerenic or valeric acid. For anxiety, 100 mg of aqueous or aqueous-ethanolic extract has been used before a stressful event.[93] For insomnia, studied doses have ranged from 400 to 900 mg of an aqueous or aqueous-ethanolic extract (corresponding to 1.5-3 g of herb), taken 30 to 60 minutes before going to bed. The more scientifically valid trials have used 600 mg daily, taken 1 hour before bedtime.[91,94] Valerian has historically been used in the form of a tea (1.5-3 g root steeped for 5-10 minutes in 150 mL boiling water), although this formulation has not been studied in RCTs.

Adverse Effects, Interactions, Pharmacokinetics. See Appendix A.

HERBAL THERAPIES WITH NEGATIVE EVIDENCE

Tea (Camellia sinensis)

Grade D: *Fair negative scientific evidence*

Levotheanine (L-theanine) is a predominant amino acid found in green tea. Preliminary research on the effects of this amino acid compared with alprazolam (Xanax), a benzodiazepine, on experimentally induced anxiety found no benefit.[95] Green tea is a source of caffeine and may reduce the sedative effects of benzodiazepines.

HERBAL THERAPIES WITH LIMITED EVIDENCE

Ginkgo (Ginkgo biloba)

Ginkgo biloba special extract Egb 761 has been suggested as beneficial in patients who have adjustment disorder with anxious mood. Researchers have proposed that ginkgo may be efficacious in elderly patients with anxiety related to cognitive decline.[96]

Herbs with Possible Sedating Properties*

HERB	SPECIFIC THERAPEUTIC USE(S)†	HERB	SPECIFIC THERAPEUTIC USE(S)†
Aconite	Anxiety, insomnia	Eucalyptus oil	Stress
American pennyroyal	Anxiety	Euphorbia	Stress
		Garlic	Stress
Anise	Anxiety, insomnia	Germanium	Stress
Ashwagandha	Nervous exhaustion, insomnia	Ginseng	Aggression, anxiety, stress, insomnia
Asparagus	Anxiety	Goldenseal	Anxiety
Astragalus	Insomnia	Guarana	Stress (heat)
Bay leaf	Anxiety	Hawthorn	Anxiety, insomnia
Belladonna	Anxiety	Holy basil	Stress
Betony	Anxiety, nervous disorders, stress, tension	Hyssop	Anxiety, stress
Black cohosh	Sleep disorders	Ignatia	Anxiety, hysteria, nervous disorders, insomnia
Black haw	Nervous disorders		
Black horehound	Anxiety, nervous disorders, insomnia	Jimson weed	Stress
		Ladies mantle	Sleep disorders
Blue cohosh	Nervous disorders	Lady's slipper	Anxiety, nervous disorders, stress (emotional), insomnia
Boswellia	Insomnia		
Boxwood	Stress	Lemongrass	Anxiety, nervous disorders, stress, sleep disorders (jet lag)
Bugleweed	Nervous disorders, insomnia		
Butterbur	Anxiety, insomnia	Maca	Anxiety
Calamus	Anxiety (neurosis), stress reduction, insomnia, sleep disorders	Mistletoe	Anxiety, insomnia, sleep disorders
		Mugwort	Anxiety, stress, insomnia
Calendula	Anxiety, insomnia	Muira puama	Anxiety, nervous exhaustion, stress
California poppy	Nervousness, insomnia	Nux vomica	Anxiety, stress (emotional), insomnia
Cardamom	Stress	Perilla	Stress
Catnip	Sleep disorders	Raspberry	Anxiety
Chasteberry	Anxiety, nervous disorders	Reishi mushroom	Nervous exhaustion, tension, insomnia
Codonopsis	Stress		
Coleus	Insomnia	Rhodiola	Anxiety, stress, insomnia
Cowslip	Anxiety	Rooibos	Nervous disorders, insomnia
Daisy	Anxiety, insomnia, sleep disorders, jet lag	Scotch broom	Stress
		Sea buckthorn	Stress (caused by cold conditions)
Danshen	Insomnia, stress	Skunk cabbage	Anxiety
Datura wrightii	Stress	Spirulina	Anxiety
Deer velvet	Stress	Sweet almond	Anxiety
Dong quai	Anxiety, stress	Sweet woodruff	Nervousness, insomnia
Eastern hemlock	Stress	Tansy	Anxiety, nervous disorders
Elder	Stress, insomnia	Yohimbe	Panic disorder, insomnia
Elecampane	Stress, sleep disorders		

*This is not an all-inclusive or comprehensive list of herbs with sedating properties; other herbs and supplements may possess these qualities. A qualified health care provider should be consulted with specific questions or concerns regarding potential sedative agents.
†Based on expert opinion, anecdote, case reports, and/or preliminary trial evidence.

Skullcap (Scutellaria spp.)

Preliminary research suggests that a single dose of skullcap may be effective in reducing anxiety; duration of action appeared to be less than 2 hours, and impact on energy and cognition was minimal.[97]

ADJUNCT THERAPIES

Anxiety

1. Depression is often accompanied by anxiety. The use of herbal agents (e.g., St. John's wort) may be beneficial for mild to moderate anxiety *and* depression (see Chapter 5).

However, these agents should be used with extreme caution because of harmful interactions with certain medications, which can have severe consequences (see Appendix A).

2. Anxiety is a common psychiatric disturbance in patients with Parkinson's disease (PD).[98] This anxiety may be a psychological reaction to the stress of the illness.[99] Controlling PD symptoms may improve anxiety symptoms. Cowhage, an herb that contains levodopa, is used to treat PD. Cowhage in divided doses of 22.5 to 67.5 g may improve PD symptoms[100-102] (see Chapter 3).

3. Sleep deprivation may cause anxiety disorders. Valerian may reduce the time to fall asleep (sleep latency) and improve the quality of sleep in addition to improving symptoms of anxiety.

Insomnia

1. Depression is a common complaint among patients with insomnia.[103] St. John's wort is often used to treat depressive disorders (see Chapter 6) but should be used with extreme caution because of potential harmful interactions with certain medications, which can have severe consequences. (see Appendix A).

2. Menopausal hot flashes may lead to sleep disturbances. Soy *(Glycine max)* products containing isoflavones may help reduce the number of hot flashes and other menopausal symptoms and consequently improve sleep (see Chapter 21).

3. Melatonin is a neurohormone produced in the brain by the pineal gland, from the amino acid tryptophan. Synthetic melatonin supplements have been used for a variety of medical conditions, most notably for disorders related to sleep. Evidence supports the use of melatonin for jet lag and other sleep disorders, such as delayed sleep phase syndrome and work shift disorder.[104]

INTEGRATIVE THERAPY PLAN

Anxiety

- Discuss the patient's anxiety symptoms and how his or her anxiety disorder has been classified (e.g., generalized anxiety disorder, panic disorder, obsessive compulsive disorder).
- Determine if the patient is seeking professional treatment for the anxiety disorder.
- Inquire if the patient has a family history of anxiety or depressive disorders.
- Determine if the patient is taking any other therapy for anxiety or depressive disorders.
- If the patient is interested in trying an herbal product, consider discussing kava, which has been shown to be effective for anxiety. Its effects may be similar to benzodiazepine drugs; 105 to 210 mg of kavalactones (standardized to 70% kavalactones) for less than 4 weeks has been used for anxiety. However, there is serious concern about safety, and although kava is still available in the United States, the FDA has issued warnings to consumers and physicians. Kava may cause liver damage, but it is not clear what dose or duration of use is correlated with liver toxicity.
- Inform the patient that there is good evidence to support the use of lavender aromatherapy for anxiety. Typically, 2 to 4 drops is added to 2 to 3 cups of boiling water, followed by inhalation of the vapors.
- Depression may be accompanied by anxiety. St. John's wort is a popular herbal remedy for depressive disorders, and it may also provide benefit in anxiety symptom reduction; 900 mg (standardized to 0.3% hypericin) once or twice daily for 2 to 4 weeks has been used in patients with generalized anxiety disorder. St. John's wort appears to be an inducer of cytochrome P450. Induction of drug metabolism increases the breakdown of some drugs and may reduce their blood levels and therapeutic effects.
- Caution is warranted when using herbal anxiolytics with other sedative medications, such as benzodiazepines and CNS depressants, because of the risk of additive sedative effects.

Insomnia

- Discuss the patient's symptoms of insomnia, including fatigue, poor concentration, irritability, and anxiousness.
- Determine if the patient's insomnia is caused by a medical condition, such as sleep apnea, restless leg syndrome, or stress.
- Inquire if the patient takes any therapies that may cause insomnia, such as beta-2 agonists (bronchodilators), decongestants, theophylline, antidepressants, thyroid medications, or stimulants.
- Ask if the patient uses any nonprescription drugs, including alcohol, caffeine, or nicotine.
- Determine if the patient is having daytime problems caused by insomnia, such as anxiety, irritability, fatigue, or poor concentration and focus.
- Inform the patient that valerian has a long history of use for sleep. It may improve sleep quality and sleep latency for up to 4 to 6 weeks. A dose of 600 mg daily, taken 30 minutes to 1 hour before bedtime, may be used for insomnia. However, there is a potential risk of hepatotoxicity with the use of valerian.
- Educate the patient that many practitioners believe chamomile possesses sedative properties and frequently recommend it. However, chamomile should not be used in patients with allergies to ragweed, marigolds, or daisies.
- Caution is warranted when using hypnotic herbs with medications such as benzodiazepines and CNS depressants because of the risk of additive sedative effects.

Case Studies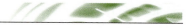

CASE STUDY 4-1

MJ is a 62-year-old man with increasing anxiety. He complains of heart palpitations and difficulty concentrating or sleeping.

MJ works as a retail-chain manager and is apprehensive about losing his job after another drop in quarterly profits. MJ presents to the pharmacy requesting information on "natural and safe" therapies such as valerian, ginkgo, and chamomile. He also takes saw palmetto for benign prostatic hypertrophy (BPH). How should you counsel?

Answer: Valerian, ginkgo, and chamomile have each been used for anxiety. Evidence supports the use of valerian for both anxiety and sleep disturbances. You may suggest to MJ to start with 400 mg of valerian 30 to 60 minutes before going to sleep. It may also help in reducing his anxiety. Additionally, valerian is generally well tolerated. Ask MJ if he is taking any other medications or dietary supplements, and determine if any will interact with valerian. Supportive evidence is lacking for the use of ginkgo or chamomile for anxiety or sleep disorders. However, chamomile is often used and recommended by many practitioners for sleep and relaxation. It may also be recommended to MJ with proper monitoring.

CASE STUDY 4-2

EK is a 21-year-old college student who has been unable to perform well on tests because of anxiety. EK has heard that kava may help his anxiety. He currently takes phenytoin (Dilantin) for epilepsy. How do you respond?

Answer: Kava has traditionally been used for anxiety. However, this is an example of how historical use of an herb does not mean that it is without dangers. In the case of EK, kava should not be used. Phenytoin has shown the potential to induce liver damage (1% of patients taking phenytoin), and hepatotoxicity has been documented with kava use. Taking two hepatotoxic agents can increase the chance of liver damage.

CASE STUDY 4-3

JO is a 45-year old woman complaining of anxiety and insomnia. She has a 4-year history of mild to moderate major depression and is taking 600 mg of St. John's wort daily. She has never taken prescription antidepressants. She asks you if she should take more St. John's wort and if any other herbs can help. How do you counsel?

Answer: You may explain to JO that she may increase her St. John's wort dose to 900 mg daily for anxiety, but that she should also consult her physician to monitor her. In regard to her sleep problem, you may suggest valerian, 600 mg 1 hour before bedtime. When valerian is used with St. John's wort, additive sedative effects may occur. Given her age, JO could possibly be experiencing premenopausal symptoms that may contribute to her insomnia; JO may benefit from soy (*Glycine max*) products containing isoflavones, which may help reduce the number of hot flashes and other menopausal symptoms, and consequently improve sleep. Recommend that JO explore psychotherapy.

References for Chapter 4 can be found on the Evolve website at http://evolve.elsevier.com/Ulbricht/herbalpharmacotherapy/

Review Questions

1. All the following are herbal treatment options for anxiety *except*:
   a. Lemon balm
   b. Kava
   c. Bitter orange
   d. Lavender

2. Kava has been associated with a risk of:
   a. Cancer
   b. Liver damage
   c. Diabetes
   d. Hypertension

3. Which of the following should *not* be recommended to a patient with insomnia who has endometriosis?
   a. Valerian
   b. Hop
   c. Lavender
   d. Lemon balm

4. True or false: Gotu kola is related to the cola nut and contains caffeine.

5. Rosemary aromatherapy is often used to treat which of the following conditions?
   a. Mood enhancement
   b. Alteration in pain perception
   c. Increase in alertness
   d. All of the above

6. Which daily dose of bacopa syrup for 1 month has been used for anxiety?
   a. 300 mL, representing 2 g of dry crude extract
   b. 30 mL, representing 2 g of dry crude extract
   c. 3 mL, representing 12 g dry crude extract
   d. 30 mL, representing 12 g of dry crude extract

7. True or false: The most common use of St. John's wort is for the treatment of anxiety.

8. Kava may affect what part of the brain?
   a. Brainstem
   b. Cerebral cortex
   c. Limbic system
   d. Basal ganglia

Answers are found in the Answers to Review Questions section in the back of the text.

5 Depressive Disorders

Outline

OVERVIEW
    Types of Depressive Disorders
        Major Depression
        Atypical Depression
        Dysthymia
        Adjustment Disorders
        Bipolar Disorder
        Seasonal Affective Disorder
        Postpartum Depression
        Premenstrual Dysphoric Disorder
    Signs and Symptoms
        Mood Changes
        Loss of Interest
        Sleep Disturbances and Fatigue
        Changes in Thought Patterns
        Other Physical Symptoms
        Depression in Children and Elderly Persons
    Diagnosis

SELECTED HERBAL THERAPIES
    Chasteberry *(Vitex agnus-castus)*
    Coleus *(Coleus forskohlii)*
    Ginkgo *(Ginkgo biloba)*
    Guarana *(Paullinia cupana)*
    Lavender *(Lavandula angustifolia)*
    Sage *(Salvia officinalis)*
    St. John's Wort *(Hypericum perforatum)*
HERBAL THERAPIES WITH LIMITED EVIDENCE
ADJUNCT THERAPIES
INTEGRATIVE THERAPY PLAN
CASE STUDIES
REVIEW QUESTIONS

Learning Objectives

- Recognize symptoms of depression and other depressive disorders.
- Discuss the herbs used for depression and other depressive disorders.
- Identify the mechanism of action and pharmacokinetics of antidepressant herbs.
- Recognize major adverse effects and drug interactions associated with antidepressant herbs.
- Discuss approaches for the management of depression using herbal agents.
- Describe adjunct herbal therapies for depression.
- Educate patients regarding an integrative pharmacotherapy plan.

OVERVIEW

Depression, a type of depressive disorder, is a psychiatric illness presenting as a marked change in both emotional and physical symptoms. Unlike normal emotional experiences of sadness, loss, or passing mood states, depressive disorders are persistent and can significantly interfere with an individual's thoughts, behavior, mood, activity, and physical health.

Depressive disorders affect approximately 18.8 million American adults, or about 9.5% of the U.S. population age 18 years and older, in any given year.[1] These statistics include not only major depressive disorders (severe depression) but also other forms of depressive illness, including *dysthymic disorder* (mild to moderate depression) and *bipolar disorder* (manic-depressive disorder). Among all medical illnesses, major depression is the leading cause of disability in the United States and many other developed countries.

Children and teenagers can also suffer from depression. Depression in younger persons is defined as an illness that causes feelings of depression that persist and interfere with the person's ability to function. Approximately 5% of children and adolescents in the general population have depression at any given time.[1] Children who experience stress, loss, or anxiety disorders are at a higher risk for depression. Problems with attention, learning, or conduct may also occur in children with depression.

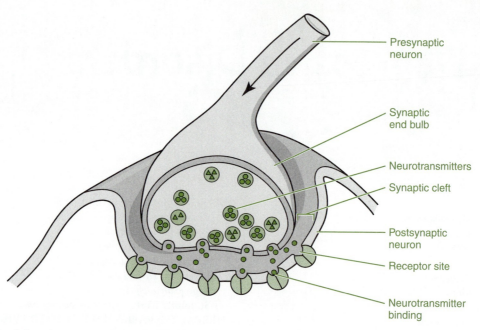

Figure 5-1 Synaptic cleft and neurotransmitter action. (Modified from Salvo S: *Massage therapy: principles and practice*, ed 2, St Louis, 2003, Saunders-Elsevier.)

Without treatment, the symptoms of depressive disorders can last for weeks, months, or years. Appropriate treatment, typically through counseling and/or antidepressant medication, can help improve symptoms in most people with depression. Antidepressants elicit their response through effects on levels of neurotransmitters in the brain, including serotonin, dopamine, and norepinephrine (Figure 5-1). There are many receptor subtypes for each of these neurotransmitters, and some of these subtypes may play a greater role in the treatment of depression than others. Neurotransmitter levels may be altered by blocking the mechanism by which these receptors are taken up into cells ("receptor reuptake") or by blocking enzymes that break down neurotransmitters (e.g., monoamine oxidase).

Types of Depressive Disorders

Major Depression

Major depression lasts more than 2 weeks. Symptoms may include overwhelming feelings of sadness and grief, loss of interest or pleasure in activities usually enjoyed, and feelings of worthlessness or guilt. This type of depression may result in poor sleep, a change in appetite, severe fatigue, and difficulty concentrating. Suicidal thoughts may become frequent in severe depression.[1]

Atypical Depression

Individuals with atypical depression, as opposed to major depression, experience improved mood when "something good happens." In addition, two of the following symptoms occur in patients who have atypical depression: increased appetite or weight gain (vs. reduced appetite or weight loss of "typical" depression), excessive sleeping (vs. insomnia), "leaden" paralysis (severe form of fatigue or tiredness), and sensitivity to rejection.[1]

Dysthymia

Dysthymia is a less severe form of depression (mild to moderate) than major depression, but it is longer in duration. Signs and symptoms usually are not disabling, and periods of mild depression can alternate with short periods of feeling normal. Dysthymia, however, may predispose a person to major depression. To be diagnosed with dysthymia, the first 2 years of depressed mood cannot include any episodes of major depression. In addition, no underlying causes of depressed mood, such as general medical conditions (e.g., premenstrual syndrome, menopause, coronary heart disease) or substance abuse, may be present. The symptoms of dysthymia and the associated signs of depression cause significant distress or impairment in social, occupational, and other important areas of functioning. When a major depressive episode occurs in addition to dysthymia, health care professionals may refer to the resultant condition as *double depression*.[1]

Adjustment Disorders

Having a loved one die, losing a job, or receiving a diagnosis of cancer or another disease can cause an individual to feel tense, sad, overwhelmed, or angry. Eventually, most people come to terms with the lasting consequences of life stresses, but some do not and develop an adjustment disorder. Adjustment disorders are forms of depression that occur when the response to a stressful event or situation causes signs and symptoms of depression. Some people develop an adjustment disorder in response to a single event (e.g., parent or spouse dying), whereas in others, it stems from a combination of stressors. Adjustment disorders can be acute (lasting less than 6 months) or chronic (longer than 6 months). Physicians classify adjustment disorders based on the primary signs and symptoms of depression.[1]

Bipolar Disorder
Alternating episodes of elation (mania) and depression are hallmarks of a condition known as *bipolar* or *manic-depressive* disorder. Mania affects judgment, causing individuals to make unwise decisions. Some people have bursts of increased creativity and productivity during the manic phase. The number of episodes at either extreme may not be equal. Some people may have several episodes of depression before having another manic phase, or vice versa.[1]

Seasonal Affective Disorder
Seasonal affective disorder (SAD) is a pattern of depression that is related to a lack of sunlight. SAD usually occurs in the winter. It may cause headaches, irritability, and a low energy level. Because it generally occurs seasonally, SAD is not considered a chronic depressive disorder.[1]

Postpartum Depression
According to the American College of Obstetricians and Gynecologists, about 10% of new mothers experience postpartum depression within the first 6 months after giving birth. It is widely believed that hormonal changes during this time can trigger depressive symptoms. For women with postpartum depression, feelings such as sadness, anxiety, and restlessness can be strong enough to interfere with daily tasks. Rarely, a more extreme form of depression known as *postpartum psychosis* can develop. Symptoms of this psychosis include a fear of harming oneself or one's baby, confusion, disorientation, hallucinations, delusions, and paranoia.[1]

Premenstrual Dysphoric Disorder
Premenstrual dysphoric disorder (PMDD) occurs when depressive symptoms, such as crying, tiredness, and sadness, occur 1 week before menstruation and disappear after menstruation.[1] As with postpartum depression, these mood fluctuations are attributed to hormonal changes.[1]

Signs and Symptoms
The symptoms of depression represent a significant change from how a person functioned before the illness, and symptoms can be mild, moderate, or severe. Initial episodes of depression may not be obvious if their onset is gradual.

Mood Changes
Mood changes are the most obvious signs of depression. The individual may feel sad, helpless, or hopeless and may have crying spells; depressed individuals may also seem restless, agitated, irritable, and easily annoyed. Feelings of worthlessness and excessive guilt are common symptoms of depression.

Loss of Interest
In depression, individuals may lose interest in (or no longer receive pleasure from) previously enjoyed activities. If the individual was sexually active before developing depression, he or she may notice decreased interest in having sexual relations (loss of libido).

Sleep Disturbances and Fatigue
Sleeping too much or difficulty sleeping may be a sign of depression. Waking in the middle of the night or early in the morning and not being able to get back to sleep are typical symptoms. Constant weariness and lack of energy are common signs of depression. The individual may feel as tired in the morning as when going to bed the night before.

Changes in Thought Patterns
The individual may have trouble concentrating and making decisions or have difficulties with memory. The individual may have a persistent negative view of his or her situation in life and the future. Individuals may have thoughts of death or dying. Suicidal thoughts may accompany depression. Anyone who has suicidal feelings, talks about suicide, or attempts suicide should be taken seriously and should receive immediate help from a mental health specialist. Certain warning signs (e.g., pacing, agitated behavior, frequent mood changes, sleeplessness for several nights), actions or threats of assault, physical harm or violence, threats or talk of death or suicide, withdrawal from activities and relationships, putting affairs in order (e.g., saying goodbye to friends, giving away prized possessions, writing a will), a sudden brightening of mood after a period of being depressed, and unusually risky behavior may be indicators of serious depression and the possibility of suicidal ideation.

Other Physical Symptoms
Depression can also cause a wide variety of physical complaints, such as gastrointestinal problems (indigestion, constipation, diarrhea), headache, and backache. An increased or reduced appetite and unexplained weight gain or loss may indicate depression.

Depression in Children and Elderly Persons
Children, adolescents, and elderly persons may react differently to depression than young or middle-aged adults. In these groups, symptoms may take different forms or may be masked by other conditions. Children may feign physical illnesses, worry that a parent is going to die, perform poorly in school, refuse to go to school, or exhibit behavioral problems. Elderly persons may be preoccupied with the physical

symptoms of depression, including aches and pains, rather than their emotional difficulties.

Diagnosis

To diagnose depression, the physician must first rule out all other disease possibilities. Typically, the diagnosis begins with a medical history, including questions about the duration, severity, and characteristics of symptoms. The physician asks about diet, stress, any medications currently being taken, and changes in sleep patterns. Questionnaires such as the Patient Health Questionnaire (PHQ)-9 may be used to determine the level of depression. The Hamilton Rating Scale for Depression (HAM-D, HRSD) is a multiple-choice questionnaire that may be used by physicians to rate depression severity; in addition, it can be used to measure the patient's progress over the course of treatment.[2] Guidelines for diagnosing depressive disorders are also defined in *Diagnostic and Statistical Manual of Mental Disorders* (DSM).[3]

SELECTED HERBAL THERAPIES

Note

To help make this educational resource more interactive, all pharmacokinetics, adverse effects, and interactions data have been compiled in Appendix A. Safety data specifically related to pregnancy and lactation are listed in Appendix B. Please refer to these appendices when working through the case studies and answering the review questions.

Depression is a serious illness, and individuals should be evaluated by their physicians and by mental health professionals before self-medicating with any herbal therapy.

Chasteberry (Vitex agnus-castus)

Grade C: *Unclear or conflicting scientific evidence (premenstrual dysphoric disorder)*

Mechanism of Action

Chasteberry has multiple active constituents, including flavonoids and iridoids, that may contribute to its therapeutic effects.[4] Chasteberry has been shown to affect various neurotransmitters and hormones; it has been reported to modulate stress-induced prolactin secretion through dopamine.[5-8]

Scientific Evidence of Effectiveness

Chasteberry has been used for treatment of premenstrual syndrome (PMS), and it may also be beneficial for premenstrual dysphoric disorder (PMDD), a mood disorder and severe form of PMS.[9,10] One clinical trial found that chasteberry was comparable to fluoxetine in relieving symptoms of PMDD.[11] Patients in both groups improved in the outcomes measured, including Penn Daily Symptom Report (DSR), HAM-D, and Clinical Global Impression–Severity of Illness and Improvement (CGI-SI, CGI-I) scales, after 8 weeks.[11]

Dose

Chasteberry, 20 to 40 mg daily for 8 weeks, was comparable to fluoxetine, 20 to 40 mg daily for 8 weeks, in relieving symptoms of PMDD.[11]

Adverse Effects, Interactions, Pharmacokinetics. See Appendix A.

Coleus (Coleus forskohlii)

Grade C: *Unclear or conflicting scientific evidence (depression)*

Mechanism of Action

Depressed patients may have reduced cyclic adenosine monophosphate (cAMP). Forskolin, the major active constituent found in *Coleus forskohlii*, may act as an activator of adenylate cyclase that directly raises levels of the second messenger cAMP.[12,13]

Scientific Evidence of Effectiveness

One preliminary study found that intravenous forskolin, given in a 75-minute infusion to four depressed patients, improved mood.[14]

Dose. Insufficient available evidence.

Adverse Effects, Interactions, Pharmacokinetics. See Appendix A.

Ginkgo (Ginkgo biloba)

Grade C: *Unclear or conflicting scientific evidence (depression, seasonal affective disorder)*

Mechanism of Action

Ginkgo biloba extract has been reported to restore brain levels of catecholamines (norepinephrine and dopamine), serotonin, and plasma corticosterone to near-normal levels.[15] Ginkgo has also been found to inhibit *monoamine oxidase* (MAO) activity in animals,[16] but this action has not been confirmed in subsequent animal research.[17] There is some evidence that gingko does not induce significant changes in human brain MAO-A or MAO-B, measured by positron emission tomography (PET).[18]

Scientific Evidence of Effectiveness

Ginkgo has been studied as a preventive therapy in patients with a history of SAD. In a double-blind trial, 27 subjects were randomized to receive either ginkgo or placebo for a 10-week period. Outcome measures included the Montgomery-Asberg Depression Rating Scale and subject self-ratings. Ginkgo was not found to be significantly effective in preventing the development of SAD symptoms.[19]

In another randomized controlled trial (RCT), 40 elderly patients with depression who had failed *tricyclic antidepressant* (TCA) therapy were given either 240 mg of ginkgo or placebo daily while continuing their prior antidepressant regimens. Particularly, these patients had also been clinically diagnosed with mild to moderate cerebral dysfunction. After 8 weeks of therapy, small but significant changes were reported in HAM-D scores, as well as in measures of cognitive function.[20] Notably, ginkgo may help decrease sexual side effects, such as loss of libido, in individuals taking antidepressants and may improve sleep in patients with major depression.[21]

Dose

Ginkgo, 240 mg daily for 8 to 10 weeks, has been used. In a small sample group, 120 mg of ginkgo (administered daily) did not induce significant changes in human brain MAO-A or MAO-B.[18]

Adverse Effects, Interactions, Pharmacokinetics. See Appendix A.

Guarana (Paullinia cupana)

Grade C: *Unclear or conflicting scientific evidence (mood enhancement)*

Mechanism of Action

The mechanism of action of guarana in depression is not well understood. However, guarana contains caffeine, which may stimulate the central nervous system and increase norepinephrine and epinephrine secretion.

Scientific Evidence of Effectiveness

In animals, crude lyophilized extracts of guarana seeds and fruit (containing known stimulants) exhibited an antidepressant effect, comparable with that of imipramine.[22]

Dose. Insufficient available evidence.

Adverse Effects, Interactions, Pharmacokinetics. See Appendix A.

Lavender (Lavandula angustifolia)

Grade C: *Unclear or conflicting scientific evidence*

Mechanism of Action. Insufficient available evidence.

Scientific Evidence of Effectiveness

In patients with mild to moderate depression, oral lavender tincture monotherapy (1:5 in 50% alcohol, 60 drops daily) appears to be slightly less effective than imipramine (100 mg daily). Lavender also appeared to have some additive antidepressant effect when administered with imipramine.[23] Alcohol in tinctures may confound these results and may be inadvisable in depressed patients, except in low concentrations.

Dose. Insufficient available evidence.

Adverse Effects, Interactions, Pharmacokinetics. See Appendix A.

Sage (Salvia officinalis)

Grade A: *Strong scientific evidence (mood and cognition enhancement)*

Mechanism of Action

Sage has a history of use for mood modulation; however, its mechanism of action is not well understood. It has been found to possess in vitro cholinesterase-inhibiting properties, which may contribute to its effects on mood and cognition.[24,25]

Scientific Evidence of Effectiveness

Sage has long been suggested to improve memory and mood. Several RCTs provide good evidence for the use of sage for these purposes, even in stressful situations.[26-28] In one RCT, 300-mg and 600-mg doses were found to decrease anxiety, improve alertness, and provide calmness, as assessed by Bond-Lader mood scales, State-Trait Anxiety Inventory (STAI), and Defined Intensity Stress Simulator (DISS).

Dose

Sage is sold as dried leaves, tinctures, fluid extracts, and essential oils. None of these preparations has been standardized. For mood enhancement, dried sage leaf, 300 or 600 mg in single daily doses, has been used with beneficial results.[26]

Adverse Effects, Interactions, Pharmacokinetics. See Appendix A.

St. John's Wort (Hypericum perforatum)

Grade A: *Strong scientific evidence*

Mechanism of Action

The exact mechanism by which St. John's wort exerts its antidepressant effects is not well understood. St. John's wort appears to inhibit serotonin, norepinephrine, and dopamine synaptic reuptake.[29-32] Hyperforin is believed to be the active component, with approximately the equivalent efficacy of standard TCAs and similar potency in serotonin, norepinephrine, and dopamine systems.[29] Although not definitive, efficacy in behavioral paradigms of depression (learned helplessness, behavioral despair) has been correlated with hyperforin content.[33]

Animal studies have noted a dose-dependent potentiation of serotonin-mediated behaviors, with greater effect when a hyperforin-enriched (38.8% hyperforin) carbon dioxide (CO_2)

extract was administered. In contrast, the ethanolic extract (4.5% hyperforin) potentiated dopamine-mediated behaviors.[34] In addition, significant downregulation of beta-receptor density and an increase in 5-HT$_2$ (serotonin) receptors has been demonstrated in animal cortex after treatment with *Hypericum* extract.[29] Also, the numbers of both 5-HT$_1$ A and 5-HT$_2$ A receptors was significantly increased compared with controls.[35] The effect on serotonergic receptors has been variable, according to the specific extract; a methanolic extract led to a significant increase in serotonin receptor density, compared with a (nonsignificant) decrease in receptor density found with a hyperforin-enriched CO_2 extract.[29] A neuroendocrine study conducted in healthy adults demonstrated an increase in cortisol with 600 mg of oral *Hypericum* extract, suggesting central norepinephrine or serotonin neurotransmitter activity.[36]

Nonetheless, the mechanism of St. John's wort activity may be different from standard antidepressants.[37] MAO inhibition with St. John's wort may be noncompetitive, via sodium channels, and may result in an enhancement of intracellular sodium concentrations.[38-40]

Antidepressant activity by St. John's wort may be caused by changes in gene expression in a discrete brain region, based on a study evaluating 66 genes differentially regulated in rat hypothalamus.[41]

Scientific Evidence of Effectiveness

St. John's wort has been reported to be more effective than placebo and equally effective as TCA in the short-term management of mild to moderate depression (1-3 months).[42-53] This conclusion is supported by overlapping meta-analyses and a Cochrane review of multiple trials over the last two decades, as well as several short-term, randomized trials.[54-56] Comparisons to selective serotonin reuptake inhibitor (SSRI) antidepressants have provided limited equivalence data to date.[46,57-61] Questions have been raised regarding the methodological quality of available studies, which have examined heterogeneous patient populations and inconsistently used standardized symptom rating instruments, including HAM-D and CGI scales. Negative results have been published for two well-conducted trials of St. John's wort for major depression; however, one trial did not include a reference-agent arm (comparison was only made to placebo),[62] and the other trial yielded negative results for an SSRI and St. John's wort.[63] Therefore, these results cannot be considered conclusive. Overall, evidence supports the efficacy of St. John's wort for mild to moderate depression, but the evidence for major depression is equivocal.

Dose

St. John's wort products are often standardized to 0.3% hypericin extract, although there has been a movement within the manufacturing industry to standardize to hyperforin (usually 2%-5%). Standardization of extracts may not be clinically relevant in predicting effectiveness, because the active ingredients in St. John's wort have not been definitively determined.

DEPRESSION

- As a starting dose, 300 mg of standardized 0.3% hypericin extract has been taken orally three times daily (may be standardized to 2%-5% hyperforin as well).
- As a maintenance dose, 300 to 600 mg daily may be sufficient, although this has not been extensively studied. A liquid form standardized to contain equivalent amounts of hypericin (as previously noted) may also be taken three times daily.[64-69]

Adverse Effects, Interactions, Pharmacokinetics. See Appendix A.

HERBAL THERAPIES WITH LIMITED EVIDENCE

Ashwagandha *(Withania somnifera)*

Manufacturers of ashwagandha claim that it may be used to stabilize mood. Ashwagandha exhibited an antidepressant effect, comparable with that of the TCA imipramine (Tofranil), in an animal study.[70]

 Ayurveda

> Early evidence suggests that a traditional Ayurvedic formula containing extracts of four Indian herbs, Ashvatha, Kapikachu, Dhanvayasa, and Bhuriphali (the GS-02 formulation), may have benefits similar to conventional antidepressant medication.[1]

 Bach Flower Remedies

> Depression is one of the major uses of Bach flower remedies. Currently, there is a lack of high-quality clinical trials that have investigated this subject; however, two case reports indicate positive results with this therapy in conjunction with psychotherapy.[71]

Damiana *(Turnera diffusa)*

Damiana has traditionally been used to relieve anxiety and depression, especially if linked to a sexual component. It is often used as a tonic to improve overall wellness.[1]

Kava *(Piper methysticum)*

Kava is a popular herb to use for anxiety. As a drink, users claim that it has tranquilizing and uplifting effects. In animal studies, kava has been reported to alter dopaminergic or serotonergic tissue levels.[72-74]

Kola Nut *(Cola acuminata)*

Caffeine is the active ingredient in kola nut. It is believed that consuming kola nut tea may help improve symptoms of temporary depression, although clinical evidence is lacking.

Licorice (*Glycyrrhiza glabra*)

The isoflavan constituents of licorice, glabridin and 4'-O-methylglabridin (4'-OMeG), and the isoflavene constituent, glabrene, were found to inhibit serotonin reuptake, which shows the potential benefit for depression.[75]

 Herbs and Supplements with Possible SSRI Effects*†

Ephedra	Passion flower
Evening primrose oil	Sepia
Fenugreek	St. John's wort
Ginkgo	Tyrosine
Hops	Valerian
Hydrazine sulfate	White horehound
Kali bromatum	Yohimbe bark extract
Lemon balm	

*This is not an all-inclusive or comprehensive list of herbs with selective serotonin reuptake inhibitor (SSRI) properties; other herbs and supplements may possess these qualities. A qualified health care provider should be consulted with specific questions or concerns regarding potential SSRI effects or interactions of agents.
†Based on expert opinion, anecdote, case reports, and/or preliminary trial evidence.

 Herbs and Supplements with Possible MAOI Effects*†

Avocado	Hydrazine sulfate
Betel nut	*Kali bromatum*
California poppy	Kava
Chaparral	Mace
Ephedra	Passion flower
Evening primrose oil	Red pepper
Fenugreek	Sepia
Ginkgo	St. John's wort
Ginseng	Valerian
Hops	Yohimbe

*This is not an all-inclusive or comprehensive list of herbs with monoamine oxidase inhibitor (MAOI) properties; other herbs and supplements may possess these qualities. A qualified health care provider should be consulted with specific questions or concerns regarding potential MAOI effects or interactions of agents.
†Based on expert opinion, anecdote, case reports, and/or preliminary trial evidence.

ADJUNCT THERAPIES

1. Depression can present with a variety of symptoms and may lead to loss of sleep and even insomnia. Agents such as melatonin, valerian, and lavender may provide benefit for sleep disturbances. Many people with depression also have anxiety. Valerian may also help with these symptoms (see Chapter 4). Some patients feel a lack of energy and inability to focus. Caffeine products such as guarana and tea as well as *ginseng* may help in boosting energy (see Chapter 5).
2. Sexual desire may be reduced in patients with depression; many antidepressant medications may also cause sexual dysfunction. Natural products such as yohimbe and damiana have been used traditionally to increase libido, and may help revitalize sexual desire in depression.[1]
3. Depression may also present with physical symptoms such as backache and headache. Devil's claw has traditionally been used as an antiinflammatory and pain reliever for joint diseases, back pain, and headache. Several human studies support the use of devil's claw for these uses (see Chapter 9).
4. Stomach aches, indigestion, or changes in bowel habits may also occur with depression. Psyllium contains a high level of soluble dietary fiber and is the main ingredient in many common laxatives. Probiotics, found in yogurts and other foods, may also provide benefit for stomach complaints (see Chapter 24).
5. Depressive symptoms may be associated with the development of Alzheimer's disease and impaired cognitive function. *Ginkgo biloba* has been found to provide benefits in patients with early-stage Alzheimer's disease and multiinfarct dementia and may be as helpful as acetylcholinesterase inhibitor drugs such as donepezil (Aricept) (see Chapter 10).

INTEGRATIVE THERAPY PLAN

- Determine if the patient is being treated by a health care professional for the depressive symptoms or if the patient is attempting to self-treat the symptoms.
- Determine if the patient has had a complete mental and physical examination.
- Perform a complete medication review to determine if any drug may be precipitating or worsening a depressive episode.
- Determine if the patient has ever thought about self-harm or suicide. If so, the patient should be referred immediately to an appropriate health care professional.
- Inquire if the patient is receiving antidepressant treatment. If so, ask if the patient is experiencing adverse effects such as sedation or sexual dysfunction. Some herbal therapies, such as, ginkgo, may help reduce sexual side effects and improve sleep. Keep in mind that there is some concern that ginkgo may increase the risk of bruising and bleeding.
- St. John's wort has been found to be safe and effective for treatment of mild to moderate depression. It has been shown to be as effective as TCAs. It remains unclear if St. John's wort is as effective as SSRIs (e.g., fluoxetine). A typical starting dose of 300 mg of standardized 0.3% hypericin extract has been taken orally three times daily (may be standardized to 2%-5% hyperforin). Maintenance doses range from 300 to 600 mg daily. Ensure that the

Herbs and Supplements with Possible Antidepressant Effects*

HERB	SPECIFIC THERAPEUTIC USE(S)†	HERB	SPECIFIC THERAPEUTIC USE(S)†
Acerola	Depression	Hop	Depression, mood disorders
Aconite	Depression, mania	Hyssop	Depression
American pennyroyal	Mania	Ignatia	Depression, mood disorders
Anise	Depression		
Bael fruit	Depression (major)	Khat	Depression
Bamboo	Postpartum depression	Lady's slipper	Depression (mild)
Black cohosh	Depression	Lemon balm	Depression
Black currant	Depression	Maca	Depression
Black horehound	Depression	Mangosteen	Depression
Bupleurum	Depression	Milk thistle	Depression
Calamus	Depression	Mistletoe	Depression
Cardamom	Depression	Mugwort	Depression
Cat's claw	Depression	Muira puama	Depression
Chamomile	Postpartum depression	Noni	Depression
Chasteberry	Depression (menopausal)	Nux vomica	Depression
Chia	Depression	Organic food	Depression
Cinnamon	Depression	Perilla	Depression
Dong quai	Mood disorders	Rhodiola	Depression, mania, mood disorders
Ephedra	Depression		
Flaxseed and flaxseed oil	Depression	Rose hip	Depression
		Salvia divinorum	Bipolar disorder, depression
Germanium	Depression	Skullcap	Depression
Ginger	Depression	Spirulina	Depression, mood disorders
Ginseng	Depression, mood disorders	Thyme	Depression
Goji	Depression	Tribulus	Mood disorders
Gotu kola	Depression, mood disorders	Valerian	Depression, mood disorders
Hoodia	Mood disorders	Yohimbe	Depression

*This is not an all-inclusive or comprehensive list of herbs with antidepressant properties; other herbs and supplements may possess these qualities. A qualified health care provider should be consulted with specific questions or concerns regarding potential antidepressant agents.
†Based on expert opinion, anecdote, case reports, and/or preliminary trial evidence.

product being considered is from a reputable and trusted manufacturer. St. John's wort has been associated with several significant drug interactions, including antiretroviral medications and digoxin. If St. John's wort is the patient's treatment of choice, it should be done under the guidance of a health care professional.

- Patients with PMDD may benefit from herbal treatment with chasteberry. Due to the dopaminergic effects of chasteberry, it could theoretically interfere with the actions of medications for Parkinson's disease and antipsychotic drugs. However, clinical evidence of chasteberry-drug interactions is lacking.
- Family members and friends should be involved, whenever possible, to evaluate and assess the patient's response to treatment.
- Monitor for compliance to antidepressant therapy.
- The cost of treating depression, including the cost of medications, should be considered. Herbal agents (e.g., St. John's wort) may prove just as effective (but at less cost) as prescription drugs. Insurance coverage varies from plan to plan.

Case Studies

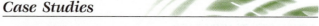

CASE STUDY 5-1

While standing at the pharmacy counter, 31-year-old KB complains of being depressed. She cannot sleep and has no desire to do anything. Further discussion reveals that KB has taken imipramine for several years with success. However, she was recently weaned off the medication because she did not like the side effects and wanted to try something "natural." KB does not take any other medications. How should you counsel?

Answer: First, advise KB to speak with a physician or mental health professional before self-medicating. St. John's wort has been shown to be effective with mild side effects in general. If KB wants to try St. John's wort, she should be advised on the dose. For a starting dose, suggest 300 mg of standardized 0.3% hypericin extract by mouth three times daily (may be standardized to 2%-5% hyperforin as well). For maintenance therapy 300 to 600 mg daily may be adequate. Follow-up of symptoms and potential side effects by a health care professional is advisable. Because KB is also having difficulty sleeping, you may also want to suggest melatonin or chamomile tea.

CASE STUDY 5-2

LH is 33 years old and suffers from PMDD. She has severe mood swings, irritability, and backaches. Her doctor gave her a prescription for fluoxetine, but she would rather try an herbal product. She also takes oral contraceptives (OCs). She asks you if there is anything that works as well as fluoxetine. How should you respond?

Answer: Chasteberry was comparable to fluoxetine (both 20-40 mg daily for 8 weeks) for relieving symptoms of PMDD. LH should be cautioned on the potential interaction between chasteberry and OCs. Chasteberry may increase plasma levels of estrogens and progesterone, thereby interfering with hormone therapy. Advise LH to speak with her doctor about monitoring her hormone levels. You may also want to recommend that she use a barrier method of birth control. For her backaches, you may suggest devil's claw, traditionally used as an antiinflammatory and pain reliever for back pain and headache.

CASE STUDY 5-3

VE is a 38-year-old man who complains of being depressed, which began shortly after he was diagnosed HIV positive, about 2 years ago. He is currently taking highly active antiretroviral therapy (HAART), consisting of didanosine, ritonavir, saquinavir, and zidovudine. He is also taking a short course of azithromycin for a recent pneumonia. He asks about using St. John's wort for the depression. How do you counsel?

Answer: Although St. John's wort may be beneficial for patients with depression, it is not an ideal option for VE. Concurrent use of St. John's wort and protease inhibitors should be avoided because of the induction of cytochrome P450 3A4 metabolism and the risk of treatment failure.

References for Chapter 5 can be found on the Evolve website at http://evolve.elsevier.com/Ulbricht/herbalpharmacotherapy/

Review Questions

1. St. John's wort appears to inhibit the reuptake of which neurotransmitter(s)?
   a. Norepinephrine
   b. Dopamine
   c. Serotonin
   d. All the above

2. True or false: Research suggests that lavender tincture alone may be beneficial to treat symptoms of depression.

3. St. John's wort has been reported to cause which of the following side effects?
   a. Sexual dysfunction
   b. Photosensitivity
   c. Headache
   d. All the above

4. Which herb has been reported to inhibit monoamine oxidase?
   a. Ginger
   b. Elder
   c. Ginkgo
   d. Lavender

5. Which is the recommended maintenance dose of St. John's wort for depression?
   a. 30 to 60 mg daily
   b. 3 to 6 g daily
   c. 300 to 600 mg three times daily
   d. 300 to 600 mg daily

6. True or false: Research suggests that ginkgo is effective in preventing the development of seasonal affective disorder.

7. All the following statements are true *except*:
   a. Short-term studies suggest that St. John's wort is more effective than TCAs for severe depression.
   b. Negative and equivocal results have been published in trials of St. John's wort for major depression, in addition to other positive studies.
   c. St. John's wort may alter the activity of cytochrome P450 enzymes.
   d. St. John's wort may cause serotonin syndrome.

8. Ginkgo may cause which of the following?
   a. Increased risk of bleeding
   b. Hypertensive crisis when ingested with tyramine-containing foods such as wine or cheese
   c. Increased insulin levels
   d. All the above

9. True or false: Chasteberry may be beneficial for premenstrual dysphoric disorder (PMDD).

10. Sage may improve which of the following symptoms?
    a. Anxiety
    b. Bloating
    c. Backache
    d. Uncontrollable crying

Answers are found in the Answers to Review Questions section in the back of the text.

6 Physical and Cognitive Enhancement

Outline

OVERVIEW
   Uses for Herbal Stimulants
      Attention Disorders
      Narcolepsy
      Chronic Fatigue Syndrome
      Fatigue and Low Energy
      Athletic Performance
      Weight Loss
SELECTED HERBAL THERAPIES
   Astragalus *(Astragalus membranaceus)*
   Betel Nut *(Areca catechu)*
   Cordyceps *(Cordyceps sinensis)*
   Evening Primrose *(Oenothera biennis)*
   Garcinia *(Garcinia cambogia)*
   Ginkgo *(Ginkgo biloba)*
   Ginseng *(Panax* spp.)
   Guarana *(Paullinia cupana)*
   Kiwi *(Actinidia deliciosa, Actinidia chinensis)*
   Papaya *(Carica papaya)*
   Pycnogenol *(Pinus pinaster* subsp. *atlantica)*
   Rhodiola *(Rhodiola rosea)*
   Sandalwood *(Santalum album)*
   Tribulus *(Tribulus terrestris)*
HERBAL THERAPIES WITH LIMITED EVIDENCE
ADJUNCT THERAPIES
INTEGRATIVE CARE PLAN
CASE STUDIES
REVIEW QUESTIONS

Learning Objectives

- Recognize the herbs used for cognitive and physical enhancement.
- Understand the evidence behind herbs used for cognitive and physical enhancement and the development of dependency.
- Identify the mechanism of action and pharmacokinetics of herbs that stimulate the central nervous system.
- Discuss the adverse effects and major drug interactions associated with stimulant herbs.
- Inform patients about adjunct therapies for physical and cognitive enhancement.
- Educate patients regarding an integrative pharmacotherapy plan.

OVERVIEW

Central nervous system (CNS) stimulants, also called psychomotor stimulants or uppers, are drugs that speed up physical and mental processes; thus, they are often used to enhance mental or physical performance. They may temporarily make patients feel more alert and improve mood.[1]

Stimulants may be used to treat certain medical conditions, such as attention-deficit disorder (ADD), attention-deficit hyperactivity disorder (ADHD), fatigue, and narcolepsy. Some stimulants have been used as appetite suppressants, although the safety of this use remains controversial. Examples of CNS stimulants include amphetamines, such as methylphenidate (Ritalin); amphetamine mixed salts (Adderall); caffeine (coffee, tea); nicotine (cigarettes, cigars); and cocaine.[1]

The CNS effects of amphetamines are caused by release of catecholamines (norepinephrine and dopamine) from presynaptic storage sites in the nerve terminals, increasing the amounts available at the postsynaptic receptor (Figure 6-1).[2] Catecholamine receptors are present throughout the CNS. Increased norepinephrine and dopamine concentrations in the brain are thought to be responsible for the increased attention span and concentration in patients treated with stimulants.[3]

The physiological and psychological effects of CNS stimulants vary depending on the specific drug.[4] In general, short-term use may cause side effects such as anxiety, insomnia, dry mouth, depersonalization, euphoria, increased heartbeat, crying, dysphoria, decreased appetite, hyperventilation, irritability, depression, nervousness, paranoia, mood swings, restlessness, shaking, or trembling. Long-term use of stimulants may cause side effects such as difficulty breathing, dizziness, changes in mood, and increased or pounding heartbeat.

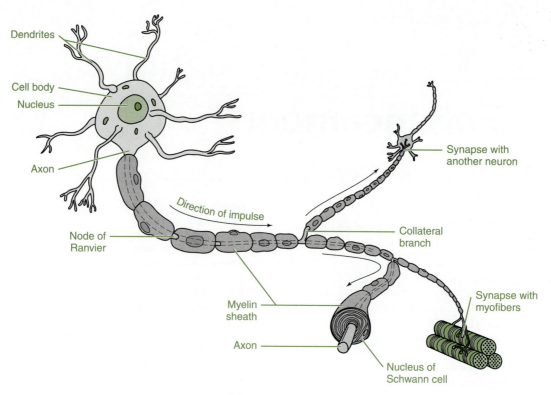

Figure 6-1 A typical neuron. (Modified from Fehrenbach MJ, ed: *Dental anatomy coloring book*, St Louis, 2008, Saunders-Elsevier.)

Some stimulant drugs are controlled substances, regulated by the Controlled Substance Act (CSA) enacted by Congress in 1970.[5] This law classified controlled substances into five categories or *schedules*:

Schedule I: Schedule I drugs have little medicinal value but a high potential for abuse. Therefore, these drugs are very rarely prescribed for medical conditions. Schedule I stimulants include aminoxaphen (Aminorex), cathinone, fenethylline (Captagon), methcathinone, methylaminorex, and amphetamine variants (e.g., 3,4-methylenedioxymethamphetamine).

Schedule II: Schedule II drugs also have a high abuse potential. Patients are likely to become psychologically and/or physically dependent on these drugs. Unless it is an emergency, prescriptions for schedule II drugs must be made in writing and signed by a healthcare professional. If it is a medical emergency, the healthcare professional must provide written confirmation of a verbal prescription within 72 hours. Prescriptions for schedule II drugs cannot be renewed. Examples of schedule II stimulants include dextroamphetamine (Dexedrine), methamphetamine (Desoxyn), methylphenidate (Ritalin), phenmetrazine (Preludin), and biphetamine. Cocaine, commonly used illegally, also falls under this category.

Schedule III: Schedule III drugs are less likely to be abused than schedule I and II drugs. Healthcare professionals can give verbal or written prescriptions and up to five renewals within 6 months. Examples of class III stimulants include benzphetamine (Didrex), chlorphentermine, clortermine, and phendimetrazine tartrate (Plegine or Prelu 2).

Schedule IV: Schedule IV drugs are less likely to be abused than schedule III drugs. Healthcare professionals can give verbal or written prescriptions and up to five renewals within 6 months. Examples of schedule IV stimulants include armodafinil (Nuvigil), norpseudoephedrine, diethylpropion hydrochloride (Tenuate), fencamfamin, fenproporex, phentermine (Fastin, Lonamin, or Adipex), mazindol (Sanorex or Mazanor), mefenorex, modafinil (Provigil), pipradrol, and sibutramine (Meridia).

Schedule V: This schedule includes one class of stimulants called pyrovalerones. These drugs are less likely to be abused than schedule IV stimulants. These drugs are regulated according to state legislation; in some areas, a prescription may not be needed.

Many stimulants are used recreationally for no medical purposes. *Substance abuse* refers to the recreational use of drugs, regardless of whether they are legal or illegal. CNS stimulants that are commonly abused include nicotine, caffeine, methamphetamine, and cocaine; other commonly abused drugs include alcohol, heroin, and marijuana. Abused drugs can be taken by mouth, injected into a vein, snorted through the nose, inhaled, or smoked.[4,5]

Stimulant abuse can lead to serious and potentially life-threatening health conditions. For example, nicotine (a stimulant found in tobacco products) temporarily makes patients feel euphoric or energized. However, nicotine is a highly addictive drug, and the tar in cigarettes increases a smoker's risk of lung cancer and emphysema.

Methamphetamine may also create feelings of pleasure, increased energy, and euphoria.[4,5] Methamphetamine can be smoked, injected, inhaled, or taken orally. When used recreationally, methamphetamine is often called chalk, crystal, glass, ice, meth, speed, or Tina. Because methamphetamine is stronger, longer lasting, and even more addictive than most other types of stimulants, it is often abused.

Cocaine, derived from the coca plant, is a CNS stimulant that is frequently abused.[1,4,5] The hydrochloride salt form of cocaine can be snorted in powder form or dissolved in water and injected into a vein. "Crack" is cocaine that has not been neutralized by an acid to make the hydrochloride salt.[4,5] Because it is cocaine in its "free" basic form, crack is often referred to as *freebase*, and its use is called *freebasing*. This form of cocaine looks like a rock crystal, and individuals who use crack typically heat it and inhale the vapors.

When addicted individuals stop using stimulants, withdrawal symptoms often develop and generally include irritability, headaches, nausea, vomiting, and mood swings.[5] The severity of symptoms varies, depending on the specific drug. For example, individuals who abuse methamphetamines experience severe withdrawal symptoms that may even be life threatening, including intense cravings for the drug, psychotic reactions, anxiety, moderate to severe depression, intense hunger, irritability, fatigue, mental confusion, and insomnia.

Uses for Herbal Stimulants

Attention Disorders

Attention-deficit hyperactivity disorder, also known as attention deficit disorder (ADD), is a psychiatric condition characterized by ongoing inattention, distractibility, impulsivity, and hyperactivity. ADHD is one of the most commonly diagnosed psychiatric disorders in children and adolescents. ADHD becomes apparent in some children in the preschool and early school years; it is thought to affect about 9.2% of boys and 2.9% of girls of school age. About 60% of children diagnosed with ADHD retain the disorder as they mature. Adults with ADHD are diagnosed under the same criteria as children.[6] Although an estimated 4.4% of adults are affected by ADHD, it often goes unrecognized in the adult population.

Methylphenidate (Ritalin) is commonly prescribed to treat ADHD, as are amphetamine mixed salts (Adderall), dextroamphetamine (Dexedrine, Dextrostat), benzphetamine (Didrex), and lisdexamfetamine (Vyvanse).[1-3,6] These stimulants help improve attention and concentration, thereby decreasing restlessness and distraction in patients with ADHD; these medications may also help stabilize emotions. These medications are typically used in combination with social, educational, and psychological therapies.[1-3,6]

Signs and Symptoms

The symptoms of ADHD fall into two broad categories: inattention and hyperactive-impulsive behavior. These symptoms often continue throughout life if untreated.

INATTENTION. Inattention may be described as excessive distractibility; this may manifest as failure to pay close attention to details, difficulty staying focused, and appearing not to listen when addressed. Procrastination is also a symptom of ADHD, as patients may avoid tasks that require a high amount of mental effort and organization, and appear unable to initiate or finish many activities. ADHD patients may seem forgetful, and may fail to follow instructions, or frequently lose items required to facilitate tasks or activities (e.g., school supplies). Household activities (e.g., cleaning, paying bills) may be difficult. Other symptoms include difficulty falling asleep, frequent emotional outbursts, and becoming easily frustrated.

HYPERACTIVE-IMPULSIVE BEHAVIOR. Hyperactive-impulsive symptoms involve frequent restlessness. This may manifest as fidgeting with the hands or feet, or squirming while sitting. Children with hyperactive impulsive behavior often have difficulty in quiet play, may get up from their seats inappropriately, and may run or climb excessively. Impulsive behavior also includes excessive speech or answering questions before speakers finish; individuals with ADHD often fail to wait their turns, and may interrupt the speech or activities of others. Impulsive spending may lead to financial difficulties.

Diagnosis

Diagnosis of ADHD is mainly based on observed symptoms and behavior.[6] A positive diagnosis is usually made only if the person has experienced six of the signs and symptoms previously listed for at least 3 months. Symptoms must appear consistently in varied environments (not only at home or school) and must interfere with general functioning.

CLINICAL TESTING. The American Academy of Pediatrics Clinical Practice Guideline for children with ADHD states that a diagnosis should be based on the following three criteria:

1. Explicit guidelines from the *Diagnostic and Statistical Manual of Mental Disorders (DSM)*, the clinical reference for psychiatric illnesses, are used (see box).[5] The Conner's Rating Scale is often used.
2. It is important to obtain information about the child's symptoms in more than one setting. This is accomplished by obtaining a personal medical and family history from parents, teachers, and the patient.
3. Coexisting conditions are also identified, which may make the diagnosis more difficult or complicate treatment planning. This is done with psychological and intelligence testing.

Diagnostic Criteria for Attention-Deficit/Hyperactivity Disorders

A. Either (1) or (2):

(1): Six (or more) of the following symptoms of inattention have persisted for at least 6 months to a degree that is maladaptive and inconsistent with developmental level:

Inattention
- (a) often fails to give close attention to details or makes careless mistakes in schoolwork, work, or other activities
- (b) often has difficulty sustaining attention in tasks or play activities
- (c) often does not seem to listen when spoken to directly
- (d) often does not follow through on instructions and fails to finish schoolwork, chores, or duties in the workplace (not due to oppositional behavior or failure to understand instructions)
- (e) often has difficulty organizing tasks and activities
- (f) often avoids, dislikes, or is reluctant to engage in tasks that require sustained mental effort (e.g., schoolwork or homework)
- (g) often loses things necessary for tasks or activities (e.g., toys, school assignments, pencils, books, or tools)
- (h) is often easily distracted by extraneous stimuli
- (i) is often forgetful in daily activities

(2): Six (or more) of the following symptoms of hyperactivity-impulsivity have persisted for at least 6 months to a degree that is maladaptive and inconsistent with developmental level:

Hyperactivity
- (a) often fidgets with hands or feet or squirms in seat
- (b) often leaves seat in classroom or in other situations in which remaining seated is expected
- (c) often runs about or climbs excessively in situations in which it is inappropriate (in adolescents or adults, may be limited to subjective feelings of restlessness)
- (d) often has difficulty playing or engaging in leisure activities quietly
- (e) is often "on the go" or often acts as if "driven by a motor"
- (f) often talks excessively

Impulsivity
- (a) often blurts out answers before questions have been completed
- (b) often has difficulty awaiting turn
- (c) often interrupts or intrudes on others (e.g., butts into conversations or games)

B. Some hyperactive-impulsive or inattentive symptoms that caused impairment were present before age 7 years.
C. Some impairment from the symptoms is present in two or more settings (e.g., at school [or work] and at home).
D. There must be clear evidence of clinically significant impairment in social, academic, or occupational functioning.
E. The symptoms do not occur exclusively during the course of a Pervasive Developmental Disorder, Schizophrenia, or other psychotic disorder and are not better accounted for by another mental disorder (e.g., Mood Disorder, Anxiety Disorder, Dissociative Disorder, or a Personality Disorder).

Code based on type:

314.01 Attention-Deficit/Hyperactivity Disorder, Combined Type: If both criteria A1 and A2 are met for the past 6 months.

314.00 Attention-Deficit/Hyperactivity Disorder, Predominantly Inattentive Type:
If criterion A1 is met but criterion A2 is not met for the past 6 months

314.01 Attention-Deficit/Hyperactivity Disorder, Predominantly Hyperactive-Impulsive Type:
If criterion A2 is met but criterion A1 is not met for the past 6 months

Coding note: For individuals (especially adolescents and adults) who currently have symptoms that no longer meet full criteria, "In Partial Remission" should be specified.

From American Psychiatric Association: *Diagnosis and statistical manual of mental disorders*, ed 4, text revision, Washington, DC, 2000, American Psychiatric Association.

Narcolepsy[1]

Patients with narcolepsy, a condition that causes individuals to have sudden attacks of deep sleep or an uncontrollable desire to sleep, may also receive stimulants.[1] These drugs help narcoleptic patients stay awake during the day. Modafinil (Provigil) is less addictive and better tolerated than other older types of stimulants. However, depending on the severity of the disease, some patients may need treatment with methylphenidate or other types of amphetamines.

Signs and Symptoms

Patients with narcolepsy are excessively tired throughout the day. Individuals can fall asleep at any time, even during conversations, or any place throughout the day. These sleep attacks may last from a few minutes to a half hour. Individuals also experience decreased alertness and concentration.

About 70% of narcoleptic patients have periodic episodes of *cataplexy*, which is a sudden and temporary loss of muscle tone. This condition, which may last from a few seconds to a few minutes, may cause symptoms that range from slurred speech and drooling to complete muscle weakness. Laughter or strong emotions, especially excitement and sometimes fear or anger, typically trigger cataplexy. Some patients may experience cataplexy only a few times a year, whereas others may have symptoms several times a day.

Sleep paralysis may occur while the individual is falling asleep or awakening. This temporary inability to move typically lasts a few seconds to several minutes. Patients may feel scared because they are often aware of what is happening, even though they cannot move. Some may experience hallucinations if they are partially awake when they start dreaming. Additional symptoms may include restless nighttime sleep or sleepwalking.

Diagnosis

If narcolepsy is suspected, the patient may be required to spend the night at a sleep center, where specialists observe the patient's sleep patterns and behavior. Electrodes may be placed on the patient's scalp for *polysomnography*, which measures the electrical activity of the brain and heart, as well as muscle and eye movements. Patients may also be asked to fill out a sleep questionnaire called the Epworth Sleepiness Scale, to rank their degree of tiredness during certain activities. A *multiple sleep latency test* may also be performed at a sleep center, with the patient taking several naps about 2 hours apart. Narcoleptic patients will fall asleep quickly and enter rapid eye movement (REM) sleep almost immediately.[1]

Chronic Fatigue Syndrome[7]

Chronic fatigue syndrome (CFS) is a disorder that causes extreme fatigue. The condition does not improve with bed rest. The flulike symptoms associated with the disorder may last for years. The U.S. Centers for Disease Control and Prevention (CDC) acknowledged the disease in 1988. However, the cause still remains unknown, and no method currently exists to measure the severity of the condition. Also, since little is known about the disease, few treatment options are available. CFS may occur after an infection. It may develop during or shortly after a period of high stress. It may also develop gradually with no clear starting point. The illness may develop at any point in life, however, it is most prevalent among individuals who are 40 to 59 years old. Occasionally, CFS is seen in members of the same family. However, there is no scientific evidence to suggest that CFS is contagious. Instead, researchers suspect that there may be a familial predisposition or genetic link to the disease. More research is needed to confirm these claims.

Women are diagnosed with CFS two to four times more often than men, according to researchers. However, it is unclear whether CFS affects more women or if women report the condition to their doctors more than men.

According to the CDC, about one million Americans have CFS. This disease affects more Americans than multiple sclerosis, lupus, lung cancer, or ovarian cancer.[1]

The cause of CFS remains unknown. However, researchers have suggested some possible causes, which include iron deficiency anemia, hypoglycemia (low blood sugar), history of allergies, viral infections (such as Epstein-Barr virus), immune system dysfunction, and hypotension, as well as changes in the levels of hormones produced in the hypothalamus, pituitary glands, and adrenal glands.

The disease may be caused by inflammation in the nervous system pathways, which occurs in reaction to the autoimmune process. However, unlike other autoimmune diseases (e.g., rheumatoid arthritis, lupus), CFS cannot be detected in the blood. Other researchers suggest that CFS occurs when a viral illness is complicated by a dysfunctional immune system.

Signs and Symptoms

Symptoms of CFS are similar to common viral infections; however, CFS symptoms may last anywhere from months to years.[7] Some individuals recover completely from the disorder while other patients' symptoms become progressively worse. Symptoms may also subside and then reappear later. Individuals meet the diagnostic criteria for CFS when they experience unexplained persistent fatigue for 6 months or longer with at least four of the eight primary symptoms, according to the International Chronic Fatigue Syndrome Study Group, which was brought together by the CDC. The eight primary symptoms of CFS include loss of memory or concentration, sore throat, painful and enlarged lymph nodes, muscle soreness, joint pain (without swelling or redness), headache, sleep disturbance, and extreme exhaustion. Individuals with CFS may also experience a wide range of symptoms that are not part of the official diagnostic criteria. Additional symptoms may include abdominal pain, alcohol intolerance, bloating, chest pain, chronic cough, diarrhea, dizziness, dry eyes or mouth, earache, irregular heartbeat, jaw pain, morning stiffness, nausea, night sweats, psychological problems (such as depression and anxiety disorders), shortness of breath, tingling sensation, and weight loss. Some people with CFS may develop a low blood pressure (hypotensive) disorder that causes fainting.

Diagnosis

In general, it is often difficult to diagnose CFS because it shares the symptoms of many other diseases, and there is currently no diagnostic or laboratory procedure that can confirm a diagnosis. In fact the CDC estimates that less than 20% of individuals who have CFS have been diagnosed. It is customary to first try to rule out other possible causes of fatigue, such as infections, immune disorders, tumors, muscle or nerve diseases (e.g., multiple sclerosis), endocrine diseases (e.g., hypothyroidism), drug dependence, heart disease, liver disease, kidney disease, or psychiatric or psychological illnesses (such as depression). A diagnosis is confirmed if the patient has experienced unexplained persistent fatigue for 6 months or longer with at least four of the eight primary symptoms described by the International Chronic Fatigue Syndrome Study Group.

Fatigue and Low Energy

Caffeine is a stimulant that is found in coffee and other beverages, including tea, soft drinks, and energy drinks, as well as in pill form (e.g., NoDoz). Caffeine is used to decrease fatigue and improve energy by increasing alertness, reducing sleepiness, enhancing mental performance, and improving mood.[1]

Athletic Performance

Athletic performance, also called *exercise performance,* describes an individual's ability to use various muscles to stay physically fit. An individual's athletic performance can be measured in terms of cardiovascular endurance, muscular strength, and exercise capacity. Energy drinks, or energy boosters, are beverages that contain stimulants, vitamins, and/or minerals. Many contain high levels of sugar as well as caffeine. Few studies have evaluated the safety or efficacy of energy drinks.[1]

Weight Loss

A common side effect of central nervous system (CNS) stimulants is decreased appetite. For this reason, several stimulants that have low risks for abuse and dependency have been prescribed to help treat obesity. Examples of these lower-risk drugs include dexfenfluramine, sibutramine, phentermine, fenfluramine, mazindol, diethylpropion, and fenproporex.[8] However, stimulants generally cause limited weight loss because patients eventually develop tolerances to chronic treatment.

Many stimulants are unsafe when taken as appetite suppressants (see Appendix A). Therefore, stimulants should only be taken to lose weight under the strict supervision of a qualified health care professional.

SELECTED HERBAL THERAPIES

Note

To help make this educational resource more interactive, all pharmacokinetics, adverse effects, and interactions data have been compiled in Appendix A. Safety data specifically related to pregnancy and lactation are listed in Appendix B. Please refer to these appendices when working through the case studies and answering the review questions.

Astragalus *(Astragalus membranaceus)*

Grade C: *Unclear or conflicting scientific evidence (athletic performance)*

Mechanism of Action

The mechanism of action of astragalus for fatigue improvement in athletes has not been determined. Astragalus has been found to have antioxidant effects and may be linked to enhanced recovery from exercise-induced fatigue.[9-19]

Scientific Evidence of Effectiveness

Astragalus is typically used in combination with other herbs; therefore it is difficult to determine if astragalus is effective as a monotherapy.

Clinical trials have investigated the effect of an astragalus-containing product, Huangqi Jianzhong Tang, in athletes.[19-20] This product was found to increase time to exhaustion, positively influence anaerobic threshold, and enhance recovery from fatigue.[19]

Dose

The dose of astragalus to boost athletic performance has not been determined.

Adverse Effects, Interactions, Pharmacokinetics. See Appendix A.

Betel Nut *(Areca catechu)*

Grade C: *Unclear or conflicting scientific evidence (stimulant)*

Despite widespread recreational use, because of documented toxicity associated with acute or chronic chewing or oral consumption, betel nut cannot be considered safe for human use, particularly when used chronically or in high doses.

Mechanism of Action

Betel nut use usually involves a combination of three ingredients: the nut of the betel palm *(Areca catechu),* part of the *Piper betel* vine, and lime. Although all three ingredients may contribute to stimulant effects, most experts attribute the psychoactive effects to the alkaloids found in betel nut.

In feline spinal neurons, the alkaloids arecaidine and guvacine, found in betel nut, were found to inhibit the uptake of gamma-aminobutyric acid (GABA), an amino acid that functions as an inhibitory neurotransmitter in the CNS. Arecaidine inhibited uptake of GABA when slices of cat cerebellum were used. The effect of electrophoretic GABA on the firing of cerebellar Purkinje cells was enhanced by electrophoretically applied arecaidine. When arecaidine was administered intravenously, there was no effect on GABA-mediated synaptic inhibition, prolonged spinal (presynaptic) inhibition, dorsal root potentials, or basket cell inhibition of Purkinje cells.[21,22]

Scientific Evidence of Effectiveness

Betel nut has not been systematically evaluated in humans, but it is often used recreationally for stimulant effects.

Dose

Betel nut can be chewed alone but is more often chewed as a *quid,* or a combination of ingredients. Ingredients other than betel nut may include calcium hydroxide, water, catechu gum, cardamom, cloves, anise seeds, cinnamon, tobacco, nutmeg, and gold or silver metal. These ingredients are often wrapped in a betel leaf, which is sucked in the lateral gingival pocket.

Adverse Effects, Interactions, Pharmacokinetics. See Appendix A.

Cordyceps (Cordyceps sinensis)

Grade C: *Unclear or conflicting scientific evidence (athletic performance)*

Mechanism of Action. Insufficient available evidence.

Scientific Evidence of Effectiveness

Although studies on exercise performance are conflicting and mainly anecdotal, Chinese athletes have used cordyceps for performance enhancement with some success.[23] In 1993, two female Chinese athletes who broke world records in the track and field competition at the Stuttgart World Championships for the 1500-, 3000-, and 10,000-meter runs admitted using cordyceps supplements. Chinese scientists also support the use of cordyceps in aging and longevity.[24] Patients who took cordyceps (CordyMax) reported beneficial effects in exercise performance, including an increase in maximal oxygen consumption.[25]

Dose

CordyMax contains 525 mg of a dried extract of cordyceps standardized to contain at least 0.14% adenosine. The extract is made from cultivated *Cordyceps mycelia*. The manufacturers recommend taking two capsules, two to three times daily. The traditional recommendation is to include 3 to 9 g daily in a hot tea or cooled meal. As an athletic performance enhancer, 3 g daily of fermented cordyceps (CordyMax) for 6 weeks has been found to increase aerobic capacity in healthy elderly subjects.[25]

Adverse Effects, Interactions, Pharmacokinetics. See Appendix A.

Evening Primrose (Oenothera biennis)

Grade C: *Unclear or conflicting scientific evidence (athletic performance)*

Grade D: *Fair negative scientific evidence (ADHD)*

Mechanism of Action

The stimulatory effects of evening primrose oil (EPO) are not well understood. EPO contains an omega-6 essential fatty acid, *gamma-linolenic acid* (GLA), which is believed to be the active ingredient.[26]

Scientific Evidence of Effectiveness

One small, randomized, double-blind, placebo controlled trial reported that patients with postviral fatigue syndrome who ingested EPO and fish oil had significantly improved symptoms of fatigue and infection compared with the placebo control group.[27] However, the effects of EPO cannot be separated from any effects that may be attributable to the concomitant administration of fish oil.

Small clinical trials have found EPO to have no significant benefit in behavioral measures greater than placebo for the treatment of ADHD.[28,29] Although these studies may not have had adequate statistical power, at this time the weight of the evidence must be considered negative.

Dose

Standardized capsules of EPO contain approximately 320 mg of linoleic acid (LA), 40 mg of GLA, and 10 IU of vitamin E.[30] Preparations may also be identified according to percent content (70% LA, 9% GLA).[31] Dietary conversion of LA provides 250 to 1000 mg daily of GLA.[32]

Taking eight 500-mg capsules of EPO and fish oil daily for 3 months has been used to treat postviral fatigue syndrome. Each capsule contained 8% EPO with 73% LA and 9% GLA, 20% fish oil with 18% eicosapentaenoic acid (EPA), and 20% docosahexaenoic acid.[27]

Adverse Effects, Interactions, Pharmacokinetics. See Appendix A.

Garcinia (Garcinia cambogia)

Grade C: *Unclear or conflicting scientific evidence (athletic performance)*

Mechanism of Action

The mechanism of action of garcinia to improve exercise performance is not well understood. Garcinia has been found to have antioxidant effects and may be linked to beneficial effects in athletic performance.[33]

Scientific Evidence of Effectiveness

Garcinia cambogia is a diminutive purple fruit native to India and Southeast Asia. The rind is rich in hydroxycitric acid (HCA). HCA capsules administered for 5 days tended to decrease the respiratory exchange ratio and carbohydrate oxidation during 1 hour of exercise in a randomized controlled trial (RCT) involving six subjects.[34] Exercise time to exhaustion was significantly enhanced ($p < 0.05$).

Dose

There is no well known standardization for garcinia. To enhance athletic performance, 250 mg of HCA for 5 days has been used in clinical study.[34]

Adverse Effects, Interactions, Pharmacokinetics. See Appendix A.

Ginkgo (Ginkgo biloba)

Grade A: *Strong scientific evidence (dementia)*

Grade B: *Good scientific evidence (cerebral insufficiency)*

Grade C: *Unclear or conflicting scientific evidence (memory)*

Grade D: *Fair negative scientific evidence (cognitive enhancement)*

Ginkgo has been studied for cerebral insufficiency, memory enhancement, and mental performance, and is discussed in Chapter 10, Alzheimer's Disease.

Ginseng (Panax spp.)

Grade C: *Unclear or conflicting scientific evidence (fatigue, athletic performance)*

Mechanism of Action

The major active components of ginseng are a diverse group of steroidal saponins called *ginsenosides*, the mechanisms of which are still largely unknown.[35-37] *Panax ginseng* has higher amounts of ginsenoside Rg1 than American ginseng. Rg1 is thought to be a slight CNS stimulant and to have hypertensive, antifatigue, and anabolic effects; it is also thought to enhance mental acuity and intellectual performance. Additionally, *P. ginseng* extracts contain similar constituents as guarana.[38]

Scientific Evidence of Effectiveness

Several studies evaluating exercise performance, cognitive performance, or mental performance have found positive benefits in fatigued patients when using *P. ginseng* supplements. Limited clinical study is currently available on testing *P. ginseng* for its effects on fatigue alone. The available clinical research indicates positive results and shows that ginseng, when taken with vitamins, may help treat symptoms of fatigue.

The evidence for and against the potential exercise performance–enhancing and ergogenic activity of *P. ginseng* is highly equivocal. Many trials have found that ginseng does not improve oxygen uptake, time to exhaustion, or rating of perceived exertion during ergometer exercise. However, decades of anecdotal evidence from China supports the use of *P. ginseng* for exercise performance and stamina, and *P. ginseng* is the most common herbal supplement used by athletes in China.[39]

Dose

Ginseng extracts may be standardized to 4% to 7% total ginsenosides content.[40] Some sources indicate that ginsenosides constitute an average of 3% of the dried, whole root,[41] and that the usual concentration of ginsenosides may actually be 1% to 3%. Standardized extracts of American ginseng *(Panax quinquefolius)* are also available.[42] The *German Federal Pharmacopeia* standardizes a minimum ginsenoside content of 1.5%, calculated in terms of the ginsenoside Rg1.[43]

A dose of 200 to 400 mg *Panax ginseng* has been taken once daily for up to 8 weeks to increase exercise endurance as well as improve cognitive performance.[44-48] American ginseng supplementation has been used for 4 weeks, but it did not improve exercise endurance.[49]

Adverse Effects, Interactions, Pharmacokinetics. See Appendix A.

Guarana (Paullinia cupana)

Grade C: *Unclear or conflicting scientific evidence (cognitive enhancement; mood enhancement; weight loss)*

Mechanism of Action

The main active ingredient of guarana is caffeine, which is responsible for its stimulatory effects.[50-53] One study found that the caffeine content of 12 different guarana products (dried paste, commercial powder, and ground tablets) ranged between 0.76% and 3.75%; an aqueous extract contained 8.9% caffeine.[54]

Caffeine, a methylxanthine, is a potent CNS stimulant.[50] It is a competitive inhibitor of phosphodiesterase, the enzyme responsible for the inactivation of cyclic 3′,5′-adenosine monophosphate (cAMP). Caffeine may cause increased alertness, decreased fatigue, and increased mental ability. Through its stimulatory effects, caffeine increases gastric secretion, cardiac output, and coronary blood flow. It may also release free fatty acids from adipose tissue.

Scientific Evidence of Effectiveness

Caffeine is a popular stimulant used worldwide. Studies have found that caffeine decreases mental concentration and recall in men but increases mental concentration and recall in women.[55,56] A meta-analysis of 12 studies involving theophylline and caffeine found that neither therapy had a significant detrimental effect on cognition or behavior.[57] However, elderly patients reportedly felt more alert when administered 250 mg of caffeine versus 250 mg of theophylline.[58] A flat dose-response relationship has been found for the psychoactive effects of caffeine.[59] Caffeine may significantly improve simple reaction time but may not improve immediate memory.[60]

Caffeine may have positive effects on mood because it has been shown to increase alertness and feelings of well-being and to improve performance on sustained attention tasks and simulated driving performance.[61-63] Slow-release caffeine consumption has been correlated with a decrease in calmness and an increase in sleep onset latency.[64]

Dose

Guarana is generally standardized in terms of caffeine content.[65] The amount of caffeine varies among products and manufacturers.[66,67] For cognitive enhancement, a single dose of 150 mg of guarana dry extract, standardized to 11% to 13% alkaloid concentration, has been used.[38] For energy enhancement, one to two tablets or capsules (200-800 mg guarana extract) before breakfast or lunch, not to exceed 3 g daily, has been used.

The U.S. Food and Drug Administration (FDA) recommends that pregnant women consume less than 300 mg of caffeine daily. Caffeine passes into breast milk in small amounts and may adversely affect the nursing infant (see Appendix B).

Adverse Effects, Interactions, Pharmacokinetics. See Appendix A.

Kiwi (Actinidia deliciosa, Actinidia chinensis)

Grade C: *Unclear or conflicting scientific evidence (athletic performance)*

Mechanism of Action. Insufficient available evidence.

Scientific Evidence of Effectiveness

One study suggests that a kiwi-containing drink may have beneficial effects on athletic performance by increasing endurance.[68] In athletes riding exercise bikes, the work time to exhaustion was longer and the workload was larger when supplementing with the kiwi-containing drink than when subjects drank a placebo.

Adverse Effects, Interactions, Pharmacokinetics. See Appendix A.

Papaya (Carica papaya)

Grade C: *Unclear or conflicting scientific evidence (athletic performance [exercise recovery])*

Mechanism of Action

Papain is an enzyme found in papaya *(Carica papaya)* fruit latex. It is a member of the papain family of cysteine proteinases that includes chymopapain, caricain, bromelain, actinidin, ficin, and aleurain, as well as the lysosomal cathepsins B, H, L, S, C, and K.[69-73] Its mechanism of action for enhancing exercise recovery is not well understood.

Scientific Evidence of Effectiveness

A controlled trial assessed the effect of protease tablets on muscle soreness and contractile performance after downhill running.[74] Ten pairs of matched runners took either two protease tablets (325 mg pancreatic enzymes, 75 mg trypsin, 50 mg papain, 50 mg bromelain, 10 mg amylase, 10 mg lipase, 10 mg lysozyme, 2 mg chymotrypsin) or a placebo four times daily, starting 1 day before an exercise test and lasting a total of 4 days. On day 2 the subjects ran a 10% grade for 30 minutes at 80% of their predicted maximal heart rate. The subjects were tested for perceived muscle soreness, pressure pain threshold, and knee extension/flexion torque and power. Those taking the protease tablets showed better recovery of contractile function and diminished effects of delayed-onset muscle soreness.

Dose. Insufficient available evidence.

Adverse Effects, Interactions, Pharmacokinetics. See Appendix A.

Pycnogenol (Pinus pinaster subsp. atlantica)

Grade C: *Unclear or conflicting scientific evidence (ADHD)*

Note: Pycnogenol contains oligomeric proanthocyanidins (OPCs) as well as several other bioflavonoids. There has been some confusion in the U.S. market regarding OPC products containing Pycnogenol or grape seed extract (GSE), because one of the generic terms for chemical constituents ("pycnogenols") is the same as the patented trade name (Pycnogenol). Some GSE products were formerly erroneously labeled and marketed in the U.S. as containing "pycnogenols." Although GSE and Pycnogenol do contain similar chemical constituents (primarily in the OPC fraction), the chemical, pharmacological, and clinical literature on the two products is distinct. The term *Pycnogenol* should therefore be used only when referring to this specific proprietary pine bark extract. Scientific literature regarding this product should not be referenced as a basis for the safety or effectiveness of GSE.

Mechanism of Action

The mechanism of action of Pycnogenol for ADHD is not well understood. It has been suggested that Pycnogenol lowers stress hormone levels in children with elevated levels, which are known to increase heart rate and blood pressure, causing excitement, arousal, and irritability.[75]

Scientific Evidence of Effectiveness

In a randomized controlled study, Pycnogenol was found to improve attention and various ratings scales in children with ADHD.[75] Endpoints included standard questionnaires: Child Attention Problems (CAP) teacher rating scale, Conner's Teacher Rating Scale (CTRS), Conner's Parent Rating Scale (CPRS), and a modified Wechsler Intelligence Scale for children. Pycnogenol administration caused a significant reduction in hyperactivity and improvement in attention and visual-motor coordination and concentration in children with ADHD. A relapse of symptoms was noted in the Pycnogenol group 1 month after study termination. Beneficial effects of Pycnogenol in adults have not been noted.[76]

Dose

Pycnogenol is a proprietary patented formula. For children with ADHD, 1 mg/kg of Pycnogenol daily for 4 weeks has been used.[75]

Adverse Effects, Interactions, Pharmacokinetics. See Appendix A.

Rhodiola (Rhodiola rosea)

Grade C: *Unclear or conflicting scientific evidence (athletic performance)*

Mechanism of Action

The mechanism of action of rhodiola for exercise performance enhancement has not been determined.[77-81] Rhodiola has been found to have antioxidant effects and may be linked to enhanced athletic performance.

Scientific Evidence of Effectiveness

Rhodiola rosea has been traditionally used to prevent fatigue and enhance physical and mental performance.[82] Although *R. rosea* was extensively studied in the former Soviet Union, much of this research is presently unavailable. Unsubstantiated reports suggest that *R. rosea* increased the duration of stable and hypoxemic phases of respiration and shortened respiratory recovery in Soviet skiers. In an experimental trial, *R. rosea* reportedly increased measured working capacity and improved self-assessed ratings of perceived exertion.[83] Also, *R. rosea* extract has been shown to have beneficial effects on creatine kinase after exhausting exercise.[78] In animals, *Rhodiola* extract increased running and swimming time.[84,85]

Dose

Properly standardized *Rhodiola* extract contains a minimum of 3% rosavin and 1% salidroside. For exercise performance enhancement, 100 mg of *R. rosea* extract has been used daily for 20 days.[86] A dose of 200 mg *R. rosea* extract, standardized to 3% rosavin and 1% salidroside, has been used as an acute treatement.[87]

Adverse Effects, Interactions, Pharmacokinetics. See Appendix A.

Sandalwood (Santalum album)

Grade C: *Unclear or conflicting scientific evidence (alertness)*

Mechanism of Action. Insufficient available evidence.

Scientific Evidence of Effectiveness

Preliminary clinical study has found that the inhalation of sandalwood oil improves alertness, attentiveness, and vigor.[88] Sandalwood was also reported to elevate pulse rate and systolic blood pressure. However, sandalwood has also been shown to cause relaxation. More research is needed to clarify these findings.

Dose

The dose of sandalwood for its use as a stimulant has not been determined.

Adverse Effects, Interactions, Pharmacokinetics. See Appendix A.

Tribulus (Tribulus terrestris)

Grade C: *Unclear or conflicting scientific evidence (athletic performance)*

Mechanism of Action. Insufficient available evidence.

Scientific Evidence of Effectiveness

Tribulus has been promoted for athletic performance and muscle mass enhancement and as a testosterone booster. However, these effects have not been demonstrated in available research.[89,90] In a randomized clinical trial to assess its effect on 15 athletes engaged in resistance training, tribulus (3.21 mg/kg body weight) or placebo was randomly administered to the subjects for 8 weeks.[89] There were no changes in body weight, percentage body fat, total body water, dietary intake, or mood states in either group. Muscle endurance (determined by maximal number of repetitions at 100%-200% of body weight) increased for the bench and leg press exercises in the placebo group ($p < 0.05$; bench press, ±28.4%; leg press, ±28.6%).

Dose. Insufficient available evidence.

Adverse Effects, Interactions, Pharmacokinetics. See Appendix A.

Bach Flower Remedies

Dr. Edward Bach (1886–1936) was a British physician who believed that illness is the effect of disharmony between body and mind, and that symptoms of an illness are the external expression of negative emotional states. The term *flower remedies* refers to a set of preparations developed by Dr. Bach. *Flower essences* are also products derived from Dr. Bach's work.[1]

Bach flower remedies constitute a therapeutic system that uses specially prepared plant infusions to balance physical and emotional disturbances. It is believed that every Bach flower remedy is related to an area on the surface of the body. Negative moods purportedly change the energetic structure in these places, which may be accompanied by pain and disturbing sensations. A *flower diagnosis* may be obtained by pinpointing the appropriate area on the body map.[1]

Bach flower remedies are produced in two ways: by the sun method or the cooking method. During the *sun method*, flowers are picked on a warm summer day in full sunshine. The flowers are placed in a glass bowl with fresh water, preferably taken from a spring close to the location of the flower. The bowl is then placed in the sun for 2 to 4 hours. According to Dr. Bach, the sun transfers the vibration of the flowers into the medium of the water, which thus becomes "energetically infused." The flowers are then removed from the water, and an equal portion of alcohol is added for preservation (Bach originally used brandy). This solution is stored in a stock bottle. During treatment the remedy is usually diluted with water and is consumed as an alcohol-based preparation, although it may also be available as a cream.

Bach Flower Remedies—cont'd

The *cooking method* for Bach flower remedies is often necessary because not all flowers, shrubs, bushes, and trees bloom at a time of year with plenty of sunshine. During the cooking method, flowers and buds are picked according to the sun method and boiled down. The extract is filtered several times and then mixed with an equal portion of alcohol as a preservative.

One RCT assessed the effect of Bach flower remedies in the treatment of children (age 7-11 years) with ADHD.[91] The 40 children were diagnosed according to the *DSM* criteria and were administered either Bach flower remedies or placebo for 3 months. A teacher evaluated the children's performance at the beginning of the study and each month during the study. Although there was no statistically significant effect on the children's behavior, a correlation was found between treatment duration and improved behavior only in the Bach flower remedy group.

Available study on the safety of Bach flower remedies is lacking. Bach flower remedies do not appear to have many adverse effects and may not seem to interact with other medicines.[92]

HERBAL THERAPIES WITH LIMITED EVIDENCE

Bitter Orange (Citrus aurantium)

Similar to ephedra, bitter orange contains alkaloids that may have stimulant effects and may increase heart rate and blood pressure. Bitter orange is currently being used as a stimulant in "ephedra-free" weight loss supplements.

Dong Quai (Angelica sinensis)

Dong quai contains a coumarin stimulant, osthol, which may inhibit phosphodiesterase activity.[93] As a result, cAMP levels remain high enough to maintain an alert state.

Ephedra (Ephedra sinica)

Dietary supplements that contain ephedra have been banned in the United States since April 2004 because of unacceptable cardiovascular health risks. *Ephedra sinica,* a species of ephedra (Ma huang), contains the alkaloids ephedrine and pseudoephedrine, which have been found to induce CNS stimulation. Manufacturers claim that ephedra, an adrenaline-like stimulant, will increase energy and endurance because it may increase blood flow to muscles, resulting in greater oxygen supply to muscles. Currently, however, there is insufficient evidence to support use of ephedra for athletic performance.

Khat (Catha edulis)

Khat is a plant used in eastern Africa and southern Arabia for its stimulant effects. Its pharmacological activity has been attributed to *d*-norpseudoephedrine, also known as cathine. The isolation in 1975 of *cathinone* revived an earlier suggestion that the fresh leaves contained a substance more potent than cathine. Cathinone produces qualitatively similar locomotor stimulation in mice and comparable stereotypy in rats as amphetamine does, although cathinone is approximately half as active. The results obtained after pretreatment with reserpine or α-methyl-*p*-tyrosine, which interfere with the catecholamine system, strongly suggest that cathinone interacts with brain catecholamines by an indirect mechanism and most probably by affecting neurotransmitter release of the labile pool.[94]

Kola Nut (Cola acuminata)

Caffeine is the active ingredient in kola nut and is known to stimulate the heart and CNS. Kola nut is popularly used for mental and physical relief, especially when associated with general muscle weakness.

Maca (Lepidium meyenii)

Maca is an herb popular in South America that is used as an intended physical and mental energizer as well as to stimulate libido.[94,95] Constituents of maca have been found to stimulate the CNS.[96] Currently, human studies to support this use are lacking.

Schisandra (Schisandra chinensis)

Schisandra fruit is typically used to increase energy and physical performance and endurance. Although human trials are lacking for this use, schisandra has been shown to stimulate the nervous system, which increases reflex responses and improves mental alertness.[97]

Tea (Camellia sinensis)

Tea is a source of caffeine, a methylxanthine that is known to stimulate the CNS. It also contains theanine, an amino acid that purportedly improves alertness while decreasing anxiety. Historically, tea was used in various ceremonies and to stay alert during long meditations.

ADJUNCT THERAPIES

1. Stimulants are frequently abused medications. There is a growing concern about the safety of these agents. In general, stimulants should be used alone at the lowest effective dose. Stimulants may cause insomnia, restlessness, and nervousness. Sedative herbs such as *valerian* or *chamomile* may be used; however, these agents may antagonize the effects of stimulant herbs. *Melatonin* may also be beneficial in treating sleep disorders and restlessness.

2. Having symptoms of sleep disorders and narcolepsy may also affect mental health and cause depression. *St. John's wort* is often used for depressive disorders and is generally tolerated for 1 to 3 months.

3. Certain drugs such as clonidine, an α-2-adrenergic agonist, may be used to treat rebound symptoms of ADHD that occur in the evening, as well as impulsivity, hyperactivity, and

Herbs with Stimulant Properties*

HERB	SPECIFIC THERAPEUTIC USE(S)†	HERB	SPECIFIC THERAPEUTIC USE(S)†
Abuta	Stimulant	Hoodia	Physical enhancement
Ackee	Stimulant	Horny goat weed	Fatigue
Aconite	Stimulant, malaise	Horseradish	Stimulant
African wild potato	Chronic fatigue syndrome	Hyssop	Fatigue, stimulant
Aloe	Chronic fatigue syndrome	Lady's slipper	Stimulant
Alpinia	Stimulant	Lavender	Fatigue
American pennyroyal	Stimulant	Lemon balm	Chronic fatigue syndrome
Arnica	Stimulant, fatigue	Lemongrass	Fatigue, stimulant
Asarum	Stimulant	Licorice	Chronic fatigue syndrome
Ashwagandha	Fatigue	Lime	Stimulant
Bacopa	Fatigue	Lousewort	Fatigue (muscular)
Bay leaf	Stimulant	Lovage	Stimulant
Bilberry	Chronic fatigue syndrome	Mangosteen	CNS stimulant
Black cohosh	Malaise	Mastic	Stimulant
Black horehound	Stimulant	Mistletoe	Fatigue
Blue flag	Fatigue, stimulant	Mugwort	Fatigue, stimulant
Boneset	Stimulant	Muira puama	Stimulant, physical enhancement, fatigue
Boxwood	Fatigue	Noni	Chronic fatigue syndrome, athletic enhancement, stimulant (brain)
Buchu	Stimulant	Organic food	Chronic fatigue syndrome
Bupleurum	Fatigue	Pokeweed	Fatigue, stimulant
Calamus	Stimulant, physical enhancement	Raspberry	Fatigue, stimulant, chronic fatigue syndrome
Calendula	Fatigue	Rehmannia	Fatigue
California jimson weed	Stimulant	Reishi mushroom	Fatigue
Cardamom	Stimulant	Rose hip	Fatigue
Cat's claw	Chronic fatigue syndrome, stimulant	Safflower	Stimulant
Chicory	Stimulant	St. John's wort	Fatigue
Cornflower	Stimulant	Sea buckthorn	Fatigue
Damiana	Physical enhancement, stimulant	Seaweed, kelp, bladderwrack	Fatigue
Dandelion	Chronic fatigue syndrome, stimulant	Shiitake	Chronic fatigue syndrome, physical enhancement, fatigue, stimulant
Datura wrightii	Stimulant	Skunk cabbage	Stimulant (gastrointestinal)
Deer velvet	Physical enhancement	Spirulina	Physical enhancement, fatigue
Desert parsley	Chronic fatigue syndrome	Star anise	Stimulant
Essiac	Chronic fatigue syndrome, physical enhancement	Stinging nettle	Fatigue
Eucalyptus oil	Stimulant	Tansy	Stimulant
Euphorbia	Fatigue	Valerian	Fatigue
Fenugreek	Physical enhancement	Watercress	Stimulant
Garlic	Fatigue	Wheatgrass	Physical enhancement, malaise
Germanium	Chronic fatigue syndrome	White water lily	Fatigue
Ginger	Stimulant	Wild yam	Energy improvement
Goji	Chronic fatigue syndrome, fatigue	Yellow dock	Chronic fatigue syndrome, physical enhancement
Goldenseal	Chronic fatigue syndrome, stimulant	Yohimbe	Fatigue, physical enhancement
Gotu kola	Stimulant, physical enhancement		
Grape seed	Chronic fatigue syndrome		
Ground ivy	Stimulant		

*This is not an all-inclusive or comprehensive list of herbs with stimulant properties; other herbs and supplements may possess these qualities. A qualified health care provider should be consulted with specific questions or concerns regarding potential stimulant effects or interactions.
†Based on expert opinion, anecdote, case reports, and/or preliminary trial evidence.

aggression symptoms of ADHD.[98] Nonpharmacological behavioral therapy and psychosocial support may be advised.
4. Playing sports and enhancing athletic performance may lead to injury. Many injuries are painful because of swelling and are usually treated with antiinflammatory agents. Herbs such as pineapple (containing bromelain) and cat's claw may reduce inflammation and may be beneficial for these types of complaints.
5. Goldenseal is purported to be effective in masking the detection of illicit drugs from urinalysis; however, the mechanism of action is not clear. In vitro, goldenseal has demonstrated inconsistent interference with urine-testing methods.[99-102] A methodologically weak human trial assessing the effectiveness of goldenseal in masking marijuana and cocaine use suggests that it may be dilution of urine that causes false-negative results on urinalysis and not goldenseal itself, although conclusions of this study are not definitive.[102] It is not clear if ingestion of goldenseal conceals illegal drugs from urinalysis detection. Notably, the ethics of conducting trials to assess the efficacy of concealing illicit substances has not been adequately addressed by studies in this area.
6. Black pepper may be useful in suppressing withdrawal symptoms from stimulant use. *Piperine* is the active constituent of black pepper; sensory cues from cigarette substitutes delivered by black pepper may suppress certain smoking withdrawal symptoms, including craving for cigarettes. A randomized, placebo-controlled study assessed the effect of black pepper essential oil inhalation on cigarette smoking withdrawal symptoms in cigarette smokers.[103] Subjects were randomly assigned to puff on one of three devices: one that delivered a vapor from essential oil of black pepper, one with a mint/menthol cartridge, or one containing an empty cartridge. In the black pepper group, reported craving for cigarettes was significantly reduced compared with the other groups.

INTEGRATIVE CARE PLAN

- Discuss any relevant past or present medical conditions.
- Provide literature and scientific evidence regarding the use of appropriate herbs.
- Discuss a treatment plan individualized for the patient and his or her medical condition.
- Educate patients inquiring about physical performance enhancement products on the safety of herbal stimulants and the risks associated with them. Overconsumption of caffeine-containing products may lead to nervousness, sleeplessness, irritability, anxiety, and heart palpitations.
- For children with ADHD, Pycnogenol, a patented formula found in pine bark extract, has been shown to improve attention and coordination and reduce hyperactivity; 1 mg/kg daily was used in a clinical trial and was generally well tolerated.
- For patients concerned about binge drinking, kudzu is popularly used to reduce alcohol intake. However, inform patients that supportive scientific research is lacking.
- Ensure that a specific follow-up plan has been made.

Case Studies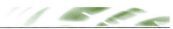

CASE STUDY 6-1

CH, a 38-year-old man, comes into the pharmacy and asks about an energy drink he wants to buy containing ginseng, guarana, and caffeine. He is going to the gym and wants something to increase his endurance. He currently takes sildenafil (Viagra) for erectile dysfunction and kava for anxiety. How should you counsel?

Answer: Energy drinks are becoming increasingly popular. They are being used by many people with different medical backgrounds and health concerns. CH should be advised not to take this energy drink because concurrent use of ginseng with kava, a hepatotoxic herb, may lead to adverse effects on the liver. Ginseng may also have additive effects when taken with sildenafil.

CASE STUDY 6-2

KG is a 30-year-old woman who comes into the pharmacy asking about weight-loss supplements. She has heard about the adverse effects of ephedra, and inquires about "ephedra-free" bitter orange. She is also drinking a large cup of coffee. How do you counsel?

Answer: Bitter orange is currently being used as a stimulant in "ephedra-free" weight loss supplements. However, bitter orange contains alkaloids that are similar to those found in ephedra, which may have stimulant effects and may increase heart rate and blood pressure. Because there are case reports of severe (and fatal) interactions between ephedra and caffeine, KG should be warned of potential interactions that may occur between bitter orange and caffeine.

CASE STUDY 6-3

BN, a 22-year-old college athlete, is looking to maximize her training. She is a sprinter, specializing in 100-meter and 200-meter races. She mentions that she previously used ephedra before it was banned. She asks you if tribulus will boost her performance. She also takes oral contraceptives (OCs). How should you counsel?

Answer: As with ephedra, tribulus has been promoted for athletic performance, and similar to ephedra, data are lacking to support this use. For BN, tribulus appears to be a safe option and has not been reported to interact with OCs. BN, however, should be warned that tribulus has been reported to cause menorrhagia (heavy menstrual bleeding).

References for Chapter 6 can be found on the Evolve website at http://evolve.elsevier.com/Ulbricht/herbalpharmacotherapy/

Review Questions

1. Which of the following has been used for postviral fatigue syndrome?
   a. Evening primrose oil
   b. Jasmine
   c. Chaparral
   d. Hops

2. Which of the following statements is *incorrect* regarding the use of borage?
   a. Borage should be used cautiously with agents that lower the seizure threshold.
   b. Gamma-linolenic acid (GLA) is a component from borage.
   c. Borage has been hypothesized as being effective for narcotic concealment.
   d. Borage may cause diarrhea and bloating.

3. Which herb has been promoted to enhance athletic performance and muscle mass?
   a. Kava
   b. Tribulus
   c. Betel nut
   d. Lavender

4. Papain may interact with which of the following?
   a. Warfarin
   b. Loperamide
   c. Cyclosporine
   d. All the above

5. True or false: The isoflavones in kudzu root extract may suppress alcohol intake and alcohol withdrawal symptoms in animals.

6. Which of the following natural products has supportive evidence for its use in ADHD?
   a. Pycnogenol
   b. Kudzu
   c. Bitter orange
   d. Aconite

7. True or false: *Rhodiola rosea* has been traditionally used for the prevention of fatigue and the enhancement of physical and mental performance.

Answers are found in the Answers to Review Questions section in the back of the text.

7 Parkinson's Disease

Outline

OVERVIEW
   Signs and Symptoms
      Primary Symptoms
      Secondary Symptoms
   Diagnosis
SELECTED HERBAL THERAPIES
   Ashwagandha *(Withania somnifera)*
   Cowhage *(Mucuna pruriens)*
   Tea *(Camellia sinensis)*

HERBAL THERAPIES WITH NEGATIVE EVIDENCE
HERBAL THERAPIES WITH LIMITED EVIDENCE
ADJUNCT THERAPIES
INTEGRATIVE THERAPY PLAN
CASE STUDIES
REVIEW QUESTIONS

Learning Objectives

- Identify signs and symptoms of Parkinson's disease.
- Understand herbal treatment strategies for patients with Parkinson's disease.
- Identify side effects caused by herbs used for Parkinson's disease.
- Recognize potential drug interactions with herbs used for Parkinson's disease.
- Counsel a patient on herbal treatment for Parkinson's disease.
- Educate patients regarding an integrative pharmacotherapy plan.

OVERVIEW

Parkinson's disease (PD) is a movement disorder that is chronic and progressive, meaning that symptoms continue and worsen over time. PD occurs when a group of cells in the substantia nigra region of the brain begin to malfunction and eventually die (Figure 7-1). These cells produce the neurotransmitter *dopamine*, which is implicated in the control of muscle movement and coordination. This loss of dopamine-producing cells decreases the amount of dopamine available in the brain. Therefore, messages from the brain telling the body how and when to move are delivered more slowly. Ultimately this leaves a person incapable of initiating and controlling movements in a normal way. PD is the most common form of *parkinsonism*, a group of movement disorders that have similar features and symptoms. Other causes of parkinsonism include viral encephalitis, degenerative disorders, structural brain disorders, head injury, drugs (e.g., antipsychotics), and toxins. When the cause of PD is unknown, it is called *idiopathic* Parkinson's disease.[1]

Because PD is associated with a reduction in dopamine-producing neurons, therapy is targeted at increasing dopamine levels in the brain and synapses, stimulating dopamine receptors with dopamine receptor agonists, or blocking dopamine metabolism and breakdown.[1]

Signs and Symptoms[1]

Parkinson's disease usually affects people over age 50. According to the American Parkinson Disease Association, more than 1.5 million people in the United States have PD. The disorder occurs in all races but is somewhat more prevalent among Caucasians. Men are affected slightly more often than women. PD is rare in people younger than age 30, and disease risk increases with age. It is estimated that 5% to 10% of patients experience symptoms before age 40.

Early symptoms of PD are subtle and occur gradually. The disease progresses more quickly in some people than in others. As the disease progresses, the shaking or tremor (which affects the majority of PD patients) may begin to interfere with daily activities.

Individuals with PD may develop various symptoms over time, but they typically develop the primary symptoms consisting of bradykinesia, tremor, and rigidity. They may also show a particular manner of walking called *parkinsonian*

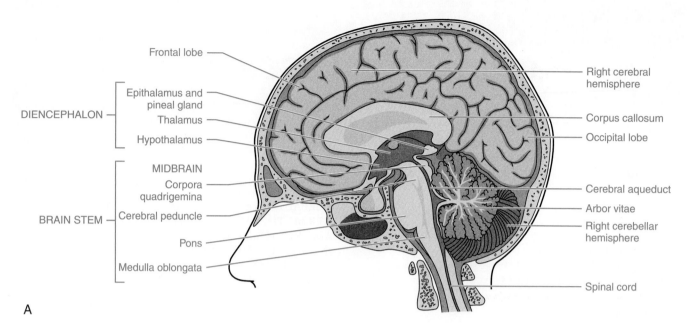

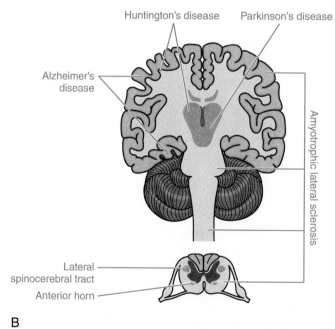

Figure 7-1 **A,** Normal central nervous system. **B,** Degenerative diseases of the brain preferentially involve various parts of the brain. Parkinson's disease is marked by changes in the substantia nigra. (*A* modified from Applegate EJ: *The anatomy and physiology learning system,* ed 3, Philadelphia, 2006, Saunders-Elsevier; *B* modified from Damjanov I: *Pathology for the health professions,* ed 3, St Louis, 2006, Saunders-Elsevier.)

gait, characterized by shuffling or taking small steps, decreased arm swinging, stooped posture, and periods of *freezing,* or inability to move. Other symptoms associated with PD include speech and swallowing difficulties and other nonmotor symptoms such as mood, cognitive, and sleep disturbances.

Primary Symptoms
Some individuals with PD experience tremor as the primary symptom, whereas others may not have tremor but instead experience balance problems. PD may progress quickly or gradually over years; many people become profoundly disabled, whereas others function relatively well. Symptoms

may vary from day to day or even from moment to moment, with no clear indication or pattern in the variation besides a possible link to disease progression or a response to PD medication.

Tremor

In the early stages of PD, approximately 70% of patients experience a slight tremor in the hand or foot on one side of the body or less often in the jaw or face. This tremor presents as a slight beating or pulsing movement in the cheek, face, or jaw. Because the Parkinson's tremor usually appears when an individual's muscles are relaxed and subsides when the muscles begin to move, it is called a *resting* tremor. As the disease progresses, tremor often spreads to the other side of the body but remains most apparent on the original side of occurrence. Hand tremors are often referred to as having a "pill-rolling" motion, because it appears the individual is rolling a pill between the thumb and fingers.

Rigidity

Rigidity is characterized by increased muscle tone and presents as stiffness or inflexibility of the muscles. In a normally functioning system, muscles stretch during movement and relax at rest. In rigidity the muscle tone of an affected limb maintains a stretched position; this results in constant stiffness without the ability to relax, sometimes resulting in pain, cramping, and a decreased range of motion. An individual with rigidity may not be able to swing the arms when walking because the muscles are too tight. "Cog wheeling" refers to the jerky movements of limbs as a constant force is applied across a joint, similar to the ratcheting of the cogs of gears as they click.[2]

Bradykinesia

Bradykinesia is characterized by slow movement and is typical in patients with PD. Individuals who have bradykinesia may walk with short, shuffling steps, called *festination* (a festinating gait).

Postural Instability

Individuals with PD often experience instability when standing or impaired balance and coordination. Postural instability combined with other symptoms (e.g., bradykinesia) increase the probability of falling in PD patients. Individuals with balance problems may have difficulty making turns or abrupt movements, and they may go through periods of *freezing*, when the individual feels stuck to the ground and has great difficulty initiating walking. The slowness and incompleteness of movement typically observed in PD patients can also affect their ability to speak and swallow.

Secondary Symptoms

Secondary symptoms of PD are typically caused by the cramping or rigidity of the muscles. The muscles in the face may become rigid, resulting in a loss of facial expression (called *masking*). There may be speech changes or a soft, whispery voice (termed *hypophonia*), difficulty swallowing, or drooling. Rigid hand muscles may cause *micrographia*, or small, cramped handwriting. Emotional disturbances may include dementia or confusion, sleep disturbances, depression and anxiety, and compulsive behavior. Skin conditions may present, including boils or eczema; patients may also experience constipation, sexual dysfunction, and urinary problems. Secondary symptoms also include pain and excessive fatigue.

Diagnosis

Because there are currently no blood or laboratory tests to detect the disease, the diagnosis of PD is based solely on medical history and neurological examination. Because of the lack of definitive testing measures, PD can be difficult to diagnose accurately. Physicians often request brain scans or laboratory tests to rule out other diseases.[1]

SELECTED HERBAL THERAPIES

Note

To help make this educational resource more interactive, all pharmacokinetics, adverse effects, and interactions data have been compiled in Appendix A. Safety data specifically related to pregnancy and lactation are listed in Appendix B. Please refer to these appendices when working through the case studies and answering the review questions.

Ashwagandha *(Withania somnifera)*

Grade C: *Unclear or conflicting scientific evidence*

Mechanism of Action. Insufficient available evidence.

Scientific Evidence of Effectiveness

Ashwagandha has been used in Ayurvedic medicine in India (see box) for hundreds of years as an "adaptogenic" herb *(rasayana)*, meaning that it is used to help the body resist physiological and psychological stress. It is purported to tone and normalize (revitalize) bodily functions. The potentially active constituents of ashwagandha include alkaloids and steroidal lactones that are collectively called *withanolides*, particularly withaferin A. Preparations are often standardized to their percentage contents of withanolides.[1,3]

There is insufficient scientific evidence to recommend the use of ashwagandha in the management of PD. Currently, clinical trial data are limited. One trial evaluated ashwagandha in an Ayurvedic combination with *Mucuna pruriens*, *Hyoscyamus reticulates*, and *Sida cordifolia* in milk. In this controlled human trial of 18 patients with PD, 13 patients received this concoction after a cleansing procedure, and five did not receive this therapy.[4] Symptomatically, the patients who received the multiherb preparation exhibited better response in tremor, bradykinesia, stiffness, and cramps. Analyses of the multiherb preparation revealed about 200 milligrams (mg) of L-dopa per dose, likely from the cowhage component; the contribution of ashwagandha was not clear. Studies evaluating ashwagandha alone are needed before a recommendation can be made.

Dose. Insufficient available evidence.

Adverse Effects, Interactions, Pharmacokinetics. See Appendix A.

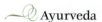

Ayurveda is a form of natural medicine that originated in ancient India more than 5000 years ago. It is an integrated system of techniques that uses diet, herbs, exercise, meditation, yoga, and massage (or "bodywork") to achieve optimal health on all levels (physical, psychological, and spiritual). In India, Ayurveda involves the eight principal branches of medicine: pediatrics, gynecology, obstetrics, ophthalmology, geriatrics, otolaryngology (ear, nose, throat), general medicine, and surgery.

Cowhage (Mucuna pruriens)

Grade C: *Unclear or conflicting scientific evidence*

Mechanism of Action

Cowhage contains about 3% to 6% levodopa (L-dopa), which is rapidly converted into dopamine by enzymes in the body. Because the symptoms of Parkinson's disease are related to insufficient dopamine, levodopa helps balance the levels of dopamine and decrease symptoms such as bradykinesia, rigidity, and tremor. Notably, because L-dopa is broken down peripherally, it is usually combined with a peripheral dopa decarboxylase inhibitor (e.g., carbidopa) to enhance its efficacy and reduce dose requirements. This approach to treatment is used in commercially available drugs for PD, which contain carefully regulated amounts of active ingredients. It has not yet been determined if cowhage should be similarly combined with other drugs, or if it independently improves symptoms of PD.[1,3]

Scientific Evidence of Effectiveness

Cowhage has long been used in traditional Ayurvedic medicine in India (see box) for treating PD. It generally contains about 3% to 6% L-dopa. Preliminary evidence shows that cowhage preparations may help improve PD symptoms, as measured by the Unified Parkinson's Disease Rating Scale.[4-6]

Dose

The exact dose of cowhage for PD has not been determined. However, specific cowhage extracts have been standardized to 3.3% L-dopa (HP-200). Doses have ranged from 22.5 to 67.5 grams (g) divided into two to five daily doses.[4-6]

Adverse Effects, Interactions, Pharmacokinetics. See Appendix A.

Tea (Camellia sinensis)

Grade C: *Unclear or conflicting scientific evidence*

The use of tea for PD, as well as many of its adverse effects and drug interactions, may be attributed to caffeine (a known stimulant), as well as to polyphenols such as green tea catechins (which are oxidized to theaflavins in black tea).

Mechanism of Action

Animal research has suggested the green tea polyphenol (—)-epigallocatechin-3-gallate (ECGC) possesses antioxidant and neuroprotective activity. Green tea polyphenols are able to cross the blood-brain barrier and may prevent dopaminergic neurodegeneration.[7] Polyphenols have been found to block the dopamine transporter, which may increase the concentration of synaptic dopamine and decrease the uptake of neurotoxins.[8]

Scientific Evidence of Effectiveness

There is a lack of clinical evidence supporting the use of tea in PD, and epidemiological studies have yielded conflicting results. Retrospective analysis of 47,351 subjects in the Nurse's Health Study and Health Professional's Follow-up Study identified 288 individuals who developed PD;[9] an inverse correlation was found between caffeine intake (from both coffee and noncoffee sources) and PD in men, whereas moderate caffeine intake was more beneficial in women (high intake was correlated with an increased incidence of disease in women). Retrospective analysis of health maintenance organization (HMO) members in Washington State between 1992 and 2000 identified 210 cases of PD[10] and found an inverse correlation between tea consumption (two or more cups daily, type unspecified) and development of PD (odds ratio, 0.4; 95% confidence interval, 0.2-0.9).

A 30-year prospective observational study found higher coffee and caffeine intake to be associated with a significantly lower incidence of PD.[11] This trend toward reduced PD risk with increased coffee consumption was also apparent in men who never smoked, were past smokers, and were current smokers at baseline ($p = 0.049$, $p = 0.22$, and $p = 0.02$, respectively).[11] Additionally, this study reported that the effects appeared to be dose related for men, but not for women. Decreased PD risk was thought to be associated with caffeine intake rather than the other nutrients contained in coffee. Conversely, tea drinking has been associated with tremors and increased PD risk[12] or with no effect on development of disease.[13-16]

Dose. Insufficient available evidence.

Adverse Effects, Interactions, Pharmacokinetics. See Appendix A.

HERBAL THERAPIES WITH NEGATIVE EVIDENCE

Kava *(Piper methysticum)*

Grade D: Fair negative scientific evidence

It is unclear whether kava is safe or effective for use in patients with Parkinson's disease. Kava has been reported to antagonize the effect of dopamine and elicit extrapyramidal effects in animal data case reports.[17-19] Therefore, kava may interfere with the effects of dopamine or dopamine agonists and exacerbate the extrapyramidal effects of dopaminergic antagonists such as droperidol, haloperidol, risperidol, and metoclopramide. Kava increases "off" periods in PD patients taking L-dopa and can cause a semicomatose state when given concomitantly with alprazolam.[20] Of note, neither high single doses nor chronic administration of kavain, from the lipophilic fraction of kava, altered dopaminergic or serotonergic tissue levels in rats.[21] Therefore, dopaminergic or serotonergic effects may reside in the water-soluble fraction of kava.[22,23] An observational study, however, noted that the extrapyramidal side effects caused by neuroleptic agents may be reduced by kava special extract WS 1490.[24] Until further research is carried out, kava is not recommended for use in PD patients.

HERBAL THERAPIES WITH LIMITED EVIDENCE

Belladonna *(Atropa* spp.)

The published literature contains limited evidence regarding the use of belladonna for treating autonomic nervous system dysfunction.[25,26] One study evaluating combination products containing belladonna found that after 1 week, patients with disturbances of the autonomic nervous system noted "very good" results with higher doses of belladonna.[25]

Ginseng *(Panax* spp.)

Ginseng may have neuroprotective properties that may help prevent various forms of neuronal cell loss, including the nigrostriatal degeneration seen in Parkinson's disease. Rodents were treated with oral ginseng before and/or after exposure to the parkinsonism-inducing neurotoxin 1-methyl-4-phenyl-1,2,3,6-tetrahydropyridine (MPTP) or its toxic metabolite, 1-methyl-4-phenylpyridinium; this treatment blocked tyrosine hydroxylase–positive cell loss in the substantia nigra brain structure, and reduced the appearance of locomotor dysfunction. It was therefore postulated that the oral administration of ginseng provides protection against neurotoxicity in rodent models of PD.[27]

Safflower *(Carthamus tinctorius)*

Safflower seed oil contains a high proportion of linoleic acid, an omega-6 unsaturated fatty acid, which is an important constituent of neuronal cell membranes and believed to have neuroprotective properties.[28] In one clinical trial, safflower decreased the neurodegeneration caused by the genetic disease Friedreich's ataxia.[29]

Yohimbe *(Pausinystalia yohimbe)*

Based on its mechanism of action, yohimbine alkaloid (an alpha-2 adrenoceptor antagonist isolated from yohimbe bark) has been suggested to improve orthostatic hypotension or other manifestations of autonomic nervous system dysfunction. Preliminary research suggests that yohimbine is useful in blood pressure regulation, including patients with Parkinson's disease.[30]

Many herbs have traditional or theoretical uses that lack sufficient evidence and therefore are not graded. See the table on herbs with neuroprotective, antitremor, antineuralgic, and/or antirigidity properties.

Herbs with Potential Therapeutic Properties for Parkinson's Disease and Associated Conditions*

HERB	SPECIFIC THERAPEUTIC USE(S)†	HERB	SPECIFIC THERAPEUTIC USE(S)†
Aconite	Catalepsy (trancelike state), neuralgia, neurological disorders	Bitter orange	Neuralgia
		Black cohosh	Neuralgia, chorea, neurological disorders
Aloe	Parkinson's disease, tic douloureux		
Alpinia	Neurological disorders	Blue cohosh	Neuralgia
Arnica	Neuralgia, neuroprotection	Bupleurum	Parkinson's disease
Asparagus	Neurological disorders	Calamus	Neuropathy
Avocado	Neuralgia	Calendula	Neurological disorders, dystrophic neurological disorders
Bacopa	Neurological disorders		
Baikal skullcap	Nerve damage	Cat's claw	Neuralgia, neuroprotection
Betony	Neuralgia	Chamomile	Neuralgia

Continued

Herbs with Potential Therapeutic Properties for Parkinson's Disease and Associated Conditions—cont'd

HERB	SPECIFIC THERAPEUTIC USE(S)†	HERB	SPECIFIC THERAPEUTIC USE(S)†
Chaparral	Neurological disorders	Lemongrass	Neuralgia
Chia	Neuroprotection	Lime	Neuralgia
Chlorella	Neurodegenerative disorders	Mastic	Neuralgia
Cinnamon	Neuralgia, neuroprotection	Mistletoe	Chorea, hypertonia
Clove	Neurodegenerative disorders	Muira puama	Ataxia, neuralgia
Codonopsis	Nerve regeneration	Mullein	Neuralgia
Cordyceps	Neurodegenerative disorders	Nux vomica	Neurological disorders, neuralgia
Devil's claw	Neuralgia	Passion flower	Neuralgia
Dong quai	Neurodegenerative disorders (age-related), neurological disorders	Peppermint	Neuralgia
		Polypodium	Neurodegenerative disorders
Elder	Neuralgia	Raspberry	Neurasthenia
English ivy	Neuropathy	Rehmannia	Neurological disorders
Eucalyptus oil	Neuralgia	Reishi mushroom	Neurasthenia
Feverfew	Neurological disorders	Rhodiola	Neurological disorders
Germanium	Neuropathy	Rosemary	Nerve regeneration
Goji	Neurological disorders	St. John's wort	Neuralgia
Grape seed	Parkinson's disease	Skunk cabbage	Chorea
Grapefruit	Parkinson's disease	Stinging nettle	Neuralgia
Guggul	Neuralgia	Tamanu	Neuralgia
Horny goat weed	Neurasthenia	Tansy	Neuralgia
Horse chestnut	Neuralgia	Thyme	Neuralgia
Horseradish	Neuralgia (facial)	Tribulus	Neurasthenia
Horsetail	Neurodermatitis	Turmeric	Neurodegenerative disorders
Kudzu	Parkinson's disease	Valerian	Neuralgia
Lavender	Neuroprotection	Yew	Nerve damage
Lemon balm	Neuralgia, neurasthenia		

*This is not an all-inclusive or comprehensive list of herbs with antitremor and antirigidity properties; other herbs and supplements may possess these qualities. A qualified health care provider should be consulted with specific questions or concerns about potential neuroprotective, antitremor, antineuralgic, and/or antirigidity effects or interactions of agents.
†Based on expert opinion, anecdote, case reports, and/or preliminary trial evidence.

ADJUNCT THERAPIES

1. Constipation is the infrequent passage of small amounts of hard, dry bowel movements, usually fewer than three times a week. It is a common complaint in people with Parkinson's disease. Bulk-forming laxatives such as psyllium (e.g., Metamucil, Fiberall) may be recommended. Patients should drink 6 to 8 glasses of water daily and should consume other medications 1 hour before or 2 hours after taking psyllium.
2. Patients with PD may be at risk for developing depression. The use of herbal agents such as St. John's wort may be beneficial for mild to moderate depression (see Chapter 6). However, they should be used with extreme caution because of potential interactions with certain medications. These interactions can have severe consequences (see Appendix A).
3. Patients with PD may have difficulty sleeping. Herbal agents such as valerian may improve the quality of sleep and reduce the time to fall asleep (sleep latency) when taken for 4 to 6 weeks (see Chapter 4). Because of potential hepatotoxicity, valerian use is cautioned in patients with preexisting liver disorders (see Appendix A).
4. Cerebellar ataxia results from the failure of part of the brain to regulate body posture and limb movements. In individuals with unsteady movements, 5-hydroxytryptophan (5-HTP or l-5-hydroxytryptophan), the precursor of the neurotransmitter serotonin, has improved coordination and the ability to stand or walk unassisted.[31,32] Other

research shows no benefit.³³,³⁴ Further research is needed before a conclusion can be drawn.

5. Choline, a rate-limiting substrate for the synthesis of the neurotransmitter acetylcholine, theoretically may be beneficial for ataxic disorders. Thus far, its use has not produced favorable effects in patients with cerebellar ataxia.³⁵,³⁶ However, the sample size in the available studies has been small; larger, well-designed studies are needed before a recommendation can be made.

INTEGRATIVE THERAPY PLAN

- Discuss Parkinson's disease symptoms and the length and severity.
- Observe the patient for tremor, rigidity, bradykinesia (slow movements), and impaired balance and coordination.
- Educate the patient regarding the various signs and symptoms of PD.
- Discuss medications or dietary supplements the patient is taking for PD or any other condition.
- Inquire about side effects the patient has experienced with other medications and any inadequate response to these medications.
- If the patient inquires about herbal therapies, or if the current therapeutic regimen is not ideal, collaboratively decide whether to explore herbal therapy within appropriate monitoring parameters. Inform the patient that cowhage contains levodopa, a frequently prescribed drug for PD, and that research suggests that it may provide some benefit. Do not recommend cowhage to patients taking L-dopa because it is duplicate therapy.
- If the patient chooses to try cowhage, suggest the doses used in clinical trials: standardized 3.3% L-dopa, 22.5 to 67.5 g divided into two to five daily doses and tested by a third-party laboratory.
- Inform the patient about adverse effects and drug interactions associated with cowhage. Cowhage may cause mild stomach upset. It may also lower blood sugar and should be used cautiously in patients with diabetes. Cowhage should also be avoided with certain drugs for psychiatric disorders (e.g., MAOI-like phenelzines such as Nardil) and with methyldopa because it may cause additive blood pressure–lowering effects.
- Because cowhage has not been used in studies with other conventional PD medications (such as carbidopa, selegiline, and amantadine, as well as catechol O-methyltransferase inhibitors), patients should discuss adjunct therapy with their primary health care providers before initiating cowhage therapy.
- Inquire and identify secondary symptoms of PD, including constipation, depression, anxiety, and sleep disturbances. If the patient is interested in using herbal products for these symptoms, inform the patient about what is known about herbal therapies (such as ashwagandha and tea) for PD.
- Inform patients that tea and ashwagandha should not be used with anticoagulants or agents that may lower blood sugar. Concurrent use may lead to additive effects.

Case Studies

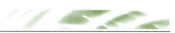

CASE STUDY 7-1

A 55-year-old man with Parkinson's disease inquires about incorporating cowhage into his current therapy. Medical history includes diabetes (8 years), controlled with glipizide (Glucotrol), and PD for 3 years, treated with levodopa/carbidopa (Sinemet). Since being diagnosed with PD, he has experienced mild psychotic symptoms, including mild illusions and vivid dreams. How should this patient be counseled?

Answer: Cowhage, which contains 3% to 6% levodopa, has been used with some success in the treatment of PD. With this in mind, it is important to realize that the patient is taking Sinemet and thus is already using levodopa, and the additional amount in cowhage may lead to added side effects and interactions. To counsel this patient, explain the rationale of duplicate therapy and that this combination cannot be advised. If the patient decides to try cowhage instead of Sinemet, emphasize that cowhage has been associated with psychosis and may worsen or advance any adverse effects, but that every patient's experience is unique. Cowhage may also lower blood sugar, and this effect may be potentiated with his use of glipizide. His blood sugar should also be carefully monitored.

CASE STUDY 7-2

Recently diagnosed with Parkinson's disease, 68-year-old RG comes to the pharmacy to pick up his prescriptions for warfarin and glipizide. He is also purchasing a gallon of tea, which he tells you will "make his mind sharper." He also says that his son mentioned an herbal product, ashwagandha, to try taking for his PD. How should you respond?

Answer: You should warn RG about the potential risks of combining warfarin with tea and ashwagandha, both of which may increase the risk of bleeding when used with anticoagulant or antiplatelet agents. Additionally, these agents may have blood sugar–lowering effects and increase the risk of hypoglycemia.

CASE STUDY 7-3

Sixty-year-old LM comes into the pharmacy to buy kava and a tea beverage. She has had some anxiety and heard from a friend that kava can help. Her medical history includes hypertension and Parkinson's disease. She is currently taking lisinopril (Zestril) and Sinemet. How should LM be counseled?

Answer: Kava has been known to worsen the symptoms of PD. Tell LM that she should not take kava for her anxiety because it may exacerbate her PD symptoms. Also, inform LM that tea contains caffeine, which may contribute to her anxiety. She may want to consider reducing her amount of caffeine consumption.

References for Chapter 7 can be found on the Evolve website at http://evolve.elsevier.com/Ulbricht/herbalpharmacotherapy/

Review Questions

1. Which constituent(s) of tea are best known for antioxidant and purported neuroprotective effects?
   a. Tannins
   b. Polyphenols, including catechins (e.g., EGCG) and theaflavins
   c. Caffeine
   d. Chlorogenic acid

2. Cowhage has been reported to induce:
   a. Hepatotoxicity
   b. Psychosis
   c. Heart attack
   d. Kidney failure

3. Ashwagandha may interact with which of the following?
   a. Repaglinide
   b. Warfarin
   c. Rivastigmine
   d. All the above

4. Which of the following should be avoided in patients with Parkinson's disease, or in patients with a history of medication-induced extrapyramidal effects?
   a. St. John's wort
   b. Garlic
   c. Kava
   d. Echinacea

5. True or false: Ashwagandha monotherapy has been shown to improve symptoms associated with Parkinson's disease.

6. Cowhage contains _____, which may contribute to its beneficial effects in Parkinson's disease.
   a. L-dopa
   b. Tyrosine
   c. Serotonin
   d. Glycine

7. According to available research, which dose of cowhage (divided into two to five daily doses) has been used in patients with Parkinson's disease?
   a. 2.5 to 6.5 grams
   b. 22.5 to 67.5 grams
   c. 22.5 to 67.5 micrograms
   d. 2.5 to 6.5 milligrams

Answers are found in the Answers to Review Questions section in the back of the text.

8 Seizure Disorders

Outline

OVERVIEW
    Types of Seizures
        Partial Seizures
        Generalized Seizures
        Other Seizures
    Signs and Symptoms
    Diagnosis
SELECTED HERBAL THERAPIES
    Bacopa *(Bacopa monnieri)*
    Euphorbia (*Euphorbia* spp.)

HERBAL THERAPIES WITH LIMITED EVIDENCE
HERBS THAT MAY CAUSE SEIZURES OR LOWER
    SEIZURE THRESHOLD
ADJUNCT THERAPIES
INTEGRATIVE THERAPY PLAN
CASE STUDIES
REVIEW QUESTIONS

Learning Objectives

- Understand herbs used for seizure disorders.
- List potential drug interactions with herbs used in seizure disorders.
- Be aware of common side effects and warnings associated with herbs used in seizure disorders.
- Counsel a patient regarding herbs used in seizure disorder.

OVERVIEW

Seizures are neurological disorders in which brain cells create abnormal electrical impulses, causing convulsions and jerking movements. In some cases, seizures cause only a loss of consciousness, a period of confusion, a staring spell, or muscle spasms. Seizures may be secondary to particular brain abnormalities or neurological disorders, or may be termed *idiopathic* (without any clear cause). Recurrent or prolonged seizures may cause brain injuries; those that last longer than 20 to 30 minutes may damage neurons. *Epilepsy* is a chronic seizure disorder, characterized by repeated episodes of seizures.

In normal neuron signal conduction, there is a balance of neurotransmitters, usually glutamate (the excitatory neurotransmitter) and gamma-aminobutyric acid (GABA, an inhibitory neurotransmitter). Sodium channels are also a target of stabilization. When the balance is changed, a seizure can occur.

Certain areas of the brain are more likely than others to be the source of a seizure. These include the *motor cortex*, which is responsible for the initiation of body movement, and the *temporal lobes*, which include an area deep in the brain called the *hippocampus* (involved in memory). These areas might be more susceptible to seizures because nerve cells in these areas are particularly sensitive to situations that can provoke abnormal electrical transmission, such as decreased oxygen levels, metabolic changes, stress, and infections.

A seizure is often divided into different parts. The *aura* is a period of warning before a seizure; individuals may experience unusual smells, visual symptoms, or unusual feelings during an aura. The seizure itself is known as the *ictus,* and the period after the seizure is called the *postictal state*. Seizure disorders are a common neurological problem. In the United States alone, more than 4 million individuals have some form of epilepsy.[1,2]

Types of Seizures

A well-recognized classification system for seizure types is the International Classification of Epileptic Seizure (Table 8-1). The type of seizure can be categorized based on location and strength of neuron firing. The two main categories of seizures are *partial* and *generalized*.[1-3]

Partial Seizures

Partial, or *focal*, seizures are those that begin in a discrete area of the brain. Partial seizures can be further subdivided into simple partial and complex partial.[1,2]

TABLE 8-1	Seizure Classification Guide			
	GENERALIZED SEIZURE (WHOLE BRAIN)		**PARTIAL SEIZURE (LOCALIZED)**	
Seizure type	Tonic-clonic	Absence	Complex	Simple
Formerly known as	Grand mal	Petit mal	Psychomotor temporal lobe	Jacksonian motor
Identifying characteristics	Affects entire body Body falls, stiffens, and jerks Loss of consciousness May cry out, bite tongue, turn pale, or stop breathing Loss of bladder and bowel control Fatigue and confusion afterward	Staring Eye blinking Eye twitching Lip smacking Jerking of hands Most common seizure in children	Altered consciousness; person may appear confused, drugged, drunk, or psychotic Lip smacking Purposeless activity or repetitive motions such as fidgeting with clothing	Jerking of one limb or side of body Person is conscious
Other information	Lasts 1 to 3 minutes	Lasts a few seconds Often thought of as daydreaming	Usually lasts 1 or 2 minutes	Person may struggle if restrained

Reprinted with permisson from Children's Hospitals and Clinics of Minnesota, Minneapolis and St. Paul. Accessed at http://xpedio02.childrensmn.org/stellent/groups/public/@manuals/@pfs/@condill/documents/policyreferenceprocedure/018297.pdf.

Simple Partial Seizures

In simple partial seizures, no change in consciousness occurs. Individuals may experience weakness, numbness, and unusual smells or tastes. Twitching of the muscles or limbs, turning the head to the side, paralysis, visual changes, or vertigo may occur. Motor symptoms that spread slowly from one part of the body to another are termed *Jacksonian epilepsy*.

Complex Partial Seizures (Temporal Lobe)

During complex partial seizures, consciousness is altered or lost during the event. Individuals may have some symptoms similar to those in simple partial seizures, but they also have some change in their ability to interact with the environment. Individuals may exhibit *automatisms* (automatic repetitive behavior), such as walking in a circle, sitting and standing repeatedly, or smacking the lips together. These symptoms are often accompanied by unusual thoughts (e.g., feeling of déjà vu), uncontrollable laughter, fear, visual hallucinations, and unusual or unpleasant odors. These symptoms are generally thought to be caused by abnormal discharges in the temporal lobe.

Generalized Seizures

Generalized seizures involve larger areas of the brain than partial seizures, often both hemispheres, from the onset. Generalized seizures are further divided into many subtypes, including tonic-clonic (grand mal), absence (petit mal), and myoclonic seizures.[1,2]

Tonic-Clonic (Grand Mal) Seizures

Tonic-clonic seizures, also called grand mal seizures, are the subtype that most people associate with seizures. Tonic-clonic are the most intense of all types of seizures. Specific movements of the arms and legs or the face may occur, with loss of consciousness. A yell or cry often precedes the loss of consciousness. Individuals may have an aura right before the loss of consciousness. Individuals will abruptly fall and begin to have jerking movements of the body and head. Drooling, biting of the tongue, and urinary incontinence may occur. When the jerking movements stop, individuals may remain unconscious for a time. The seizure usually lasts 5 to 20 minutes. Individuals often awaken confused and may sleep awhile. *Todd's paralysis* (postepileptic paralysis) is a term used to describe prolonged weakness after a seizure. Tonic-clonic seizures may also occur in *eclampsia*, a severe complication of pregnancy that is unrelated to epilepsy.[4] Eclampsia is usually preceded by *preeclampsia*, or gestational hypertension. Women with eclampsia generally do not have seizure disorders outside of pregnancy.[5]

Absence (Petit Mal) Seizures

Absence seizures (also called petit mal seizures) cause only a loss of consciousness, with no other associated motor symptoms, such as the jerking motions that occur with grand mal seizures. Usually there is no aura or warning, and the loss of consciousness is brief. Individuals may briefly stop what they are doing, stare for 5 to 10 seconds, and then continue the activity. No memory of the event exists. Subtle motor movements may accompany the alteration in consciousness. Absence seizures are characterized by staring, subtle body movements, and brief lapses of awareness.

Myoclonic Seizures

Myoclonic seizures are characterized by a brief jerking movement that arises from the central nervous system (CNS), usually involving both sides of the body. The movement may be subtle or dramatic. Myoclonic seizures usually appear as sudden jerks of the arms and legs. Many different syndromes are associated with myoclonic seizures, including juvenile myoclonic epilepsy, West syndrome, and Lennox-Gastaut syndrome. Most cases of myoclonic epilepsy occur during the first 5 years of life.

Other Seizures[1,2]

West Syndrome

West syndrome involves a group of symptoms, including infantile spasms, retardation of psychomotor development, and a particular abnormality on an electroencephalogram (EEG) known as *hypsarrhythmia,* which indicates a grossly disorganized pattern of electrical brain activity. Infantile spasms are characterized by a particular posturing of the infant's body, in which the child assumes a jackknife (or folded) position. These spasms may occur frequently over the course of the day or may be continuous. Neurological problems are ultimately found in most of these children. It is often difficult to control the seizures associated with West syndrome because of a lack of response to most anticonvulsant medications.

Lennox-Gastaut Syndrome

Lennox-Gastaut syndrome is characterized by the early onset of a common seizure type called *minor motor seizures.* These seizures include the myoclonic seizures, atypical absence seizures, and atonic seizures. *Atypical absence seizures* may involve staring and brief episodes of unconsciousness. They may occur in cycles and are associated with EEG findings different from those seen in typical absence seizures. *Atonic seizures* may be associated with sudden loss of muscle tone.

Status Epilepticus

Status epilepticus is prolonged, repetitive seizure activity that lasts more than 20 to 30 minutes. During this time the patient is unconscious. Status epilepticus is a medical emergency with a significantly poor outcome. It may result in death if not treated aggressively. Causes of status epilepticus include improper use of certain medications, poisoning, stroke, infection, trauma, cardiac arrest, drug overdose, and brain tumor.

Signs and Symptoms

Seizures can affect any process under brain coordination because of abnormal activity in brain cells. A seizure can produce temporary confusion, complete loss of consciousness, a staring spell, or uncontrollable jerking movements of the arms and legs. Symptoms vary depending on the type of seizure. In most cases an individual with epilepsy will tend to have the same type of seizure each time, so the symptoms will be similar from episode to episode. However, some individuals have many different types of seizures, with different symptoms each time.

Most people with epilepsy can live normal lives. Although epilepsy is not considered a curable disorder, it eventually disappears with age in some individuals. Most seizures do not cause brain damage. Individuals with epilepsy, especially children, may develop behavioral and emotional problems, which are sometimes the consequence of embarrassment and frustration or bullying, teasing, or avoidance in school and other social settings. For many individuals with epilepsy, the risk of seizures restricts their independence and recreational activities; some states refuse a driver's license to people with epilepsy.

Individuals with epilepsy have an increased risk of status epilepticus (a life-threatening condition) and sudden, unexplained death. Most women with epilepsy can become pregnant, but they should discuss their epilepsy and the medications they are taking with their physicians. Women with epilepsy have a 90% or greater chance of having normal, healthy babies.[1,2]

Diagnosis

Physicians will ask about the individual's history of seizures, along with other diseases, surgeries, and medications. A thorough history of recreational drug and alcohol use or abuse is equally important. It is helpful for the physician to distinguish seizure subtypes (partial or generalized); time of day of the event, including whether the seizure occurred during wakefulness or sleep; and any known triggers, such as a flickering light, severe sleep deprivation, or dehydration.

Physicians will perform a complete physical examination, including neurological examination and brain function tests. Laboratory data used to evaluate patients with seizure disorders may include computed tomography (CT) scan, magnetic resonance imaging (MRI), and electroencephalography (EEG). A complete blood panel, including drug/toxicology screening and urinalysis, are usually performed. Urine tests can determine if the individual is having a seizure because of illicit drug use (e.g., cocaine, methamphetamine). Blood tests will determine the basic functioning of the body, such as electrolyte levels (e.g., sodium, potassium) and kidney and liver function. Although it is not related to epilepsy, preeclampsia increases the risk of seizures (eclampsia) in pregnancy, and is characterized by high blood pressure and *proteinuria* (protein in the urine) in pregnant patients.[5]

SELECTED HERBAL THERAPIES

 Note

To help make this educational resource more interactive, all pharmacokinetics, adverse effects, and interactions data have been compiled in Appendix A. Safety data specifically related to pregnancy and lactation are listed in Appendix B. Please refer to these appendices when working through the case studies and answering the review questions.

Bacopa (Bacopa monnieri)

Grade C: *Unclear or conflicting scientific evidence*

Mechanism of Action

The exact mechanism by which bacopa affects epilepsy is not well understood. Bacopa has been found to reverse the expression of *N*-methyl-D-aspartate receptor 1 (NMDA R1) and glutamate receptor binding alterations to near-control levels in epileptic rats.[6,7] These data indicate that bacopa may have a neuroprotective property and may have beneficial effects in epilepsy.

Scientific Evidence of Effectiveness

Although bacopa is traditionally used in Ayurvedic medicine to treat epilepsy, high-quality clinical trials are lacking. One case study was conducted with 24 epileptic patients, including those with diagnoses complicated by cerebral palsy, mental subnormality, and schizophrenia.[8] Sixteen participants were given crude aqueous bacopa extract (2 oz daily for up to 5 months), and eight were given defatted alcoholic bacopa extract (2-4 mg/kg body weight daily for up to 5 months). Measurement outcomes included number of seizures per month and, in the case of participants with epilepsy and cerebral palsy, salivation, restlessness, aggressiveness, total hours of sleep, and destructive tendencies. After 5 months, aqueous bacopa was found to be effective in 50% of patients in alleviating seizures, whereas defatted alcoholic bacopa extract was effective in 60% of participants. The study was poorly executed with no blinding, placebo, or randomization. In those patients in whom bacopa did not reduce seizure frequency, participants used standard medications (phenytoin and phenobaritone) in conjunction with bacopa. Higher-quality research is needed before bacopa can be recommended for epilepsy.

Dose

For epilepsy, 2 oz of crude aqueous extract of bacopa has been used daily for up to 5 months, as has 2 to 4 mg/kg of defatted alcoholic bacopa extract dissolved in distilled water.[8] Researchers adjusted doses of the alcohol extract according to the degree and severity of the disease.

Adverse Effects, Interactions, Pharmacokinetics. See Appendix A.

Euphorbia (Euphorbia spp.)

Grade C: *Unclear or conflicting scientific evidence*

Mechanism of Action

It has been reported that the active alkaloid in *Euphorbia fisheriana* has anticonvulsant effects and might be useful in patients with epilepsy, but the exact mechanism of action is not known.[6,9]

Scientific Evidence of Effectiveness

Evidence is limited regarding the effect of euphorbia in patients with epilepsy. One randomized, single-blind, placebo-controlled trial of 72 patients showed that *E. fisheriana* reduced the frequency of seizures in epileptic patients compared with placebo. The effective rate of patients treated with *Euphorbia* alkaloid was 59%, versus 32% for the placebo control group.[9] The authors failed to explain the degree of improvement needed for considering an "effect" or a "marked effect," and they did not include statistical analysis. Euphorbia may have an anticonvulsant effect, but better-designed trials with a larger number of patients are needed to properly evaluate this finding.

Dose

The dose of *E. fisheriana* alkaloid for epilepsy is not clearly described.

Adverse Effects, Interactions, Pharmacokinetics. See Appendix A.

HERBAL THERAPIES WITH LIMITED EVIDENCE

Betony (*Stachys* spp.)

Betony has been regarded as a cure-all by many societies, including Greece, Italy, Spain, and Britain, as far back as 2000 years ago. Its constituents include tannins, alkaloids, and glycosides, which are typically the active ingredients in herbal remedies. Some herbalists claim betony is useful for convulsions, but scientific evidence is lacking.

Blue Cohosh (*Caulophyllum thalictroides*)

Blue cohosh has been historically used to treat epilepsy; however, seizures have been documented in infants whose mothers ingested blue cohosh during pregnancy.[10] Blue cohosh should not be recommended in people with seizure disorders.

False Hellebore (*Veratrum* spp.)

In the eighteenth and nineteenth centuries, false hellebore was prescribed for epilepsy and convulsions. However, current awareness of toxic and irritating constituents now preclude its use.

Jointed Flatsedge (*Cyperus articulatus*)

The marshland plant jointed flatsedge is commonly used in traditional medicine in Africa and Latin America to treat a wide variety of human diseases, including epilepsy. Animal and laboratory studies have found it to have anticonvulsant properties.[11-14] This may be, at least in part, caused by inhibition of NMDA-mediated neurotransmission.[11-13]

Kava (Piper methysticum)
Kava is popularly used to treat symptoms of anxiety. Kavalactones have been found to facilitate GABA transmission and bind to sodium and calcium channels, prolonging inactivation.[15-20] Laboratory and animal studies have found weak antiseizure effects;[18-21] however, kava has not been tested for seizures in humans.

Mistletoe (Viscum album)
European mistletoe has been used in traditional medicine for treating seizures. Paradoxically, high doses of mistletoe have been reported to cause seizures.

Mugwort (Artemisia vulgaris)
Mugwort has traditionally been considered a "cure-all." In orthodox medicine, mugwort was believed to be a remedy for epilepsy. Research, however, is currently lacking in this area.

Passion Flower (Passiflora incarnata)
Chrysin, a constituent of passion flower, has shown sedative and antianxiety effects; in animals it demonstrated effects (comparable to benzodiazepine) in preventing induced seizures.[22] Currently, clinical evidence is lacking.

Skullcap (Scutellaria spp.)
Skullcap has long been used as a tranquilizer and antispasmodic. In folk medicine it has been used to treat grand mal seizures. Currently, there is a lack of scientific evidence for epilepsy.

Valerian (Valeriana officinalis)
In Europe, valerian has been used traditionally as an effective treatment for epilepsy. Animal studies have found weak anticonvulsive properties.[23,24]

HERBS THAT MAY CAUSE SEIZURES OR LOWER SEIZURE THRESHOLD

Borage (Borago officinalis)
According to a review, borage may lower the seizure threshold[25]. However, in two clinical trials, borage did not cause any adverse effects.[26,27]

Evening Primrose (Oenothera biennis)
Several case reports have associated lowered seizure threshold with the use of EPO in patients with or without known seizure disorders, and possibly with the combination of EPO and anesthetics.[28,29]

Herbs with Potential Antiseizure Properties*

HERB	SPECIFIC THERAPEUTIC USE(S)†	HERB	SPECIFIC THERAPEUTIC USE(S)†
Abuta	Seizures	Cowslip	Seizures, epilepsy
Ackee	Epilepsy	Elder	Epilepsy
Aconite	Seizures, epilepsy	Eyebright	Epilepsy
African wild potato	Seizures, epilepsy	Germanium	Epilepsy
Anise	Seizures	Ginkgo	Seizures
Annatto	Seizures, epilepsy	Ginseng	Seizures
Bael fruit	Seizures	Gotu kola	Epilepsy
Bay leaf	Seizures	Jequirity	Seizures, epilepsy
Berberine	Seizures	Ladies mantle	Seizures
Bitter orange	Epilepsy	Lavender	Seizures, epilepsy
Black currant	Seizures	Lemongrass	Seizures
Black horehound	Seizures	Mullein	Seizures
Bupleurum	Epilepsy	Oleander	Epilepsy
Calamus	Seizures, epilepsy	Reishi mushroom	Seizures
Cardamom	Seizures	Skunk cabbage	Seizures, epilepsy
Cat's claw	Seizures	Tansy	Seizures, epilepsy
Chamomile	Seizures	Thyme	Epilepsy
Chasteberry	Epilepsy	Traditional Chinese Medicine	Epilepsy
Chinese medicine herbs	Epilepsy	Turmeric	Epilepsy
Cleavers	Epilepsy	Yew	Epilepsy
Coleus	Seizures, epilepsy		

*This is not an all-inclusive or comprehensive list of herbs with antiseizure properties; other herbs and supplements may possess these qualities. A qualified health care provider should be consulted with specific questions or concerns regarding potential antiepileptic effects or interactions.
†Based on expert opinion, anecdote, case reports, and/or preliminary trial evidence.

Hyssop (Hyssopus officinalis)

Based on case reports and animal studies, hyssop is a powerful convulsant and may cause tonic-clonic seizures or a generalized tonic status, possibly leading to permanent damage.[30,31]

Sage (Salvia officinalis)

Sage has been noted to cause seizures when the essential oil or tinctures are taken internally in doses of 12 drops or more.[30,31] However, aqueous sage extracts are speculated to be safer.

Water Hemlock (Cicuta spp.)

Water hemlock is a highly toxic plant. According to case reports, oral ingestion may cause an explosive illness with seizures and convulsions.[32-35]

Yohimbe (Pausinystalia yohimbe)

Yohimbine has been associated with reports of general CNS and autonomic excitation, tremulousness,[36-38] head twitching, seizure threshold changes,[39] and enhanced brain norepinephrine release (increasing resting heart rate and blood pressure).[40] Yohimbine has also been shown to dose-dependently induce clonic seizures in mice.[41] Since yohimbine crosses the blood-brain barrier, it may elicit a centrally mediated increase of sympathetic output and peripheral presynaptic transmitter release.[42] In theory, these effects may also occur with the use of yohimbe bark extract. Anecdotal reports have noted agitation, dizziness, headache, irritability, nervousness, tremors, and insomnia with the use of yohimbe bark extract.

ADJUNCT THERAPIES

1. Stress and anxiety can trigger seizure activity. Various forms of calming *meditation* have been practiced for thousands of years worldwide, with many techniques originating in Eastern religious practices. In modern times, numerous meditation types are in use, often outside of their original religious and cultural contexts. Yoga meditation may help prevent seizures in epileptic patients, although higher-quality clinical studies are needed. Several human studies report a reduction in the number of monthly seizures with the use of Sahaja yoga, when it is added to standard antiseizure drug treatment, or a yoga meditation protocol. Natural antianxiety products such as *valerian* may also be used to help with stress and anxiety.
2. *Chiropractic* is a health care discipline that focuses on the relationship between musculoskeletal structure (primarily the spine) and body function (as coordinated by the nervous system), and how this relationship affects the preservation and restoration of health. Chiropractic manipulation is thought to help decrease pressure on nerves that may be causing seizure activity; several case studies reported positive results using chiropractic to treat epilepsy.[43,44] To date, definitive evidence from controlled trials is lacking. Chiropractic manipulation should be approached cautiously in patients with underlying medical conditions, as a slight correlation has been made between cervical manipulation and ischemic stroke in some patient populations.[45]
3. Diet may also affect seizure activity. Supplementation with vitamins D, E, and B_6 may reduce seizure frequency. High-protein diets have traditionally been used by individuals with epilepsy. According to available clinical trials, the Atkins Diet, a low-carbohydrate/high-protein diet, may reduce the incidence of seizures.[46,47]
4. Seizure may also be associated with diarrhea and constipation. *Psyllium* is a source of soluble fiber and is used to treat several gastrointestinal conditions. Besides being effective as a bulk laxative for reducing constipation,[48,49] psyllium also increases fecal viscosity and improves fecal consistency and thus may benefit patients with diarrhea. Psyllium may interfere with the body's absorption of many drugs, and any epilepsy drugs or herbs should be taken 1 hour before or 4 hours after taking psyllium.

INTEGRATIVE THERAPY PLAN

- Accurate diagnosis and classification of seizure type are critical for developing optimal therapeutic strategies.
- Pharmacotherapy for epilepsy depends greatly on the individual. Identify the patient's treatment goals and whether or not the patient is experiencing side effects from conventional antiepileptic drugs.
- Keep in mind that many antiepileptic drugs are metabolized through the cytochrome P450 (CYP450) system, although through different subtypes. Drugs such as carbamazepine, phenytoin, and phenobarbital induce the activity of several CYP450 enzymes, which may lead to decreased plasma concentration and diminished efficacy of drugs. Additionally, drugs such as phenytoin are highly protein bound. Ensure proper therapeutic drug monitoring when adding any herb/supplement to conventional antiepileptic drug regimen.
- Ensure that the patient is being chronically monitored for seizure control, dosage adjustments, drug interactions, and compliance.
- Although a limited number of herbs have been studied for epilepsy, studies of herbs such as bacopa and euphorbia are promising and deserve future research. There is a lack of information regarding the combination of antiepileptic herbs with prescription drugs for epilepsy.
- Avoid using herbs that have been associated with lowered seizure threshold, including borage seed oil, evening primrose oil, and sage. Yohimbe bark extract may contain yohimbine, which has also been associated with lowered seizure threshold. Herbs such as hyssop and water hemlock have known toxicity and have been shown to induce seizures.

Case Studies

CASE STUDY 8-1

A neurologist calls the pharmacy with questions regarding bacopa for epilepsy. His patient, AR, is a 30-year-old woman who was recently diagnosed with epilepsy. She currently takes Trileptal, but her epilepsy is not well controlled. The physician tells you that his patient also wants to try an herbal agent, and he heard that bacopa may offer some benefit. He also asks you about herbal therapies for AR's anxiety. AR also takes levothyroxine for hypothyroidism. How do you respond?

Answer: Bacopa should not be recommended for this patient. Trileptal is a CYP3A inducer, and bacopa may interact with drugs metabolized by CYP450. This interaction could result in reduced levels of Trileptal and increase AR's risk of seizure. Additionally, bacopa may increase thyroid hormone levels and may interfere with thyroid agents. However, you may recommend yoga, meditation, or chiropractic manipulation for AR's anxiety. Stress and anxiety can often trigger seizure activity. These therapies have been shown to reduce anxiety as well as seizure activity and may aid in better seizure control. Certain herbal supplements have been associated with lowered seizure threshold, including borage seed and evening primrose oil, and should be avoided.

CASE STUDY 8-2

KG, a 28-year-old man recently diagnosed with epilepsy, does not want to take prescription medication because of the reported side effects. His past medical history includes hepatitis B and chronic constipation. He would like to try a herbal therapy for the epilepsy and asks you if he should try euphorbia. How do you counsel? Are there alternatives that you would recommend?

Answer: Although *Euphorbia* alkaloid has demonstrated some antiepileptic effects, it may also have harmful effects, including enhancing Epstein-Barr virus (EBV). Because KG has hepatitis and EBV may be associated with hepatitis, euphorbia should not be recommended. Psyllium, a source of soluble fiber, has been shown to be effective as a bulk laxative for reducing constipation. This agent should be recommended to KG for his constipation problem. KG should also be counseled regarding alternative methods for reducing seizures, such as yoga and meditation; chiropractic manipulation; supplementation with vitamins D, E, and B_6; and high-protein diets (e.g., Atkins Diet). However, KG should be advised to seek professional medical advice before starting any herbal or nutritional regimen. KG should also be aware of herbal supplements associated with lowered seizure threshold, including borage seed oil and evening primrose oil.

References for Chapter 8 can be found on the Evolve website at http://evolve.elsevier.com/Ulbricht/herbalpharmacotherapy/

Review Questions

1. True or false: Lavender has been shown to reverse the expression of NMDA R1 and glutamate receptor binding.

2. Which of the following agents should be used cautiously with bacopa?
   a. Chloral hydrate
   b. Methimazole
   c. Phenytoin
   d. All the above agents may interact with bacopa.

3. True or false: Although false hellebore was historically used for epilepsy, it is potentially toxic and should not be used.

4. Which species of *Euphorbia* has been reported to have anticonvulsant activity?
   a. *Euphorbia fisheriana*
   b. *Euphorbia fulgens*
   c. *Euphorbia esula*
   d. *Euphorbia tirucalli*

5. Which of the following therapies may be useful for epilepsy?
   a. Atkins Diet
   b. Vitamin E
   c. Chiropractic medicine
   d. All the above

Answers are found in the Answers to Review Questions section in the back of the text.

9 Pain

Outline

OVERVIEW
    Types of Pain
        Acute Pain
        Chronic Pain
        Nerve Pain
        Nociceptive Pain
        Psychogenic Pain
    Signs and Symptoms
        Breakthrough Pain
        Complex Regional Pain Syndrome
    Diagnosis
SELECTED HERBAL THERAPIES
    Aconite *(Aconitum napellus)*
    Arnica *(Arnica* spp.)
    Belladonna *(Atropa* spp.)
    Bromelain *(Bromeliaceae)*
    Butterbur *(Petasites hybridus)*
    Clove *(Syzygium aromaticum,* syn. *Eugenia aromaticum)*
    Coleus *(Coleus forskohlii)*
    Comfrey *(Symphytum* spp.)
    Devil's Claw *(Harpagophytum procumbens)*
    Eucalyptus *(Eucalyptus* spp.)
    Feverfew *(Tanacetum parthenium)*
    Lavender *(Lavandula angustifolia)*
    Peppermint *(Mentha x piperita)*
    Pycnogenol *(Pinus pinaster* subsp. *atlantica)*
    Reishi Mushroom *(Ganoderma lucidum)*
    Saw Palmetto *(Serenoa repens)*
    Soy *(Glycine max)*
    Turmeric *(Curcuma longa)*
    White Horehound *(Marrubium vulgare)*
    Willow *(Salix* spp.)
HERBAL THERAPIES WITH LIMITED EVIDENCE
ADJUNCT THERAPIES
INTEGRATIVE THERAPY PLAN
CASE STUDIES
REVIEW QUESTIONS

Learning Objectives

- Recognize herbs useful for treating pain.
- Understand the mechanism of action, pharmacokinetics, and scientific evidence behind herbal analgesics.
- Describe major side effects, toxicities, and drug interactions associated with herbal analgesics.
- Recommend an integrative care plan for patients with pain.

OVERVIEW

Pain is defined as an unpleasant sensory and emotional experience associated with actual or potential damage to body tissues, including the nerves, skin, organs, bones, and muscles. Although pain is the most common reason that individuals seek medical care, it is often undertreated.[1]

Pain is a result of nerve impulses being carried to a specific part of the brain that registers painful stimuli. Many endogenous hormones are involved in transmitting pain. Prostaglandins play a large role in pain and inflammation; many analgesic and antiinflammatory agents act by inhibiting their synthesis. For example, many non-steroidal antiinflammatory drugs (NSAIDS) inhibit prostaglandins by blocking the cyclooxygenase (COX) pathway resulting in antiinflammatory and analgesic effects.[1]

Pain can be classified as *acute* (immediate, short term) or *chronic* (long term, >3 months). The four most common types of pain are lower back pain, severe headache or migraine pain, neck pain, and facial ache or pain. Back pain is the leading cause of disability in Americans younger than age 45 years.[1,2] Headaches are also common. *Primary* headaches are not associated with (or caused by) other diseases; examples are migraine headaches, tension headaches, and cluster headaches. *Secondary* headaches are caused by associated diseases, such as brain tumors. The associated disease may be minor or serious and life threatening. Seven in 10 people have at least one type of headache a year.[1]

Each year 30 to 40 million Americans have pain that is unrelieved by over-the-counter (OTC) analgesics, such as acetaminophen (Tylenol), aspirin, and ibuprofen (Advil, Motrin).

According to the American Medical Association (AMA), 13 to 15 million Americans suffer from chronic, intractable, and severe pain, most of which is inadequately treated.[1,2]

The annual cost of chronic pain in the United States, including health care expenses, lost income, and lost productivity, is estimated to be $100 billion.

Types of Pain

Acute or chronic pain can also be divided into categories that help explain its origin and its effects on the body. Types of pain include nerve or neuropathic, nociceptive, and psychogenic.[1]

Acute Pain

Acute pain is a normal sensation triggered in the central nervous system (CNS) to alert the individual to possible injury. Acute pain, for the most part, results from disease, injury to tissues, or inflammation. Generally, the onset is sudden (e.g., after trauma or surgery). Acute pain is frequently accompanied by anxiety or emotional distress, which may result in acute tachycardia, increased respiratory rate and blood pressure, sweating, and dilated pupils.[1]

Chronic Pain

Chronic pain is a persistent, ongoing type of pain. Pain signals from the nervous system fire continuously, sometimes for weeks, months, or even years. It may stem from an acute injury, such as an infection or sprained muscle, or an underlying chronic condition such as arthritis or cancer. Many chronic pain conditions affect older adults. Some individuals experience chronic pain in the absence of any past injury or evidence of body damage. Pain that is not associated with a known cause is termed *idiopathic pain*.

Common chronic pain complaints include headache and lower back pain. Conditions that can lead to chronic pain include cancer and arthritis. *Neurogenic* pain (caused by damage to peripheral nerves or to CNS itself) and *psychogenic* pain (unrelated to past disease or injury or any visible sign of damage inside or outside CNS) may also be chronic.

Chronic pain may be associated with vegetative signs, such as fatigue, loss of libido, loss of appetite, and depressed mood. Pain tolerances vary considerably among individuals. Chronic pain is widely believed to represent disease itself, which can be made much worse by environmental and psychological factors or even be resistant to most medical treatments. Chronic pain can, and often does, cause severe problems for the individual.[1,2]

Nerve Pain

Nerve pain (also known as *neurogenic pain, neuropathic pain,* or *neuropathy*) is caused by pressure on nerves or on the spinal cord or by damage to nerves. Nerve pain can be caused by tumors, injury (e.g., surgical, falls), chemical damage (e.g., mercury, lead, chemotherapy), radiation therapy, or viral infections (e.g., herpes zoster).

Nerve pain can be severe and is usually described as a "burning" or "tingling" sensation. Neuropathic pain is not usually widespread; rather, it is restricted to one particular place on the body or occurs along the path of a nerve.

Nerve pain is typically more difficult to treat than other types of pain, and unique medication treatment options exist. Opioids and nonsteroidal antiinflammatory drugs (NSAIDs) are usually *not* effective in relieving nerve pain.

Phantom pain, a type of nerve pain, may also occur after amputation of a limb or other part of the body. An estimated 60% to 70% of amputees feel phantom pain. The pain may resemble squeezing, burning, or crushing sensations, but it often differs from any sensation previously experienced. For some people, phantom limb pain occurs less frequently as time passes, but for others, it persists. Massage can sometimes help, but drug therapy may be necessary.[1,3,4]

Nociceptive Pain

Most pain is nociceptive pain, typically characterized as aching, sharp, or throbbing. Pain receptors for tissue injury (called *nociceptors*) are primarily located in the skin or internal organs. Nociceptive pain is caused by an injury to bodily tissues, such as acute injury, bruising, bone fracture, crush injury, tumor invasion, or burns. Postsurgical pain is almost always nociceptive pain. The pain may be constant or intermittent, often worsening when an individual moves, coughs, laughs, or breathes deeply, or when the dressings over the surgical wound are changed. Nociceptive pain can be further divided into somatic pain and visceral pain.[1,3,4]

Somatic pain is pain caused by activation of pain receptors in cutaneous tissues (located on body surface) or deep tissues, such as muscle and bone. Common causes of somatic pain include postsurgical pain or pain related to a laceration.[1,3]

Visceral pain is caused by activation of pain receptors in the internal organs of the thoracic, abdominal, and pelvic cavities. Common causes of visceral pain include pancreatic cancer, kidney disease, and metastases in the abdomen. Visceral pain is not well localized and is usually described as "pressure-like" and causing sensations of deep "squeezing."[1,3]

Psychogenic Pain

Psychogenic pain is entirely or mostly related to a psychological disorder, such as hypochondria (health-anxiety phobia). Psychogenic pain does cause physical pain. When individuals have persistent pain with evidence of psychological disturbances and without evidence of a disorder that could cause the pain, the pain may be described as "psychogenic." Pain that is purely psychogenic is rare.

Pain complicated by psychological factors still requires treatment, often by a health care team that includes a psychologist or psychiatrist. For most individuals who have chronic psychogenic pain, the goals of treatment are to improve comfort, as well as physical and psychological function.[1,3,4]

Signs and Symptoms

Pain can occur in many locations throughout the body. Pain can be constant or intermittent. Intensity can vary from a dull ache to searing agony. The onset may be sudden or acute, with or without apparent reason, or gradual and chronic.[1-4]

Clinicians determine whether pain is acute or chronic. Acute pain begins suddenly and usually does not last long. When severe, acute pain may cause anxiety, rapid heartbeat, increased breathing rate, elevated blood pressure, sweating, and dilated pupils.[1-4] Chronic pain persists for weeks, months, or even years, and usually describes pain that persists for more than 1 month beyond the usual course of an illness or injury, pain that recurs off and on for months or years, or pain that is associated with a chronic disorder such as cancer. Usually, chronic pain does not affect the heartbeat, breathing rate, blood pressure, or pupils, but it may result in other problems, such as depression, disturbed sleep, decreased energy, loss of appetite, weight loss, and loss of libido.[2]

Breakthrough Pain

Many individuals who are being treated for chronic pain may experience a brief, often severe flare-up of pain. This flare-up is called "breakthrough" pain because it breaks through the regularly scheduled pain treatment. Typically, breakthrough pain begins suddenly, lasts up to 1 hour, and feels much like the individual's chronic pain, except it is more severe. Breakthrough pain may differ from one individual to another and is often unpredictable.[1,3]

Complex Regional Pain Syndrome

Complex regional pain syndrome (CRPS) is a chronic pain condition, with symptoms of continuous, intense pain that is disproportionate to the severity of the injury. Over time, this intense pain worsens rather than improves. CRPS usually affects one of the arms, legs, hands, or feet, and quite often the pain spreads to include the entire extremity. Typical features include dramatic changes in the color and temperature of the skin over the affected limb or body part, accompanied by intense burning pain, skin sensitivity, sweating, and swelling.[1,3]

Diagnosis

Diagnosing the underlying cause of pain can be difficult. When an individual experiences pain, a clinician may take a number of steps to assess the pain and attempt to determine its cause. Assessment of pain typically begins with a discussion of the patient's medical history and a physical examination. The medical history includes the patient's age, weight, and height, current and past medical problems, and medications taken. In the discussion portion of the pain assessment, the patient may be asked to describe the pain according to when it started, what it feels like, how bad it hurts, where it is located, and factors that improve or worsen it. The clinician may use a pain diagram or picture of the human body to evaluate the pain. The patient marks the area(s) where pain is felt on the chart.[1-4]

Clinicians may also use pain scales, which help quantify the pain intensity. A *numerical pain scale* identifies how much pain the patients are having by choosing on a 0 to 10 scale, with 0 being "no pain" and 10 being "the worst pain imaginable." A *visual analog pain scale* uses a straight line with the left end of the line representing "no pain" and the right end of the line representing the "worst pain." The patients mark where on the line they think their pain is. The *categorical pain scale* has four categories: none, mild, moderate, and severe. Patients select the category that best describes their pain. The *faces pain scale* uses six faces with different expressions on each face[5] (Figure 9-1). Patients are asked to choose the face that best reflects the level of pain they are feeling.

Pain perception is very subjective and varies from one individual to the next. During a physical examination, a clinician inspects the area of pain, looking for visual signs of causes, such as trauma and injury. Depending on the location, the clinician may test joints and muscles for strength and range of motion.[1-4] Some injuries, particularly spinal chord injuries, may result in a loss of nociceptive pain or heat sensations.

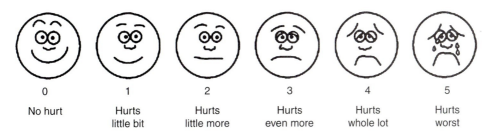

Figure 9-1 Wong-Baker Faces Pain Rating Scale. (From Wong DL, Hockenberry-Eaton M, Wilson D, et al: *Wong's essentials of pediatric nursing*, ed 6, St Louis, 2001, Mosby.)

SELECTED HERBAL THERAPIES

Note
To help make this educational resource more interactive, all pharmacokinetics, adverse effects, and interactions data have been compiled in Appendix A. Safety data specifically related to pregnancy and lactation are listed in Appendix B. Please refer to these appendices when working through the case studies and answering the review questions.

Aconite (*Aconitum napellus*)

Grade C: *Unclear or conflicting scientific evidence (postoperative pain in infants)*

Note: Based on widespread use, many experts believe aconite to be unsafe, even in recommended amounts in otherwise healthy individuals.

Mechanism of Action

There are approximately 350 species of aconite. Generally, the alkaloids aconitine, hypaconitine, mesaconitine, and jesaconitine have the strongest pharmacological and toxic effects, whereas their derivatives are weaker and less toxic.[1,6]

The analgesic and antiinflammatory mechanisms of aconite are not fully understood. Based on animal experiments, the analgesic effects of mesaconitine are mediated by central noradrenergic pathways.[7,8] Mesaconitine did not inhibit prostaglandin synthesis, and the adrenal system was not involved in antiinflammatory effects.[9]

Alkaloids from methanol extracts of crude *Aconitum carmichaeli* roots inhibited acute inflammation but were not effective against chronic inflammation in animal models. Inhibitory effects of aconitines, when induced by histamine, appear in decreasing order: aconitine > hypaconitine > mesaconitine. Their benzoylaconine analogs were effective in acute inflammation at higher doses. Their antiinflammatory effects appear in decreasing order: benzoylmesaconine > benzoylaconine > benzoyhypaconine.[10] However, because homeopathic preparations contain negligible amounts of the purported active constituents, the mechanism of action for homeopathic aconite is unclear.

Scientific Evidence of Effectiveness

Traditionally, aconite has been used to treat acute inflammatory illnesses and peripheral neuropathy pain; however, well-designed clinical trials are lacking. In one randomized controlled trial (RCT), homeopathic aconite significantly relieved postoperative pain agitation in infants who had undergone subumbilical surgeries. Fifteen minutes after administration of a single dose of homeopathic aconite, infants showed significant improvement. The action of homeopathic aconite was found to be both rapid and profound.[11]

Dose

Homeopathic preparations are made by diluting the active ingredient in a distilled water/alcohol mixture, either 1:10 or 1:100, and then vigorously shaking the mixture. The original mixture is serially diluted until the desired "potency" is obtained. Aconite homeopathic preparations of 6c to 30C have been used. A "30C" potency strength is made by diluting one part of aconite tincture to 99 parts of alcohol or water, then repeating the dilution for a total of 30 dilutions.

Adverse Effects, Interactions, Pharmacokinetics. See Appendix A.

Arnica (*Arnica* spp.)

Grade C: *Unclear or conflicting scientific evidence (analgesia; trauma: pain and wound healing)*

Mechanism of Action

The sesquiterpene lactones, helenalin and dihydrohelenalin, of arnica may be responsible for antiinflammatory and analgesic activity.[12,13] Arnica has been shown to block the action of histamine;[14] prevent the release of the immune regulator nuclear factor kappa B (NF-κB) and inhibit prostaglandin synthesis.[15] However, because homeopathic preparations contain negligible amounts of the purported active constituents, the mechanism of action for homeopathic arnica is unclear.

Scientific Evidence of Effectiveness

Homeopathic arnica is typically used to relieve postoperative pain; however, the results from clinical trials have been mixed.[16-24] Although pain measurement is highly subjective, most studies attempted to measure pain objectively by a visual analog pain scale;[17,24] however, some studies used more subjective methods.[16] Based on multiple RCTs, homeopathic arnica was reported to reduce swelling, as measured by knee circumference, and thereby reduce pain.[21] Homeopathic arnica was also shown to reduce subjective pain scores in tonsillectomy patients.[18] However, no significant differences in postoperative pain and infection management between homeopathic therapy with arnica and placebo were found in an RCT of women undergoing total abdominal hysterectomy.[23]

Dose

Note: Arnica is toxic if taken internally, except when diluted into homeopathic preparations.

Homeopathic arnica is derived by taking the alcohol tincture of fresh arnica flowers, through serial dilutions using equal proportions of ethyl alcohol and purified water, coupled with *succussion* (vigorous agitation of solution).[17] Homeopathic preparations are made by diluting the active ingredient in a distilled water/alcohol mixture, either 1:10 or 1:100, and then vigorously shaking the mixture. The original mixture is serially diluted until the desired "potency" is obtained. When the process is repeated 30 times on a 1:10 dilution it is said to be a 30X or 30D (10^{-30}) potency. When the process is repeated 30 times on a 1:100 dilution, it is said to be 30C (10^{-60}).[25]

Homeopathic treatment is usually individualized to correspond specifically to the patient's symptoms. The wide range of homeopathic potencies and treatment methodologies pose a challenge when applying standard testing and statistical procedures to the homeopathic medical model.

Studies for pain and analgesia have used various homeopathic preparations, and the concentrations of constituents tend to vary. Oral homeopathic dosages for arnica include two doses of arnica (30C potency), taken in the 24th hour preoperatively, followed by three doses each day for 5 days;[23] three tablets of arnica (D6 or D30 potency) taken sublingually every 4 hours for 2 days, followed by three times daily for 3 days;[26] arnica 30C potency two or three times daily;[20] and 1 x 5 globules of the homeopathic dilution 30X of arnica given before surgery and 3 x 5 globules administered daily thereafter.

Adverse Effects, Interactions, Pharmacokinetics. See Appendix A.

Belladonna (*Atropa* spp.)

Grade C: *Unclear or conflicting scientific evidence (headache)*

Mechanism of Action

Belladonna alkaloids are competitive inhibitors of the muscarinic actions of acetylcholine, acting at receptors located in exocrine glands, smooth and cardiac muscle, and intramural neurons.[1,6] However, because homeopathic preparations contain negligible amounts of the purported active constituents, the mechanism of action for homeopathic belladonna is unclear.

Scientific Evidence of Effectiveness

Belladonna is an herb that has been used for centuries for a variety of indications, including headache. Studies comparing belladonna-containing compounds to placebo have been small and have reported limited or no benefits in symptoms, prophylaxis, or frequency of headache.[27-29] However, this research has been of poor quality and has examined combination products containing other agents, such as ergotamine or phenobarbital (which may be efficacious in the absence of belladonna), or has used highly diluted homeopathic belladonna preparations that contain little or no active constituents.

Dose

The exact dose of belladonna for headache has not been determined.

Adverse Effects, Interactions, Pharmacokinetics. See Appendix A.

Bromelain (Bromeliaceae)

Grade B: *Good scientific evidence (antiinflammatory)*

Mechanism of Action

Bromelain is a sulfur-containing proteolytic digestive enzyme that is extracted from the stem and fruit of the pineapple plant (*Ananas comosus*, family Bromeliaceae). The mechanism of bromelain's putative antiinflammatory activity is not well understood. Bromelain may inhibit the biosynthesis of proinflammatory prostaglandins by lowering kininogen and bradykinin in serum and tissues, and it may alter prostaglandin synthesis.[30] In addition, bromelain may activate plasmin production from plasminogen and reduce kinin by inhibiting the conversion of kininogen to kinin.

Scientific Evidence of Effectiveness

The results from human clinical trials evaluating bromelain for pain and inflammation have been mixed.[31-49] Limited study has found bromelain to reduce pain and inflammation after tooth extraction.[36] However, other studies evaluating the use of bromelain after dental procedures and operations, did not report positive results.[34,36,37,41,43] There is limited evidence that bromelain may reduce inflammation, edema, pain at rest, and pain while walking after an episiotomy.[33] However, other studies evaluating bromelain for this use did not find the same results.[38,50]

Dose

Bromelain is standardized to milk-clotting unit (mcu) or gelatin-digesting unit (gdu) activity. The milk-clotting unit of measurement is officially recognized by the Food Chemistry Codex. Bromelain (Ananase), 240 mg, has been used for 5 days to treat inflammation.[37]

Adverse Effects, Interactions, Pharmacokinetics. See Appendix A.

Butterbur (*Petasites hybridus*)

Grade C: *Unclear or conflicting scientific evidence (migraine prophylaxis)*

Mechanism of Action

Extracts of butterbur have been made from the rhizomes, roots, and leaves. The sesquiterpenes (isopetasin, oxopetasin, and petasin) are believed to be the active constituents responsible for pharmacological activity.[51] Some research suggests that petasin may be the most active component.[1,6]

Potential antiinflammatory properties of butterbur extracts have been attributed to the petasin content, which has been reported to cause inhibition of lipoxygenase activity and down-regulation of leukotriene synthesis.[51] Isopetasin and oxopetasin esters in *Petasites hybridus* have also been reported to inhibit the synthesis of leukotrienes.[52] Inhibition of COX-2 and prostaglandin E_2 (PGE_2) has been reported in animal research as well.[53]

Scientific Evidence of Effectiveness

Butterbur has been traditionally used for pain relief and headache prevention. Recent preclinical studies suggest antiinflammatory and vasodilatory properties of butterbur, thereby supporting a possible mechanism of action. A small number of human trials report efficacy of butterbur for migraine prevention when taken regularly for up to 4 months.[53-57] This evidence is compelling enough to suggest benefits of butterbur for migraine prevention, although conclusive evidence warrants larger well-designed studies. Comparisons to other agents used for this purpose, such as beta blockers or feverfew, have not been conducted.

Dose

A few standardized products containing butterbur root rhizome are currently available. Products may be standardized to their specific petasin and isopetasin contents. Petadolex and Petaforce are carbon dioxide–standardized extracts from the rhizome of *P. hybridus*.[55] Petadolex is reported to contain 7.5 mg of petasin and isopetasin per 50-mg tablet.[58]

For migraine headache prophylaxis, the pyrrolizidine-free butterbur rhizome extract Petadolex (standardized to 7.5 mg of petasin and isopetasin per 50-mg tablet), administered at 50 to 75 mg twice daily for up to 4 months, has been studied.[53-56]

Adverse Effects, Interactions, Pharmacokinetics. See Appendix A.

Clove (*Syzygium aromaticum*, syn. *Eugenia aromaticum*)

Grade C: *Unclear or conflicting scientific evidence (dental pain)*

Mechanism of Action

The clove component *eugenol* is popular in dentistry for its mild anesthetic and analgesic effects; however, its mechanism of action is not well understood. Eugenol may inhibit prostaglandin biosynthesis, thereby depressing pain sensory receptors.[59]

Scientific Evidence of Effectiveness

Clove essential oil is a common dental *anodyne*, an externally-applied medicine that relieves pain by lessening pain sensitivity. Eugenol is frequently used by dentists because of its analgesic, local anesthetic, antiinflammatory, and antibacterial effects.[60] A zinc oxide and eugenol combination (ZOE) has been used as standard cement or filling in dental work.[61-66] There is some clinical evidence that a homemade clove gel is as effective as benzocaine 20% gel.[67] No significant difference was found in pain scores on the variables of a "good night's sleep" or previous local anesthesia. However, preliminary research noted that this combination was inferior to collagen paste for inflammation caused by dry socket.[68] Despite these conflicting findings, the sum of the evidence is promising. Additional research is needed.

Adverse Effects, Interactions, Pharmacokinetics. See Appendix A.

Coleus (*Coleus forskohlii*)

Grade C: *Unclear or conflicting scientific evidence (antiinflammatory action after cardiopulmonary bypass)*

Mechanism of Action

Forskolin, a component of *Coleus forskohlii*, increases levels of cyclic adenosine monophosphate (cAMP), apparently attenuating cytokine balance in favor of antiinflammatory effects.[69] Forskolin also inhibits the release of histamine from basophils and mast cells.[70]

Scientific Evidence of Effectiveness

There is preliminary clinical evidence that intraoperative administration of coleus (colforsin daropate hydrochloride) may have potent inotropic and vasodilatory activity, and may attenuate cytokine production and respiratory dysfunction after cardiopulmonary bypass (CPB).[69] Interleukin-1β, interleukin-6, and interleukin-8 levels after CPB were significantly ($p < 0.05$) lower in the coleus group compared with the group who did not receive coleus. Research suggests that coleus may be effective in treating CPB-related inflammatory responses.

Dose. Insufficient available evidence.

Adverse Effects, Interactions, Pharmacokinetics. See Appendix A.

Comfrey (*Symphytum* spp.)

Grade B: *Good scientific evidence (pain, inflammation)*

Mechanism of Action

The roots of comfrey (*Symphytum officinale*) contain toxic pyrrolizidine alkaloids, including symlandine, symphytine, and echimidine. A water-soluble hydroxycinnamate-derived polymer (>1000 kDa) from *Symphytum asperum* inhibited degranulation of azurophil granules and superoxide generation in primed leukocytes in vitro indicating antiinflammatory effects.[71] In animals a water extract of comfrey altered the production of prostaglandins, which are lipid compounds that reduce inflammation.[72]

Scientific Evidence of Effectiveness

Clinical trials investigating topical application of comfrey-containing creams have found significant reductions in inflammation and pain associated with sprains and muscle injuries.[73-77] Topical comfrey has been studied in patients with pain and swelling associated with ankle injuries.[73] Swelling, decreases in scores for pain during active motion, pain at rest, and functional impairment were significantly and clinically lower after 3 to 7 days of comfrey treatment.

Topical comfrey has also been shown to be equally as effective as topical diclofenac, a prescription NSAID; 164 patients received either topical comfrey or topical diclofenac gel four times daily for 7 days.[75] Primary variables measured included pain reaction to pressure on the injured area, spontaneous pain sensation at rest and during movement, and consumption of rescue medications. There were no significant differences between groups.

Evidence supporting oral use of comfrey is lacking.

Dose

Clinical trials and case series have used four main types of cream containing comfrey: Traumaplant, Kytta-Salbe f, Kytta-Plasma f, and Kytta-Balsam f.

For pain and inflammation, clinical trials have used 2 to 3 g of topical comfrey three or four times daily for up to 14 days.[73-77]

Adverse Effects, Interactions, Pharmacokinetics. See Appendix A.

Devil's Claw (Harpagophytum procumbens)

Grade B: *Good scientific evidence (low back pain)*

Mechanism of Action

The major constituent of devil's claw, *harpagoside,* an iridoid glycoside, appears to be responsible for its pharmacological effects. However, there have been conflicting reports regarding the antiinflammatory and analgesic effects of devil's claw. Harpagoside has been found to inhibit lipoxygenase pathways and COX, especially COX-2.[78,79] Devil's claw also helps moderate the production of tumor necrosis factor alpha (TNF-α),[80] which may contribute to its antiinflammatory effects.

Scientific Evidence of Effectiveness

There are several controlled human trials supporting the use of devil's claw for the treatment of low back pain.[81-93] However, the majority of studies are small and performed by the same authors. Devil's claw has been found to lessen low back pain, and 50 to 100 mg of harpagoside daily seems to reduce low back pain as effectively as 12.5 mg of rofecoxib (Vioxx).[90-93] Patients who used devil's claw have reportedly needed less rescue medications.[81-86]

Dose

For low back pain, 2 to 9 g of devil's claw crude extract has been taken daily.[94-96] As tablets, 600 to 2400 mg (standardized to contain 50-100 mg of harpagoside) has been taken orally three times daily.[81-93]

Adverse Effects, Interactions, Pharmacokinetics. See Appendix A.

Eucalyptus (Eucalyptus spp.)

Grade C: *Unclear or conflicting scientific evidence (headache)*

Mechanism of Action

The antiinflammatory activity of eucalyptus has been demonstrated in animal and in vitro studies,[97-106] and it may be related to antioxidant activity.[101,102] The principal component of eucalyptus, *cineole,* has been shown to inhibit cytokine production and arachidonic acid metabolism.[97,98] Eucalyptus has also been associated with analgesia in animal studies.[100]

Scientific Evidence of Effectiveness

The effects of topical eucalyptus oil on mechanisms associated with the pathophysiology of headache have been assessed in combination with peppermint oil.[107,108] The combination of peppermint oil, eucalyptus oil, and ethanol was reported to increase cognitive performance and to possess muscle-relaxing and "mental-relaxing" effects. It did not, however, have a significant effect on pain sensitivity. A significant analgesic effect with a reduction in sensitivity to headache was produced by a combination of peppermint oil/ethanol/trace eucalyptus, but not with the combination eucalyptus/ethanol/trace peppermint. These findings suggested that peppermint oil may be efficacious as a topical therapy for headache while eucalyptus is not.

Dose

Standardization data are lacking. It has been suggested that to be effective medicinally, eucalyptus leaf oil must contain 70% to 85% 1,8-cineole (eucalyptol).

Generally, external application of 5% to 20% eucalyptus in oil-based formulation, or 5% to 10% eucalyptus in alcohol-based formulation, is used. Topical use may lead to toxicity,[109] and several cases of poisoning have been reported after eucalyptus oil ingestion.[110-112]

Adverse Effects, Interactions, Pharmacokinetics. See Appendix A.

Feverfew (Tanacetum parthenium)

Grade B: *Good scientific evidence (migraine headache prophylaxis)*

Mechanism of Action

In the 1980s, feverfew was proposed as an inhibitor of prostaglandin synthesis,[113,114] with observed inhibition of COX and lipoxygenase activity.[115,116] In vitro inhibition of prostaglandin synthetase–mediated PGE_2 production from arachidonic acid was reported by the feverfew constituents parthenolide, michefuscalide, and chrysanthenyl acetate.[117] Extracts of feverfew leaves and commercially available powdered leaves produced dose-dependent inhibition of the generation of thromboxane B_2 (TXB_2) and leukotriene B_4 (LTB_4) by stimulated rat and human leukocytes.[118]

Scientific Evidence of Effectiveness

Feverfew leaves have long been used orally for the treatment or prevention of migraine headaches. Several controlled human trials in this area have had mixed results.[119-128] Overall, these studies suggest that feverfew taken daily as dried-leaf capsules may reduce the incidence of attacks in patients who experience chronic migraine headaches. Nausea and vomiting were less severe during feverfew administration compared with placebo.[121] There is limited clinical evidence that feverfew freeze-dried leaves, but not ethanolic extracts, reduced the frequency and severity of migraine headache.[120]

Adverse Effects, Interactions, Pharmacokinetics. See Appendix A.

Lavender (Lavandula angustifolia)

Grade C: *Unclear or conflicting scientific evidence (perineal discomfort after childbirth)*

Mechanism of Action

The analgesic effects of lavender are not well understood. According to limited animal study, lavender leaf and essential oil appear to have antiinflammatory and analgesic effects.[129]

Scientific Evidence of Effectiveness

Lavender has been evaluated as an additive to bathwater to relieve pain in the perineal area (between vagina and anus) in women after childbirth.[130] Subjects were divided into three groups: group 1 added a natural lavender oil extract to baths, group 2 added a synthetic lavender oil to baths, and the third group used an unspecified control substance that had U.S. Food and Drug Administration (FDA) "Generally Recognized As Safe" status. This trial found no significant differences in perineal relief among the groups.

Dose

For perineal discomfort after childbirth, 6 drops of lavender oil has been studied as a bath additive, but the dose was not shown to be effective (no specific brand).[130] In addition, ¼ to ½ cup of whole dried lavender flowers added to hot bathwater may be used.

Adverse Effects, Interactions, Pharmacokinetics. See Appendix A.

Peppermint (Mentha x piperita)

Grade B: *Good scientific evidence (tension headache)*

Mechanism of Action

Menthol, which exerts a direct, antinociceptive effect, has been identified as a principal active component of peppermint oil.[131,133] Menthol stimulates cold-sensitive receptors and produces a prolonged cold sensation at the application site.[107,132-134]

Scientific Evidence of Effectiveness

Preliminary trials have evaluated topical peppermint oil in patients with tension headache.[107,134] Compared with placebo, the topical peppermint oil solution significantly alleviated the symptoms of tension headache (p <0.01) after 15 minutes; no statistically significant difference has been found between 1000 mg of acetaminophen and 10% peppermint in ethanol solution.[134]

A combination product of peppermint and eucalyptus was reported to increase cognitive performance and to possess muscle-relaxing and "mental relaxing" effects. However, it did not have a significant effect on pain sensitivity.[107]

Adverse Effects, Interactions, Pharmacokinetics. See Appendix A.

Pycnogenol (Pinus pinaster subsp. atlantica)

Grade C: *Unclear or conflicting scientific evidence (cramps/muscular pain)*

Note: Pycnogenol contains oligomeric proanthocyanidins (OPCs) as well as several other bioflavonoids. There has been some confusion in the U.S. market regarding OPC products containing Pycnogenol or grape seed extract (GSE), because one of the generic terms for chemical constituents ("pycnogenols") is the same as the patented trade name (Pycnogenol). Some GSE products were formerly erroneously labeled and marketed in the United States as containing "pycnogenols." Although GSE and Pycnogenol do contain similar chemical constituents (primarily in the OPC fraction), the chemical, pharmacological, and clinical literature on the two products is distinct. The term *Pycnogenol* should therefore be used only when referring to this specific proprietary pine bark extract. Scientific literature regarding this product should not be referenced as a basis for the safety or effectiveness of GSE.

Mechanism of Action

The mechanism of action of Pycnogenol for pain and inflammation is not well understood but may be related to its antioxidant effects. Pycnogenol has been shown to inhibit transcription factor NF-κB and activator protein-1 (AP-1) in lipopolysaccharide-stimulated RAW 264.7 cells. As a result, Pycnogenol reduced gene expression and formation of interleukin-1.[135]

Scientific Evidence of Effectiveness

Pycnogenol has been shown to help prevent cramps, muscular pain at rest, and pain after/during exercise in normal subjects, in athletes prone to cramps, in patients with venous disease, in those with intermittent claudication, and in diabetic patients with microangiopathy.[136] Additional high-quality trials are needed to make a firm recommendation.

Dose

Pycnogenol is a proprietary patented formula. For cramps and muscular pain, 200 mg has been taken daily in divided doses.[136]

Adverse Effects, Interactions, Pharmacokinetics. See Appendix A.

Reishi Mushroom (Ganoderma lucidum)

Grade C: *Unclear or conflicting scientific evidence (pain relief for postherpetic neuralgia and herpes zoster)*

Mechanism of Action. Insufficient available evidence.

Scientific Evidence of Effectiveness

Administration of hot-water–soluble extracts of *Ganoderma lucidum* decreased pain in two female patients with postherpetic neuralgia and two male patients with severe pain of herpes zoster infection.[137] Two women (Case 1 and Case 2) with herpes zoster were treated with 6.4 g of dry reishi extracts (equivalent to 36 g dry weight) in three divided doses daily. No other treatment was used. In Case 1, pain dramatically decreased 4 days after the onset of therapy. She stopped taking reishi after about 45 days of treatment. Months later a mild form of the pain recurred, so she initiated therapy with the extract. Within 2 days the pain decreased and was almost gone in 10 days. In Case 2 the initial dose did not decrease the woman's severe pain. She doubled her reishi intake to 12.8 g dry powder extract (equivalent to 72 g of dry reishi) daily, and after 10 days her pain was reduced on a three-point pain scale from 3 to 2. When the extract was stopped, the pain recurred. The extract was resumed, and within 60 days her pain scores were 1, and within 9 months, she was pain free. Two male patients who received the 6.4-g dose of reishi for the treatment of herpes zoster experienced pain relief and complete remission without the need for additional treatments.

Dose

The exact dose of reishi for pain relief has not been determined.

Adverse Effects, Interactions, Pharmacokinetics. See Appendix A.

Saw Palmetto (Serenoa repens)

Grade C: *Unclear or conflicting scientific evidence (prostatitis/chronic pelvic pain syndrome [CPPS])*

Mechanism of Action

Saw palmetto is often used for benign prostatic hyperplasia (BPH), and its mechanism of action may involve testosterone-altering and antiinflammatory effects. Saw palmetto has been shown to inhibit 5α-reductase activity on testosterone in vitro, thereby preventing the conversion of testosterone to dihydrotestosterone (DHT).[138-141] Antiinflammatory properties may be based on the ability of saw palmetto to inhibit lipoxygenase and COX in vitro,[142,143] as well as the ability to inhibit mast cell accumulation in vivo.[144]

Scientific Evidence of Effectiveness

The available scientific evidence on saw palmetto as a prostatitis treatment has produced conflicting results and has evaluated saw palmetto as part of combination therapies, making it difficult to isolate the effects of saw palmetto alone.[144-148] Patients with prostatitis/chronic pelvic pain syndrome (CPPS) who received saw palmetto, 325 mg daily for 1 year, did not experience improvements in their quality of life, pain domains, or urination.[145] In contrast, patients treated with finasteride, 5 mg daily for 1 year, had significant and long-lasting improvement in all parameters except voiding.[145]

Dose

A standardized extract of saw palmetto containing 80% to 95% sterols and fatty acids (liposterolic content) has been recommended. For prostatitis/CPPS, 320 mg of prostamol (*Sabal serrulata* plant extract) has been used.[146]

Adverse Effects, Interactions, Pharmacokinetics. See Appendix A.

Soy (Glycine max)

Grade C: *Unclear or conflicting scientific evidence (cyclical breast pain)*

Mechanism of Action

Soy's potential to relieve breast pain may result from isoflavones, a type of phytoestrogen.[1,6] Phytoestrogens may exert estrogenic effects. Because breast pain corresponds with hormone cycles, it is possible that isoflavones may have an effect.

Scientific Evidence of Effectiveness

There is limited preliminary evidence that soy intake may reduce cyclical breast pain in women.[149] Patients who drank soy milk (34 g of soy protein daily) for 3 months experienced relief of breast pain.

Dose

For mastalgia, 34 g of soy protein taken daily for 3 months may be beneficial.[149]

Adverse Effects, Interactions, Pharmacokinetics. See Appendix A.

Turmeric (Curcuma longa)

Grade C: *Unclear or conflicting scientific evidence (inflammation)*

Mechanism of Action

Turmeric has been associated with the inhibition of TNF-α, interleukin-8, monocyte inflammatory protein-1, interleukin-1β, and monocyte chemotactic protein-1.[150] Turmeric and its constituent, *curcumin*, have been found to inhibit lipoxygenase and COX in rat tissues and in vitro,[151-153] as well as TXB_2[154] and LTB_4 formation.[153,155] Based on animal research, oral administration of curcumin may reduce expression of several cytokines, chemokines, and proteinases.[156] In rat macrophages, curcumin has been shown to inhibit the incorporation of arachidonic acid into membrane lipids, as well as PGE_2, LTB_4, and LTC_4, but did not affect the release of arachidonic acid.[157]

Scientific Evidence of Effectiveness

In vitro and animal studies have demonstrated antiinflammatory activity of turmeric and its constituent curcumin. Multiple mechanisms have been implicated, including effects on prostaglandins and cytokines. In a clinical trial of 40 subjects with postoperative inflammation after hernia or hydrocele repair, 400 mg of curcumin was compared to placebo or 100 mg of phenylbutazone three times daily for 5 days.[158] Curcumin and phenylbutazone were found to significantly reduce edema and tenderness compared with placebo.[158] Details of outcome measurements were not clear.

Dose

For inflammation, 400 mg of curcumin has been taken three times daily for 5 days, with 500 mg of ampicillin four times daily, given concurrently.[158]

Adverse Effects, Interactions, Pharmacokinetics. See Appendix A.

White Horehound (Marrubium vulgare)

Grade C: *Unclear or conflicting scientific evidence (pain)*

Mechanism of Action

Processed white horehound contains 0.3% to 1% of the bitter principle marrubiin, diterpene alcohols, alkaloids, bitter lactones, flavonoids, saponins, sterols, tannins, vitamin C, and 0.06% of volatile oils.[159-162] Marrubiin does not exist in the fresh plant but is formed from premarrubiin during processing.[163,164]

The exact analgesic mechanism of white horehound remains to be determined, but does not appear to involve the inhibition of COX or opioid receptors. In vivo models of pain in mice report significant analgesic activity of the hydroalcoholic extract of white horehound and antinociceptive effects of marrubiin.[164,165] An in vitro study of white horehound demonstrated concentration-dependent, noncompetitive antagonism and concentration-dependent muscle contractions induced by several agonists of smooth muscle tissue.[166]

Scientific Evidence of Effectiveness

White horehound has traditionally been used in the management of pain associated with menstruation. There is preliminary supportive evidence from animal studies.[164-165] Currently, human studies are lacking in this area.

Dose

The dose of white horehound for pain has not been clearly established.

Adverse Effects, Interactions, Pharmacokinetics. See Appendix A.

Willow (Salix spp.)

Grade B: *Good scientific evidence (lower back pain)*

Grade C: *Unclear or conflicting scientific evidence (headache)*

Mechanism of Action

The active constituents of willow bark are the salicylates, which are chemical precursors to the well-known analgesic aspirin (acetylsalicylate). In addition to salicylates, willow bark contains glycosides, tannins, and flavonoids. Salicin, the principle salicylate found in willow bark, appears to have a similar mechanism of action as aspirin, and has been shown to inhibit COX-2–mediated prostaglandin release. Willow bark may also act as a weak inhibitor of proinflammatory cytokines.[167]

Scientific Evidence of Effectiveness

Willow bark from certain *Salix* species contains salicin, which has been historically used to treat many different kinds of pain, including rheumatic pain, back pain, toothache, headache, and menstrual cramps. Only some *Salix* species are high in salicin content. These species include *Salix alba* L. (white willow), *Salix fragilis*, *Salix purpurea* (purple willow), *Salix daphnoides*, and *Salix pentandra*.

There is promising evidence that willow bark reduces low back pain. An RCT examined the use of 120 or 240 mg of salicin or placebo in 210 patients with low back pain. In the fourth and final week of the study, 39% of the group taking 240 mg of salicin were pain free for at least 5 days, compared with 21% in the 120-mg group and only 6% in the placebo group.[168] There is evidence that 240 mg daily of willow bark may be as effective as rofecoxib (Vioxx) for lower back pain.[169]

A salicin topical cream has been investigated clinically for the treatment and prophylaxis of migraine and tension-type headache.[170] Of the 34 patients receiving salicin, 28 found salicin effective, with an average rating of 7.42 on the 10-point scale ($p < 0.001$). Although this study that the topical salicin cream was more effective than placebo for the treatment of headache, several methodological flaws prevent any conclusion. The dose of salicin is unclear, and the results may have been confounded by the combination of salicin with the APPM and standard headache agents.

Dose

Assalix, a proprietary preparation, is standardized to 15.2% salicin, corresponding to 240 mg of salicin per tablet.[171] From 120 to 240 mg daily of the salicin constituent of willow bark may reduce pain. It may take up to 1 week for pain relief.[168]

Adverse Effects, Interactions, Pharmacokinetics. See Appendix A.

HERBAL THERAPIES WITH LIMITED EVIDENCE

Camphor *(Cinnamomum camphora)*

Camphor is typically used as a topical analgesic and anesthetic. It acts similarly to menthol by producing a cooling feeling on the skin. It can be found in products such as Vicks' VapoRub.

Cat's Claw *(Uncaria spp.)*

Cat's claw has a long history of use in South America and is believed to reduce inflammation and promote wound healing. Cat's claw produced dose-related pain relief in several models of chemical and thermal pain through mechanisms that involve an interaction with serotonin receptors.[172]

Dandelion *(Taraxacum officinale)*

Dandelion's therapeutic effects have historically been attributed to the bitter constituents found in roots and leaves.[173] Research in laboratory animals suggests that dandelion root may possess antiinflammatory properties; sesquiterpene lactones may be responsible for this activity.[174] well-conducted human studies are lacking on the antiinflammatory properties of dandelion.

Dong Quai *(Angelica sinensis)*

Dong quai has been used for various types of pain, including neuropathic pain, menstrual migraine headache, and dysmenorrhea (painful menstruation).[175] Currently, there is a lack of scientific evidence to support the use of dong quai alone for pain.

Euphorbia *(Euphorbia spp.)*

Ethanol extracts of whole plant *Euphorbia prostrata* and its partitioned fractions may demonstrate antiinflammatory properties, as seen in carrageenan animal models.[176] Furthermore, acute inflammatory studies of fractions using histamine- and bradykinin-induced pedal edema indicated a selective inhibition of histamine-induced edema, suggesting suppression of the first phase of the acute inflammatory reaction.

Eyebright *(Euphrasia officinalis)*

Limited evidence from animal research suggests that several iridoid glycosides isolated from eyebright, particularly *aucubin*, possess antiinflammatory properties comparable to those of indomethacin. The mechanism of action may be the inhibition of thromboxane-synthase.[177,178] The clinical relevance in humans is unclear, as clinical observations or controlled trials are currently lacking in this area.

Stinging Nettle *(Urtica dioica)*

Stinging nettle has been used historically to treat muscle pain and arthritis. Stinging nettle leaf exhibited its ability to slow the inflammatory cytokine response caused by endotoxins.[179]

Herbs with Potential Analgesic or Antiinflammatory Properties*

HERB	SPECIFIC THERAPEUTIC USE(S)†	HERB	SPECIFIC THERAPEUTIC USE(S)†
Abuta	Pain (dental)	Alpinia	Inflammation, pain
Acacia	Inflammation	Andiroba	Pain
Acai	Inflammation	*Andrographis paniculata* Nees, Kan Jang, SHA-10	Inflammation
Ackee	Pain, headache		
African wild potato	Inflammation		
Alfalfa	Inflammation	Angel's trumpet	Anesthesia, pain
Alkanna	Inflammation	Anise	Inflammation, musculoskeletal pain, pain
Allspice	Musculoskeletal pain		

Continued

Herbs with Potential Analgesic or Antiinflammatory Properties*—cont'd

HERB	SPECIFIC THERAPEUTIC USE(S)†	HERB	SPECIFIC THERAPEUTIC USE(S)†
Annatto	Pain, inflammation, headache	Bulbous buttercup	Pain (anodyne), headache
Aristolochia spp.	Inflammation	Bupleurum	Pain, inflammation, musculoskeletal pain, epigastric pain, headache
Arnica	Pain, inflammation		
Arrowroot	Inflammation (mucous membranes)		
Asafoetida	Inflammation	Burdock	Pain, inflammation, headache
Asarum	Pain, anesthesia, pain, headache	Cajeput oil	Anesthesia
Ash	Pain, inflammation	Calamus	Inflammation
Asparagus	Inflammation	Calendula	Inflammation, pain, headache
Astragalus	Inflammation, musculoskeletal pain	California jimson weed	Pain (anodyne), anesthesia, arthritis, inflammation
Avocado	Inflammation (oral)	Cardamom	Inflammation
Babassu	Inflammation, pain	Carqueja	Pain, inflammation
Bacopa	Pain, inflammation	Cascara sagrada	Pain
Bael fruit	Inflammation, pain	Cat's claw	Pain, musculoskeletal pain
Baikal skullcap	Inflammation	Chamomile	Inflammation, headache
Bamboo	Inflammation, pain, headache	Chaparral	Pain, inflammation
Barberry	Inflammation	Chasteberry	Inflammation
Bay leaf	Pain, inflammation, migraine	Chia	Inflammation
Bellis perennis	Pain, inflammation, migraine	Chicory	Inflammation, headache
Berberine	Inflammation, headache	Chlorella	Inflammation
Betony	Inflammation, pain, headache	Chrysanthemum	Anesthesia, inflammation
Birch	Inflammation	Cinnamon	Pain, anesthesia, inflammation, musculoskeletal pain
Bitter almond	Pain, inflammation, local anesthesia		
Bitter melon	Pain	Cleavers	Inflammation
Bitter orange	Pain, musculoskeletal pain, headache	Coltsfoot	Inflammation
		Cordyceps	Inflammation
		Cornflower	Inflammation
Black bryony	Pain, inflammation	Couch grass	Inflammation
Black cohosh	Inflammation, musculoskeletal pain, pain, headache	Cramp bark	Inflammation
		Cranberry	Inflammation
Black currant	Inflammation, pain	Damiana	Inflammation, headache
Black pepper	Inflammation, pain	Danshen	Inflammation
Black tea	Pain, headache	Datura wrightii	Pain (anodyne), anesthesia, arthritis, inflammation
Blessed thistle	Inflammation		
Bloodroot	Pain, anesthesia, inflammation, migraine	Deer velvet	Inflammation
		Eastern hemlock	Inflammation
Blue cohosh	Inflammation, pain (pregnancy)	Echinacea	Pain, migraine
Blue flag	Inflammation, pain, headache, migraine	Elder	Inflammation, headache, migraine
Boldo	Inflammation, pain, headache	Elecampane	Pain, headache
Boneset	Inflammation, musculoskeletal pain, headache, migraine	English ivy	Inflammation
		Ephedra	Inflammation
		Evening primrose	Inflammation, pain
Borage seed oil	Inflammation	Fenugreek	Pain, inflammation, musculoskeletal pain
Boswellia	Pain, inflammation		
Bromelain	Inflammation, pain	False hellebore	Pain
Buchu	Inflammation, musculoskeletal pain	False pawpaw	Inflammation (mouth and throat)

Herbs with Potential Analgesic or Antiinflammatory Properties*—cont'd

HERB	SPECIFIC THERAPEUTIC USE(S)†	HERB	SPECIFIC THERAPEUTIC USE(S)†
False pennyroyal	Musculoskeletal pain, headache	Lesser celandine	Inflammation
Germanium	Inflammation	Licorice	Inflammation
Garcinia	inflammation	Lime	Headache
Garlic	inflammation, headache	Lingonberry	Inflammation
Ginger	Pain, headache, migraine	Lotus	Inflammation
Ginkgo	Migraine	Mangosteen	Inflammation
Ginseng	Pain, inflammation, headache, migraine	Marshmallow	Inflammation, musculoskeletal pain
Goji	Inflammation	Mastic	Musculoskeletal pain
Goldenrod	Pain, inflammation, headache (topically)	Meadowsweet	Pain, inflammation, headache
		Milk thistle	Inflammation
Goldenseal	Anesthesia, inflammation, musculoskeletal pain, pain, headache	Mistletoe	Headache
		Morus nigra	Pain
		Muira puama	Pain
Gotu kola	Inflammation, pain	Mugwort	Headache
Grape seed	Inflammation, pain (acroparesthesia)	Mullein	Pain (anodyne), inflammation, headache, migraine
Greater celandine	Pain, inflammation	Neem	Pain, inflammation
Green tea	Headache	Noni	Pain, inflammation, chronic pain, musculoskeletal pain, headache
Ground ivy	Inflammation, headache		
Guarana	Migraine		
Guggul	Pain	Nopal	Inflammation
Gumweed	Pain	Nux vomica	Pain, inflammation, headache, migraine
Hibiscus	Pain (antinociceptive)		
Holy basil	Pain, inflammation, headache	Oleander	Inflammation
Hops	Pain, inflammation	Oregano	Musculoskeletal pain, headache
Horny goat weed	Pain, inflammation, musculoskeletal pain	Organic food	Pain, chronic pain, headache, migraine
Horseradish	Pain (anodyne), inflammation, musculoskeletal pain headache	Pagoda tree	Inflammation
		Passion flower	Pain (chronic)
		Perilla	Inflammation
Hyssop	Inflammation	Pokeweed	Inflammation (upper and lower respiratory tract), headache
Jequirity	Pain (anodyne), inflammation, headache		
		Polypodium leucotomos	Inflammation
Jiaogulan	Inflammation	Pomegranate	Headache
Jointed flatsedge	Headache	Populus	Inflammation
Jojoba	Inflammation	Quassia	Pain
Juniper	Pain, inflammation	Raspberry	Pain, inflammation
Kava	Pain, anesthesia, inflammation, migraine	Red yeast rice	Inflammation
		Rehmannia	Inflammation, pain (bone cancer)
Khella	Inflammation	Rhodiola	Inflammation, headache
Kudzu	Inflammation, musculoskeletal pain, pain, headache, migraine	Rhubarb	Headache
		Rooibos	Headache
Labrador tea	Pain, headache	Rose hip	Inflammation, headache
Ladies mantle	Inflammation	Rosemary	Pain, inflammation
Lady's slipper	Pain	Safflower	Inflammation, Inflammation after tooth extraction (dry socket), pain
Lemon balm	Pain, migraine, tension headache		
Lemongrass	Pain, inflammation, musculoskeletal pain, headache		
		Sage	Inflammation

Continued

Herbs with Potential Analgesic or Antiinflammatory Properties*—cont'd

HERB	SPECIFIC THERAPEUTIC USE(S)†	HERB	SPECIFIC THERAPEUTIC USE(S)†
Salvia divinorum	Pain	Thyme	Inflammation (colon), headache
Sarsaparilla	Inflammation	Tree tobacco	Inflammation, headache
Scotch broom	Inflammation, musculoskeletal pain	Tribulus	Inflammation, pain, headache
		Tylophora	Inflammation
Sea buckthorn	Pain, inflammation	Usnea	Pain, inflammation, headache
Shepherd's purse	Inflammation	Valerian	Musculoskeletal pain (spasm/tension), pain, headache, migraine
Shiitake	Inflammation (kidney)		
Skunk cabbage	Headache		
Slippery elm	Inflammation	Verbena	Inflammation
Spirulina	Inflammation	Wasabi	Pain
St. John's wort	Inflammation, pain (dental), pain	Water hemlock	Headache
Star anise	Pain	Watercress	Inflammation
Stevia	Inflammation	Wheatgrass	Pain (abdominal)
Strawberry	Inflammation	White oak	Inflammation
Sweet basil	Inflammation	White water lily	Inflammation
Sweet woodruff	Inflammation	Wild yam	Inflammation
Tamanu	Pain, inflammation	Yarrow	Inflammation
Tangerine	Inflammation	Yerba santa	Inflammation
Tansy	Inflammation, migraine	Yew	Pain, headache
Tea tree oil	Inflammation, musculoskeletal pain	Yohimbe	Anesthesia
		Yucca	Inflammation

*This is not an all-inclusive or comprehensive list of herbs with analgesic or antiinflammatory properties; other herbs and supplements may possess these qualities. A qualified health care provider should be consulted with specific questions or concerns regarding potential analgesic or antiinflammatory effects or interactions.
†Based on expert opinion, anecdote, case reports, and/or preliminary trial evidence.

ADJUNCT THERAPIES

1. *Acupuncture*[1] is widely used throughout the world and is one of the main pillars of traditional Chinese medicine (TCM). Acupuncture involves penetrating the skin with thin, solid, metallic needles that are manipulated by the hands or by electrical stimulation. The placement of these needles by an acupuncturist purportedly manipulates the body's energy, or *qi*, so healing can take place. Evidence from well-designed systematic review of randomized controlled trials (RCTs) supports the use of acupuncture for pain or discomfort associated with gastrointestinal (GI) endoscopic procedures. Acupuncture may also be effective for dental pain.

2. *Chiropractic*[1] is a health care discipline that focuses on the relationship between musculoskeletal structure (primarily the spine) and body function (as coordinated by the nervous system), and how this relationship affects the preservation and restoration of health. The broad term *spinal manipulative therapy* incorporates all types of manual techniques, including chiropractic. Multiple clinical studies have examined the effects of spinal manipulation in patients with acute or chronic neck pain. Overall, however, the quality of studies has been poor, and reviews of this topic have been unable to form clear or convincing conclusions. Better-quality clinical research on the use of chiropractic for neck pain is necessary before a firm conclusion can be drawn. Although chiropractic helps many people with back pain (including lower back pain), there is not enough reliable scientific evidence to conclude whether chiropractic techniques are beneficial in the management of back pain when compared to conventional approaches, such as medication and surgery. Chiropractic has also been studied in lumbar disc herniation and whiplash injuries, with mixed results.

3. Various forms of hypnosis, trance, and altered states of consciousness have played roles across cultures throughout history. *Hypnotherapy*[1] has been studied in the management of pain, including low back pain, surgery-related pain, cancer-related pain, dental procedure–related pain, burn pain, repetitive strain injury, temporomandibular joint disorders, sickle cell disease–related pain, irritable bowel syndrome, oral mucositis, tension headache, and chronic pain from various causes. Various hypnotherapy approaches have been used, and the optimal technique or duration of treatment is unclear.

4. *Music* is used to influence physical, emotional, cognitive, and social well-being and improve quality of life for healthy people, as well as those who are disabled or ill. It may involve either listening to or performing music, with or without the presence of a music therapist. Music therapy[1] helps in a wide range of pain conditions, primarily by its ability to improve mood, encourage relaxation, and elevate pain threshold. There is evidence of benefit of music therapy for pain in cancer, neonates in intensive care, burn care, general postsurgical patients, hospice patients, osteoarthritis, postanesthesia care, open-heart surgery recovery, and coronary artery bypass graft surgery. Results are not universal; however, studies found no or unclear benefits in stroke patients during upper-extremity joint exercises, tissue biopsy or port placement or removal in cancer, musculoskeletal trauma, inguinal hernia surgery, and abdominal hysterectomy. Thus, music therapy may be less helpful with more severe pain.

5. *Therapeutic touch*[1] may reduce pain and improve joint mobility in people with osteoarthritis, decrease pain and anxiety caused by burns, and improve chronic muscle and joint pain in elderly patients. Preliminary research reports that patients treated with therapeutic touch may need less pain medication after surgery. However, most studies of therapeutic touch have not been well designed, and therapeutic touch has not been clearly compared to common pain treatments such as pain-relieving drugs.

6. A physical therapist can apply a variety of treatments, such as heat, ice, ultrasound, electrical stimulation, and muscle-release techniques, to areas where pain originates. As pain improves, the physical therapist can teach the individual specific exercises to increase flexibility, strengthen the back and abdominal muscles, and improve posture. Regular use of these techniques may help prevent pain from coming back. Exercise may correct current back problems, help prevent new back complications, and relieve back pain, particularly after an injury. Proper exercise strengthens back muscles that support the spine and strengthens the abdomen, arms, and legs, reducing strain on the back. Exercise also strengthens bones and reduces the risk of falls and injuries.

7. Capsaicin, the active component of chili peppers (*Capsicum* spp.), is found in FDA-approved topical preparations for treating pain. Capsaicin binds to nociceptors (C fibers) in the skin, causing a "hot" sensation through the release of substance P; the subsequent depletion of substance P, and possibly degradation of nerve fibers, leads to reduced sensitivity desensitization with repeated application.[180] This feature of capsaicin led to its use as a topical treatment for muscle soreness, post-herpetic neuralgia, diabetic neuropathy, and osteoarthritis.[181] In a review of six RCTs (656 patients total) for neuropathic pain and three RCTs (368 patients) for musculoskeletal conditions,[182] 0.075% topical capsaicin had a relative benefit of 1.4 (95% confidence interval 1.2 to 1.7) compared to placebo, while 0.025% capsaicin used for musculoskeletal disorders had a relative benefit of 1.5 (95% confidence interval 1.1 to 2.0). Local adverse events occurred in about $1/2$ of the patients treated with capsaicin. While the overall evidence suggests that capsaicin has poor to moderate efficacy for treating musculoskeletal or neuropathic pain, capsaicin was suggested to be possibly beneficial in patients with refractory pain, or as an adjunct therapy for other analgesics.

INTEGRATIVE THERAPY PLAN

- A thorough pain assessment is crucial for effective pain management.
- Determine if the pain is acute or chronic.
- Identify the source of the pain.
- Ask the patient to describe the pain and when it started.
- Ask the patient what makes the pain better or worse, and if the pain intensity has changed.
- Discuss the patient's fears of pain therapy, including unwanted side effects, addiction and tolerance, and medication costs.
- Encourage the use of regimens for breakthrough pain, because evidence is lacking to support the use of any herb for that type of pain.
- Discuss the various herbal agents that have scientific evidence to support their use as pain relievers and antiinflammatory agents.
- Review the patient's medication record, and identify any relevant herb-drug interactions.
- Various study results on the antiinflammatory actions of *bromelain* are promising, with minimal adverse effects reported. Bromelain may affect individuals with bleeding disorders or those taking medications that decrease clotting, such as aspirin or warfarin (Coumadin).
- *Willow bark* is also used as an antiinflammatory, and good evidence supports its use for lower back pain. Willow bark contains salicin, a chemical similar to aspirin, which is thought to be responsible for its pain-relieving and antiinflammatory effects. Because willow bark contains salicin, it should not be used by people who are allergic or sensitive to salicylates (e.g., aspirin). Willow bark should also be avoided in patients taking blood-thinning agents.
- *Devil's claw* exhibits antiinflammatory properties, possibly via COX-2 inhibition, and may be useful for pain and headache. Potential side effects include GI upset, hypotension, and cardiac effects. Specifically, devil's claw may possess inotropic and negative chronotropic properties based on animal data. Devil's claw should be avoided in patients taking blood-thinning agents.
- *Feverfew* may be recommended to patients for migraine headache prophylaxis. Preclinical studies reported anti-

inflammatory and blood vessel dilatory effects. Feverfew may cause an increase in bleeding, and it should not be used in patients allergic to plants in the aster family, including ragweed, marigolds, daisies, and chrysanthemums.
- For women experiencing pain related to childbirth, *lavender* may be a safe option as a bath additive. In general, however, pain related to pregnancy should not be treated with herbal agents because of a lack of known effects to the mother and fetus.
- Discuss adjunct therapies such as capsaicin, acupuncture, hypnosis, therapeutic touch, or music therapy to help with pain relief.

Case Studies

CASE STUDY 9-1

RA is 49-year-old man with a history of lower back pain. He has been treated over time with various modalities, including NSAIDs and chiropractic treatment. He tells you that he previously took Vioxx, but since it was taken off the market, he has not tried any other drug. He also adds that he does not like the "cracking" sound when he goes to the chiropractor. RA has a history of type 2 diabetes and takes metformin, 1000 mg twice daily; he also has depression, for which he takes St. John's wort. What should you recommend?

Answer: Devil's claw exhibits antiinflammatory properties, possibly via COX-2 inhibition, and may be useful for lower back pain. It has been shown to reduce low back pain as well as rofecoxib (Vioxx). You may recommend that RA take 50 to 100 mg of harpagoside (active principle of devil's claw) daily. Anecdotal evidence indicates devil's claw may lower blood sugar. You should recommend that RA monitor his blood sugar regularly. Notably, St. John's wort may have antiinflammatory effects and theoretically may have additive effects when used with devil's claw. You may also want to suggest adjuvant therapy with acupuncture, hypnosis, or therapeutic touch. Using one of these modalities may provide additional pain relief.

CASE STUDY 9-2

DS is a 47-year-old man who experiences migraine headaches. He has a history of allergy to salicylates. His daughter recommended that he try willow bark. He also takes garlic and niacin for high cholesterol and low HDL (high-density lipoprotein) levels. How should you counsel?

Answer: Willow bark should not be recommended to DS. Willow bark contains salicin, a chemical similar to aspirin, and people with salicylate allergies should not use willow bark. Additionally, willow bark may increase the risk of bleeding when used with garlic (herb with possible anticoagulant effects). As an alternative herb, you may recommend *butterbur*. It has been used for migraine headache prophylaxis. When used prophylactically for migraine headaches, a pyrrolizidine-free butterbur rhizome extract standardized to 7.5 mg of petasin and isopetasin per 50-mg tablet (Petadolex), dosed at 50 to 75 mg twice daily for up to 4 months, has been studied. Efficacy of butterbur for migraine prevention has been reported when taken regularly for up to 4 months. Interactions between garlic and niacin have not been reported. You may also want to suggest that DS try adjuvant therapy with acupuncture or hypnosis, to help further prevent migraine headaches.

CASE STUDY 9-3

MB is a 27-year-old female nurse who works nights. She comes into your pharmacy and complains about her pain after a tooth extraction. She currently takes melatonin to help her sleep. She read that bromelain may help with the pain. How should you counsel her?

Answer: The results from human clinical trials evaluating bromelain for pain and inflammation have been mixed. Limited clinical study has found bromelain to reduce pain and inflammation after tooth extraction, which may be beneficial for MB. Bromelain, 240 mg for 5 days, may be recommended. However, she should be counseled on the potential interaction between bromelain and melatonin, a supplement often used for sleep disorders. Bromelain may cause additive sedative effects, and MB should be advised to be cautious.

References for Chapter 9 can be found on the Evolve website at http://evolve.elsevier.com/Ulbricht/herbalpharmacotherapy/

Review Questions

1. True or false: Bromelain may inhibit the biosynthesis of proinflammatory prostaglandins by lowering kininogen and bradykinin in serum and tissues and may alter prostaglandin synthesis.

2. Which active component of clove may be responsible for its anesthetic and analgesic effects?
   a. Forskolin
   b. Eugenol
   c. Harpogaside
   d. Salicin

3. Which natural product should be used cautiously with other agents that may cause photosensitivity?
   a. Dong quai
   b. Devil's claw
   c. Feverfew
   d. Both a and c

4. Dong quai has been used for which type of pain?
   a. Menstrual pain
   b. Cancer-related pain
   c. Myofascial pain
   d. None of the above

5. White horehound may interact with which of the following?
   a. Citalopram
   b. Digoxin
   c. Levothyroxin
   d. All of the above

6. What components of dandelion are thought to be responsible for its antiinflammatory activity?
   a. Caffeic acid
   b. Vitamin K
   c. Sesquiterpene lactones
   d. Fiber

7. Willow bark should be avoided in patients with which type of allergy?
   a. Daisy
   b. Peanut
   c. Aspirin
   d. Gluten

8. True or false: Soy protein may help relieve breast pain in women.

Answers are found in the Answers to Review Questions section in the back of the text.

10 Alzheimer's Disease and Related Disorders

Outline

OVERVIEW
  Signs and Symptoms
    Stages of Alzheimer's Disease
    Mild Symptoms
    Moderate Symptoms
    Severe Symptoms
  Diagnosis
    Medical History
    Blood Tests
    Mental Status Evaluation
    Brain Scans
    Genetic Testing
SELECTED HERBAL THERAPIES
  Astragalus *(Astragalus membranaceus)*
  Bacopa *(Bacopa monnieri)*
  Bupleurum *(Bupleurum* spp.)
  Cranberry *(Vaccinium macrocarpon)*
  Ginkgo *(Ginkgo biloba)*
  Ginseng *(Panax* spp.)
  Grape Seed *(Vitis* spp.)
  Guarana *(Paullinia cupana)*
  Jojoba *(Simmondsia chinensis)*
  Khat *(Catha edulis)*
  Lavender *(Lavandula angustifolia)*
  Lemon Balm *(Melissa officinalis)*
  Peppermint *(Mentha x piperita)*
  Polypodium *(Polypodium leucotomos)*
  Rhodiola *(Rhodiola rosea)*
  Rhubarb *(Rheum* spp.)
  Sage *(Salvia officinalis)*
  Soy *(Glycine max)*
  Tea *(Camellia sinensis)*
  Turmeric *(Curcuma longa)*
HERBAL THERAPIES WITH NEGATIVE EVIDENCE
ADJUNCT THERAPIES
INTEGRATIVE THERAPY PLAN
CASE STUDIES
REVIEW QUESTIONS

Learning Objectives

- Identify signs and symptoms of Alzheimer's disease and related conditions.
- Understand herbal treatment strategies for patients with Alzheimer's disease and related conditions.
- Identify side effects caused by herbs used for Alzheimer's disease and related conditions.
- Recognize potential interactions with herbs used for Alzheimer's disease and related conditions.
- Counsel a patient on herbal treatment for Alzheimer's disease.

OVERVIEW

Alzheimer's disease (AD) is a progressive neurological disorder that results in the loss of cognitive functions, primarily memory, judgment, reasoning, movement coordination, and pattern recognition. AD may progress from mild forgetfulness and cognitive impairment to widespread loss of mental abilities. In advanced AD, people become dependent on others for every aspect of their care.[1-3]

Alzheimer's disease is the most common form of *dementia*, which includes neurodegenerative disorders that cause impaired cognitive and behavioral functioning. Other forms of dementia include *vascular dementia* (caused by lack of blood flow to the brain) and *mixed dementia* (presence of both AD and vascular dementia). *Creutzfeldt-Jakob disease* is an infectious form of dementia characterized by rapidly declining memory and cognition; it is caused by pathological proteins called *prions*, which are acquired by consuming infected animals, such as cattle with "mad-cow" disease.[1-3]

It is estimated that about 5 million Americans suffer from AD, and about 360,000 people are newly diagnosed every year. Age is the most important risk factor for AD. It affects about 10% of people age 65 and older, and the number doubles about every 5 to 10 years after age 65. Half the population age 85 and older may have AD. According to the Centers for Disease Control and Prevention (CDC) Alzheimer's disease was ranked the seventh leading cause of death in 2008. The time course of the disease varies by individual, ranging from 5 to 20 years, and death usually results from secondary illnesses such as pneumonia.[1-3]

An estimated 24 million people have general dementia worldwide.[1-3] Every 72 seconds in the United States, someone develops Alzheimer's disease. By 2050, the estimated range of AD prevalence will be 13 to 16 million older Americans, unless a cure or prevention is found.[4,5] There is currently no known cure or effective treatment for AD, although researchers have made progress in understanding the disease mechanisms and treatments.

The direct and indirect costs of AD and other dementias amount to more than $148 billion annually in the United States alone.[5] The financial cost of caring for an AD patient can be overwhelming, estimated to exceed $50,000 per individual in direct annual medical expenses.[6] Medicare and other health care insurance plans may help offset the costs for individuals and caregivers.

Research continues to elucidate the pathophysiology of Alzheimer's disease. The neurotransmitter acetylcholine may be important in the pathogenesis of AD, as low levels of acetylcholine in the brain have been associated with AD; restoring these levels may slow the progression of AD.[1-3]

In addition to cholinergic dysfunction, beta-amyloid deposition, oxidative stress, and inflammation may also contribute to the etiology of AD.[7] Alzheimer's disease appears to occur from the formation of a peptide known as *beta-amyloid* or *amyloid beta*. Beta-amyloid clusters into amyloid plaques (senile plaques) on the blood vessels and on the outside surface of neurons of the brain, which ultimately cause neural degeneration.[8]

In AD patients, inflammation occurs in susceptible regions of the brain. Inflammatory mediators, such as glial cells and cytokines, are increased and may contribute to amyloid plaque formation.[9] Free radicals may result in oxidative stress, damage, and tissue inflammation in the brain and may contribute to the progression of AD.[10] Other abnormalities may contribute to Alzheimer's pathology as well. These include deficits in the serotonergic pathway and increased monoamine oxidase (MAO) type B activity.[11] Estrogen may also play a role by promoting neuronal growth and preventing oxidative damage.[12]

Signs and Symptoms

In general, the early symptoms of Alzheimer's disease progress slowly.[1-3] The disease course varies from person to person; however, 8 years is the average length of time from diagnosis to death. Life expectancy begins to decline rapidly 3 years after diagnosis, but some people with AD live more than a decade.

Stages of Alzheimer's Disease

Changes in the brain of individuals with AD may begin 10 to 20 years before any visible signs or symptoms appear.[1-3,13] Structural brain changes may include shrinkage of some regions of the brain; this can be detected during brain imaging, such as positron emission tomography (PET) scanning.[1-3] Such structural changes generally cause memory loss, which is often the first visible sign of AD. Over time, AD progresses through three main stages: mild (early), moderate, and severe[1-3,13] (Box 10-1).

Mild Symptoms

Individuals with mild symptoms of AD often seem healthy, but mental deterioration (such as memory impairment and confusion) are occurring progressively. Symptoms and early

BOX 10-1 Stages of Cognitive Decline: Global Deterioration Scale (GDS)

Stage 1: No cognitive decline
- Experiences no problems in daily living.

Stage 2: Very mild cognitive decline
- Forgets names and locations of objects.
- May have trouble finding words.

Stage 3: Mild cognitive decline
- Has difficulty traveling to new locations.
- Has difficulty handling problems at work.

Stage 4: Moderate cognitive decline
- Has difficulty with complex tasks (finances, shopping, planning dinner for guests).

Stage 5: Moderately severe cognitive decline
- Needs help to choose clothing.
- Needs prompting to bathe.

Stage 6: Severe cognitive decline
- Needs help putting on clothing.
- Requires assistance bathing; may have a fear of bathing.
- Has decreased ability to use the toilet or is incontinent.

Stage 7: Very severe cognitive decline
- Vocabulary becomes limited, eventually declining to single words.
- Loses ability to walk and sit.
- Becomes unable to smile.

Data from Reisberg B, Ferris SH, de Leon MJ, et al: Global Deterioration Scale for assessment of primary degenerative dementia, *Am J Psychiatry* 139:1136-1139, 1982.

signs of AD may include difficulty learning (and remembering) new information as well as depressive symptoms (such as sadness, decreased interest in usual activities, and loss of energy). The individual is usually still able to perform most activities (such as driving a car) but may become lost going to familiar places.[1-3]

Moderate Symptoms
In persons with moderate symptoms of AD, the neurological damage in the brain worsens and spreads to other areas that control language, reasoning, sensory processing, and thought.[1-3] During this stage, signs and symptoms of AD become more severe, and behavioral problems may become more obvious.[1-3] Signs and symptoms may include forgetting old facts, continually repeating stories, and asking the same questions repetitively. The individual may become *confabulatory*, or make up stories to fill memory gaps. Individuals have difficulty performing regular tasks, such as keeping a checkbook, shopping for groceries, following written notes, managing finances, planning meals, and taking medication on schedule. They may easily become agitated and restless and may make repetitive movements (e.g., rocking back and forth, rubbing hands). Persons with moderate AD may wander off and thus may require close supervision. They may start to have difficulty remembering family and friends. Deficiencies in intellect and reasoning, along with a lack of concern for appearance, hygiene, and sleep, become more noticeable. Paranoia, delusions, and hallucinations may occur.

Severe Symptoms
In the advanced stage of AD there is widespread damage to the brain's nerve cells or *neurons*.[1-3] Individuals with severe AD may have difficulty walking and often develop complications from other illnesses (e.g., pneumonia). Signs of severe AD may include groaning, screaming, mumbling, or speaking incoherently. Patients with severe AD may refuse to eat and may cry out inappropriately. At this point, patients may even be bedridden and may require full-time care. Individuals with severe or advanced symptoms fail to recognize the faces of family members or caregivers. For friends, family members, and caregivers, this can be the most difficult stage. *Apraxia* (inability to perform physical tasks such as dressing and eating) and *aphasia* (loss of ability in comprehension of spoken or written language) are typically seen. During this stage, patients have great difficulty with all essential activities of daily life.

Diagnosis
Because early symptoms of Alzheimer's disease progress slowly, diagnosis is difficult and often delayed.[1-3] Criteria for the diagnosis of AD have been established by the National Institute of Neurological and Communicative Disorders and Stroke and the Alzheimer's Disease and Related Disorders Association (NINCDS-ADRDA),[2,3,14] as well as in the

---

BOX 10-2 Common Criteria for Dementia

1. Memory impairment
2. At least one of the following:
   - Apraxia
   - Agnosia
   - Disturbance
3. The disturbance in 1 and 2 significantly interferes with work, social activities, or relationships.
4. Disturbance does not occur exclusively during delirium.

ADDITIONAL CRITERIA FOR DEMENTIA TYPE
Dementia of the Alzheimer's Type
Gradual onset and continuing cognitive decline
Not caused by identifiable medical, psychiatric, or neurological condition

Vascular Dementia:
Focal neurological signs or laboratory evidence of cerebrovascular condition

Dementia Due to Other Medical Conditions
Evidence from history, physical examination, or laboratory findings of a specific medical condition causing cognitive deficits (HIV disease, head trauma, Parkinson's disease, Huntington's chorea, Pick's disease, Creutzfeldt-Jakob disease)

Data from American Psychiatric Association: *Diagnostic and statistical manual of mental disorders,* 4th edition *(DSM-IV),* Washington, DC, 1994, APA Press.

Diagnostic and Statistical Manual of Mental Disorders (DSM)[15] (Box 10-2).

Small, undetected strokes, in which a lack of oxygen to the brain causes neurological damage, can lead to vascular dementia.[1-3] Individuals with Parkinson's disease, a degenerative nerve disorder, may also develop dementia. Depression can also cause lapses in memory. Furthermore, many older adults are taking multiple medications that may decrease their ability to think clearly.

Medical History
Questions in the medical history focus on general health and current medications. Past medical problems (including physical trauma, diseases, and surgeries) are also discussed. Family members usually are involved in the medical history process.[14,15]

Blood Tests
Blood tests are ordered to determine the patient's basic health. A complete blood count (CBC) can detect thyroid problems, electrolyte imbalances (e.g., abnormal levels of sodium and

potassium), and vitamin deficiencies and can help evaluate immune health.[14,15]

Mental Status Evaluation

A mental status evaluation (MSE) screens memory, problem-solving abilities, attention spans, counting skills, and language skills. Recall tests are also used. Physicians may list familiar objects and then ask a patient to repeat them immediately and again 5 minutes later. Common tools used to assess mental status and cognitive dysfunction include the Clock Drawing Test, Mini-Mental State Examination (MMSE), Alzheimer's Disease Assessment Scale–Cognitive Subscale (ADAS-Cog), Geriatric Evaluation by Relative's Rating Instrument (GERRI), and the Functional Assessment Staging (FAST).

In some cases, clinicians may more extensively assess memory, problem-solving abilities, attention spans, counting skills, and language. This is especially helpful in early diagnosis of AD. Physicians use formal psychological tests to determine if an individual's mental abilities are as expected for the person's age and education. The patterns of any mental deficits observed during neuropsychological testing can help physicians determine possible causes of dementia.[13-15]

Brain Scans

Physicians may use brain scans to pinpoint visible abnormalities in the brain. Several types of brain scans are available, including computed tomography (CT), magnetic resonance imaging (MRI), and PET. A CT scan uses x-rays to take many pictures of the brain. Using a computer, these images are then combined to provide a detailed picture. A CT scan can often show changes in brain structure. MRI scans for AD diagnosis display a cross section of the brain using radio waves and strong magnets instead of radiation. A contrast dye may be injected, although it is not used often. PET scans involve the injection of a radioactive isotope into the blood that goes to the brain. Images can then be analyzed for changes in function and structure of the brain. PET scans may take longer than CT scans, and the patient is placed inside a confining tube. CT, MRI, and PET scans are performed at a clinic or hospital. Some individuals receive mild sedatives, such as alprazolam (Xanax) or midazolam (Versed). These medications may cause drowsiness. Therefore, it is not recommended that the individuals drive after taking sedatives. Instead, patients should be driven by friends or family members.[14,15]

Genetic Testing

Mutations in three genes have been linked to AD: *APP* (which codes for the amyloid precursor protein), *PS1* (which codes for the presenilin 1 protein), or *PS2* (which codes for presenilin 2).[1-3] Because of the discovery of genes associated with developing Alzheimer's disease, genetic testing may be used in the future as a routine diagnostic tool or for determining the risk of developing AD.

SELECTED HERBAL THERAPIES

 Note

To help make this educational resource more interactive, all pharmacokinetics, adverse effects, and interactions data have been compiled in Appendix A. Safety data specifically related to pregnancy and lactation are listed in Appendix B. Please refer to these appendices when working through the case studies and answering the review questions.

Astragalus (*Astragalus membranaceus*)

Grade C: *Unclear or conflicting scientific evidence (cognitive function)*

Mechanism of Action

Astragalus has been shown to increase M-cholinergic receptor density in senile rats, which suggests that astragalus may have a role in combating brain senility.[16] Astragalus constituents, particularly the flavonoids, exert significant cellular antioxidant effects, which appear to be protective against neurological disorders.[17]

Scientific Evidence of Effectiveness

Clinical evidence suggests that a mixture containing *Astragalus membranaceus*, *Bupleurum chinense*, *Scutellaria baicalensis*, *Codonopsis pilosula*, *Ligustrum lucidum*, *Lophatherum gracile*, and thread of ivory may aid in mental performance of children with low intelligence quotients (IQs).[18] However, because astragalus was studied in combination with other herbs, its individual effects cannot be assessed. Additional clinical trials that use astragalus as a monotherapy are required before a firm conclusion can be made.

Dose

The dose of *Astragalus* used for mental performance has not been clearly established.

Adverse Effects, Interactions, Pharmacokinetics. See Appendix A.

Bacopa (*Bacopa monnieri*)

Grade B: *Good scientific evidence (cognitive function)*

Grade C: *Unclear or conflicting scientific evidence (memory)*

Mechanism of Action

Bacopa is considered a *nootropic* agent, which refers to a class of agents that may improve cognition.[19,20] Evidence suggests that bacosides A and B may aid in cognitive performance.[21,22] Although the mechanism of action has not been clearly determined, bacopa may alter and improve acetylcholine and glutamate levels.[19-21] It may also modulate muscarinic receptor binding.[21]

Scientific Evidence of Effectiveness

Although bacopa is traditionally used in Ayurvedic medicine to enhance memory, high-quality clinical trials are lacking. There is some evidence that bacopa improves cognition in healthy children.[20] Improvements in learning rate, memory consolidation, and decreased forgetfulness have also been noted in healthy males and females receiving bacopa treatment.[21] On the contrary, one randomized controlled trial of adults between ages 40 and 65 did not report positive results for bacopa on memory. Rate of forgetting newly acquired information, visual short-term memory, everyday memory function, and retrieval of preexisting knowledge were not affected by bacopa use.[23]

Dose

For cognitive function, 300 mg of Keenmind *Bacopa monnieri* extract has been used for 12 weeks.[21]

Adverse Effects, Interactions, Pharmacokinetics. See Appendix A.

Bupleurum (*Bupleurum* spp.)

Grade C: *Unclear or conflicting scientific evidence (brain injury)*

Mechanism of Action

The mechanisms by which bupleurum may improve brain injury have not been determined. Bupleurum has been found to have antiinflammatory and antioxidant properties that may contribute to its beneficial effects.[24-27]

Scientific Evidence of Effectiveness

A combination containing *Bupleurum chinense*, *Scutellaria baicalensis*, *Astragalus membranaceus*, *Codonopsis pilosula*, *Ligustrum lucidum*, *Lophatherum gracile*, and thread of ivory was assessed in one study as a treatment for children with minimal brain dysfunction.[28] However, the individual effects of bupleurum cannot be assessed because it was combined with other ingredients. Additional clinical studies that use bupleurum as a monotherapy are needed before a firm conclusion can be made.

Dose

A safe or effective dose of bupleurum has not been determined. Bupleurum is typically taken in combination formulas with other ingredients and has not been thoroughly studied as a monotherapy for neurological dysfunction.

Adverse Effects, Interactions, Pharmacokinetics. See Appendix A.

Cranberry (*Vaccinium macrocarpon*)

Grade C: *Unclear or conflicting scientific evidence (memory)*

Mechanism of Action

The exact mechanism of action of cranberry has not been determined. Cranberry possesses antioxidant properties, which may theoretically help improve cognition and memory.[29,30]

Scientific Evidence of Effectiveness

According to the available clinical evidence, ingestion of cranberry juice for 6 weeks does not enhance memory in older adults with no history of dementia or neurocognitive impairments. A randomized controlled trial (RCT) analyzed 50 patients to determine if cranberry juice improved neurophysiological function in cognitively intact older adults.[31] Participants underwent many standardized neuropsychological tests at baseline and again after 6 weeks. No significant improvements were noted in overall ability to remember, thinking abilities/processes, moods, energy levels, or overall health.

Dose

The dose of cranberry for memory improvement has not been clearly established.

Adverse Effects, Interactions, Pharmacokinetics. See Appendix A.

Ginkgo (*Ginkgo biloba*)

Grade A: *Strong scientific evidence (dementia)*

Grade B: *Good scientific evidence (cerebral insufficiency)*

Grade C: *Unclear or conflicting scientific evidence (memory)*

Grade D: *Fair negative scientific evidence (cognitive function)*

Mechanism of Action

Ginkgo contains flavonoid constituents that serve as free-radical scavengers and have been shown to reduce oxidative stress in human models.[32-40] This mechanism is hypothesized to reduce oxidative cellular damage in Alzheimer's disease and has prompted theories that ginkgo may have favorable effects on reperfusion injury.[41-47] MAO inhibition by ginkgo has been reported in animals[48] but has not been confirmed by subsequent animal research.[49] Limited human study has not demonstrated significant changes in human brain MAO type A or B, measured by PET after 1 month of 120 mg of ginkgo daily.[50] Neuroprotective properties have been attributed to inhibition of age-related decline of adrenergic and cholinergic receptors.[51-54] Ginkgo has also been found to increase serotonin levels, increase muscarinic binding sites, and increase serum levels of acetylcholine and norepinephrine.[55]

Scientific Evidence of Effectiveness

DEMENTIA. Research has produced an abundance of in vitro, in vivo, and clinical trial data examining ginkgo as a therapy for dementia and cognitive impairment. Although many trials have been published to date (mostly preliminary studies), almost all have methodological deficiencies, including vague classification, pseudorandomization, improper blinding, limited sample size, and inadequate description of dropouts and treatment effects.[56-81] Pooled analyses of research in this area report significant benefits over placebo with small effect sizes using ginkgo at doses less than 200 mg daily over 12 to 54 weeks.[76,82] Because of the heterogeneity of studies and broad inclusion criteria of many trials, it is difficult to formulate firm conclusions about which specific patient groups or diagnoses may benefit from ginkgo. Significant improvements have been noted in age-related memory impairment, activities of daily living, and quality of life. It remains unclear if there is any difference in effect between the 120-mg and 240-mg daily dosing regimens of ginkgo for these indications.

Some authors allude to the preferable side effect profile of ginkgo compared with drugs such as cholinesterase inhibitors,[83] although the availability of direct comparison is limited. one review[84] compared historical results from ginkgo trials[78,79] to four trials of acetylcholinesterase inhibitors (donepezil, tacrine, rivastigmine, metrifonate). Acetylcholinesterase inhibitors and ginkgo yielded similar improvements in dementia symptoms on the same validated scale (ADAS-Cog) compared with placebo. It was suggested that ginkgo may be as equally effective as acetylcholinesterase inhibitors. However, baseline characteristics of patients across trials were dissimilar, and adequacy of blinding and randomization varied among studies.

Preliminary evidence from a retrospective case-control study suggests possible protective effects of ginkgo against the development of Alzheimer's disease, although these results are preliminary.[85]

CEREBRAL INSUFFICIENCY. Multiple clinical trials have been conducted to evaluate ginkgo for cerebral insufficiency.* This condition, which is diagnosed more often in Europe than in the United States, is characterized by a complex of symptoms, including impaired concentration, confusion, absentmindedness, decreased physical performance, fatigue, headaches, dizziness, depression, and anxiety. The diagnosis is often made clinically. The etiology of cerebral insufficiency is believed to be decreased cerebral circulation caused by fixed atherosclerotic disease. In Europe, ginkgo is often used to treat these symptoms when they are suspected manifestations of cerebral insufficiency. Meta-analyses and clinical reviews have demonstrated efficacy but suffer from significant methodological limitations, including inconsistent inclusion criteria, inadequate blinding in studies, and inaccurate translation of foreign-language articles.

Ginkgo administration at 112 to 160 mg daily in three divided doses for up to 12 weeks has been shown to improve concentration and functional status and reduce headaches, dizziness, depression, and anxiety in patients with cerebral insufficiency. Few trials document imaging or other studies that confirm vascular compromise. Therefore, it is difficult to discern if subjects' symptoms are truly caused by poor cerebral circulation rather than other etiologies, such as early Alzheimer's disease or multiinfarct dementia (for which there is evidence of efficacy). Nonetheless, there is good support in the literature for this syndrome, as defined symptomatically.

MEMORY (AGE-ASSOCIATED MEMORY IMPAIRMENT). A nonspecific syndrome, age-associated memory impairment (AAMI) likely results from one of several pathophysiological etiologies. Some patients may have early manifestations of Alzheimer's disease or multiinfarct dementia, conditions for which ginkgo has been shown to yield some benefit. However, it is unclear if ginkgo helps improve symptoms of AAMI, because results from available studies are mixed.[59,75,108-111] Modest improvements have been reported in visual memory and speed of response in nondemented patients with AAMI.[118,111] However, another study reported no significant benefits in terms of psychometric functioning (detectability against the intensity of the stimulus) or activities of daily living.[59]

MEMORY (IN HEALTHY PATIENTS). A well-designed 2002 trial demonstrated no benefits of ginkgo, 120 mg daily, on multiple measures of memory and concentration after 6 weeks of therapy in older individuals,[119] as assessed by various tests, including tests of learning and memory (California Verbal Learning Test, Logical Memory subtest of Wechsler Memory Scale–Revised, Visual Reproduction Subscale, Memory Questionnaire, and a global evaluation completed by a spouse or companion); attention and concentration (Digit Symbol subscale of Wechsler Adult Intelligence Scale–Revised, Stroop Test, Digit Span, Mental Control test); expressive language (Controlled Category Fluency test, Boston Naming Test); and mental status (MMSE).[112-117] However, prior evidence from smaller, less rigorous studies suggests that ginkgo in doses of 240 mg or greater daily for up to 6 weeks may play a role in general enhancement of memory and other cognitive functions in healthy individuals. Therefore, although it remains unclear if higher doses of ginkgo are effective, it seems unlikely that 120 mg has significant benefits.

COGNITIVE FUNCTION (POSTPRANDIAL). Supplementation with ginkgo (mean dose, 184.5 mg daily [range, 130-234 mg daily]) has been found to be ineffective at alleviating symptoms of the postlunch dip in mental alertness or at enhancing taste and smell function.[118]

Dose

A standardized extract of ginkgo leaves is a well-defined product and contains approximately 24% flavone glycosides (primarily quercetin, kaempferol, and isorhamnetin) and

---

*References 58, 60, 63, 66, 67, 69, 72, 86-107.

6% terpene lactones (2.8%-3.4% ginkgolides A, B, and C and 2.6%-3.2% bilobalide). Products that utilize standardized extracts referred to as *EGb 761* should contain 24% *Ginkgo biloba* flavone glycosides and 6% terpenoids. Products that utilize standardized extracts referred to as *LI 1370* should contain 25% *Ginkgo biloba* flavone glycosides and 6% terpenoids.

DEMENTIA. Doses of 120 to 240 mg daily in three divided doses have been studied.[69,76,80] Ginkgo treatment has been evaluated up to 1 year.[79,80]

CEREBRAL INSUFFICIENCY. Ginkgo administration at doses of 120 to 160 mg daily in three divided doses for up to 12 weeks has resulted in improved concentration and functional status, as well as reduced headaches, dizziness, depression, and anxiety.*

MEMORY (HEALTHY INDIVIDUALS). Doses of 240 to 360 mg of ginkgo daily in three divided doses have been studied,[119-125] as has 40 mg aqueous extract twice daily.[126] LI 1370 (60 mg daily)[127] and Ginkgoba (40 mg three times daily) for 6 weeks have also been studied.[112-117]

MEMORY (AGE-ASSOCIATED MEMORY IMPAIRMENT). Ginkgo extract EGb 761 (160 mg or 240 mg daily) for 12 weeks has been studied for AAMI, but no significant effects were found.[59]

Adverse Effects, Interactions, Pharmacokinetics. See Appendix A.

Ginseng (*Panax* spp.)

Grade B: *Good scientific evidence (cognitive function)*

Grade C: *Unclear or conflicting scientific evidence (senility)*

Mechanism of Action

Ginseng is typically used to invigorate weak bodies and help restore homeostasis. Research suggests that *ginsenosides* and *ginseng saponins,* active constituents of ginseng, may have beneficial effects on aging and neurodegenerative diseases. Ginseng's ability to improve cognitive performance may result from a modulatory effect on neurotransmission. Ginsenosides Rb1 and Rg1, the most abundant ginsenosides in ginseng root, may modulate acetylcholine release and reuptake and the number of choline uptake sites, especially in the hippocampus.[128] They also increase choline acetyltransferase levels in rodent brains.[129,130]

Scientific Evidence of Effectiveness

MENTAL PERFORMANCE. Several trials of varying methodological quality suggest some *adaptogenic* effect (i.e., improvement of performance in the absence of illness) of *Panax ginseng* at doses of 200 to 400 mg of standardized extract G115 daily.[123,131-138] Enhanced cognitive performance has been reported even with single doses of ginseng.[139] Several trials used fixed combinations with other herbs (e.g., gingko) or multivitamins.[123,131,132,138] Better abstract thinking and tendency toward faster simple reactions have been reported.[134] Mental performance has been assessed using standardized measurements of reaction time, concentration, learning, math, and logic. Benefits have been seen both in healthy young people and in older ill patients. Future research should focus on determining whether such effects might be specific to clearly defined subgroups and whether longer treatment duration adds benefit.

SENILITY. Studies have reported the effects of *Panax ginseng* on elderly patients, including quality of life, mental performance, and senility. Positive outcomes in elderly individuals presenting symptoms of senile dementia have been reported.[140-142] Improved functioning of the adrenal cortex has also been noted.[140] However, the studies had flaws in methodological design or did not use standardized extracts.

Dose

Ginseng extracts may be standardized to 4% to 7% total ginsenosides content.[143-144] Some sources indicate that ginsenosides constitute an average of 3% of the dried, whole root,[145] and that the usual concentration of ginsenosides can actually be 1% to 3%. Standardized extracts of American ginseng (CNT-2000) are also available.[146] The German Federal Pharmacopeia standardizes a minimum ginsenoside content of 1.5%, calculated in terms of Rg1.[147]

COGNITIVE FUNCTION. Doses of 200 to 400 mg of ginseng daily have been used.[123,131,136,148,149]

MEMORY. Ginseng doses of 160 mg twice daily (for a total of 320 mg daily) for 14 weeks have been taken.[132]

SENILITY. A dose of 50 mg of ginseng-rhizome saponin has been taken three times daily.[140]

Adverse Effects, Interactions, Pharmacokinetics. See Appendix A.

Grape Seed (*Vitis* spp.)

Grade C: *Unclear or conflicting scientific evidence (agitation in dementia)*

Note: Grape seed extract (GSE) and Pycnogenol are not the same, even though both contain oligomeric proanthocyanidins (OPCs). Pycnogenol is a patented nutrient supplement extracted from the bark of the European coastal pine *Pinus maritima*.

Mechanism of Action

The active components of GSE are OPCs. The antioxidant properties of OPCs have made products containing these extracts candidate therapies for a wide range of human disease.

Scientific Evidence of Effectiveness

Grape seed oil is a popular (nonscented) carrier oil used in aromatherapy. Data are mixed as to whether grape seed oil aromatherapy may benefit agitation in dementia. It is unclear

---

*References 58, 60, 63, 66, 67, 69, 72, 86-107.

whether administration by cutaneous application of essential oils versus through the air only may determine effects. One study found no benefit of lavender oil, thyme oil, or grape seed (unscented) oil in treating agitation in patients with dementia.[150] Agitation was assessed every 2 days using a modified Cohen-Mansfield Agitation Inventory. Olfactory functioning was assessed with structured olfactory identification and discrimination tasks, as well as with qualitative behavioral observation during those tasks. Grape seed was used as the control in this study, and additional studies are warranted to assess the effects of grape seed in aromatherapy or another route of administration.

Dose

The dose of grape seed for agitation in dementia has not been determined.

Adverse Effects, Interactions, Pharmacokinetics. See Appendix A.

Guarana *(Paullinia cupana)*

Grade C: *Unclear or conflicting scientific evidence (cognitive function)*

Mechanism of Action

The mechanism of action of guarana for cognitive enhancement is not well understood. The main active ingredient of guarana is caffeine, which may be responsible for these effects.

Scientific Evidence of Effectiveness:

In available studies, guarana has not been shown to alter cognitive function or arousal. However, several studies have analyzed the effects of caffeine, which is thought to be the main active constituent of guarana. One study found caffeine to decrease mental concentration in males while increasing mental concentration in females.[151] Similar results were found with recall.[152] A meta-analysis of 12 studies on theophylline and caffeine found that neither therapy has significant detrimental effects on cognition or behavior.[153] However, elderly patients felt more alert when administered 250 mg of caffeine versus 250 mg of theophylline.[154] A dose-response relationship has been found for the psychoactive effects of caffeine.[155] Caffeine may significantly improve simple reaction time, but may not improve immediate memory.[156]

Dose

Guarana is generally standardized in terms of the content of caffeine, which is widely accepted as the active ingredient.[157] The amount of caffeine varies among products and manufacturers.[158,159] For cognitive enhancement, a single dose of 150 mg guarana dry extract, standardized to 11% to 13% alkaloid concentration, has been used.[131]

Adverse Effects, Interactions, Pharmacokinetics. See Appendix A.

Jojoba *(Simmondsia chinensis)*

Grade C: *Unclear or conflicting scientific evidence (dementia)*

Mechanism of Action

The mechanism of action of jojoba for improving memory has not been determined. Jojoba has been found to have anti-inflammatory effects that may be linked to enhanced mental performance.[160]

Scientific Evidence of Effectiveness

Jojoba oil is traditionally used as a carrier or massage oil. Limited research has examined the effects of massage with jojoba oil on symptoms of dementia. Available clinical research has compared the effects of lavender aromatherapy to jojoba oil massage on cognitive function, emotion, and aggressive behavior in individuals with Alzheimer's dementia; no differences were found in cognitive functioning between groups.[161] However, lavender aromatherapy improved emotion and aggressive behavior to a greater extent than jojoba oil massage. In this study, jojoba massage was considered to be a control group.[161] Currently, available evidence is insufficient to suggest that jojoba oil would have a beneficial effect on symptoms of dementia.

Adverse Effects, Interactions, Pharmacokinetics. See Appendix A.

Khat *(Catha edulis)*

Grade C: *Unclear or conflicting scientific evidence (cognitive function)*

Mechanism of Action

Cathinone, an alkaloid structurally related to amphetamine, has been found to be the main constituent of khat. Cathinone is a central nervous system (CNS) stimulant, and its effects are mediated through monoamine neurotransmitter systems.[162]

Scientific Evidence of Effectiveness

Two vague trials that evaluated khat in cognitive function did not find beneficial results.[163,164] One study found that khat negatively affected cognitive function. Three groups of flight attendants were assessed: (1) daily khat chewing ($N = 25$), (2) occasional khat chewing ($N = 39$), and (3) non–khat chewing ($N = 24$). Measurements included an electroencephalographic (EEG) frequency analysis and four psychometric tests that measured decision-speed and perceptual-visual memory. There was no consistent correlation in the EEG frequency analysis and the scores of the psychometric testing. The psychometric tests showed a significantly lower score in both groups of khat users compared with nonusers, and daily users scored significantly lower than occasional users.

Dose. The dose of khat for cognitive function is unclear.

Adverse Effects, Interactions, Pharmacokinetics. See Appendix A.

Lavender (Lavandula angustifolia)

Grade C: *Unclear or conflicting scientific evidence (dementia)*

Mechanism of action
Caffeic acid, a constituent of lavender, has been demonstrated to possess antioxidant effects in vitro, which may provide benefit for dementia and cognition.[165]

Scientific Evidence of Effectiveness
Available clinical research has compared the effects of lavender aromatherapy to jojoba oil massage on cognitive function, emotion, and aggressive behavior in individuals with Alzheimer's dementia; no differences were found in cognitive functioning between groups. However, lavender aromatherapy improved emotion and aggressive behavior to a greater extent than jojoba oil (control) massage.[161]

Dose
The dose of lavender used to treat dementia has not been clearly established.

Adverse Effects, Interactions, Pharmacokinetics. See Appendix A.

Lemon Balm (Melissa officinalis)

Grade C: *Unclear or conflicting scientific evidence (cognitive function; agitation in dementia)*

Mechanism of Action
The exact mechanism by which lemon balm may improve cognitive performance has not been clearly determined. Lemon balm has displayed cholinesterase enzyme inhibition and may play a part in Alzheimer's disease.[166-168]

Scientific Evidence of Effectiveness
COGNITIVE PERFORMANCE. Clinical evidence suggests that standardized lemon balm extract may have some effect on particular self-reported measures of mood and cognition through cholinergic activities.[166-168] Lemon balm, 60 drops daily (1:1 in 45% alcohol, standardized to contain 500 mcg/mL citral) for 16 weeks, improved cognitive function in patients with mild to moderate Alzheimer's disease, as measured by the ADAS-Cog and Clinical Dementia Rating–Sum of the Boxes (CDR-SB).[169]

AGITATION IN DEMENTIA. Preliminary evidence also suggests that aromatherapy using essential oil of lemon balm lotion can effectively reduce agitation in people with severe dementia when applied to the face and arms twice daily.[170]

Dose
For cognitive improvement, Alzheimer's patients have taken 60 drops of lemon balm extract (1:1 in 45% alcohol, standardized to contain 500 mcg/mL citral) daily for 16 weeks.[169]

For agitation in dementia, aromatherapy with essential oil of lemon balm lotion applied to the face and arms twice daily has been used in clinical study.[170]

Adverse Effects, Interactions, Pharmacokinetics. See Appendix A.

Peppermint (Mentha x piperita)

Grade C: *Unclear or conflicting scientific evidence (vigilance improvement in brain injury [aromatherapy])*

Mechanism of Action
It is unclear how peppermint may improve brain injury. Peppermint has been shown to have antiinflammatory[171] and antioxidant[172] activity, which may contribute to its beneficial effects for this use.

Scientific Evidence of Effectiveness
Preliminary evidence suggests potential benefit of the scent of peppermint oil in vigilance (alertness) in patients who experienced attention maintenance difficulty after brain injury, as well as in normal subjects.[173]

Dose
The dose of peppermint oil for brain injuries has not been clearly established.

Adverse Effects, Interactions, Pharmacokinetics. See Appendix A.

Polypodium (Polypodium leucotomos)

Grade C: *Unclear or conflicting scientific evidence (dementia)*

Mechanism of Action
The mechanism of *Polypodium leucotomos* in Alzheimer's disease is not well understood but may be related to its antioxidant and antiinflammatory activity.[174-178] In vitro and animal research using *P. leucotomos* extract (anapsos) has demonstrated free radical–scavenging activity[174-175] and cytokine inhibition.[176-178]

Scientific Evidence of Effectiveness
There is insufficient human data to recommend for or against the use of *P. leucotomos* extract (also referred to as "anapsos") in the management of dementia. Anapsos was studied as a therapy for dementia in an RCT of 45 patients with mild to moderate senile dementia of the vascular or the Alzheimer type.[179] Patients were randomized to receive anapsos 360 mg, 720 mg, or placebo daily. Results showed that anapsos 360 mg daily improved cognitive performance, cerebral blood

perfusion, and brain bioelectrical activity in patients with senile dementia. These effects of anapsos were more marked in demented patients with mild mental deterioration and/or with dementia of the Alzheimer type. Improvements were not as significant with the 720 mg daily dose.

Dose

There is no widely accepted standardization for the preparation of *Polypodium leucotomos* extract. A dose of 360 mg of anapsos (*P. leucotomos* extract) daily showed improvement in cognitive performance, cerebral blood perfusion, and brain bioelectrical activity in patients with senile dementia.

Adverse Effects, Interactions, Pharmacokinetics. See Appendix A.

Rhodiola (Rhodiola rosea)

Grade C: *Unclear or conflicting scientific evidence (cognitive function)*

Mechanism of Action

The mechanism of action of rhodiola for improving learning and memory capacity has not been determined. Rhodiola has been found to have antiinflammatory[180] and antioxidant effects[181-185], which may be linked to enhanced mental performance. A single dose of *Rhodiola rosea* before maze training facilitated learning and memory in animals.[186]

Scientific Evidence of Effectiveness

Evidence suggests that supplementation with rhodiola improves mental performance in healthy night-shift workers.[187] Rhodiola treatment (170 mg daily) resulted in significant improvement in mental performance tests after 2 weeks. The mental performance tests included speed of visual and audio perception, attention capacity, and short-term memory. There was no significant effect during the second 2-week period, but longer night duty was suggested to be a potential reason. Another study reported beneficial results of a repeated low-dose regimen (50 mg twice daily) of rhodiola extract on fatigue in students under stress during examinations.

Dose

SHR-5 is a standardized rhodiola extract that contains rosavin (3.6%), salidroside (1.6%), and *p*-tyrosol (<0.1%).[187] For mental performance (during fatigue), 170 mg of *Rhodiola rosea* extract (SHR-5) has been used twice daily for up to 20 days.[188]

Adverse Effects, Interactions, Pharmacokinetics. See Appendix A.

Rhubarb (Rheum spp.)

Grade C: *Unclear or conflicting scientific evidence (memory; senility)*

Mechanism of Action

The mechanism of action of rhubarb for improving memory capacity has not been determined. Rhubarb has been found to have antiinflammatory and antioxidant effects, which may be linked to enhanced mental performance.[189,190]

Scientific Evidence of Effectiveness

Rhubarb has a role in traditional Chinese medicine (TCM). Rhubarb combination herbal products used in TCM have been shown to improve memory in senile patients.[191] However, it is difficult to determine if the effects are attributed to rhubarb alone or to other products in the combination.

Dose

The dose of rhubarb for memory enhancement has not been clearly established.

Adverse Effects, Interactions, Pharmacokinetics. See Appendix A.

Sage (Salvia officinalis)

Grade A: *Strong scientific evidence (cognitive function)*

Grade B: *Good scientific evidence (Alzheimer's disease)*

Mechanism of Action

The mechanism of action of sage in AD and cognitive improvement is not well understood. Sage has been found to possess in vitro cholinesterase-inhibiting properties, which may contribute to its effects on cognition in AD.[167,192-194]

Scientific Evidence of Effectiveness

COGNITIVE FUNCTION. Sage has long been suggested to improve memory and mood. Several RCTs provide good evidence for the use of sage for these purposes.[195-197] In clinical study, 300-mg and 600-mg doses of sage were found to improve alertness, as assessed by the Bond-Lader mood scale.[195] Tildesley et al.[196] evaluated the effects of sage essential oil and reported improvements in the "speed of memory" factor, as assessed by the Cognitive Drug Research (CDR) computerized test. Mood was consistently improved, as well as self-rated "alertness, calmness, and contentedness," following a 50-mcL dose. In young adults a 50-mcL dose significantly improved immediate word recall, supporting the use of small doses of sage for short-term memory.[197]

ALZHEIMER'S DISEASE. Because of its potential anticholinergic effects,[191] sage has been evaluated for AD. *Salvia lavandulaefolia* and *Salvia officinalis* may provide beneficial effects in cognitive function in AD patients when used for up to 16 weeks.[191,198] Clinical study has found that an ethanolic extract of sage (*S. officinalis*) prevented deterioration of cognition over 16 weeks, as measured by the AD assessment scale and clinical dementia rating.[198] Other study reported that the administration of essential oil of Spanish sage (*S. lavandulaefolia*) reduced Neuropsychiatric Inventory (NPI) scores (an AD assessment tool) and vigilance task performance.[191]

Dose

COGNITIVE FUNCTION. A single daily dose of 25 or 50 mcL of the essential oil of Spanish sage (*Salvia lavandulaefolia*) has been used.[196,197]

ALZHEIMER'S DISEASE. Three daily doses of 50 mcL of the essential oil of Spanish sage (*S. lavandulaefolia*) has been used.[191] Single daily doses of 60 drops of an ethanolic extract of sage (*S. officinalis*) has also been used for AD; the extract was made by combining 1 kg of dried leaves in 1 L of 45% ethanol.[198]

Adverse Effects, Interactions, Pharmacokinetics. See Appendix A.

Soy (Glycine max)

Grade C: *Unclear or conflicting scientific evidence (cognitive function)*

Mechanism of Action

The soy isoflavones daidzein and genistein act as weak agonists at estrogen receptors in the brain.[199-201] These receptors may play an important role in mental function by enhancing neuronal survival and shaping neuronal connections in the hippocampus, an area involved with memory.[201,202]

Scientific Evidence of Effectiveness

Clinical trials evaluating supplementation with soy isoflavones for cognitive function have reported conflicting results.[203,204] Postmenopausal women (age 55 to 75 years) not receiving estrogen therapy demonstrated improved visual memory after taking 110 mg of soy daily for 6 months.[203] A 10-week study found that healthy male and female adults who were supplemented with soy had improved memory and mental flexibility (learning rule reversals).[204] However, another clinical study evaluating postmenopausal women (age 60 to 75 years) found no difference between groups taking 25.6 g of soy protein powder (containing 99 mg total isoflavones, 52 mg genistein, 41 mg daidzein, and 6 mg glycetein) or total milk protein powder daily for 12 months.[205]

Dose

Although research is conflicting, 60 to 100 mg daily of soy isoflavones may provide benefit in cognitive function and memory.[204-205]

Adverse Effects, Interactions, Pharmacokinetics. See Appendix A.

Tea (Camellia sinensis)

Grade C: *Unclear or conflicting scientific evidence (memory, cognitive function)*

Mechanism of Action

Some of the effects of tea may be attributed to caffeine, a known CNS stimulant that may improve cognition and increase alertness and thought.[151-156,206,207] Tea (black, green, or various other kinds of tea made from *Camellia sinensis*) contains various constituents (including catechins, theophylline, and tannins) with antioxidant properties that may also help improve cognition.[151-156,208-210]

Scientific Evidence of Effectiveness

Ingestion of black tea (300 mg caffeine daily) has been associated with rapid increases in alertness and information-processing capacity. Tea drinking throughout the day has been reported to help sustain alertness. However, effects of tea may not result entirely from caffeine; other factors either intrinsic to the beverage (e.g., sensory attributes) or the presence of other biologically active substances (e.g., epigallocatechin) may play a role in mediating the responses.[211] Lower doses of caffeine (60 mg) consumed in tea have been found to speed up reaction time in healthy males; however, accuracy of performance in cognitive function testing did not improve.[212]

Dose

For cognitive performance, 300 mg of caffeine from tea has been taken three times daily.[211]

Adverse Effects, Interactions, Pharmacokinetics. See Appendix A.

Turmeric (Curcuma longa)

Grade C: *Unclear or conflicting scientific evidence (cognitive function)*

Mechanism of Action

Curcumin from turmeric has demonstrated antioxidant and antiinflammatory effects and may reduce beta-amyloid and plaque burden, which may prevent cognitive decline.[213,214]

Scientific Evidence of Effectiveness

Preliminary evidence suggests that curry, which contains turmeric as a spice, improved cognitive function, as measured by MMSE scores,[215] when consumed "occasionally" and "often to very often." Additional studies are warranted before a recommendation can be made.

Dose

The dose of turmeric used to improve cognitive function has not been clearly established.

Adverse Effects, Interactions, Pharmacokinetics. See Appendix A.

Ayurveda

Similar to other traditions of nature-based medicine, Ayurveda teaches that vital energy, referred to as *prana*, is the basis of all life and healing. As prana circulates throughout the human body, it is governed by the five elements: *earth, air, fire, water,* and *ether*. In Ayurveda, these terms represent subtle qualities of prana energy and how it purportedly expresses itself in the human body. According to Ayurveda, health is a state of balance and harmony among the five elements, and illness occurs when there is imbalance or lack of harmony. The five elements combine with one another into pairs called *doshas*. There are three doshas: *vata* (ether and air), *pitta* (fire and water), and *kapha* (earth and water).

Alzheimer's disease is thought to be caused by an imbalance of vata energy, the "kinetic" principle. Ayurvedic herbs, such as bacopa or "Brahmi," have been used to treat AD. There is some evidence that Ayurvedic bacopa improves cognition in children.[20] Improved learning rates, memory consolidation, and decreased forgetting have also been noted in healthy males and females.[21] Clinical studies using Ayurvedic medicine on AD are lacking.

 Traditional Chinese Medicine

Traditional Chinese medicine (TCM) herbal combinations have been used to treat dementia and reportedly improve cognitive function and activities of daily living. The compound Tong Jiang Oral Liquid with Da Huang (rhubarb root) improved memory in senile patients better than Qi Yin oral liquid without Da Huang.[191]

HERBAL THERAPIES WITH NEGATIVE EVIDENCE

Bitter Orange *(Citrus aurantium)*

Grade D: *Fair negative scientific evidence (agitation in dementia)*

Aromatherapy interventions with bitter orange *(Citrus aurantium)* did not reduce combative, resistive behaviors in individuals with dementia.[216]

ADJUNCT THERAPIES

1. Currently, no known cure exists for Alzheimer's disease (AD), so the goal of treatment is to slow its progression. Various prescription drugs, dietary supplements, and complementary modalities may play a role in delaying AD. These agents may also be beneficial as adjuncts to standard treatment.
2. Inflammation is believed to contribute to damage from AD. Antiinflammatory drugs (e.g., NSAIDs), particularly cyclooxygenase (COX)-2 inhibitors, may reduce levels of beta-amyloid peptide and may have a protective effect on the development of AD.[217] Linoleic and alpha linolenic acids have also been found to inhibit COX-2 and may help reduce AD risk.
3. Hydroxymethylglutaryl–coenzyme A (HMG-CoA) reductase inhibitors, or *statins,* may also reduce the risk of AD. Several recent studies have observed a reduced risk of AD with statin use.[218-221] However, it remains unclear if statins prevent neurodegeneration, promote neuroregeneration, or prevent primary factors (such as plaque formation) that underlie AD pathology.

Herbs with Potential Therapeutic Properties for Alzheimer's Disease and Associated Conditions*

HERB	SPECIFIC THERAPEUTIC USE(S)†	HERB	SPECIFIC THERAPEUTIC USE(S)†
Abuta	Delirium	Cat's claw	Alzheimer's disease, memory, dementia
Aconite	Agitation	Chamomile	Delirium tremens (DTs)
African wild potato	Delirium	Chasteberry	Dementia
Aloe	Alzheimer's disease	Chlorella	Alzheimer's disease, cognitive function
Alpinia	Dementia		
Anise	Cognitive function	Club moss	Alzheimer's disease
Aristolochia spp.	Alzheimer's disease	Codonopsis	Brain injury (anoxic) memory, senility
Ashwagandha	Cognitive function, senility, dementia	Cordyceps	Alzheimer's disease, memory, senility (weakness)
Black pepper	Alzheimer's disease	Danshen	Brain injury (anoxic)
Blessed thistle	Memory		
Calamus	Cognitive function/memory, senility, learning	Deer velvet	Memory

Continued

Herbs with Potential Therapeutic Properties for Alzheimer's Disease and Associated Conditions* —cont'd

HERB	SPECIFIC THERAPEUTIC USE(S)†	HERB	SPECIFIC THERAPEUTIC USE(S)†
Elder	Alzheimer's disease	Noni	Brain injury, senility
Eyebright	Memory	Organic food	Alzheimer's disease, cognitive funciton
Fo-ti	Memory, learning	Perilla	Memory
Garlic	Senility	Pycnogenol	Alzheimer's disease
Goji	Alzheimer's disease, agitation	Raspberry	Agitation
Gotu kola	Alzheimer's disease, memory	Red clover	Cognitive function
Grapefruit	Alzheimer's disease	Rehmannia	Dementia
Honeysuckle	Agitation	Rosemary	Memory
Horny goat weed	Alzheimer's disease, cognitive function, memory	Rutin	Brain injury (cerebral function disorders)
Kava	Brain injury	Safflower	Alzheimer's disease (prevention), cognitive function, memory
Lady's slipper	Delirium tremens		
Lemongrass	Agitation	Salvia divinorum	Alzheimer's disease, dementia
Lotus	Agitation	Sea buckthorn	Senility
Maca	Cognitive function	Spirulina	Brain injury, memory
Mugwort	Agitation	Valerian	Memory
Muira puama	Alzheimer's disease, memory, cognitive function	Yohimbe bark extract	Alzheimer's disease, cognitive function

*This is not an all-inclusive or comprehensive list of herbs with neuroprotective, antitremor, antineuralgic, and/or antirigidity properties; other herbs and supplements may possess these qualities. A qualified health care provider should be consulted with specific questions or concerns regarding potential neuroprotective, antitremor, antineuralgic, and/or antirigidity effects or interactions of agents.
†Based on expert opinion, anecdote, case reports, and/or preliminary trial evidence.

4. *Omega-3 fatty acids* are a type of polyunsaturated fatty acid (PUFA). Research has linked certain types of omega-3s to a reduced risk of heart disease and stroke. Research suggests that high levels of omega-3s may help reduce the risk of dementia or cognitive decline. Docosahexaenoic acid (DHA) is the primary omega-3 in the brain found in the fatty membranes that surround nerve cells, especially at the junctions where cells connect to one another. According to a 2006 systematic review by the Cochrane Collaboration, larger clinical trials are needed to determine if omega-3 supplements prevent cognitive decline or dementia.[222] However, the authors found enough laboratory and epidemiological studies to conclude that this is a promising area of research. Theories about why omega-3s might influence dementia risk include their beneficial effects on the heart and blood vessels, antiinflammatory effects, and support and protection of nerve cell membranes. Preliminary evidence also suggests that omega-3s may be beneficial for patients with depression or bipolar disorder (manic depression). Laboratory evidence suggests that omega-3s may stimulate the growth of the branches that connect one cell to another. As a result, this may help increase the brain's ability to process, store, and retrieve information.

5. *Vitamin E* has been proposed and evaluated for the prevention or slowing of dementia (including Alzheimer's type), based on its antioxidant properties and findings of low vitamin E levels in some individuals with dementia. There is some evidence that all-*rac*-α-tocopherol (synthetic vitamin E) is similar in effects to a common drug for AD, selegiline (Eldepryl), in slowing cognitive decline in patients with moderately severe AD; no additive effect was observed when used in combination with selegiline.[223]

6. *Coenzyme Q10* (CoQ10) is produced by the human body and is necessary for the basic functioning of cells. Promising preliminary evidence suggests that CoQ10 supplementation may slow dementia in animal models of AD.[224] Clinical trials are warranted.

7. *Huperzine A* is a moss extract that has been used in TCM for centuries. It has been shown to act similar to cholinesterase inhibitors, one class of FDA-approved Alzheimer medications, and thus is promoted as a treatment for AD. Limited evidence from small studies suggests that huperzine A may be as effective as approved drugs such as donepezil (Aricept) and rivastigmine (Exelon). In spring 2004 the National Institute on Aging (NIA) launched the first large U.S. clinical trial to assess the efficacy of

huperzine A in mild to moderate AD. However, a recent systematic review found insufficient evidence to support using huperzine A in AD treatment.[225] Because current formulations of huperzine A are dietary supplements, they are unregulated and manufactured with no uniform standards. Concomitant use with FDA-approved Alzheimer drugs such as donepezil may increase the risk of serious side effects.

8. *Phosphatidylserine* is a lipid that is the primary component of the membranes that surround nerve cells. In AD, nerve cells degenerate for unknown reasons. Phosphatidylserine may alter the cell membrane and help prevent neuron degeneration. Using phosphatidylserine derived from cows, preliminary trials produced promising results. However, most trials included small samples of participants, and studies were discontinued in the 1990s over concerns about "mad-cow disease." Since then, some animal studies have used phosphatidylserine derived from soy. In 2000, a small clinical trial reported that phosphatidylserine produced encouraging results in 18 subjects with age-associated memory impairment.[226] However, larger, well-designed trials are needed to determine if this is a viable treatment.

9. *Art therapy* allows the opportunity to exercise the eyes and hands, improve eye-hand coordination, and stimulate neurological pathways from the brain to the hands. Art therapy may be an effective means of improving quality of life in elderly persons.[227]

10. Maintaining mental and physical fitness may also delay the onset of dementia.[228,229] Some researchers believe that lifelong mental and physical exercise and learning may promote the growth of additional synapses (connections between neurons) and delay the onset of dementia. Other researchers argue that advanced education gives a person more experience with the types of memory and thinking tests used to measure dementia. Doing crossword puzzles, reading books, and increasing social activities are recommended by health care providers.

11. Adjunct therapeutic interventions are also directed at treating agitation, psychosis, anxiety, and depression in AD patients. There is good scientific evidence to support the use of *aromatherapy* for agitation and anxiety in patients with dementia.[161] *Music therapy* has also been found to reduce aggressive or agitated behavior in people with Alzheimer's dementia.[230]

INTEGRATIVE THERAPY PLAN

- Perform a thorough baseline assessment using the criteria of the National Institute of Neurological and Communicative Disorders and Stroke and the Alzheimer's Disease and Related Disorders Association (NINCDS-ADRDA).
- Obtain history and current status from the patient and caregiver.
- Assess the patient's behavior. With the patient and caregiver, determine what behavioral problems occur and when, how often, and how they are involved in the situation.
- Routine laboratory tests and physical and psychiatric examinations should be performed at baseline and regularly throughout the course of the disease to rule out other disorders that may cause dementia (e.g., vitamin B12 deficiency, hypothyroidism) and to identify complicating physiological issues (e.g., electrolyte problems from dehydration), which can worsen in dementia.
- Obtain information regarding prescription and dietary supplement use, history of alcohol or other substance use, and family medical history, as well as any history of trauma, depression, or head injury.
- Use the Global Deterioration Scale (GDS) to stage the diagnosis of Alzheimer's disease.
- Inquire about medication effects and inadequate response to a medication. Advise that a medication log be used to track all the medications used by the patient, including all current prescription drugs, over-the-counter medications, and vitamins or herbal supplements.
- Pharmacotherapy should be geared at decreasing the rate of cognitive decline as well as improving quality of life, mood, and behavior. Counsel the patient and caregiver regarding integrative therapies and potential risks and interactions.
- Cholinesterase inhibitors, such as donepezil (Aricept), are regarded as first-line pharmacotherapy for mild to moderate Alzheimer's disease. Also, educate the patient and family regarding the use of NSAIDs and statin agents that may help reduce AD risk.
- Ginkgo may provide benefits in patients with early-stage AD and multiinfarct dementia and may be as effective as acetylcholinesterase inhibitors (donepezil). Ginkgo may cause bleeding, especially in sensitive individuals, such as those taking medications for bleeding disorders (including warfarin [Coumadin]).
- Implement pharmacological and nonpharmacological strategies to manage neuropsychiatric and behavioral symptoms of AD. Music therapy or aromatherapy may reduce such symptoms and may be used with conventional medications.
- Counsel the patient, family, and caregiver regarding prognosis and limitations of treatment. Refer the family to local resources such as the Alzheimer's Association to obtain detailed information regarding support services.

Case Studies

CASE STUDY 10-1

RF is a 69-year-old man who comes to your pharmacy with his daughter to pick up his prescription for warfarin following a hip replacement. She asks you about ginkgo for her father because he is beginning to have difficulty recalling recent events and he keeps repeating himself. RF denies any memory problems. He also takes atorvastatin for hyperlipidemia and echinacea to prevent colds. How should you counsel?

Answer: If a patient is taking warfarin, ginkgo should not be used to help with cognitive function and dementia. Similarly, ginseng, which has also been shown to modestly improve thinking and learning, should not be used by patients using blood-thinning medications.

Bacopa, or "Brahmi," is used in Ayurvedic medicine and widely used in India for enhancing memory. Although bacopa is traditionally used to enhance cognition, high-quality research is lacking. Limited studies have found some evidence that bacopa improves cognition. If RF decides to try bacopa, you may recommend he try 300 mg of *Bacopa monnieri* extract for 12 weeks. Bacopa is generally well tolerated but may cause palpitations, nausea, dry mouth, thirst, and fatigue.

Bacopa has not been reported to interact with warfarin or other anticoagulant medications; however, warfarin has a narrow therapeutic range, and caution should always be observed when this drug is administered to any patient and when any other drug or dietary supplement is added. RF should notify his physician immediately if he notices signs of bleeding, including prolonged bleeding from cuts, nosebleeds, bleeding gums, or unusual bruising.

If the patient decides to take bacopa, an interaction is possible between this herb and RF's echinacea. Both bacopa and echinacea may interfere with cytochrome P450 activity, and caution is warranted.

In this case, maintaining mental fitness may delay onset of dementia for RF. Doing crossword puzzles, reading books, and increasing social activities are recommended by health care providers.

CASE STUDY 10-2

GP, a 76-year-old fair-skinned man with mild Alzheimer's disease, comes into your pharmacy with his daughter to pick up his prescription for glipizide and donepezil (Aricept) and to buy a bottle of St. John's wort. He tells you that he is becoming quite depressed as he gets older and begins to become a burden on his family. His daughter inquires about ginkgo to help her father's memory. How should you counsel?

Answer: Overall, research suggests that ginkgo benefits people with early-stage AD and may be as helpful as donepezil (Aricept). For dementia, doses of 120 to 240 mg daily in three divided doses have been used for up to 1 year. However, cholinergic effects (e.g., salivation, urination) may potentially be precipitated when used with drugs such as donepezil.

Although St. John's wort may improve GP's symptoms of depression, a potentially harmful interaction may occur between St. John's wort and glipizide. Both glipizide, a drug used for type 2 diabetes, and St. John's wort may cause photosensitivity; their combined use increases the risk of a photosensitivity reaction. Because GP is fair skinned, he may be more susceptible to photosensitization. St. John's wort may also have the potential to alter blood sugar levels. As an alternative intervention, suggest that GP use music therapy, which may help promote wellness and relieve symptoms of depression.

Ginkgo may alter blood sugar, but interactions with antidiabetes agents are not clear. GP should be advised to monitor his blood sugar closely if he decides to try ginkgo. He should also be monitored closely by a health care professional because medication adjustments may be necessary. If GP decides to take ginkgo, inform him and his daughter that ginkgo is generally well tolerated. Minor adverse effects, including headache, nausea, and stomach complaints, have been reported. GP should also be counseled regarding the risk of bleeding with ginkgo use. If any unusual bleeding occurs, his physician should be notified immediately. Ginkgo should be stopped before some surgical or dental procedures.

Maintaining mental fitness may also delay onset of dementia. Some researchers believe that lifelong mental exercise and learning may promote the growth of additional synapses, the connections between neurons, and delay the onset of dementia. Other researchers argue that advanced education gives a person more experience with the types of memory and thinking tests used to measure dementia. Doing crossword puzzles, reading books, and increasing social activities are recommended by health care providers.

CASE STUDY 10-3

About 5 years have passed, and GP's daughter from Case Study 10-2 returns to the pharmacy and tells you that her father now resides at an assisted-living facility. GP has become verbally abusive and often displays angry, emotional outbursts when the nurses try to help him. At other times, he seems withdrawn and indifferent. She asks you if there is anything other than "adding a drug" to help her father. How should you counsel?

Answer: Many patients with Alzheimer's disease exhibit disruptive and violent behaviors. Aromatherapy, using essential oil of lemon balm lotion, has been shown to reduce agitation in people with severe dementia when applied to the face and arms twice daily. Lavender aromatherapy may also improve emotion and aggressive behavior in individuals with Alzheimer's dementia. Music therapy may also help promote wellness and relieve symptoms of depression. GP's withdrawn behavior may not respond to medications unless the patient is oversedated. Art therapy may help the patient exercise his eyes and hands, improve hand-eye coordination, and stimulate neurological pathways from the brain to the hands. This intervention may help improve GP's quality of life.

References for Chapter 10 can be found on the Evolve website at http://evolve.elsevier.com/Ulbricht/herbalpharmacotherapy/

Review Questions

1. True or false: Cathinone, an alkaloid structurally related to amphetamine, has been found to be the main constituent of ginseng.

2. Which of the following mechanisms has been reported with ginkgo?
   a. Reduction of oxidative cellular damage
   b. MAO inhibition
   c. Increased levels of serotonin and norepinephrine
   d. All the above

3. Ginkgo may interact with which of the following drugs?
   a. Clopidogrel
   b. Carbamazepine
   c. Nifedipine
   d. All the above

4. What dose of bacopa may be recommended for enhancing memory?
   a. 30 mcg daily for 12 weeks
   b. 3000 mg daily for 12 weeks
   c. 300 mg daily for 12 weeks
   d. 30 g daily for 12 weeks

5. True or false: Enhancement of cognitive performance has been exhibited by even single doses of ginseng.

6. Which of the following mechanisms may contribute to soy's beneficial effects in Alzheimer's disease?
   a. Soy isoflavones (daidzein and genistein) act as weak agonists at estrogen receptors in the brain.
   b. Soy prevents the formation of amyloid beta into amyloid plaques and therefore prevents the death of neurons.
   c. Soy inhibits acetylcholinesterase.
   d. Soy blocks the neurotransmitter glutamate.

7. Which of the following natural products may be used for agitation in patients with dementia?
   a. Lavender
   b. Khat
   c. Ginseng
   d. Gingko

Answers are found in the Answers to Review Questions section in the back of the text.

11 Hypertension

Outline

OVERVIEW
    Signs and Symptoms
        Malignant Hypertension
        Preeclampsia
    Diagnosis
SELECTED HERBAL THERAPIES
    Black Currant *(Ribes nigrum)*
    Evening Primrose *(Oenothera biennis)*
    False Hellebore *(Veratrum* spp.*)*
    Flax *(Linum usitatissimum)*
    Garlic *(Allium sativum)*
    Ginseng *(Panax* spp.*)*
    Hibiscus *(Hibiscus* spp.*)*
    Onion *(Allium cepa)*
    Pycnogenol *(Pinus pinaster* subsp. *atlantica)*
    Reishi Mushroom *(Ganoderma lucidum)*
    Rhubarb *(Rheum* spp.*)*
    Safflower *(Carthamus tinctorius)*
    Sea Buckthorn *(Hippophae rhamnoides)*
    Soy *(Glycine max)*
    Stevia *(Stevia rebaudiana)*
HERBAL THERAPIES WITH LIMITED EVIDENCE
ADJUNCT THERAPIES
INTEGRATIVE THERAPY PLAN
CASE STUDIES
REVIEW QUESTIONS

Learning Objectives

- Develop a systematic approach to using herbal therapy in patients with hypertension.
- Know potential interactions with antihypertensive herbs.
- Describe some of the common side effects associated with antihypertensive herbs.
- Discuss with patients ways to decrease blood pressure using an herbal treatment plan as well as adjunct therapies.

OVERVIEW

Each time the heart beats, it pumps blood through blood vessels to supply oxygen and nutrients to the body's muscles, organs, and tissues. Blood pressure is the force of blood pushing against the walls of arteries. Over the course of a day, an individual's blood pressure rises and falls transiently many times in response to various stimuli. Elevated blood pressure over a sustained period is referred to as *hypertension*.[1] Almost one third of American adults has high blood pressure. Approximately two thirds of Americans older than 65 years have high blood pressure, and an estimated 71.8% are aware of their condition. Of all people with high blood pressure, 61.4% are under current treatment, 35.1% have it under control, and 64.9% do not have it controlled.[2]

High blood pressure is easily detected and usually controllable; however, from 1994 to 2004 the mortality rate from high blood pressure increased 15.5%, and the actual number of deaths rose 41.8%.[2] Non-Hispanic blacks are more likely to have high blood pressure than non-Hispanic whites. Within the African-American community, those with the highest rates of hypertension are more likely to be middle aged or older, overweight or obese, physically inactive, and diabetic. In 2004 the mortality rates per 100,000 population from high blood pressure were 15.6 for white males, 49.9 for black males, 14.3 for white females, and 40.6 for black females.[2]

The World Health Organization (WHO) estimates that the prevalence of hypertension exceeds 10% in developed nations.[3] High blood pressure increases the risk of *coronary heart disease* (CHD) and *cerebrovascular accident* (CVA or stroke), which are the leading causes of death among Americans.[2]

To maintain a normal blood pressure, there must be a balance between the amount of resistance in blood vessels and the output of the heart. The kidneys and sympathetic nervous system are thought to play a major role in this balance. As with other muscle contractions in the body, the dilation and contraction of smooth muscles in the blood vessels depend on the electrolytes sodium, potassium, and calcium;

the neurotransmitters epinephrine and norepinephrine also play a role. An increase or decrease in blood pressure can result not only from direct stimulation of the blood vessels but also from fluid volume as well. Volume depletion by diuretics stimulating the elimination of sodium in the kidneys has been shown to decrease blood pressure. The kidneys also can lower blood pressure through the renin-angiotensin system. The kidney excretes renin in response to a decrease in sodium or a signal from the sympathetic nervous system. The renin then helps to create the angiotensin component, a strong blood vessel constrictor. Blocking the renin-angiotensin system may decrease the kidneys' ability to increase blood pressure.[1]

Signs and Symptoms

Hypertension is called the "silent killer" because an individual can have it for years without knowing it. Hypertension rarely causes symptoms at first but is a risk factor for many other conditions, including kidney disease and CHD, which may lead to stroke (also known as *cardiovascular accident* or CVA) or heart attack (also known as *myocardial infarction* or MI).

Hypertension can also cause vertigo, tinnitus, dimmed vision, fatigue, palpitations, impotence, and fainting; however, these symptoms are relatively rare. Extremely elevated blood pressure can cause a headache on awakening or, even more rarely, nosebleed, nausea, or vomiting.

Malignant Hypertension

Malignant hypertension can be life threatening and has recognizable symptoms that require immediate treatment. Symptoms include blurred vision, headache, confusion, anxiety, drowsiness, fatigue, and weakness or numbness in the arms, legs, face, or other areas. Other physical symptoms of malignant hypertension may include nausea, vomiting, chest pain, shortness of breath, cough, and decreased urine output.

Preeclampsia

Preeclampsia is characterized by the triad of hypertension, edema, and proteinuria (protein in the urine) and is also known as *pregnancy-induced hypertension*. It can cause serious complications for the mother and baby. Preeclampsia can decrease the supply of blood and oxygen available to the mother and developing child and may result in conditions such as a lower birth weight and neurological damage. The mother is at risk for kidney problems, seizures (eclampsia), strokes, breathing problems, and even death. The cause of preeclampsia is not known, but is thought to involve soluble factors secreted by the placenta.[4] Preeclampsia usually occurs during the second half of the pregnancy, and affects about 5% of pregnant women.

Diagnosis

Blood pressure is measured with a stethoscope and an inflatable arm cuff with a pressure-measuring gauge called a sphygmomanometer. A blood pressure reading, given in millimeters of mercury (mm Hg), has two numbers. The first, or upper, number measures the pressure in the arteries when the heart beats *(systolic pressure)*. The second, or lower, number measures the pressure in the arteries between beats when the chambers of the heart are filling with blood *(diastolic pressure)*.

In general, "lower is better" with respect to blood pressure. However, very low blood pressure *(hypotension)* can sometimes be a cause for concern. The latest blood pressure guidelines, issued in 2003 by the National Heart, Lung, and Blood Institute, divide measurements into four general categories: *normal* (<120/80 mm Hg), *pre-hypertension* (120-139 systolic and 80-89 diastolic), *stage 1 hypertension* (140-159 systolic and 90-99 diastolic), and *stage 2 hypertension* (160 or higher systolic and 100 or higher diastolic). To obtain accurate measurements, the readings should be evaluated based on the average of two or more blood pressure readings.

Blood pressure readings are usually taken when sitting or lying down and relaxed. Patients should be advised not to drink coffee or smoke cigarettes 30 minutes before having blood pressure taken, wear short sleeves, and go to the bathroom before the reading (because having a full bladder can affect blood pressure). Patients should also sit for 5 minutes before the test.

SELECTED HERBAL THERAPIES

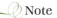

Note
To help make this educational resource more interactive, all pharmacokinetics, adverse effects, and interactions data have been compiled in Appendix A. Safety data specifically related to pregnancy and lactation are listed in Appendix B. Please refer to these appendices when working through the case studies and answering the review questions.

Black Currant (Ribes nigrum)

Grade C: *Unclear or conflicting scientific evidence (hypertension)*

Mechanism of Action

Black currant has been found to contain phenolic compounds, flavonoids (anthocyanins, proanthocyanidins), and the seeds contain the essential fatty acids gamma-linolenic acid (GLA) and alpha-linolenic acid (ALA).[5-8] The exact mechanism of black currant for lowering blood pressure is not well understood but may be attributed to GLA component and potential angiotensin II receptor inhibition.[9,10] GLA has been found to decrease central venous blood pressure in both normotensive and hypertensive animal studies.[11-14] This effect may be caused by angiotensin II receptor inhibition.[15]

Scientific Evidence of Effectiveness

The effects of black currant seed oil supplementation on resting blood pressure and cardiovascular reactivity to psychological stress in borderline hypertensive males has shown evidence that GLA-rich fatty acid preparations are likely to influence cardiovascular control, although the mechanism of action remains to be clarified.[16] In clinical study, subjects given black currant seed oil have shown improvement in blood pressure reactivity and diastolic and systolic blood pressure over those given placebo.[16] The sample size was relatively small (n = 27) and consisted only of males, so further studies are needed to determine if similar effects occur in the larger population and in females.

Adverse Effects, Interactions, Pharmacokinetics. See Appendix A.

Evening Primrose (Oenothera biennis)

Grade C: *Unclear or conflicting scientific evidence (preeclampsia [pregnancy-induced hypertension])*

Mechanism of Action

Evening primrose oil (EPO) contains the omega-6 essential fatty acid GLA, which is thought to be the active ingredient. Essential fatty acids are building blocks for a number of molecules in the body, including prostaglandins. GLA has been found to decrease central venous blood pressure in both normotensive and hypertensive animal studies.[11-14] This effect may be caused by angiotensin II receptor inhibition.[15,17]

Scientific Evidence of Effectiveness

Basic scientific research has suggested that prostaglandins play a role in the pathology of preeclampsia. Because of the proposed effect of EPO on prostaglandin metabolism, it has been theorized that EPO therapy may benefit or prevent this condition. Currently, there are limited trials of EPO for this application. Available studies have not been adequately powered or methodologically sound enough to support a recommendation for or against EPO for this indication.[18-21] Preliminary evidence suggests that the combination of EPO and fish oil may be equally as efficacious as magnesium oxide for preeclampsia,[21] but definitive evidence from adequately powered trials is lacking.

Dose

The dose of evening primrose oil for preeclampsia has not been determined.

Adverse Effects, Interactions, Pharmacokinetics. See Appendix A.

False Hellebore (Veratrum spp.)

Grade C: *Unclear or conflicting scientific evidence (hypertension, preeclampsia)*

Note: False hellebore (particularly the species *Veratrum viride*, or American hellebore) was studied during the late 1940s and early 1950s as a hypotensive agent in essential hypertension, hypertension during renal dysfunction, and eclamptic toxemia during pregnancy.[5,22-36] However, because of the cardiotoxic effects associated with the genus *Veratrum*, it is not considered safe for use.[37-49]

Mechanism of Action

In laboratory studies the isolated steroidal compounds from false hellebore significantly influenced arterial pressure responses; decreased mean aortic pressure; caused renal, femoral, and mesenteric vasodilation; and decreased the heart rate.[50-52] False hellebore alkaloids do not seem to affect cardiac output significantly, suggesting diminished arteriolar resistance.[23] The isolated constituent *O*-acetyljervine has been reported to have beta-agonist activity in laboratory studies.[53]

Several reports suggest that both oral use and parenteral use of the isolated alkaloids found in false hellebore cause a fall in mean arterial pressure without a reduction in cardiac output.[22,23] Early reports suggested that the alkaloids caused vasodilation, and it was later found that an isolated alkaloid also had beta-adrenergic blocking activity.[24,45] *Atropine* abolishes the bradycardia induced by the isolated alkaloids of American hellebore, but only partially reverses the hypotensive effects.[23] No postural hypotension was noted with the administration of the isolated alkaloids.[24,33]

Scientific Evidence of Effectiveness

Limited research has shown a small magnitude of benefit for hypertension. Patients who received intramuscular (IM) injections of false hellebore experienced a fall in mean arterial pressure and an increase in cardiac output.[23] Beneficial results have also been noted in pregnancy-induced hypertension (preeclampsia) and in patients with renal dysfunction.[33-35,54,55] However, other herbs and prescription drugs may treat these conditions more effectively with fewer toxic side effects.

Dose

Note: Doses are based on historical use and early clinical trials. *Veratrum* species should not be administered to humans because of the toxic effects associated with its use. Based on available research, only homeopathic preparations of false hellebore, which contain negligible amounts of the active and toxic constituents, are recommended for human use at this time.

False hellebore was used historically by preparing pharmaceutical dosage forms extracted from the root and rhizome, including tinctures, fluid extracts, and powders. In the late 1940s, research on false hellebore focused on the isolation and standardization of steroidal alkaloids. Well-known standardization values are lacking for false hellebore as a dietary supplement.

Homeopathic preparations of American hellebore are made by diluting the alcohol tincture of fresh root/rhizome with a distilled water/alcohol mixture, either 1:10 or 1:100, and then vigorously shaking the mixture, a process called *succussion.* The original mixture is serially diluted until the desired potency is obtained. When the process is repeated 30 times on a 1:10 dilution, it is said to be of 30X or 30D (10^{-30}) potency. When the process is repeated 30 times on a 1:100 dilution, it is said to be 30C (10^{-60}). Homeopathic treatment is usually individualized to correspond specifically to the patient's symptoms. The wide range of homeopathic potencies and treatment methodologies pose a challenge when applying standard testing and statistical procedures to the homeopathic medical model.

For hypertension, IM injection of 2.5 mg/mL Veratrone (0.2-1.0 mL) has been used.[23] For preeclampsia, 0.2 mL of Veratrone has been used.[33]

Adverse Effects, Interactions, Pharmacokinetics. See Appendix A.

Flax *(Linum usitatissimum)*

Grade C: *Unclear or conflicting scientific evidence (hypertension)*

Mechanism of Action

Flaxseed is composed of multiple chemical constituents, the mechanisms of which are slowly being elucidated. Studies have attributed different properties to the plant, seed, oil, and individual plant components. The plant, seed, and oil contain polyunsaturated fatty acids (PUFAs), including alpha-linolenic acid (ALA) and linoleic acid. They also contain monounsaturated fatty acids (MUFAs), such as oleic acid. ALA and linoleic acid are both essential fatty acids, meaning they cannot be synthesized by the human body and must be derived from the diet.[56-58] ALA is a precursor to eicosapentaenoic acid (EPA)[59-60] and docosahexaenoic acid (DHA). EPA and DHA have been associated with decreased risk of cardiovascular disease.[61] Preliminary evidence suggests that higher levels of linolenic acid in human adipose tissues may correlate with lower blood pressure.[62]

Scientific Evidence of Effectiveness

Flaxseed and its derivative flaxseed oil/linseed oil are rich sources of the essential fatty acid ALA, which is the parent compound to all omega-3 fatty acids, and may lower blood pressure. Flaxseed-supplemented diets have had mixed effects on blood pressure in animal studies.[62,63] Limited evidence suggests that 2 weeks of flaxseed supplementation of 60 mL lowers blood pressure.[64] At this time, however, insufficient data exist to recommend for or against this use of flaxseed.

Dose

Flaxseed products are not standardized based on specific chemical components, but rather are evaluated with a number of identity and quality tests. Tests may include microscopic and macroscopic inspection and organoleptic evaluation. Flaxseed is approximately 35% oil, of which 55% is ALA.[61,65-68] From 58% to 60% of flaxseed is omega-3 fatty acid, and 18% to 20% is omega-6 fatty acid. Flaxseed and linseed oil contain 30% to 45% unsaturated fatty acids, and approximately 8% of the plant contains soluble fiber mucilage.[69] The plant also contains 20% protein. Flaxseed oil is composed of 73% PUFAs, 18% MUFAs, and 9% saturated fatty acids.

Adverse Effects, Interactions, Pharmacokinetics. See Appendix A.

Garlic *(Allium sativum)*

Grade C: *Unclear or conflicting scientific evidence (hypertension)*

Mechanism of Action

Chemical analysis conducted in the 1800s attributed garlic's activity to the sulfur-containing garlic oil. In the mid-1900s the strong-smelling liquid was named "allicin."[70] The sulfur compound *alliin* (*S*-allyl-L-cysteine sulfoxide) produces allicin (diallyl thiosulfinate) through the enzyme *allinase* when the bulb is crushed or ground. However, allicin is not considered to be the major active constituent, as previously believed. Some or all of the sulfur-containing moieties, including allicin, are thought to exert some pharmacological effect. The magnitude of effect attributed to each constituent is not clear.

Vasorelaxant properties of garlic have been noted in multiple preclinical studies.[71-73] Cutaneous microperfusion is increased in humans after ingestion of 600 mg of garlic,[74-76] and vasodilation of conjunctival arterioles and venules occurs at 900 mg.[77] Garlic may act on the nitric oxide system[78-80] and exert effects on the elastic properties of vasculature,[81] yielding changes in systemic blood pressure.[82]

Scientific Evidence of Effectiveness

Numerous studies have reported small mean reductions in systolic and diastolic blood pressure associated with the use of oral garlic versus placebo. In general, mean differences have been less than 10 mm Hg (<10%). The majority of studies have been small (<100 subjects), with incomplete descriptions of methodology and results. Blood pressure measurements have often not been measured as primary outcomes, and in many cases, specific blood pressure numbers were not provided. Methods and timing of measurement have been variable.

A meta-analysis of eight trials reported a small, 7.7–mm Hg mean reduction of systolic blood pressure with a standardized dehydrated garlic formulation (Kwai), 600 to 900 mg daily.[81] However, another systematic review of 27 studies was not able to pool studies because of heterogeneity of results, although most studies reported small reductions in systolic blood pressure of variable significance.[83,84] Preliminary data suggest that dehydrated garlic products such as Kwai may be more efficacious than garlic oil.[85] Also, enteric-coated formulations may be more effective than non–enteric-coated products (e.g., Kwai) because they were designed to deliver garlic powder directly to the stomach. Overall, it appears that oral garlic may exert a small blood pressure–lowering effect, although the available evidence is weak. It is unclear whether effects might be more pronounced in individuals who are hypertensive versus normotensive.

Dose

The Lichtwer Pharma GmbH (Berlin) standardized powder product Kwai has often been used in studies utilizing fresh garlic and is standardized to 1.3% alliin content. Other trials have used a standardized preparation that contains 220 mg of garlic powder and produces 2.4 mg of allicin in vitro.[86] U.S. Pharmacopeia–grade garlic must contain 0.3% (powdered) to 0.5% (fresh, dried) allicin, whereas European pharmacopeia–grade garlic must yield no less than 0.45% allicin.

A dose of 600 to 900 mg daily of dehydrated garlic powder that is not enteric-coated in three divided doses has been used for hypertension in multiple clinical trials.

Adverse Effects, Interactions, Pharmacokinetics. See Appendix A.

Ginseng (*Panax* spp.)

Grade C: *Unclear or conflicting scientific evidence (hypertension)*

Mechanism of Action

The hypotensive effects of ginseng in humans[87,88] and animals[89] may be caused by a relaxing effect on smooth muscle induced by certain ginseng saponins known as ginsenosides (e.g., Rb1).[90-93] This might also explain the improvement in symptoms of coronary artery disease, including typical electrocardiographic (ECG) changes, such as repolarization disturbances.[94] Calcium could play a role in the cardiovascular effects of ginseng.[92,95] Ginsenosides Rb1 and Rg1 appear to have vasodilatory effects, possibly mediated by the proportion of nitric acid release,[93] where enhanced nitric oxide synthesis from the endothelium of the lung, heart, kidney, and corpus cavernosum promotes vasodilation.[96]

Scientific Evidence of Effectiveness

Preliminary research suggests that ginseng may lower both systolic and diastolic blood pressure.[87,97,98] One clinical trial with 140 subjects assessed the effects of two dosages of *Panax ginseng* on risk factors of cardiovascular disease.[96] For 3 weeks, subjects received 4.5 g of ginseng daily, 3 g of *P. ginseng* daily, or placebo. Results did not reveal any significant effects between the 3 g and 4.5 g of ginseng. Because of this outcome, results of the subjects receiving ginseng at either dose were combined in an analysis. A total of 103 subjects then received ginseng, with the remaining receiving a placebo. Blood pressure reductions by ginseng were noted. On average, systolic readings decreased by a mean of 7 points, and diastolic readings decreased by a mean of 10 points.

Dose

The dose of ginseng for hypertension has not been determined. One clinical trial used two dosages (3 g and 4.5 g) of ginseng for 2 weeks, but did not produce significant effects over placebo.[97]

Adverse Effects, Interactions, Pharmacokinetics. See Appendix A.

Hibiscus (*Hibiscus* spp.)

Grade B: *Good scientific evidence (hypertension)*

Mechanism of Action

The mechanisms underlying the hypotensive effects of hibiscus are not well understood. Hibiscus contains significant amounts of anthocyanins, which are flavonoid pigments with antioxidant effects. The vasorelaxant and hypotensive effects of hibiscus have been observed in isolated animal tissue.[99] Cardioprotective activities and inhibition of angiotensin I–converting enzyme have been demonstrated in animals.[100]

Scientific Evidence of Effectiveness

Hibiscus has been used for centuries by Ayurvedic and Chinese medical practitioners. There is clinical evidences that extracts of hibiscus may lower the systolic and diastolic pressure in patients with mild to moderate hypertension.[101,102] In other study, hibiscus standardized extract exhibited comparable hypotensive effects as captopril (Capoten), an inhibitor of angiotensin-converting enzyme (ACE).[101]

Dose

There is no well-known standardization for hibiscus. An herbal infusion (tea made by steeping herbs in hot water) prepared with 10 g of dried calyx (outer floral leaves) from *Hibiscus sabdariffa* combined with water (9.6 mg of anthocyanin content), daily before breakfast for 4 weeks, reduced blood pressure.[102]

Adverse Effects, Interactions, Pharmacokinetics. See Appendix A.

Onion (*Allium cepa*)

Grade C: *Unclear or conflicting scientific evidence (hypertension)*

Mechanism of Action

The exact mechanism by which onion reduces blood pressure is not well understood. Onion is rich in the antioxidant *quercetin*,[103-116] which has vasoprotectant effects that may account for onion's beneficial cardiovascular effects.

Scientific Evidence of Effectiveness

Onions are featured prominently in the Mediterranean diet, which has been shown to lower blood pressure.[117] A clinical trial found that onion–olive oil capsules significantly lowered systolic blood pressure both immediately and 1 week after administration.[118] Because of the use of a combination of onion and olive oil, the effects of onion alone cannot be determined. More research is needed in this area using onion as a monotherapy.

Dose

The dose of onion for hypertension has not been determined.

Adverse Effects, Interactions, Pharmacokinetics. See Appendix A.

Pycnogenol (*Pinus pinaster* subsp. *atlantica*)

Grade C: *Unclear or conflicting scientific evidence (hypertension)*

Note: Pycnogenol contains oligomeric proanthocyanidins (OPCs) as well as several other bioflavonoids. There has been some confusion in the U.S. market regarding OPC products containing Pycnogenol or grape seed extract (GSE), because one of the generic terms for chemical constituents ("pycnogenols") is the same as the patented trade name (Pycnogenol). Some GSE products were formerly erroneously labeled and marketed in the United States as containing "pycnogenols." Although GSE and Pycnogenol do contain similar chemical constituents (primarily in the OPC fraction), the chemical, pharmacological, and clinical literature on the two products is distinct. The term *Pycnogenol* should therefore be used only when referring to this specific proprietary pine bark extract. Scientific literature regarding this product should not be referenced as a basis for the safety or effectiveness of GSE.

Mechanism of Action

Pycnogenol is a proprietary mixture of water-soluble bioflavonoids extracted from the bark of French maritime pine (*Pinus pinaster* subsp. *atlantica*). The main constituents are phenolic compounds, generally divided into monomers (catechin, epicatechin, and taxifolin) and condensed flavonoids (procyanidins and proanthocyanidins).[119] Pycnogenol has been reported to have vasorelaxant activity.[120] It also has been shown to inhibit angiotensin-converting enzyme (ACE) activity in vivo and reduce systolic and diastolic blood pressure in rats.[121]

Scientific Evidence of Effectiveness

Pycnogenol reduced systolic blood pressure significantly, but the lowering of diastolic blood pressure did not reach statistical significance when compared to placebo in clinical study.[122] In another study, Pycnogenol improved endothelial function in hypertensive patients and reduced the need for nifedipine (Procardia), a calcium channel blocker, in a statistically significant manner.[123]

Dose

A daily dose of 100 to 200 mg of Pycnogenol resulted in a reduced need for nifedipine and decreased systolic blood pressure in mildly hypertensive patients.[122,123] Because of its astringent taste and potential to cause occasional minor stomach discomfort, Pycnogenol may be taken with or after meals.

Adverse Effects, Interactions, Pharmacokinetics. See Appendix A.

Reishi Mushroom (*Ganoderma lucidum*)

Grade C: *Unclear or conflicting scientific evidence (hypertension)*

Mechanism of Action

Terpenes (hydrocarbons) in reishi, such as ganoderic acids B, D, F, H, K, S, and Y and ganoderal A and B, have ACE inhibitory activity.[124,125] Mycelium isolated from reishi mushrooms has a hypotensive effect.[126] Reishi mushroom extract has decreased diastolic and systolic blood pressure, accompanied by an inhibition of renal efferent sympathetic nerve activity. The extract did not result in a decreased heart rate, although there was dose-dependent induced hypotension. Thus, the decrease in blood pressure from reishi might theoretically be attributed to the sympatholytic activity of reishi mycelium on the central nervous system.

Scientific Evidence of Effectiveness

Ancient Chinese monks purportedly used the reishi mushroom to calm their minds for meditation. Theoretically, the physiological effects of decreasing blood pressure may have led to the calming effect precipitated by the ingested reishi. A double-blind trial evaluated the effects of *lin zhi* (reishi) in patients with stage II hypertension.[127] The results yielded a change over a 4-week period, with the greatest drop in systolic and diastolic blood pressure becoming apparent after the first week. Improvements were also seen in capillary loop density, diameter, and red blood cell velocity.

Dose

Standardization of reishi extracts might not be clinically relevant in predicting effectiveness because the active ingredient in *Ganoderma lucidum* has not been fully determined. However, the dose of *G. lucidum* is often based on its content of polysaccharide peptides and triterpenes. These doses can be extracted from spores or the whole–fruiting body preparation; it is uncertain which is more beneficial in hypertension. Oral doses of 150 to 300 mg three or four times daily have been standardized to contain 10% to 12.5% polysaccharides and 4% triterpenes per dose. The New Zealand product Ganopoly, used in some clinical trials, contains 600 mg extract of *G. lucidum* per capsule, with 25% (w/w) crude polysaccharides, which is equivalent to 30 g fruiting body of *G. lucidum*.[128]

Extract of reishi (lin zhi) has been used clinically for hypertension at 55 mg daily for 4 weeks.[127]

Adverse Effects, Interactions, Pharmacokinetics. See Appendix A.

Rhubarb (*Rheum* spp.)

Grade C: *Unclear or conflicting scientific evidence (preeclampsia)*

Mechanism of Action

The procyanidins B-5 3,3′di-O-gallate and C-13,3′3″-tri-O-gallate isolated from rhubarb have been shown to inhibit ACE activity in vitro.[129] These tannins did not inhibit the activities of other proteases, such as trypsin, chymotrypsin, leucine, aminopeptidase, carboxypeptidase A, and urinary kallikrein.

Scientific Evidence of Effectiveness

Preliminary evidence suggests that rhubarb may be beneficial in the treatment of preeclampsia.[130,131] Rhubarb has been administered (0.75 g by mouth daily for 9-10 weeks) from the 28th week of gestation until delivery and significantly lowered the rate of pregnancy-induced hypertension.

Dose

The exact dose of rhubarb for decreasing blood pressure has not been determined; however, rhubarb (0.75 g by mouth daily for 9-10 weeks) significantly lowered blood pressure induced by pregnancy.[130,131]

Adverse Effects, Interactions, Pharmacokinetics. See Appendix A.

Safflower (*Carthamus tinctorius*)

Grade C: *Unclear or conflicting scientific evidence (hypertension)*

Mechanism of Action

The mechanism by which safflower reduces blood pressure is not well understood. However, according to laboratory studies, safflower oil may be involved in synthesis of prostaglandins, which are responsible for vascular regulation and inflammatory responses and may affect hypertension.[132-135]

Scientific Evidence of Effectiveness

Clinical trials evaluating safflower oil for hypertension have yielded mixed results. Studies have not reported significant effects on blood pressure.[136-139] However, an increased plasma renin activity in normotensive first-degree relatives of hypertensive patients has been noted.[139]

Dose

The dose of safflower oil for hypertension has not been determined.

Adverse Effects, Interactions, Pharmacokinetics. See Appendix A.

Sea Buckthorn (*Hippophae rhamnoides*)

Grade C: *Unclear or conflicting scientific evidence (hypertension)*

Mechanism of Action

The mechanism by which sea buckthorn reduces blood pressure is not well understood. It has been shown to block the angiotensin signal pathway.[140,141]

Scientific Evidence of Effectiveness

Sea buckthorn may be a promising herbal agent for hypertension. It has been shown to reduce elevated blood pressure in animal[141] and human studies. Patients receiving sea buckthorn did not experience an increase in heart rate or blood pressure after exercise. More research is needed before a recommendation can be made.

Dose

The dose of sea buckthorn for hypertension has not been determined.

Adverse Effects, Interactions, Pharmacokinetics. See Appendix A.

Soy (*Glycine max*)

Grade C: *Unclear or conflicting scientific evidence (hypertension)*

Mechanism of Action

The mechanism by which soy reduces blood pressure is not clear. Decreases in blood pressure were shown to be related to urinary genistein excretion but not daidzein (soy isoflavones).[142]

Scientific Evidence of Effectiveness

Consuming soy products, including soy nuts and soy milk, is believed to help prevent and treat high blood pressure. Patients with mild to moderate essential hypertension who consumed soy milk (500 mL twice daily for 3 months) experienced a reduction in blood pressure.[142] Research is ongoing to better understand soy's effects on blood pressure.

Adverse Effects, Interactions, Pharmacokinetics. See Appendix A.

Stevia (Stevia rebaudiana)

Grade B: *Good scientific evidence (hypertension)*

Mechanism of Action

Stevioside is a constituent of stevia that has exhibited antihypertensive effects in animal studies.[143-148] Stevioside may promote vascular relaxation by inhibiting calcium influx into blood vessels.[145-146]

Scientific Evidence of Effectiveness

Randomized controlled studies (RCTs) have investigated stevia administration for up to 2 years with significant, lasting decreases in blood pressure in hypertensive patients.[143,147] Other studies, evaluating stevia in divided doses, found no significant changes in blood pressure compared with placebo. Nonetheless, stevia appears to have some benefit, and more research is warranted to compare its effectiveness with the current standard of care or to determine if it is beneficial as an adjunct therapy.

Dose

Stevia at oral doses of 250 to 500 mg three times daily for up to 2 years decreased blood pressure in hypertensive patients.[142-146]

Adverse Effects, Interactions, Pharmacokinetics. See Appendix A.

HERBAL THERAPIES WITH LIMITED EVIDENCE

Coleus (Coleus forskohlii)

Forskolin is the major active constituent of coleus. *Coleonol*, a distereoisomer of forskolin, has been shown to lower blood pressure in animal studies.[149,150] Forskolin lowered blood pressure in the absence of adrenergic blockade, suggesting that it relaxes vascular smooth muscle.[150]

Hawthorn (Crataegus spp.)

Hawthorn is used to treat various cardiovascular problems, including heart failure. Animal studies have demonstrated hawthorn's hypotensive effects,[151-153] but human studies are lacking.

Indian Snakeroot (Rauwolfia serpentina)

Of the many species commonly known as Indian snakeroot, *Rauwolfia serpentina* is primarily used in herbal medicine. One of the alkaloids isolated from this plant's root is *reserpine*, a prescription drug used to control hypertension.

Mistletoe (Viscum album)

Mistletoe has been used in folk medicine as a blood pressure regulator. At low doses, mistletoe is said to reduce blood pressure, but at high doses it may raise blood pressure. Human and animal studies are lacking to support these claims.

Olive (Olea europaea)

Olive leaves come from the olive tree *(Olea europaea)*, a native of the Mediterranean. Although olives and olive oil are used as foods, olive leaf is primarily used medicinally or as a tea. It has been found to reduce diastolic blood pressure in rats.[154] However, supportive clinical evidence is lacking.

ADJUNCT THERAPIES

1. Improving the *diet* with low-fat and low-sodium foods and adding certain supplements may also play a role in reducing high blood pressure. Omega-3 fatty acids are essential fatty acids found in some plants and fish. Experts recommend a balance of omega-6 and omega-3 fatty acids for health. Multiple human trials report small reductions in blood pressure with intake of omega-3 fatty acids. DHA

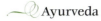 Ayurveda

> Ayurveda means "science of life" and stems from the ancient body of spiritual teachings known as the Vedas. Some medical historians believe Ayurveda was also the original basis for Chinese medicine. Ayurveda is an integrated system of specific theories and techniques employing diet, herbs, exercise, meditation, yoga, and massage or bodywork. The goal of Ayurveda is to achieve optimal health on all levels: physical, psychological, and spiritual.
>
> In India, Ayurveda involves the eight principal branches of medicine: pediatrics, gynecology, obstetrics, ophthalmology, geriatrics, otolaryngology (ear, nose, and throat), general medicine, and surgery. It is used by 80% of the Indian population today, although it exists side by side with conventional medicine. There are more than a quarter-million practitioners of Ayurveda in India, and entire hospitals are based on this approach to medicine.
>
> Ayurveda made its way to the West mainly through Europe, where it still has a strong presence. However, in modern times and particularly in Western countries, the practice of Ayurveda is less focused on its spiritual roots than on its use as a form of complementary or alternative medicine.
>
> *Abana* is a combination herbal and mineral formulation that has been traditionally used in Ayurveda for cardiovascular health. Abana contains various medicinal plants, including arjuna *(Terminalia arjuna)*, ashwagandha *(Withania somnifera)*, guduchi *(Tinospora cordifolia)*, Indian gooseberry *(Emblica officinalis)*, hundred husbands *(Asparagus racemosus)*, gotu kola *(Centella asiatica)*, muskroot *(Nardostachys jatamansi)*, saffron *(Crocus sativus)*, myrobalan *(Terminalia chebula)*, and licorice *(Glycyrrhiza glabra)*. Preliminary evidence suggests that abana may reduce blood pressure.[1] Further research is needed to confirm these results.

(docosahexaenoic acid) may have greater benefits than EPA (eicosapentaenoic acid). However, daily high intake of omega-3 fatty acids may be necessary to obtain clinically relevant effects, and risk of bleeding is increased at this dose level.

2. Several studies have found that introducing *calcium* to the system can have hypotensive effects. These studies indicate that high calcium levels lead to sodium loss in the urine and decreased parathyroid hormone (PTH) levels, both of which reduce blood pressure. In another study, however, these results did not hold true for middle-aged patients with mild to moderate essential hypertension. In the Dietary Approaches to Stop Hypertension (DASH) study, three servings daily of calcium-enriched low-fat dairy products reduced systolic and diastolic blood pressure, indicating that a calcium intake at the recommended level may be helpful in preventing and treating moderate hypertension. Treatment of high blood pressure should only be done under supervision of a qualified health care professional.

3. *Coenzyme Q10* (CoQ10) is produced by the human body and is necessary for basic cellular function. Preliminary research suggests that CoQ10 causes small decreases in blood pressure (systolic and possibly diastolic). Low blood levels of CoQ10 have been found in people with hypertension, although it is not clear if CoQ10 "deficiency" is a cause of high blood pressure.

4. *Rutin* is an antioxidant that naturally occurs in various plants (e.g., apple peels, black tea, rue, tobacco, buckwheat). Quercetin (a flavonoid found in rutin) and rutin are used as vasoprotectants and are ingredients in numerous multivitamin preparations and herbal remedies. The flavonoids found in rutin have documented effects on capillary permeability (leakage) and edema (swelling) and have been used for the treatment of disorders of the venous and microcirculatory (capillary) systems. Overall, the results of clinical studies suggest a benefit of rutin for venous hypertension.

5. Regular physical activity can help lower blood pressure and keep weight under control. Individuals should strive for at

Herbs with Possible Hypotensive Properties*†

HERB		HERB	
Abuta	Cinnamon	Horny goat weed	Rhodiola
Aconite	Clove	Horseradish	Rooibos
Alpinia	Codonopsis	Hyssop	Rosemary
Annatto	Coltsfoot	Kudzu	Saw palmetto
Aristolochia spp.	Comfrey	Ladies mantle	Scotch broom
Asafoetida	Cordyceps	Lavender	Shepherd's purse
Asarum	Cramp bark	Lemon balm	Shiitake
Astragalus	Dandelion	Lemongrass	Spirulina
Bamboo	Danshen	Lotus	Stinging nettle
Barberry	Deer velvet	Maitake mushroom	Traditional Chinese Medicine
Berberine	Dong quai	Morus nigra	
Betony	Elecampane	Mugwort	Tribulus
Bilberry	Fenugreek	Myrcia	Turmeric
Black cohosh	Fo-ti	Neem	Uva ursi
Bloodroot	Germanium	Noni	Valerian
Boldo	Ginger	Nopal	Verbena
Bromelain	Ginkgo	Organic food	Wheatgrass
Buchu	Goji	Passion flower	White horehound
Cajeput oil	Goldenrod	Perilla	Yarrow
Cat's claw	Goldenseal	Psyllium	Yerba santa
Chia	Gotu kola	Red yeast rice	
Chrysanthemum	Gymnema	Rehmannia	

*This is not an all-inclusive or comprehensive list of herbs with hypotensive properties; other herbs and supplements may possess these qualities. A qualified health care provider should be consulted with specific questions or concerns regarding potential hypotensive effects or interactions of agents.
†Based on expert opinion, anecdote, case reports, and/or preliminary trial evidence.

Herbs and Supplements with Possible Hypertensive Properties*†

HERB	
Andrographis paniculata Nees, Kan Jang, SHA-10	Lavender
Bloodroot	Rehmannia
Cramp bark	Scotch broom
Ginger	Shepherd's purse
Grape seed	Yohimbe

*This is not an all-inclusive or comprehensive list of herbs with hypertensive properties; other herbs and supplements may possess these qualities. A qualified health care provider should be consulted with specific questions or concerns regarding potential hypertensive effects or interactions of agents.
†Based on anecdotal or historical reports, preclinical data, or human studies.

least 30 to 45 minutes three to five times per week. *Yoga* is an ancient system of relaxation, exercise, and healing with 2000-year-old origins in Indian philosophy. Several human studies support the use of yoga in the treatment of high blood pressure, when practiced for up to 1 year. It is not clear if yoga is better than other forms of exercise for blood pressure control; better research is needed in this area. Yoga practitioners sometimes recommend that patients with high blood pressure avoid certain positions, such as headstands or shoulder stands, which may increase blood pressure.

INTEGRATIVE THERAPY PLAN

- Ask the patient about lifestyle habits such as smoking, alcohol consumption, exercise routine, dietary intake, and family history of hypertension.
- Carefully and accurately perform blood pressure measurements with the patient seated and with the arm positioned level to the heart. Before blood pressure is taken, the patient should sit quietly for 5 minutes.
- Document the patient's height and weight.
- There is good evidence regarding the hypotensive effect of stevia. At oral doses of 250 to 500 mg three times daily for up to 2 years, stevia decreased blood pressure in hypertensive patients.
- Hibiscus has been shown to work as well as the ACE inhibitor captopril. Hibiscus may be taken as a tea daily before breakfast. It should be avoided in patients allergic to hibiscus and in women attempting to conceive.
- Garlic may exert a weak antihypertensive effect, but it should not be used with anticoagulants or antiplatelets because of multiple accounts of associated bleeding.
- Pycnogenol (100-200 mg daily) resulted in a reduced need for the calcium channel blocker nifedipine. Pycnogenol may also be beneficial in patients with elevated systolic blood pressure.
- Antihypertensive herbs and supplements may be beneficial as adjuncts to conventional drug therapy but should be done with caution and regular blood pressure monitoring.
- Monitor for complications or signs of progressive disease complications as well as adverse effects or potential interactions with natural products.
- Encourage patients to follow a low-fat, low-cholesterol, and low-sodium diet. Patients should restrict sodium intake to 2.3 g of sodium or 6 g of sodium chloride daily to assist with reducing blood pressure. Advise patients to avoid canned soups and frozen dinners, which are high in sodium.
- Urge the patient to follow a regular exercise regimen to assist in reducing blood pressure. Exercising 30 to 45 minutes three to five times per week is recommended.
- Educate patients regarding the signs of low blood pressure, including lightheadedness, dizziness, and fainting.

Case Studies

CASE STUDY 11-1

JR is a 55-year-old man who has a 5-year history of refractory hypertension. He asks if there is anything else he can do about his blood pressure; he currently takes nifedipine, captopril, and doxazosin, but his blood pressure is regularly in the 150s/90s. He also takes saw palmetto for benign prostatic hypertrophy (BPH). He comes into your pharmacy and inquires about stevia. How should you counsel?

Answer: Stevia appears to have some benefit for the treatment of hypertension. However, stevia may act as a calcium channel blocker and interfere with nifedipine. If JR decides to try stevia, you should suggest to JR's physician to alter his current regimen. Because calcium channel blockers and diuretics may interact with stevia, a beta blocker such as atenolol may be used for additional blood pressure control. Saw palmetto also has hypotensive effects, but even with this product, his hypertension is not controlled.

Stevia, 250 to 500 mg orally three times daily, has been used in clinical trials. Although generally well tolerated, stevia occasionally has been reported to cause nausea, abdominal fullness, myalgia, muscle weakness, and dizziness. JR should be monitored carefully on initiation of therapy because the degree of blood pressure reduction is difficult to predict. Signs of hypotension include dizziness, especially when standing from a crouched or sitting position or rising from bed, and tachycardia. He should also understand that there is no promise of any additional hypotensive effects.

JR should also be counseled regarding exercise and a low-fat, low-sodium diet. He may also want to consider adding supplements such as omega-3 fatty acids or coenzyme Q10 to assist with blood pressure control.

CASE STUDY 11-2

FL is a heavyset 49-year-old man with a 6-month history of type 2 diabetes. He is currently taking metformin and gymnema for blood sugar control. He also takes cat's claw for arthritis. At his last doctor's visit, FL had a slight increase in blood pressure, slightly above target range, for patients with diabetes. A neighbor who practices traditional Chinese medicine suggested that FL try lin zhi extract to help keep his hypertension under control. How should you counsel?

Answer: Lin zhi extract, or *reishi*, has antihypertensive properties and may help FL with controlling his blood pressure. However, reishi may complicate his diabetes regimen by causing additive hypoglycemic effects. If FL decides to try reishi, he should monitor his blood sugar levels closely and be aware of the signs and symptoms of hypoglycemia, including tremors, sweating, and increased heart rate. Although generally well tolerated, reishi occasionally may cause skin rash, dizziness, and headache. A clinical trial reported using 55 mg of reishi daily for 4 weeks to reduce hypertension. *Cat's claw* contains the compound rhynchophylline, which may cause hypotension and may cause additive effects when used with reishi.

Advise FL to be aware of the signs of hypotension, including lightheadedness, dizziness, and fainting. FL should also be counseled on regular physical activity of at least 30 minutes a day. Yoga may also be an option for exercise and potential blood pressure control. He should also be counseled on a low-fat, low-sodium diet.

CASE STUDY 11-3

PM is a 55-year-old woman who comes to the pharmacy requesting information on natural products for high blood pressure. On questioning, PM states that she has been self-testing her blood pressure on her mother's machine and has seen her blood pressure increase in the last month. You have her test it in the pharmacy and her BP is found to be 130/82 mm Hg. When asked if she takes any other drugs, herbs, or supplements, she mentions that she is using a soy product for menopausal symptoms. Other than that, PM states that she is in good health. How should you advise?

Answer: Based on current guidelines, PM may have "prehypertension." Studies suggest that *hibiscus* may help patients with mild to moderate hypertension and may be a reasonable option for PM. Hibiscus may be taken as a tea daily before breakfast, and it may take a few weeks before an effect is seen. Hibiscus is generally well tolerated. *Soy* is a phytoestrogen, and hibiscus may also have estrogenic activity. The clinical significance is unclear; therefore, if PM decides to start hibiscus, she should monitor for any unusual additive estrogenic effects, such as weight gain, water retention, breast tenderness, and fatigue. PM should continue to have her blood pressure monitored regularly. Signs of hypotension include dizziness, especially when standing from a crouched or sitting position or rising from bed, and tachycardia. She should also understand that there is no promise of hypotensive effects with hibiscus.

References for Chapter 11 can be found on the Evolve website at http://evolve.elsevier.com/Ulbricht/herbalpharmacotherapy/

Review Questions

1. Hibiscus was reported to lower blood pressure equally as well as:
   a. Candesartan
   b. Captopril
   c. Propranolol
   d. Verapamil

2. Which of the following statements is true about hibiscus?
   a. Has exhibited antifertility activity
   b. Is commonly used in wound healing
   c. Is used internally as a laxative
   d. May be nephrotoxic

3. Hibiscus may interact with which of the following?
   a. Propranolol
   b. Acetaminophen
   c. Chloroquine
   d. All of the above

4. True or false: Pycnogenol may decrease diastolic blood pressure in patients with high blood pressure.

5. Which of the following is true of Pycnogenol?
   a. Pycnogenol may lower glucose levels and should be used cautiously with hypoglycemic agents
   b. Pycnogenol should be used cautiously in conjunction with anticoagulants because of its potential to decrease coagulation.
   c. Grape seed extract and Pycnogenol are synonymous
   d. a and b

6. True or false: Stevia should not be recommended for short-term use because of the risk of adverse effects.

7. What dose of garlic has been used in clinical trials for hypertension?
   a. 600 to 900 mg daily in three divided doses
   b. 6 to 9 mg four times daily
   c. 60 to 90 mg twice daily
   d. 600 to 900 mg three times daily

8. Rhubarb contains what poisonous chemical?
   a. Formic acid
   b. Dimethyl sulfate
   c. Oxalic acid
   d. Sulfuric acid

9. Which of the following is true of reishi mushroom?
   a. Ancient Chinese monks utilized reishi to calm their minds for meditation.
   b. Reishi has been shown to have angiotensin converting enzyme (ACE) inhibitory activity
   c. The active ingredients in *Ganoderma lucidum* have been fully determined and standardized
   d. a and b

10. All the following statements about Pycnogenol are true *except*:
    a. Pycnogenol has vasorelaxant properties.
    b. Pycnogenol may exert its effects on blood pressure through the renin-angiotenisin system.
    c. Pycnogenol (100-200 mg daily) resulted in reduced need for nifedipine.
    d. It is recommended to avoid taking Pycnogenol with meals.

Answers are found in the Answers to Review Questions section in the back of the text.

12 Congestive Heart Failure and Diuresis

Outline

OVERVIEW
  Signs and Symptoms
  Diagnosis
SELECTED HERBAL THERAPIES
  Aconite *(Aconitum napellus)*
  Ashwagandha *(Withania somnifera)*
  Astragalus *(Astragalus membranaceus)*
  Coleus *(Coleus forskohlii)*
  Dandelion *(Taraxacum officinale)*
  Ginseng *(Panax* spp.)
  Goldenseal *(Hydrastis canadensis)*
  Hawthorn *(Crataegus* spp.)
  Horsetail *(Equisetum* spp.)
  Oleander *(Nerium oleander, Thevetia peruviana)*
  Passion Flower *(Passiflora incarnata)*
  Rutin ($C_{27}H_{30}O_{16}$)
HERBAL THERAPIES WITH LIMITED EVIDENCE
ADJUNCT THERAPIES
INTEGRATIVE THERAPY PLAN
CASE STUDIES
REVIEW QUESTIONS

Learning Objectives

- List the herbs used for congestive heart failure.
- Know the side effects associated with herbs used for congestive heart failure.
- List potential drug interactions with herbs used for congestive heart failure.
- Counsel patients on herbs used for congestive heart failure, and be able to recommend an integrative care plan.

OVERVIEW

Congestive heart failure (CHF) is a condition in which the heart cannot adequately pump blood throughout the body, or cannot prevent blood from accumulating in the lungs (Figure 12-1). CHF may be caused by weak cardiac muscle, which in turn may be caused by myocardial infarction (MI, heart attack). Coronary artery disease can lead to ischemic cardiomyopathy, a common cause of CHF. Other problems, such as defects in the heart structure or increased blood pressure and volume, may also lead to heart failure.

According to the American Heart Association (AHA), almost 5 million individuals experience CHF, and about 550,000 new cases are diagnosed each year in the United States. Heart failure becomes more prevalent with age, and the number of cases is expected to grow as the overall age of the general population and the baby-boomer generation increases. The condition affects 1% of people age 50 years or older and about 5% of those age 75 years or older. African Americans experience CHF twice as often as Caucasians. Approximately 10% of patients diagnosed with CHF die within 1 year, and about 50% die within 5 years of diagnosis.[1-3]

The goal of therapy for patients with CHF is to increase the output of the heart. This can be done by decreasing fluid volume using diuretics, decreasing blood pressure using antihypertensives, or increasing the strength of the heart muscle contraction using inotropic agents (Figure 12-2). Several types of medications have proved useful in the treatment of CHF, including angiotensin-converting enzyme (ACE) inhibitors, angiotensin receptor blockers (ARBs), beta-adrenergic blockers, digoxin, diuretics, and aldosterone antagonists. To maintain a normal blood pressure, there must be a balance between the amount of resistance in blood vessels and the output of the heart. The kidneys and sympathetic nervous system are thought to play a major role in this balance.

As with other muscle contractions throughout the body, the dilation and contraction of blood vessels depend on the electrolytes sodium, potassium, and calcium; the neurotransmitters epinephrine and norepinephrine also play a role. An increase or decrease in blood pressure can result not only

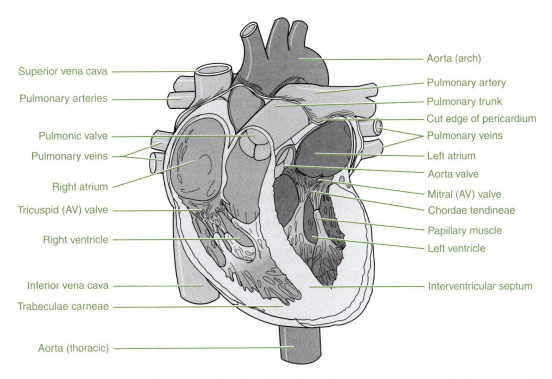

Figure 12-1 Heart (internal view). (Modified from Fehrenbach MJ, editor: *Dental anatomy coloring book*, St Louis, 2008, Saunders-Elsevier.)

from direct stimulation of blood vessels, but also from fluid volume. Volume depletion by diuretics stimulating the elimination of sodium in the kidneys has been shown to decrease blood pressure. The kidneys can also lower blood pressure through the renin-angiotensin system. The kidneys excrete renin in response to decreases in sodium or signals from the sympathetic nervous system. The renin then helps to create the angiotensin component, a strong blood vessel constrictor. Blocking the renin-angiotensin system may result in decreasing the kidneys' ability to increase blood pressure.[1]

Signs and Symptoms

Congestive heart failure is a chronic condition and generally occurs slowly. Blood backup (congestion) may occur in the liver, abdomen, lower extremities, and lungs. The backed-up blood causes symptoms such as shortness of breath, fatigue, and leg swelling. Other symptoms develop as the body tries to compensate for the heart's reduced ability to pump blood, causing the heart to beat faster, which results in thickening of the heart wall muscle and stretching of the ventricles to accommodate more blood. Damage to the ventricles may cause them to pump "out of sync," further reducing the efficient delivery of blood to the body.

Symptoms of CHF include the following:

- A dry, hacking cough, shortness of breath, and lung congestion as the blood backs up in the lungs; wheezing and spasms of the airways similar to asthma[1,2]
- Confusion, sleepiness, and disorientation; dizziness, fainting, fatigue, or weakness
- Fluid buildup, especially in the legs, ankles, and feet
- Increased urination at night
- Nausea; abdominal swelling, tenderness, or pain (from fluid buildup in body and blood backup in liver)
- Weight gain (from fluid buildup)
- Weight loss (as nausea decreases appetite and body fails to absorb food well)
- Rapid breathing, restlessness, and anxiety

Diagnosis

To determine the best course of therapy, physicians often assess the stage of heart failure according to the New York Heart Association (NYHA) functional classification system (Table 12-1).[3] This system relates symptoms to daily activities and quality of life.

SELECTED HERBAL THERAPIES

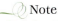 Note

To help make this educational resource more interactive, all pharmacokinetics, adverse effects, and interactions data have been compiled in Appendix A. Safety data specifically related to pregnancy and lactation are listed in Appendix B. Please refer to these appendices when working through the case studies and answering the review questions.

The use of diuretics is vital and regarded as first-line treatment in patients with CHF. Diuretics are often used to relieve congestive symptoms in the heart and control fluid

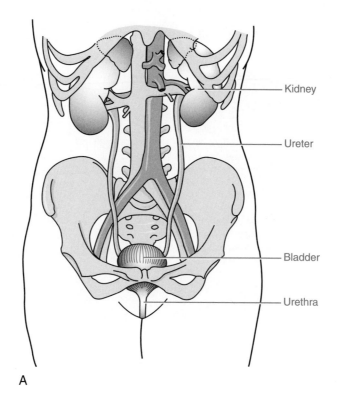
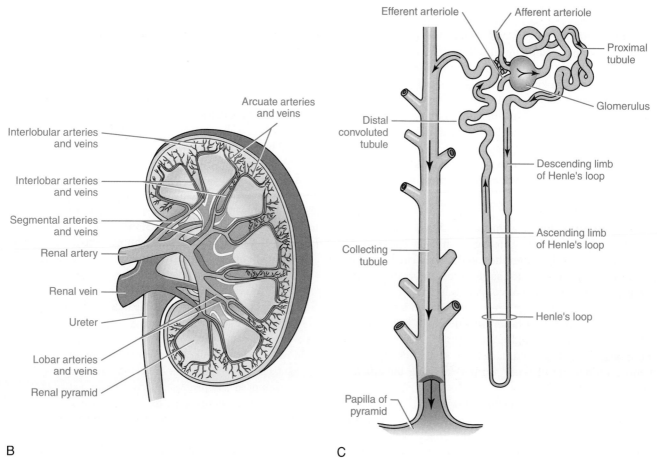

Figure 12-2 **A,** Urinary system (frontal view). **B,** Section through a kidney demonstrating blood flow and urine output. **C,** Structures of a nephron. (*A* modified from Fehrenbach MJ, editor: *Dental anatomy coloring book,* St Louis, 2008, Saunders-Elsevier; *B* modified from Thibodeau GA, Patton KT: *Anatomy & physiology,* ed 5, St Louis, 2003, Mosby; *C* modified from Brundage DJ: *Renal disorders,* St Louis, 1992, Mosby.)

TABLE 12-1 Stages of Heart Failure (NYHA Classification)

CLASS	PATIENT SYMPTOMS
I (mild)	No limitation of physical activity. Ordinary physical activity does not cause undue fatigue, palpitation, or dyspnea (shortness of breath).
II (mild)	Slight limitation of physical activity. Comfortable at rest, but ordinary physical activity results in fatigue, palpitation, or dyspnea.
III (moderate)	Marked limitation of physical activity. Comfortable at rest, but less than ordinary activity causes fatigue, palpitation, or dyspnea.
IV (severe)	Unable to carry out any physical activity without discomfort. Symptoms of cardiac insufficiency at rest. If any physical activity is undertaken, discomfort is increased.

From Heart Failure Society of America http://www.abouthf.org.

retention. Some of the following herbs have not been studied specifically for CHF but have been found to promote water excretion.[4]

Aconite (Aconitum napellus)

Grade C: *Unclear or conflicting scientific evidence (heart failure)*

Note: The toxic effects associated with the administration of aconite, including renocardiovascular disease and left ventricular dysfunction, limit its ability to be used clinically as an agent to treat heart failure. Aconite has been repeatedly associated with adverse cardiovascular events.[5-19] For this reason, use of aconite is not recommended.

Mechanism of Action

There are approximately 350 species of aconite. Generally, the alkaloids aconitine, hypaconitine, mesaconitine, and jesaconitine have the strongest pharmacological and toxic effects, whereas their derivatives are weaker and less toxic. Aconite has been shown to have positive inotropic, positive chronotropic, vasodilatory, and diuretic effects,[20] which may involve the anterior hypothalamus and surrounding muscarinic receptors.[21]

Scientific Evidence of Effectiveness

A double-blind, placebo-controlled study was conducted in 35 patients with left ventricular failure to evaluate the effects of aconite tuber.[20] Patients received all previous medications prescribed and aconite (aconiti tuber), 250 mg four times daily for 7 months. In the eighth month, patients received identical-looking placebo capsules, then were switched back to aconite for the ninth month. According to the NYHA classification, the percentage of left ventricular shortening and the cardiac output were significantly increased during the 7 months of aconite treatment ($p < 0.05$). During the placebo month, all parameters, except for left atrium empty index, were significantly deteriorated, but again improved during the ninth month, at which time the patients were given aconite in place of placebo. All parameters pertaining to renal function were significantly improved after 6 months of aconite treatment, including creatinine clearance, potassium clearance, sodium clearance, and chloride clearance. Aconite showed positive inotropic, positive chronotropic, vasodilatory, and diuretic effects. However, despite positive findings, aconite is highly toxic and has been implicated in numerous cases of poisoning.[1] Therefore, aconite use is not recommended in clinical practice.

Dose

The dose of aconite for heart failure has not been clearly established. In clinical study, patients with left ventricular failure received aconite (aconiti tuber), 250 mg four times daily for 7 months as adjunct therapy.[20] The toxic effects associated with the administration of aconite may limit its potential as an agent to treat heart failure.

Adverse Effects, Interactions, Pharmacokinetics. See Appendix A.

Ashwagandha (Withania somnifera)

Grade C: *Unclear or conflicting scientific evidence (diuresis)*

Mechanism of Action

Ashwagandha has purported diuretic effects, although its mechanism of action is not well understood.

Scientific Evidence of Effectiveness

Ashwagandha has been used as a diuretic agent in folk medicine in the Canary Islands and has been shown to increase the rate of water excretion in animal study; it exhibited diuretic effects in mice, some of which were comparable to that of hydrochlorothiazide, a prescription diuretic.[22] In a case series, 12 patients were administered powdered roots of ashwagandha, and significant increases in urine volume and urine sodium levels compared to baseline were reported.[23]

Dose

The dose of ashwagandha for CHF has not been determined. However, diuretic effects were observed in patients taking powdered roots for 30 days by mouth.[23]

Adverse Effects, Interactions, Pharmacokinetics. See Appendix A.

Astragalus (Astragalus membranaceus)

Grade C: *Unclear or conflicting scientific evidence (heart failure)*

Mechanism of Action

Experimental studies indicate that astragalosides affect cardiovascular function at the cellular, isolated tissue, and whole-body levels in both animals and humans. In isolated working rat hearts, *Astragalus* extract produced positive inotropic actions at higher doses and negative inotropic effects at low doses.[24] Astragalus also produced hypotensive actions through peripheral vasodilation in healthy and hypertensive animals.[25,26] Astragalus significantly reduced arterial pressure in the rat model of renal hypertension and improved cardiac function in experimental CHF.[27] This effect was confirmed by a report that astragalus improved left ventricular systolic function and potentiated the cardiotonic, diuretic, and natriuretic renal responses to atrial natriuretic peptide in rats with experimentally induced chronic heart failure.[28] There is in vitro evidence that astragalus may also stimulate angiogenesis and revascularization in ischemic myocardium[29] and amnion, and promote vascular endothelial cell proliferation and DNA synthesis.[30] Astragalus has been suggested to increase sodium pump activity in erythrocytes.[31]

Scientific Evidence of Effectiveness

A clinical trial was conducted in CHF patients with NYHA Class II to IV.[32] Clinical heart function, total effective rate, left ventricular ejection fraction (LVEF), fractional shortening of left ventricular short axis (FS), ratio of maximum blood flow between advanced and early atrial systole (E/A), stroke volume (SV), cardiac output (CO), and cardiac index (CI) all improved in astragalus-treated patients. Other human studies report similar positive findings associated with symptomatic improvement with astragalus use in patients with CHF.[29,33-38]

Dose

For heart failure, an intravenous (IV) drip of 30 to 40 mL of astragalus (equivalent to 60-80 g crude drug) in 500 mL of 5% glucose solution has been used once daily for 14 to 20 days.[32,34] The oral dose of astragalus for CHF has not been established.

Adverse Effects, Interactions, Pharmacokinetics. See Appendix A.

Coleus (Coleus forskohlii)

Grade B: *Good scientific evidence (cardiomyopathy)*

Mechanism of Action

Coleus species have been used in Asian traditional medicine for several indications. Since the 1970s, research has predominantly concentrated on forskolin, a root extract of *Coleus forskohlii*. Forskolin stimulates the cellular production of cyclic adenosine monophosphate (cAMP), and most research tested this effect on cAMP as a starting point for an in-depth study of the pharmacological profile of forskolin. The antithrombotic[39,40] and inotropic[41] actions of forskolin may explain its beneficial effects in cardiomyopathy, a common cause of CHF.

Although most studies have used isolated forskolin extract, it is believed that the whole coleus plant may also be effective, due to the presence of multiple compounds that may act synergistically. Other important constituents of coleus are caffeic acid and its derivatives, such as rosmarinic acid, because these compounds have been shown to have antioxidant effects.[42]

Scientific Evidence of Effectiveness

A small number of studies suggest that forskolin may improve cardiovascular function in patients with cardiomyopathy.[43-45] Given intravenously, forskolin was an effective vasodilator[43] and showed positive hemodynamic effects in patients with dilated cardiomyopathy.[44] Forskolin also reduced cardiac preload and afterload values and blood pressure, which increased cardiac output.[45]

Dose

No standard has been rigorously tested in human trials, although anecdotally, coleus products are most frequently standardized to 10% to 18% forskolin content. Case studies of cardiomyopathy patients have used 0.5 to 4 mcg/kg/min of IV forskolin with proposed hemodynamic benefits.[43-45] Effects appear to be dose dependent.

Adverse Effects, Interactions, Pharmacokinetics. See Appendix A.

Dandelion (Taraxacum officinale)

Grade C: *Unclear or conflicting scientific evidence (diuresis)*

Mechanism of Action

The mechanism of action of the diuretic effects of dandelion is not well understood. Constituents of dandelion include sesquiterpene lactones, artemetin, quercetin, luteolin, luteolin-7-O-beta-D-glucopyranoside, caffeic acid, esculetin, stigmasterol, and taraxasteryl acetate.[46] Dandelion leaves and roots have a high potassium content.[47] Sesquiterpene lactones may be responsible for dandelion's diuretic effects.[48]

Scientific Evidence of Effectiveness

The German Commission E (a committee of scientists, toxicologists, physicians, and pharmacists formed by the German government in 1978 to determine if herbs sold in Germany are safe and effective) has approved the use of dandelion as a diuretic based on its traditional use. However, animal studies are mixed,[47,49,50] and human data are lacking to clarify these conflicting results.

Dose

The dose of dandelion for CHF has not been clearly established.

Adverse Effects, Interactions, Pharmacokinetics. See Appendix A.

Ginseng (*Panax* spp.)

Grade C: *Unclear or conflicting scientific evidence (congestive heart failure)*

Mechanism of Action

The exact mechanism of ginseng in CHF is not well understood. There has been conflicting research on the effect of ginseng on blood pressure. The hypotensive effects in humans[51,52] and animals[53] may be caused by a relaxing effect on smooth muscle induced by certain ginsenosides (e.g., Rb1).[54-59] This might also explain the improvement of symptoms of coronary artery disease, including typical electrocardiographic (ECG) changes, such as repolarization disturbances.[58] Calcium may play a role in the cardiovascular effects of ginseng.[56,59] Ginsenosides Rb1 and Rg1 appear to have vasodilatory effects, possibly mediated by the proportion of nitric acid release,[54] in which enhanced nitric oxide synthesis from the endothelium of the lung, heart, kidney, and corpus cavernosum contributes to the vasodilation.[60] Other researchers, however, have described hypertensive effects of ginseng.[61,62] The total saponins of *Panax notoginseng* may improve myocardial relaxation secondary to enhanced calcium pump activity and inhibited intracellular calcium overload.[63]

Scientific Evidence of Effectiveness

Clinical research involving patients with NYHA Class IV CHF found that *Panax ginseng* and digoxin displayed synergism for treatment of CHF, and *P. ginseng* alone was an effective and safe adjuvant without reported side effects. *P. ginseng* at 2 g alone (five 0.4-g tablets three times daily) and at 2 g plus 0.25 mg of digoxin both resulted in improved hemodynamic and biochemical parameters.[64]

Dose

Ginseng extracts may be standardized to 4% to 7% total ginsenoside content.[65,66] Some sources indicate that ginsenosides constitute an average of 3% of the dried whole root,[67] and that the usual concentration of ginsenosides may be 1% to 3%. Standardized extracts of American ginseng (CNT-2000) are also available.[68] The German Federal Pharmacopeia standardizes a minimum ginsenoside content of 1.5%, calculated in terms of the ginsenoside Rg1.[69]

The exact dose of *P. ginseng* for CHF has not been determined, although 2 g alone (five 0.4-g tablets three times daily) and 2 g with 0.25 mg of digoxin have been used in NYHA Class IV patients.[64]

Adverse Effects, Interactions, Pharmacokinetics. See Appendix A.

Goldenseal (*Hydrastis canadensis*)

Grade B: *Good scientific evidence (heart failure)*

Mechanism of Action

Efficacy studies regarding goldenseal are limited to one of its main constituents, *berberine*, and few clinical studies have evaluated the use of goldenseal itself in humans. Because of the small amount of berberine actually available from goldenseal preparations (0.5%-6.0%), it is difficult to extrapolate the available evidence regarding berberine salts to the use of goldenseal. Another active constituent found in goldenseal is *hydrastine*.

Berberine has been shown to significantly improve systemic and pulmonary vascular resistance, right atrial and left ventricular end-diastolic pressures, cardiac index, and LVEF in patients with CHF.[70] Intravenous berberine raised left ventricular end-diastolic pressure in anesthetized dogs with embolized left main coronary arteries.[71] Berberine has exhibited positive inotropic effects in dogs and prevents or reverses ouabain (poison)–induced ventricular arrhythmias.[71-73] In animal experiments, berberine restored ventricular arrhythmias and atrial fibrillation to normal sinus rhythm.[73-76] Berberine at 0.2 to 0.7 mg/kg/min increases cardiac output and decreases total peripheral resistance and heart rate in animals; doses of 0.02 mg/kg/min only increase cardiac output.[77]

Scientific Evidence of Effectiveness

Goldenseal is currently one of the five top-selling herbal products in the United States. However, little scientific evidence regarding its efficacy or toxicity is available. Goldenseal can be found in dietary supplements, eardrops, feminine cleansing products, cold/flu remedies, allergy remedies, laxatives, and digestive aids.

Human studies suggest that berberine, in addition to a standard prescription drug regimen for CHF that includes ACE inhibitors, digoxin, diuretics, and nitrates, may improve quality of life and cardiac function, decrease vascular resistance and incidence of premature ventricular contractions (PVCs), and improve mortality rate, specifically in patients with CHF secondary to ischemic or idiopathic dilated cardiomyopathy.[78-79] Further research is necessary before a firm conclusion can be drawn regarding berberine's comparative effects with other established drugs for this indication that are often added to standard therapy, such as beta blockers or spironolactone.

In a case series of 12 patients with refractory CHF who received an IV infusion of berberine, either 0.02 or 0.2 mg/kg/min for 30 minutes, several statistically significant changes were observed at the higher dose, including 48% decrease in systemic vascular resistance, 41% decrease in pulmonary vascular resistance, 28% decrease in right atrial pressures,

32% decrease in left ventricular end-systolic pressures, 45% increase in cardiac index, a 45% increase in stroke volume, and a 56% increase in LVEF.

Dose

Published analyses of various commercially available goldenseal-containing products by high-performance liquid chromatography (HPLC) have not found consistency in the content of hydrastine or berberine, the proposed active constituents of goldenseal, with hydrastine concentrations ranging from 0% to 2.93% and berberine from 0.82% to 5.86%.[80,81]

The dose of goldenseal for CHF has not been firmly established. A daily oral dose of 1.2 g berberine (0.3 g four times daily) has been taken for 8 weeks in conjunction with conventional therapy (ACE inhibitors, digoxin, diuretics, nitrates), and beneficial effects have been noted. The maximum dose was 0.5 g four times daily.[79]

In a case series evaluating the acute effects of berberine on refractory CHF, 0.2 mg/kg/min for 30 minutes had reported beneficial effects.[70]

Adverse Effects, Interactions, Pharmacokinetics. See Appendix A.

Hawthorn (*Crataegus* spp.)

Grade B: *Good scientific evidence (congestive heart failure)*

Mechanism of Action

Hawthorn is a flowering shrub of the rose family, common in Europe. Because of widespread hybridization, the different species of *Crataegus* are difficult to distinguish. Multiple species are typically found in hawthorn preparations, including *Crataegus laevigata*, *C. oxyacantha*, and *C. monogyna*. Major pharmacologically active components in hawthorn are believed to be flavonoids, such as hyperoside and vitexin, and procyanidins.

Animal and in vitro studies suggest that flavonoids and other pharmacologically active compounds found in hawthorn may synergistically improve the performance of damaged myocardium. Furthermore, they may prevent or reduce symptoms of coronary artery disease.

Administration of hawthorn extract has been shown to decrease blood pressure and total peripheral resistance, economize myocardial function, and decrease cardiac preload in healthy subjects.[82,83] More specifically, hawthorn extract has shown an inotropic effect on myocardial tissue isolated from patients with terminal left ventricular heart failure.[84] The inotropic effects of hawthorn may be caused by inhibition of 3′,5′-cAMP diesterase,[85] rather than beta-sympathomimetic activity.[86]

Scientific Evidence of Effectiveness

Hawthorn's use in cardiovascular disease dates back to the first century AD. Numerous well-conducted human clinical trials have demonstrated efficacy of a specific, standardized hawthorn leaf and flower extract, WS 1442 or LI 132, in NYHA Class I to III heart failure.[87-101] Hawthorn extract has been found to improve ejection fraction and exercise tolerance and reduce symptoms of dyspnea and fatigue in patients with NYHA Class II heart failure.[89,93-95,101-104] Additionally, hawthorn extract WS 1442 was given in combination with preexisting diuretic therapy and improved exercise tolerance and reduced subjective symptoms in patients with NYHA Class III heart failure. Maximum effect was noted after 16 weeks of combined diuretic therapy and 1800 mg of WS 1442 daily.[105]

The therapeutic equivalence of hawthorn extracts to drugs considered "standard of care" for heart failure (ACE inhibitors, diuretics, beta blockers) remains to be established, as does the effect of concomitant use of hawthorn with these drugs. Equivalence study has found hawthorn comparable to captopril, but the study may not have been adequately powered to detect small differences between therapies.[101]

The results of an international multicenter, randomized, placebo-controlled trial investigating the long-term effect of hawthorn therapy on mortality and prognosis of patients with CHF are not yet clear.[100] However, a retrospective analysis of another clinical trial (randomized, double blind, placebo controlled) found that WS 1442 had no clinically significant effects in CHF patients.[106]

Dose

For CHF, extracts of specific standardized hawthorn leaf and flower extract (WS 1442 or LI 132) at doses of 160 to 900 mg daily have been used in two or three divided doses for 4 to 8 weeks.[87-101] Another study used WS 1442 at daily doses of 900 mg for 6 months.[106]

Adverse Effects, Interactions, Pharmacokinetics. See Appendix A.

Horsetail (*Equisetum* spp.)

Grade B: *Good scientific evidence (diuresis)*

Mechanism of Action

Horsetail purportedly has diuretic effects, although the mechanism of action is not well understood. Constituents of horsetail include petrosins (onitin), flavone glycosides (isoquercitrin, equisetrin, galuteolin), saponins (equisetonin), sterols (β-sitosterol, campestrol, isofucosterol),[107] tannins, and caffeic acid derivatives,[108-110] in addition to silica and silicic acids. Diuretic properties may be caused by equisetonin and flavonoids.[111]

Scientific Evidence of Effectiveness

The use of horsetail in humans has been reported to cause a mild but statistically significant diuretic effect. In a study of 34 patients with a history of forming uric acid kidney stones, horsetail (dose not clearly reported) caused an increase in diuresis compared with baseline after 8 to 12 weeks of use.[111] Another study evaluating an oral infusion of horsetail (*Equisetum bogotense*), 0.75 g daily for 2 consecutive days, in healthy subjects reported a mild diuretic effect, evidenced by a positive water balance difference in 87.5% of subjects. Significant decreases in urinary excretion of potassium, sodium, and chloride were also noted.[112]

Various *Equisetum* spp., including *E. hyemale, E. fluviatile, E. giganteum,* and *E. myriochaetum*, exhibited diuretic effects in mice, some of which were stronger than furosemide and hydrochlorothiazide.[113]

Dose

The dose of horsetail for CHF has not been clearly established. Oral infusion of horsetail (*E. bogotense*), 0.75 g daily for 2 consecutive days, has been used in clinical study.[112] A starting dose of 300 mg three times daily, up to a maximum of 6 g daily, is sometimes recommended.

Adverse Effects, Interactions, Pharmacokinetics. See Appendix A.

Oleander (Nerium oleander, Thevetia peruviana)

Grade C: *Unclear or conflicting scientific evidence (congestive heart failure)*

Note: All parts of the oleander plant, including flowers, leaves, and nectar, are considered toxic and are not recommended for consumption.

Mechanism of Action

Both common oleander *(Nerium oleander)* and yellow oleander *(Thevetia peruviana)* contain cardiac glycosides with mechanisms of action similar to ouabain and digoxin. *Nerium oleander* contains oleandrin, digitoxigenin, nerriin, and folinerin. Yellow oleander contains thevetin A, thevetin B, nerifolin, thevetoxin, peruvoside, and ruvoside. The pharmacological mode of action of the cardiac glycosides is through inhibition of the sodium/potassium-dependent adenosine triphosphatase (ATPase) pump, resulting in elevation of intracellular levels of calcium and sodium, with decreased intracellular/increased extracellular potassium levels. The intracellular accumulation of calcium appears to provide the basis for increased myocardial contractility.[114]

Scientific Evidence of Effectiveness

Cardiac glycosides found in oleander have been staples of CHF therapy in China and Russia for decades. In the available studies from the 1930s, oleander was reported to improve symptoms of CHF, including heart rate and dyspnea, and to decrease venous pressure, edema, and diuresis.[115-119] Oleander preparations exist in other countries, most notably China, as therapies for heart failure and are available in 100-mcg tablets.

High-quality comparative studies to other, better-tolerated cardiac glycoside preparations do not appear to exist for oleander. Notably, cardiac glycosides have not been shown to improve mortality in CHF patients, although well-tolerated and widely used drugs such as digoxin have been demonstrated to alleviate symptoms and reduce frequency of hospitalization.

Dose

The dose of oleander for CHF has not been determined.

Adverse Effects, Interactions, Pharmacokinetics. See Appendix A.

Passion Flower (Passiflora incarnata)

Grade C: *Unclear or conflicting scientific evidence (congestive heart failure [exercise capacity])*

Mechanism of Action

Among the more than 400 species of *Passiflora*, there are many substances with potential pharmacological activity, although not all have been identified or isolated from *Passiflora incarnata*. The principal constituents are up to 2.5% flavonoids, including vitexin, isovitexin, coumarin, apigenin, umbelliferone, and maltol. Harmala alkaloids, including harman, harmaline, harmine, and harmalol, have been reported but may be in subtherapeutic quantities. Passion flower fruit (skin and pericarp) contains a great amount of lycopene, whereas the content of other carotenoids is very low or almost nonexistent.[120]

The effects of passion flower on heart failure are poorly understood. Animal studies of various *Passiflora* spp. suggest antianxiety and anticonvulsant effects, which may be mediated by benzodiazepine receptors.[121-123] Effects independent of benzodiazepine receptors are also possible.[124] Passion flower may also have antihypertensive effects, which may be partially caused by the vasodilatory effect of polyphenols such as luteolin.[125]

Scientific Evidence of Effectiveness

There is insufficient available evidence to recommend for or against passion flower for the treatment of exercise capacity or dyspnea in patients with CHF. Although researched in clinical study with a passion flower–hawthorn combination product, this indication is not a typical clinical use of passion flower.[104] Effects may have been attributable to hawthorn, which is used often in Europe for CHF and may be beneficial in preventing heart failure, as shown in several initial randomized trials.

Dose

For CHF, an extract containing both passion flower (140 mg) and hawthorn has been taken for 6 weeks.[104]

Adverse Effects, Interactions, Pharmacokinetics. See Appendix A.

Rutin ($C_{27}H_{30}O_{16}$)

Grade B: *Good scientific evidence (diuresis)*

Mechanism of Action

Rutins are flavonoids that serve as the chemical precursors for *oxerutins,* a group of synthetic bioflavonoids. Oxerutins belong to a group of edema-protective agents that possess antiexudative and membrane-protective activities.[126] *O-*(beta-hydroxyethyl)-rutoside and tri-(hydroxyethyl)-rutoside decreased edema induced by sodium retention and increased diuresis of sodium and potassium when given orally and intravenously to rats.[127] The antiedematous effect appears to be dose responsive.[128]

Scientific Evidence of Effectiveness

Various rutin compounds may be useful in reducing edema or excess swelling caused by fluid retention[129-140] and may also help prevent edema.[131,133,134] Rutin may work best when administered with vitamin C and other flavonoids.[141]

Several controlled clinical trials report that the rutin derivative hydroxymethylrutoside is effective in the treatment of symptoms of venous insufficiency, including heavy legs, edema, paresthesia, and cramps.[126,132,142-153] Rutin reduced pain, cramps, restless legs, and swelling significantly compared with placebo.[150]

Dose

Venoruton (oxerutins) is a standardized mixture of *O-*(beta-hydroxyethyl)-rutosides used for the relief of edema and related symptoms in patients with chronic venous insufficiency.[151] For edema, 500 to 1000 mg twice daily for up to 6 months has been used.[132,152,153]

Adverse Effects, Interactions, Pharmacokinetics. See Appendix A.

 Traditional Chinese Medicine

> *Chinese medicine* is a broad term encompassing many different modalities and traditions of healing that share a common heritage of technique or theory rooted in ancient Chinese philosophy (Taoism). Clinical symptoms of CHF fall under traditional Chinese disease categories of "heart palpitations" *(xin ji),* "water swelling *(shui zhong),* "phlegm rheum" *(tan yin),* and "heart impediment" *(xin bi).* Traditional Chinese medicine (TCM) uses a well-defined theory and emphasizes herbal medicine supplemented by acupuncture. Herbs are usually given in the form of manufactured or processed pills, extracts, capsules, tinctures, or powders, in contrast to the raw and dried form favored in ethnic TCM. These practices have historically been used in the treatment of CHF.[1]

HERBAL THERAPIES WITH LIMITED EVIDENCE

Foxglove *(Digitalis purpurea, Digitalis lanata)*

Note: Digitalis is considered unsafe when used orally and therefore cannot be recommended.

Foxglove is a source of *digitoxin,* a cardiac glycoside, and is a member of the *Digitalis* genus. Foxglove is currently rarely used because of its toxicity profile and cases of poisoning and the availability of pure digoxin and digitoxin. Digitalis has been shown to increase cardiac contractility, reduce conduction at the atrioventricular node, decrease heart rate, and increase cardiac output.[154-156]

Horse Chestnut *(Aesculus hippocastanum)*

Horse chestnut is widely used in Europe for chronic venous insufficiency, a syndrome characterized by lower extremity edema, varicosities, pain, pruritus, atrophic skin changes, and ulcerations. In animal study, aescine and aesculine, active principles of horse chestnut, have displayed moderate diuretic activity, increasing the renal loss of sodium, chloride, and potassium.[157]

Scotch Broom *(Cytisus scoparius)*

Grade C: Unclear or conflicting scientific evidence (diuretic)

Scotch broom preparations, particularly those made from the flower, have been used traditionally as diuretics and to remove the fluid in the lungs occurring in CHF. Based on preliminary study, sparteine has been shown to have curare-like properties and extend heart rate without affecting the force of contraction. Scotch broom contains tyramine and sparteine, which according to secondary sources, may alter blood pressure (increase or decrease). The diuretic effect of scotch broom may be due to the flavone glycosides, scoparoside, and scoparin. There is particular concern about the potential toxicity of scotch broom because of the presence of small amounts of the toxic alkaloids sparteine and isosparteine, which are found in both the flowers and herb (above-ground parts of the plant).

Stinging Nettle *(Urtica dioica)*

Stinging nettle is traditionally used for urination disorders, and animal study evaluating the aerial parts of nettle reported diuretic and natriuretic effects.[158]

Tea *(Camellia sinensis)*

Tea is a source of caffeine, a known stimulant and diuretic.[159]

Herbs with Potential Cardiotonic Properties*

HERB	SPECIFIC THERAPEUTIC USE(S)†	HERB	SPECIFIC THERAPEUTIC USE(S)†
Abuta	Diuretic	Devil's claw	Diuretic
Agave	Diuretic	Dong quai	Diuretic, congestive heart failure
Agrimony	Diuretic	Eastern hemlock	Diuretic
Alfalfa	Diuretic	Elder	Diuretic
Alizarin	Diuretic	Ephedra	Diuretic
Aloe	Congestive heart failure	False pennyroyal	Diuretic
Alpinia	Diuretic	Garcinia	Diuretic
Anise	Diuretic	Garlic	Diuretic
Annatto	Diuretic	Ginkgo	Congestive heart failure
Arnica	Diuretic	Globe artichoke	Diuretic
Asarum	Diuretic	Goldenrod	Diuretic
Asparagus	Diuretic	Gotu kola	Diuretic
Bacopa	Diuretic	Grape seed	Diuretic
Barberry	Congestive heart failure	Ground ivy	Diuretic
Bay leaf	Diuretic	Guarana	Diuretic
Bee pollen	Diuretic	Gumweed	Diuretic
Belladonna	Diuretic	Gymnema	Diuretic
Bellis perennis	Diuretic	Horseradish	Diuretic
Betel nut	Diuretic	Hyssop	Diuretic
Betony	Diuretic	Jequirity	Diuretic
Birch	Diuretic	Jewelweed	Diuretic
Black currant	Diuretic	Juniper	Diuretic
Black horehound	Diuretic	Kava	Diuretic
Blessed thistle	Diuretic	Khella	Diuretic
Bloodroot	Diuretic	Labrador tea	Diuretic
Blue cohosh	Diuretic	Ladies mantle	Diuretic
Blue flag	Diuretic	Lavender	Diuretic
Boldo	Diuretic	Lemongrass	Diuretic
Boneset	Diuretic	Licorice	Diuretic
Boswellia	Diuretic	Lime	Diuretic
Bromelain	Diuretic	Lovage	Diuretic
Buchu	Diuretic, congestive heart failure	Marshmallow	Diuretic
Bugleweed	Diuretic	Mastic	Diuretic
Bupleurum	Pulmonary edema	Meadowsweet	Diuretic
Burdock	Diuretic	Morus nigra	Diuretic
Butterbur	Diuretic	Mullein	Diuretic
Calendula	Diuretic	Nopal	Diuretic
Chamomile	Diuretic	Polypodium	Diuretic
Chaparral	Diuretic	Raspberry	Diuretic
Chicory	Diuretic	Red clover	Diuretic
Cinnamon	Diuretic	Rehmannia	Diuretic
Cleavers	Diuretic	Rhubarb	Diuretic
Club moss	Diuretic	Rose hip	Diuretic
Couch grass	Diuretic	Rosemary	Diuretic
Cranberry	Diuretic	Saw palmetto	Diuretic
Damiana	Diuretic	Shepherd's purse	Diuretic
Danshen	Left ventricular hypertrophy	Skullcap	Diuretic

Continued

Herbs with Potential Cardiotonic Properties—cont'd

HERB	SPECIFIC THERAPEUTIC USE(S)†	HERB	SPECIFIC THERAPEUTIC USE(S)†
Skunk cabbage	Diuretic	Tansy	Diuretic
Slippery elm	Diuretic	Thyme	Diuretic
Sorrel	Diuretic	Tribulus	Diuretic
Squill	Diuretic	Valerian	Diuretic, congestive heart failure
St. John's wort	Diuretic	Watercress	Diuretic
Star anise	Diuretic	White horehound	Diuretic
Stinging nettle	Diuretic	Yew	Diuretic
Sweet woodruff	Diuretic		

*This is not an all-inclusive or comprehensive list of herbs with cardiotonic properties; other herbs and supplements may possess these qualities. A qualified health care provider should be consulted with specific questions or concerns regarding potential cardiotonic effects or interactions.
†Based on expert opinion, anecdote, case reports, and/or preliminary trial evidence.

Uva Ursi (Arctostaphylos uva-ursi)

Uva ursi is derived from the bearberry tree, and the leaves contain hydroquinone derivatives, mainly *arbutin*,[160,161] which is thought to have diuretic properties. Increased urine flow has been noted in animal study.[162]

ADJUNCT THERAPIES

1. Congestive heart failure is a serious condition, and managing CHF involves many factors. The goal of developing a pharmaceutical and lifestyle program should include strengthening cardiac function, reducing symptoms, and slowing down cardiac remodeling. A complementary approach may involve lifestyle changes and dietary supplements along with herbal or conventional therapy to help slow the progression of CHF and improve quality of life.
2. Lifestyle changes can help reduce symptoms such as fatigue, shortness of breath, and edema (swelling). These modifications may include dietary changes (e.g., restricted salt intake of <2000 mg daily), abstaining from alcohol, quitting smoking, and exercising regularly (under physician supervision).
3. During CHF, the heart changes shape and becomes larger and thinner. This process, known as *cardiac remodeling*, causes reduced quality of life in many patients. Some dietary supplements may help improve function, increase energy and blood flow, and reduce swelling of the heart.
4. *Coenzyme Q10* (CoQ10) may decline in patients with CHF. Scientific studies have shown that CoQ10 used in combination with vitamins and minerals,[163] hawthorn, and magnesium[164] has benefits for patients with CHF. It has been reported to improve ejection fraction, cardiac output, and systolic function.[167] CoQ10 may also improve exercise capacity and quality of life[166].
5. Similar to CoQ10, *creatine*, L-*carnitine*, and *taurine* may be decreased in patients with CHF. By increasing levels of these nutrients, patients with CHF may experience fewer symptoms, better cardiac function, and less cardiac remodeling. Several studies report that creatine supplementation is associated with improved heart muscle strength, body weight, and endurance in CHF patients.
6. Heart health may also be related to antioxidant levels. Oxidative stress may be a mechanism of disease progression in CHF. *Antioxidants* such as vitamins C and E and alpha-lipoic acid may reduce damage to the heart and improve cardiac function. However, available human studies are limited and insufficient to support or negate the use of antioxidants for CHF.
7. *Fish oil* may be another beneficial addition to a CHF regimen. Although not well studied in patients with CHF, fish oil has been shown to reduce the risk of nonfatal heart attack, fatal heart attack, sudden death, and mortality (death from any cause) in patients with cardiovascular disease.[167-173]
8. Angiotensin-converting enzyme (ACE) inhibitors are widely prescribed for heart failure and may cause unwanted side effects. These drugs are often associated with nonproductive cough (occurs in about 10% of patients). Taking *iron* orally seems to inhibit cough associated with ACE inhibitors. Iron has been reported to reduce the production of nitric oxide, which is known to have inflammatory effects on bronchial cells in the lungs.[174] *Peppermint, fennel, white horehound, honey*, and *aromatherapy* may also be useful in reducing cough.

INTEGRATIVE THERAPY PLAN

- Discuss the patient's heart failure symptoms, including shortness of breath, persistent coughing or wheezing, swelling in the legs and feet, tiredness, confusion, fatigue, increased heart rate, and weight gain.
- Ensure that patients with heart failure are receiving appropriate therapy, including ACE inhibitors, ARBs, beta blockers, digoxin, diuretics, and aldosterone antagonists.
- Educate the patient regarding *hawthorn*, a widely used herb for treating NYHA Class I or II heart failure. It is still unclear whether hawthorn is comparable to standard-of-care drugs

for heart failure; the effect of concurrent use of hawthorn with these drugs is also unclear. Despite previous evidence supporting its effectiveness in CHF, hawthorn was found to be ineffective in a recent retrospective study. Hawthorn appears to be safe and well tolerated but should be used under medical supervision. Hawthorn is a potentially beneficial treatment for patients who will not or cannot take prescription drugs. It may also provide additive benefits to prescription drug therapy. Recommended hawthorn doses use standardized extracts (WS 1442 or LI 132) at doses of 160 to 900 mg daily in two or three divided doses for 4 to 8 weeks.

- Other herbs, such as astragalus and ginseng, and constituents, such as berberine, may also be potentially beneficial in CHF patients, but more scientific support is needed before a recommendation can be made.
- Educate the patient regarding the importance of adherence to the CHF medication regimen. Also, advise the patient to restrict salt and fluid intake and to monitor weight.

Case Studies

CASE STUDY 12-1

VB is a 72-year-old woman who comes into the pharmacy and asks you where she can find glucosamine/chondroitin. You notice that she is having difficulty breathing after walking the short distance from her car. As the pharmacist, you ask to speak to her in the consultation area. You then ask if being out of breath is normal for her. She responds that recently, when she goes on her daily walks, she cannot make it around the block without being out of breath and feeling tired. Six months ago, she was able to walk farther without a problem. She tells you that she has heart failure, high blood pressure, and osteoarthritis, but she does not want to see any doctor or take any prescription medications. She has been controlling her blood pressure with diet and mild exercise (walking); taking glucosamine/chondroitin for osteoarthritis; and using Metamucil to help with chronic constipation. Her blood pressure is 139/88 mm Hg and heart rate 90 beats/min. She has no visible edema. How do you counsel VB?

Answer: VB has a history of heart failure, which is currently not being treated because of her objections to prescription drugs. On inspection, VB does not appear to be in acute distress. Her heart rate and blood pressure are at the high end of normal. It appears that VB has subjective (e.g., shortness of breath) and objective (e.g., elevated heart rate) signs and symptoms of worsening CHF.

Appropriate drug treatment for CHF includes an ACE inhibitor, diuretic, digoxin, and vasodilator. However, VB does not want to take prescription medications, so appropriate alternative treatments should be discussed. Some herbs, such as hawthorn, may help improve symptoms of CHF. Hawthorn has been found to relax the blood vessels to lower blood pressure, increase blood flow to the heart, and control heart rate. Hawthorn may also help improve exercise tolerance.

For heart failure, extracts of specific standardized hawthorn leaf and flower extract (WS 1442 or LI 132) at doses of 160 to 900 mg daily have been used in two or three divided doses for 4 to 8 weeks. Higher doses may cause abnormally low blood pressure. Advise VB to monitor blood pressure regularly at home and to follow up with you in approximately 4 weeks to see if symptoms have improved.

Supplements, such as CoQ10, creatine, L-carnitine, and taurine, may also be added as a part of complementary treatment.

Remind VB that CHF is a serious health condition that can lead to hospitalization. Uncontrolled CHF may be fatal. Patients with CHF can live symptom-free lives if they work with physicians and other health care professionals.

CASE STUDY 12-2

RW is a 71-year-old man who asks about using goldenseal. His past medical history includes NYHA Class IV CHF, type 2 diabetes, and hypertension. He currently takes furosemide, enalapril, spironolactone, and glipizide for these conditions. His conditions are uncontrolled. How do you respond and counsel?

Answer: Stage IV heart failure is severe and limits daily life. Although RW's current medications will help with some symptoms and mortality, his heart is becoming very weak and damaged. A component of goldenseal, berberine, has been shown to be beneficial in CHF patients; however, because of the small amount of berberine actually available in goldenseal preparations, it is difficult to extrapolate the available evidence regarding berberine salts to the use of goldenseal. Adding a daily dose of 1.2 g of goldenseal may offer a small benefit, but RW's cardiologist should determine if the risks outweigh the benefits. You may also want to talk to RW's cardiologist about adding a beta blocker.

CASE STUDY 12-3

NS is a 58-year-old retired nurse's aide with increasing shortness of breath and noticeable leg edema. Six months ago, she was diagnosed with NYHA Class I CHF. She smokes between one and two packs of cigarettes daily. NS has been taking hawthorn under physician supervision. She visits her physician, who advises her to take a diuretic. NS insists on taking only natural products. Her physician calls you for assistance and asks about horsetail. How should you counsel?

Answer: Horsetail is an herb with diuretic properties. However, NS is a smoker, and because horsetail contains small amounts of nicotine, additive effects are possible when used with cigarettes. You should tell her physician about this potential interaction. You may also want to suggest trying grape seed, which also has good evidence to support its use as a diuretic. Notably, neither herb has been studied in CHF. Caution and monitoring should be advised.

References for Chapter 12 can be found on the Evolve website at http://evolve.elsevier.com/Ulbricht/herbalpharmacotherapy/

Review Questions

1. True or false: Numerous well-conducted human clinical trials have demonstrated safety and efficacy of hawthorn leaf and flower in New York Heart Association (NYHA) Class IV heart failure (characterized by inability to carry on any physical activity without discomfort).

2. Hawthorn should be used cautiously with which of the following conditions?
   a. Low blood pressure
   b. Asthma
   c. Chronic fatigue syndrome
   d. All the above

3. Hawthorn doses of _____ have been shown to be effective in the treatment of mild to moderate CHF, improving exercise capacity and alleviating symptoms of cardiac insufficiency.
   a. 160 to 900 mg daily
   b. 160 to 900 g daily
   c. 160 to 900 mg twice daily
   d. 160 to 900 g twice daily

4. True or false: Oleander is a poisonous plant that contains numerous toxic compounds, which may cause serious adverse effects and possibly death.

5. Goldenseal and/or berberine may interact with which of the following?
   a. Warfarin
   b. Doxycycline
   c. Timolol
   d. All the above

6. What compounds in horsetail promote fluid loss?
   a. Pectin and saponin glycosides
   b. Equisetonin and flavonoids
   c. Sesquiterpene lactones
   d. Sarsaponin and cyanogenic glycosides

7. What are the active components of grape seed extract?
   a. Catechins
   b. Oligomeric proanthocyanidins
   c. Cysteine sulfoxides
   d. Anthraquinones

8. True or false: Ashwagandha has been shown in vitro to stimulate sodium and potassium excretion in a dose-dependent manner.

9. Which of the following drugs may interact with dandelion?
   a. Triamterene
   b. Warfarin
   c. Insulin
   d. All the above

10. Diuretic effects of scotch broom may be attributed to which constituents?
    a. Solanine and scoparoside
    b. Solanine and psilocybin
    c. Scoparin and scoparoside
    d. Sparteine and scoparoside

Answers are found in the Answers to Review Questions section in the back of the text.

13 Angina

Outline

OVERVIEW
   Signs and Symptoms
   Diagnosis
      Physical Examination and Tests
      Cardiac Stress Test
      Carotid Ultrasonography
      Arteriography
      Computed Tomographic Angiography
      Magnetic Resonance Imaging
SELECTED HERBAL THERAPIES
   Danshen *(Salvia miltiorrhiza)*
   Dong Quai *(Angelica sinensis)*
   Ginseng *(Panax* spp.)
   Hawthorn *(Crataegus* spp.)
   Kudzu *(Pueraria lobata)*
   Reishi Mushroom *(Ganoderma lucidum)*
   Safflower *(Carthamus tinctorius)*
   Tribulus *(Tribulus terrestris)*
HERBAL THERAPIES WITH LIMITED EVIDENCE
ADJUNCT THERAPIES
INTEGRATIVE THERAPY PLAN
CASE STUDIES
REVIEW QUESTIONS

Learning Objectives

- Know the herbs that possess antianginal properties.
- Understand data currently available to support herbal treatment selection for angina.
- Explain the mechanisms of action, adverse effects, and interactions associated with antianginal herbs.
- Educate patients regarding integrative pharmacotherapy plans and adjunct therapies.

OVERVIEW[1-3]

The term *angina pectoris* describes chest pain that occurs when the heart cells do not receive enough oxygen. Angina is classified as stable or unstable angina. *Stable angina* is precipitated by activity, when the heart is working harder and there is a greater demand for oxygen-rich blood to reach the heart. *Unstable angina* typically occurs at rest. This type is serious if left untreated and may lead to a heart attack.

Angina is the most common symptom of *coronary artery disease* (CAD), also known as *coronary heart disease* (CHD). CAD occurs when the coronary arteries, which supply oxygen-rich blood to the heart muscle, gradually become narrowed or blocked by plaque deposits. When arteries become narrowed, this condition is known as *stenosis*. The plaques are a combination of fatty material, calcium, scar tissue, and proteins; these deposits decrease the space through which blood can flow, thus reducing its flow. As platelets attach to the narrowed area, blood clots may form around the plaque, and the artery narrows even further. In some cases the blood clot breaks apart, and blood supply is restored. In other cases the blood clot *(coronary thrombus)* may completely block the blood supply to the heart muscle *(coronary occlusion)*. This lack of blood flow, called *ischemia,* can "starve" some of the heart muscle and lead to angina. A *myocardial infarction* (MI), or heart attack, results when blood flow is completely blocked, usually by a blood clot forming over a plaque that has ruptured. Unhealthy habits, such as a diet high in cholesterol and other fats, smoking, and lack of exercise, accelerate the deposit of fat and calcium within the inner lining of the coronary arteries (see Chapter 14).

CAD is the most common form of heart disease, and affects about 14 million men and women in the U.S. population. CAD is also the leading cause of death in men and women in the United States, and claims more lives than the other seven leading causes of death combined.

Nitrates remain important agents for the treatment of stable and unstable angina pectoris. These agents induce coronary vasodilation and dilate peripheral veins. This reduces venous return to the heart and decreases heart size, which lowers myocardial oxygen demand. Nitrates are available as a sublingual tablet, long-acting oral tablet, topical ointment, spray, patch, or intravenous preparation. Sublingual tablets or sprays are used to shorten or prevent an anticipated angina attack. Long-acting nitrates are indicated for long-term management of angina.

Platelet inhibitors, such as aspirin or clopidogrel (Plavix), may also be recommended; however, patients should be aware that these drugs may increase the risk of bleeding. Beta blockers such as metoprolol (Lopressor, Toprol) may be prescribed to help decrease the heart rate and blood pressure, thereby reducing the heart's demand for oxygen. Calcium channel blockers such as amlodipine (Norvasc) or diltiazem (Cardizem) may also be prescribed. These medications slow the heart rate and dilate the coronary blood vessels. Angiotensin-converting enzyme (ACE) inhibitors such as lisinopril (Prinivil, Zestril) or ramipril (Altace) may be prescribed to help dilate the blood vessels and increase oxygen to the heart. Satins, or hydroxymethylglutaryl coenzyme A (HMG-CoA) reductase inhibitors, such as atorvastatin (Lipitor) or lovastatin (Mevacor), may be prescribed to help lower cholesterol levels. HMG-CoA reductase inhibitors may cause liver problems or muscle pain.

If the patient's arteries are severely blocked, they may need to be expanded using balloon angioplasty (also called percutaneous transluminal coronary angioplasty, or PCTA) and stent placement. A balloon catheter is inserted in or near the blockage and then inflated to open the blood vessel and restore blood flow. In some cases a stent is also placed where the blockage occurred; this helps keep the artery open. Several types of balloons, stents, and catheters are available to treat the plaque inside the vessel. Some of these surgical tools contain anticlotting medications. The physician chooses the type of procedure based on individual patient's needs. Common complications include *restenosis* (renarrowing of the artery), bleeding, and infection.

Patients with significant CAD may undergo a procedure called *coronary artery bypass graft* (CABG) surgery, in which one or more blocked blood vessels are bypassed by a *graft*, or transplant of healthy arteries or veins. This helps restore normal blood flow to the heart. These grafts usually come from the patient's own arteries and veins located in the chest, leg, or arm. The graft goes around the clogged artery to create new pathways for oxygen-rich blood to flow to the heart. Problems associated with CABG include heart attack (MI), stroke, blood clots, sternal wound infection, and death. Infections are most often associated with obesity, diabetes, or previous CABG. Some patients may develop swelling in the tissue around the heart, called *postpericardiotomy syndrome,* a few days to 6 months after surgery. Symptoms typically include fever and chest pain. The incision in the chest or the graft site may be itchy, sore, numb, or bruised after surgery. Some patients report memory loss or loss of mental clarity after CABG.

Signs and Symptoms

Angina refers to a painful feeling in the chest, which may be described as discomfort, heaviness, pressure, aching, burning, numbness, fullness, or squeezing. Angina usually begins in the chest, but it can also start or spread to different areas of the body, such as down the left arm (most common site), to the left shoulder, to the neck or lower jaw, to the midback, or down the right arm. If these symptoms begin suddenly or last only a few seconds, it is less likely to be angina. Angina can be mistaken for indigestion or heartburn, and the pain can be difficult to pinpoint. The chest pain associated with angina usually begins at a low level, then gradually increases over several minutes to a peak. Angina that occurs during activity usually decreases when the activity is stopped. Angina may also be caused by the use of drugs (e.g., cocaine, amphetamines), exposure to cold temperatures, anger, smoking, or eating a heavy meal.

Diagnosis
Physical Examination and Tests

The diagnosis of angina is primarily based on symptoms. Laboratory tests, chest x-ray, and a stress test may also be helpful in diagnosing the heart disease. Risk factors for stroke are evaluated, including high blood pressure, high cholesterol levels, calcium levels, diabetes, medications, elevated levels of homocysteine and C-reactive protein (CRP, a marker of inflammation), and obesity.

Cardiac Stress Test

A stress test determines how well the blood is flowing to the heart during exercise compared with resting. The patient either walks on a treadmill or is given an intravenous medication that stimulates exercise, such as dipyridamole (Persantine), that simulates exercise while connected to an electrocardiograph (ECG) machine. A nuclear stress test involves the injection of radioactive isotopes (most often technetium or Tc 99m sestamibi) to visualize blood flow to and from the heart.

Carotid Ultrasonography

Carotid ultrasonography (US) evaluates blood flow using a wandlike device, called a *transducer,* that sends high-frequency sound waves into the neck to determine if there is any narrowing or clotting in the carotid arteries.

Arteriography

An arteriogram (or angiogram) provides images of the arteries in the heart, brain, kidneys, and many other parts of the body not normally visible in x-ray films. A catheter is inserted through a small incision, usually in the groin area. The catheter is manipulated through the major arteries and into the carotid or vertebral artery. A dye is then injected through the catheter to provide images of the arteries.

Computed Tomographic Angiography

In computed tomographic angiography (CTA) a dye is injected into the blood, and x-ray beams create a three-dimensional image of the blood vessels in the neck and brain. CTA is used to look for aneurysms or blood vessel malformations and to evaluate arteries for narrowing. CT scanning, which is done without dye, can provide images of the brain and show hemorrhages, but without as much detailed information on the blood vessels.

Magnetic Resonance Imaging

Magnetic resonance imaging (MRI) uses a strong magnetic field to generate a three-dimensional view of the brain. This test is sensitive for detecting an area of brain tissue damaged by an ischemic stroke (lack of blood flow and oxygen to the brain). Magnetic resonance angiography (MRA) uses this magnetic field and a dye injected into the veins to evaluate arteries in the neck and brain.

SELECTED HERBAL THERAPIES

 Note

To help make this educational resource more interactive, all pharmacokinetics, adverse effects, and interactions data have been compiled in Appendix A. Safety data specifically related to pregnancy and lactation are listed in Appendix B. Please refer to these appendices when working through the case studies and answering the review questions.

There is a lack of evidence to support the use of any herb or supplement for acute angina attacks.

Danshen (Salvia miltiorrhiza)

Grade C: *Unclear or conflicting scientific evidence (cardiovascular disease/angina)*

Mechanism of Action

Although the potential mechanisms have not been confirmed, danshen may have antioxidant effects[4-8] and has been shown to decrease endothelin levels, which are elevated in patients with CHD.[7,9] Danshen may also benefit lipoprotein levels.[8] In animals, treatment with a salvianolic acid B–rich fraction of *Salvia miltiorrhiza* induced apoptosis in the neointima of the vascular system.[10] In animal study, danshen increased the coronary flow rate in isolated rat hearts, offering protection.[11] Constituents of danshen root, particularly protocatechualdehyde and 3,4-dihydroxyphenyl-lactic acid, are believed to be responsible for its vascular effects.

Scientific Evidence of Effectiveness

As an ancient Chinese medicine, danshen has traditionally been used in combination with other herbs to treat cardiovascular disease. There is limited clinical evidence that danshen may provide benefits in patients with disorders of the heart and blood vessels, including cardiac chest pain (angina). Studies have shown danshen to relieve chest pain, prolong exercise duration, and delay the time of onset of exercise angina.[12-15] Danshen was also reported to be as effective as isosorbide dinitrate (Isordil) in relieving symptoms in patients with chronic stable angina.[14] However, studies have been small and of weak methodological strength. Nonetheless, this research provides preliminary evidence that danshen may be beneficial in patients with angina.

Dose

No specific dose or standardized preparation of danshen is widely accepted for cardiovascular disorders.

Adverse Effects, Interactions, Pharmacokinetics. See Appendix A.

Dong Quai (Angelica sinensis)

Grade C: *Unclear or conflicting scientific evidence (angina pectoris/coronary artery disease)*

Mechanism of Action

The mechanism of dong quai in angina is not well understood. The compound *n*-butylidenephthalide, isolated from *Angelica sinensis,* has demonstrated vasorelaxation and increased coronary blood flow in animal studies.[16,17]

Scientific Evidence of Effectiveness

Preliminary evidence from animal studies suggests that *n*-butylidenephthalide may be beneficial in the treatment of angina without increasing blood pressure.[16,17] Human studies are lacking.

Dose

The dose of dong quai for angina has not been determined.

Adverse Effects, Interactions, Pharmacokinetics. See Appendix A.

Ginseng (Panax spp.)

Grade C: *Unclear or conflicting scientific evidence (coronary artery disease)*

Mechanism of Action

Because ginseng has been studied in combination with other agents, it is difficult to extrapolate its mechanism of action for angina.

Scientific Evidence of Effectiveness

Several studies from China report that ginseng in combination with various other herbs, including ophiopogon root *(Ophiopogonis japonicus)* and magnolia vine *(Schisandra chinensis),* may reduce CAD symptoms (e.g., anginal chest pain) and may improve ECG abnormalities.[18-21] However, because ginseng has not been studied as a monotherapy for angina, it is difficult to determine if these effects are attributable solely to ginseng.

Dose
The dose of ginseng for CAD has not been determined.

Adverse Effects, Interactions, Pharmacokinetics. See Appendix A.

Hawthorn (Crataegus spp.)

Grade C: *Unclear or conflicting scientific evidence (coronary artery disease/angina)*

Mechanism of Action
The mechanism of action by which hawthorn reduces angina is not well understood. Increased myocardial perfusion and performance have been observed in animals after they were exposed to hawthorn.[22,23]

Scientific Evidence of Effectiveness
A randomized, double-blind trial of 46 patients was conducted to evaluate the effects of hawthorn on angina.[24] Patients received 100 mg of *Crataegus pinnatifida* extract orally three times daily or placebo for 4 weeks. With the exception of nitroglycerin (NTG) during angina episodes, no beta blockers, calcium antagonists, or antianginal drugs were used, and digoxin, diuretics, or antihypertensive drugs were continued. After 4 weeks of treatment, angina improved in 91% of patients in the hawthorn group, versus only 37% ($p < 0.01$) in the placebo group. Accordingly, 45% of the hawthorn group completely stopped NTG, versus 25% of the placebo group. An additional 35% of the hawthorn group reduced intake of NTG, versus 11% in the placebo group ($p < 0.01$). ECG findings improved in 46% of hawthorn subjects, versus 3% of placebo group ($p < 0.01$). These results suggested that hawthorn may effectively prevent angina in CAD patients. However, most patients did not receive beta blockers or ACE inhibitors regularly, often considered the standard of care, so the results may not be applicable to patients taking these drugs.

Dose
The dose of hawthorn for angina has not been clearly established.

Adverse Effects, Interactions, Pharmacokinetics. See Appendix A.

Kudzu (Pueraria lobata)

Grade C: *Unclear or conflicting scientific evidence (cardiovascular disease/angina)*

Mechanism of Action
The exact mechanism of action of kudzu for angina is not completely understood. Early preclinical and animal research suggests kudzu has a protective effect against myocardial ischemia and may improve cardiac function.[25-35] Animal research suggests that puerarin, one of kudzu's isoflavones, may reduce both systolic and diastolic blood pressure and diminish myocardial oxygen consumption.[36] Puerarin may have vasorelaxant properties, possibly by blocking beta-adrenergic receptors.[37-39]

Scientific Evidence of Effectiveness
Puerarin injection has been widely used to treat CHD and angina pectoris. One clinical study[40] demonstrated the efficacy of puerarin in treating patients with unstable angina. Frequency of angina events, consumed doses of nitrates, heart rate, blood pressure, rest electrocardiogram (ECG), and myocardial oxygen consumption were observed before and after drug therapy in the puerarin group (21 cases) and control group (18 cases). Reductions in the frequency of angina events, consumed doses of nitrates, and improved abnormal rest ECG were observed in the puerarin group. It also appeared to be more effective in reducing myocardial oxygen consumption and increasing exercise duration compared with the control group. Puerarin injection may also be effective in unstable angina when used in combination with conventional treatments; however, there is currently a lack of evidence that puerarin has better or worse effects than other conventional treatments.[41] Evidence on the use of oral kudzu for angina is also lacking.

Dose
The dose of kudzu for angina has not been determined.

Adverse Effects, Interactions, Pharmacokinetics. See Appendix A.

Reishi Mushroom (Ganoderma lucidum)

Grade C: *Unclear or conflicting scientific evidence (coronary heart disease)*

Mechanism of Action. Insufficient available evidence.

Scientific Evidence of Effectiveness
A randomized, double-blind, placebo-controlled trial was conducted in 170 patients with confirmed CHD.[42] Treatment with an unclear dose of ganopoly, a *Ganoderma lucidum* polysaccharide extract, improved primary symptoms (e.g., chest pain, palpitation, angina pectoris, shortness of breath) in a significantly higher percentage of patients compared with patients who received placebo, although the degree of improvement is unknown and difficult to measure. Because the study was conducted with an unknown dosage, the evidence is questionable.

Dose
The dose of reishi for angina has not been determined.

Adverse Effects, Interactions, Pharmacokinetics. See Appendix A.

Safflower (Carthamus tinctorius)

Grade C: *Unclear or conflicting scientific evidence (coronary artery disease/angina pectoris)*

Mechanism of Action. Insufficient available evidence.

Scientific Evidence of Effectiveness
A randomized controlled trial assessed the effect of safflower yellow injection in treating angina pectoris.[43] A total of 448 patients with angina pectoris were enrolled and divided into two groups: 336 in the test group treated with safflower yellow injection and 112 in the control group treated with *Salvia* injection by intravenous drip once daily for 14 days. Angina symptoms, ECG, and therapeutic effect improved significantly compared with the control group.

Adverse Effects, Interactions, Pharmacokinetics. See Appendix A.

Tribulus (Tribulus terrestris)

Grade C: *Unclear or conflicting scientific evidence (angina)*

Mechanism of Action
The exact mechanism of tribulus is not well understood; however, it has been shown to dilate coronary arteries and improve blood circulation.[44]

Scientific Evidence of Effectiveness
According to preliminary evidence, tribulus may be beneficial treatment for angina. Subjects who took tribulus experienced a greater angina pectoris remission rate compared with the control group.[44] Further research is needed before a recommendation can be made.

Dose
The dose of tribulus for CAD has not been determined.

Adverse Effects, Interactions, Pharmacokinetics. See Appendix A.

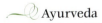 Ayurveda

There is some evidence that Ayurveda's comprehensive purification and detoxification regimen, known as *panchakarma*, may lead to increased vasoactive intestinal peptide (VIP, a vasodilator), acute reduction in total cholesterol, reduction in lipid peroxide (a measure of free-radical damage), and a significant reduction in anxiety in heart disease patients. *Abana* is a combination herbal and mineral formulation traditionally used in Ayurveda for cardiovascular health. Its main ingredients are *Terminalia arjuna, Withania somnifera, Terminalia chebula, Phyllanthus emblica, Nardostachys jatamansi, Tinospora cordifolia, Glycyrrhiza glabra, Zingiber officinale,* and *Nepeta hindostana*. Preliminary studies suggest that abana may reduce the frequency and severity of angina pain.[1]

Arjuna (Terminalia arjuna) is a type of bark powder traditionally used as an antiischemic and cardioprotective agent in high blood pressure and ischemic heart disease. It may be a safe and effective antiangina agent comparable to isosorbine mononitrate and better tolerated. However, further research is needed before a recommendation can be made.[1]

 Traditional Chinese Medicine

Traditional Chinese medicine (TCM) consists of herbs, acupuncture, food therapy, massage, and therapeutic exercise that are used to treat and prevent diseases.[1] TCM herbal formulas have been reported to reduce symptoms of stable and unstable angina. Certain natural products, such as kudzu, may be used to relieve myocardial ischemia and reduce myocardial oxygen consumption; herbs such as danshen may be used for their antiplatelet/anticoagulant action; and herbs such as ginseng may be used to relieve the symptom of chest pain.[45] However, research designs have been weak, and more studies of better quality are needed before recommendations can be made.

HERBAL THERAPIES WITH LIMITED EVIDENCE

Terminalia (Terminalia arjuna)

Terminalia is commonly used in Ayurvedic medicine, and has been shown to reduce post-MI angina, improve left ventricular ejection fractions, and decrease left ventricular mass when used as a short-term adjunct to conventional therapy, compared with standard therapy alone.[46,47]

 Herbs with Possible Antianginal Properties*

HERB	HERB
Arnica	Elecampane
Astragalus	Fo-ti
Bael fruit	Ginkgo
Bilberry	Horny goat weed
Blue flag	Khella
Bromelain	Scotch broom
California jimson weed	Sea buckthorn
Chia	Stinging nettle
Cinnamon	Tamarind
Coleus	Valerian
Comfrey	Yohimbe
Datura wrightii	

*This is not an all-inclusive or comprehensive list of herbs with antianginal properties; other herbs and supplements may possess these qualities. A qualified health care provider should be consulted with specific questions or concerns regarding potential antianginal effects of agents or interactions.
†Based on expert opinion, anecdote, case reports, and/or preliminary trial evidence.

ADJUNCT THERAPIES

1. *Kundalini yoga* is one of many traditions of yoga that share common roots in ancient Indian philosophy. It is comprehensive in that it combines physical poses with breath-control exercises, chanting (mantras), meditation, prayer, visualization, and guided relaxation. A case series report suggests that breathing techniques used in Kundalini yoga may help people with angina pectoris reduce symptoms and the need for medication. A specific breathing technique of Kundalini yoga reputed to help prevent heart attacks was examined to determine its effects on heart function. The technique is as follows: one breath per minute of respiratory exercise, with slow inspiration for 20 seconds, breath retention for 20 seconds, and slow expiration for 20 seconds. This occurs for 31 consecutive minutes. The technique was found to stabilize the heart's electrical wave patterns, which may have preventive value in heart health.[48,49]
2. The practice of *acupuncture*, or the insertion of needles into various points on the body, originated in China 5000 years ago. Some research also suggests that acupuncture may help reduce distress and symptoms of angina, but this has not been consistently shown in other studies.[50-54]
3. Early research suggests that *relaxation therapy* may reduce frequency of angina episodes, need for medication, and physical limitations.
4. Studies suggest that taking *supplements* such as coenzyme Q10, L-carnitine, and omega-3 fish oils may reduce symptoms of angina and may improve exercise tolerance.[55-65]

INTEGRATIVE THERAPY PLAN

- Discuss the patient's angina symptoms, including where and when symptoms occur.
- Discuss the patient's risk factors for coronary artery disease (CAD), including cigarette smoking, diabetes mellitus, dyslipidemia, and hypertension.
- Discuss the patient's family history of CAD.
- Encourage the use of nitrates for the prophylaxis and treatment of angina. Sublingual or aerosol nitroglycerin should be used to abort episodes of angina.
- Tell the patient that there is a lack of evidence to support the use of any herb or supplement for acute angina attacks.
- Inform the patient that there is a lack of strong supportive evidence for the use of any herb in the treatment of angina. However, promising herbal agents for the treatment of angina are kudzu, hawthorn, reishi, and safflower. Each of these herbs should be used cautiously when combined with other drugs used for cardiovascular disease, including antihypertensives and anticoagulants. Doses of these herbs for the treatment of angina have not been determined.
- Encourage patients to exercise and to follow a low-fat diet.

Case Studies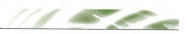

CASE STUDY 13-1

RF is a 60-year-old electrician who comes into your pharmacy and tells you that he has been experiencing occasional angina episodes, ranging from one to three episodes, usually while he is working. Current medications include atenolol (50 mg daily), hydrochlorothiazide (HCTZ, 25 mg daily), and nitroglycerin (NTG, 0.4 mg as needed). He does not smoke but drinks about four to five beers daily. He asks you if there is a natural product he can add to help relieve these episodes. How should you counsel?

Answer: Kudzu may reduce the frequency of angina events. However, it has the potential to cause additive blood pressure–lowering effects with the atenolol and HCTZ and additive vasodilatory effects with the NTG. The oral dose of kudzu to reduce angina symptoms has not been determined. Kudzu should only be taken under the supervision and monitoring of a health care professional. Moreover, since the U.S. Centers for Disease Control (CDC) defines "heavy drinking" as consuming an average of more than two drinks daily (for men) and one drink daily (for women), RF should be advised to cut back on his alcohol intake.

CASE STUDY 13-2

GE is a 68-year-old man with a 4-year history of chronic stable angina. He has been using sublingual NTG tablets, 0.4 mg as needed, and isosorbide dinitrate, 40 mg three times daily. He also takes a garlic supplement to lower his cholesterol. He has been experiencing two or three angina episodes per week. His daughter told him that hawthorn may help his chest pain. How should you counsel?

Answer: Hawthorn has been shown to be beneficial in angina and CAD. You may recommend 100 mg of Crataegus pinnatifida extract orally three times daily. This dose has been used in clinical trials and has been studied with NTG. Caution is warranted, however, when using hawthorn with garlic. Concurrent use may increase the risk of bleeding. Any unusual bruising or bleeding should be reported immediately. Taking hawthorn should be done under the strict supervision of GE's physician.

CASE STUDY 13-3

DS is a 56-year-old woman with a 30-year history of smoking and a 40-year history of type 1 diabetes. She currently takes metoprolol for chronic angina, insulin (Humalog, Lantus), and a phytoestrogen supplement. She also recently started having chest pains a few times a week, then started taking kudzu, which she read may help. Although her chest pains have lessened, her glucose levels have been off lately, and she has been having more hot flashes than usual. She asks for your advice. How should you counsel?

Answer: Concurrent use of herbs may mimic, enhance, or counteract the effects of drugs or other herbs and supplements. The recently added kudzu may lower blood glucose levels, interfere with phytoestrogen therapy, and cause additive blood pressure–lowering effects. You may want to counsel DS on discontinuing the kudzu, because it is interacting with various agents. You should also counsel DS regarding smoking cessation. Smoking will increase her chance of death from heart disease.

⊖ References for Chapter 13 can be found on the Evolve website at http://evolve.elsevier.com/Ulbricht/herbalpharmacotherapy/

Review Questions

1. All the following natural products have clinical evidence to support their use in angina *except:*
   a. Hawthorn
   b. Reishi mushroom
   c. Kava
   d. Safflower

2. True or false: Kudzu has been reported to reduce frequency of angina events, reduce need for nitrates, and improve abnormal rest ECG.

3. Danshen may alter which of the following?
   a. Lipids
   b. Coagulation panel
   c. Digoxin levels
   d. All the above

4. All the following statements are true *except:*
   a. Safflower contains linoleic acid, which is rapidly excreted into human breast milk.
   b. Injection of safflower oil has been shown to reduce symptoms of angina pectoris in patients with coronary artery disease.
   c. Injection of safflower yellow has been shown to reduce symptoms of angina pectoris in patients with coronary artery disease.
   d. Safflower may cause allergic reactions in patients sensitive to daisies.

5. All the following statements are true *except:*
   a. Ginseng, as a monotherapy, may reduce symptoms of coronary artery disease, such as anginal chest pain.
   b. Danshen has been reported to be as effective as isosorbide dinitrate (Isordil) in relieving symptoms of angina.
   c. Reishi mushroom has been well tolerated for up to 16 months.
   d. Hawthorn has not been tested against standard-of-care drugs.

6. Which of the following is true of hawthorn?
   a. Hawthorn has not been associated with any adverse effects.
   b. Hawthorn safety has been systematically evaluated in patients.
   c. There is good evidence supporting the use of hawthorn to treat angina.
   d. Because of in vitro evidence of thromboxane A_2 inhibition, hawthorn should be used cautiously with anticoagulants/antiplatelets such as warfarin.

7. True or false: A breathing technique of Kundalini yoga has been shown to be beneficial for heart health.

Answers are found in the Answers to Review Questions section in the back of the text.

14 Ischemic Disease and Heart Rhythm Disorders

Outline

OVERVIEW
    Myocardial Infarction (Heart Attack)
        Types of Myocardial Infarction
        Signs and Symptoms
        Diagnosis
    Cerebrovascular Accident (Stroke)
        Types of Stroke
        Signs and Symptoms
        Diagnosis
    Arrhythmia (Dysrhythmia)
        Types of Arrhythmia
        Tachycardias
        Bradycardias
        Premature Heartbeats
        Syncope (Fainting)
        Signs and Symptoms
        Diagnosis
SELECTED HERBAL THERAPIES
    Aconite (*Aconitum napellus*)
    Arnica (*Arnica* spp.)
    Astragalus (*Astragalus membranaceus*)
    Betel nut (*Areca catechu*)
    Danshen (*Salvia miltiorrhiza*)
    Flax (*Linum usitatissimum*)
    Garlic (*Allium sativum*)
    Ginkgo (*Ginkgo biloba*)
    Horny Goat Weed (*Epimedium grandiflorum*)
    Policosanol
    Pomegranate (*Punica granatum*)
    Quercetin
    Resveratrol
    Safflower (*Carthamus tinctorius*)
    Sea Buckthorn (*Hippophae rhamnoides*)
    Squill (*Urginea maritima,* syn. *Scilla maritima*)
    Tea (*Camellia sinensis*)
HERBAL THERAPIES WITH NEGATIVE EVIDENCE
HERBAL THERAPIES WITH LIMITED EVIDENCE
HERBS THAT MAY CAUSE ARRHYTHMIA
ADJUNCT THERAPIES
INTEGRATIVE THERAPY PLAN
    Myocardial Infarction and Stroke
    Arrhythmia
CASE STUDIES
REVIEW QUESTIONS

Learning Objectives

- Define characteristics of myocardial infarction, stroke, and arrhythmia.
- Discuss herbs that may be used for myocardial infarction, stroke, and arrhythmia.
- Review data currently available to support herbal treatment selection for myocardial infarction, stroke, and arrhythmia.
- Explain mechanisms of action, adverse effects, and interactions associated with herbs used for myocardial infarction, stroke, and arrhythmia.
- Educate patients regarding integrative pharmacotherapy plans.

CHAPTER 14 Ischemic Disease and Heart Rhythm Disorders

OVERVIEW

Myocardial Infarction (Heart Attack)

Myocardial infarction (MI), commonly known as *heart attack*, occurs when the supply of blood and oxygen to an area of heart muscle is blocked (Figure 14-1).[1-3] A *thrombus* is a blood clot in an intact blood vessel. In a large vessel, a thrombus decreases blood flow through that vessel. In a small blood vessel, blood flow may be completely cut off, resulting in *ischemia* (lack of blood) and the death of tissue supplied by that vessel. If the clot completely stops the blood flow in the coronary artery, an MI develops. If a thrombus dislodges and becomes free floating, it is an *embolus*; this free-floating clot may travel to other parts of the body. If treatment is not started quickly, the affected area of heart muscle begins to die. This injury to the heart muscle can lead to serious complications and may even be fatal. A person can survive a heart attack, but part of the heart muscle may be damaged. This may result in shortness of breath and chest pain (angina) on exertion or at rest, and may also increase the risk for another MI.

Sudden death from MI can result from an arrhythmia called *ventricular fibrillation*.[1-3] However, the survival rate for U.S. patients hospitalized with MIs is 90% to 95%, a significant improvement related to improvements in emergency medical response and treatment strategies.[1-3] In general, a heart attack can occur at any age, but its incidence rises with age and depends on predisposing risk factors. Approximately 50% of all MIs in the United States occur in people younger than 65 years of age, but as the baby-boomer population ages, this percentage will probably shift, and more people age 65 and older may be affected.

Ischemic heart disease remains the leading cause of death in the United States as well as in most industrialized nations. Approximately 800,000 people in the United States are affected annually, and 250,000 die before arrival at a hospital. Approximately every 65 seconds, an American dies of a heart-related medical emergency. The World Health Organization (WHO) estimated that in 2002, 12.6% of deaths worldwide were from ischemic heart disease.[1-4]

Types of Myocardial Infarction

There are several types of heart attacks. *Acute coronary syndrome* (ACS) refers to three types of coronary artery disease that are associated with sudden rupture of plaque inside the coronary arteries: unstable angina, non–ST-segment elevation myocardial infarction (NSTEMI), or ST-segment elevation myocardial infarction (STEMI). The location of the blockage, the length of time that blood flow is blocked, and the amount of damage that occurs determines the type of ACS. Figure 14-2 is an algorithm for evaluation and management of patients suspected of having ACS.[5]

Unstable Angina

Angina pectoris is a type of chest pain that occurs when the heart cells do not receive enough oxygen (see chapter 13). Unstable angina can occur more frequently, occur more easily at rest, feel more severe, or last longer than stable angina. Although this type of angina can often be relieved with oral medications, it is unstable and may progress to a heart attack. More intense medical treatment or a procedure usually is required. Unstable angina is a type of ACS and should be treated as a medical emergency.[1-3]

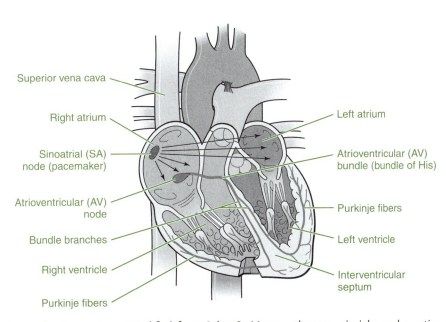

Figure 14-1 The heart's conduction system. (Modified from Salvo S: *Massage therapy: principles and practice*, ed 2, St Louis, 2003, Mosby.)

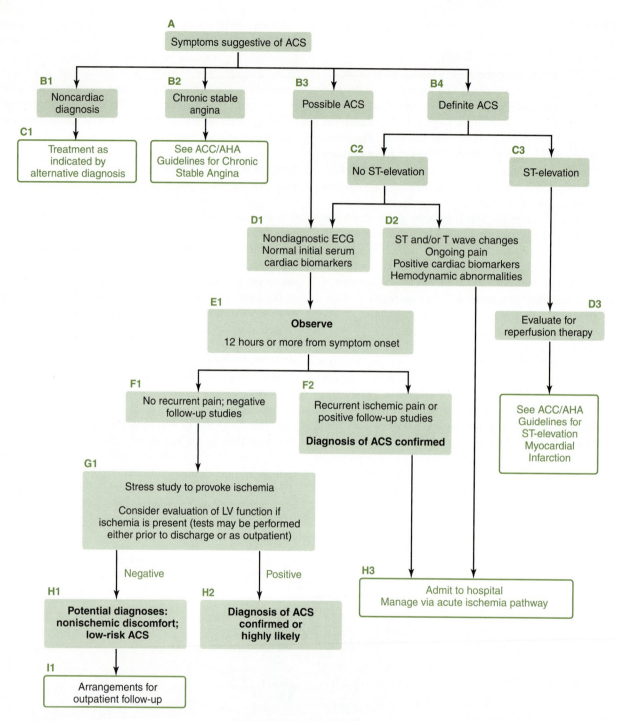

Figure 14-2 Algorithm for evaluation and management of patients suspected of having acute coronary syndrome (ACS). ACC/AHA, American College of Cardiology/American Heart Association; ECG, electrocardiogram; LV, left ventricular. (Modified from the ACC/AHA 2007 guidelines for the management of patients with unstable angina/non-ST-elevation myocardial infarction, Circulation 116[7]:148.)[5]

Non–ST-Segment Elevation Myocardial Infarction

This myocardial infarction does not cause changes on an electrocardiogram (ECG). However, chemical markers in the blood, including C-reactive protein (CRP), creatine kinase MB (CK-MB), and troponin, indicate that damage has occurred to the heart muscle. In NSTEMI the blockage may be partial or temporary, so the extent of the damage to the heart is relatively minimal.[1-3]

ST-Segment Elevation Myocardial Infarction

The STEMI type of heart attack is caused by prolonged ischemia. It affects a large area of the heart muscle, causing changes on the electrocardiogram (ECG), as well as in blood levels of the key chemical markers.[1-3]

Atherosclerosis

Atherosclerosis is the hardening and narrowing of the arteries. It is caused by the slow buildup of plaque on the inside of walls of the arteries. Plaque is made up of fat, cholesterol, calcium, and other substances found in the blood. As plaque builds up, it causes the inside of the artery to narrow, and it may eventually restrict blood flow.

Coronary Artery Disease

Coronary artery disease (CAD), also known as *coronary heart disease* (CHD), occurs when the coronary arteries gradually become narrowed or blocked by plaque deposits. Depending on where the blockage occurs, this can lead to a heart attack or stroke. Sometimes an MI is the first sign of CAD. Some individuals with CAD and ischemia have no symptoms; this is called "silent ischemia." In rare cases a patient may have a "silent heart attack," which is an MI without symptoms.

Signs and Symptoms

Classic symptoms of MI include chest pain or pressure, jaw pain, or extension of pain into the arms or shoulder (especially the left arm). Pain may also occur in the back or upper abdomen; gastrointestinal problems (such as heartburn, indigestion, nausea, or vomiting) are also common. Other symptoms may include unexplained shortness of breath, unexplained sweating, heart palpitations, anxiety, a sudden feeling of illness, and general lethargy.

Sometimes a heart attack is the first sign of CAD. According to the Framingham Heart Study, more than 50% of men and 63% of women who died suddenly of CAD (mostly from heart attack) had no previous symptoms of this disease, and approximately 25% of all MIs occur without chest pain or other symptoms.[1-3] These silent MIs can occur more frequently in people with diabetes. Symptoms of a silent heart attack can include discomfort in the chest, arms, or jaw that seems to go away after resting; shortness of breath; and tiring easily.

Diagnosis

Electrocardiograms, blood tests, and imaging studies are used to diagnose MI.[1-3] An ECG is performed during the initial evaluation and triage of patients with suspected acute MI. It indicates if an MI is in progress or has already occurred. Blood tests detect evidence of myocardial cell death. Cardiac enzymes are considered the "gold standard" for diagnosing MI and are obtained at regular intervals starting on admission and performed consecutively for about 2 days. Other laboratory studies include tropinin and myoglobin levels, complete blood count (CBC), chemistry profile, and lipid profile. Cardiac enzymes are compared with ECG and physical examination findings. An echocardiogram may be useful in determining which portion of the heart the MI affected and which coronary arteries are likely occluded. Other helpful diagnostic tools include chest radiography and myocardial perfusion imaging.

Cerebrovascular Accident (Stroke)

A stroke, or cerebrovascular accident (CVA), is similar to a heart attack but affects the brain instead of the heart. A stroke involves the sudden interruption of blood flow and oxygen to areas in the brain and can cause brain damage and loss of function. A stroke develops suddenly, usually in a matter of minutes, and causes symptoms such as paralysis, numbness or weakness (often affecting one side of the body), confusion, dizziness, speech problems, and loss of vision. Symptoms vary depending on where the CVA occurs in the brain and the extent of brain damage.

Strokes are medical emergencies, and prompt treatment could mean the difference between life and death. Early treatment can also minimize damage to the brain and reduce the risk of disability. In the United States, strokes are leading causes of adult disability and the third-leading cause of death; only heart disease and cancer cause more deaths annually. Men are 1.25 times more likely to have strokes than women, yet 60% of deaths from stroke occur in women. An estimated 80% of CVAs are preventable, which would save approximately 600,000 Americans annually.[1-3,6]

Types of Strokes

Ischemic Stroke

About 80% of CVAs are ischemic strokes.[1-3,6] Blood clots or other particles such as cholesterol may block arteries to the brain and cause ischemia. This deprives the brain cells of necessary oxygen and nutrients and may lead to cell death within minutes. The most common ischemic strokes include thrombotic stroke and embolic stroke.

Thrombotic Stroke

The thrombotic type of ischemic stroke occurs when a thrombus forms in one of the arteries that supply blood to the brain. Areas damaged by atherosclerosis are highly susceptible to developing a blood clot. Carotid arteries that carry blood to the brain are susceptible. An ischemic stroke may also be caused by *stenosis*, or narrowing of the artery, which is caused by a buildup of plaque.

Embolic Stroke

An embolic stroke is a type of ischemic stroke that occurs when a thrombus or other particle forms in a blood vessel away from the brain and travels through the blood, eventually to lodge in narrower brain arteries (embolus). Emboli may often be caused by irregular beating in the heart's two upper chambers *(atrial fibrillation)*. This abnormal heart rhythm can lead to stagnant blood flow and the formation of blood clots.

Hemorrhagic Stroke

Hemorrhagic stroke occurs when a blood vessel in the brain leaks or ruptures. Hemorrhages can result from a number of conditions that affect the blood vessels, including *aneurysms* (abnormal dilation or bulging of an artery) and uncontrolled hypertension. A less common cause of hemorrhage is the rupture of an *arteriovenous malformation* (AVM), or a malformed tangle of thin-walled blood vessels present at birth. The two types of hemorrhagic stroke are intracerebral hemorrhage and subarachnoid hemorrhage.

In intracerebral hemorrage, a blood vessel in the brain bursts and spills into the surrounding brain tissue, damaging cells. Brain cells beyond the leak are deprived of oxygen and are also damaged. Hypertension is the most common cause of intracerebral hemorrhagic stroke, causing small arteries inside the brain to become fragile and susceptible to tearing and rupture.

In subarachnoid hemorrhage bleeding starts in a large artery on or near the membrane surrounding the brain and spills into the space between the surface of the brain and skull. A subarachnoid hemorrhage is often signaled by a sudden, severe headache, sometimes called a "thunderclap" headache. This type of stroke is typically caused by the rupture of an aneurysm, which can develop with age or result from a genetic predisposition. After a subarachnoid hemorrhage, vessels may go into *vasospasm,* in which arteries near the hemorrhage widen and narrow erratically, causing brain cell damage by further restricting or blocking blood flow to portions of the brain.

Signs and Symptoms

Signs and symptoms of a stroke include sudden numbness or weakness of the face, arm or leg, especially on one side of the body; sudden confusion; trouble speaking or understanding; sudden trouble seeing in one or both eyes; sudden difficulty walking, dizziness; loss of balance or coordination; and sudden, severe headache with no known cause.

For most people, stroke has no warning. One possible indicator of a future stroke is a *transient ischemic attack* (TIA). A TIA is a temporary interruption of blood flow to some part of the brain. TIA signs and symptoms are similar to stroke but last a shorter time (usually several minutes to 24 hours), then disappear with no apparent permanent effects. Individuals who have had a TIA are at a very high risk of stroke.[1-3,6]

Diagnosis

Several types of physical examinations and tests may be performed in the diagnosis of stroke. Risk factors of stroke are evaluated, including high blood pressure, high cholesterol levels, diabetes, medications, elevated levels of homocysteine, and obesity. Stroke symptoms are documented after the occurrence, often using scoring systems such as the National Institutes of Health Stroke Scale, Cincinnati Stroke Scale, and Los Angeles Prehospital Stroke Screen. These tests ask medical history questions and measure left-sided and right-sided paralysis.[1-3,6]

Carotid ultrasonography evaluates blood flow using a wandlike device *(transducer)* that sends high-frequency sound waves into the neck. Narrowing or clotting in the carotid arteries can be determined.

Arteriography views arteries in the brain not normally able to be seen in x-ray films. A catheter is inserted through a small incision, usually in the groin area. The catheter is manipulated through the major arteries and into the carotid or vertebral artery. A dye is then injected through the catheter to provide x-ray images of the arteries.

In computed tomographic angiography (CTA) a dye is injected into the blood, and x-ray beams create a three-dimensional image of the blood vessels in the neck and brain. CTA is used to look for aneurysms or AVMs and to evaluate arteries for narrowing. CT scanning, which is done without dye, can provide images of the brain and show hemorrhages, but without as much detailed information about the blood vessels.

Magnetic resonance imaging (MRI) uses a strong magnetic field to generate a three-dimensional view of the brain. This test is sensitive for detecting an area of brain tissue damaged by an ischemic stroke. Magnetic resonance angiography (MRA) uses this magnetic field and a dye injected into the veins to evaluate arteries in the neck and brain.

Arrhythmia (Dysrhythmia)

The majority of MIs are accompanied by abnormal heart rhythms, also called *arrhythmia* or *dysrhythmia*.[1,7] When the heart beats, the electrical impulses that cause it to contract must follow a precise pathway through the heart. Any change in the normal conduction will disrupt the heart rhythm and may cause the heart to pump blood less effectively.[1,2]

Each day, a normal heart contracts about 100,000 times, at a rate of 60 to 100 times a minute. Not all heart rhythm variations indicate disease; changes in rate brought about by variations in activity, diet, medications, and age are common. For example, during exercise it is normal to develop sinus tachycardia as the heart speeds up to provide body tissues with more oxygen-rich blood. During intense exercise, a heart may speed up to 160 to 180+ beats per minute. Running up a flight of stairs or being startled by a noise account for normal increases in heart rate as well.[1,2] The rapid-fire contractions in all these situations are faster than the normal resting heart rate but generally pose little or no danger.

In arrhythmias the heartbeats may be too slow (bradycardia, <60 beats/min), too rapid (tachycardia, >100 beats/min), too early (premature contraction), or irregular (atrial or ventricular fibrillation). In most people, arrhythmias are minor and are not dangerous. A small number of people, however, have arrhythmias that are dangerous and require treatment.

The rhythm of the heart is normally generated and regulated by pacemaker cells within the *sinoatrial* (SA) *node,* which is located within the wall of the right atrium of the heart. SA nodal pacemaker activity normally governs the rhythm of the atria and ventricles. Normal rhythm is very regular, with minimal fluctuation. Furthermore, atrial contraction is normally followed by ventricular contraction. When this rhythm becomes irregular, or when the frequency of the atrial and ventricular beats are different, this is called an arrhythmia. In general, arrhythmias that start in the ventricles are more serious than those that start in the atria.[1,2]

Heart cells are voltage dependent and rely on a careful balance of sodium, potassium, and calcium, which move in and out of cells to cause muscle contraction. The signals that carry out the contractions rely not only on sodium, potassium, and calcium channels but also on beta receptors that affect heart rate.

About 14 million people in the United States have arrhythmias. During a 24-hour period, about 20% of healthy adults are likely to have multiple types of premature ventricular beats. The most common arrhythmias are atrial fibrillation and atrial flutter. As many as 2 million Americans are living with atrial fibrillation. The number of atrial arrhythmias is highly related to age and the presence of underlying heart disease. The prevalence approaches 30% after open-heart surgery.[1,2]

Types of Arrhythmia

Arrhythmias are classified not only by where they originate (atria or ventricles) but also by the speed of the resulting heart rate.

Tachycardia refers to a fast heart rate, greater than 100 beats a minute. When the heart beats too quickly, the ventricles do not have enough time to fill with blood and cannot effectively pump blood to the rest of the body. The lack of oxygen can prove deadly and gives rise to symptoms, including the heart skipping a beat or palpitations, dyspnea, dizziness, syncope, temporary blind spots, angina, and even death.

Bradycardia refers to a slow heartbeat, or a resting heart rate less than 60 beats a minute. Some bradycardias do not produce any symptoms; others do and warrant treatment. When the heart beats too slowly, not enough oxygen-rich blood flows throughout the body. Symptoms of bradycardia include fatigue and weakness, dizziness, lightheadedness, syncope, and dyspnea. *Tachycardia* and *bradycardia* are general terms that refer to a number of specific conditions, which are discussed below.

Tachycardias

Atrial Fibrillation

Atrial fibrillation is a common arrhythmia and affects mainly older people (60 years and older). It results from normal wear and tear on the heart muscle, as well as from cardiovascular problems such as hypertension (high blood pressure). During atrial fibrillation the electrical activity of the atria becomes uncoordinated. The atria beat so rapidly, as fast as 350 to 600 beats per minute, that instead of producing a single, forceful contraction, they fibrillate (quiver). Atrial fibrillation can be intermittent (paroxysmal), lasting a few minutes to an hour or more before returning to a regular heart rhythm. It can also be chronic, causing an ongoing problem. Atrial fibrillation is seldom a life-threatening arrhythmia, but over time it can be the cause of more serious conditions, such as stroke (CVA).

Atrial Flutter

Atrial flutter is similar to atrial fibrillation. Both can coexist in the heart, coming and going in an alternating manner. The key distinction is that the more organized and rhythmic electrical impulses are called atrial *flutter*. These occur because atrial flutter, unlike atrial fibrillation, arises from a short circuit. In typical atrial flutter, this short circuit exists in the right atrium. This is an important distinction because typical right atrial flutter is more amenable to some forms of treatment, such as catheter ablation.

Supraventricular Tachycardia

Supraventricular tachycardia (SVT) is a broad term that includes many forms of arrhythmia originating above the ventricles (supraventricular). SVTs usually cause a burst of rapid heartbeats that begin and end suddenly and can last from seconds to hours. These often start when the electrical impulse from a premature heartbeat begins to circle repeatedly through an extra pathway. SVT may cause the heart to beat 160 to 200 times a minute. Although generally not life threatening in an otherwise normal heart, symptoms from the racing heart may feel quite uncomfortable. These arrhythmias are common in young people.

WOLFF-PARKINSON-WHITE SYNDROME. One cause of SVT is known as Wolff-Parkinson-White syndrome. This arrhythmia is caused by an extra electrical pathway between the atria and the ventricles. This pathway may allow electrical current to pass between the atria and the ventricles without passing through the *atrioventricular* (AV) *node*, leading to short circuits and rapid heartbeats.

Ventricular Tachycardia

Ventricular tachycardia (VT) is a fast, regular beating of the heart caused by abnormal electrical impulses originating in the ventricles. Often, VTs are caused by a short circuit around a scar from a previous MI and can cause the ventricles to contract more than 200 beats per minute. Most VT occurs in individuals with some form of heart-related problem, such as scars or damage within the ventricle muscle from CAD or MI. Some VTs last for 30 seconds or less (called *unsustained*) and are usually harmless, although they cause inefficient heartbeats. Still, an unsustained VT may be a predictor of more serious ventricular arrhythmias, such as longer-lasting *(sustained)* VT. An episode of sustained VT is a medical emergency. It may be associated with palpitations, dizziness, fainting, or possibly death. Without prompt medical treatment, sustained VT often degenerates into ventricular fibrillation. Rarely, VT occurs in an otherwise normal heart, when it is much less dangerous, although the condition still needs medical attention.

Ventricular Fibrillation

About 300,000 Americans die every year of sudden cardiac death believed to be caused by ventricular fibrillation (VF).[1,2] With VF, rapid, chaotic electrical impulses cause the ventricles to quiver uselessly instead of pumping blood. Without an effective heartbeat, the blood pressure falls rapidly, cutting off blood supply to vital organs, including the brain. Most individuals lose consciousness within seconds and require immediate medical assistance, including cardiopulmonary resuscitation (CPR). The chances of survival may be prolonged if CPR is delivered until the heart can be shocked back into a normal rhythm with a device called a *defibrillator*. Without CPR or defibrillation, death results in minutes. Most cases of VF are linked to some form of heart disease; they are frequently triggered by MI.

Long-QT Syndrome

Long-QT syndrome can be acquired or inherited. When the QT interval is prolonged, ventricle cells may not have recovered in time to conduct the next heartbeat properly. In older adults, this rare arrhythmia may be triggered by certain medications, including antibiotics, antidepressants, antihistamines, diuretics, heart medications, cholesterol-lowering drugs, diabetes medications, as well as some antifungal and antipsychotic drugs, which may affect the heart's electrical function. Individuals with long-QT syndrome are prone to palpitations and fainting spells and may have an increased risk of sudden death. Beta blockers are the drugs of choice for patients with long-QT syndrome.[1,2]

Bradycardias

Sick Sinus

If the pacemaking sinus node is not sending impulses properly, the heart rate may be too slow, or it may speed up and slow down intermittently. If the sinus node is functioning properly, sick sinus can be caused by an impulse block near the sinus node that is slowing, disrupting, or completely blocking conduction.

Conduction Block

Conduction block of the heart's electrical pathways can occur in or near the AV node or along pathways that conduct impulses to each ventricle. Depending on the location and type of block, the impulses between the atria and ventricles may be slowed or partially or completely blocked. If the signal is completely blocked, certain cells in the AV node or ventricles are capable of initiating a steady, although usually slower, heartbeat. Some blocks may cause no signs or symptoms, and others may cause skipped beats or bradycardia. Even without signs or symptoms, a conduction block is usually detectable on an ECG. Since some blocks are caused by heart disease, an ECG showing a block may be an early sign of heart problems.

Premature Heartbeats

Premature heartbeats can originate in either the atria or the ventricles. Although it is often described as a skipped heartbeat, a premature heartbeat is actually an extra beat between two normal heartbeats. Premature heartbeats occurring in the ventricles come before the ventricles have had time to fill with blood following a regular heartbeat.

This type of arrhythmia is typically caused by stimulants, such as caffeine from coffee, tea, soft drinks, over-the-counter (OTC) cold remedies containing pseudoephedrine, and some asthma medications. If they occur regularly, premature heartbeats may indicate a more serious problem.

Syncope (Fainting)

Fainting, or syncope, is a sudden loss of consciousness. It most often occurs when the blood pressure is too low (hypotension) and the heart does not pump a normal supply of oxygen to the brain. Typically, a fainting spell lasts only a few seconds or minutes, and then the individual regains consciousness. Syncope is a common problem that affects 1 million people in the United States every year.[1,2] About one third of the population will faint at least once during their lifetime. A single fainting spell usually is not serious. It may be explained by factors such as stress, grief, overheating, dehydration, exhaustion, or illness.

Signs and Symptoms

Many arrhythmias cause no signs and symptoms other than irregular heart rhythm (which may or may not be noticeable). Some of the most common signs include palpitations, changes in the speed or "patter" of the heartbeat (too slow, too rapid, irregularity, feeling of pauses between beats), anxiety, weakness, dizziness, lightheadedness, near-fainting, sweating, shortness of breath, and chest pain.

Diagnosis

Cardiac cycles (or heartbeats) are triggered by electrical impulses, which may be detected via electrodes by an electrocardiograph machine. An electrocardiogram or ECG (commonly referred to as EKG, from the German "Elektrokardiogramm") is a graphical representation of these electrical impulses and may be used to identify an abnormal heart rhythm. In a normal cardiac cycle, the P wave (which represents atrial contraction) precedes the QRS wave complex (which corresponds to ventricular depolarization). The QRS complex is followed by the T wave, which denotes the repolarization of the ventricles in preparation for the next cardiac cycle. U waves are detectable in 50% to 75% of ECGs; these follow the T wave and are thought to indicate papillary muscle or Purkinje fiber repolarization. The amplitude and duration of these waves (as well as the durations of the intervals between them) may be diagnostic of a number of cardiac conditions. For example, an elevated ST segment (between the QRS complex and the T wave) may be indicative of MI. Alterations in ECG readings may also represent damaged heart muscle, which may occur after MI.

Sound waves may be used to create a moving image of a beating heart, called an *echocardiogram* (echo), which is similar to an ultrasound. Thus, echocardiograms may also be referred to as "cardiac ultrasounds." Both ECGs and echocardiograms are widely used to diagnose a variety of cardiovascular conditions, including MI and arrhythmia. Echocardiograms may also be used to identify physical abnormalities that contribute to arrhythmias.

SELECTED HERBAL THERAPIES

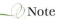
Note
To help make this educational resource more interactive, all pharmacokinetics, adverse effects, and interactions data have been compiled in Appendix A. Safety data specifically related to pregnancy and lactation are listed in Appendix B. Please refer to these appendices when working through the case studies and answering the review questions.

Aconite (*Aconitum napellus*)

Grade C: *Unclear or conflicting scientific evidence (arrhythmia)*

Note: Based on widespread use, many experts believe aconite to be unsafe, even in recommended amounts in otherwise healthy individuals.

Mechanism of Action

Aconite is a highly toxic plant that has been used historically as a poison. In very low doses, it has also been used historically to treat a number of conditions. Aconite may induce several cardiac effects, including bradycardia, hypertension, hypotension, and tachycardia. These may be mediated by α-adrenergic and serotonergic pathways and are largely attributed to the alkaloids aconitine, hypaconitine, mesaconitine, and jesaconitine. Aconite-induced bradycardia is thought to involve the hypothalamus and surrounding muscarinic receptors.[8,9] Aconite induces vasoconstriction, which contributes to hypertensive effects; tachycardic effects are thought to be mediated by β-adrenergic receptors.[10] The constituent *higenamine* has been shown to have positive inotropic effects in guinea pig papillary muscles.[11] High doses of aconite have positive chronotropic effects in rats, whereas low doses may have either positive or negative chronotropic effects; these may result in bradycardia, tachycardia, arrhythmia, or hypertension.[12] Aconite may produce extremely rapid tachycardia, flutter, and fibrillation by spontaneously inducing slow depolarization.[13]

Scientific Evidence of Effectiveness

Clinical studies involving aconite are limited; however, a specific constituent of aconite (higenamine) has been shown to improve bradyarrhythmias in patients with coronary heart disease.[14] These conclusions need to be validated in randomized controlled trials (RCTs) before clinical applications are justified. The toxic effects of aconitine may limit its ability to be used clinically as an agent to treat bradycardias.

Dose

A safe and effective dose of aconite for bradyarrhythmia has not been determined.

Adverse Effects, Interactions, Pharmacokinetics. See Appendix A.

Arnica (*Arnica* spp.)

Grade C: *Unclear or conflicting scientific evidence (stroke)*

Mechanism of Action

The sesquiterpene lactones of arnica, including helenalin and dihydrohelenalin, have been shown to inhibit human platelet aggregation[15] and reduce serum lipids in animals.[16] These constituents have also been shown to inhibit nuclear factor kappa B (NF-κB)–mediated inflammation,[17,18] histamine-induced vascular permeability,[19] and neutrophil migration.[20]

Scientific Evidence of Effectiveness

Despite the basic scientific evidence, clinical studies thus far do not show significant effects of arnica on coagulation. Some studies have used arnica in homeopathic preparations, in which the concentrations of the active ingredients are so low (or even nonexistent) that they are unlikely to achieve the effects. There is limited evidence that homeopathic concentrations of arnica may increase bleeding time in healthy male volunteers.[21] However, there is also contradictory evidence that homeopathic concentrations of arnica have no significant effects over placebo in stroke victims.[22]

Dose

The dose of homeopathic arnica for stroke (CVA) has not been determined.

Adverse Effects, Interactions, Pharmacokinetics. See Appendix A.

Astragalus (*Astragalus membranaceus*)

Grade C: *Unclear or conflicting scientific evidence (coronary artery disease)*

Mechanism of Action

Astragalus constituents, particularly the flavonoids, exert significant cellular antioxidant effects, which appear to be protective against cardiovascular, hepatic, pulmonary, and renal pathological changes.[23,24] Similarly, astragalus appears to protect cells against hypoxic challenges. *Astragaloside IV* has been reported to protect human endothelial cells and intestinal epithelial cells against reperfusion injury in vitro after hemorrhagic shock.[25] Cellular protection from anoxia has also been observed in cultured neurons[26] and in mouse brain after transient focal ischemia.[27] Astragaloside IV has also been reported to inhibit platelet aggregation, decrease plasminogen activation, and facilitate intravascular lysis of fibrin clots in humans and in animal disease models.[28,29] In a model of ototoxicity, astragalus protected cells from pathological injury through enhanced DNA and RNA synthesis.[30]

Experimental studies indicate that astragalosides affect cardiovascular function at the cellular, isolated-tissue, and whole-body level in both animals and humans. In isolated working rat hearts, astragalus extract produced positive inotropic actions at higher doses and negative inotropic effects at low doses.[31] Astragalus also produces hypotensive actions through peripheral vasodilation in healthy and hypertensive animals.[32,33] Astragalus significantly reduced arterial pressure in a rat model of renal hypertension and improved cardiac function in experimental congestive heart failure.[34] This effect was confirmed by another study, in which astragalus improved left ventricular systolic function and potentiated the cardiotonic, diuretic, and natriuretic renal response to atrial natriuretic peptide in rats with experimentally induced chronic heart failure.[35] In vitro evidence indicates that astragalus may also stimulate angiogenesis and revascularization in ischemic myocardium[36] and amnion[37] and promote vascular endothelial cell proliferation and DNA synthesis.[37] Astragalus may increase sodium pump activity in erythrocytes[38] and lower cholesterol.[39]

Scientific Evidence of Effectiveness

Most clinical studies suggest that astragalus may exert beneficial antioxidant and antilipidemic actions, as well as improve immune responses in acute MI.[40-46] However, because of design and analysis limitations of most studies, the clinical efficacy data are inconclusive.

Dose

Astragalus products are available standardized to 70% polysaccharides, 0.3% astragaloside content, or 0.5% triterpenoids glycoside content, according to secondary sources. For CAD, astragalus (20 g) was administered three times daily in one study.[41] Powdered dried whole astragalus root has been used at 1 to 3 g daily, according to secondary sources.

Astragalus fluid extract (1:1 water or alcohol whole-root extract in 25% ethanol) has been administered in doses of 2 to 4 mL three or four times daily. Other general dosing regimens have included (1) 250 to 500 mg of astragalus extract four times daily, (2) boiling-water extract of up to 60 g of dried astragalus root daily, and (3) powdered–astragalus root capsules at 500 to 1000 mg three times daily.

Adverse Effects, Interactions, Pharmacokinetics. See Appendix A.

Betel Nut (Areca catechu)

Grade C: Unclear or conflicting scientific evidence (stroke)

Note: Despite widespread recreational use, betel nut cannot be considered safe for human use (particularly when used chronically or in high doses) because of documented toxicity associated with acute or chronic chewing and oral consumption.

Mechanism of Action

Betel nut contains a number of related pyridine alkaloids, notably *arecoline*, which may range in concentration from 0.1% to 0.9%. In high concentrations, arecoline may inhibit neutrophil functions. Betel nut extracts stimulate the production of prostaglandin E_2 (PGE_2) and induce cyclooxygenase-2 (COX-2) messenger ribonucleic acid (mRNA) in human gingival keratinocytes in vitro, providing a potential explanation for the oral inflammation seen in betel nut users. However, cytotoxicity appears to occur independently from prostaglandin alterations.[47] Areca II-5-C, a fraction isolated from betel, showed angiotensin-converting enzyme (ACE) inhibitory activity in vitro.[48] Areca nut extracts lowered concentrations of cholesterol and triglycerides significantly in rats fed a diet containing cholesteryl oleate.[49]

Scientific Evidence of Effectiveness

A small number of poor-quality studies have been conducted in patients recovering from thromboembolic CVA (stroke).[50,51] Recovery of various measures of functional status have been reported to improve statistically significantly faster in subjects ingesting an aqueous extract of betel nut versus those not using betel nut. It is unclear whether these results may be caused by central nervous system (CNS) stimulant or cholinergic activity. Because of methodological weaknesses with the available data, as well as the known risks associated with betel use, it is not clear if the potential benefits outweigh the risks.

Dose

The dose of betel nut for stroke has not been determined.

Adverse Effects, Interactions, Pharmacokinetics. See Appendix A.

Danshen (Salvia miltiorrhiza)

Grade C: Unclear or conflicting scientific evidence (ischemic stroke)

Mechanism of Action

Given the number of potentially active ingredients in danshen, the mechanism by which danshen imparts benefit is not clear. However, its effects may be caused, at least in part, by its antioxidant effects. In a study of patients with ischemic infarction, danshen decreased levels of lipid peroxide and apolipoprotein (apo) B-100 and increased levels of superoxide dismutase and apo A-1 in serum.[52] In animals, danshen decreased cerebral cortex levels of vasoactive intestinal peptide (VIP), which plays a role in ischemia.[53] Other animal studies suggest danshen offers cellular protection during stroke.[54-62]

Scientific Evidence of Effectiveness

In animals, danshen offers cellular protection during stroke[54-62] and pretreatment and treatment with danshen for focal cerebral ischemia reduced infarct volume and significantly improved neurological function.[63] However, treatment after stroke had negative effects on function. Because of limited evidence from human trials,[52,64,65] unclear safety, and more proven treatments for ischemic stroke, danshen is not recommended as a primary treatment for stroke. Moreover, interactions between danshen and warfarin have been noted.[66]

Dose

Note: Treatment with danshen after ischemia may aggravate brain injury.

Danshen is often combined with other herbs. Oral dosing of danshen alone has not gained strong evidence for efficacy; therefore, no specific dose can be recommended. There is no widespread consensus about the safe or efficacious dosing of intravenous (IV) danshen. Dosing is available from poor-quality studies only and is not adequately reported in all studies. An IV dose of 8 mL danshen (16 g of the herb diluted in 500 mL of a 10% glucose solution) daily for 1 to 4 weeks has been used to treat ischemic stroke.[64]

Adverse Effects, Interactions, Pharmacokinetics. See Appendix A.

Flax *(Linum usitatissimum)*

Grade C: *Unclear or conflicting scientific evidence (atherosclerosis/coronary artery disease)*

Mechanism of Action

Flaxseed is composed of multiple chemical constituents, the mechanisms of which are slowly being elucidated. Flaxseed is approximately 35% oil, of which 55% is alpha-linolenic acid (ALA).[67-71] Approximately 60% of flaxseed oil is omega-3 fatty acid, and 18% to 20% is omega-6 fatty acid. Flaxseed and linseed oil contain 30% to 45% unsaturated fatty acids, and approximately 8% of the plant contains soluble fiber mucilage.[72] The plant also contains 20% protein. Flaxseed oil is composed of 73% polyunsaturated fatty acids (PUFAs), 18% monounsaturated fatty acids, and 9% saturated fatty acids.

It is thought that the antioxidant properties of flaxseed may exert a beneficial effect on atherosclerotic plaque formation. Omega-3 fatty acids have been shown to suppress oxygen-free radicals from neutrophils and monocytes, as well as the production of interleukin-1 (IL-1), tumor necrosis factor (TNF), and leukotriene B_4 (LTB_4).[73] Lignans can act as platelet-activating factor (PAF) receptor antagonists and inhibit the production of oxygen free radicals by neutrophils.[67,74]

Flaxseed oil has been demonstrated to inhibit platelet aggregation.[75] Increased bleeding time is associated with the ALA component of both flaxseed and flaxseed oil.[76] Diets high in ALA have been reported to improve arterial compliance.[77]

Scientific Evidence of Effectiveness

It has been proposed that flaxseed may exert a beneficial effect on atherosclerotic plaque formation or cardiovascular outcomes, based on purported antioxidant and lipid-lowering properties.[78,79] There is a paucity of strong human data in this area. However, there is promising evidence regarding the role of n-3 PUFAs and ALA for improving outcomes in individuals with CAD. In addition, animal studies suggest beneficial effects of flaxseed on atherosclerotic plaque formation. ALA-rich diets, such as the Mediterranean diet, have been associated with improved outcomes in patients who have already had an MI.[80] Despite this evidence, it remains unclear if flaxseed supplementation improves human cardiovascular endpoints, and dosing regimens are not established.

Dose

Flaxseed products are not standardized based on specific chemical components, but rather are evaluated with a number of identity and quality tests. Tests may include microscopic and macroscopic inspection and organoleptic evaluation (see Mechanism of Action).

Patients who had survived a recent (<3 months) MI and who received 1 g of n-3 PUFAs daily for 2 years had a reduction in death, nonfatal MI, and stroke.[81]

Adverse Effects, Interactions, Pharmacokinetics. See Appendix A.

Garlic *(Allium sativum)*

Grade C: *Unclear or conflicting scientific evidence (atherosclerosis)*

Mechanism of Action

Currently, garlic is one of the most widely used herbal compounds in the United States, with ongoing research in several areas related to cardiovascular health, oncology, and infectious diseases. Garlic's mechanism of action appears to be related to many compounds and not only to allicin, as previously believed.[82-85] The European Scientific Cooperative on Phytotherapy (ESCOP) lists the following indications for garlic: prophylaxis of atherosclerosis, treatment of elevated blood lipids, improvement of circulation in peripheral arterial vascular disease, upper respiratory tract infections, and catarrhal conditions.[86] In addition, the World Health Organization (WHO) lists the following uses for garlic as supported by clinical data: adjuvant for dietary management for hyperlipidemia, prevention of age-dependent atherosclerosis, and possibly mild hypertension.[87]

Garlic appears to exert numerous effects on the cardiovascular system, and atherosclerosis in particular, beyond the reduction of serum lipids. The multiple protective effects of garlic may include inhibition of platelet aggregation and enhancement of fibrinolysis.[88-90]

Garlic and its derived compound, *ajoene*, have demonstrated inhibition of platelet aggregation in vitro and in vivo[91-102] and reduction of platelet-dependent thrombus formation.[103-104] Antiplatelet activity may also be attributable to adenosine, allicin, and paraffinic polysulfides.[105] Several preclinical studies and controlled human trials have reported impaired platelet aggregation associated with oral garlic use.[92,106-112] Raw garlic has been shown to inhibit platelet COX in vitro.[93] Dose-dependent inhibition of COX in human placental villi was observed with garlic and with allicin-negative (acid-washed) garlic.[113] However, boiling garlic before administration appears to reduce or abolish the antiplatelet effects.[93,102]

Increased fibrinolytic activity, involving fibrinogen and plasminogen, may account for some degree of garlic's anticlotting effects.[84,114-116] Both raw garlic and cooked garlic, as well as essential oil from raw garlic, have demonstrated significant increases in fibrinolytic activity in humans.[117,118] An increase in fibrinolytic activity in patients with ischemic heart disease was found to be maintained after 7 to 8 weeks of continued therapy.[119,120]

Scientific Evidence of Effectiveness

There is limited evidence regarding the effects of garlic on the prevention or treatment of atherosclerosis. A small number of studies have explored this issue and reported favorable results, although overall these studies have been poorly designed and reported, including unclear descriptions of randomization, blinding, plaque measurement methods, and statistical analysis.[121,122] In patients with past MIs, garlic may reduce the reinfarction rate, though further study is warranted.

Dose

The Lichtwer Pharma GmbH (Berlin) standardized powder product Kwai has often been used in studies utilizing fresh garlic and is standardized to 1.3% allicin content. Other trials have used a standardized preparation that contains 220 mg of garlic powder and produces 2.4 mg of allicin in vitro.[124] U.S. Pharmacopeia–grade garlic must contain 0.3% (powdered) to 0.5% (fresh, dried) allicin, whereas European Pharmacopeia–grade garlic must yield no less than 0.45% allicin.

An ESCOP 1997 monograph recommends 3 to 5 mg of allicin daily (1 clove, or 0.5-1.0 g dried powder) for prophylaxis of atherosclerosis.[86] A WHO 1999 monograph recommends 2 to 5 g of fresh garlic, 0.4 to 1.2 g of dried garlic powder, 2 to 5 mg of garlic oil, 300 to 1000 mg of garlic extract, or other formulations corresponding to 2 to 5 mg of allicin.[87]

Adverse Effects, Interactions, Pharmacokinetics. See Appendix A.

Ginkgo (Ginkgo biloba)

Grade C: Unclear or conflicting scientific evidence (acute ischemic stroke)

Mechanism of Action

Flavonoids (glycosides) and terpenoids (ginkgolide, bilobalide) are considered to be ginkgo's primary active components.[125-129] Most studies have been conducted with the standardized ginkgo preparation EGb 761 (24% ginkgo flavone glycosides, 6% terpenoids), or LI 1370 (25% ginkgo flavone glycosides, 6% terpenoids). Ginkgo has been found to have vasodilatory effects, which have been attributed to stimulation of endothelium-derived relaxing factor (EDRF) and prostacyclin release. Studies suggest that ginkgo inhibits nitric oxide, and arachidonic acid metabolism causing vascular relaxation.[130-133] Ginkgo ingestion has also been demonstrated to reduce the levels of thiobarbituric acid reacting (TBAR) substances[134] and malondialdehyde[135] in human platelets. In a controlled single-blind study of 10 healthy human subjects[136] and a controlled crossover study of patients with known claudication,[137] ginkgo was shown to increase blood capillary flow significantly and decrease erythrocyte aggregation.

Scientific Evidence of Effectiveness

It has been postulated that ginkgo therapy may be beneficial after acute ischemic stroke because of vascular and antioxidant properties.[138] However, the limited available evidence suggests that ginkgo does not elicit clinical improvements in patients after ischemic CVAs. In clinical study, patients with computed tomographic (CT) evidence of acute ischemic infarction were given ginkgo, 40 mg four times daily for 4 weeks.[139] At 2 and 4 weeks, no difference was noted between the ginkgo and placebo groups in scores on the validated Matthew's neurological assessment scale.

Dose

The dose of ginkgo for acute ischemic stroke has not been determined.

Adverse Effects, Interactions, Pharmacokinetics. See Appendix A.

Horny Goat Weed (Epimedium grandiflorum)

Grade C: Unclear or conflicting scientific evidence (atherosclerosis)

Mechanism of Action

Epimedium is traditionally used to treat cardiovascular disease. It has been suggested to lower blood lipids, have free radical–scavenging activity, and adjust balance between prostacyclin (PGI_2) and thromboxane A_2 (TXA_2).[8]

Scientific Evidence of Effectiveness

Limited clinical study suggests that *Epimedium* may improve symptoms associated with ischemic cardiocerebrovascular diseases.[140] After *Epimedium* treatment the total and marked effective rates were 96.7% and 39.5%, respectively. The ECG improved in 70% of patients with coronary heart disease (CHD) and in 75% of those with cerebral arteriosclerosis. However, further well-designed clinical trials are required before a conclusion can be made.

Dose

The dose of horny goat weed for atherosclerosis has not been determined.

Adverse Effects, Interactions, Pharmacokinetics. See Appendix A.

Policosanol

Grade B: *Good scientific evidence (coronary heart disease)*

Mechanism of Action

Policosanol is a natural mixture of higher aliphatic primary alcohols, isolated and purified from sugar cane (*Saccharum officinarum*) wax.[141-143] There is strong scientific evidence for policosanol's effects in hypercholesterolemia and platelet aggregation inhibition. Policosanol has a protective effect on the development of atherosclerotic lesions[144] and reduces several other CHD risk factors, including blood pressure[145,146] and lipid peroxidation.[147-149]

Scientific Evidence of Effectiveness

The effects of policosanol supplementation on exercise-ECG testing responses have been studied in patients with CHD.[150] Beneficial changes were noted in functional capacity, rest and exercise angina, cardiac events, and maximum oxygen uptake. The effect was even more significant when policosanol was administered with aspirin. Although this represents early compelling evidence, further research is necessary before a clear conclusion can be reached.

Dose

For CHD, 5 to 40 mg of policosanol daily has been studied with favorable results.[151,152]

Adverse Effects, Interactions, Pharmacokinetics. See Appendix A.

Pomegranate (*Punica granatum*)

Grade C: *Unclear or conflicting scientific evidence (atherosclerosis)*

Mechanism of Action

Several mechanisms of action have been hypothesized for the antiatherogenic effects exhibited by pomegranate juice, which contains a significant amount of polyphenols. Mice treated with pomegranate juice have significantly reduced macrophage-mediated oxidation of low-density lipoprotein (LDL). Pomegranate juice also reduced the size of atherosclerotic lesions and foam cell numbers in mice.[153] Compound 25, an isolated antioxidant compound from pomegranate, reduced both copper sulfate ($CuSO_4$)–induced LDL oxidation and atherosclerotic lesions in mice. Pomegranate juice and compound 25 reduced plasma lipid peroxide concentrations by 17% and 25%, respectively. The cellular degradation rate of LDL oxidized by peritoneal macrophages was reduced by 25% and 34% for whole-pomegranate juice and compound 25, respectively.[154] Consumption of pomegranate juice also resulted in other LDL modifications, including prolongation of LDL oxidation time, reduction of LDL aggregation, and reduction of LDL retention (entrapment of LDL in arterial walls) in vitro.[153]

Collagen-induced platelet aggregation was significantly decreased in platelet-rich plasma obtained from healthy men consuming pomegranate juice for 2 weeks compared to baseline. This effect may be caused by the interaction of constituents in pomegranate juice and collagen binding sites on platelet surfaces, or by the free radical–scavenging ability of pomegranate.[153]

Scientific Evidence of Effectiveness

Although pomegranate juice has usually been consumed for atherosclerosis, evidence of its effectiveness is inconclusive. Pomegranate juice did not cause significant changes in lipid profiles of healthy men or animals. Ex vivo collagen-induced platelet aggregation was significantly decreased in platelet-rich plasma obtained from men who received pomegranate juice, suggesting a protective effect against atherosclerosis.[153] Pomegranate juice decreased serum ACE activity and lowered blood pressure in elderly hypertensive patients.[155] Pomegranate juice supplementation decreased size of atherosclerotic lesions and foam cell numbers in atherosclerotic apolipoprotein E–deficient (E0) mice.[153]

Dose

For atherosclerosis, 50 mL of pomegranate juice was administered by mouth daily for 2 weeks.[156] In another study, subjects consumed 1 L of pomegranate juice daily for 5 days.[156]

Adverse Effects, Interactions, Pharmacokinetics. See Appendix A.

Quercetin

Grade C: *Unclear or conflicting scientific evidence (cardiovascular disease)*

Mechanism of Action

Quercetin is a major flavonol, one of the almost 4000 polyphenolic compounds (flavonoids) that occur ubiquitously in foods of plant origin. It mainly occurs in plants as glycosides, such as *rutin* (quercetin rutinoside) in tea. Quercetin consumption has exhibited an inhibitory effect on development of aortic atherosclerotic lesions and on atherogenic modifications of LDL injury by inhibiting lipoprotein oxidation or directly protecting cells from oxidized LDL.[157-159] The effects may be mediated by the metabolites of quercetin.[160]

Scientific Evidence of Effectiveness

Laboratory and animal studies suggest that flavonoids may effectively reduce cardiovascular disease risk. Such effects include inhibition of the oxidation and cytotoxicity of LDL as well as general antioxidant effects. Quercetin has been associated with risk reduction for CHD,[161,162] stroke, cancers, and other medical conditions, but strong evidence to support any of these associations is lacking.

Dose

Healthy men and women with cholesterol levels of 4.0 to 7.2 mmol/L consumed four capsules daily of a quercetin-containing supplement (1.0 g quercetin daily) for 28 days. Quercetin intakes were approximately 50-fold greater than the dietary intakes associated with lower CHD mortality on the basis of epidemiological studies.[163]

Adverse Effects, Interactions, Pharmacokinetics. See Appendix A.

Resveratrol

Grade C: *Unclear or conflicting scientific evidence (cardiovascular disease)*

Mechanism of Action

Resveratrol can exist as both *cis* and *trans* isomers. The *trans* isomer is thought to be the more active one, that is, the isomer responsible for the beneficial effects of red wine on decreasing the risk of cardiovascular disease. Subsequently, a large percentage of research performed is done using the *trans* isomer.

Resveratrol may offer cardioprotective effects through various mechanisms. Resveratrol has been shown to strongly inhibit nitric oxide (NO) generation in activated macrophages in vitro,[164] as well as to increase endothelial NO synthase expression.[165-167] Also, data suggest that resveratrol suppresses the aberrant expression of various cytokines in vascular cells in vitro.[168] Resveratrol inhibits the activity of COX-2.[169] Also in vitro, resveratrol has been shown to inhibit angiogenesis.[170] Resveratrol administration before ischemia attenuates ischemic/reperfusion damage of isolated Langendorff perfused rat hearts.[171] In isolated arteries from female guinea-pigs, resveratrol induced vasorelaxation.[172] In isolated endothelium-intact rat aorta, resveratrol inhibited the contractile response to noradrenaline.[173]

Resveratrol has been suggested to have oxygen-scavenging activity.[174] In rats, short-term administration of resveratrol inhibited renal lipid peroxidation induced by ischemia and reperfusion in both the cortex and the medulla, through an NO-dependent mechanism.[175] Preincubation of human platelets with resveratrol has a protective effect against the oxidation of platelet thiols induced by peroxynitrite (ONOO-).[176] Resveratrol has also been suggested to increase peroxidase activity.[177]

Laboratory studies suggest that resveratrol has antiaggregating and antithrombin activity.[166,168,178-184] Resveratrol significantly inhibited the adhesion of activated platelets[185] as well as the aggregation of stimulated platelets in vitro and in animal models.[178,179,182,186-190]

Scientific Evidence of Effectiveness

Limited available study has examined the effects of a combination therapy including resveratrol on risk factors for cardiovascular disease. Through alterations in lipoprotein metabolism, oxidative stress, and inflammatory markers, intake of the combination product beneficially affected key risk factors for CHD in both premenopausal and postmenopausal women.[191] The effects of resveratrol cannot be adequately assessed from this trial using a combination regimen, because of the possible confounding effects of the other constituents.

Dose

The dose of resveratrol for cardiovascular disease has not been determined.

Adverse Effects, Interactions, Pharmacokinetics. See Appendix A.

Safflower (Carthamus tinctorius)

Grade C: *Unclear or conflicting scientific evidence (atherosclerosis/coronary artery disease)*

Mechanism of Action

Safflower oil is high in oleic acid. It is lower in saturates and higher in monounsaturates than olive oil. In the U.S. diet, safflower oil has been frequently substituted for oils with higher saturated fat content, because monounsaturated fat may have a beneficial effect on the risk of CHD.[192] The cardioprotective effects of safflower oil may result from its ability to inhibit platelet aggregation, as demonstrated in human studies.[193-197]

Scientific Evidence of Effectiveness

In clinical studies, safflower oil has reduced blood pressure and improved anticoagulation and fibrinolytic function.[193,198,199] Safflower oil has been shown to increase oxidation of LDL and had lower thiobarbituric acid–reactive substances (TBARS) compared with fish oil.[200,201]

Dose

The dose of safflower for atherosclerosis is not well understood.

Adverse Effects, Interactions, Pharmacokinetics. See Appendix A.

Sea Buckthorn (Hippophae rhamnoides)

Grade C: *Unclear or conflicting scientific evidence (cardiovascular disease)*

Mechanism of Action

Sea buckthorn contains numerous constituents that may have beneficial effects in heart disease prevention, including vitamin E, carotenoids, flavonoids, sterols, PUFAs, free amino acids, and flavonols (especially pentamethylquercetin, syringetin, isorhamnetin, quercetin, kaempherol, and myricetin).[202-206] The total flavones of sea buckthorn display inhibitory effects on ACE activity and on angiotensin II formation in vitro.[207] In healthy mice, flavonoids from sea buckthorn significantly reduced serum cholesterol and serum triglyceride levels.[205,208] Similar effects were not observed in human studies,[203,206,209] although an increase in HDL levels was noted in limited available study.[210] Sea buckthorn has also shown antiplatelet effects.[203,211]

Scientific Evidence of Effectiveness

Studies have been conducted using different formulations of sea buckthorn to improve cardiovascular conditions;[212,213] however, the details of these trials were not clearly reported.

Dose

The dose of sea buckthorn for cardiovascular disease has not been determined.

Adverse Effects, Interactions, Pharmacokinetics. See Appendix A.

Squill (*Urginea maritima*, syn. *Scilla maritima*)

Grade C: *Unclear or conflicting scientific evidence (coronary artery disease)*

Mechanism of Action

According to secondary sources, *scillitoxin* and *scillipicrin* in squill are cardiac substances with effects similar to digoxin, including positive inotropic and negative chronotropic effects. Squill may have additional cardiovascular properties that include reducing left ventricular diastolic pressure and reducing pathologically elevated venous pressure.

Scientific Evidence of Effectiveness

Squill has been observed to have cardiokinetic constituents.[214] A 1-mg dose of methylproscillaridin, a glycoside of squill, demonstrated an increase in the maximum rate of pressure development in the left ventricle compared to placebo.[215] These preliminary results suggest that squill may have some cardiac effects. However, more clinical research is needed to determine the clinical significance of squill in CAD.

Dose

The dose of squill for CAD has not been determined.

Adverse Effects, Interactions, Pharmacokinetics. See Appendix A.

Tea (*Camellia sinensis*)

Grade C: *Unclear or conflicting scientific evidence (heart attack prevention)*

Mechanism of Action

Tea flavonoids may reduce the risk of platelet aggregation or endothelial dysfunction, proposed to be beneficial against blockage of arteries in the heart.[8] However, the mechanisms of action remain unclear; clinical evidence suggests that non-flavonoid constituents may contribute to the cardioprotective effects of tea. The long-term effects of tea consumption on cardiovascular risk factors, such as cholesterol levels, blood pressure, and atherosclerosis, are not known.

Scientific Evidence of Effectiveness

Numerous epidemiological, cohort, and case-control studies show that diets containing tea and other dietary flavonoids are inversely associated with cardiovascular disease and stroke.[216] The purported cardioprotective and antithrombotic effects of tea have been attributed to flavonoids; however, clinical research suggests that other constituents (or perhaps other lifestyle factors) may be responsible for the risk reduction observed in epidemiological studies.[217]

Dose

Tea (450 mL to 900 mL daily) was administered to patients with CAD for 4 weeks to examine its effects on platelet aggregation.[217]

Adverse Effects, Interactions, Pharmacokinetics. See Appendix A.

Traditional Chinese Medicine

Traditional Chinese medicine (TCM) is a broad term encompassing many different modalities and traditions of healing. TCM places strong emphasis on herbal medicine. There are more than 2000 different kinds of herbs used in TCM; about 400 are frequently used, often in combination with other herbs or ingredients (see Chapter 31).

Some herb combinations have been found to improve some markers of CHD and to reduce symptoms of stable and unstable angina. TCM herb combinations have also been used in stroke and to stabilize arrhythmia after viral myocarditis (inflammation of heart). Despite a long history of efficacy, research on TCM is limited.

In TCM, therapies for ischemic diseases can be grouped into four broad categories based on mechanism of action: antiinflammatory drugs, antithrombotic drugs, neuroprotective drugs, and drugs associated with TCM philosophical principles. The latter group is least conducible to well-controlled clinical research; however, the other three categories contain several herbs with some evidence of efficacy from theory, basic science, or animal studies.

Continued

Traditional Chinese Medicine—cont'd

Willow bark (*Salix* spp.), an herb used in TCM, has documented antiinflammatory activities. A major constituent of willow bark extract is salicylic acid, which is a precursor to the well-known antiinflammatory/antithrombotic aspirin[218-230]. Other TCM herbs with thrombotic effects include ligusticum root (*Ligusticum* spp.),[221] danshen (*Salviae miltiorrhizae*),[66,217] dong quai (*Angelica sinensis*),[222] ginseng (*Panax* spp.),[223] stephania (*Stephania tetrandrae*),[224] and Chinese peony (*Paeoniae* spp.).[225] TCM herbs with putative neuroprotective effects include gastrodia (*Gastrodiae* spp.),[226] danshen,[227] and ginseng.[228] Of note, ginseng has been associated with menometrorrhagia (uterine bleeding) and tachychardia.[229]

HERBAL THERAPIES WITH NEGATIVE EVIDENCE

Evening Primrose (Oenothera biennis)

Grade D: *Fair negative scientific evidence (cardiovascular health)*

Preliminary research of evening primrose oil shows a lack of significant beneficial effects on cardiovascular function and health.[230]

HERBAL THERAPIES WITH LIMITED EVIDENCE

Bilberry (Vaccinium myrtillus)

Bilberry contains several compounds belonging to the flavonoid class of organic compounds, including anthocyanins[231,232] and resveratrol, another type of flavonoid.[233,234] Flavonoids have been shown in vitro to possess a number of biological properties, including inhibition of prostacyclin synthesis, reduction of capillary permeability and fragility, free radical scavenging, inhibition of a wide range of enzymes, impairment of coagulation and platelet aggregation, and anticarcinogenicity.[235,236] Anthocyanins have been shown to inhibit platelet aggregation in vitro.[237-241]

Bilberry has been used traditionally to treat symptoms of vascular disease, including CAD. However, there is limited human research in this area. Preliminary evidence from numerous in vitro and animal studies has suggested that bilberry extracts may be useful in the prevention of vascular disease.[242-244] Bilberry extracts have been shown to decrease platelet aggregation and may reduce oxidation of LDL.[245-249] In animal studies, *Vaccinium myrtillus* anthocyanoside (VMA) extract was shown to reduce microvascular impairment after reperfusion[250] and to reduce vascular permeability in the setting of hypertension.[243] Decreases in lipid deposition

Herbs with Potential Antiischemic or Antiarrhythmic Properties*

HERB	SPECIFIC THERAPEUTIC USE(S)†	HERB	SPECIFIC THERAPEUTIC USE(S)†
Abuta	Palpitations	Feverfew	Myocardial injury
Agrimony	Cardiotonic	Fo-ti	Cerebral ischemia
Annatto	Cardiotonic	Ginseng	Ischemia-reperfusion injury prevention, stroke, myocardial injury, palpitations
Ashwagandha	Stroke		
Bacopa	Cardiotonic	Goldenseal	Arrhythmia
Bael fruit	Cardiotonic, palpitations	Hawthorn	Arrhythmia
Barberry	Arrhythmia	Katuka	Myocardial infarction
Black cohosh	Palpitations	Kava	Cerebral ischemia, stroke
Bloodroot	Palpitations	Khella	Myocardial infarction (recovery), arrhythmia
Calamus	Arrhythmia		
Cat's claw	Stroke, arrhythmia	Kudzu	Cerebral ischemia
Chia	Stroke, myocardial infarction, ischemic injury	Lavender	Arrhythmia
		Lemon balm	Palpitations
Chicory	Tachycardia	Lime	Palpitations
Cinnamon	Arrhythmia	Lotus	Cardiotonic, palpitations
Codonopsis	Myocardial injury, palpitations	Mangosteen	Cardiotonic
Cordyceps	Arrhythmia	Milk thistle	Ischemic injury
Devil's claw	Arrhythmia	Mistletoe	Tachycardia
Dong quai	Stroke, arrhythmia, palpitations	Muira puama	Stroke
Elecampane	Myocardial infarction	Myrcia	Cardiotonic
Essiac	Paralysis	Neem	Cardiac arrhythmia
False hellebore	Cerebrovascular accident (stroke), arrhythmia, heart rate reduction (homeopathic)	Nopal	Ischemic injury
		Oleander	Cardiotonic

Herbs with Potential Antiischemic or Antiarrhythmic Properties—cont'd

HERB	SPECIFIC THERAPEUTIC USE(S)†	HERB	SPECIFIC THERAPEUTIC USE(S)†
Pycnogenol	Cerebral ischemia, myocardial ischemia/reperfusion injury, cardiac mitral valve prolapse	Shiitake	Stroke prevention (cerebral hemorrhagic)
		Skullcap	Stroke, myocardial ischemia
Rhodiola	Stroke, arrhythmia	Sweet woodruff	Arrhythmia
Rosemary	Ischemic heart disease	Valerian	Nervous tachycardia
Seaweed	Fatty heart	White horehound	Arrhythmia

*This is not an all-inclusive or comprehensive list of herbs with antiischemic or antiarrhythmic properties; other herbs and supplements may possess these qualities. A qualified health care provider should be consulted with specific questions or concerns regarding potential adverse effects of antiischemic or antiarrhythmic agents or interactions with other therapies.
†Based on expert opinion, anecdote, case reports, and/or preliminary trial evidence.

and intimal proliferation have also been demonstrated in VMA-treated animals.[251] These studies suggest that there may be a vasoprotective role for VMA in ischemic diseases. However, supportive clinical evidence is lacking.

Chamomile (Matricaria recutita, syn. Matricaria suaveolens, Matricaria chamomilla, Anthemis nobilis, Chamaemelum nobile, Chamomilla chamomilla, Chamomilla recutita)

Chamomile has been used medicinally for thousands of years and is widely used in Europe. It is a popular treatment for numerous ailments, including sleep disorders, anxiety, digestion and intestinal conditions, skin infections and inflammation (including eczema), wound healing, infantile colic, teething pains, and diaper rash.[8] In the United States, chamomile is best known as an ingredient in herbal tea preparations used as a mild sedative. Chamomile contains *coumarin*, a widespread plant compound that is the chemical precursor to warfarin and other anticoagulants;[252-253] however, the specific effects of chamomile on coagulation are unclear.

Foxglove (Digitalis purpurea, Digitalis lanata)

Traditionally, foxglove (*Digitalis purpurea*) has been used to treat atrial fibrillation or atrial flutter.[254] However, because of its toxicity profile and cases of poisoning, foxglove is not considered safe;[8] furthermore, with advent of newer pharmacotherapies for cardiac disorders, the use of digitalis has declined.[254]

Meadowsweet (Filipendula ulmaria)

Meadowsweet has historically been used to treat stomach complaints, inflammatory conditions, and symptoms of the common cold. Two prominent constituents of meadowsweet, salicylates and a plant form of heparin, are theoretically responsible for much of its pharmacological activity.[218,255] Many of the uses and side effects of meadowsweet correlate with those of pharmaceutical preparations of salicylates and heparin.[8]

Although meadowsweet shares chemistry, history, and proposed uses with the drug aspirin,[218,255] its efficacy and place in pharmacotherapy compared with aspirin have not been evaluated in well-designed clinical studies.

Red Clover (Trifolium pratense)

Red clover has been shown to improve vascular endothelial function in diabetic postmenopausal women,[256] but not in healthy postmenopausal women.[257] Further study is warranted to determine the effects of red clover on cardiovascular parameters.

Scotch Broom (Cytisus scoparius)

Scotch broom herb has been taken by mouth traditionally for a variety of conditions related to the heart or blood circulation, including arrhythmias (tachycardia), peripheral edema, pulmonary edema, congestive heart failure, hypotension, and cardiomyopathy. The effects of scotch broom have been attributed to the alkaloid *sparteine*, which is present in small amounts. Sparteine is a class 1a antiarrhythmic agent and may affect the electrical conductivity of heart muscle (similar to other class 1a antiarrhythmic drugs such as quinidine).[8] However, sparteine is not approved by the U.S. Food and Drug Administration (FDA) for use in treating arrhythmias.

In spite of the known cardiovascular effects of sparteine,[258-262] there is limited clinical evidence regarding scotch broom use in humans. It is not clear if sparteine found in the plant form has clinically meaningful effects. These potential properties of scotch broom may be dangerous in individuals with heart disease or those who are taking cardiac medications.

Willow (*Salix* spp.)

Willow bark from certain *Salix* species contains *salicin* (salicylic acid), which is mildly analgesic and has been used historically to treat many different types of pain.[218-220] In several European countries, willow bark is approved for use in treating fever, pain, inflammation, and a variety of other complaints. Salicylic acid is a chemical precursor to acetylsalicylic acid, known commonly as aspirin, which is currently used not only as an analgesic and antipyretic, but also to prevent MI, CVA, and colorectal cancer.[219] Some herbalists recommend willow bark extract as a natural substitute for aspirin for these same benefits. In Germany, willow bark is often taken along with aspirin to enhance therapeutic effects while minimizing side effects.

HERBS THAT MAY CAUSE ARRHYTHMIA

This section is not an all-inclusive or comprehensive discussion of herbs that may cause arrhythmia; other herbs and supplements may possess these qualities. A qualified health care practitioner should be consulted with specific questions or concerns.

Ephedra (*Ephedra sinica*)

Lethal cardiac arrhythmias have been associated with the use of ephedrine alkaloids (ephedra).[263,264] All ephedra products are banned in the United States because of multiple serious cardiovascular adverse effects associated with its use. Caffeine has been shown to potentiate the effects of ephedra.[265-267]

Ginseng (*Panax* spp.)

A 39-year-old woman was using both topical and oral ginseng (species not indicated) for "cosmetic reasons." An ECG revealed sinus tachycardia with occasional atrial premature beats. After 10 days of not using ginseng, the arrhythmia stopped.[229]

Guarana (*Paullinia cupana*)

An increased risk of ventricular premature beats is associated with high consumption of caffeine, the active constituent of guarana. There have been numerous case reports of arrhythmias associated with guarana use.[268-271] Death from intractable ventricular fibrillation was reported in a 25-year-old woman with previously diagnosed mitral valve prolapse who had a postmortem caffeine level of 19 mcg/mL from a guarana-containing drink.[268]

ADJUNCT THERAPIES

1. An integrative approach to prevent myocardial infarction (MI, heart attack) and cerebrovascular accident (CVA, stroke) may involve diet changes, dietary supplements, exercise, and relaxation techniques. Furthermore, because some foods and supplements may contribute to arrhythmia, these should be avoided as well. Certain lifestyle choices may thus significantly decrease cardiovascular disease risk.

2. Hyperlipidemia (also known as dyslipidemia, high cholesterol, or hypercholesterolemia) refers to unhealthy levels of cholesterol in the blood (see Chapter 16). Hyperlipidemia is considered a major risk for both stroke and coronary heart disease (CHD), which includes MI. Sources of soluble fiber, such as barley, oats, and psyllium, may help reduce serum cholesterol. Soy consumption may also help to improve cholesterol levels. For foods containing soy protein, the FDA has approved the use of health claims regarding the benefits of soy in lowering the risk of CHD. Other supplements with good scientific evidence for improving cholesterol include β-glucan, β-sitosterol, niacin, omega-3 fatty acids, fish oil, and alpha-linolenic acid (ALA).

3. Coronary heart disease is often referred to as coronary artery disease (CAD). The most common symptom of CAD is angina pectoris, which results from insufficient oxygen to the heart cells. Angina is described as a feeling of discomfort (heaviness, pressure, aching, burning, numbness, fullness, squeezing, or pain) in the chest. Nitrates remain important agents for treating angina. Some herbs, such as kudzu (*Pueraria lobata*) and hawthorn (*Crataegus* spp.), may also provide some relief in angina; however, strong evidence is lacking, and the antianginal mechanisms remain unclear. Herbs traditionally used to treat angina include ginseng, puncture vine (*Tribulus terrestris*), and terminalia (*Terminalia arjuna*). Chronic stable angina may be accompanied by secondary carnitine deficiency, for which L-carnitine supplementation is effective.

4. Hypertension is also considered a major risk factor for both heart disease and stroke (see Chapter 11). Strong evidence supports the role of omega-3 fatty acids, fish oil, and ALA, found in some plants and fish, in reducing blood pressure. Hibiscus (*Hibiscus* spp.) and stevia (*Stevia rebaudiana*) also possess hypotensive properties and have been used traditionally to treat hypertension. Alternative modalities that may lower blood pressure with good supporting evidence include Qi gong and yoga.

5. As a central role in numerous biological processes, *magnesium* is essential for the health of many organisms. Dietary magnesium may be derived from numerous sources, even tap water. Epidemiological studies have associated high magnesium intake with reduced risk of cardiovascular disease.[272] As a mild calcium antagonist, magnesium is given intravenously to treat acute-onset atrial fibrillation, purportedly with fewer side effects than other calcium antagonists or amiodarone.[273] The epidemiological evidence strongly suggests that magnesium intake may directly affect cardiovascular risk factors; however,

clinical studies have yielded inconsistent results. The association between reduced cardiovascular disease risk and high magnesium intake may simply result from healthy dietary choices.[272]

6. Several aromatic herbs, such as black pepper *(Piper nigrum)* and peppermint *(Mentha x piperita)*, have been used to treat secondary symptoms in recovering stroke patients. Nasal inhalation of black pepper has been suggested to improve symptoms of swallowing dysfunction after stroke.[274] Peppermint oil has been used with other oils (as aromatherapy) to reduce hemiplegic shoulder pain in stroke patients[275] and may improve cognitive function after brain injury.[276] More studies are needed to assess the effectiveness of both black pepper and peppermint aromatherapy in stroke recovery.

7. *Cerebral insufficiency* is a term often used to describe decreased blood flow to the brain caused by clogged arteries (e.g., ischemic stroke). Ginkgo is often used to improve cognitive function, and there is some evidence that ginkgo supplementation may improve short-term memory and concentration and reduce dizziness, headaches, and mood disturbances in patients with cerebral insufficiency (see Chapter 10).

8. *Ischemic cardiomyopathy* is a term used to describe CAD that has progressed to congestive heart failure (CHF). Forskolin, an active constituent of coleus *(Coleus forskohlii)*, has antithrombotic[277,278] and inotropic[279] actions that may explain its beneficial effects in cardiomyopathy, a common cause of CHF. A small number of studies suggest that forskolin may improve cardiovascular function in patients with cardiomyopathy.[280-282] Although most studies have used isolated forskolin extract, it is believed that the whole coleus plant may also be effective, because of the presence of multiple compounds that may act synergistically. Other important constituents of coleus are caffeic acid and its derivatives, such as rosmarinic acid; these compounds have been shown to have antioxidant effects.[283]

INTEGRATIVE THERAPY PLAN

Myocardial Infarction and Stroke

- All individuals should undergo blood pressure monitoring at routine medical visits. Individuals age 20 and older should also have their blood lipid profiles (total cholesterol, HDL cholesterol, LDL cholesterol, and triglycerides) measured at least once every 5 years.
- Discuss the patient's family history of heart disease or stroke.
- Discuss modifiable risk factors associated with cardiovascular disease and stroke, including hyperlipidemia, hypertension, diabetes, obesity, physical activity, and smoking.
- Preventive measures for hypertension and hyperlipidemia include a healthy diet and regular exercise. Diets high in fiber and omega-3 fatty acids, yet low in saturated fats (especially *trans* fats) and cholesterol, will help maintain healthy blood lipid levels. Regular exercise and weight reduction will also help to maintain healthy blood pressure and cholesterol levels.
- Patients with elevated blood pressure and lipid levels may consider supplementing their diets with foods high in soluble fiber and omega-3 fatty acids, such as chia and flaxseed.[284] Recommended adult servings for chia and flaxseed are 2 to 3 tablespoons daily. Soluble fiber, such as that found in flaxseed and chia, may help lower cholesterol. These agents should be taken with plenty of water. In general, prescription drugs should be taken 1 hour before or 2 hours after taking flaxseed and chia.
- Strong evidence supports the cholesterol-lowering effects of garlic. Garlic may have additional cardioprotective effects, but these are unclear. Nonetheless, the World Health Organization lists the following uses for garlic as supported by clinical data: adjuvant for dietary management for hyperlipidemia, prevention of age-dependent atherosclerosis, and possibly mild hypertension.
- There is a strong correlation between magnesium intake and reduced risk of cardiovascular disease, including MI, stroke, and arrhythmia. Although this correlation may occur because diets high in magnesium also tend to be higher in healthier food choices, magnesium supplementation may be considered.
- Caution patients about herbal remedies for the treatment of stroke and related conditions. These include arnica, betel nut, and danshen. Unclear or insufficient evidence exists to support their safety or efficacy.
- Because MI and stroke are medical emergencies, professional medical intervention should be sought. In the event of MI or stroke, integrative therapies should not be used in place of professional medical treatment.
- A dose of 160 to 325 mg of aspirin should be given on day 1 of acute MI and continued indefinitely on a daily basis.

Arrhythmia

- Discuss the patient's range of symptoms and those that may be attributed to an arrhythmia.
- Ask if the patient has been experiencing any palpitations, lightheadedness, dyspnea, angina, syncope, exercise intolerance, or sensation of rapid pulse.
- Ensure that blood pressure and pulse are measured.
- Inquire about any family history of arrhythmia and cardiac disease.
- Ask the patient about ingestion of any toxic substance, including plants, herbs, mushrooms, drugs, and other possibly poisonous agents.
- Discuss the potential side effects of drug therapy and treatment complications.

- Educate the patient that evidence is lacking to support the use of any herb for the treatment of arrhythmias.
- Discuss that certain herbs may cause arrhythmias, such as ginseng, ephedra, and guarana.

Case Studies

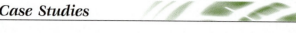

CASE STUDY 14-1

FH is a 47-year-old man who visited his family physician 2 weeks ago because of an occasional "flip-flop" sensation in his chest. An ECG revealed sinus tachycardia (116 beats/min) and occasional premature ventricular contractions (PVCs). His blood pressure was slightly elevated (144/92 mm Hg). His physician recommended that he quit his usual coffee consumption (3-5 cups daily) and return in 1 month for a reevaluation. Despite 2 weeks without coffee, FH still experiences an occasional flip-flop. He takes ginseng and horny goat weed to "put lead in his pencil." He also ingests one or two cans of a guarana-containing energy drink daily. He asks if an herbal remedy will clear up his flip-flop. When queried, FH replies that he did not inform his physician about his use of herbs, because they were "just herbs and not drugs." How should you counsel?

Answer: Although no herb has been shown to treat cardiac arrhythmias effectively, a number of substances (e.g., caffeine) may cause them. FH may not be aware that guarana is an extremely rich source of caffeine; it contains up to three times the amount of caffeine contained in coffee. Furthermore, energy drinks often do not list the amount of caffeine. FH's other supplements may also contribute to heart rhythm disorders. Both ginseng (American ginseng, Asian ginseng, Chinese ginseng, Korean red ginseng, *Panax ginseng*) and horny goat weed (*Epimedium grandiflorum*) may affect heart rate. Potentially worsening FH's situation, each of the herbs he is ingesting may elevate blood pressure.

FH should be advised to discontinue his herbal remedies and energy drinks. Doing so may help resolve the tachycardia and cardiac arrhythmia by the time he returns to his physician for a follow-up. FH may also reduce his blood pressure by cutting back on caffeine intake and eliminating certain supplements that may contribute to heart rhythm disorders.

CASE STUDY 14-2

TL is a 54-year-old man who presents at the pharmacy with a prescription for hydrochlorothiazide (HydroDiuril), digoxin (Lanoxin), warfarin (Coumadin), atorvastatin (Lipitor), and glipizide (Glucotrol). He appears to be about 50 pounds overweight. He explains that he was recently released from the hospital for the treatment of an acute myocardial infarction (MI). He adds that his physician has been experiencing some difficulty in regulating his warfarin dosage. TL smoked two packs of cigarettes a day for many years; however, since his MI, he "has seen the light" and has cut back to one pack a day. When asked if he is taking any other medications, he replies that he is just taking a "safe herbal product" (astragalus) because a friend told him it would reduce his chance of another MI. How do you counsel?

Answer: Astragalus (*Astragalus membranaceus*) has no proven efficacy for coronary artery disease. It does possess some hypoglycemic properties and may potentiate the effect of glipizide. It also possesses some diuretic and hypotensive properties; thus, astragalus may potentiate the effect of hydrochlorothiazide. It also might lower lipid levels and may augment the effect of atorvastatin. Countering these possible benefits, astragalus possesses some anticoagulant properties and may be part of the reason his physician has difficulty in regulating TL's warfarin dosage. If astragalus is used, the dosage must be standardized.

Garlic (*Allium sativum*) is currently the most widely used herbal product in the United States. According to available data, garlic is more likely to augment the effect of atorvastatin than astragalus. Garlic may have antiatherosclerotic effects by inhibiting platelet aggregation and enhancing fibrinolysis. Similar to astragalus, garlic may increase the anticoagulant effect of warfarin. Therefore, if garlic is used, his prothrombin time must be closely monitored, and TL should take a daily standardized dose of garlic. It also may decrease serum glucose levels.

Chia (*Salvia hispanica*) is taken for cardiovascular disease prevention. Chia seeds are a good source of omega-3 and omega-6 unsaturated fatty acids, dietary fiber, and folic acid.[284] Organic compounds found in chia seeds (kaempferol and quercetin) may contribute to chia's antioxidant effects. Salba is a chia product that the manufacturer (Core Naturals) claims to be selectively bred to maximize nutrient value; furthermore, Salba is reported to contain more omega-3 fatty acids than typical chia seeds. Chia is reported to have some antihypertensive properties and may interact with warfarin, augmenting its effect.

Because all the aforementioned herbs can potentiate warfarin, their ingestion might be postponed until warfarin therapy is discontinued. If warfarin is to be continued indefinitely, precautions must be taken with any of these herbs.

Beyond herbal remedies, TL must make extensive lifestyle changes if he wants to lower his chances for another MI. He must adopt a strict exercise program and quit smoking altogether. If he does not quit, chances are he will soon be back up to his two-pack-a-day habit. If he is successful in a healthy regimen, TL may not need to visit your pharmacy with a handful of prescription refills to treat his (largely) self-inflicted diseases.

CASE STUDY 14-3

SN wheels an elderly Vietnamese woman, TN, up to the pharmacy counter and hands you a prescription for propranolol (Inderal). TN is an obvious stroke victim with left-sided facial weakness. You notice that TN's teeth and gums are stained purple. An argument ensues between TN and SN. You cannot follow the conversation because they are both speaking Vietnamese. SN soothes the old woman and explains that she is TN's daughter-in-law and that TN only takes herbal remedies. She is bitterly opposed to any prescription medication. SN states that TN is already taking danshen to help prevent stroke. You ask if the purple stains are caused by chewing betel nuts. SN replies that TN has chewed betel nut all her life and refuses to quit. How do you counsel?

Answer: Danshen *(Salvia miltiorrhiza)* is a traditional Chinese medicine used for the treatment of cardiovascular disease. It should not be used in combination with propranolol because danshen can induce CYP activity; thus, it will interact with propranolol, which is metabolized by cytochrome P450. The beneficial effects of danshen are currently unclear or conflicting. Chia currently appears to be more efficacious; however, it also can induce CYP activity.

Arnica *(Arnica chamissonis, A. cordifolia, A. fulgens, A. latifolia, A. montana, A. sororia)* is another herbal remedy (used in minute homeopathic doses) for stroke. Arnica may reduce the efficacy of propranolol and other hypertensive agents; it is also highly toxic, and its use is not advised.

Of concern is TN's chronic chewing of betel nuts *(Areca catechu)*. Betel nut chewing dates back thousands of years in Asia; it is a mild CNS stimulant. It has documented toxicity and cannot be considered safe for human ingestion. Individuals chewing betel nuts have experienced dyspnea, pulmonary edema, angina, tachycardia, palpitations, ventricular arrhythmias, and hemodynamic instability (hypotension/hypertension). Constituents of betel nut are potentially carcinogenic. Chronic use has been associated with squamous cell carcinoma, precancerous oral lesions, and oral submucosal fibrosis. TN's chronic betel nut chewing may have been a contributing factor to her stroke.

You are obviously dealing with an extremely noncompliant patient. Your best course of action is to explain all the potential risks to SN in the hope that TN will forego her traditional herbs and try therapies that have more evidence of safety and efficacy.

References for Chapter 14 can be found on the Evolve website at http://evolve.elsevier.com/Ulbricht/herbalpharmacotherapy/

Review Questions

1. Salicylic acid is a precursor to which common medication?
   a. Acetaminophen (Tylenol)
   b. Ibuprofen (Advil)
   c. Aspirin (Bayer)
   d. Lovastatin (Monacolin K)

2. Which of the following statements is *false* concerning the use of flaxseed or its constituents?
   a. Both flaxseed and flaxseed oil contain alpha-linolenic acid (ALA).
   b. Flaxseed contains fiber and protein, whereas flaxseed oil does not.
   c. Flaxseed may interact with oral contraceptives.
   d. Flaxseed oil contains omega-3 fatty acids, but not omega-6 fatty acids.

3. The sesquiterpene lactones (SLs) of *Arnica montana* (including helenalin and 11,13-dihydrohelenal) have been shown to inhibit which of the following?
   a. Platelet aggregation
   b. Serum lipids
   c. Inflammation
   d. All the above

4. Which of the following constituents of flaxseed may contribute to its cholesterol-lowering effects?
   a. Fiber
   b. Omega-6 fatty acids only
   c. Statins
   d. None of the above

5. Which of the following herbs are natural sources of salicylic acid?
   a. Chia *(Salvia hispanica)*
   b. Meadowsweet *(Filipendula ulmaria)*
   c. Both a and b
   d. None of the above

6. Which of the following has been used traditionally to treat stroke?
   a. Golden chia
   b. Plants of the genus *Salvia*
   c. Danshen
   d. All the above

7. Betel nut is associated with which of the following?
   a. Oral cancer
   b. Cervical dysplasia
   c. Cholinergic activity
   d. All the above

8. True or false: The toxic effects associated with the administration of aconite limit its ability to be used clinically as an agent to treat bradycardia.

9. All the following have potential antiarrhythmic properties *except*:
   a. Bloodroot
   b. Mistletoe
   c. Devil's claw
   d. Echinacea

10. True or false: All arrhythmias are abnormal.

Answers are found in the Answers to Review Questions section in the back of the text.

15 Coagulation Disorders

Outline

OVERVIEW
   Hemostasis
      Vessel Wall
      Platelets
      Coagulation Cascade
      Fibrinolysis
   Coagulopathy
      Insufficient Clotting
      Excessive Clotting
   Signs and Symptoms
      Increased Bleeding
      Increased Clotting
   Diagnosis
      Disorders of Excessive Bleeding
      Disorders of Excessive Clotting
SELECTED HERBAL THERAPIES
   Daisy *(Bellis perennis)*
   Garlic *(Allium sativum)*
   Ginger *(Zingiber officinale)*
   Grape Seed *(Vitis* spp.)
   Policosanol
   Pycnogenol *(Pinus pinaster* subsp. *atlantica)*
   Rhubarb *(Rheum* spp.)
   Rutin $(C_{27}H_{30}O_{16})$
   Turmeric *(Curcuma longa)*
   Yohimbe *(Pausinystalia yohimbe)*
HERBAL THERAPIES WITH LIMITED EVIDENCE
ADJUNCT THERAPIES
INTEGRATIVE THERAPY PLAN
CASE STUDIES
REVIEW QUESTIONS

Learning Objectives

- Identify herbs that may increase the risk of bleeding.
- Identify herbs that may increase clotting.
- Describe mechanisms by which herbal agents may affect coagulation.
- Recognize herbs that affect clotting and their potential interactions with other herbs, supplements, and medications.

OVERVIEW[1,2]

Coagulation is a process in which blood clots form. A blood clot is composed of proteins (clotting factors) and platelets (a type of blood cell), and forms at the site of blood vessel injury to stop bleeding. Blood clots are critical for maintaining the integrity of the vasculature, which is known as *hemostasis*. Coagulation disorders occur when too much or too little coagulation occurs. If coagulation is excessive, it may result in pathological blood clots that interfere with normal blood flow; this condition is known as *thrombosis*. If a thrombus dislodges and travels to another part of the body, it is known as an *embolus*. A common complication of thrombosis is embolism, which may lead to ischemic disease, as in myocardial infarction (MI or heart attack) or cerebrovascular accident (CVA or stroke) (Figure 15-1). In other coagulation disorders, clot formation may be delayed or inadequate, which may lead to excessive bleeding or *hemorrhage*. Both excessive clotting and delayed clotting range from mild to severe; at times, clotting disorders may even be life threatening.

Hemostasis

Hemostasis is a complex process, and involves four major components: the vessel wall, platelets, the coagulation cascade, and fibrinolysis.

Vessel Wall

Vascular endothelial cells produce various hemodynamic factors that are essential for vascular tone, such as *prostacyclin* (PGI_2) and *nitric oxide* (NO). When a blood vessel is injured, production of these factors decreases, causing the surrounding

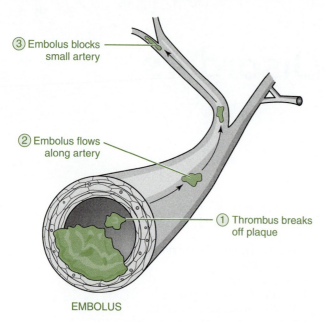

Figure 15-1 Embolus. (Modified from Gould B: *Pathophysiology for the health professions*, ed 2, Philadelphia, 2002, Saunders.)

vascular smooth muscle to contract. This resulting vasoconstriction slows blood flow and facilitates clot formation. *Collagen*, which lies beneath the surface of blood vessels, is also exposed by injury to the vessel wall. The exposed collagen binds the platelets and plays a critical role in their activation.

Platelets

Platelets are anucleated thrombocytes that normally circulate in the bloodstream. The principal function of platelets is to prevent bleeding. The decreased levels of prostacyclin and NO cause the platelets to adhere to the vessel wall. The exposed collagen at the site of injury also induces platelet aggregation, because platelets have collagen-specific binding proteins on their cell surfaces. Primary hemostasis results in a hemostatic plug, which may form within seconds of an injury and acts as a temporary plug to control bleeding.

Once the platelets have aggregated, they change in shape from round to ragged, attracting more platelets and the clotting factor *thrombin*. Some blood clots are visible and appear as bruises on the skin. The formation of a blood clot also requires a specific stepwise process known as the coagulation cascade, which involves thrombin, other clotting factors, and platelets. Vitamin K, which is central to proper clot formation, is also involved.

Coagulation Cascade

In addition to platelets, the coagulation process involves a concert of various protein factors (Figure 15-2). Coagulation factors are usually designated by a Roman numeral in the inactive form, and by a Roman numeral followed by an "a" when activated. The factors *prothrombin* (formerly factor II), *thrombin* (factor IIa), *fibrinogen* (I), and *fibrin* (Ia) no longer use the Roman numeral designation because their names have become commonplace in medical practice. The coagulation cascade consists of three parts: the *extrinsic* (tissue factor) pathway; *intrinsic* (contact activation) pathway; and the *common* pathway. These three pathways have been historically separated based on study of the clotting cascade in vitro. In the human body, however, the process is more complex, and hemostasis is achieved primarily though the extrinsic and common pathways. Nonetheless, the clotting cascade is typically discussed according to these three theoretical pathways.

Each pathway of the coagulation cascade involves a different sequence of coagulation factors and their activation. The extrinsic pathway involves the factors III, VII, and X. The intrinsic pathway involves factors VIII, IX, X, XI, and XII.

These two pathways lead to the activation of factor X, which marks the beginning of the common pathway. In addition to factor X, the common pathway involves factors V, XIII, thrombin, and fibrin. Thrombin plays a major role in several aspects of the coagulation cascade; its principle role is to convert the inactive fibrinogen protein into fibrin. Without the formation of fibrin, the clot formed from platelet aggregation and clumping would not be strong enough to achieve hemostasis. In the final step of the coagulation cascade, thrombin converts fibrinogen (bound to the platelet surface receptor glycoprotein IIa-IIIb complex) to its active form, fibrin. Multiple fibrin molecules bind many platelets together to form a hemostatic plug, which stops blood loss from the injured vessel.

The activation of a coagulation factor depends on a variety of cofactors. *Vitamin K* has been identified as necessary for the activation of factors VII, IX, X, prothrombin, and proteins C and S. Therefore, dietary intake of vitamin K is essential for the coagulation cascade, and drugs that affect clotting (such as the anticoagulant warfarin (Coumadin) may be significantly affected by fluctuations in vitamin K intake.

Fibrinolysis

Beside coagulation, hemostasis also involves clot dissolution, or *fibrinolysis*. This occurs once the blood vessel is healed, and it involves other blood factors that are specifically released to break down the fibrin clot. The protein *plasmin* is the primary enzyme responsible for breaking down the clot. The cells that line the blood vessels release plasminogen-activating factors, including tissue plasminogen activator and urokinase, which convert the inactive protein *plasminogen* into plasmin. The clot is then dissolved into the blood. Fibrinolysis is also involved in the body's regulation of the coagulation cascade to prevent excessive coagulation clotting. Enzymes regulating the cascade include protein C, protein S, antithrombin, tissue factor pathway inhibitor, α_2-macroglobulin, and heparin cofactor II. These enzymes break down the activated coagulation factors so that they are no longer active.[3]

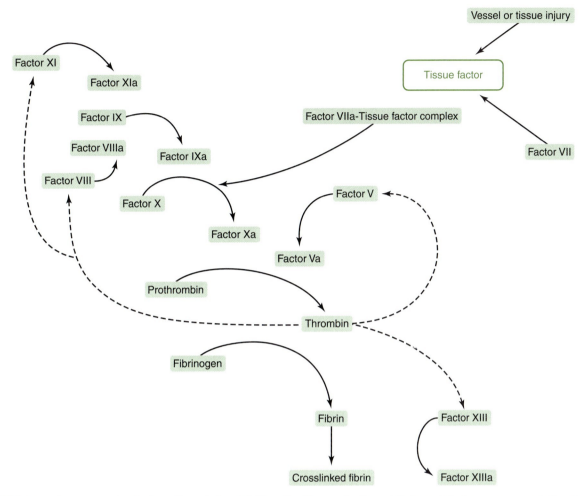

Figure 15-2 Coagulation cascade. (Redrawn from Cohen, M: The role of low-molecular-weight heparin in the management of acute coronary syndromes, *J Am Coll Cardiol* 41(4SupplS):55S-61S, 2003.)

Coagulopathy

Abnormalities in the clotting process may lead to coagulation disorders, collectively referred to as *coagulopathies*. These disorders may be chronic genetic conditions (e.g., hemophilia) or may be temporary conditions triggered by surgery, severe injuries, medications, or other medical conditions (most notably heart disease).

Insufficient Clotting

An impaired coagulation process may lead to hemorrhagic or bleeding disorders. When blood does not clot effectively, even a minor injury to a blood vessel may lead to a hemorrhage. Patients with impaired clotting may also have spontaneous bleeding with no history of trauma.

Insufficient clotting may result from defects in the proteins involved in the coagulation cascade. One example is *hemophilia*, a bleeding disorder caused by defective forms of clotting factor VIII or IX. About 70% of cases of hemophilia are inherited, and 30% result from spontaneous mutations during embryonic development. Some individuals are not born with mutations but develop hemophilia later in life; *acquired hemophilia* is thought to be an autoimmune disorder that attacks clotting-factor proteins. Acquired hemophilia is typically seen in older individuals, over age 50.[4]

In addition to clotting-factor defects, platelet disorders may also result in insufficient clotting and increased bleeding. Platelets normally produce the protein von Willebrand factor (vWF), which helps them adhere to the blood vessel walls. In *von Willebrand disease*, platelets produce insufficient levels of this protein, resulting in platelet dysfunction and prolonged bleeding time. *Bernard-Soulier syndrome* is caused by a deficiency of the cell surface glycoprotein Ib/IX, and platelets fail to adhere properly at sites of injury. In *alpha-granule deficiency* (gray platelet syndrome), the lack of platelet alpha granules also impairs platelet adhesion and aggregation. In *dense granule deficiency* (delta storage pool deficiency), the platelets lack storage granules for factors involved in platelet activation. Various disorders, including *May-Hegglin anomaly, Alport syndrome,* and *Wiskott-Aldrich* syndrome, may cause low platelet count and increased bleeding time.

Excessive Clotting

When a blood vessel is partially or fully blocked by a clot, *thrombosis* occurs. Depending on where the blockage occurs, it can interfere with normal blood flow and may even be fatal. For example, if arteries in the heart are blocked, thrombosis may lead to a heart attack. If a blockage occurs in an artery that supplies the brain, a *thrombotic stroke* may occur.

In some cases a thrombus that forms in a vessel may detach from the vessel wall, and travel freely in the blood. This free-floating clot is called an *embolus*. Eventually, this embolus may lodge in an artery or vein, called a *thromboembolus*. Thromboembolic diseases are defined by where the embolus lodges. For example, if the embolus lodges in the pulmonary arteries (which carry deoxygenated blood from the heart to the lungs), the condition is called a *pulmonary embolism*. If the embolus lodges in an artery supplying the brain, an *embolic stroke* may occur.

Of all the blood vessels, the veins in the legs are most often affected by excessive clotting, because of their low position relative to the heart and the relatively slow movement of blood in veins compared with arteries. This potentially life-threatening condition is called *deep vein thrombosis* (DVT). This is considered a potentially dangerous condition because fragments of the blood clot can break off and travel to the heart, then via the pulmonary arteries to the lungs, causing a pulmonary embolism. Clots that form on heart valves or in the arterial circulation can travel to the brain and cause an embolic stroke.[5]

Signs and Symptoms

In general, patients with coagulation disorders have either increased bleeding or increased clotting. However, patients may have symptoms of both bleeding and clotting with a coagulopathy known as *disseminated intravascular coagulation* (DIC), a severe condition associated with infection, pregnancy, or malignancy.

Increased Bleeding

Patients with increased bleeding may have a history of easy bleeding and bruising from minor accidents, heavy menstrual flow in women (menorrhagia), nosebleeds (epistaxis), or bleeding of the gums. Disorders of the coagulation cascade may produce bleeding into tissues, (such as into joint spaces or the abdominal cavity). In contrast, bleeding caused by platelet disorders is typically located in the skin or mucous membranes (e.g., bleeding gums, nosebleeds) and tends to occur immediately after a traumatic injury.

Increased Clotting

In coagulation disorders of excessive clotting, symptoms may depend on which blood vessels are blocked with clots. For example, a blocked blood vessel in an arm or leg may cause swelling and pain. The area of local inflammation may also become itchy and reddish brown in color (similar to a bruise). When this occurs, the skin may be easily injured, often resulting in an ulcer. Fragments of blood clots from the veins in the legs, abdomen, or pelvis can travel through the bloodstream to the lungs, where they can block major arteries. The blockage depends entirely on the size of the embolus relative to the vessel diameter. A large embolus can block a major pulmonary vessel, whereas a small embolus can block a smaller, peripheral vessel. Sudden death may occur with major vessel blockage. Small-vessel blockages may be asymptomatic or may cause chest pain or hemoptysis (coughing up blood). Blocked blood vessels in the lungs result in pulmonary embolism. Symptoms may include shortness of breath, wheezing, chest pain, increased heartbeat, leg swelling, dizziness, or hemoptysis. If blood vessels in the liver are blocked, symptoms may include yellowing of the skin and eyes (jaundice) and abdominal tenderness.

If blood vessels in the brain become blocked, the patient may have a stroke. Symptoms may include sudden onset of numbness or weakness, difficulty speaking, confusion, difficulty seeing with one or both eyes, headache, dizziness, and imbalance.[5] If arteries to the heart become clogged, the patient may have a heart attack. Symptoms may include chest pain or pressure, shortness of breath, nausea, and weakness, as well as pain radiating to the arms, neck, or jaw. Small areas (such as on the fingers or toes) may turn black if clots restrict blood flow to these areas.[6]

Diagnosis

Disorders of Excessive Bleeding

Patients with bleeding disorders may be asked about family histories of coagulopathies. Patients should also be asked about medication use, including nonsteroidal antiinflammatory drugs (NSAIDs) and certain herbal supplements (such as garlic or ginseng) that are known to affect bleeding. A thorough physical examination should be performed to note the location of bleeding and to detect signs of deep tissue bleeding including joint or abdominal pain. Patients with severe bleeding may have signs of anemia, such as pale skin and a rapid heart rate (tachycardia), or they may be in hemorrhagic shock, with low blood pressure, tachycardia, and evidence of organ failure (confusion, loss of consciousness, lack of urine output).

Initial laboratory tests that may be used to evaluate a bleeding disorder include platelet count, vWF levels, prothrombin time (PT), and activated partial thromboplastin time (aPTT).

Platelet Count

The normal platelet range depends on the laboratory methods used. Typically the range is 150 to 400×10^9/L. A decreased platelet count may suggest a platelet deficiency as the underlying cause; however, clinically apparent bleeding does not usually occur until the platelet count drops significantly below normal, usually less than 5×10^7/L. *Thrombocytopenia*, (low platelet count) may be secondary to various causes, including a transient or progressive autoimmune disorder, infection, bone marrow failure syndrome, or other malignancy. A normal platelet count does not rule out abnormal platelet function as the underlying cause of bleeding. If platelet dysfunction is suspected, a platelet aggregation study can be performed. This in vitro study evaluates the ability of an individual's platelets to aggregate in response to different stimuli and can be used to detect inherited and acquired platelet disorders.

Von Willebrand Factor Levels

Von Willebrand factor (vWF) is released by platelets and vessels and helps platelets attach to an injured vessel wall. Deficiency of vWF is the most common inherited coagulation disorder. Patients may have normal platelet counts, but because vWF is not present to aid in the formation of a platelet plug, they may have spontaneous and excessive bleeding. A vWF deficiency is diagnosed based on measurements of vWF in the blood and an abnormal platelet aggregation study.

Prothrombin Time

The PT is a measure of the extrinsic and common coagulation pathways. This includes plasma factors VII, X, and V; prothrombin; and fibrinogen. The PT is also reported as the *international normalized ratio* (INR), which is a ratio of the patient's PT to a laboratory control value. The INR was developed by the World Health Organization (WHO) to account for variations in PT results that occur from laboratory to laboratory when monitoring anticoagulant medications such as warfarin. Normal PT values depend on the methods of individual laboratories. A normal PT value is generally between 10 and 13 seconds, and a normal INR is 1.

Activated Partial Thromboplastin Time

The aPTT tests the factors of the intrinsic and common coagulation pathways, including prekallikrein; high-molecular-weight kininogen; prothrombin; fibrinogen; and factors XII, XI, IX, VIII, X, and V. The normal range of aPTT depends on the laboratory methods and reagents used and is usually 28 to 34 seconds.

A coagulation factor deficiency or inhibitor may prolong the PT or aPTT. A *coagulation factor inhibitor* is a molecule (e.g., antibody) that binds to a normal factor and prevents it from functioning. Prolongation of the PT and aPTT generally does not occur until one or more factors are at least 70% deficient or inactive.

Mixing Study

To determine the difference between a factor deficiency and an inhibitor, a mixing study can be performed. The patient's plasma is mixed with normal plasma in a 1:1 ratio. If the patient's abnormality is caused by a factor deficiency, the normal plasma should provide the necessary factors, and the PT or aPTT should be normal after mixing. If the patient's disorder is caused by an inhibitor, the inhibitor will also prevent the factor(s) in the normal plasma from functioning, and the PT and aPTT will remain abnormally high after mixing.

Tests for Specific Clotting Factor Deficiencies

If a specific factor deficiency is suspected, laboratory evaluation focuses on this factor or genetic mutations associated with the factor deficiency. Causes of bleeding that may not be detected by platelet count, PT, or aPTT include factor VIII deficiency, von Willebrand disease, and rare disorders of fibrinolysis. If suspected in a patient with normal laboratory values, specific testing for the disorder can be performed.

Disorders of Excessive Clotting

Excessive clotting often leads to medical situations requiring immediate medical attention before a diagnosis can be made. Patients should be questioned about a history of clotting or a family history of blood disorders. Other factors that can increase a patient's risk of clotting include prolonged stasis (impaired circulation), which may result from decreased activity after major surgery or pregnancy; oral contraceptive use; severe infection; high serum levels of homocysteine; and malignancy.

Physical examination findings depend on the location of the clot(s); the symptoms previously discussed may be present. Immediate care for a patient with a thrombus or thromboembolus is often directed at removal of the clot. The method used largely depends on the size and location of the clot. For example, with DVT, heparin therapy is initiated to prevent further clotting. Warfarin (Coumadin) therapy may also be initiated, but may take a week or more to become fully effective, as the clots are not removed but dissolve in time. Invasive intervention usually occurs with events such as an acute coronary occlusion. Once the patient is stabilized, further workup of the underlying coagulation disorder can proceed. Further evaluation is warranted in patients with no obvious predisposing factor, with a history of more than one clot, with a family history of recurrent clots, or with a stroke or heart attack before age 50 years.[5]

Abnormalities of several clotting factors may underlie disorders of excessive clotting. Mutations in the prothrombin gene or elevated levels of clotting factors (e.g., VII, XI, IX, VIII, vWf) may lead to excessive clotting. If an inherited or acquired hypercoagulable state is suspected, testing for the specific factor can be performed. Depending on the factor, tests may include evaluating the factor's level of activity in the patient's blood or genetic testing for abnormal genes.

Clotting disorders may also affect fibrinolysis, including deficiencies in protein C or S or antithrombin.

SELECTED HERBAL THERAPIES

 Note

To help make this educational resource more interactive, all pharmacokinetics, adverse effects, and interactions data have been compiled in Appendix A. Safety data specifically related to pregnancy and lactation are listed in Appendix B. Please refer to these appendices when working through the case studies and answering the review questions.

Daisy (Bellis perennis)

Grade C: Unclear or conflicting scientific evidence (mild postpartum bleeding)

Mechanism of Action

The hemolytic activity of preparations made from the leaves, roots, and capitula of daisy (*Bellis perennis*) change depending on the time of year that capitula is collected, peaking in summer months.[7,8] The mechanisms of the hemostatic effects attributed to daisy extract are not fully understood.

Scientific Evidence of Effectiveness

Traditionally, homeopathic *B. perennis* has been used for bruising, bleeding, and recovery from surgery. However, there is limited evidence supporting the use of daisy for treating bleeding disorders. In an available study using a homeopathic combination of arnica and *B. perennis* for postpartum bleeding, the treatment group had higher hemoglobin levels.[9] However, because homeopathic preparations contain little (if any) of the purported active ingredient(s), the scientific basis for any observed effect is unclear.

Dose

There is currently no well-known standardization of *Bellis perennis*. However, *B. perennis* preparations have been used as homeopathic preparations, as well as in traditional herbal preparations. Homeopathic treatment is usually individualized to correspond specifically to the patient's symptoms. The wide range of homeopathic potencies and treatment methodologies pose a challenge when applying standard testing and statistical procedures to the homeopathic medical model. The dose of daisy for mild postpartum bleeding has not been determined.

Adverse Effects, Interactions, Pharmacokinetics. See Appendix A.

Garlic (Allium sativum)

Grade C: Unclear or conflicting scientific evidence (antiplatelet effects)

Mechanism of Action

PLATELET EFFECTS. Garlic and its derived compound, *ajoene*, have inhibited platelet aggregation in vitro and in vivo[10-20] and reduced platelet-dependent thrombus formation.[21,22] Several preclinical studies and controlled human trials have reported impaired platelet aggregation associated with oral garlic use.[11,23-29] In clinical trials[25,26] 800 mg of garlic daily for 4 to 12 weeks was linked to a decrease in platelet aggregation in patients with peripheral vascular disease. In addition, research has demonstrated inhibition of platelet aggregation in men with hypercholesterolemia, in healthy subjects, in patients with coronary artery disease (CAD),[30-34] and in subjects with cerebrovascular risk factors.[25,28] In contrast, low dietary garlic did not have similar effects.[35] However, most studies have not provided concrete evidence. Comparisons to established antiplatelet agents have not been adequately assessed; furthermore garlic doses are not established, duration of effect is not clear, and clinical outcomes are not known.

Cyclooxygenase (COX), an enzyme needed to produce various biological mediators (e.g., prostaglandin, prostacyclin, thromboxane), has been shown to be inhibited by raw garlic in vitro.[13] Dose-dependent COX inhibition in human placental villi was observed with garlic and with allicin-negative (acid-washed) garlic.[36] Antiplatelet activity may be attributable to garlic constituents such as adenosine, allicin, and paraffinic polysulfides.[37] Compared to raw garlic, a boiled aqueous garlic extract has demonstrated approximately a 50% decrease in the inhibition of platelet aggregation at identical concentrations,[13,20] suggesting that cooking garlic may reduce antiplatelet effects. Raw garlic has been shown to reduce serum thromboxane B_2 in animal and human research at a dose of 1 clove per day.[30,38,39] However, boiling garlic before administration appears to reduce or abolish this effect,[31] again suggesting a negative impact of cooking on garlic's antiplatelet activity.

FIBRINOLYTIC EFFECTS. Increased fibrinolytic activity, involving fibrinogen and plasminogen, may account for some degree of garlic's anticoagulation effects.[40-43] Both raw garlic and cooked garlic, as well as essential oil from raw garlic, have demonstrated significant increases in fibrinolytic activity in humans.[44,45] Increased fibrinolytic activity in patients with ischemic heart disease was maintained after 7 to 8 weeks of therapy.[46,47] However, another study reported that fibrinolytic activity returned to pretreatment levels after 12 weeks of continuous garlic therapy.[47]

Scientific Evidence of Effectiveness

The effects of garlic on platelet aggregation have been assessed in several human trials. Although these studies overall have not produced unequivocal results garlic does appear to possess platelet-inhibiting properties. Dosing, safety, comparison to other agents, duration of effects, and clinical outcomes are not known, and the potential benefits of using garlic for this purpose are not clear. Because garlic has been associated with several cases of bleeding, therapy should be used cautiously—particularly in patients using other agents that may promote bleeding (e.g., warfarin).

Several preclinical studies and controlled human trials have reported impaired platelet aggregation associated with oral garlic use.[11,23-29] In clinical trials, 800 mg of garlic daily led to a decrease in platelet aggregation in patients with peripheral vascular disease.[25,26] In most cases, platelet aggregation has been measured by assessing the effects of garlic on adenosine diphosphate (ADP)–induced platelet aggregation.

Again, garlic has been associated with several case reports of bleeding and may increase fibrinolytic activity[43] and prolong clotting time.[48,49] Garlic has also been associated with a case of an increase in a previously stabilized INR when used concomitantly with warfarin (Coumadin).[50,51]

Dose

For the treatment of thrombotic disease, 10 g of raw garlic daily[49] and 800 mg powdered garlic tablets[25,26] for up to 2 months have been used in clinical studies.

Adverse Effects, Interactions, Pharmacokinetics. See Appendix A.

Ginger (*Zingiber officinale*)

Grade C: *Unclear or conflicting scientific evidence (antiplatelet agent)*

Mechanism of Action

The "pungent principles," or nonvolatile constituents, of ginger are considered to be responsible for its flavor, aromatic properties, and pharmacological activity.[52] These include (6)-gingerol (usually <1% of root's weight);[53] (6)-shagaol, a dehyroxylated analog of (6)-gingerol; (6)- and (10)-dehydrogingerdione; (6)- and (10)-gingerdione; (6)-paradol; vallinoids; galanals A and B; and zingerone. Other compounds present include carbohydrates, fats, minerals, oleoresins, vitamins, waxes, and zingibain (a proteolytic enzyme). The rhizome of ginger contains pungent vanillyl ketones, including (6)-gingerol and (6)-paradol, and has been reported to possess strong antiinflammatory activity as well as anti–tumor-promoting properties.[54]

Ginger has been shown to inhibit platelet aggregation[55-57] and to decrease platelet thromboxane production in vitro.[57-59] (8)-Gingerol, (8)-shogaol, (8)-paradol, and gingerol analogs (1 and 5) exhibited antiplatelet activities.[57] However, its effects in vivo are not entirely clear. Although some evidence suggests that ginger may decrease platelet aggregation[60] and decrease thromboxane levels,[61] other studies have suggested that ginger does not affect platelet count,[62] platelet aggregation,[62,63] thromboxane levels,[64] fibrinolytic activity,[63] or bleeding time.[62]

Scientific Evidence of Effectiveness

In theory, because ginger has been observed to inhibit thromboxane synthetase, and decreased platelet aggregation has been reported in clinical trials,[65] the concurrent use of ginger with agents that predispose to bleeding could enhance their effect and increase the risk of bleeding.[55,56,66,67] Case reports and reviews also note ginger as an anticoagulant.[68-72] One case study reported overanticoagulation in a patient receiving long-term phenprocoumon therapy after taking ginger, which suggests an anticoagulant effect that may be additive with coumarins.

Dose

The dose of ginger for antiplatelet effects has not been determined. However, there is limited evidence that thromboxane levels may be decreased by ginger ingestion (5 g daily for 7 days).[61]

Adverse Effects, Interactions, Pharmacokinetics. See Appendix A.

Grape Seed (*Vitis* spp.)

Grade C: *Unclear or conflicting scientific evidence (inhibition of platelet aggregation)*

Note: Grape seed extract (GSE) and Pycnogenol are not the same, even though they both contain oligomeric proanthocyanidins (OPCs). Pycnogenol is a patented nutrient supplement extracted from the bark of European coastal pine *Pinus maritima*.

Mechanism of Action

Grape seed extract has been demonstrated to inhibit platelet aggregation, enhance NO release, and prevent platelet superoxide production.[73,74] In vitro study comparing GSE to the antiplatelet agent resveratrol found that GSE reduced platelet adhesion, aggregation, and generation of oxygen in blood platelets significantly more than resveratrol.[75] Intravenous injection of the grape seed constituent proanthocyanidin prevented thrombus formation in mice.[76]

Scientific Evidence of Effectiveness

For the effect of GSEs on platelet aggregation and coagulation, clinical evidence is lacking. There is some evidence that flavanol-rich GSE may decrease platelet aggregation in male smokers.[77] There is clinical evidence of a strong but not statistically significant trend toward increased ADP-induced closure time in postmenopausal women after 8 weeks of GSE treatment.[78]

Dose

The dose of grape seed for antiplatelet effects has not been determined. However, one study suggested antithrombotic effects in patients taking 400 mg GSE by mouth for 8 weeks.[78]

Adverse Effects, Interactions, Pharmacokinetics. See Appendix A.

Policosanol

Grade A: *Strong scientific evidence (platelet aggregation inhibition)*

Mechanism of Action

Policosanol reduced serum levels of thromboxane in animals and humans and inhibited platelet aggregation in hypertensive patients and healthy volunteers.[79-86] Inhibition was most effective against induction by collagen and arachidonic acid, but also occurred with ADP and epinephrine stimulation.

Scientific Evidence of Effectiveness

Various studies have investigated the effect of policosanol on platelet aggregation;[81,84,85,87,88] most suggest policosanol inhibits platelet aggregation. Studies with healthy volunteers showed that policosanol inhibited platelet aggregation[80,84,85,88] and production of thromboxane B_2.[88] Policosanol was found to be as effective as aspirin in preventing platelet aggregation.[84] A similar study in type II hypercholesterolemic patients found that policosanol inhibited platelet aggregation.[87] These results were seen at doses of 10 to 40 mg daily. The effects of policosanol in patients with thrombotic disease are not known.

Dose

A policosanol dose of 10 to 40 mg has been taken daily to inhibit platelet aggregation.[81,84,85,87,88] Most often, doses of 10 or 20 mg have been used for 4 to 6 weeks.

Adverse Effects, Interactions, Pharmacokinetics. See Appendix A.

Pycnogenol (*Pinus pinaster* subsp. *atlantica*)

Grade C: *Unclear or conflicting scientific evidence (gingival bleeding/plaque; platelet aggregation (smokers); prevention of blood clots during long airplane flights)*

Note: Pycnogenol contains oligomeric proanthocyanidins (OPCs) as well as several other bioflavonoids. There has been some confusion in the U.S. market regarding OPC products containing Pycnogenol or grape seed extract (GSE) because one of the generic terms for chemical constituents of GSE ("pycnogenols") is the same as the patented trade name (Pycnogenol). Some GSE products formerly were erroneously labeled and marketed in the United States as containing "pycnogenols." Although GSE and Pycnogenol do contain similar chemical constituents (primarily in the OPC fraction), the chemical, pharmacological, and clinical literature on the two products is distinct. The term *Pycnogenol* should therefore be used only when referring to this specific proprietary pine bark extract. Scientific literature regarding this product should not be referenced as a basis for the safety or effectiveness of GSE.

Mechanism of Action

In vitro study showed that ethanol-dissolved Pycnogenol enhanced acetylsalicylic acid's (aspirin's) platelet inhibition effects.[89] The constituents responsible for these actions and their mechanisms are not well understood.

Scientific Evidence of Effectiveness

Preliminary human studies suggest that Pycnogenol treatment may be effective in decreasing the number of thrombotic events (DVT and superficial vein thrombosis) during long-duration airplane flights.[90] Edema following long flights was reduced in asymptomatic subjects compared with placebo.[91] Other human studies report reduced platelet aggregation in smokers who received Pycnogenol supplements,[92,93] without affecting bleeding time,[104] and with no effect seen in nonsmokers.[93] Pycnogenol chewing gum significantly reduced gingival bleeding compared with regular chewing gum.[94] Further research is needed to confirm the safety and efficacy of Pycnogenol in patients with known thrombotic risks.

Dose

Pycnogenol is a proprietary patented formula. Because of its astringent taste and occasional minor stomach discomfort, Pycnogenol may be taken with or after meals.[95]

For gingival bleeding/plaque, 5 mg of Pycnogenol in chewing gum (six pieces daily) has been used for 14 days.[94]

The dose of Pycnogenol for platelet aggregation has not been determined. To prevent blood clots during long flights, studies have used two 100-mg Pycnogenol capsules taken 2 to 3 hours before flight with 250 mL of water, two capsules taken 6 hours later with 250 mL of water, and one capsule taken the next day.[90,91]

Adverse Effects, Interactions, Pharmacokinetics. See Appendix A.

Rhubarb (*Rheum* spp.)

Grade C: *Unclear or conflicting scientific evidence (upper gastrointestinal bleeding; hemorrhage [nephritic syndrome])*

Mechanism of Action

In a DIC rat model, oral rhubarb reduced erythrocyte deformability and decreased platelet count and fibrinogen levels after 4 hours, compared with untreated rats.[96] The constituents responsible for this antithrombotic effect are unknown.

Scientific Evidence of Effectiveness

UPPER GASTROINTESTINAL BLEEDING. Rhubarb has been used in traditional Chinese medicine for many gastrointestinal disorders, including upper gastrointestinal bleeding (UGIB). Relatively low-quality studies suggest that rhubarb may be beneficial in reducing UGIB. In clinical trials, rhubarb supplementation achieved hemostasis in patients with UGIB[97,98] in an average of 2.8 days[97] and with a higher efficacy and faster cure rate than conventional treatment.[99,100] Rhubarb was equivalent to cimetidine (Tagamet) treatment in UGIB patients.[101] Rhubarb improved symptoms in patients with bleeding gastric ulcers.[102]

HEMORRHAGE (NEPHRITIC SYNDROME). Available clinical evidence suggests that a combination of rhubarb and sanchi powder seemed to reduce the hemorrhagic effects of nephritic syndrome more than dicynonum.[103] Higher-quality studies are necessary to confirm the use of rhubarb in bleeding disorders.

Dose

For UGIB, clinical studies have used 3 g of alcoholic extract tablets or powder, or 6 mL of rhubarb syrup, two to four times daily for up to 2 weeks.[97-99] The exact dose of rhubarb for hemorrhage (nephritic syndrome) has not been determined.

Adverse Effects, Interactions, Pharmacokinetics. See Appendix A.

Rutin ($C_{27}H_{30}O_{16}$)

Grade C: *Unclear or conflicting scientific evidence (thrombosis, retinal vein occlusion)*

Mechanism of Action

Studies have confirmed the antierythrocyte aggregation effect of *troxerutin*,[104] a constituent of rutin, and suggest a favorable effect on blood fibrinolytic activity.[105] Acute endothelial cell desquamation and enhanced platelet function caused by smoking cigarettes were not prevented by rutoside supplementation in one study.[106]

Clinical study showed that O-(β-hydroxyethyl)-rutoside (HR) produced a significant decrease in venous capacitance, with increased venous tone and decreased venous distensibility.[107] At the end of follow-up, the troxerutin-treated group had diminished progression of ischemia and decreased red blood cell (RBC) aggregability compared with the controls. Troxerutin demonstrated profibrinolytic activities in pharmacological studies.[108]

Scientific Evidence of Effectiveness

THROMBOSIS. Limited clinical evidence suggests that the standardized rutoside mixture Venoruton in combination with elastic compression or thrombectomy, may offer benefit in superficial venous thrombosis compared with these treatments alone.[109]

RETINAL VEIN OCCLUSION. For the treatment of retinal vein occlusion, troxerutin significantly improved visual acuity, macular threshold, retinal circulation times, and macular edema.[107] Patients also had diminished progression of ischemia and decreased RBC aggregability.

Dose

Venoruton is available in different releasing formulations.[110,111] Rutosides (e.g., Venoruton) or oxerutins are a standardized mixture of hydroxyethyl derivatives of rutin, of which tri-7,3′,4′-hydroxyethylrutoside (tri-HR, or troxerutin, CAS 7085-55-4) is the qualitatively major component, at approximately 38%.[112]

For postthrombotic syndrome, 1200 mg of HR capsules have been taken daily for 8 weeks.[113] For superficial vein thrombosis, 1 g of Venoruton has been taken three times daily in combination with elastic compression for 8 weeks.[114] For retinal vein occlusion, 7 g of troxerutin powder have been used daily.[115]

Adverse Effects, Interactions, Pharmacokinetics. See Appendix A.

Turmeric (*Curcuma longa*)

Grade C: *Unclear or conflicting scientific evidence (blood clot prevention)*

Mechanism of Action

Curcumin, the active constituent in turmeric, inhibits thromboxane A_2 without affecting the synthesis of prostaglandin I2 (PGI_2, prostacyclin).[116] Curcumin also inhibits platelet aggregation.[117,118] Turmeric appears to inhibit arachidonic acid incorporation into platelet phospholipids, degradation of phospholipids, and COX.[119,120]

Scientific Evidence of Effectiveness

Preclinical evidence suggests that turmeric has antiplatelet activity.[116-118,121] There is insufficient clinical evidence regarding the effect of turmeric on coagulation in humans.

Dose

The dose of turmeric for blood clot prevention has not been determined.

Adverse Effects, Interactions, Pharmacokinetics. See Appendix A.

Yohimbe (*Pausinystalia yohimbe*)

Grade C: *Unclear or conflicting scientific evidence (inhibition of platelet aggregation)*

Mechanism of Action

In doses of 4-mg, 8-mg, and 12-mg, yohimbine was found to inhibit epinephrine-induced platelet aggregation ex vivo.[122] The lowest dose of yohimbine that significantly inhibited platelet aggregation was 8 mg, and the inhibitory effect lasted 10 hours with the 12-mg dose. Consistent with these findings, yohimbine has also been shown to bind the α_2-adrenoceptor responsible for noradrenaline-induced platelet aggregation.[123] Evidence also indicated that the binding capacities of ^{3}H-yohimbine on intact human platelets were considerably lower than ^{3}H-dihydroergocryptine, an ergot alkaloid derivative.

Scientific Evidence of Effectiveness

Preclinical studies report that yohimbine alkaloid, isolated from yohimbe bark, may inhibit platelet aggregation. Research in humans is limited, and it is unclear if these platelet effects are beneficial in the management of coagulation disorders.[123]

Dose

The exact dose of yohimbine for coagulation disorders has not been determined in clinical studies.

Adverse Effects, Interactions, Pharmacokinetics. See Appendix A.

HERBAL THERAPIES WITH LIMITED EVIDENCE

Breviscapine *(Erigeron breviscapus)*

New breviscapine (NB) is the soluble sodium and calcium salts of the flavonoid breviscapine (4′-scutellarin-7-glucuronide), extracted from the Chinese herb *Erigeron breviscapus*. It has been demonstrated to inhibit platelet thromboxane B_2 production[124] and promote the release of tPA and thrombomodulin.[125] Additional study is warranted to examine NB's effect on coagulation in vivo.

Fenugreek *(Trigonella foenum-graecum)*

Fenugreek preparations may contain coumarin derivatives that may increase PT or INR and may increase the risk of bleeding.[126,127] In animals, a fenugreek extract was shown to inhibit platelet aggregation.[128]

Marjoram *(Origanum majorana)*

In vitro studies demonstrated the ability of marjoram to inhibit platelet adhesion.[129] Clinical research is lacking.

Rosemary *(Rosmarinus officinalis)*

Rosemary showed significant antithrombotic activity in preclinical studies.[130] Further research is needed to elucidate these effects.

Savory *(Satureja spp.)*

Summer savory *(satureja hortensis)* has been demonstrated to inhibit platelet adhesion in vitro.[129] Its effect on hemostasis in vivo is unclear.

Seaweed

Many distinct types of marine algae are known collectively as *seaweed*; these contain a variety of high-molecular-weight polysaccharides, including fucoidans and fucans. Fucoidans isolated from bladderwrack *(Fucus vesiculosus)* have been found in vitro to enhance the heparin cofactor II–thrombin reaction through the formation of a ternary complex with both substances.[131-133] An additional ex vivo analysis using human plasma has demonstrated the ability of fucoidan to prolong aPTT.[3]

Fucoidans isolated from bladderwrack have stronger anticoagulant properties than those isolated from other brown seaweed or kelp species, including *Sargassum muticum* and *Laminaria digitata*, because of higher contents of fucose and sulfate.[134,138] Animal and in vitro studies have demonstrated the anticoagulant properties of fucoidans isolated from bladderwrack in vitro and in rabbits. More recent studies have confirmed the anticoagulant properties of fucoidans from bladderwrack and other brown seaweeds, including *Ascophyllum nodosum*, *Laminaria religiosa*, and *Pelvetia caniculata*.[131,134-136] Bladderwrack fucoidan was demonstrated to increase the rate of heparin cofactor II–thrombin inhibition, resulting in anticoagulant effects in vitro.[131] Fucans with higher fucose and sulfate levels, such as those isolated from bladderwrack, were found to have more potent anticoagulant properties than fucans with low sulfate and fucose concentrations.[134] Fucoidan extract from *L. religiosa* was demonstrated to have greater antithrombin activity than heparin and activated plasminogen.[135] Fucoidan derivatives isolated from bladderwrack stimulated tissue plasminogen activator (tPA)–induced clot lysis through the activation of plasminogen, and slowed the rate of fibrin polymerization in vitro; intravenous fucoidan, administered weekly to hyperlipidemic rats, also decreased the size of hepatic vein thrombi induced by endotoxin.[136]

In the 1860s it was discovered that some seaweeds are hypermetabolic thyroid stimulants, attributed primarily to its iodine constituent. Based on this effect, bladderwrack has been included as a component of numerous weight loss formulas. Bladderwrack has also been shown in preclinical studies to possess anticoagulant and hypoglycemic properties.[131-138] However, a literature review reveals that clinical evidence is lacking in support of (or against) its efficacy for any use. The active ingredients of bladderwrack have not all been fully identified, and little research exists on its components. Therefore, most pharmacological activities attributed to bladderwrack are generally recognized for brown seaweed species and are not specific to bladderwrack.

Tarragon *(Artemisia dracunculus)*

In vitro studies showed that tarragon prevented platelet adhesion[129]; further research is needed to evaluate the effect in humans and in hypercoagulable states.

Thyme *(Thymus vulgaris)*

In vitro studies have shown that thyme has antithrombotic activity.[130] Additional study is necessary to determine its effects in humans.

Willow *(Salix spp.)*

Willow bark from certain *Salix* species contains salicin (salicylic acid), which is a chemical precursor to acetylsalicylic acid (aspirin).[139] Aspirin has known anticoagulant effects and is widely used to prevent MI and stroke.[140] Some herbalists recommend willow bark extract as a natural substitute for aspirin for these same benefits. In Germany, willow bark is often taken with aspirin to enhance therapeutic effects while minimizing side effects.[141]

Herbs and Supplements that May Increase Risk of Bleeding or Clotting*

HERB	SPECIFIC THERAPEUTIC USE(S)†	HERB	SPECIFIC THERAPEUTIC USE(S)†
Abuta	Hemorrhage (bleeding)	Ginseng	Anticoagulant
Acacia	Anticoagulant	Goldenrod	Hemorrhage (internal bleeding)
Acerola	Hemorrhage (retinal bleeding), anticoagulant	Goldenseal	Hemorrhage (antiheparin), anticoagulant, blood circulation
Aconite	Hemorrhage (bleeding), anticoagulant, phlegmasia alba dolens or milk leg syndrome	Green tea	Hemorrhage (bleeding of gums or tooth sockets)
African wild potato	Hemorrhage (bleeding)	Guggul	Hemorrhage (bleeding)
Agrimony	Hemorrhage (bleeding)	Horny goat weed	Anticoagulant
Alfalfa	Hemorrhage (procoagulant)	Horse chestnut	Anticoagulant (pulmonary embolism, deep venous thrombosis)
Alpinia	Anticoagulant	Horseradish	Anticoagulant
Andrographis paniculata	Anticoagulant	Horsetail	Hemorrhage (bleeding)
Annatto	Hemorrhage (bleeding) anticoagulant	Jequirity	Anticoagulant
Apricot	Hemorrhage (bleeding)	Jiaogulan	Hemorrhage (subarachnoid hemorrhage), anticoagulant
Arnica	Anticoagulant (pulmonary embolism, thrombophlebitis)	Kudzu	Anticoagulant (pulmonary embolism)
Astragalus	Hemorrhage (bleeding), anticoagulant	Lemongrass	Anticoagulant
Babassu	Anticoagulant	Lime	Hemorrhage (intestinal bleeding)
Bael fruit	Hemorrhage (bleeding)	Meadowsweet	Anticoagulant
Bear's garlic	Anticoagulant	Milk thistle	Hemorrhage (bleeding)
Bilberry	Hemorrhage (bleeding gums)	Mistletoe	Hemorrhage (bleeding), malignant hematologic disease
Black currant	Anticoagulant	Myrcia	Hemorrhage (bleeding)
Black haw	Hemorrhage (bleeding)	Nopal	Hemorrhage (bleeding)
Blessed thistle	Hemorrhage (bleeding)	Onion	Anticoagulant
Boldo	Anticoagulant	Oregano	Anticoagulant
Bromelain	Anticoagulant (fibrinolysis)	Populus	Anticoagulant
Burdock	Anticoagulant	Psyllium	Hemorrhage (bleeding)
Calamus	Blood circulation (ischemia)	Raspberry	Hemorrhage (bleeding)
Calendula	Anticoagulant	Red yeast rice	Blood circulation
Cat's claw	Hemorrhage (bleeding)	Rehmannia	Anticoagulant
Chamomile	Anticoagulant	Reishi mushroom	Anticoagulant
Chia	Anticoagulant	Rose hip	Anticoagulant
Chlorella	Hemorrhage (bleeding)	Rosemary	Anticoagulant
Cinnamon	Anticoagulant,	Safflower	Anticoagulant, blood circulation
Clove	Anticoagulant	Sage	Hemorrhage (bleeding gums), anticoagulant
Codonopsis	Blood circulation		
Coleus	Anticoagulant	Sassafras	Anticoagulant
Coltsfoot	Anticoagulant	Scotch broom	Hemorrhage, bleeding gums, hemophilia
Cordyceps	Hemorrhage (bleeding)	Sea buckthorn	Anticoagulant, blood circulation
Cowhage	Anticoagulant	Shepherd's purse	Hemorrhage (bleeding)
Danshen	Anticoagulant (antiphospholipid syndrome)	Shiitake	Hemorrhage (cerebral hemorrhage), anticoagulant
Desert parsley	Anticoagulant	Skunk cabbage	Hemorrhage (bleeding)
Dong quai	Hemorrhage (bleeding hemorrhoids), anticoagulant	Sorrel	Hemorrhage (bleeding)
Flax	Anticoagulant	Soy	Anticoagulant

Continued

Herbs and Supplements that May Increase Risk of Bleeding or Clotting—cont'd

HERB	SPECIFIC THERAPEUTIC USE(S)†	HERB	SPECIFIC THERAPEUTIC USE(S)†
Stinging nettle	Hemorrhage (bleeding)	Willow bark	Anticoagulant
Strawberry	Anticoagulant	White oak	Hemorrhage (bleeding gums)
Tamanu	Hemorrhage (internal bleeding), anticoagulant	White water lily	Hemorrhage (bleeding)
Usnea	Anticoagulant	Yarrow	Hemorrhage (bleeding), anticoagulant
Wasabi	Anticoagulant	Yew	Anticoagulant
Wheatgrass	Blood circulation		

*This is not an all-inclusive or comprehensive list of herbs that affect bleeding time; other herbs and supplements may possess these qualities. A qualified health care provider should be consulted with specific questions or concerns regarding the potential effects of agents or interactions.
†Based on expert opinion, anecdote, case reports, and/or preliminary trial evidence.

ADJUNCT THERAPIES

1. Because *vitamin K* is involved in the coagulation cascade, low levels in the blood may lead to an increased risk of bleeding. Therefore, patients should consume healthy and balanced diets that are rich in vitamin K. Vitamin K is found in green, leafy vegetables such as spinach, broccoli, asparagus, watercress, cabbage, and cauliflower. It is also found in bananas, green peas, beans, olives, canola, soybeans, meat, cereals, and dairy products. Vitamin K is necessary for normal clotting of blood in humans. Specifically, vitamin K is required for the liver to make factors that are necessary for coagulation, including factor II (prothrombin), factor VII (proconvertin), factor IX (thromboplastin component), and factor X (Stuart factor). Other clotting factors that depend on vitamin K are proteins C, S, and Z.

2. Because dietary intake of vitamin K can affect anticoagulant function, inconsistent levels of vitamin K in the diet may make it difficult to control anticoagulant stability. *Warfarin* is an anticoagulant that inhibits vitamin K–dependent clotting factors. If a person's blood becomes too "thin," bleeding management should be under strict medical supervision and may include oral or injected vitamin K to help reverse the effects of warfarin.

3. Another therapy is *mesoglycan,* which is a glycosaminoglycan found in aortic acid and made from the aorta of animals (e.g., sheep, cows). Mesoglycan is said to prevent recurrent deep vein thrombosis (DVT); however, research does not support these claims. According to available study, oral mesoglycan with compression stockings did not reduce the recurrence of DVT.[142]

INTEGRATIVE THERAPY PLAN

- Interview the patient to determine the history of the bleeding or clotting problem and, with hemostatic disease, how long the bleeding has occurred. Ask whether the bleeding predominantly occurs in mucosal and skin locations, or whether bleeding episodes have occurred in deep tissue structures such as the abdomen or joints.
- Question patients with thrombotic disease about the location of previous or current clots and associated symptoms.
- Discuss the patient's medical history and family history of thrombosis or bleeding. Some clotting factor abnormalities, such as hemophilia, are genetic and may be hereditary.
- Initial evaluation involves measurements of platelet count, prothrombin time (PT), and activated partial thromboplastin time (aPTT). Hemoglobin and/or hematocrit may also be warranted if there is a suspicion of anemia. The results will help with further workup, which may include evaluation for platelet abnormalities, coagulation deficiencies or inhibitors, or factor deficiencies that result in a prothrombotic state.
- The laboratory values that should be monitored regularly in patients with bleeding disorders depend on the exact diagnosis and treatment and may include a complete blood count (CBC), a platelet count, PT, aPTT, international normalized ratio (INR), and a hemoglobin/hematocrit.
- Identify any habits relevant to hemostasis, including excessive alcohol use, consumption of vitamin K in the diet, sedentary lifestyle, and nutritional deficiencies.
- Identify other risks factors for thrombosis, such as obesity, pregnancy, and malignancy.
- Discuss with the patient all the medications being taken, including anticoagulants such as warfarin (Coumadin) and NSAIDs (aspirin). Also, any herbs or dietary supplements that the patient is taking should be discussed. Those that increase the risk of bleeding should be identified.
- Currently, no known herbal or alternative therapies are known to effectively treat hemostasis or hypercoagulable states. Only policosanol has strong evidence of effective inhibition of platelet aggregation, but this evidence comes primarily from studies of healthy adults, and its

effects in patients with excessive clotting are unknown. Because of the serious risks associated with poorly treated hemostatic or thrombotic disease, patients should continue therapy with conventional prescription therapy.
- If herbs or supplements are added that may affect platelet aggregation or coagulation, patients should discuss this with their physician before beginning supplementation and should have their clinical and laboratory parameters monitored closely.
- Immediate care for a patient with a thrombus or thromboembolus is often directed at removal of the clot. The method used largely depends on the clot's size and location. For example, with DVT, heparin therapy is initiated to prevent further clotting. Warfarin therapy may also be initiated, but may take a week or more to become fully effective. Invasive intervention usually occurs with events such as an acute coronary occlusion. Once the patient is stabilized, further workup of the underlying coagulation disorder can proceed. Further evaluation is warranted in patients with no obvious predisposing factor, a history of more than one clot, a family history of recurrent clots, or a stroke or heart attack before age 50.
- Patients who are already receiving coagulation therapy should not drastically change their eating habits unless they consult their health care providers first. Significant changes in vitamin K consumption may have an impact on the effectiveness of treatment.
- Regular exercise may help reduce the risk of blood clots. Sitting still for extended periods may slow blood flow, causing blood to accumulate in the veins, especially in patients who are at risk of developing blood clots.
- Patients who are sitting on airplanes for several hours should stand up and stretch every hour. If possible, walk up and down the aisle a few times during a flight to increase blood flow. Patients on long car, bus, or train trips are likewise advised to get up every couple of hours and stretch their legs. Avoid crossing the legs because that may increase the pressure on the blood vessels.
- Weight control may help prevent blood clots from forming. Obese patients are more likely to develop blood clots because the extra weight puts pressure on the veins and reduces blood flow.

Case Studies

CASE STUDY 15-1

FP is a 52-year-old man who presents to your clinic with complaints of cramping in his left calf when he walks farther than two blocks. His physician diagnosed him with intermittent claudication and gave him a prescription for clopidogrel (Plavix), but he would rather try an herbal agent. Past medical history includes hypertension and hyperlipidemia. FP is currently taking enalapril (Vasotec) and atorvastatin (Lipitor) and smokes one pack of cigarettes a day. He has no known drug allergies. He occasionally takes yohimbe for sexual dysfunction and ginseng for energy. How would you counsel this patient?

Answer: Because the patient is both hypertensive and hyperlipidemic and has atherosclerotic vascular disease, he has increased risks for myocardial infarction and stroke. Anticoagulant agents may decrease the risk of blood clots and help prevent blockages.

There is good evidence that policosanol inhibits platelet aggregation. If FP wants to try policosanol, he should be warned of its potential additive effects with his current medications. Policosanol has antihypertensive and antilipidemic effects and may theoretically act synergistically with his enalapril and atorvastatin. Yohimbe also has antiplatelet activity, and its combination with policosanol may overanticoagulate this patient. In addition, small doses of yohimbe have been associated with hypertension, and high doses have caused hypotension. Yohimbe contains small amounts of yohimbine, a toxic alkaloid. Because of the potential for serious side effects and interactions, the U.S. Food and Drug Administration (FDA) does not consider yohimbine safe for over-the-counter (OTC) sale. Because yohimbe bark may contain clinically significant amounts of yohimbine alkaloid, similar risks may apply. Notably, many yohimbe bark products contain only low levels of yohimbine that may not carry these risks, although most yohimbe bark products are not standardized to yohimbine content.

Given FP's history of hypertension and current treatment with enalapril, he should monitor his blood pressure carefully, with a treatment goal of less than 140/90 mm Hg.

FP's use of ginseng should also be discussed. Ginseng has been associated with hypertension, hypotension, edema, chest pain, palpitations, and tachycardia. Interference with the anticoagulant warfarin has also been reported; thus, ginseng may theoretically increase the risk of thrombosis. Additionally, ginseng has been reported to interact with angiotensin-converting enzyme (ACE) inhibitors and antilipemic agents. Blood pressure and cholesterol levels should be monitored while using ginseng.

CASE STUDY 15-2

KL is a 42-year-old woman who comes into your pharmacy with questions regarding herbal supplements to increase her energy. Ever since her 70-year-old mother died from a massive myocardial infarction (MI) 1 year ago, KL has had severe anxiety about her own cardiac risks and has begun to feel "exhausted from worry." On questioning, you find that she has no additional family members with cardiovascular disease and no significant medical history.

KL has recently begun exercising daily and eating a low-fat diet in an effort to reduce her cardiac risk. She takes no medications and does not drink alcohol or smoke. After a visit with her physician, she was disappointed that he did not provide any prescription medication to help decrease her risk of a MI. After her subsequent Internet reading on OTC treatment for heart health, KL began taking aspirin, yohimbe, garlic, and Pycnogenol.

KL appears very pale and is breathing quickly. You notice several bruises on her forearms; she does report a recent history of easy bruising and bleeding gums when she brushes her teeth. You recommend she visit her physician for evaluation.

KL comes back the next week and tells you that her doctor performed laboratory tests and informed her she was anemic. How would you counsel this patient?

Answer: KL a relatively healthy patient, with no significant risk factors for anemia or bleeding. It is unlikely that the herbs are responsible for the anemia. A healthy patient can replace the small blood loss from the gums. The iron in blood contained in bruises is reabsorbed and reused. KL most likely has another problem causing the anemia: a bleeding ulcer. With anemia, her physician would have initiated an intense workup (or referred her to a colleague) to determine the source of bleeding and underlying cause. Aspirin, yohimbe, garlic, and Pycnogenol have all been shown to have antiplatelet activity. Aspirin and Pycnogenol are the two supplements with the most scientific evidence of effect on platelet aggregation. Yohimbe and garlic have less evidence, but in KL the synergistic effects of these supplements may have led to overanticoagulation. At this point, you cannot counsel KL on exactly which herb or combination is to blame, but she should stop taking all of them and may need iron supplementation.

You should also counsel KL about a healthy lifestyle to reduce cardiovascular disease. Her mother's MI at age 70 does not imply an increased risk for KL, who has no other significant family or personal history that would place her at increased risk of cardiovascular disease.

CASE STUDY 15-3

PM is a 65-year-old man who comes to the pharmacy counter with questions about his current medications: atenolol (Tenormin, 50 mg daily) and hydrochlorothiazide (Dyazide, 25 mg daily); a 6-month course of warfarin (Coumadin, 4 mg daily) was also initiated. He has a history of hypertension and DVT after hip replacement surgery 5 months ago. PM tells you that he bruises every time he bumps into anything, and after having his routine laboratory tests yesterday, the nurse said his INR was 5.0, which indicates that he is at risk of bleeding (goal INR, 2.0-3.0). He is wondering why his INR, which has been maintained around 2.0 consistently for the previous 5 months, has suddenly become too high. How would you counsel this patient?

Answer: PM had a significant risk factor for venous thrombosis: surgery with prolonged immobilization. He recently began taking garlic and turmeric for cancer prevention, but he may not be aware that these herbal supplements also have antiplatelet activity. Both are contraindicated in patients taking anticoagulants because of potential exacerbations of the drug's effect. Garlic has been reported to cause bleeding. Turmeric theoretically may also increase the risk of hemostatic instability because of its in vitro antiplatelet effects.

PM should be counseled to stop taking both supplements and to inform his physician that he has been taking them. PM should also avoid certain foods, such as spinach and bananas, which are high in vitamin K. Inconsistent vitamin K intake may also contribute to hemostatic instability during warfarin therapy.

If PM discontinues warfarin at a future date, he may then cautiously begin supplementation. He should do this under careful supervision and laboratory monitoring.

References for Chapter 15 can be found on the Evolve website at http://evolve.elsevier.com/Ulbricht/herbalpharmacotherapy/

Review Questions

1. Which of the following statements about garlic is *false*?
   a. It increases fibrinolytic activity.
   b. It has been reported to cause intraoperative bleeding.
   c. It may significantly decrease the plasma levels of protease inhibitors.
   d. It has been reported to cause hyperthyroidism.

2. Which of the following laboratory parameters may be affected by garlic supplementation?
   a. Serum potassium
   b. Serum glucose
   c. Urinary ketones
   d. Serum albumin

3. Drugs that may *potentially* interact with ginger include which of the following?
   a. Procainamide
   b. Digoxin
   c. Isotretinoin
   d. a and b

4. Grape seed extract has all the following effects *except*:
   a. Enhanced nitric oxide release
   b. Prevention of superoxide production
   c. Increased O_2 production
   d. Reduced platelet aggregation

5. True or false: In general, policosanol increases the rate of adverse glycemic events in diabetic patients.

6. Which statement about Pycnogenol is true?
   a. It decreases the effect of salicylates in vitro.
   b. Pycnogenol may increase platelet aggregation.
   c. Pycnogenol treatment may be effective in preventing deep vein thrombosis and superficial vein thrombosis.
   d. All of the above statements are true.

7. True or false: Turmeric inhibits the degradation of platelet phospholipids and the incorporation of arachidonic acid into platelet membranes.

8. Which of the following statements about yohimbe is *true*?
   a. It binds to the α_2-adrenoreceptor on platelets.
   b. It is rapidly absorbed after oral administration.
   c. It has a half-life of approximately 24 hours.
   d. It is safe to take during pregnancy.

9. True or false: The FDA has determined yohimbine to be safe for over-the-counter sale.

10. Which of the following drugs is likely safe to take with grape seed extract?
    a. Allopurinol
    b. Methotrexate
    c. Cimetidine
    d. Enalapril

Answers are found in the Answers to Review Questions section in the back of the text.

16 Lipid Disorders

Outline

OVERVIEW
  Signs and Symptoms
  Diagnosis
    Total Cholesterol Levels
    Lipoprotein Levels
    Triglyceride Levels
    Treatment Categories
SELECTED HERBAL THERAPIES
  Alfalfa (*Medicago sativa*)
  Ashwagandha (*Withania somnifera*)
  Astragalus (*Astragalus membranaceus*)
  Avocado (*Persea americana*)
  Barley (*Hordeum vulgare*)
  Beet (*Beta vulgaris*)
  Beta-Glucan (β-Glucan)
  Beta-sitosterol (β-Sitosterol), Sitosterol
    (22,23-Dihydrostigmasterol, 24-Ethylcholesterol)
  Borage (*Borago officinalis*)
  Carob (*Ceratonia siliqua*)
  Chia (*Salvia hispanica*)
  Cordyceps (*Cordyceps sinensis*)
  Danshen (*Salvia miltiorrhiza*)
  Elder (*Sambucus nigra*)
  Fenugreek (*Trigonella foenum-graecum*)
  Flax (*Linum usitatissimum*)
  Garlic (*Allium sativum*)
  Ginseng (*Panax* spp.)
  Globe Artichoke (*Cynara scolymus*)
  Goldenseal (*Hydrastis canadensis*)
  Grapefruit (*Citrus* x *paradisi*)
  Grape Seed (*Vitis* spp.)
  Guggul (*Commiphora mukul*)
  Gymnema (*Gymnema sylvestre*)
  Lemongrass (*Cymbopogon* spp.)
  Milk Thistle (*Silybum marianum*)
  Nopal (*Opuntia* spp.)
  Omega-3 Fatty Acids, Alpha-Linolenic Acid
  Policosanol
  Psyllium (*Plantago* spp.)
  Pycnogenol (*Pinus pinaster* subsp. *atlantica*)
  Red Clover (*Trifolium pratense*)
  Red Yeast Rice (*Monascus purpureus*)
  Reishi Mushroom (*Ganoderma lucidum*)
  Rhubarb (*Rheum* spp.)
  Safflower (*Carthamus tinctorius*)
  Soy (*Glycine max*)
  Spirulina (*Arthrospira* spp.)
  Sweet Almond (*Prunus amygdalus dulcis*)
  Tea (*Camellia sinensis*)
  Turmeric (*Curcuma longa*)
  White Horehound (*Marrubium vulgare*)
  Wild Yam (*Dioscorea villosa*)
  Yucca (*Yucca schidigera*)
HERBAL THERAPIES WITH NEGATIVE EVIDENCE
HERBAL THERAPIES WITH LIMITED EVIDENCE
ADJUNCT THERAPIES
INTEGRATIVE THERAPY PLAN
CASE STUDIES
REVIEW QUESTIONS

Learning Objectives

- Describe the impact of cholesterol on cardiovascular risk.
- Understand herbal approaches used to manage hypercholesterolemia.
- Recognize major adverse effects associated with cholesterol-lowering herbs.
- Screen for potential interactions with cholesterol-lowering herbs.
- Counsel a patient regarding cholesterol-lowering herbs.

OVERVIEW

The term *lipid disorders* (also known as dyslipidemia or hyperlipidemia) refers to unhealthy levels of lipids in the blood. Dyslipidemia most often refers to elevated plasma cholesterol and triglyceride levels; however, a low serum level of *high-density lipoprotein* cholesterol (also known as "good cholesterol") is also a form of dyslipidemia. If left untreated, lipid disorders may lead to atherosclerosis, myocardial infarction (MI or heart attack), or cerebrovascular accident (CVA or stroke).[1]

Cholesterol is a soft, waxy, fatty substance that is an essential component of the cells in the body, as well as a precursor to several hormones. Cholesterol may be obtained through the diet, particularly in animal products (e.g., meats, eggs, dairy). However, the majority of the cholesterol needed by the body is produced by the body itself, primarily in the liver. Cholesterol synthesis is a naturally occurring process that produces membranes for all cell types, including those in the brain, nerves, muscles, skin, liver, intestines, and heart. Cholesterol is primarily synthesized in many cells and tissues from *acetyl coenzyme A* (acetyl CoA) through the hydroxymethylglutaryl (HMG)–CoA reductase pathway. Acetyl CoA is also an important precursor to the neurotransmitter acetylcholine. Cholesterol is also converted into steroid hormones, such as the male and female sex hormones (androgens and estrogens, respectively) and the adrenal hormones (cortisol, corticosterone, and aldosterone). In the liver, cholesterol is one of the main components of bile, which aids in the digestion of food (especially fats). Cholesterol is also a precursor to vitamin D, a key nutrient for the skeletal, endocrine, and immune systems.

Cholesterol and other fats are transported in the blood by *lipoproteins*. The two main types of lipoproteins are *low-density lipoprotein* (LDL, also known as *LDL cholesterol* or LDL-C) and *high-density lipoprotein* (HDL or HDL-C). LDL carries cholesterol into the bloodstream, and HDL carries it back to the liver for storage. *Very-low-density lipoprotein* (VLDL or VLDL-C) is converted into LDL in the bloodstream. Each form of lipoprotein contains a specific combination of cholesterol, proteins, and fats *(triglycerides)*. Unused calories from food are converted into triglycerides and stored in fat cells; of all types of cholesterol, VLDL cholesterol contains the highest amount of triglyceride.

Excessive amounts of LDL can block the arteries and increase the risk of heart attack and stroke; thus, LDL is often referred to as "bad cholesterol." A high LDL level is a major risk factor for heart disease (heart failure, stroke). On the other hand, HDL is believed to remove excess cholesterol from arteries, thus slowing the buildup of *plaque* (composed of cholesterol, other fatty substances, fibrous tissue, calcium) in the arteries. High levels of HDL are associated with lower risks of heart attack and stroke.[2]

Lipid disorders can cause plaque deposits to form and accumulate in the arteries; these may become deposited on the artery walls if the blood does not flow properly. As the artery walls thicken, the passageway for blood narrows. The development of plaque and blockage in the arteries involves several steps. When the endothelium is damaged by oxidation, cholesterol particles, proteins, and other substances may deposit into the damaged wall and form plaque. More cholesterol and other substances incorporate into the plaque, which grows and causes *stenosis* (narrowing of artery). Over time, plaque deposits may grow large enough to interfere with blood flow through the artery.[3] If uncontrolled, buildup of plaque in the arteries results in atherosclerosis or coronary artery disease (CAD). When arteries in the legs are blocked, leg pain or cramping may occur. When arteries supplying the heart with blood (coronary arteries) are blocked, *angina* (chest pain; see Chapter 13) or MI may occur. When arteries that supply the brain are blocked, stroke may occur.

If platelets gather in a narrowed artery, they may form a clot that further restricts blood flow. A blood clot, or *thrombus*, may break off and travel through the body. This type of clot, known as an *embolism*, may then become lodged in vessels of the leg, brain, or (less often) lungs (see Chapter 15).

According to a 2006 report by the American Heart Association (AHA), 71.3 million people in the United States have one or more forms of cardiovascular disease.[4] The most prevalent conditions are hypertension (65 million), coronary heart disease (CHD, 13.2 million), stroke (5.5 million), heart failure (5 million), and congenital heart defects (1 million). The highest prevalence occurs in women between ages 65 and 74. The World Health Organization (WHO) reports that high cholesterol contributes to 56% of cases of CHD worldwide and causes about 4.4 million deaths each year.[5]

Generally, people who live in countries where blood cholesterol levels are lower, such as Japan, have lower rates of heart disease. Conversely, countries with very high cholesterol levels (such as Finland) have very high rates of CHD. However, some populations with similar total cholesterol levels have very different heart disease rates, suggesting that other factors (e.g., diet, genetics, smoking) also influence CHD risk.

Signs and Symptoms

High cholesterol levels may lead to specific physical symptoms over time. These may include thickening of tendons from accumulation of cholesterol (called *xanthoma*), yellowish patches around the eyelids (called *xanthelasma*), and white discoloration of the outer edges of the cornea from cholesterol deposits (called *arcus senilis*).

A high serum cholesterol level causes the arteries to narrow and can slow (or even block) blood flow to the heart. This reduced blood supply prevents the heart from receiving enough oxygen. In addition to heart attacks, chronic high cholesterol can also lead to angina (chest pain), stroke (including transient ischemic attacks), atherosclerosis, and peripheral artery disease (PAD).

Diagnosis

Recommendations for cholesterol screening and treatment have been provided by the National Institutes of Health (NIH) and are summarized in the National Cholesterol Education

Program (NCEP).[6,7] These guidelines recommend that all adults have their cholesterol levels checked at least once every 5 years. Patients with CHD or other forms of atherosclerosis are at the highest risk for heart attack (MI) and stroke (CVA). These patients may benefit the most from cholesterol reduction therapy and should have a full lipid profile performed annually. A lipid profile includes measuring total cholesterol, LDL, VLDL, HDL, triglycerides, and lipoprotein levels. For the most accurate measurements, patients should fast for 9 to 12 hours before the blood sample is taken.

Total Cholesterol Levels

Total serum cholesterol levels (in milligrams per deciliter) fall into one of three categories[6,7]: (1) *desirable* (<200 mg/dL), (2) *borderline high risk* (200-239 mg/dL), or (3) *high risk* (≥240 mg/dL). For children and adolescents (2-19 years old), total cholesterol levels are categorized as *acceptable* (<170 mg/dL), *borderline* (170-199 mg/dL), or *high* (≥200 mg/dL). If the total cholesterol is less than 200 mg/dL, the risk of heart attack is relatively low unless there are other risk factors, such as smoking, previous MI, or high blood pressure. About one third of American adults are in the borderline-high-risk group (200-239 mg/dL), whereas almost one half of adults have total cholesterol levels below 200 mg/dL. Not everyone with a borderline cholesterol level is at increased risk. For example, premenopausal women who lack other risk factors for a heart attack may have high HDL levels, which increases their total cholesterol count. However, if the total cholesterol level is 240 mg/dL or more, an individual is at high risk of heart attack and stroke. In general, people who have a total cholesterol level of 240 mg/dL have twice the risk of CHD as those with a level of 200 mg/dL. About 20% of the U.S. population have high blood cholesterol levels.

Lipoprotein Levels

Low-density lipoprotein cholesterol (bad cholesterol) is a major risk factor for developing atherosclerosis and CAD.[2] LDL levels of less than 100 mg/dL are optimal for patients at risk for heart disease.[6,7] If individuals have other risk factors for heart disease (e.g., previous MI), LDL levels of less than 70 mg/dL are optimal. LDL levels can also be *near optimal* (100-129 mg/dL), *borderline high* (130-159 mg/dL), *high* (160-189 mg/dL), and *very high* (≥190 mg/dL). LDL cholesterol levels for children are classified as *acceptable* (<110 mg/dL), *borderline* (110-129 mg/dL), and *high* (≥130 mg/dL). On the contrary, HDL (good cholesterol) is protective against heart disease, so higher levels of HDL are more desirable. HDL levels of 60 mg/dL or more help to lower the risk for developing heart disease. HDL levels of less than 40 mg/dL are considered major risk factors for developing heart disease.

Triglyceride Levels

Triglycerides (TGs) are a type of fat that exists in both food and the blood. After eating food, TGs are stored in fat cells. Hormones then control the release of TGs to meet the body's energy needs. High TG levels can increase heart disease risk. TG levels that are borderline high (150-199 mg/dL) or high (≥200 mg/dL) may require treatment.[6,7]

Treatment Categories

Lipid profiles may be used to assess cardiovascular disease risk. This is typically broken down into treatment categories, ranging from category I (very high risk) to category V (low risk):[8]

Category I (Very High Risk)

Individuals in category I are at the highest risk of heart attack. Patients who have existing heart disease are classified as category I if they also have one or more of the following: diabetes or renal dysfunction, other severe risk factors (e.g., smoking, high blood pressure), risk factors for metabolic disorders (e.g., TGs >200 mg/dL; HDL <40 mg/dL), or previous MI or unstable angina. In those with highest cardiovascular disease risk, the LDL goal is less than 100 mg/dL (ideally, ≤70 mg/dL).

A cholesterol-lowering diet, called the *therapeutic lifestyle changes* (TLC) *diet,* should be initiated to help reduce category I risk, even if the LDL level is less than 100 mg/dL. The TLC diet is a low-saturated-fat, low-cholesterol eating plan that calls for less than 7% of calories to come from saturated fat (e.g., in animal products) and less than 200 mg of dietary cholesterol daily.

If the LDL level is 100 mg/dL or greater, drug treatment is typically started at the same time as the TLC diet. If LDL is below 100 mg/dL, drug treatment may also be started together with the TLC diet. The physician will also determine if the risk is "very high," for example, if the individual has had a recent heart attack or has both heart disease and diabetes.

Category II (High Risk)

Individuals are classified as "high risk" if they have one or more of the following: (1) history of heart disease, such as heart attack, angina, or previous heart surgery (e.g., angioplasty, bypass); (2) current heart disease, diabetes, or kidney disease; or (3) other risk factors, such as smoking, high blood pressure, family history of heart disease, or greater than 20% MI risk in the next 10 years. For individuals with Category II risk, the target LDL level is less than 130 mg/dL (ideally, <100 mg/dL).

If the LDL level is 130 mg/dL or higher, treatment with the TLC diet should be initiated. If LDL is 130 mg/dL or more after 3 months of following the TLC diet, drug treatment is started along with the TLC diet. If LDL is less than 130 mg/dL, individuals should follow the "heart-healthy diet for all Americans," which permits slightly more saturated fat and cholesterol than the TLC diet.

Category III (Moderately High Risk)

Individuals in the moderately high-risk category have two or more risk factors for heart disease, such as advanced age, smoking, high blood pressure, or family history of premature heart disease, and a 10% to 20% chance of developing heart disease in the next 10 years. For individuals with category III risk, the LDL goal is less than 130 mg/dL. If the LDL level is 130 mg/dL or higher, the TLC diet is initiated. If LDL is 160 mg/dL or greater after following the TLC diet for 3 months, drug treatment may be started along with the TLC diet. If LDL is less than 130 mg/dL, the heart-healthy diet for all Americans is used.

Category IV (Moderate Risk)

Individuals in the moderate-risk category have two or more risk factors for heart disease, such as age, smoking, high blood pressure, or family history, but a chance of less than 10% of having heart disease in the next 10 years. For individuals with category IV risk, the LDL goal is less than 160 mg/dL (ideally, <130 mg/dL). If LDL is 160 mg/dL or higher, the TLC diet is started. If LDL is still 160 mg/dL or more after 3 months of following the TLC diet, drug treatment may be started along with the TLC diet to lower LDL, especially if LDL is 190 mg/dL or greater. If LDL is less than 160 mg/dL, the heart-healthy diet for all Americans is used.

Category V (Low Risk)

Individuals in the low-risk category have no more than one risk factor for heart disease.

SELECTED HERBAL THERAPIES

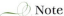
Note
To help make this educational resource more interactive, all pharmacokinetics, adverse effects, and interactions data have been compiled in Appendix A. Safety data specifically related to pregnancy and lactation are listed in Appendix B. Please refer to these appendices when working through the case studies and answering the review questions.

Alfalfa (Medicago sativa)

Grade C: *Unclear or conflicting scientific evidence (atherosclerosis; hyperlipidemia)*

Mechanism of Action

Multiple animal studies suggest that alfalfa may lower cholesterol and triglyceride levels, possibly without altering HDL.[9-14] Saponins in alfalfa may decrease intestinal absorption and increase fecal excretion of cholesterol.[9,15]

Scientific Evidence of Effectiveness

HYPERLIPIDEMIA. Two small case series have reported that alfalfa decreases total cholesterol and LDL levels.[16,17] HDL levels remained unchanged.[17] The AHA Step 1 diet was maintained throughout the study.

ATHEROSCLEROSIS. Currently available evidence for the use of alfalfa in atherosclerosis is limited to animal studies. Ingestion of alfalfa is associated with regression of atherosclerotic plaque in animals.[18-20] Human data are lacking.

Dose

For hyperlipidemia, 40 g of heated-prepared seeds has been used three times daily with food.[16] In three volunteers, ingestion of 160 g of alfalfa daily for 3 weeks, followed by 80 g daily for another 3 weeks, resulted in decreased plasma cholesterol levels.[17]

Adverse Effects, Interactions, Pharmacokinetics. See Appendix A.

Ashwagandha (Withania somnifera)

Grade C: *Unclear or conflicting scientific evidence (hypercholesterolemia)*

Mechanism of Action

Ashwagandha has been reported to possess antioxidant properties[21,22] and to prevent lipid peroxidation in animal studies.[23-25] These properties may contribute to its cholesterol-lowering effects.

Scientific Evidence of Effectiveness

In a case series, 12 patients who received powdered roots of ashwagandha showed significant decreases in serum total cholesterol levels, triglycerides, LDL, and VLDL.[26] Additional clinical evidence is warranted.

Dose

In a case series, patients with mild hypercholesterolemia took powdered roots of ashwagandha (dosage unclear) for 30 days by mouth.[26]

Adverse Effects, Interactions, Pharmacokinetics. See Appendix A.

Astragalus (Astragalus membranaceus)

Grade C: *Unclear or conflicting scientific evidence (coronary artery disease)*

Mechanism of Action

The hypocholesterolemic action of astragalus is not well understood. Polysaccharide fractions of *Astragalus* have been reported to have hypolipidemic actions in vitro and in both normal and diabetic animals.[27]

Scientific Evidence of Effectiveness

Currently, human studies evaluating the hypocholesterolemic effects of astragalus are lacking. A combination of *Astragalus mongholicus* and *Angelica sinensis* significantly lowered cholesterol, triglycerides, LDL, and VLDL in rats.[28]

Dose

For CAD, 20 g of *Astragalus* has been used three times daily.[29]

Adverse Effects, Interactions, Pharmacokinetics. See Appendix A.

Avocado (Persea americana)

Grade B: *Good scientific evidence (hypercholesterolemia)*

Mechanism of Action

The cholesterol-lowering effects of avocado may result from its monounsaturated fatty acid content, specifically oleic acid.[30] Avocado is also a rich source of β-sitosterol, which has strong scientific evidence for reducing hypercholesterolemia (see Beta-Sitosterol).

Scientific Evidence of Effectiveness

Various clinical trials have been performed to investigate effects of avocado on serum lipids.[31-36] All the studies substituted some of the initial fat in the diet with fat from avocado, which appeared to lower total cholesterol, LDL cholesterol, triglycerides, and apolipoprotein B (apo B).[31-35] It also appeared to raise HDL levels.[30,31,34] The longest study was only 12 weeks, and most of the studies were poorly controlled for possible confounding factors such as exercise.

Dose

Studies have shown that 0.5 to 1.5 avocados consumed daily for 2 to 4 weeks can decrease serum lipids.[30,34,35] One study used 300 g of avocado daily for 7 days as a substitute for other lipids.[30] Avocado-enriched diets, in which 75% of fat comes from avocado, have been used for 2 to 4 weeks for hypercholesterolemia.

Adverse Effects, Interactions, Pharmacokinetics. See Appendix A.

Barley (Hordeum vulgare)

Grade B: *Good scientific evidence (hyperlipidemia)*

Mechanism of Action

Plasma lipid-lowering effects of barley have been attributed to high levels of *beta-glucan*, a water-soluble fiber.[36] The beta-glucan component of barley is believed to slow gastric emptying time, prolong the feeling of fullness, and stabilize blood sugar levels. An additional contributory factor may be *d*-alpha-tocotrienol, which works in the liver to inhibit cholesterol production.[37] In chicks, high-protein barley flour (HPBF)–based diets increased body weight (18%), suppressed HMG-CoA reductase (−36%), impaired fatty acid synthetase (−40%), and decreased serum triglyceride (−9%) and cholesterol levels (−23%).[38]

Scientific Evidence of Effectiveness

Several small clinical studies suggest that high-fiber barley, barley bran flour, and barley oil elicit small reductions in serum cholesterol levels by increasing cholesterol excretion.[39-41] Strong evidence supports the use of barley along with a cholesterol-lowering diet in patients with mild hypercholesterolemia. Barley consumption appears to reduce total and LDL cholesterol but does not appear to affect triglycerides or HDL.[40,42] The U.S. Food and Drug Administration (FDA) has approved health claims that two dietary fibers (beta-glucan and psyllium) may reduce the risk of CHD.[43]

Dose

Barley has been used in various doses and forms to treat hyperlipidemia. These have included the following: a "barley diet" for 6 weeks,[40] 3 g of barley oil extract or 30 g of barley bran flour for 30 days,[41] muffins with either easily absorbed barley endosperm (containing 7 g of beta-glucan) or barley in a less absorbable form (5 g beta-glucan) for unclear duration,[42] barley enriched with beta-glucan (8.1-11.9 g daily scaled to body weight) for unclear duration,[44] and boiled barley/rice (1:1 by weight) twice daily for 2 to 4 weeks.[45]

Adverse Effects, Interactions, Pharmacokinetics. See Appendix A.

Beet (Beta vulgaris)

Grade C: *Unclear or conflicting scientific evidence (hyperlipidemia)*

Mechanism of Action

Research in animals suggests that the cholesterol-lowering effects of sugar beet fiber may be partly caused by byproducts of bacterial fermentation in the intestines.[46] Short-chain fatty acids, especially acetic acid, have been identified as the compounds potentially responsible for the cholesterol-lowering effects. However, the exact mechanism of these effects is not well understood.

Scientific Evidence of Effectiveness

Increased dietary fiber intake is recommended based on findings that support its antilipemic effects and potential benefits for reducing the risk of cardiovascular disease. Beet pulp and pectin have been studied and used as sources of dietary fiber in humans.[47-50] Despite these findings, controlled clinical trials evaluating the effects of sugar beet fiber have yielded inconsistent results.[47-53]

Dose

There is no well-known standardization for any part of the beet plant, including the beetroot, leaves, pulp, or pulp fiber, for human consumption. For high cholesterol, 26 to 30 g has been taken daily by mouth for 4 to 12 weeks.[48,49]

Adverse Effects, Interactions, Pharmacokinetics. See Appendix A.

Beta-Glucan (β-Glucan)

Grade A: **Strong scientific evidence (hyperlipidemia)**

Mechanism of Action

Beta-glucan is a soluble fiber derived from the cell walls of algae, bacteria, fungi, yeast, and plants. Notable plant sources of beta-glucan are barley and oats. Soluble fibers may increase the viscosity of food mass in the small intestine and lead to the formation of a thick, watery layer adjacent to the intestinal mucosa. This layer may act as a physical barrier to reduce the absorption of nutrients and bile acids and prevent cholesterol absorption.[54-55]

Scientific Evidence of Effectiveness

Beta-glucan is typically used for its cholesterol-lowering effects. The FDA has approved health claims that dietary fiber (including beta-glucan) may reduce the risk of CHD.[43] In 1997 the FDA approved oat bran to be registered as the first cholesterol-reducing food, at 3 g of beta-glucan daily.[56] Numerous controlled trials have examined the effects of oral beta-glucan on cholesterol.[43,45,55-69] Small reductions in total and LDL cholesterol have been reported.[55,57,58,61-69] Total and LDL cholesterol were reduced by 6% and 9%, respectively, in a group of patients who received oat beta-glucan (0.75 L daily for 5 weeks).[58] Little to no significant changes have been noted in triglyceride or HDL levels.[57,58,64,65]

Dose

For hypercholesterolemia, 3-g to 16-g doses of beta-glucan daily have been used.[44,56,58,62-66,69,70] The FDA approved and recommends that 3 g of beta-glucan daily is needed to reduce cholesterol levels.[56]

Adverse Effects, Interactions, Pharmacokinetics. See Appendix A.

Beta-Sitosterol (β-Sitosterol), Sitosterol (22,23-Dihydrostigmasterol, 24-Ethylcholesterol)

Grade A: **Strong scientific evidence (hypercholesterolemia)**

Mechanism of Action

Beta-sitosterol is one of the most common dietary phytosterols (plant sterols) found and synthesized exclusively by plants.[71-83] Beta-sitosterol and its glucoside (a glycoside derived from glucose) are structurally related,[75,82,84,85] found in the tissues and plasma of healthy individuals, and excreted in the feces.[86-88] Other phytosterols include *campesterol* and *stigmasterol*.[71,74,76,77,80,89,90] Stanols are saturated derivatives of sterols.[91] Beta-sitosterol is classified as a "noncholesterol sterol," or neutral sterol. However, it is structurally similar to cholesterol and is the main plant sterol in the Western diet.[62,74,92-97]

Beta-sitosterol may lower cholesterol levels by interfering with the intestinal absorption of cholesterol and increasing bile acid secretion. Another possible mechanism for its ability to lower cholesterol is inhibition of sterol reductase, which has been demonstrated in vitro.[97] Sterol reductase is an essential enzyme in the process of cholesterol biosynthesis.[62,96,98-101] In vitro studies suggest that plant sterols limit cholesterol ester availability in cells, leading to increased degradation of apoB-100 and apoA-48. This would result in the decreased production of VLDL from the liver and chylomicrons from the intestine, precursors of LDL and chylomicron remnants, respectively.[102]

Scientific Evidence of Effectiveness

Many animal and human studies have demonstrated that supplementation of beta-sitosterol into the diet decreases total serum cholesterol and LDL cholesterol.[81,96,98-100,103-160] Margarines enriched with phytosterol esters, including beta-sitosterol, have been marketed for their cholesterol-lowering effects.* Beta-sitosterol supplementation has reduced total cholesterol by 6% to 13% and LDL cholesterol levels by 8% to 23%.†

High-density lipoprotein cholesterol has been shown in clinical trials to increase by about 5% to 15% with beta-sitosterol supplementation,[99,148] although not as effectively as bezafibrate.[165] Data from other clinical trials contradict this and suggest that beta-sitosterol does not increase HDL.‡

Dose

Standardization of beta-sitosterol products is lacking.[101,166,167] For hypercholesterolemia, the oral dose range is 1.5 to 6 g daily in divided doses administered before meals.[101,158,168-170] Higher beta-sitosterol doses of 6 to 18 g daily have also been used.[130,150] Margarine and salad dressings enriched with phytosterol esters have also been shown to reduce total and LDL cholesterol when consumed daily as 1.6 to 9 g of phytosterols daily.[99,104,112,124,125,158] Children 5 to 13 years old have taken 1.5 to 2.3 g daily in divided doses.[103,152,171]

Adverse Effects, Interactions, Pharmacokinetics. See Appendix A.

Borage (*Borago officinalis*)

Grade C: **Unclear or conflicting scientific evidence (hyperlipidemia)**

Mechanism of Action

Borage's main constituent of interest is gamma-linolenic acid (GLA), which is likely responsible for its cholesterol-lowering effects.[172,173]

Scientific Evidence of Effectiveness

According to a clinical study, an unspecified source of GLA decreased plasma triglyceride levels and increased HDL cholesterol concentration.[173] Another clinical trial non-specifically found that

---

*References 91, 99-101, 104, 112, 120, 124, 135, 142, 157, 158, 161.
†References 80, 91, 99, 100, 104, 105, 112, 119, 120, 122, 125, 127, 128, 130, 135, 143, 148, 150, 152, 155, 158, 160, 162-164
‡References 90, 119, 120, 128, 137, 145, 152, 155, 158.

supplement oils. This area is very promising, but more research

Dose
The dose of borage seed oil for hyperlipidemia is unclear. One

Carob (Ceratonia siliqua)

cholesterol turnover by decreasing the absorption of bile acids

Scientific Evidence of Effectiveness

4 of carob treatment, then remained relatively constant.[176]

+4.5%,[184] whereas other studies have shown no effect.[176]

Dose
For hypercholesterolemia, 15 g of carob daily, incorporated in

Adverse Effects, Interactions, Pharmacokinetics. See Appendix A.

Chia (Salvia hispanica)

Grade B: *Good scientific evidence (cardiovascular disease prevention/atherosclerosis)*

Mechanism of Action
Various constituents of chia, particularly the omega-3 fatty acids and soluble fiber, are thought to benefit lipid parameters. Chia seed positively influenced serum lipid parameters in animals.[179] Rats fed chia had significantly improved fatty acid ratios in plasma.

lesterol, LDL, and triglycerides and increase HDL.[179] Salba who claim they selectively breed their product to maximize omega-3 fatty acids than typical dark-colored chia seeds. Clinical evidence suggests that Salba has the potential to reduce cardiovascular risk factors in type 2 diabetic patients. Blood lipid profile and glycemic control were not affected by Salba

Willebrand factor were also decreased. Although Salba had no

suggested to reduce cardiovascular risk factors.[180]

Adverse Effects, Interactions, Pharmacokinetics. See Appendix A.

Cordyceps (Cordyceps sinensis)

LDL oxidation.[181-183] Also, cultured cordyceps was shown to

Scientific Evidence of Effectiveness
The polysaccharides in cordyceps have been shown to lower total plasma cholesterol and triglyceride levels in normal

porarily lower cholesterol levels by an average of 70% and triglycerides by 9.2%.

Dose
To lower cholesterol and triglycerides, 999 mg was administered three times daily (total of 2997 mg) for 4 to 8 weeks.[185]

Adverse Effects, Interactions, Pharmacokinetics. See Appendix A.

Danshen (Salvia miltiorrhiza)

Grade C: *Unclear or conflicting scientific evidence (hyperlipidemia)*

Both EPA and DHA have been associated with decreased risk of cardiovascular disease.[216,217] The fiber portion of flaxseed has been proposed to exert lipid-lowering effects by enhancing gastric emptying time, altering transit time, interfering with bulk-phase diffusion of fat, and increasing excretion of bile acids.[218] Flaxseed may exert a beneficial effect on atherosclerotic plaque formation because of the antioxidant properties of lignans and omega-3 fatty acids.[217]

Scientific Evidence of Effectiveness

Flaxseed is approximately 35% oil, of which 55% is ALA.[219-223] Flaxseed contains 58% to 60% omega-3 fatty acid, 18% to 20% omega-6 fatty acid, 30% to 45% unsaturated fatty acids, and approximately 8% of the plant contains soluble fiber mucilage.[224] The plant also contains 20% protein. Flaxseed oil is composed of 73% PUFAs, 18% MUFAs, and 9% saturated fatty acids.

Flaxseed and flaxseed oil have been reported to possess lipid-lowering properties in vitro and in animals.[217,219,225] Multiple poor-quality human studies have administered flaxseed products and measured effects on lipids, with mixed results.[224,226-236] Flaxseed preparations have reduced total and LDL cholesterol levels in normal and hypercholesterolemic patients.[224,226-230] Flaxseed does not appear to alter HDL or triglyceride levels.[227] Flaxseed was also found to improve lipid profile without altering biomarkers of bone metabolism in postmenopausal women.[226,227] Consumption of muffins containing 50 g of flaxseed daily for 4 weeks reduced total cholesterol by 6% and LDL by 9%.[228] Reduction in total cholesterol levels is somewhat less than that reported with other agents, such as HMG-CoA reductase inhibitors (statins).[226] Flaxseed has been shown to reduce LDL levels significantly compared with sunflower seeds.[227] Other studies, however, have reported no change in lipids.[231-236]

Dose

Flaxseed products are not standardized based on specific chemical components, but rather are evaluated with a number of identity and quality tests. Tests may include microscopic and macroscopic inspection and organoleptic evaluation. For hypercholesterolemia, preparations providing 20 to 50 g of flaxseed have been used.[226-229] Flaxseed is usually incorporated into baked goods.

Adverse Effects, Interactions, Pharmacokinetics. See Appendix A.

Garlic (Allium sativum)

Grade B: *Good scientific evidence (hyperlipidemia)*

Grade C: *Unclear or conflicting scientific evidence (familial hyperlipidemia; atherosclerosis)*

Mechanism of Action

The hypocholesterolemic action of garlic is not well understood, although a few mechanisms have been proposed. Garlic's lipid-lowering effects may result from inhibition of HMG-CoA reductase or other enzymes,[237-244] possibly through the diallyl disulfide and trisulfide components of garlic.[245,246] Other suggested mechanisms include increased loss of bile salts in feces and mobilization of tissue lipids into circulation,[247] because garlic has a profound effect on postprandial hyperlipidemia.[248] Wild garlic *(Allium ursinum)* has shown similar efficacy to garlic *(Allium sativum)* in decreasing hepatocyte cholesterol synthesis in vitro.[249,250] Aged garlic extract and its constituents have been shown to inhibit Cu^{2+}-induced oxidative modification of LDL.[251] Aged garlic extract and its constituent, *S*-allylcysteine, have been found to protect vascular endothelial cells from injury caused by oxidized LDL.[252]

Animal and human cell lines have demonstrated reductions in vascular tissue lipids,[253,254] fatty streak formation, and atherosclerotic plaque size.[253,255-260] The mechanism of action may include reduced lipoprotein oxidation, as demonstrated in vitro[251,252,261] and in vivo,[262] possibly caused by organosulfur compounds in garlic.[263] However, this hypothesis has been in dispute based on a 6-month trial in moderately hypercholesterolemic volunteers that failed to demonstrate any effects of garlic supplementation on lipoprotein oxidation.[264]

Scientific Evidence of Effectiveness

HYPERLIPIDEMIA. Oral tablets containing dehydrated garlic powder appear to elicit modest reductions in total cholesterol compared with placebo (<20 mg/dL) when taken short term (4-12 weeks). Effects were unclear after 20 weeks. Small reductions in LDL (by <10 mg/dL) and triglycerides (by <20 mg/dL) may also occur in the short term, although results have been variable. HDL values have not changed significantly. Numerous controlled trials have examined the effects of oral garlic on serum lipids. Most studies have been small (<100 subjects) with poorly described design and results, and most have reported nonsignificant modest benefits of garlic therapy. Several overlapping meta-analyses of pooled studies reported significant mean decreases in total cholesterol between 4 and 12 weeks; these studies also reported reductions in LDL and triglycerides of varying significance.[265-269] The statistical significance of these effects disappears after 20 weeks,[265] possibly because of low statistical power. Criticisms of existing trials include frequent use of the non-enteric-coated preparations, which may allow for degradation of alliinase by gastric acid; however, scant reliable data exist on the efficacy of enteric-coated preparations.[270,271] Also, preliminary evidence indicates that aged garlic extract may elicit superior resistance to LDL oxidation than fresh garlic.[272] The long-term maintenance of effects remains unclear, and ultimate effect on cardiovascular morbidity and mortality is not known.

FAMILIAL HYPERLIPIDEMIA. One small study of familial hyperlipidemia in children did not demonstrate significant effects on lipids, although this trial was not designed to detect small effects.[273] Therefore, small reductions in total and LDL cholesterol may occur but may not be of significant clinical benefit. Further research is warranted.

ATHEROSCLEROSIS. A few studies have suggested that garlic may be beneficial in preventing or treating atherosclerosis,[274,275] though the evidence thus far has been weak. Further research is warranted.

Dose

The optimal dose and preparation for maximal benefit are not clear. For hyperlipidemia, most studies have used 900 mg daily of non-enteric-coated dehydrated garlic powder tablets (Kwai) standardized to 1.3% alliin in three divided doses.

The European Scientific Cooperative on Phytotherapy (ESCOP) recommends 3 to 5 mg of allicin daily (equivalent to 1 clove, or 0.5-1.0 g dried powder) for atherosclerosis prophylaxis.

Adverse Effects, Interactions, Pharmacokinetics. See Appendix A.

Ginseng (Panax spp.)

Grade C: *Unclear or conflicting scientific evidence (coronary artery disease; hyperlipidemia)*

Mechanism of Action

The major active components of ginseng are a diverse group of steroidal saponins known as *ginsenosides* (e.g., F1, F2, F3, R0, Ra1, Ra2, Rb1, Rb2, Rb3, Rc, Rd, Rd2, Re, Rf, Rg1, Rg2, Rg3, Rh1, Rh2, Rh3, Rs4).[276,277,278] Their lipid-lowering effects may be attributed to the stimulation of cholesterol enzymes, such as lipoprotein lipase, which may enhance lipid metabolism.[279,280] Ginsenoside Re may reduce cholesterol, but Rb1 may raise it.[279]

Scientific Evidence of Effectiveness

Some evidence suggests that *P. ginseng* may reduce cholesterol levels;[280-282] however, studies have been of lower methodological strength. One study of five normal and six hyperlipidemic subjects found that ginseng reduced liver cholesterol concentrations, decreased atherogenic index, elevated HDL levels, and decreased triglycerides.[281] Serum cholesterol was not significantly altered in this study.[281] Another trial in postmenopausal women found that a low dose of 500 mg for 12 weeks demonstrated no significant differences in serum cholesterol, HDL, or triglyceride concentrations.[282]

Dose

Ginseng extracts, such as the brand G115, may be standardized to 4% to 7% total ginsenosides content.[283,284] Some sources indicate that ginsenosides constitute an average of 3% of the dried, whole root,[285] and that the usual concentration of ginsenosides can actually be 1% to 3%. Standardized extracts of *P. quinquefolius* (CNT-2000) are also available.[286] The German Federal Pharmacopeia standardizes a minimum ginsenoside content of 1.5%, which is calculated in terms of the ginsenoside Rg1.[287] An evaluation of commercial ginseng products showed a wide variance in panaxoside content.[288] One study of 50 commercial ginseng products found that ginsenoside content varied from 1.9% to 9.0%.[289] A proprietary ginseng product, Cold-fX, is a powdered aqueous extract from the dried root of American ginseng *(P. quinquefolius)*. According to the manufacturer, this product contains consistent levels of *poly*-furanosyl-pyranosyl-saccharides (>90%) and has obtained FDA Investigational New Drug clearance for the conduct of a Phase II clinical trial.[290]

For hyperlipidemia, 6 g of *P. ginseng* extract has been taken daily for 8 weeks.[280]

Adverse Effects, Interactions, Pharmacokinetics. See Appendix A.

Globe Artichoke (Cynara scolymus)

Grade B: *Good scientific evidence (hyperlipidemia)*

Mechanism of Action

Phenolic acids found in artichoke include chlorogenic acid, cynarin, and caffeic acid. The antiatherosclerotic action of artichoke is thought to be the product of two mechanisms of action: (1) an antioxidant effect that reduces LDL oxidation[291] and (2) inhibition of cholesterol synthesis.[292] Globe artichoke extract has been shown to decrease cholesterol synthesis by inhibiting the action of HMG-CoA reductase.[293] Cyanoroside and its constituent, luteolin, may be responsible for inhibition of cholesterol synthesis, while cynarin did not show any effect on cholesterol synthesis.[293]

Scientific Evidence of Effectiveness

In vitro and animal studies have shown *cynarin* and artichoke extracts to reduce serum cholesterol and triglyceride levels.[294-296] In clinical studies, artichoke has demonstrated lipid-lowering effects, with reductions noted in total and LDL cholesterol levels as well as LDL/HDL ratio.[297-300] The effects of globe artichoke on triglycerides have been mixed.[297-300] HDL levels have tended to decrease.[298] Although the lipid-lowering effects of artichoke extract are supported by in vitro and animal studies, and small to moderate beneficial effects are reported in humans, the evidence is still somewhat equivocal. Artichoke may work best in people with higher cholesterol levels.[297,301]

Dose

For hypercholesterolemia, doses have included 320 to 1920 mg of standardized extract (Hepar-SL forte) daily for 4 to 12 weeks;[297,298,302,303] 10 to 20 mL of fresh artichoke juice daily for 6 weeks;[304,305] and 500 mg daily of the isolated artichoke constituent, cynarin.[300]

Adverse Effects, Interactions, Pharmacokinetics. See Appendix A.

Goldenseal (Hydrastis canadensis)

Grade C: *Unclear or conflicting scientific evidence (hypercholesterolemia)*

Mechanism of Action

It is unclear whether berberine can effectively lower cholesterol. Berberine, the main active constituent of goldenseal, has been found to upregulate low-density lipoprotein receptor (LDLR) expression independent of sterol regulatory element binding proteins, but dependent on extracellular signal-regulated kinase (ERK) activation.[306] Berberine elevates LDLR expression through a posttranscriptional mechanism that stabilizes messenger RNA (mRNA).[306]

Scientific Evidence of Effectiveness

Preliminary clinical evidence indicates that berberine may reduce triglycerides, serum cholesterol, and LDL cholesterol.[306,307] Serum cholesterol was reduced by 29%, triglycerides by 35%, and LDL by 25% in a clinical trial of 32 subjects.[306] HDL was not affected.[307]

Dose

There is no well-known standardization for goldenseal, though it is sometimes standardized to its alkaloid constituents (including berberine). For hypercholesterolemia, 0.5 g of berberine has been used twice daily for 3 months.[306,307]

Adverse Effects, Interactions, Pharmacokinetics. See Appendix A.

Grapefruit (Citrus x paradisi)

Grade C: *Unclear or conflicting scientific evidence (heart disease)*

Mechanism of Action

Active constituents of grapefruit include flavonoids such as naringin and furanocoumarins (bergamottin).[308,309] Grapefruit may lower cholesterol, but the mechanism of action is not well understood. Grapefruit is high in *pectin*, a soluble fiber, and contains antioxidants that may be responsible for its cholesterol-lowering effects.

Scientific Evidence of Effectiveness

Grapefruit pectin supplementation has been shown to inhibit hypercholesterolemia in animals.[310] Promising but inconclusive clinical evidence supports the use of grapefruit pectin in heart disease prevention. In subjects with hypercholesterolemia, grapefruit pectin supplementation decreased plasma cholesterol by 7.6%, LDL by 10.8%, and LDL/HDL ratio by 9.8%.[316]

Dose

For high cholesterol, 15 g of grapefruit pectin has been taken in divided doses with meals for 16 weeks.[311]

Adverse Effects, Interactions, Pharmacokinetics. See Appendix A.

Grape Seed (Vitis spp.)

Grade C: *Unclear or conflicting scientific evidence (hypercholesterolemia)*

Note: Grape seed extract (GSE) and Pycnogenol are not the same, even though they both contain oligomeric proanthocyanidins (OPCs). Pycnogenol is a patented nutrient supplement extracted from the bark of European coastal pine *Pinus pinaster* subsp. *atlantica*.

Mechanism of Action

The proposed active components of GSE, the OPCs are responsible for the red color of grapes and belong to a large category of plant chemicals called flavonoids. GSE has demonstrated antioxidant activity, which may contribute to its potential cholesterol-lowering effects.[312-316] In healthy subjects, GSE has been shown to exert reducing effects on oxidized LDL.[317]

Scientific Evidence of Effectiveness

Clinical, animal, and basic science research has focused on the effects of OPCs on lipid metabolism and atherosclerosis and on GSE's antioxidant activity as a basis for this "cardioprotective effect." In one study of hypercholesterolemic subjects, only a combination product of chromium and GSE was found to decrease LDL compared with placebo; HDL levels were unchanged, with no difference in triglyceride concentrations.[318] Researchers also noted a trend toward decreasing the circulating autoantibodies to oxidized LDL in two groups receiving GSE.

Dose

According to anecdotal reports, grape seed preparations may be standardized to contain 40% to 80% OPCs or 95% polyphenols per dose. Different commercial preparations vary slightly in their composition, and the source of OPCs may also differ (either grape seed or pine bark extract).

In healthy individuals, tablets containing 200 to 400 mg GSE (calculated as proanthocyanidin) reduced oxidized LDL after 12 weeks of administration.[317]

Adverse Effects, Interactions, Pharmacokinetics. See Appendix A.

Guggul (Commiphora mukul)

Grade C: *Unclear or conflicting scientific evidence (hyperlipidemia)*

Mechanism of Action

Guggul (gum guggul) is a resin produced by the mukul mirth tree. *Guggulipid* is extracted from guggul using ethyl acetate. The preparation produced by extraction with petroleum ether is called fraction A. Typical guggulipid preparations contain

2.5% to 5% of the plant sterols *guggulsterones E* and *Z*; these two components reportedly exert effects on lipids.[319,320] Guggulsterones, particularly guggulsterone (4,17[20]-pregnadiene-3,16-dione), reportedly antagonize the nuclear hormone receptors, farsenoid X receptor (FXR), and the bile acid receptor (BAR), which are involved with cholesterol metabolism and bile acid regulation.[321-323] Guggulsterone does not exert its lipid effects on mice lacking FXR. Also, guggul may inhibit lipogenic enzymes and HMG-CoA reductase in the liver,[324,325] increase uptake of cholesterol by the liver through stimulation of LDL receptor binding,[320] directly activate the thyroid gland,[326-329] and increase biliary and fecal excretion of cholesterol.[325]

Scientific Evidence of Effectiveness

Before 2003, scientific evidence suggested that guggulipid significantly reduced serum total cholesterol, LDL, and triglycerides and increased HDL.[321,330-339] However, most published studies were small and methodologically weak. In August 2003 a well-designed trial reported small but significant increases in serum LDL levels associated with the use of guggul compared with placebo.[340] No significant changes in total cholesterol, HDL, or triglycerides were measured. These results were consistent with two previous case reports.[341,342] This evidence suggests that guggul is ineffective for treating hypercholesterolemia; however, because of the previous research and historical use, further conclusive evidence is necessary before a definitive conclusion can be reached. There is a lack of reliable research comparing guggul preparations with HMG-CoA reductase inhibitors (statins) or evaluating long-term effects of guggul on cardiac morbidity or mortality outcomes.

Dose

Doses of 500 to 1000 mg of guggulipid (standardized to 2.5% guggulsterones) taken two or three times daily have been used both clinically and in research. An equivalent dose of commercially prepared guggulsterone is 25 mg three times daily or 50 mg twice daily by mouth.[330,337,338] A higher dose has been studied (2000 mg three times daily, standardized to 2.5% guggulsterones) but may be associated with a greater risk of hypersensitivity skin reactions.[340]

Adverse Effects, Interactions, Pharmacokinetics. See Appendix A.

Gymnema (*Gymnema sylvestre*)

Grade C: *Unclear or conflicting scientific evidence (hyperlipidemia)*

Mechanism of Action

The mechanism by which gymnema potentially reduces cholesterol is not well understood. Gymnema may lower cholesterol through decreasing cholesterol synthesis, increasing cholesterol metabolism, or decreasing intestinal fat absorption.[343]

Scientific Evidence of Effectiveness

Reductions in levels of serum triglycerides (TGs), total cholesterol, VLDL, and LDL have been observed in animals after administration of gymnema.[344,345] One study of gymnema in type 2 diabetic patients reported decreased cholesterol and TG levels as a secondary outcome.[346] In addition to baseline conventional oral hypoglycemic agents, gymnema extract GS4 (400 mg daily) was administered for 18 to 20 months to 22 patients. The control group continued receiving conventional drug therapy alone without GS4 and was followed for 12 months. Although this study was designed to evaluate the effects of gymnema on serum glucose levels, the measurement of plasma lipids was a secondary outcome. In the treatment group, statistically significant reductions in plasma lipid levels were observed compared with baseline, including cholesterol (18% reduction), TGs (16% reduction), and free fatty acids (22% reduction). Lipid levels in patients on conventional drug therapy alone remained unchanged.

Dose

An ethanolic acid–precipitated extract from gymnema, labeled GS4, has been used in human trials.[346,347] GS4 has since been patented as "ProBeta" by researchers.

A dose of 200 mg of GS4 extract, taken orally twice daily, was found to lower cholesterol and TG levels.[346]

Adverse Effects, Interactions, Pharmacokinetics. See Appendix A.

Lemongrass (*Cymbopogon* spp.)

Grade C: *Unclear or conflicting scientific evidence (atherosclerosis/hyperlipidemia)*

Mechanism of Action

Lemongrass oil is rich in nonsterol end products of plant mevalonate metabolism.[359] These products include the monoterpenes geraniol and citral, which may suppress cholesterol synthesis.[348]

Scientific Evidence of Effectiveness

One study on the effects of lemongrass oil in hypercholesterolemic subjects found no significant difference from baseline in cholesterol levels after 90 days of lemongrass oil (140-mg capsule daily).[348]

Dose

The dose of lemongrass for atherosclerosis/hyperlipidemia has not been determined.

Adverse Effects, Interactions, Pharmacokinetics. See Appendix A.

Milk Thistle (*Silybum marianum*)

Grade C: *Unclear or conflicting scientific evidence (hyperlipidemia)*

Mechanism of Action

A standard milk thistle extract contains 70% silymarin, a mixture of flavonolignans (silydianin and silychristine), and silibinin. According to in vitro assays, the silymarin component is primarily responsible for the biological effects.[8] Silmaryin inhibits lipid peroxidation, which may contribute to the potential cholesterol-lowering effects of milk thistle.[349-351] In vitro and animal studies also suggest this effect may be attributed to regulation of lipid metabolism and inhibition of cholesterol synthesis in the liver.[355,356]

Scientific Evidence of Effectiveness

Preliminary clinical studies have not consistently found that silymarin lowers cholesterol levels.[357,358] An open clinical study noted small reductions in total cholesterol in 14 hyperlipidemic outpatients treated with 420 mg of silymarin daily for 7 months; decreased HDL cholesterol was also observed.[357] In another study of 15 cholecystectomy (gallbladder removal) patients, those who received silymarin (420 mg daily for 1 month) experienced a significant decrease in biliary cholesterol concentration compared with the placebo group, suggesting decreased hepatic cholesterol synthesis.[358]

Dose

Milk thistle capsules, tinctures, and powders are often standardized to contain 70% to 80% silymarin. One of the most studied and used milk thistle products is Legalon (Madeus, Gemany).

For hypercholesterolemia, 420 mg of silymarin has been taken daily.[357,358]

Adverse Effects, Interactions, Pharmacokinetics. See Appendix A.

Nopal (*Opuntia* spp.)

Grade C: *Unclear or conflicting scientific evidence (hyperlipidemia)*

Mechanism of Action

The potential cholesterol-lowering effects of nopal (also called *prickly pear*) are likely attributable to its fiber content, which includes pectin.[359] Fiber has the potential to prevent the absorption of carbohydrates and lipids from the gut.

Scientific Evidence of Effectiveness

Preliminary studies in animal models suggest a hypolipidemic effect of nopal.[360-362] Methodologically weak studies suggest a potential lipid-lowering activity of nopal in humans.[359,363-365] In a case series of 10 patients with heterozygous familial hypercholesterolemia, nopal reduced total and LDL cholesterol levels after 6 weeks.[363] No effects have been noted on HDL or triglycerides.[363]

Dose. Insufficient available evidence.

Adverse Effects, Interactions, Pharmacokinetics. See Appendix A.

Omega-3 Fatty Acids, Alpha-Linolenic Acid

Grade C: *Unclear or conflicting scientific evidence (hypertriglyceridemia)*

Grade D: *Fair negative scientific evidence (hypercholesterolemia)*

Mechanism of Action

Dietary sources of omega-3 fatty acids (also called n-3 fatty acids) include fish oil and certain plant and nut oils. Fish oil contains the omega-3 fatty acids docosahexaenoic acid (DHA) and eicosapentaenoic acid (EPA), and some nuts (e.g., English walnuts) and vegetable oils (canola, soybean, flaxseed/linseed, olive) contain alpha-linolenic acid (ALA), which is the parent compound of all omega-3 fatty acids, including EPA and DHA. It is thought that the antioxidant properties of omega-3 fatty acids may exert a beneficial effect on atherosclerotic plaque formation. Omega-3 fatty acids from flaxseed have been shown to suppress oxygen free radicals from neutrophils and monocytes, as well as the production of interleukin-1 (IL-1), tumor necrosis factor (TNF), and leukotriene B_4 (LTB_4).[366]

Based on studies examining fish oil, omega-3 fatty acids are utilized in the liver for the synthesis of phospholipids, which are located on the surface of lipoproteins.[367] In most studies reporting reductions in total and LDL cholesterol, however, saturated fat intake was lowered when switching from a control diet to a fish oil diet. When fish oil was administered to subjects consuming constant levels of saturated fat, there was no effect on total cholesterol levels.[368] Nevertheless, there were reports that even under such rigorously controlled conditions (e.g., at low and high fixed concentrations of saturated fatty acids), fish oil was capable of lowering plasma total cholesterol, VLDL, and LDL.[369-371] The decrease in triglycerides (TGs) associated with fish oil dietary consumption or supplementation has been confirmed in numerous human trials.[372-386] Fish oils are thought to lower TGs by decreasing secretion of VLDLs, increasing VLDL apoB secretion, and possibly by increasing VLDL clearance, decreasing VLDL size, and reducing TG transport. Fish oils appear to decrease synthesis of VLDL by inhibiting 1,2-diacylglycerol-sterol *o*-acyltransferase or phosphatidate phosphatase.

Although ALA is the parent compound of all omega-3 fatty acids, including the EPA and DHA found in fish oil, only a small percentage of ALA (<10%) is converted to EPA and DHA, making this an inefficient source of omega-3 fatty acids in the body. A recent systematic review, which examined data from 14 randomized controlled trials (RCTs) of omega-3 fatty acids (as fish oil supplements or diets rich in omega-3 fatty acids), as well as one prospective cohort study, concluded that fish oil (but not ALA) had favorable outcomes on cardiovascular disease.[387] A larger systematic review of 41 RCTs (36,913 participants) and 41 cohort studies suggested that omega-3 fatty acids did not clearly affect cardiovascular risk factors and did not differ whether from fish or plant sources.[388]

Scientific Evidence of Effectiveness

HYPERTRIGLYCERIDEMIA. There is strong scientific evidence from human trials that omega-3 fatty acids from fish or fish oil supplements (EPA + DHA) significantly reduce blood TG levels.[389-394] Benefits appear to be dose dependent, with effects at doses as low as 2 g of omega-3 fatty acids daily. Higher doses have greater effects, and 4 g daily can lower TG levels by 25% to 40%. Effects appear to be additive with HMG-CoA reductase inhibitor (statin) drugs such as simvastatin,[395] pravastatin,[396,397] and atorvastatin.[398] The effects of fish oil on hypertriglyceridemia are similar in patients with or without diabetes[394] and in those with kidney disease receiving dialysis. It is not clear how fish oil therapy compares with other agents used for hypertriglyceridemia, such as fibrates (e.g., gemfibrozil, fenofibrate) or niacin/nicotinic acid. Furthermore, it is not as clear whether omega-3 fatty acids from plant sources are as effective.

HYPERCHOLESTEROLEMIA. Fish oil supplements also appear to cause small improvements (increases) in HDL by 1% to 3%. However, worsening (increases) of LDL by 5% to 10% are also observed. For individuals with high blood levels of total or LDL cholesterol, therefore, significant improvements will likely not be seen and a different treatment may be more beneficial. Whether ALA significantly affects TG levels is unclear, with conflicting evidence.

C-reactive protein (CRP), an acute-phase protein reactant and a marker for inflammation, may be useful in predicting the future of cardiovascular events such as heart attack and stroke.[399] The data on fish oils and CRP are mixed.[400,401] Whereas omega-3 fatty acids from both plants (ALA) and fish (EPA + DHA) have been shown to reduce CRP in some studies, others have shown no effect. There is growing evidence that reducing CRP improves cardiovascular outcomes, although additional research is pending in this area. Although statin drugs, weight reduction, smoking cessation, and cyclooxygenase (COX-2) inhibitors all appear to reduce CRP, the evidence regarding fish oil remains equivocal.

Dose

In the 2003 recommendations, AHA reports that supplementation with 2 to 4 g of EPA plus DHA each day can lower TGs by 20% to 40%.[402] Because of the risk of bleeding from omega-3 fatty acids, particularly at doses greater than 3 g daily), a physician should be consulted before starting treatment with supplements.

Adverse Effects, Interactions, Pharmacokinetics. See Appendix A.

Policosanol

Grade A: *Strong scientific evidence (hypercholesterolemia)*

Mechanism of Action

Policosanol is a natural mixture of higher aliphatic primary alcohols, isolated and purified from sugar cane wax. Policosanol is believed to decrease total and LDL cholesterol and increase HDL by inhibiting cholesterol synthesis and increasing LDL processing.[403] Policosanol may lower cholesterol by inhibiting hepatic cholesterol synthesis before mevalonate generation, but direct inhibition of HMG-CoA reductase activity is thought to be unlikely.[404-407] Policosanol may exert its hypocholesterolemic effects by downregulating expression of HMG-CoA reductase,[404,408] by decreasing its de novo synthesis, or by stimulating its degradation.[409] Even at high concentrations, however, policosanol fails to downregulate HMG-CoA reductase by more than 50%.[410] It has also been shown in vitro that policosanol activates adenosine monophosphate (AMP)–kinase (which suppresses cholesterol synthesis), thus reducing cholesterol levels.[411] Animal studies suggest that LDL catabolism may possibly be enhanced through receptor-mediated mechanisms,[412] but the precise mechanism of action is not well understood.[412]

Scientific Evidence of Effectiveness

Numerous studies, including well-designed trials, have analyzed the effects of policosanol on cholesterol levels. Cholesterol-lowering effects have been demonstrated in virtually all studies.[413-437] Lipid profile improvements with the use of policosanol have been noted in healthy volunteers, patients with type II hypercholesterolemia, type 2 diabetic patients with hypercholesterolemia, postmenopausal women with hypercholesterolemia, and patients with combined hypercholesterolemia and abnormal liver function tests.[415,438] Policosanol has demonstrated effects equal to or better than simvastatin, pravastatin, lovastatin, probucol, or acipimox, and has been reported to have fewer side effects than these drugs in patients with type II hypercholesterolemia.[416-420,430,439] One meta-analysis found that although plant sterols, plant stanols, and policosanol are well tolerated and safe, policosanol is more effective than plant sterols and stanols for LDL reduction and has a more favorable effect on lipid profile, approaching antilipemic drug efficacy.[421]

There is a plausible and well-described mechanism supporting the use of policosanol for cholesterol-lowering effects. However, most human studies have been conducted in Cuba and many have been conducted by the same researchers. At this time, the evidence supporting the efficacy of this agent is compelling, although greater acceptance in the U.S. market may require stronger clinical evidence from independent studies.

Dose

Cuban-manufactured policosanol is a mixture of alcohols isolated and purified from sugar cane. It consists of 66% octacosanol, 12% triacontanol, and 7% hexacosanol. Other alcohols (15%), including tetracosanol, heptacosanol, nonacosanol, dotriacontanol, and tetratriacontanol, are minor components.[440]

For hypercholesterolemia, daily doses of policosanol have ranged from 5 to 40 mg.*

Adverse Effects, Interactions, Pharmacokinetics. See Appendix A.

Psyllium (*Plantago* spp.)

Grade A: *Strong scientific evidence (hypercholesterolemia)*

Mechanism of Action

The soluble fiber found in psyllium is proposed to affect cholesterol absorption.[442-448] One proposed hypocholesterolemic effect of psyllium is "displacement" of dietary fat by soluble fiber.[449-451] Psyllium in the diet may thus reduce the amount of cholesterol available for absorption. Psyllium has been shown to increase fecal excretion of bile acids and cholesterol, bind bile acids and cholesterol in the intestines, allow less circulation for reabsorption, and cause the liver to use more cholesterol to make bile acids; the fatty acids *propionate* and *acetate* are produced from soluble fiber by bacteria in the colon and may also indirectly inhibit cholesterol biosynthesis in the liver.[450]

Scientific Evidence of Effectiveness

Psyllium has been well studied as a "nonsystemic" lipid-lowering agent.[443,452-485] A meta-analysis of eight studies found that consumption of 10.2 g of psyllium daily lowered serum total cholesterol by 4%, LDL by 7%, and the ratio of apoB to apoA-I by 6%, relative to placebo, in subjects already consuming a low-fat diet. The meta-analysis found no effect on serum HDL or triacylglycerol concentrations. Compared with conventional antilipidemic agents such as lovastatin (which lowers total cholesterol by 30%, LDL by 40%, and triglycerides by 20%), the effect of psyllium on lipids is minimal; its use as the sole therapy in patients with moderate to severe hypercholesterolemia is not recommended.[486] As an adjunct to the AHA Step 1 diet therapy, however, psyllium may be useful.[486] Psyllium may be suitable when combined with low-fat diet therapy in individuals with mild to moderate hypercholesterolemia.[453] The FDA has approved health claims that two dietary fibers (beta-glucan and psyllium) may reduce the risk of coronary heart disease.[487]

Dose

Psyllium products may contain husks of *Plantago ovata* seeds or the seeds themselves; the husks are more frequently used. Amounts of psyllium in products are generally reported as total grams. Seed preparations contain approximately 47% soluble fiber by weight, and husk preparations generally contain 67% to 71% soluble fiber and 85% total fiber by weight.[443,454]

To lower cholesterol, 3.4 to 45 g daily of psyllium, in two to three divided doses for 8 to 12 weeks, may be recommended. * Studies using psyllium-enriched cereals or other food products have generally used preparations providing 3 to 12 g daily of soluble fiber for up to 8 weeks.[462,477,488]

Because taking psyllium may cause choking, the FDA requires products to be labeled with directions to take psyllium with at least 8 ounces (a full glass) of water or other fluid.

Adverse Effects, Interactions, Pharmacokinetics. See Appendix A.

Pycnogenol (*Pinus pinaster* subsp. *atlantica*)

Grade C: *Unclear or conflicting scientific evidence (hypercholesterolemia)*

Note: Pycnogenol contains oligomeric proanthocyanidins (OPCs) as well as several other bioflavonoids. There has been some confusion in the U.S. market regarding OPC products containing Pycnogenol or grape seed extract (GSE) because one of the generic terms for chemical constituents ("pycnogenols") is the same as the patented trade name (Pycnogenol). Some GSE products were formerly erroneously labeled and marketed in the United States as containing "pycnogenols." Although GSE and Pycnogenol do contain similar chemical constituents (primarily in the OPC fraction), the chemical, pharmacological, and clinical literature on the two products is distinct. The term *Pycnogenol* should therefore be used only when referring to this specific proprietary pine bark extract. Scientific literature regarding this product should not be referenced as a basis for the safety or effectiveness of GSE.

Mechanism of Action

Pycnogenol is a proprietary mixture of water-soluble bioflavonoids extracted from the bark of French maritime pine (*Pinus pinaster* subsp. *atlantica*). The main constituents are phenolic compounds, which may be further categorized as monomers (catechin, epicatechin, taxifolin) and condensed flavonoids (procyanidins, proanthocyanidins).[489] The exact mechanism by which Pycnogenol may reduce cholesterol levels is not fully understood, but it may result from its antioxidant effects. Pycnogenol has been shown to increase cell viability and reduce lipid peroxidation in vitro.[490]

Scientific Evidence of Effectiveness

In a study evaluating the efficacy of Venostasin (horse chestnut seed extract) and Pycnogenol in the treatment of chronic venous insufficiency, Pycnogenol was found to reduce blood levels of total and LDL cholesterol; no affect was noted on HDL levels.[491]

---

*References 413-420, 422-424, 428, 430-435, 438, 439, 441.

*References 442-445, 452, 454-457, 460, 466, 474, 475, 477, 478, 481-484, 488.

Dose
A dose of 360 mg of Pycnogenol, taken daily for 4 weeks, was found to reduce total and LDL cholesterol.[491]

Adverse Effects, Interactions, Pharmacokinetics. See Appendix A.

Red Clover (Trifolium pratense)

Grade C: *Unclear or conflicting scientific evidence (hypercholesterolemia)*

Mechanism of Action
Red clover is a legume like soy (also a legume) that contains *phytoestrogens,* plant-based compounds that are structurally similar to estradiol and capable of binding to estrogen receptors as agonists or antagonists. The mechanisms for the potential cholesterol-lowering effects of red clover are not fully understood but may be caused by estrogenic effects of the red clover isoflavones *genistein* and *daidzein,* phytoestrogens that are also found in soy.

Scientific Evidence of Effectiveness
The available clinical evidence of red clover's lipid-lowering effect remains inconclusive. Clinical studies have produced largely negative evidence.[492-494] No significant changes in total cholesterol, LDL, or triglycerides have been reported during red clover supplementation in premenopausal and postmenopausal women.[495-497] HDL levels significantly increased after red clover supplementation of 28.5, 57, and 85.5 mg.[498]

Soy protein, another source of isoflavones, has been reported to reduce serum lipid levels by up to 10%. However, soy proteins contain higher levels of genistein and daidzein than red clover and contain other potentially active ingredients (saponins, pectins, essential fatty acids). Preliminary evidence suggests that soy protein is superior to isolated red clover isoflavones for reduction of serum lipid levels.[8]

Dose
To reduce cholesterol levels, daily doses of 28.5, 57, or 85.5 mg of red clover isoflavones (Rimostil) have been taken for 6 months.[498] A dose of 80 mg of red clover isoflavones (Promensil) has also been taken daily for 4 months.[496,498]

Adverse Effects, Interactions, Pharmacokinetics. See Appendix A.

Red Yeast Rice (Monascus purpureus)

Grade A: *Strong scientific evidence (hypercholesterolemia)*

Grade C: *Unclear or conflicting scientific evidence (coronary heart disease)*

Note: Red yeast rice is a product of the yeast *Monascus purpureus* grown on rice and is a dietary staple in some Asian countries. It contains several compounds collectively known as *monacolins,* substances known to inhibit cholesterol synthesis. One of these, monacolin K, is a potent inhibitor of HMG-CoA reductase, the liver enzyme responsible for regulating cholesterol production (and the target of pharmaceutical intervention). This active ingredient is also known as the prescription drug lovastatin (Mevacor), which is approved by the FDA for the treatment of high cholesterol. Of note, lovastatin can cause severe muscle problems that could result in kidney damage. In 2007 the FDA issued a warning to consumers to avoid red yeast rice products promoted on the Internet because these products were found to contain lovastatin. Although red yeast rice is still available in the United States, it is fermented using a different process, and the active ingredient has been removed. Its ability to lower cholesterol is now questionable.

Mechanism of Action
Monacolin is considered the active compound in red yeast rice's cholesterol-lowering effects. Monacolin K, an inhibitor of cholesterol synthesis, is the secondary metabolite of the *Monascus* species and is affected by the cultivation environment and method.[499] Monacolin K was first noted to be a specific inhibitor of HMG-CoA reductase in 1980.[500] Total monacolin content of proprietary supplements of red yeast rice range from 0% to 0.58% by weight (0.15-3.37 mg per capsule),[501] but monacolin K amounts have been shown to differ among products.[502] The commercial product Cholestin (Pharmanex), when it included red yeast rice, contained 0.4% naturally occurring HMG-CoA reductase inhibitors, including the most abundant, monacolin K.[501]

Besides HMG-CoA reductase inhibition, mechanisms proposed for the cholesterol-lowering effects of red yeast rice include inhibition of cholesterol absorption (sterol components), increased clearance of cholesterol, and antioxidant effects.[503] The red yeast rice product Cholestin was shown to inhibit cholesterol biosynthesis in vitro.[504]

Scientific Evidence of Effectiveness
HYPERCHOLESTEROLEMIA. Overall, results suggest that red yeast rice products decrease levels of total and LDL cholesterol and triacylglycerol in subjects with mild to moderate hypercholesterolemia.[505-521] In one study, presented at the Annual Conference on Cardiovascular Disease Epidemiology and Prevention, 187 patients (116 men, 71 women) were given red yeast rice (2.4 g daily) for 8 weeks, after being on the AHA Step 1 diet for 4 weeks; they had significant reduction in total cholesterol (16.4%), LDL (21.0%), triglycerides (24.5%), and total/HDL cholesterol ratio (17.7%). In addition, HDL was significantly increased by 14.6%.[522] However, because the cholesterol-lowering effects likely result from the monacolin content, it is questionable whether approved red yeast rice products (which do not contain monacolins) have similar effects.

CORONARY HEART DISEASE. Results from human trials suggest that red yeast rice use may improve blood flow through increased dilation of blood vessels and reduced levels of the inflammatory molecule C-reactive protein (CRP).[510,523] Further information is required to determine the effect of red yeast rice supplementation on cardiovascular disease symptoms and mortality, especially with products that do not contain monacolins.

Dose

There is no well-known standardization for red yeast rice. However, a few red yeast rice extract products report total monacolin content, primarily monacolin K.[501] Before removing its red yeast rice ingredients, Cholestin was standardized to contain 0.4% total HMG-CoA reductase inhibitors (9.6 mg daily in recommended dosage of 2400 mg daily) and greater than 0.8% unsaturated fatty acids.[524]

Food may enhance bioavailability of lovastatin (monacolin K). Therefore, patients may want to take red yeast rice with food. A dose of 1200 mg of concentrated red yeast powder capsules has been taken orally two times daily with food for 8 weeks. The average consumption of naturally occurring red yeast rice in Asia has been reported as 14 to 55 g daily.

Red yeast rice (xuezhikang), 1200 to 2400 mg, has been taken daily for 2 to 6 weeks and has been found to reduce serum CRP and improve flow-mediated dilation.[510,523,525]

Adverse Effects, Interactions, Pharmacokinetics. See Appendix A.

Reishi Mushroom (Ganoderma lucidum)

Grade C: *Unclear or conflicting scientific evidence (coronary heart disease)*

Mechanism of Action

In animals, reishi has been shown to regulate lipid metabolism, enhance antioxidation, and reduce lipid peroxidation in rats with hyperlipidemia.[526] *Triterpenes,* found in reishi, appear to be responsible for the inhibition of cholesterol absorption and synthesis. Cholesterol biosynthesis is inhibited by the rate-limiting enzyme HMG-CoA reductase. Oxygenated triterpenes are inhibitors of HMG-CoA in vitro. Ganodermic acid (a terpene) and its derivatives, especially sterol VI, potently inhibited cholesterol synthesis in vitro.[527] Further, lanosterol 14α-demethylase, which converts 24,25-dihydrolanosterol to cholesterol, can be inhibited by the 26-oxygenosterols from *Ganoderma lucidum*.[528]

Scientific Evidence of Effectivenes

Few human studies examining reishi's effects on lowering cholesterol have been conducted. One randomized controlled trial reported that Ganopoly, a *G. lucidum* polysaccharide extract, improved major symptoms of CHD, including decreasing serum cholesterol levels.[529]

Dose

Standardization of extracts may not be clinically relevant in predicting effectiveness because the active ingredient in *G. lucidum* has not been fully determined. However, the dose of reishi is often based on its content of polysaccharide peptide and triterpene. These doses can be extracted from spores or the whole-fruiting body preparation. The New Zealand product Ganopoly contains 600 mg of *G. lucidum* extract per capsule and 25% (w/w) crude polysaccharides, equivalent to 30 g fruiting body of *G. lucidum*.[530] A dose of 1800 mg three times daily has been used for CAD.[531]

Adverse Effects, Interactions, Pharmacokinetics. See Appendix A.

Rhubarb (Rheum spp.)

Grade C: *Unclear or conflicting scientific evidence (hypercholesterolemia)*

Mechanism of Action

Rhubarb stalk powder contains 74% fiber and exhibits a bile salt–binding property, which may be responsible for its purported cholesterol-lowering effects.[532-534]

Scientific Evidence of Effectiveness

In mice, dried ground rhubarb stalk fiber decreased plasma concentrations of cholesterol, triglycerides, and hepatic total cholesterol.[535] In hypercholesterolemic men, rhubarb stalk fiber supplementation significantly lowered the serum total cholesterol (8%) and LDL (9%); however, HDL remained unchanged.[532] Similarly, hypercholesterolemic men who received the combination product qing-shen tiao-zhi tablets (containing *Rheum palmatum* and *Alismatics orientalis*) also had decreases in total cholesterol, LDL, and triglycerides.[536]

Dose

For hypercholesterolemia, 27 g of ground rhubarb fiber stalk daily for 4 weeks was shown to lower cholesterol levels.[532]

Adverse Effects, Interactions, Pharmacokinetics. See Appendix A.

Safflower (Carthamus tinctorius)

Grade C: *Unclear or conflicting scientific evidence (familial hyperlipidemia; hypercholesterolemia; atherosclerosis)*

Mechanism of Action

Safflower oil is a good source of *linoleic acid,* an essential unsaturated fatty acid. Clinical evidence suggests that cholesterol synthesis is lower in individuals consuming diets rich in coconut fat and safflower oil than in individuals consuming diets rich in butter; this effect might be associated with lower production rates of apoB–containing lipoproteins.[537] Hepatic accumulation of cholesterol, possibly resulting from the combination of enhanced cholesteryl ester transfer to apoB–containing lipoproteins and increased hepatic uptake of cholesterol, may contribute to the cholesterol-lowering effect of high–oleic acid safflower oil (MUFA) and safflower oil (PUFA) in cholesteryl ester transfer protein (CETP) transgenic mice.[538]

Scientific Evidence of Effectiveness

FAMILIAL HYPERLIPIDEMIA. Safflower oil significantly reduced total cholesterol, LDL, and total apoB levels in patients receiving a safflower (omega-6 fatty acid)–enriched diet, compared with a basal diet high in saturated fat.[539] Normal subjects and patients with familial combined hyperlipidemia had similar responses to the diet, including a marked decrease in triglycerides.[539]

HYPERCHOLESTEROLEMIA. Ingestion of certain fats is known to affect various serum lipid levels; however, the effects of safflower oil are not entirely clear. Some studies suggest that safflower oil may decrease serum total cholesterol, LDL, apoB, and malondialdehyde-LDL,[537,538,540-544] whereas others indicate that safflower oil increases some serum lipids, including cell cholesterol in the plasma and triglyceride-rich lipoproteins.[545-548] Other studies have shown that safflower oil does not significantly affect any lipid/lipoprotein values.[544,549-556] Futher research is needed to resolve these conflicting results.

ATHEROSCLEROSIS. Safflower oil has been shown in clinical studies to increase oxidation of LDL and lower thiobarbituric acid reactive substances (TBARS) compared with fish oil.[557,558]

Dose

A dose of 14 g daily of linoleic acid for 6 weeks has been shown to decrease LDL.[545] A dose of 97 g of safflower oil daily for 14 days has also been used to decrease cholesterol.[559]

A dose of 15 g of safflower oil daily has been used for atherosclerosis in postmenopausal women (duration not noted).[557,558]

Adverse Effects, Interactions, Pharmacokinetics. See Appendix A.

Soy (Glycine max)

Grade A: *Strong scientific evidence (hypercholesterolemia; cardiovascular disease)*

Mechanism of Action

Soy contains phytoestrogens (the isoflavones genistein and daidzein) that may be responsible for its cholesterol-lowering properties.[560] This has not been clearly demonstrated in clinical studies, however, and the mechanism behind the cholesterol-lowering effects of soy remains controversial. It is not known whether products containing isolated soy isoflavones have the same effects as regular dietary intake of soy protein.

Scientific Evidence of Effectiveness

HYPERCHOLESTEROLEMIA. Soy is a member of the pea family and has been a dietary staple in Asian countries for at least 5000 years. Adding soy protein to the diet can moderately decrease blood levels of total and LDL cholesterol by up to 10%.[560] Small reductions in triglycerides may also occur, whereas HDL levels do not seem to be significantly altered.[560] The greatest effects appear to occur in people with elevated cholesterol levels, and benefits last as long as the diet is continued. Total replacement of dietary animal proteins with soy protein yields the greatest benefits.[561] People consuming low-cholesterol diets experience further reductions in cholesterol levels by adding soy to the diet.[561]

CARDIOVASCULAR DISEASE. Research suggests that cholesterol-lowering effects of dietary soy may theoretically reduce cardiovascular risk.[562] However, dietary soy protein has not been shown to affect long-term cardiovascular outcomes (e.g., MI, stroke). Studies have shown that soy has antihypertensive effects[563] and antihyperglycemic properties in patients with type 2 diabetes, although the evidence is not definitive. Although the addition of soy to a healthful diet with regular exercise may theoretically improve cardiovascular outcomes, this has not been definitively proved.

To decrease the risk of coronary heart disease (CAD), the FDA recommends at least 25 g of soy daily. The FDA has approved the use of health claims stating that soy food products decrease the risk of CAD if they contain at least 6.25 g of soy protein per serving and meet other criteria, such as low fat and low sodium. Foods that may carry this health claim include soy beverages, tofu, tempeh, soy-based meat alternatives, and some baked goods.[564]

Dose

To lower cholesterol, the FDA recommends at least 6.25 g of soy per serving (total of 25 g daily).[564]

Adverse Effects, Interactions, Pharmacokinetics. See Appendix A.

Spirulina (Arthrospira spp.)

Grade C: *Unclear or conflicting scientific evidence (hypercholesterolemia)*

Mechanism of Action

Spirulina contains *C-phycocyanin,* a metalloprotein that has been shown to have hypocholesterolemic activity in rats.[565] Cholesterol-lowering activity of spirulina has been found to depend on the degree of fecal steroid excretion.[566] Additionally, spirulina contains gamma-linolenic acid (GLA), an essential fatty acid, which may prevent the accumulation of cholesterol in the body.[567]

Scientific Evidence of Effectiveness

Animal studies have found spirulina to be effective at decreasing serum cholesterol and triglyceride levels.[567-570] Encouraging preliminary evidence from several small trials suggests possible efficacy in humans.[567,571,572] Spirulina was associated with decreased total and LDL cholesterol,[571,572] as well as triglycerides and free fatty acids.[571]

Dose

For high cholesterol, clinical studies have used 2 to 4.2 g of spirulina daily for up to 8 weeks.[571,572]

Adverse Effects, Interactions, Pharmacokinetics. See Appendix A.

Sweet Almond (Prunus amygdalus dulcis)

Grade B: *Good scientific evidence (hypercholesterolemia)*

Mechanism of Action

The hypocholesterolemic action of sweet almond is not entirely clear. One possible mechanism by which sweet almond lowers LDL is through enhancement of LDL receptor activity when monounsaturated fatty acids replace saturated fatty acids in the diet.[573]

Scientific Evidence of Effectiveness

Almonds have been reported to lower LDL and total cholesterol levels.[573-577] In a randomized trial of 45 individuals,[574] an almond-based diet was compared with an olive oil–based diet or a dairy-based diet; in the almond group, statistically significant reductions were observed for total cholesterol, LDL, and total/HDL cholesterol ratio, whereas HDL values remained unchanged. Significant changes were not observed in the olive oil group. Total and HDL cholesterol increased significantly in the dairy-based group.

Dose

Whole almonds have been studied in hyperlipidemic patients in doses ranging from 84 to 100 g daily, with no reported side effects.[574,575]

Adverse Effects, Interactions, Pharmacokinetics. See Appendix A.

Tea (Camellia sinensis)

Grade C: *Unclear or conflicting scientific evidence (hypercholesterolemia; hypertriglyceridemia)*

Mechanism of Action

The mechanism by which green tea potentially lowers cholesterol is not well understood. *Catechins* may prevent cardiovascular diseases by preventing LDL oxidation, through free radical–quenching and metal-chelating abilities, or by recycling other antioxidants such as vitamin E. Catechins appear to interfere with several stages of the inflammatory process involved in atherosclerosis and may influence hemostatic parameters and reduce thrombosis.[578]

The use of green tea for lipid disorders, as well as many of its adverse effects and drug interactions, may be attributable to its caffeine content. One study found that the combination of 20 mg of ephedrine and 200 mg of coffee three times daily for 8 weeks decreased plasma triglycerides (TGs) in a sample of obese females.[579] However, another trial found that French-pressed coffee did not raise TG levels.[580] It remains unclear whether any effects may be attributed to caffeine or other coffee constituents, or whether these effects may be extrapolated to green tea.

Scientific Evidence of Effectiveness

HYPERCHOLESTEROLEMIA. In a randomized placebo-controlled trial, green tea extract (75 mg theaflavins, 150 mg green tea catechins, and 150 mg other tea polyphenols), taken for 12 weeks, was found to reduce total serum and LDL cholesterol by 11.3% and 16.4%, respectively, in adults with mild to moderate hypercholesterolemia.[581]

HYPERTRIGLYCERIDEMIA. Preliminary evidence suggests that green tea may decrease postprandial TG levels in individuals with hypertriglyceridemia. Moderate (224 mg) and high (674 mg) tea catechins reduced postprandial TG levels in healthy adults.[582] Use of a green tea extract did not affect fasting plasma TG levels.[583] Stronger evidence is needed before green tea can be recommended for the treatment or prevention of hypertriglyceridemia.

Dose

The dose of green tea for hypercholesterolemia or hypertriglyceridemia has not clearly been determined, although theaflavin-enriched extract (75 mg theaflavins, 150 mg green tea catechins, 150 mg other polyphenols) for 12 weeks has been used.[581]

Adverse Effects, Interactions, Pharmacokinetics. See Appendix A.

Turmeric (Curcuma longa)

Grade C: *Unclear or conflicting scientific evidence (hypercholesterolemia)*

Mechanism of Action

Turmeric contains the polyphenolic compound *curcumin* (diferuloylmethane), which is responsible for its bright-yellow color and is believed to be its principal pharmacological agent. Turmeric appears to enhance the activity of hepatic cholesterol-7α-hydroxylase and increase cholesterol catabolism.[584-586] The turmeric constituents—demethoxycurcumin, bisdemethoxycurcumin, and acetylcurcumin—also appear to inhibit lipid peroxidation, as demonstrated in rat tissues and liver microsomes.[587]

Scientific Evidence of Effectiveness
In animal models of hyperlipidemia, oral turmeric has been shown to reduce total and LDL cholesterol levels.[584-586] In a case series the effect of curcumin administration on serum lipids was examined in 10 healthy human volunteers.[588] Subjects received 500 mg of oral curcumin daily for 7 days, which was associated with a significant 29% increase in HDL levels and a significant 12% decrease in total cholesterol. This preliminary evidence is encouraging; however, evidence from controlled clinical research is lacking.

Dose
Oral curcumin 500 mg daily for 7 days was reported to decrease total cholesterol and increase HDL.[588]

Adverse Effects, Interactions, Pharmacokinetics. See Appendix A.

White Horehound (Marrubium vulgare)

Grade C: *Unclear or conflicting scientific evidence (hypercholesterolemia)*

Mechanism of Action
The mechanism by which white horehound may lower cholesterol is not well understood. However, *marrubinic acid*, a constituent of white horehound, has been found to stimulate secretion of bile.[589,590]

Scientific Evidence of Effectiveness
In one study evaluating patients with type 2 diabetes, white horehound treatment was associated with reduced cholesterol and triglycerides (4.16% and 5.78%, respectively).[591]

Dose. Insufficient available evidence.

Adverse Effects, Interactions, Pharmacokinetics. See Appendix A.

Wild Yam (Dioscorea villosa)

Grade C: *Unclear or conflicting scientific evidence (hypercholesterolemia)*

Mechanism of Action
The plants considered to be true yams are defined by the constituent *diosgenin*. Multiple animal studies have found that diosgenin decreases intestinal cholesterol absorption and reduces total serum cholesterol levels,[592-599] although the exact mechanism is unknown.

Scientific Evidence of Effectiveness
Diosgenin, a constituent of wild yam, decreased intestinal cholesterol absorption and reduced total serum cholesterol levels in animal studies.[592-601] One study showed that administering vitamin C may enhance the cholesterol-lowering effects of clofibrate and diosgenin.[601] In a case series, seven elderly adults treated with up to eight wild yam pills daily for 6 weeks (individual doses not stated) experienced significant decreases in serum triglycerides and phospholipids, increased serum HDL, and unchanged total serum cholesterol.[602] This study supported the results of a vaguely described 1970s case series, in which patients with ischemic heart disease were treated with yam and reportedly showed significant decreases in serum triglycerides, without significant changes in total cholesterol levels.[603]

Dose
Typical standardization of wild yam products is to 10% diosgenin per dose. Clinical studies of wild yam are lacking; however, there are several traditionally used preparations. Some experts recommend 2 to 4 g or 1 to 2 tsp of dried root daily in two or three divided doses. In capsule form, doses have included 250 mg of wild yam one to three times daily or 450 to 900 mg daily of dioscorea extract from wild yam. Other anecdotal doses include 2 to 4 mL of liquid tinctures (1:1 in 45% alcohol) daily in three to five divided doses.

Adverse Effects, Interactions, Pharmacokinetics. See Appendix A.

Yucca (Yucca schidigera)

Grade C: *Unclear or conflicting scientific evidence (hypercholesterolemia)*

Mechanism of Action. Insufficient available evidence.

Scientific Evidence of Effectiveness
There is limited evidence that yucca may reduce blood lipids. A 6:4 (v/v) blend of partially purified *Yucca schidigera* and *Quillaja saponaria* extract filtrates (0.9 mg daily for 4 weeks) decreased the total and LDL cholesterol levels of hypercholesterolemic patients.[604]

Dose
The dose of yucca for hypercholesterolemia has not been determined.

Adverse Effects, Interactions, Pharmacokinetics. See Appendix A.

HERBAL THERAPIES WITH NEGATIVE EVIDENCE

Acacia (Acacia senegal)

Grade D: *Fair negative scientific evidence*

Gum arabic, derived from *Acacia senegal*, has been studied for the treatment of hypercholesterolemia. Animal studies suggest that acacia may decrease LDL cholesterol.[605] However, in one clinical study, acacia did not yield favorable results; 5 g twice daily for 4 weeks did not affect plasma lipid levels.[606]

HERBAL THERAPIES WITH LIMITED EVIDENCE

Capsicum (*Capsicum* spp.)

The active ingredient in peppers of the *Capsicum* genus is a pungent substance known as *capsaicin*. Capsicum is popularly and traditionally considered a circulatory stimulant and is claimed to improve capillary strength, but human clinical trials are lacking. However, the oleoresin of *Capsicum annuum* has been shown to prevent the accumulation of cholesterol and triglycerides in gerbils.[607]

Hawthorn (*Crataegus* spp.)

Hawthorn has an extensive history of use in cardiovascular disease. Monomeric catechins and oligomeric procyanidins from hawthorn berries are thought to contribute to its hypocholesterolemic effect. The hypocholesterolemic effect was noted to result from an upregulation of hepatic LDL receptors, causing greater influx of plasma cholesterol into the liver. Hawthorn also prevented the accumulation of cholesterol in the liver by enhancing cholesterol degradation to bile acids and by simultaneously suppressing cholesterol biosynthesis.[608]

Hyssop (*Hyssopus officinalis*)

The use of hyssop as an herbal remedy is mentioned in the Old and New Testaments of the Bible. Although not typically used or recommended for hypercholesterolemia, in vitro and in vivo studies show that both oleanolic acid and ursolic acid, constituents of hyssop, have antihyperlipidemic properties.[609]

Resveratrol

Resveratrol, a naturally occurring hydroxystilbene identified in more than 70 plant species (including nuts, grapes, pine trees, certain vines) is thought to play a role in the prevention of heart disease. The "French paradox" has directed attention in recent years to resveratrol's potential health benefits in humans. The French paradox suggests that due to frequent consumption of red wine (a good source of resveratrol), French citizens have lower coronary heart disease mortality than those with similar risk profiles in other industrialized countries. Laboratory tests have noted that resveratrol may help prevent cardiovascular disease, possibly by inhibiting lipid peroxidation of LDL and preventing the cytotoxicity of oxidized LDL.[610,611] Observational studies have also noted correlations in the consumption of wine with a decrease in cardiovascular disease risk; currently, however, high-quality trials are lacking to support resveratrol for this indication.

ADJUNCT THERAPIES

1. The main goal of cholesterol-lowering treatment is to reduce the risk of developing heart disease or having a heart attack. The higher the risk, the lower the LDL goal should be. The two main ways to lower cholesterol are *therapeutic lifestyle changes* (TLC) and drug therapy. TLC includes a cholesterol-lowering diet (called the TLC diet), physical activity, and weight management. TLC is appropriate for anyone whose LDL cholesterol is above his or her target number and goal. Drug treatment with cholesterol-lowering drugs can be used together with TLC treatment to help lower LDL Prevention of elevated cholesterol may be started if an individual is at risk for high cholesterol levels or heart disease.

2. The *TLC diet* is a low-saturated fat, low-cholesterol eating plan. Less than 7% of calories should come from saturated fat (as in animal products), and the diet should contain less than 200 mg of dietary cholesterol daily. The TLC diet recommends only enough calories to maintain a desirable weight and to avoid weight gain. If LDL is not decreased enough by reducing intake of saturated fat and cholesterol, the patient can increase consumption of dietary soluble fiber, such as psyllium and beta-glucan. Soluble fiber is found in cereals, breads, and supplements and may help to increase HDL and decrease LDL. Certain food products that contain plant sterols (a cholesterol-lowering component in many plants) can also be added to the TLC diet to boost its LDL-lowering power. Drinking green tea may help lower cholesterol and promote weight loss. Chromium picolinate may help to balance sugar metabolism and decrease cravings for sweets.

3. Regular physical activity for at least 30 minutes on most (if not all) days is recommended for those who can tolerate exercise. A brisk 30-minute walk, three to four times a week, can positively impact cholesterol levels. Exercise can help raise HDL while lowering LDL and triglycerides, and is especially important for those who are overweight and have a large waist circumference. Stretching exercises such as tai chi, yoga, and Qi gong have also been found to improve cardiovascular health and to help lower cholesterol levels, as well as blood pressure (another risk factor for cardiovascular disease).[612-616]

4. *Coenzyme Q10* (CoQ10) supplementation may also be beneficial in patients with lipid disorders. This fat-soluble substance is produced by the human body and is necessary for the basic functioning of cells. CoQ10 levels are reported to decrease with age and tend to be low in patients

Herbs with Potential Hypolipemic or Hypolipidemic Effects*

HERB	SPECIFIC THERAPEUTIC USE(S)†	HERB	SPECIFIC THERAPEUTIC USE(S)†
Abuta	Hypercholesterolemia	Ginkgo	Hyperlipidemia
Acerola	Hypercholesterolemia	Goji	Hyperlipidemia
African wild potato	Hypercholesterolemia	Hibiscus	Hypercholesterolemia
Aloe	Hyperlipidemia	Holy basil	Hypercholesterolemia
Alpinia	Hyperlipidemia	Hops	Hyperlipidemia
Annatto	Hypercholesterolemia	Horny goat weed	Hypercholesterolemia
Arnica	Hyperlipidemia	Hyssop	Hyperlipidemia
Bael fruit	Hyperlipidemia	Jiaogulan	Hypercholesterolemia
Banaba	Hyperlipidemia, hypertriglyceridemia	Katuka	Hyperlipidemia
		Khella	Hyperlipidemia
Bilberry	Hyperlipidemia	Licorice	Hypercholesterolemia
Bitter melon	Hypercholesterolemia	Lotus	Hyperlipidemia
Black horehound	Hypercholesterolemia	Maitake mushroom	Hypercholesterolemia
Boswellia	Hyperlipidemia	Neem	Hyperlipidemia
Bupleurum	Hypercholesterolemia, hyperlipidemia	Perilla	Hypercholesterolemia, hypertriglyceridemia
Calamus	Hyperlipidemia	Rehmannia	Hyperlipidemia
Cat's claw	Hypercholesterolemia	Rose hip	Hypercholesterolemia
Chicory	Hyperlipidemia, hypertriglyceridemia	Rosemary	Hypercholesterolemia
		Sea buckthorn	Hyperlipidemia
Chlorella	Hypercholesterolemia	Seaweed	Hyperlipidemia
Cinnamon	Hypercholesterolemia	Shiitake mushroom	Hypercholesterolemia
Clove	Hyperlipidemia	Skullcap	Hyperlipidemia
Dandelion	Hypercholesterolemia	Tamarind	Cholesterol metabolism disorders
Devil's claw	Hyperlipidemia		
Dogwood	Hyperlipidemia	Tribulus	Hypercholesterolemia
Dong quai	Hypercholesterolemia	Yellow dock	Hypercholesterolemia
Euphorbia	Hyperlipidemia	Yerba santa	Hypercholesterolemia
Evening primrose	Hypercholesterolemia	Yohimbe	Hypercholesterolemia
Fo-ti	Hypercholesterolemia		
Ginger	Hypercholesterolemia		

*This is not an all-inclusive or comprehensive list of herbs with hypolipemic or hypolipidemic properties; other herbs and supplements may possess these qualities. A qualified health care provider should be consulted with specific questions or concerns regarding the potential effects or interactions.
†Based on expert opinion, anecdote, case reports, and/or preliminary trial evidence.

with some chronic diseases such as heart conditions. Supplementing with CoQ10 may reduce angina and improve exercise tolerance in patients with clogged heart arteries. It may also reduce adverse effects associated with statin therapy, including reduced heart function.
5. Studies suggest that *acupuncture* may help reduce cholesterol levels and improve heart health, although the mechanism of action is unclear.[8] In addition, liver cleansing and milk thistle supplements are sometimes used to remove toxins that may contribute to elevated cholesterol levels. However, supportive scientific evidence is unclear.
6. *Niacin*, also known as nicotinic acid or vitamin B_3, is approved by the FDA for treating hyperlipidemia. Prescription niacin typically comes in strengths of 500 mg or higher. Dietary supplements containing niacin are usually available in strengths of 250 mg or less. Niacin is not extensively discussed in this chapter because it is not an herb. It should be noted that niacin is first-line therapy for patients with isolated low HDL cholesterol.

A common side effect of immediate-release niacin is flushing or hot flashes. Most people develop a tolerance to flushing, which can sometimes be decreased by taking the drug during or after meals or by using aspirin

30 minutes before taking niacin. Additionally, niacin may be unsafe for use in certain populations, such as those with hepatic disease or dysfunction. Niacin has been implicated in hepatotoxicity.[617-638]

INTEGRATIVE THERAPY PLAN

- Individuals age 20 and older should have their cholesterol levels measured at least once every 5 years. A complete lipid profile should be performed to measure total cholesterol, HDL cholesterol, LDL cholesterol, and triglycerides.
- Discuss the patient's family history of heart disease to help assess cardiovascular disease risk.
- Initial therapy for cholesterol disorders should include therapeutic lifestyle changes, including saturated fat and cholesterol restriction, regular exercise, and weight reduction. For patients in whom lifestyle changes fail to control lipid disorders, lipid-lowering medications (e.g., statins) may be prescribed.
- Patients who have not responded to standard cholesterol-lowering medications may consider combination therapy with a natural product such as psyllium, beta-glucan, or soy. Patients should be monitored closely for potential adverse effects and drug interactions.
- Soluble fiber, such as that found in psyllium and barley, may help lower cholesterol. These agents should be taken with plenty of water. In general, prescription drugs should be taken 1 hour before or 2 hours after taking psyllium or barley. Doses of 3.4 to 45 g daily of psyllium, in two to three divided doses for 8 to 12 weeks, have been used in clinical trials.
- There is strong supportive evidence for the use of soy to help lower total and LDL cholesterol and triglycerides. Total replacement of dietary animal proteins with soy protein has yielded the greatest benefits. The FDA has approved a health claim stating that soy products (containing at least 6.25 g of soy protein per serving, one-fourth the effective level of 25 g daily) may reduce the risk of coronary heart disease by lowering blood cholesterol levels. Caution is advised for women with hormone-sensitive conditions, because soy contains phytoestrogens and may have estrogenic effects.
- Beta-sitosterol is one of the most prevalent dietary phytosterols (plant sterols) found in plants, as in fruits, vegetables, soybeans, breads, peanuts, and peanut products. Many human and animal studies have demonstrated that supplementation with beta-sitosterol decreases total and LDL cholesterol.
- There is strong scientific evidence from human trials that omega-3 fatty acids from fish or fish oil supplements significantly reduce blood triglyceride levels. Fish oil supplements also appear to elicit small improvements in HDL; however, increases (worsening) in LDL have also been observed. The AHA reports that supplementation with 2 to 4 g of EPA plus DHA daily can lower triglycerides by 20% to 40%. Because of the risk of bleeding from omega-3 fatty acids, particularly at doses greater than 3 g daily, a physician should be consulted before starting treatment with supplements.
- Guggul may help reduce serum total cholesterol, LDL, and triglycerides and may increase HDL. Doses of 500 to 1000 mg of guggulipid (standardized to 2.5% guggulsterones) two or three times daily have been used in clinical trials. Concurrent use of guggul with other anticoagulant drugs may increase the risk of bleeding.
- Warn patients about purchasing red yeast rice from other countries over the Internet. These unregulated products may contain lovastatin, the cholesterol-lowering ingredient in the prescription drug Mevacor, which has numerous documented adverse effects (e.g., muscle damage, kidney failure). Legitimate red yeast products, which are formulated to contain no lovastatin, are of questionable efficacy for cholesterol reduction.

Case Studies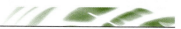

CASE STUDY 16-1

KB is a 48-year-old Caucasian man who was prompted to have a cholesterol evaluation following his father's recent death from heart attack. KB's first lipid panel revealed total cholesterol of 220 mg/dL, LDL 164 mg/dL, triglycerides 125 mg/dL, and HDL 26 mg/dL. KB was counseled by his physician about diet and exercise. His most recent lipid profile revealed total cholesterol of 209 mg/dL, LDL 158 mg/dL, triglycerides 123 mg/dL, and HDL 39 mg/dL. His medical history includes hypertension of 5 years' duration and diabetes for 2 years. KB's current medications include extended-release glipizide (5 mg twice daily) for diabetes, hydrochlorothiazide (25 mg daily) and lisinopril (10 mg daily) to manage hypertension. He also takes low-dose aspirin to reduce CVD risk, fish oil to help lower cholesterol, and bilberry to improve his overall health. He denies smoking and drinks an occasional beer socially. He asks you if there are any additional natural products he can use to help further reduce his cholesterol levels. How should you counsel?

Answer: Based on KB's cholesterol levels and his risk factors, he is at "borderline high risk." Because his father died from heart disease, KB has an increased risk of having a heart attack. As a man, he is at a greater risk for heart attack than age-matched women. Because KB's total and LDL cholesterol are elevated and HDL is borderline low, a natural product to consider is beta-sitosterol, shown to reduce total and LDL cholesterol as well as to elevate HDL. The recommended dose is 1.5 to 6 g daily in divided doses before meals.[101,158,168-170] On a cautionary note, beta-sitosterol and bilberry may both cause lower blood sugar levels; therefore, KB should be counseled regarding the signs of low blood sugar, which include hunger, shakiness, perspiration, dizziness, sleepiness, confusion, anxiousness, and weakness. Advise KB to monitor his blood closely. Because both aspirin and fish oil have anticoagulant effects, concomitant use may increase the risk of bleeding. KB should be warned of this potential interaction. KB may also ask his doctor about niacin, which is FDA-approved for treating hyperlipidemia. Because niacin may be hepatotoxic, caution shoud be used when used with other hepatotoxic agents (such as acetaminophen and alcohol).

CASE STUDY 16-2

SH is a 56-year-old postmenopausal woman. She has a mean LDL cholesterol of 200 mg/dL after a 4-month trial of the TLC diet. She has a family history of cardiovascular problems. Her 80-year-old father has hypertension and type 2 diabetes, and her mother died at age 60 from a heart attack. SH has no siblings and no hypertension or diabetes. However, SH has epilepsy, for which she has been receiving a stable dose of carbamazepine. She also has mild depression, for which she takes St. John's wort. She smokes one pack of cigarettes a day. Her mean HDL cholesterol is 57 mg/dL and triglycerides 80 mg/dL. She is physically active and maintains a normal weight. She complains of daily hot flashes and night sweats. She recently started taking black cohosh for these symptoms, but states that it does not seem to work. She asks you if there are any other natural products she can try. How should you counsel her?

Answer: Although heart disease is more prevalent in men, it is more likely to be fatal in women. In fact, heart disease is the leading cause of death among women, especially after menopause. SH has high cholesterol, which is a major risk factor for heart disease. Studies have shown strong evidence supporting the use of soy to lower cholesterol. The addition of soy protein to the diet can moderately decrease blood levels of total and LDL cholesterol. Dietary soy protein has not been shown to affect long-term cardiovascular outcomes (e.g., MI, stroke). The FDA has approved health claims that soy products (at least 25 g daily) may reduce the risk of coronary heart disease by lowering blood cholesterol levels. Foods that may carry this health claim include soy beverages, tofu, tempeh, soy-based meat alternatives, and possibly some baked goods. As a food product, soy is generally regarded as safe. The most frequent adverse effects related to soy are allergic reactions and gastrointestinal difficulties (bloating, nausea, constipation).

Soy products containing isoflavones have been studied for the reduction of menopausal symptoms such as hot flashes. The scientific evidence is mixed in this area; although several human trials suggest reductions in hot flashes and other menopausal symptoms, more recent research suggests little benefit. Red clover also contains isoflavones that act as phytoestrogens and may benefit menopausal symptoms. However, the research to support red clover is not as strong as that for soy. Because soy and the black cohosh she is taking may both have estrogenic activity, caution is warranted when using these products in combination. Advise SH to consult her physician if she experiences breast tenderness, water retention, or weight gain.

Because the patient is on a stable dose of carbamazepine, dose should not be changed. However, SH should be warned against taking natural products that have been documented to lower seizure threshold, such as evening primrose oil (EPO). SH has a family history of hypertension, a risk factor for CVD. Advise SH to monitor her blood pressure, and to seek medical advice if it is high. Because smoking is another CVD risk factor, advise SH to quit smoking.

CASE STUDY 16-3

MG is a 65-year-old man who weighs 220 pounds. He has recently lost 10 pounds after starting an exercise regimen and a low-fat diet. His daily medications include 10 mg atorvastatin for hypercholesterolemia, 10 mg enalapril for hypertension, 325 mg aspirin, and a multivitamin. His father had a heart attack at age 58, and his postmenopausal sister has hypercholesterolemia and takes a statin. MG reports not smoking or drinking alcohol. His most recent lipid profile is total cholesterol 190 mg/dL, triglycerides 220 mg/dL, HDL 30 mg/dL, and LDL 110 mg/dL. MG is interested in natural products that may help lower cholesterol, particularly red yeast rice products available on the Internet. What is your assessment of MG, and what natural products should you suggest to him?

Answer: MG's total and LDL cholesterol levels are being controlled with atorvastatin. However, according to NCEP guidelines, MG has high triglyceride levels. MG should be counseled regarding diet and exercise. Additionally, there is strong scientific evidence from human trials that omega-3 fatty acids from fish or fish oil supplements (EPA + DHA) significantly reduce blood triglyceride levels. Benefits appear to be dose dependent, with effects at doses as low as 2 g of omega-3 fatty acids daily. Effects also appear to be additive with HMG-CoA reductase inhibitor drugs such as atorvastatin, which MG is currently taking. However, because statin drugs have numerous documented adverse effects (e.g., kidney and muscle damage), MG should avoid taking nephrotoxic agents and should be monitored for muscle damage. He should also avoid unregulated red yeast rice products, which may contain lovastatin (another HMG-CoA reductase inhibitor). Because MG is already taking a statin, additional sources of statins may increase the risks of associated adverse effects.

Patients with high triglyceride levels frequently have low HDL levels. Fish oil supplements also appear to cause small improvements in HDL. However, increases (worsening) in LDL have also been observed. MG should be advised to monitor his lipid levels closely.

The AHA reports that supplementation with 2 to 4 g of EPA plus DHA daily can lower triglycerides by 20% to 40%.[402] Because of the risk of bleeding from omega-3 fatty acids, particularly at doses greater than 3 g daily, a physician should be consulted before starting treatment with supplements, especially since MG is also taking aspirin, which increases bleeding risk as well.

Additionally, fish liver oil products contain the fat-soluble vitamins A and D. Because oil-containing supplements may increase the absorption of fat-soluble vitamins, fish oil products may increase the risk of vitamin A or D toxicity when taken with these vitamins. Because MG takes a multivitamin regularly, you should discuss the potential risks with him.

⊖ **References for Chapter 16 can be found on the Evolve website at http://evolve.elsevier.com/Ulbricht/herbalpharmacotherapy/**

Review Questions

1. True or false: The U.S. Food and Drug Administration (FDA) has approved health claims that two dietary fibers (beta-glucan and psyllium) may reduce the risk of coronary heart disease (CHD).

2. Recommended doses of guggul for hyperlipidemia are:
   a. 5 to 10 mg
   b. 50 to 100 mg
   c. 500 to 1000 mg
   d. 0.5 to 1 mg

3. Which of the following statements is *true* concerning the use of psyllium or its constituents?
   a. Psyllium should not be taken within 1 hour of taking medications or other oral agents.
   b. Psyllium is systemically absorbed.
   c. Psyllium products are considered to be unsafe during all three trimesters of pregnancy.
   d. There is not enough scientific evidence to support the use of psyllium in reducing cholesterol levels.

4. True or false: Safflower oil is a good source of linoleic acid, an essential unsaturated fatty acid.

5. Which constituents of reishi appear to be responsible for inhibition of cholesterol absorption and synthesis?
   a. Flavones
   b. Coumarins
   c. Triterpenes
   d. None of the above

6. Barley should be avoided in patients with which of the following conditions?
   a. Phenylketonuria
   b. Allergy or hypersensitivity to grass or wheat
   c. Hypertension
   d. Lupus

7. Which substances in red yeast rice are known to inhibit cholesterol synthesis?
   a. Phenolic diterpenes
   b. Polyphenols
   c. Hydroxybenzenes
   d. Monacolins

8. True or false: The FDA approved a health claim that soy products may reduce the risk of CHD by lowering blood cholesterol levels.

9. Which of the following constituents of hyssop may contribute to its cholesterol-lowering effects?
   a. Camphene and thujone
   b. Geraniol and borneol
   c. Pinene and limonene
   d. Oleanolic acid and ursolic acid

10. True or false: The oleoresin of hawthorn has been shown to prevent the accumulation of cholesterol and triglycerides.

11. Which of the following isoflavone(s) may be responsible for the cholesterol-lowering properties of red clover?
    a. Genistein
    b. Glycitein
    c. Daidzein
    d. Both a and c

12. To lower cholesterol, which of the following doses of psyllium should be recommended based on clinical evidence of efficacy?
    a. 4 to 12 mg daily in two or three divided doses for 8 to 12 weeks
    b. 34 to 40 mcg daily in two or three divided doses for 8 to 12 weeks
    c. 3.4 to 45 g daily in two or three divided doses for 8 to 12 weeks
    d. 0.34 to 0.45 mg daily in two or three divided doses for 8 to 12 weeks

13. True or false: Fenugreek has been shown to reduce total and LDL cholesterol levels and to increase HDL levels.

Answers are found in the Answers to Review Questions section in the back of the text.

17 Respiratory Disorders

Outline

OVERVIEW
    Asthma
        Signs and Symptoms
        Diagnosis
    Chronic Obstructive Pulmonary Disease
        Signs and Symptoms
        Diagnosis
    Allergic Rhinitis
        Signs and Symptoms
        Diagnosis
    Cystic Fibrosis
        Signs and Symptoms
        Diagnosis
    Pulmonary Fibrosis
        Signs and Symptoms
        Diagnosis
    Pulmonary Hypertension
        Signs and Symptoms
        Diagnosis
SELECTED HERBAL THERAPIES
    Belladonna *(Atropa* spp.*)*
    Borage *(Borago officinalis)*
    Boswellia *(Boswellia serrata)*
    Bromelain (Bromeliaceae)
    Butterbur *(Petasites hybridus)*
    Cat's Claw *(Uncaria* spp.*)*
    Coleus *(Coleus forskohlii)*
    Cordyceps *(Cordyceps sinensis)*
    Danshen *(Salvia miltiorrhiza)*
    Dong Quai *(Angelica sinensis)*
    English Ivy *(Hedera helix)*
    Ephedra *(Ephedra sinica)*
    Eucalyptus *(Eucalyptus* spp.*)*
    Ginkgo *(Ginkgo biloba)*
    Ginseng *(Panax* spp.*)*
    Kiwi *(Actinidia deliciosa, Actinidia chinensis)*
    Mistletoe *(Viscum album)*
    Onion *(Allium cepa)*
    Peppermint *(Mentha x piperita)*
    Perilla *(Perilla frutescens)*
    Pycnogenol *(Pinus pinaster* subsp. *atlantica)*
    Rhodiola *(Rhodiola rosea)*
    Safflower *(Carthamus tinctorius)*
    Stinging Nettle *(Urtica dioica)*
    Tea *(Camellia sinensis)*
    Tylophora *(Tylophora indica)*
HERBAL THERAPIES WITH NEGATIVE EVIDENCE
HERBAL THERAPIES WITH LIMITED EVIDENCE
ADJUNCT THERAPIES
INTEGRATIVE THERAPY PLAN
CASE STUDIES
REVIEW QUESTIONS

Learning Objectives

- Understand herbs used to manage asthma and other respiratory disorders.
- Know the adverse effects, drug interactions, and dosing associated with herbs used in respiratory disorders.
- Be able to devise an integrative care plan for the patient with a respiratory disorder.

OVERVIEW[1-3]

Respiratory disorders, are diseases of the lungs, and include asthma, chronic obstructive pulmonary disease (COPD), emphysema, and allergic rhinitis. Respiratory disorders also include lung cancers and infections. Lung disease can affect people of all ages and both genders, and is the fourth leading cause of death in the United States. In infants, respiratory disorders account for more deaths than any other group of disorders.

Asthma

Asthma is a chronic, inflammatory lung disease. In people with asthma the air passages within the lungs become swollen, restricting the amount of air that can pass through the trachea. Asthmatic patients have recurrent breathing problems and a tendency to cough and wheeze. According to the American Lung Association (ALA), approximately 20 million Americans have asthma, resulting in about 5000 deaths each year. There is no cure for asthma, but many medications and behavioral changes may help manage the condition.

According to a 2002 National Health Interview Survey, asthma has been diagnosed in 9 million people under the age of 19 in the United States. Asthma rates in children younger than 5 years have increased more than 160% between 1980 and 1994. One study found a strong correlation between obesity and asthma, but no similar relationship between obesity and allergies. Some researchers believe this is the result of increased physical exertion of the lungs in obese individuals.

The various asthmatic conditions cause airway obstruction and inflammation, which are partly reversible by medication. The symptoms are usually similar, with the main difference being the cause of the asthma. Classifications of asthma include the following:

- **Allergic (extrinsic) asthma.** Allergic immune responses trigger what is known as allergic asthma, which causes airway inflammation and obstruction. Agents that induce allergies are called *allergens*. Inhaled allergens, such as dust mites, mold spores, pollen, and pet dander, may trigger allergic asthma. It is the most common form of asthma, and accounts for more than half of all cases.
- **Nonallergic (intrinsic) asthma.** Nonallergic asthma is not triggered by allergens, but rather factors such as anxiety, stress, exercise, cold air, dry air, hyperventilation, and viruses.
- **Exercise-induced asthma.** When the airway becomes constricted during vigorous physical activity, the condition is known as exercise-induced asthma.
- **Cough-variant asthma.** A chronic, persistent cough without shortness of breath is known as cough-variant asthma.
- **Occupational asthma.** Poor or compromised air quality in work environments may result in what is called occupational asthma.

Because asthma is an *inflammatory* process, several cells (mostly immune system–mediated cells) have been implicated in the disease process. There are three major parts of the immune response involved in asthma: antibodies, inflammatory cells, and inflammatory mediators. The antibody *immunoglobulin E* (IgE) is involved in most allergic reactions; IgE activation can result in shortness of breath, inflammation, and airway obstruction. The major inflammatory cells involved in asthma are *mast cells, basophils,* and *eosinophils*. Mast cells, which can be found in the lungs, mediate the inflammatory response that is triggered by IgE. The inflammatory eosinophils are closely associated with all types of asthma and can be found in various parts of the lungs and respiratory system. When these inflammatory cells are activated, inflammatory mediators are released. The mediators most often involved in asthma include *histamine,* which is released by activated basophils and mast cells. Other mediators include inflammatory *cytokines* such as *leukotrienes, prostaglandins,* and others. This inflammatory process contributes to airway restriction and bronchospasm, which are caused by tightening of the muscles surrounding the respiratory system. This tightening is achieved by the binding of *catecholamines* (such as epinephrine and norepinephrine) to beta-2 receptors in the lungs and airway.

Signs and Symptoms

Symptoms of asthma include *bronchospasm* (abnormal contraction of the bronchi, which obstructs the airway), coughing (constant or intermittent), wheezing or whistling sounds when exhaling, shortness of breath or rapid breathing, chest tightness or pain, and fatigue. Infants may have trouble feeding and may grunt during suckling.

Asthma symptoms may appear at any time in life. Those who develop asthma as adults, as late as age 50 or older, have what is known as *adult-onset asthma*. Unlike children, who usually experience intermittent symptoms, individuals with adult-onset asthma are more likely to experience persistent symptoms. The cause of adult-onset asthma is unknown. However, some evidence suggests that allergy and asthma may be genetically determined, or related to early childhood development. In addition, obesity, which has both genetic and environmental influences, appears to increase significantly the risk of developing asthma as an adult.

Diagnosis

Spirometry is a noninvasive way to evaluate the air capacity of the lungs. The person breathes into a mouthpiece connected to an instrument called a spirometer, which records the amount and rate of air breathed in and out over a specified time. The most common measurements used for interpretation are forced expiratory volume after 1 second (FEV_1), forced vital capacity (FVC), and forced expiratory flow at 25% to 75% of maximal lung volume (FEF_{25-75}). These are expressed as percentages of what is predicted for normal lung function.[3,4]

In patients with asthma, physicians are also able to measure the volume of air exhaled before and after use of a bronchodilator (e.g., albuterol). During this procedure the spirometer measures the airflow when the patient exhales. This measurement is then compared to the average lung capacity for the individual's age and racial group. After the patient inhales medicine from a short-acting bronchodilator, the procedure is repeated. If there is an increase in lung capacity, the asthma symptoms likely can be controlled.[4]

Chronic Obstructive Pulmonary Disease

Chronic obstructive pulmonary disease (COPD) is a type of lung disease that involves damage to or obstruction of the airways of the lungs, which makes it difficult to breathe. COPD is a general term referring to a group of chronic lung conditions, including chronic bronchitis and emphysema, and possibly asthma or asthmatic bronchitis. Although chronic bronchitis and emphysema may occur separately, patients often have both diseases simultaneously.[5]

The U.S. Centers for Disease Control and Prevention (CDC) reports that COPD affects up to 24 million Americans. The main risk factor for COPD is smoking, and researchers estimate that smoking causes 80% to 90% of COPD deaths. COPD is most likely to develop in cigarette smokers, but cigar, pipe, and marijuana smokers also are susceptible.[5] The risk of COPD is directly related to the number of years a person smokes and the amount smoked. The ALA reports that COPD is the fourth leading cause of death in the United States. COPD patients typically die from complications, such as severe lung infections, heart problems, or lung cancers. Female smokers are almost 13 times more likely to die from COPD than women who never smoked, and male smokers are almost 12 times more likely to die from COPD than men who never smoked.[3]

Signs and Symptoms[3-5]

Symptoms of COPD usually develop gradually over many years and typically worsen over time. Some patients may develop chronic bronchitis or emphysema, whereas others may have both diseases.

Patients with COPD for many years may develop a bluish discoloration of the lips and nail beds. This condition, called *cyanosis*, occurs when there is not enough oxygen in the blood. Some patients may develop headaches in the morning because of the body's inability to remove carbon dioxide from the blood. Many people with COPD also experience weight loss because their bodies use more energy to breathe than those without COPD.

Chronic Bronchitis

Symptoms of chronic bronchitis include chronic cough, increased mucus that is yellow-greenish in color, frequent clearing of the throat, wheezing, and shortness of breath. Patients typically experience fatigue because the body has to work harder to obtain enough oxygen.

Emphysema

Shortness of breath (or *dyspnea*), especially during activity, is one of the earliest symptoms of emphysema. As the disease progresses, shortness of breath becomes constant, even during rest. Individuals with emphysema are likely to feel tired because of the physical difficulty in breathing and the lack of oxygen.

Other

Other symptoms of COPD include distress resulting from the inability to obtain enough air, wheezing, chronic mucus production, exhaling through pursed (puckered) lips or grunting before exhaling, and needing to lean forward to breathe while sitting. Individuals with emphysema are often thin and have very pink skin. Individuals with advanced disease may have the characteristic "barrel chest" from the increase in lung size.

Diagnosis

Pulmonary function tests (PFTs) can detect COPD before symptoms are apparent. These noninvasive tests measure how much air the lungs can hold and airflow into and out of the lungs. PFTs also measure oxygen and carbon dioxide exchange in the lungs and include spirometry and lung volume testing (Table 17-1).[4]

Allergic Rhinitis[1,2]

Rhinitis is inflammation of nasal mucous membranes. Allergic rhinitis (commonly called "hay fever") occurs when the immune system overreacts to inhaled allergens, such as mold, pollen, animal dander, or dust mites. Once the allergen is inhaled through the nose, white blood cells of an allergic individual produce IgE, which attaches to the allergen. This triggers the release of histamine and other inflammatory chemicals that cause allergic rhinitis symptoms, such as postnasal drip (excess mucus in nose and throat causing the sensation of mucus dripping in the back of nose) and nasal congestion.

Signs and Symptoms

Symptoms of allergic rhinitis vary greatly among individuals. Common symptoms include cough; headache; itchy nose, mouth, throat, and skin; nosebleeds; impaired smell; watery eyes; sore throat; wheezing; fever; cross-reactivity allergy to some fruits; pinkeye; postnasal drip; and swelling of the nasal tissues (which can cause headaches). Some patients, especially those with vasomotor rhinitis, sneeze when moving from a cold room to a warmer one.

Diagnosis

A medical history is performed to determine whether the patient's symptoms vary depending on the time of day or season. An allergen-specific IgE blood test called the *radioallergosorbent test* (RAST) can help determine if a patient with allergy symptoms (e.g., runny nose, watery eyes, hives) is allergic to particular allergens. The blood sample is exposed to suspected allergens (e.g., dust mites, pollen, animal dander)

TABLE 17-1	Classification of the Severity of COPD	
STAGE	SPIROMETRY	SYMPTOMS
Mild	$FEV_1/FVC \leq 70\%$ $FEV_1 \geq 80\%$ predicted	Breathlessness with strenuous exercise, when hurrying, or walking up slight hill
Moderate	$FEV_1/FVC \leq 70\%$ $50\% \leq FEV_1 < 80\%$ predicted	Breathlessness causing patient to stop or walk slower after walking about 100 meters on level ground
Severe	$FEV_1/FVC < 70\%$ $30\% \leq FEV_1 < 50\%$ predicted	Patient too breathless to leave the house, breathless after changing clothes, or presence of chronic respiratory failure, or clinical signs of right heart failure

Data from Celli B, MacNee W: ATS/ERS Task Force. Standards for the diagnosis and treatment of patients with COPD: a summary of the ATS/ERS position paper, *Eur Respir J* 23:932-946, 2004; American Thoracic Societ:. Standards for the diagnosis and care of patients with chronic obstructive pulmonary disease, *Am J Respir Crit Care Med* 152:S77-S121, 1995; Siafakas NM, Vermeire P, Pride NB, et al: Optimal assessment and management of chronic obstructive pulmonary disease (COPD), The European Respiratory Society Task Force, *Eur Respir J* 8:1398-1420, 1995.
COPD, Chronic obstructive pulmonary disease; FEV_1, forced expiratory volume in 1 second; FVC, forced vital capacity.

to determine whether the patient has developed allergen-specific IgE antibodies.

Cystic Fibrosis[1,3,6]

Cystic fibrosis (CF), also called *mucoviscidosis*, is a life-threatening inherited disorder that causes severe lung damage and nutritional deficiencies. CF causes the body to produce abnormally thick and sticky mucus, saliva, sweat, and digestive enzymes. In healthy individuals, these secretions serve as lubricants in the body. In CF patients, however, the secretions are so thick that they plug up tubes and passageways in the body. The lungs and pancreas are the organs most frequently affected.

Cystic fibrosis is most common among Caucasians. Researchers estimate that 1 in every 3500 Caucasians in the United States is born with CF. About 1 in every 15,000 African Americans, 1 in 9200 Hispanics, and 1 in 31,000 Asian Americans are born with CF in the United States.

Complications of CF, including lung infections and nutritional deficiencies, can be fatal. The average life expectancy of CF patients is 35 years.

Signs and Symptoms

Symptoms of CF vary among patients. Some patients may experience severe symptoms that affect the lungs as well as the digestive and reproductive systems. Others may experience milder symptoms that affect fewer parts of the body. In some cases, severity of symptoms may change as patients age.

In newborns the first sign of CF may be a blockage of the intestines. Healthy babies normally pass greenish black stools, called meconium, during their first 2 days of life. However, if the infant has CF, the meconium may be too thick to move through the intestines. Other signs and symptoms may include oily stools, failure to grow, and frequent lung infections.

Children and adults with CF typically have increased amounts of salt in their sweat. Parents may taste the salt when they kiss their children's skin; thus, the term "salty kiss" is often used to refer to CF. Other symptoms in children and adults may include oily stools, thick sputum, coughing, difficulty breathing, and wheezing. Patients with CF often have bowel obstructions, which may lead to protrusion of part of the rectum through the anus. Almost all patients eventually experience enlargement or rounding of the fingertips or toes (*clubbing*), resulting from chronic low blood-oxygen levels.

Less common symptoms may include abnormal growths (polyps) in the nasal passageway and cirrhosis of the liver caused by inflammation or obstruction of the bile ducts. Children over 4 years old may experience displacement of one part of the intestine into another part.

Diagnosis

Most patients with CF are diagnosed by age 2. In general, genetic testing is not needed to confirm a diagnosis. Instead, genetic testing is primarily used to determine if the individual is a carrier of the disease.

A less expensive test, called a *sweat test,* measures the amount of salt in the patient's sweat and is considered the standard diagnostic tool for CF. In this test, a sweat-producing chemical is applied to the patient's arm or leg; an electrode is then attached to the area. A painless electrical current passes through the electrode, which causes a warm or tingling feeling in the patient. Several minutes later, the provider collects two samples of sweat to be analyzed in a laboratory. Two sweat samples are tested at the same time to ensure that the results are accurate. If there are high levels of salt in the sample, the patient is diagnosed with CF. The sweat test may not be accurate in newborns, who may be unable to produce enough sweat during the first few months of life; thus it is generally not performed until the patient is several months old.

Pulmonary Fibrosis[1,3]

Pulmonary fibrosis, also known as *interstitial lung disease* (ILD), is a general term that encompasses more than 100 chronic lung disorders that damage the *interstitium* (the tissue located between the air sacs of the lungs). The disease affects the lungs in three ways: the lung tissue is damaged; the interstitium becomes inflamed; and fibrosis (scarring) begins in the alveoli and interstitium, causing the lung to become stiff and making breathing difficult. This scarring of the lung tissue is irreversible, and many patients never regain full use of their lungs.

Signs and Symptoms

Dyspnea is the most common symptom of ILD. Patients may also experience a dry cough without sputum production. When the disease is severe and prolonged, heart failure and swelling of the legs may occur. Less common symptoms of ILD include wheezing, weight loss, cyanosis of the skin or mucous membranes, and clubbing of the fingers.

Diagnosis

Diagnosis is made by using high-resolution computed tomography (HRCT) scan, PFTs, exercise tests, bronchoscopy (transbronchial biopsy), bronchoalveolar lavage (BAL), chest radiography, video-assisted thoracoscopic surgery, and blood gas studies.

Pulmonary Hypertension[1,3]

Pulmonary hypertension results from constriction or tightening of the blood vessels that supply the lungs. As a result, it becomes difficult for blood to pass through the lungs, which in turn makes it more difficult for the heart to pump blood. This causes the heart to enlarge and fluid to accumulate in the liver and tissues. Pulmonary hypertension is a complication in many patients with advanced lung disease, including those with COPD.

Signs and Symptoms

Patients with pulmonary hypertension may experience chronic fatigue, shortness of breath, chest pain, palpitations, fainting, edema, and fluid in the abdomen or legs.

Diagnosis

An echocardiogram (echo) may be used to determine if a patient has pulmonary hypertension. This noninvasive test uses sound waves to create an image of the heart, allowing the physician to determine the size and thickness of the heart muscle.

SELECTED HERBAL THERAPIES

 Note

To help make this educational resource more interactive, all pharmacokinetics, adverse effects, and interactions data have been compiled in Appendix A. Safety data specifically related to pregnancy and lactation are listed in Appendix B. Please refer to these appendices when working through the case studies and answering the review questions.

Warning: No herbal agent should replace a rescue inhaler and should not be used in acute exacerbations.

Belladonna (*Atropa* spp.)

Grade C: *Unclear or conflicting scientific evidence (prevention of airway obstruction)*

Mechanism of Action

Belladonna alkaloids are competitive inhibitors of the muscarinic actions of acetylcholine. They act at receptors located in exocrine glands, smooth and cardiac muscle, and intramural neurons. Anticholinergic agents such as belladonna may relax smooth muscles of the airway and reduce mucus production.[1,7]

Scientific Evidence of Effectiveness

Although the known mechanisms of anticholinergic agents such as belladonna are compelling and have been accepted as a treatment in chronic asthma, efficacy and research are equivocal.[8] Belladonna may be more effective for chronic asthma.[9] Individuals using a homeopathic 30C concentration of belladonna reported no effect on relieving asthma symptoms.[10]

One study on treatment of airway obstruction during sleep in infants demonstrated a beneficial effect of belladonna. Twenty infants age 4 to 46 weeks with a history of "breath-holding spells" received an oral tincture of belladonna equivalent to 0.01 mg/kg body weight of atropine.[11] Belladonna induced cessation of obstructed-breathing episodes in 10 infants.

Dose

To prevent airway obstruction, a controlled trial administered an oral tincture of belladonna, in a dose equivalent to 0.01 mg/kg of atropine, at bedtime to infants.[11]

Adverse Effects, Interactions, Pharmacokinetics. See Appendix A.

Borage (*Borago officinalis*)

Grade B: *Good scientific evidence (acute respiratory distress syndrome)*

Grade C: *Unclear or conflicting scientific evidence (asthma; cystic fibrosis)*

Mechanism of Action

Borage seed oil is a source of *gamma-linolenic acid* (GLA). GLA has shown some immunosuppressant activity that may be helpful in reducing asthma symptoms. GLA is broken down into di-homo-GLA (DGLA), which may be converted to prostaglandin E_1 (PGE_1), a hormone-like substance with antiinflammatory properties.[12] PGE_1 analogs have also been shown to inhibit gastric acid secretion and to increase duodenal bicarbonate secretion, improving fat and nutrient absorption in CF.[13,14]

Scientific Evidence of Effectiveness

ACUTE RESPIRATORY DISTRESS SYNDROME (ARDS). A study in mice demonstrated that supplementation of specific lipids during sepsis-induced ARDS may improve cardiopulmonary function and reduce proinflammatory eicosanoid synthesis and lung inflammation.[15] One clinical study found similar positive results.[16] Further research may be necessary to confirm these findings and determine optimal dosing.

ASTHMA. There is some clinical evidence that borage seed oil may suppress some immunological responses in asthma patients. Borage seed oil was found to increase DGLA in polymorphonuclear (PMN) phospholipids and to suppress *leukotriene B_4* (LTB_4), a potent inducer of bronchoconstriction and asthma, without reaching significance in asthma scores.[17]

CYSTIC FIBROSIS. Preliminary evidence in CF patients indicates that borage seed oil may have some benefits.[13] Small increases in vital capacity (VC) and FEV_1 were noted after administration of 1500 mg of borage oil daily for 4 weeks in nine CF patients. A positive correlation was found between change in VC and change in linoleic acid content of serum cholesteryl esters and arachidonic acid content of serum phospholipids.

Dose

For asthma, 2 g of GLA (borage seed oil) has been taken daily for 12 months.[17]

For cystic fibrosis, 1500 mg of borage seed oil (330 mg GLA) has been taken daily for 4 weeks.[13]

Adverse Effects, Interactions, Pharmacokinetics. See Appendix A.

Boswellia (Boswellia serrata)

Grade B: Good scientific evidence (asthma)

Mechanism of Action

Multiple pentacyclic triterpenic acids, referred to as *boswellic acids*, have been isolated from resins of the *Boswellia* species and identified as major antiinflammatory components of boswellia gum resin extract.[18-27] Acetyl-11-keto-β–boswellic acid has been identified as one of the primary antiinflammatory pentacyclic triterpenes in *Boswellia* resin extract. Animal studies have shown that it inhibits the release of LTB_4.[18,28-33] Additional studies have found that boswellia inhibits *human leukocyte elastase* (HLE), which is involved in the pathogenesis of emphysema, CF, chronic bronchitis, and ARDS.[28,29]

Scientific Evidence of Effectiveness

Boswellia is known in Ayurvedic medicine as *salai guggal*, and has been proposed as a potential chronic asthma therapy, based on its known properties as an inhibitor of leukotriene biosynthesis.[18,28,29,32] One randomized controlled trial (RCT) reported improvements in FEV_1, FVC, number of asthma exacerbations, and wheezing after 41 days of boswellia therapy.[34] Although baseline characteristics among patients in this study were not comparable, the existing data provide good initial evidence in favor of this use of boswellia. Future studies are warranted to assess the long-term efficacy and safety of boswellia, the temporality of effects, and the efficacy of boswellia versus standard therapies.

Dose

Boswellia capsules (300 to 1200 mg) have been taken daily in three divided doses.[34]

Adverse Effects, Interactions, Pharmacokinetics. See Appendix A.

Bromelain (Bromeliaceae)

Grade C: Unclear or conflicting scientific evidence (COPD)

Mechanism of Action

Bromelain has purported antiinflammatory effects, which may be of benefit in COPD. Bromelain may inhibit the biosynthesis of proinflammatory prostaglandins by lowering kininogen and bradykinin in serum and tissues, and it may alter prostaglandin synthesis.[35] In addition, bromelain may activate plasmin production from plasminogen and reduce kinin by inhibiting the conversion of kininogen to kinin.

Scientific Evidence of Effectiveness

Preliminary research suggests that bromelain (Traumanase) may be beneficial in patients with COPD.[36] Results showed improvement in FEV_1 outcome.

Dose

The exact dose of bromelain for COPD has not been determined.

Adverse Effects, Interactions, Pharmacokinetics. See Appendix A.

Butterbur (Petasites hybridus)

Grade B: Good scientific evidence (allergic rhinitis prevention)

Grade C: Unclear or conflicting scientific evidence (asthma)

Mechanism of Action

Extracts of butterbur have been made from the rhizomes, roots, and leaves. Sesquiterpenes found in butterbur (isopetasin, oxopetasin, and petasin) are believed to be the active constituents responsible for its pharmacological activity.[37] Some research suggests that petasin may be the most active component.[1,7]

Potential antiinflammatory properties of butterbur extracts have been attributed to the petasin content, reported to cause inhibition of lipoxygenase activity and downregulation of leukotriene synthesis.[37] Isopetasin and oxopetasin esters in

Petasites hybridus have also been reported to inhibit the synthesis of leukotrienes.[38] Inhibition of cyclooxygenase (COX-2) and prostaglandin E_2 (PGE_2) has also been reported in animal research.[39]

Scientific Evidence of Effectiveness

ALLERGIC RHINITIS PREVENTION. Preclinical studies report that butterbur extract has antiinflammatory and leukotriene-inhibiting properties, which suggests a mechanism of action in the prevention of allergic rhinitis exacerbations in susceptible individuals.[37,40] Though several clinical studies have examined butterbur for allergic rhinitis prevention,[41-44] the overall evidence has been weak. Comparisons of butterbur to prescription drugs, such as fexofenadine (Allegra) and cetirizine (Zyrtec), have reported similar efficacy. Because of small sample size, short duration, and variable outcome measures, these studies can be considered "exploratory" but not definitive. Nonetheless, the results do suggest benefits of butterbur for allergic rhinitis prevention. Definitive studies are warranted, especially since the long-term safety of butterbur use (beyond 12 to 16 weeks) is not clear.

ASTHMA. Butterbur was used historically to treat asthma, particularly in ancient Greece. Preliminary clinical research suggests possible benefits.[45,46] A small study evaluated 16 atopic asthmatic patients with FEV_1 of 4 (78% of age-matched predicted value) who received butterbur as add-on therapy to inhaled corticosteroids.[45] Adenosine monophosphate (AMP) bronchoprovocation was assessed as the primary outcome of the study, with additional measurements of exhaled nitric oxide, serum eosinophil cationic protein, and peripheral blood eosinophil count. All primary and secondary outcomes were reported as significantly superior in the butterbur group ($p < 0.05$).

In another study, 80 subjects (64 adults, 16 children) with active asthma symptoms (coughing, difficulty breathing, chest tightness, difficulty exhaling, wheezing, expectoration) were given an extract of butterbur (Petadolex).[46] The mean number, duration, and severity of asthma attacks decreased, and peak expiratory flow rate (PEFR), FEV_1, and all measured symptoms improved during butterbur therapy. During the study, 21.3% of patients reported experiencing an asthma attack. After 2 months of treatment, the mean number of asthma attacks in each group decreased by 50%. Because no placebo arm was included, it is unclear to what extent the improvement in both groups was caused by a "placebo effect," or if the asthma resolved over time.

Dose

Currently, a few standardized products of butterbur root rhizome are available. Products may be standardized to their specific petasin and isopetasin contents. Petadolex and Petaforce are standardized high-pressure carbon dioxide (CO_2) extracts from the rhizome of *P. hybridus*.[45] Petadolex is standardized to contain 7.5 mg each of petasin and isopetasin per 50-mg tablet.[46]

Dosing for asthma is unclear due to insufficient clinical evidence of efficacy. One small study used 50 mg of standardized butterbur (Petaforce) in two divided doses daily in patients taking inhaled corticosteroids.[47] A clinical study used 150 mg of standardized butterbur daily in three divided daily doses (Petadolex) for 2 to 4 months.[46]

For allergic rhinitis, 50 mg of butterbur (Petadolex, standardized to contain 7.5 mg of petasin and isopetasin in each 50-mg tablet) has been used twice daily.[41-43] A larger study used one tablet of CO_2 extract standardized to 8.0 mg of total petasin per tablet (Tesalin) taken four times daily.[44] A smaller study reported effectiveness for two standardized tablets taken three times daily.[48]

Adverse Effects, Interactions, Pharmacokinetics. See Appendix A.

Cat's Claw (*Uncaria* spp.)

Grade C: *Unclear or conflicting scientific evidence (allergies)*

Mechanism of Action

The exact mechanism of action of cat's claw in allergies is not well understood. Cat's claw has been found to have antiinflammatory and immunostimulant effects, which may benefit allergy symptoms.[49-54]

According to in vitro and clinical studies, the antiinflammatory properties of cat's claw may result from the ability to inhibit tumor necrosis factor alpha (TNF-α) and to a lesser extent PGE_2 production.[49-51,53] An in vitro analysis corroborated this mechanism of action and found that cat's claw is a remarkably potent TNF-α inhibitor.[51] Another in vitro study characterized the antioxidative and antiinflammatory properties of *Uncaria tomentosa* and *Uncaria guianensis*.[54] The plants contain alkaloids and flavanols, and both species showed effective antioxidant and antiinflammatory activities, although *U. guianensis* was more potent than *U. tomentosa*. Presence of oxindole or pentacyclic alkaloids in these species does not appear to influence antioxidant and antiinflammatory properties. However, these constituents have been found to enhance the cellular immune system.[52]

Based on secondary sources, cat's claw may also have antihistamine effects.

Scientific Evidence of Effectiveness

Open-label pilot studies in Europe assessed the effects of cat's claw in patients with allergic respiratory diseases.[55] A 10-year follow-up revealed that some patients experienced improvements. No side effects were noted. Controlled studies are warranted to demonstrate effectiveness.

Dose. Insufficient available evidence.

Adverse Effects, Interactions, Pharmacokinetics. See Appendix A.

Coleus (Coleus forskohlii)

Grade B: *Good scientific evidence (asthma)*
Grade C: *Unclear or conflicting scientific evidence (breathing aid for intubation)*

Mechanism of Action

Forskolin is the major active constituent found in *Coleus forskohlii*. Forskolin has been shown to produce a concentration-dependent inhibition of histamine release from pulmonary mast cells exposed to IgE, with concurrent increases in intracellular levels of cyclic AMP (cAMP). Forskolin appears to modulate the release of mediators of immediate-hypersensitivity reactions through the activation of adenylate cyclase in human basophils and mast cells.[56]

Bronchospasm induced in sensitized guinea pigs was prevented in a dose-dependent manner by intravenous or intratracheal administration of forskolin. In vitro, forskolin inhibited contractions of lung parenchyma provoked by histamine, leukotriene D_4, or antigens.[57]

Scientific Evidence of Effectiveness

ASTHMA. Forskolin has been used for many years to treat respiratory disorders such as asthma. Small clinical trials report promising results for this use.[58-60] In a small RCT, inhaled forskolin relieved bronchoconstriction in patients with asthma.[65] FEV_1 and airway conductance were significantly increased.[58] These effects of forskolin have been compared to fenoterol, a beta-2 receptor agonist, which appears to have a stronger effect.[58,60]

BREATHING AID FOR INTUBATION. Prophylactic bronchodilator treatment with intravenous (IV) coleus (colforsin daropate) before tracheal intubation resulted in lower airway resistance and greater dynamic lung compliance after placement of the endotracheal tube.[61] More research is needed before a recommendation can be made.

Dose

According to anecdotal reports, coleus products are most frequently standardized to 10% to 18% forskolin content. For bronchospasm, 10 mg of forskolin powder, inhaled from a Spinhaler, has been used.[58]

As a breathing aid for intubated patients, the effective dose of coleus has not been determined.

Adverse Effects, Interactions, Pharmacokinetics. See Appendix A.

Cordyceps (Cordyceps sinensis)

Grade C: *Unclear or conflicting scientific evidence (asthma)*

Mechanism of Action

The mechanism of action of cordyceps is not well understood, but may involve immunomodulating properties. Cordyceps has been shown to increase T-helper cells, prolong survival of lymphocytes, enhance TNF-α and interleukin-1 (IL-1) production, and increase the activity of natural killer (NK) cells.[62-66]

Scientific Evidence of Effectiveness

One study reports a 20.2% reduction in symptoms associated with asthma with the use of cordyceps.[67] Details of this study are not entirely clear.

Dose

The dose of cordyceps for asthma has not been determined.

Adverse Effects, Interactions, Pharmacokinetics. See Appendix A.

Danshen (Salvia miltiorrhiza)

Grade C: *Unclear or conflicting scientific evidence (asthmatic bronchitis)*

Mechanism of Action

The exact mechanism by which danshen affects asthma remains unclear. Danshen has demonstrated antiinflammatory effects. It has been found to reduce cytokine levels, including IL-6, IL-8, and TNF-α.[68]

Scientific Evidence of Effectiveness

Clinical evidence suggests that danshen may improve breathing and lessen coughing and wheezing in patients with chronic asthmatic bronchitis.[69] Patients with asthmatic bronchitis who received routine management plus danshen injection (3 g/2 mL) for 10 days showed improved pulmonary function, lower arterial CO_2 partial pressure ($Paco_2$), elevated arterial oxygen partial pressure (Pao_2), and enhanced immune function compared with placebo.

Dose

The effective dose of danshen for asthmatic bronchitis has not been determined. However, a danshen injection of 3 g per 2 mL has been used for 10 days.[69]

Adverse Effects, Interactions, Pharmacokinetics. See Appendix A.

Dong Quai (Angelica sinensis)

Grade C: *Unclear or conflicting scientific evidence (pulmonary hypertension)*

Mechanism of Action

The ligustilide constituent of dong quai appears to have antiasthmatic effects, but the exact mechanism has not been determined.[70,71]

Scientific Evidence of Effectiveness

Various human trials have studied the effects of dong quai injection (either alone or in combination with other natural products) in COPD and pulmonary hypertension.[72-74] Dong quai injection may improve pulmonary hemodynamics in patients with COPD complicated by pulmonary hypertension. A 25% *A. sinensis* injection has been shown to improve pulmonary hemodynamics by influencing the metabolism of endothelin-1 (ET-1), angiotensin-II (AT-II), and endogenous digitalis-like factor (EDF) and by increasing Pao_2.[72,73] Additive benefit may be achieved when combined with *nifedipine*.[73]

Dose

A dose of 25% *Angelica sinensis*, 250 mL in IV drip once daily for 10 days (alone or in combination with nifedipine) has been used in patients with COPD complicated by pulmonary hypertension.[72,73]

Adverse Effects, Interactions, Pharmacokinetics. See Appendix A.

English Ivy *(Hedera helix)*

Grade C: *Unclear or conflicting scientific evidence (asthma; chronic obstructive pulmonary disease)*

Mechanism of Action

English ivy is traditionally known as an herbal expectorant. However, available research regarding its mucolytic and secretolytic activity is limited.

Scientific Evidence of Effectiveness

English ivy has been studied in children with bronchial asthma.[75-80] Formulations in drops, syrup, and suppositories have been used; these may improve respiratory function, as measured by body plethysmography and spirometry.[76-78] Several studies noted improved lung function (FEV_1) in children with severe, reversible chronic respiratory tract diseases (obstructive or nonobstructive).[76] However, these studies have been lacking in methodological design overall. They did not assess long-term efficacy and tolerance, and did not compare English ivy to conventional agents.

Dose

The dose of English ivy for asthma or COPD has not been clearly established.

Adverse Effects, Interactions, Pharmacokinetics. See Appendix A.

Ephedra *(Ephedra sinica)*

Grade B: *Good scientific evidence (asthmatic bronchoconstriction)*

Grade C: *Unclear or conflicting scientific evidence (allergic rhinitis)*

Note: All dietary supplements that contain a source of ephedrine alkaloids such as ephedra have been banned by the U.S. Food and Drug Administration (FDA). However, products regulated as drugs that contain chemically synthesized ephedrine are not dietary supplements and are not covered by this rule. These include drugs used for the short-term treatment of asthma, bronchitis, and allergic reactions.[81]

Mechanism of Action

Ephedra has been used traditionally as a decongestant and to treat asthma. The primary constituents of ephedra, *ephedrine* and *pseudoephedrine*, are plant alkaloids responsible for its bronchodilating action; pseudoephedrine (Sudafed) is approved by the FDA as a decongestant. Both ephedrine and pseudoephedrine are sympathomimetics that act directly and indirectly on the sympathetic nerves. Its bronchodilating effects are the result of relaxation of bronchial smooth muscle through direct stimulation of beta-2 receptors.[1,7]

Scientific Evidence of Effectiveness

ASTHMATIC BRONCHOCONSTRICTION. Numerous trials have reported the efficacy of ephedrine as a bronchodilator. The use of ephedrine to treat asthma in children was first reported in Western medicine in 1927;[82] its clinical effectiveness and side effects, (which have included fatalities) were subsequently reported in several studies.[82-86] Synthetic forms of ephedrine were used to treat asthma in the United States until the advent of more specific beta-agonist medications. Studies showed an improvement in bronchodilator activity, as measured by increased PEFR and reduced bronchial resistance.[87-96] Ephedrine has been administered safely along with theophylline.[87] Despite this evidence of efficacy for ephedrine, the nonprescription dietary supplement ephedra does not appear to be a safe alternative therapy for asthmatic bronchoconstriction because of the variable concentrations of ephedrine in commercial preparations of ephedra and numerous reports of serious adverse effects.

ALLERGIC RHINITIS. An RCT has shown promising results with a 1% ephedrine saline nasal wash in the treatment of allergic rhinitis.[97] The mechanism of action is not clear, although local vasoconstriction may play a role. Although effects in this study reportedly lasted for 2 to 4 weeks, a theoretical concern is that tolerance might develop. Notably, saline nasal washes alone have been demonstrated as effective. Further study is warranted in this area, with a long-term comparison to saline monotherapy and nasally inhaled corticosteroids.

Dose

The most appropriate dose of ephedra for asthma that can be considered effective and safe is controversial. Amounts of ephedra in various products are inconsistent.

Adverse Effects, Interactions, Pharmacokinetics. See Appendix A.

Eucalyptus (*Eucalyptus* spp.)

Grade C: *Unclear or conflicting scientific evidence (asthma)*

Mechanism of Action

The monoterpene cyclic ether eucalyptol (1,8-cineole) is the isolated active agent of eucalyptus oil. Preparations may contain up to 80% of 1,8-cineole.[98] Antiinflammatory activity of eucalyptus oil has been demonstrated in animal models,[99,100] possibly related to its proposed antioxidant activity.[101] In laboratory studies, 1,8-cineole was found to be a strong inhibitor of cytokines, which may make it beneficial for airway inflammation in bronchial asthma.[102,103]

Scientific Evidence of Effectiveness

Eucalyptus is licensed in Germany as a medicinal tea for bronchitis or throat inflammation and has been approved by the German Commission E for *catarrh* (mucus membrane inflammation) of the respiratory tract.

Eucalyptus oil is typically used as a decongestant and expectorant for upper respiratory tract infections or inflammation. The oil is found in numerous over-the-counter (OTC) cough and cold lozenges, as well as in inhalation vapors or topical ointments. Initial research reports that long-term systemic therapy with eucalyptol may decrease the amount of oral corticosteroids required in steroid-dependent asthma.[104] Comparison is still needed with other agents used in asthma, such as leukotriene inhibitors, salmeterol, and inhaled corticosteroids.

Dose

To be medicinally effective, some suggest that eucalyptus leaf oil must contain 70% to 85% 1,8-cineole (eucalyptol). For asthma, the eucalyptol constituent of eucalyptus oil has been given in doses of 200 mg three times daily.[104]

Adverse Effects, Interactions, Pharmacokinetics. See Appendix A.

Ginkgo (*Ginkgo biloba*)

Grade C: *Unclear of conflicting scientific evidence (interstitial pulmonary fibrosis)*

Mechanism of Action

Ginkgolides inhibit receptor binding of platelet-activating factor (PAF), which may mediate beneficial clinical effects.[105-117] PAF is proinflammatory, induces platelet aggregation, and contracts bronchial smooth muscle.[118] Ginkgo has been found to increase corticosteroid secretion in rats.[119]

Scientific Evidence of Effectiveness

Preliminary evidence from animal and human studies suggests that ginkgo may be beneficial in patients with interstitial pulmonary fibrosis.[120,121] Therapeutic outcomes were similar between ginkgo extract (1 g three times daily) and prednisone (30 mg daily).[120] Clinical symptoms, pulmonary function, and PaO_2 were improved after ginkgo use.

Dose

For interstitial pulmonary fibrosis, an experimental dose of ginkgo extract of 1 g three times daily for 3 months has been used.[120]

Adverse Effects, Interactions, Pharmacokinetics. See Appendix A.

Ginseng (*Panax* spp.)

Grade C: *Unclear or conflicting scientific evidence (chronic obstructive pulmonary disease; respiration)*

Mechanism of Action

A ginsenoside-induced, nitric oxide (NO)–mediated relaxation effect has been observed in vitro in bronchial smooth muscle.[122] This was supported by a study that examined the bronchodilatory effects of ginseng.[123] Promotion of NO release also may be a mechanism in the vasorelaxation and prevention of oxygen free-radical injury in pulmonary endothelium by ginsenosides.[124]

Scientific Evidence of Effectiveness

CHRONIC OBSTRUCTIVE PULMONARY DISEASE. An RCT found that *Panax ginseng* was superior to placebo in improving pulmonary functions, including FEV_1, in patients with COPD.[125] Another RCT tested a combination product containing three herbs, of which *P. ginseng* was the main ingredient.[126] Significant improvements were seen in all outcomes, including PFTs (FEV_1, VC), global clinical assessment of effectiveness, and the Borg symptom score (10-point scale in which patient rates symptoms of breathlessness and muscle fatigue after exercise tests; higher scores indicate worse symptoms).

RESPIRATION. One study reports effectiveness of a Chinese soup containing *P. ginseng* and other herbs in the management of respiratory function in severely burned patients.[127] The direct effects on improving respiratory function were not well established, but overall survival seemed to improve.

Dose

Ginseng extracts may be standardized to 4% to 7% total ginsenosides content.[128,129] Some sources indicate that ginsenosides constitute an average of 3% of the dried, whole root,[130] and that the usual concentration of ginsenosides can actually be between 1% and 3%. Standardized extracts of American ginseng (CNT-2000) are also available.[131] The German Federal Pharmacopeia standardizes a minimum ginsenoside content of 1.5%, calculated in terms of the ginsenoside Rg1.[132]

For COPD, 200 mg of ginseng extract in oral capsules (Ginsana, 200 mg) has been taken along with current medical treatment.[125]

Adverse Effects, Interactions, Pharmacokinetics. See Appendix A.

Kiwi (Actinidia deliciosa, Actinidia chinensis)

Grade C: *Unclear or conflicting scientific evidence (prevention of respiratory problems)*

Mechanism of Action

Kiwi contains high amounts of the dietary antioxidant vitamin C, which has been hypothesized to protect against oxidation-induced inflammation.[133] Also, evidence indicates that asthmatic patients may have low plasma and leukocyte concentrations of vitamin C.[134,135]

Scientific Evidence of Effectiveness

Currently, sufficient data are lacking on the therapeutic benefit of kiwi in the prevention of lung conditions. One survey study suggests that kiwi and other fruits high in vitamin C may have a protective effect, especially on wheezing, among children already susceptible to such symptoms.[136] Subjects who ate kiwi or other citrus fruit at least one to two times per week had improved respiratory symptoms compared to subjects who ate citrus or kiwi fruit less than once a week. Symptoms that improved included shortness of breath with wheezing, nocturnal cough, chronic cough, and noncoryzal rhinitis.

Dose

Intake of kiwi fruit or other citrus fruit at least once or twice a week has been associated with beneficial effects on wheezing and other respiratory problems.[136]

Adverse Effects, Interactions, Pharmacokinetics. See Appendix A.

Mistletoe (Viscum album)

Grade C: *Unclear or conflicting scientific evidence (recurrent respiratory disease)*

Mechanism of Action

Mistletoe's beneficial effects in respiratory disease may result from its purported immune-modulating effects. Mistletoe has been shown to increase the number and activity of various types of white blood cells (WBCs). Increased secretion of immune system–enhancing cytokines (e.g., TNF, IL-1, IL-6) by WBCs has been observed after exposure to mistletoe.[137-144]

Scientific Evidence of Effectiveness

Clinical studies evaluating a fermented extract of European mistletoe, Iscador, reported beneficial effects on the immune status and clinical symptoms in immunocompromised children with recurrent respiratory disease.[145,146] Treatment with mistletoe resulted in marked clinical improvement in tiredness, emotional instability, headaches, sweating, and muscle and joint pain. Compared with baseline values, use of mistletoe was associated with a significant elevation of lymphocyte subsets (CD4/CD3, CD3/CD8, CD3/CD19, CD3–/CD16+CD56+), a lower PHA-stimulated lymphocyte response, an increase in NK cell activity for the duration of therapy, and lower phagocytic cell counts and incidents of phagocytosis.[145]

Dose

In children (5 to 14 years of age) suffering recurrent respiratory infections due to radioactive fallout exposure, *Viscum album* preparations (either Iscador M or P were injected subcutaneously at individual doses of 0.001 mg to 1.0 mg, twice weekly for 5 weeks.[146]

Adverse Effects, Interactions, Pharmacokinetics. See Appendix A.

Onion (Allium cepa)

Grade C: *Unclear or conflicting scientific evidence (allergies)*

Mechanism of Action

The mechanism of onion for allergy symptoms is not well understood. Onion may contain antiinflammatory substances or have antiallergic properties.[147]

Scientific Evidence of Effectiveness

One small study in atopic and nonatopic subjects challenged with subcutaneous injections found that topical application of an alcoholic onion extract significantly reduced allergic responses, such as wheels and flares.[147] More research is needed in this area to establish the efficacy and dosing of topical onion extracts.

Dose

The exact dose of onion for allergy symptoms has not been determined. However, topically applied 5% alcohol/onion extract reduced late skin reactions.[147]

Adverse Effects, Interactions, Pharmacokinetics. See Appendix A.

Peppermint (Mentha x piperita)

Grade C: *Unclear or conflicting scientific evidence (asthma)*

Mechanism of Action

The principal active components of peppermint oil include *menthol*, which has a direct, antinociceptive effect.[148] Menthol stimulates cold-sensitive receptors and produces a prolonged cold sensation at the application site.[149-151] Menthol inhalation decreased the sensation of respiratory discomfort during loaded breathing, possibly from stimulation of cold receptors in the upper airway.[152] In addition, inhaled peppermint oil induced rapid, positive changes in patients with infiltrative pulmonary tuberculosis, including its regression.

Scientific Evidence of Effectiveness

Preliminary research suggests that menthol in peppermint may help to improve airway hyperresponsiveness in cases of mild asthma.[153] The small size of this trial, with no difference between the placebo and treatment groups, makes it difficult to draw any conclusions about the use of peppermint oil or menthol in asthma.

Dose

For mild chronic asthma, nebulized menthol (10 mg twice daily for 4 weeks) has been used.[153]

Adverse Effects, Interactions, Pharmacokinetics. See Appendix A.

Perilla (Perilla frutescens)

Grade C: *Unclear or conflicting scientific evidence (asthma)*

Mechanism of Action

The exact mechanism by which perilla improves pulmonary function is not well understood. Perilla seed oil may be beneficial in asthma because it has been shown to supress the production of leukotrienes B_4 (LTB_4) and C_4 (LTC_4) by leukocytes in vitro.[154]

Scientific Evidence of Effectiveness

Preliminary evidence suggests some benefit of perilla oil for symptoms of asthma.[154,155] In one study, 14 asthmatic subjects were divided randomly into two equal groups: one consumed perilla seed oil–rich supplements and the other consumed corn oil–rich supplements for 4 weeks.[154] LTB_4 and LTC_4 decreased in subjects with perilla supplementation. Also, significant increases in peak expiratory flow (PEF), FVC, FEV_1, and rate of airflow at 25% of the forced vital capacity (V(25)) were found in subjects who received perilla seed oil.[156] Studies comparing perilla oil with other standards of care are needed.

Dose

For asthma, 10 to 20 g of perilla seed oil has been taken daily for 4 weeks.[154]

Adverse Effects, Interactions, Pharmacokinetics. See Appendix A.

Pycnogenol (Pinus pinaster subsp. atlantica)

Grade B: *Good scientific evidence (asthma)*

Note: Pycnogenol contains oligomeric proanthocyanidins (OPCs) as well as several other bioflavonoids. There has been some confusion in the U.S. market regarding OPC products containing Pycnogenol or grape seed extract (GSE) because one of the generic terms for chemical constituents ("pycnogenols") is the same as the patented trade name (Pycnogenol). Some GSE products were formerly erroneously labeled and marketed in the United States as containing "pycnogenols." Although GSE and Pycnogenol do contain similar chemical constituents (primarily in the OPC fraction), the chemical, pharmacological, and clinical literature on the two products is distinct. The term Pycnogenol should therefore be used only when referring to this specific proprietary pine bark extract. Scientific literature regarding this product should not be referenced as a basis for the safety or effectiveness of GSE.

Mechanism of Action

The mechanism of action of Pycnogenol in asthma is not well understood but may be related to its antioxidant and antiinflammatory effects.[157-170]

Scientific Evidence of Effectiveness

Randomized controlled trials have examined Pycnogenol in children and adults.[171,172] Taking Pycnogenol in combination with conventional medications was found to decrease asthma symptoms and the need for rescue medications in children age 6 to 18 years with mild to moderate asthma.[173] Pycnogenol has not been compared with other agents used for asthma.

Dose

Pycnogenol is a proprietary patented formula. Because of its astringent taste and occasional minor stomach discomfort, Pycnogenol may be taken with or after meals.[174] For children with asthma, 1 mg/lb body weight of Pycnogenol has been taken daily (in two divided doses).[173]

Adverse Effects, Interactions, Pharmacokinetics. See Appendix A.

Rhodiola (Rhodiola rosea)

Grade C: *Unclear or conflicting scientific evidence (lung disease [acute injury])*

Mechanism of Action. Insufficient available evidence.

Scientific Evidence of Effectiveness

Results from one clinical trial investigating the effect of composite rhodiola on lung protection during extracorporeal circulation suggested improvement and protection against major risk factors, including ARDS.[175] Further studies are required to determine mechanism of action and optimal dosing.

Dose

In patients with acute lung injury, 4 g of rhodiola was administered 7 to 10 days before surgery and 5 to 7 days after surgery.[175]

Adverse Effects, Interactions, Pharmacokinetics. See Appendix A.

Safflower (Carthamus tinctorius)

Grade C: *Unclear or conflicting scientific evidence (cystic fibrosis)*

Mechanism of Action
Patients with CF and pancreatic insufficiency usually have decreased linoleic acid from reduced absorption of nutrients.[176,177] Safflower oil is a good source of linoleic acid that may help build cell membranes and may play a role in lung function.

Scientific Evidence of Effectiveness
The results from clinical trials evaluating the effects of safflower oil on plasma fatty acid composition are mixed. Increases in serum and cellular fatty acid[178,179] levels and higher tissue linoleate levels have been noted.[176,177,180-182] Clinical status, including sweat electrolytes, clinical scores, and oxygen saturation, has not been shown to improve.[176,177,181,182]

Dose
Although some trials have standardized safflower oil to 74% linoleic acid, consensus on safflower or safflower oil's standardization is lacking.[183,184] For CF, 102 to 132 mg/kg of safflower oil has been taken daily for 6 weeks.[185]

Adverse Effects, Interactions, Pharmacokinetics. See Appendix A.

Stinging Nettle (Urtica dioica)

Grade C: *Unclear or conflicting scientific evidence (allergic rhinitis)*

Mechanism of Action
Polysaccharides in stinging nettle have demonstrated anti-inflammatory and immunomodulatory activity.[186-192] Some of the polysaccharides isolated from the aqueous extract fraction of stinging nettle stimulated T-lymphocyte proliferation or influenced the complementary system.[186,187] The water-soluble fraction of stinging nettle leaf extract (IDS 23; Rheuma-Hek, Germany) demonstrated inhibition of leukotriene and prostaglandin synthesis,[189] reduction of TNF-α and IL-1β in lipopolysaccharide-stimulated human whole blood,[191] and inhibition of nuclear factor kappa B (NF-κB). The NF-κB family of transcription factors is critical for the inducible expression of many genes involved in inflammatory responses.[192]

Scientific Evidence of Effectiveness
For many years, a freeze-dried preparation of *Urtica dioica* has been prescribed by physicians and sold over the counter to treat allergic rhinitis. There is preliminary evidence to support this use.[193] However, controlled clinical trials are needed to support the use of nettle in the treatment of allergic rhinitis.

Dose
Nettle preparations are not widely standardized. For allergic rhinitis, 600 mg of freeze-dried nettle at the onset of symptoms for 1 week has been used.[193]

Adverse Effects, Interactions, Pharmacokinetics. See Appendix A.

Tea (Camellia sinensis)

Grade C: *Unclear or conflicting scientific evidence (asthma)*

Mechanism of Action
Theophylline is a constituent of tea (including green tea and black tea), and is widely prescribed as a treatment for asthma. Much of the effect of tea is caused by the caffeine constituent. Caffeine is part of a group of compounds known as *methylxanthines*, which also includes theophylline, a drug used for respiratory disorders. Caffeine, as with theophylline, relaxes bronchial smooth muscle because of its similar chemical structure and its ability to inhibit phosphodiesterase enzyme activity, resulting in increased intracellular concentrations of cAMP.[194,195]

Scientific Evidence of Effectiveness
Theophylline has been widely used as an accepted treatment for asthma; however, it is not clear if the concentrations of theophylline found in tea are sufficient to reach pharmacological efficacy. Research has shown that caffeine improves bronchodilation.[196-198] However, it is not clear if tea use has significant benefits in people with asthma.

Dose
The effective dose of tea for asthma has not been determined.

Adverse Effects, Interactions, Pharmacokinetics. See Appendix A.

Tylophora (Tylophora indica)

Grade C: *Unclear or conflicting scientific evidence (asthma)*

Mechanism of Action
The antiasthmatic effects of tylophora are unclear, but may be related to increased activity of the adrenal gland through direct action of tylophora on the adrenal cortex.[199] Another possible mechanism may involve suppression of the anaphylactic response of *Tylophora indica* on mucous membranes, thereby reducing nasobronchial response to inhaled allergens by a reflex mechanism.[200] Tylophora has also been shown to inhibit acetylcholine and histamine.[201,202]

Scientific Evidence of Effectiveness

Tylophora indica has been used extensively for asthma in traditional Ayurvedic medicine. Available studies of tylophora for asthma show conflicting results.[200-205] Preliminary trials have reported relief in asthma symptoms.[203,204] However, a randomized, double-blind study found no significant difference between tylophora and placebo in symptom scores and pulmonary function.[205] *T. indica* was compared to ephedrine hydrochloride, theophylline, or phenobarbitone, and no significant differences were found.[206]

Dose

Doses of 250 mg once to three times daily (standardized to 0.1% tylophorine per dose) and 30 to 60 mg twice daily (standardized to 0.15% tylophorine) have been reported anecdotally. For asthma, one clinical trial reported using 350 mg of *Tylophora* leaf placed in a capsule and given once daily for 7 days.[210] Another clinical trial reported using 0.5 mg of alkaloid *Tylophora* in powder form given once daily to asthmatic patients for 6 days.[207] The patients were instructed to place the powder on their tongues to allow the powder to mix with the saliva, then swallow with ½ oz of water.

Adverse Effects, Interactions, Pharmacokinetics. See Appendix A.

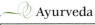 Ayurveda

> Ayurvedic medicine has been used traditionally to treat asthma. Boswellia *(Boswellia serrata)*, known in Ayurveda as *salai guggal*, has good scientific evidence to support its effectiveness in treating asthma (see Boswellia). Tylophlora is also a traditional asthma treatment in Ayurveda (see Tylophora). Another Ayurvedic herb, Devadaru *(Cedrus deodara)*, may have antispasmodic effects and reduce symptoms in bronchial asthma, particularly for patients with shorter histories of asthma and lower frequencies of attacks.[207]

 Traditional Chinese Medicine

> In traditional Chinese medicine (TCM), herbs are almost always administered in combination formulas consisting of several herbs that balance each other's effects and enhance treatment success. An available case study provided some initial objective data on the formula "Invigorating Kidney," which includes goji *(Lycium chinense,* 9 g) combined with 15 g each *Viscum coloratum, Psoralea corylifolia, Eucommia ulmoides,* and *Tussilago farfara,* and 9 g each *Artemisia capillaris* and *Pogostemon cablin.* Results showed that this formula may reverse airway obstruction.[208] This research does not provide any data about one herb specifically, but it is worthwhile for its contribution to the scientific literature on TCM herbalism.

HERBAL THERAPIES WITH NEGATIVE EVIDENCE

Evening Primrose (Oenothera biennis)

Grade D: *Fair negative scientific evidence (asthma)*

The active ingredient in evening primrose oil (EPO) is thought to be gamma-linolenic acid (GLA), one of the omega-6 essential fatty acids. Essential fatty acids are the building blocks for a number of molecules in the body and are essential in the creation of leukotrienes and prostaglandins. GLA has been shown to be a precursor to PGE_1, an effective bronchodilator.[209] Despite the theory that EPO may be beneficial in asthmatic patients, clinical trials have found that it does not control asthma symptoms.[209-211] In one clinical trial, no significant differences were found between patients with atopic asthma who received eight EPO capsules daily and those who received placebo for two 8-week periods.[209] The available evidence does not support the efficacy of EPO for treating asthma.

HERBAL THERAPIES WITH LIMITED EVIDENCE

Anise (Pimpinella anisum)

Anise is native to the eastern Mediterranean and is one of the oldest known spice plants used for culinary purposes as well as medicinal indications, including asthma, bronchitis, and whooping cough. Bronchodilating effects may be caused by anise's inhibitory effects on muscarinic receptors.[212] Human clinical trials are currently lacking.

Comfrey (Symphytum spp.)

Comfrey has been historically used for a variety of symptoms, including for asthma and respiratory conditions. According to in vitro and animal studies, comfrey has displayed antiinflammatory effects and may help tissue repair.[213-215] However, comfrey is not safe for oral use because of the potential for liver toxicity.

Lobelia (Lobelia inflata)

Lobelia is traditionally used for bronchitis, asthma, and whooping cough. The alkaloid *lobeline,* an active ingredient in lobelia,[216] has similar effects to nicotine, is considered a nicotine substitute, and is found in smoking-cessation products. However, clinical research does not support this use.[217]

Milk Thistle (Silybum marianum)

A flavonoid complex of milk thistle called silymarin can be extracted from the seeds of milk thistle and is believed to be the biologically active component. "Milk thistle" and "silymarin" are often used interchangeably. Silymarin was shown to have protective effects in the early phase of allergic asthma and to decrease histamine-induced bronchoconstriction.[218]

Mullein (Verbascum thapsus)

Mulleins have been used in natural medicine for centuries and are among the oldest known medicinal plants. They are most often used for inflammation in various areas of the body, including the respiratory tract. The most frequently reported use is for respiratory tract conditions such as bronchitis and asthma. Mullein's effects may result from its ability to reduce the amount of mucus formation and act as an expectorant.[219-221]

Quercetin

Quercetin is one of about 4000 polyphenolic compounds called *flavonoids*, which are antioxidants that occur ubiquitously in foods of plant origin, such as red wine, onions, tea, apples, berries, and brassica vegetables (cabbage, broccoli, cauliflower, turnips). It is also found in *Ginkgo biloba*, St. John's wort, and American elder. It mainly occurs in plants as glycosides, such as rutin (quercetin rutinoside) in tea.

Quercetin has displayed antiinflammatory properties.[222,223] Preliminary evidence suggests that quercetin may work similar to cromolyn, a drug used to treat wheezing and difficulty breathing caused by asthma. Similarly, quercetin has been shown to inhibit antigen-stimulated histamine from mast cells. These effects may be caused by quercetin's ability to inhibit antigen-stimulated histamine release from mast cells.[223]

Sanicle (Sanicula europea)

Sanicle has been used orally for mild respiratory inflammation and catarrh, according to secondary sources. Limited human evidence from an available case report suggests potential favorable results of a *Sanicula aqua* heuristic homeopathic preparation for asthma.[224]

Turmeric (Curcuma longa)

Cystic fibrosis is a progressive and ultimately fatal inherited disorder caused by a mutant CF transmembrane conductance regulator *(CFTR)* gene. In CF the mutant CFTR protein is trapped inside the cells. Curcumin treatment has been shown in mouse models to release the defective CFTR protein from the inappropriate compartment inside the cell and allow it to reach its proper destination and function normally in the cell lining of the nose and rectum.[225,226]

ADJUNCT THERAPIES

1. Although its use is not common, intravenous *magnesium sulfate* appears to improve acute asthma attacks and may be considered in emergency situations.[227-229] In patients with chronic asthma, however, magnesium does not appear to improve FEV_1 or to reduce the need for bronchodilators.[230] Inhaled magnesium does not appear to be more effective than placebo.[231] The role of oral replacement magnesium therapy is unclear.[232]
2. *Choline* may be effective when taken orally for asthma. Choline supplements seem to decrease the severity of symptoms, number of symptomatic days, and the need to use bronchodilators in asthma patients. There is some evidence that higher doses of 3 g daily might be more effective than lower doses of 1.5 g daily. Choline is generally regarded as safe, appears to be well tolerated, and may be used in combination with other agents to help relieve symptoms associated with asthma and COPD.
3. *St. John's wort* may improve symptoms of anxiety[233,234] and lead to relaxation and decreased stress. Theoretically, this herb may help reduce stress-related asthma attacks by decreasing stress "triggers." An association also exists between smoking and depression; however, St. John's wort has not been shown to aid in smoking cessation.[235]
4. Smoking is the most common cause of COPD. *Smoking cessation* (quitting tobacco smoking) is difficult and may require multiple attempts; users often relapse because of withdrawal symptoms. These symptoms may include depression, cravings, nervousness, and irritability. Nicotine is the chemical in cigarettes and other forms of tobacco that causes addiction. Several pharmacological therapies exist to help individuals stop smoking. *Nicotine replacement therapy* (NRT) and medications for decreasing the side effects of nicotine withdrawal, such as chemical imbalances in the brain and labored (difficulty) breathing, are available. NRTs deliver small, steady doses of nicotine into the body to help relieve withdrawal symptoms. These products are available in patches, gums, lozenges, nasal sprays, and inhalers and appear to be equally effective in smoking cessation. The consistent use of one of these products doubles an individual's chances of successfully quitting smoking.
5. Preliminary evidence indicates that *auricular acupressure* (pressure to points on the ear) may help with quitting smoking. Also, preliminary evidence suggests that acupressure may be a helpful adjunct therapy to assist with the prevention of relapse, withdrawal, or dependence.
6. *Yoga* is an ancient system of relaxation, exercise, and healing with origins in Indian philosophy. Preliminary research suggests that yoga may be beneficial when added to standard therapies for the treatment of drug abuse, including smoking.
7. A small amount of research has examined the use of *melatonin* to reduce symptoms associated with smoking cessation, such as anxiousness, restlessness, irritability, and cigarette craving. *Astragalus* also has been shown to have positive effects in smoking cessation.

Herbs Used for Respiratory Disorders*

HERB	SPECIFIC THERAPEUTIC USE(S)†	HERB	SPECIFIC THERAPEUTIC USE(S)†
Abuta	Asthma	Euphorbia	Respiratory disorders
Aconite	Asthma, respiratory disorders	Eyebright	Asthma, respiratory infections
Alfalfa	Asthma	False pennyroyal	Asthma, respiratory disorders
Aloe	Asthma	Feverfew	Asthma
Angel's trumpet	Asthma	Flax	Bronchial irritation
Anise	Asthma, bronchodilation, respiratory disorders	Garcinia	Bronchodilation
		Garlic	Asthma
Annatto	Asthma, respiratory disorders	Germanium	Asthma
Apricot	Asthma	Ginger	Asthma
Arnica	Asthma, respiratory disorders	Goldenrod	Asthma
Ashwagandha	Asthma, respiratory disorders	Goldenseal	Asthma, cystic fibrosis
Astragalus	Asthma, breathing difficulties	Gotu kola	Asthma
Bacopa	Asthma	Ground ivy	Asthma
Bael fruit	Asthma	Guarana	Asthma
Bamboo	Asthma	Guggul	Asthma
Barberry	Respiratory disorders	Gumweed	Asthma, bronchial irritation
Barley	Bronchodilation	Hawthorn	Asthma, breathing difficulties
Betel nut	Asthma, respiratory disorders	Holy basil	Asthma
Betony	Asthma, respiratory disorders	Honeysuckle	Asthma, breathing difficulties
Bitter melon	Respiratory infections	Horny goat weed	Asthma, respiratory disorders
Black cohosh	Asthma	Horseradish	Respiratory disorders
Black currant	Respiratory disorders	Hyssop	Asthma, respiratory tract infections
Black horehound	Bronchial irritation		
Bloodroot	Asthma, respiratory disorders	Jequirity	Asthma
Blue flag	Respiratory disorders	Katuka	Asthma
Boneset	Respiratory congestion	Kava	Asthma, respiratory tract infections
Buchu	Respiratory disorders		
Bupleurum	Asthma	Khella	Asthma, chronic obstructive pulmonary disease (COPD)
Burdock	Respiratory infections		
California jimson weed	Asthma, respiratory disorders, breathing difficulties	Labrador tea	Asthma
		Lavender	Asthma
Cardamom	Asthma	Licorice	Asthma
Chamomile	Asthma, respiratory disorders, respiratory tract infections	Lime	Asthma
		Milk thistle	Asthma
Cinnamon	Asthma, respiratory tract infections	Morus nigra	Asthma
		Mugwort	Asthma
Clove	Asthma	Mullein	Asthma
Codonopsis	Asthma, breathing difficulties	Neem	Respiratory disorders, cystic fibrosis
Coltsfoot	Asthma, emphysema		
Cramp bark	Asthma	Noni	Asthma
Damiana	Asthma, respiratory disorders	Nux vomica	Respiratory disorders
Datura wrightii	Asthma, respiratory disorders, breathing difficulties	Oleander	Asthma
		Oregano	Asthma, respiratory disorders
Desert parsley	Asthma	Organic food	Asthma
Dogwood	Respiratory disorders	Passion flower	Asthma
Echinacea	Respiratory infections	Pleurisy	Asthma
Elder	Asthma, respiratory distress	Raspberry	Asthma, respiratory disorders
Essiac	Asthma	Red clover	Asthma

Continued

Herbs Used for Respiratory Disorders*—cont'd

HERB	SPECIFIC THERAPEUTIC USE(S)†	HERB	SPECIFIC THERAPEUTIC USE(S)†
Rehmannia	Asthma	St. John's wort	Asthma
Reishi mushroom	Asthma	Star anise	Breathing difficulties
Rooibos	Asthma	Tamarind	Asthma
Rose hip	Asthma, respiratory disorders	Thyme	Asthma, breathing difficulties
Rosemary	Asthma, respiratory disorders	Turmeric	Asthma
Sage	Asthma	Valerian	Asthma, bronchospasm
Saw palmetto	Asthma	Watercress	Respiratory tract inflammation
Sea buckthorn	Asthma	White horehound	Asthma, COPD, breathing difficulties
Shiitake	Asthma	White oak	Respiratory disorders
Skunk cabbage	Asthma	White water lily	Bronchial irritation
Slippery elm	Respiratory disorders	Wild yam	Asthma
Sorrel	Respiratory inflammation	Yerba santa	Asthma
Soy	Cystic fibrosis	Yew	Respiratory disorders
Squill	Asthma, bronchitis		

*This is not an all-inclusive or comprehensive list of herbs with bronchodilating properties used for respiratory disorders; other herbs and supplements may possess these qualities. A qualified health care provider should be consulted with specific questions or concerns regarding potential bronchodilating effects of agents or interactions.
†Based on expert opinion, anecdote, case reports, and/or preliminary trial evidence.

INTEGRATIVE THERAPY PLAN

- Asthma and COPD are two different conditions, although they have similar characteristics. Asthma and COPD may coexist in the same patient; however, the similarities and differences in diagnosis, treatment, and long-term outcome must be understood.
- Perform pulmonary function tests (PFTs) to diagnose and assess asthma and COPD. PFTs may show signs of airway obstruction. However, patients with asthma may display an improvement in PFTs after the use of a bronchodilator.
- Talk to the patient with asthma or COPD regarding symptoms such as shortness of breath, coughing, and wheezing.
- Determine any environmental triggers, such as smoke, dust, perfumes, or allergens, that may set the inflammatory process in motion and cause asthma attacks.
- Identify food allergies that may worsen asthma symptoms. Food sensitivities to nuts, eggs, wheat, soy, dairy, peanuts, fish, and shellfish may induce asthma. Some people with asthma may have sensitivity to salicylates in aspirin and certain foods, including instant coffee, soy sauce, tomato pastes/sauces, beer, and honey.
- Document if the patient with COPD currently smokes and how much.
- Warn all patients that no natural product should replace a rescue inhaler and should not be used for an acute asthma attack. Short-acting inhaled bronchodilators or beta-2 agonists are preferred for quick relief. Both asthma and COPD may be treated with these agents.
- Drugs and natural products with antiinflammatory activity are preferred for long-term control therapy of asthma. For COPD, these products may not be as beneficial.
- Boswellia may be used to help manage and control changes in asthma patients. A dose of 200 to 1200 mg (capsules) by mouth three times daily may be recommended. Boswellia is generally believed to be safe when used as directed. However, it should be used cautiously with cytochrome P450 substrates and sedative agents.
- Preliminary data suggest that coleus may be a promising agent for asthma; however, more research is needed to confirm safety and efficacy in bronchial asthma.
- Ephedra contains the bronchodilators ephedrine and pseudoephedrine and has been used to treat asthma symptoms. The FDA banned the sale of ephedra products because of serious health risks, including heart attack, heart damage, breathing difficulties, and fluid retention in the lungs.
- Recommend other integrative approaches for asthma management, including acupuncture, breathing exercises, Qi gong, relaxation, and mind-body therapies. Using an integrative approach with complementary therapies may offer additional benefit in controlling symptoms and improving self-management.
- Smoking is the most common cause of COPD, and the most important step in treatment is smoking cessation, which should be strongly recommended to all patients with COPD. Nicotine is a highly addictive psychoactive drug that produces dependence. NRT and medications for decreasing the side effects of nicotine withdrawal are available,

Review Questions

1. Based on what potential mechanism has boswellia been proposed as a potential therapy for asthma?
   a. Blocking the physiological action of acetylcholine.
   b. Inhibiting the release of leukotrienes.
   c. Stimulating β_2-adrenergic receptors.
   d. None of the above.

2. What dose of boswellia has been used to treat asthma?
   a. 200 to 1200 mg three times daily
   b. 2 to 12 g twice daily
   c. 20 to 120 mg three times daily
   d. 20 to 120 g three times daily

3. Which of the following natural products have been used for cystic fibrosis?
   a. Safflower
   b. English ivy
   c. Tylophora
   d. None of the above

4. True or false: The effects of forskolin have been compared to fenoterol, a beta-2 receptor agonist, but forskolin appears to have a stronger effect.

5. Goji may affect which test results?
   a. Triglycerides
   b. International normalized ratio
   c. White blood cells
   d. All the above

6. All the following statements are true *except*:
   a. Butterbur has been shown to inhibit lipoxygenase activity and to downregulate leukotriene synthesis.
   b. Potential antiinflammatory properties of butterbur have been attributed to ephedrine content.
   c. Butterbur was used in ancient Greece to treat asthma.
   d. Raw, unprocessed butterbur plant should not be ingested because of the potential hepatotoxicity of pyrrolizidine alkaloids.

7. True or false: Pycnogenol in combination with conventional medications was found to decrease asthma symptoms and reduce the need for rescue medications in children.

8. What dose of standardized butterbur has been used in the treatment of asthma?
   a. 15 mg in three divided daily doses for 2 to 4 months
   b. 1.5 mg in three divided daily doses for 2 to 4 months
   c. 150 mg in three divided daily doses for 2 to 4 months
   d. 1500 mg in three divided daily doses for 2 to 4 months

9. What dose of perilla oil has been used to treat asthma?
   a. 10 to 20 g daily for 4 weeks
   b. 10 to 20 mg daily for 4 weeks
   c. 1 to 2 g daily for 4 weeks
   d. 10 to 20 mcg daily for 4 weeks

10. Which of the following is true about kiwi?
    a. Kiwi consumption may increase platelet aggregation.
    b. Kiwi contains a high concentration of the neurotransmitter serotonin.
    c. Kiwi may be safely used in people with banana allergies.
    d. All the above.

Answers are found in the Answers to Review Questions section in the back of the text.

18 Diabetes Mellitus

Outline

OVERVIEW
  Hyperglycemia
  Hypoglycemia
  Types of Diabetes
    Type 1 Diabetes
    Type 2 Diabetes
    Prediabetes
    Metabolic Syndrome
    Gestational Diabetes
    Maturity-Onset Diabetes of the Young
  Diagnosis
    Fasting Blood Glucose Test
    Oral Glucose Tolerance Test
    Random Blood Glucose Test
    Metabolic Syndrome
    Gestational Diabetes
    Maturity-Onset Diabetes of the Young
    Monitoring Blood Glucose
SELECTED HERBAL THERAPIES
  Alfalfa *(Medicago sativa)*
  Aloe *(Aloe vera)*
  Ashwagandha *(Withania somnifera)*
  Astragalus *(Astragalus membranaceus)*
  Banaba *(Lagerstroemia speciosa)*
  Barley *(Hordeum vulgare)*
  Beet *(Beta vulgaris)*
  Berberine
  Beta-Glucan (β-Glucan)
  Bitter Melon *(Momordica charantia)*
  Burdock *(Arctium lappa)*
  Chrysanthemum *(Chrysanthemum* spp.)
  Cinnamon *(Cinnamomum* spp.)
  Dandelion *(Taraxacum officinale)*
  Devil's Club *(Oplopanax horridus)*
  Evening Primrose *(Oenothera biennis)*
  Fenugreek *(Trigonella foenum-graecum)*
  Fig *(Ficus carica)*
  Flax *(Linum usitatissimum)*
  Ginseng *(Panax* spp.)
  Gotu Kola *(Centella asiatica)*
  Gymnema *(Gymnema sylvestre)*
  Holy Basil *(Ocimum sanctum)*
  Jackfruit *(Artocarpus heterophyllus)*
  Kudzu *(Pueraria lobata)*
  Maitake Mushroom *(Grifola frondosa)*
  Milk Thistle *(Silybum marianum)*
  Myrcia *(Myrcia* spp.)
  Nopal *(Opuntia* spp.)
  Onion *(Allium cepa)*
  Psyllium *(Plantago* spp.)
  Pycnogenol *(Pinus pinaster* subsp. *atlantica)*
  Red Clover *(Trifolium pratense)*
  Red Yeast Rice *(Monascus purpureus)*
  Reishi Mushroom *(Ganoderma lucidum)*
  Seaweed
  Soy *(Glycine max)*
  Spirulina *(Arthrospira* spp.)
  Stevia *(Stevia rebaudiana)*
  Tea *(Camellia sinensis)*
  White Horehound *(Marrubium vulgare)*
HERBAL THERAPIES WITH NEGATIVE EVIDENCE
HERBAL THERAPIES WITH LIMITED EVIDENCE
ADJUNCT THERAPIES
INTEGRATIVE CARE PLAN
CASE STUDIES
REVIEW QUESTIONS

Learning Objectives

- Understand the physiological mechanisms of prediabetes, type 1 diabetes, type 2 diabetes, and gestational diabetes.
- Identify the causes of and treatment for hypoglycemia and hyperglycemia.
- Identify natural products commonly used for diabetes and diabetes-related complications and their mechanisms of action.
- Cite scientific evidence on natural products used to treat diabetes.
- Understand the adverse effects and interactions associated with natural products used for diabetes.
- Provide an integrative care plan for patients with diabetes.

OVERVIEW[1-3]

Diabetes mellitus (commonly known simply as *diabetes*) is a metabolic disease in which the body cannot properly metabolize (break down) *glucose* in the blood. A preferred source of energy for the cells of the body, glucose may be derived from the carbohydrates found in many foods, including fruits, vegetables, and grains. In addition, the liver can synthesize glucose from noncarbohydate sources (such as protein) in a process called *gluconeogenesis*. Glucose is stored in the liver and muscles as *glycogen*, which can be converted back into glucose for use by the cells. When food sources of glucose are inadequate, the body compensates by breaking down glycogen into glucose.

Glucose metabolism is dependent on hormones produced by the *pancreas* (a large gland that lies behind the stomach), which is a part of the endocrine system. In addition to *insulin*, a major hormone in glucose metabolism, the pancreas secretes the hormones *glucagon* and *somatostatin*. These hormones are produced in the pancreas by cell groups called *islets of Langerhans*. At least five cell types exist in the islets: alpha, beta, delta, PP, and epsilon. The alpha and beta cells are particularly central to blood glucose regulation; the alpha cells secrete glucagon, and the beta cells secrete insulin. In healthy individuals, these hormones play complementary roles in the body. When the brain senses hunger, the pancreas secretes *glucagon*, which increases the supply of glucose by stimulating the conversion of stored glycogen to glucose. When the brain senses the presence of glucose in the blood, insulin increases the uptake of glucose by the cells and stimulates the conversion of glucose into glycogen, and decreases gluconeogenesis by the liver.

In diabetes, the inability to properly metabolize glucose is caused by a deficiency in the hormone *insulin*. In some forms of diabetes, insulin levels are inadequate (usually as a result of a loss of beta cell function) to facilitate the uptake of glucose into the cells. In other forms of diabetes, insulin is produced; however cells may not recognize the presence of insulin. This condition is known as *insulin resistance*. In either case, the conversion of glucose into energy within body cells is compromised, and the body resorts to other sources of energy, including protein from the muscles and fat from adipose tissue. This process requires the body to use more energy, resulting in excessive fatigue or hunger. Furthermore, because glucose in the blood is not adequately metabolized, glucose levels in the blood and urine may be elevated. Dietary intervention is often necessary to help control blood glucose levels. In cases of insufficient insulin production, injections of synthetic insulin may be necessary.

Hyperglycemia

High blood sugar, or *hyperglycemia*, is one of the defining symptoms of diabetes; it refers to excessive glucose and/or inadequate insulin in the blood. People with diabetes may develop hyperglycemia if they eat too much, do not exercise enough, or do not take their medications. Hyperglycemia may also be caused by exposure to physical stress (e.g., cold temperatures, infections) or emotional stress. Hyperglycemia is responsible for many of the devastating complications of diabetes, including vision loss from diabetic retinopathy, caused by pathological blood vessel overgrowth in the retina. A leading cause of legal blindness in the U.S. today is diabetic retinopathy. Blurry vision is not specific to diabetes, but it is frequently present with high blood sugar levels.

In hyperglycemia, the brain senses that the concentration of glucose in the blood is too high and attempts to compensate. The body attempts to regulate blood glucose levels in two ways: consuming more fluid to dilute glucose levels and increasing the excretion of glucose in the urine. These compensatory mechanisms cause the symptoms of diabetes, which include excessive thirst *(polydipsia)* and frequent urination *(polyuria)*. A large amount of body water is lost with polyuria, exacerbating polydipsia. High levels of glucose in the blood also indicate less glucose being transported into the cells. Because the cells are not receiving the energy they require, the brain signals the body to consume more food. Therefore, hyperglycemia may also lead to excessive hunger *(polyphagia)*. Despite increased caloric intake, a person with diabetes may gain very little weight or even lose weight.

If left untreated, hyperglycemia may cause serious health problems. If blood glucose level is greater than 240 mg/dL, the individual should seek medical treatment because of the risk of developing a serious and potentially life-threatening medical condition called *ketoacidosis*. Ketoacidosis occurs when toxic waste products, known as ketones, build up in the blood. Symptoms of ketoacidosis include shortness of breath, breath that smells fruity, nausea, vomiting, and dry mouth. Patients who experience these symptoms should seek immediate medical treatment, which generally involves intravenous (IV) insulin therapy. Patients also require fluid and electrolyte replacement. After treatment, patients should meet with their health care providers to determine what triggered the episode and how to prevent recurrence. Patients are encouraged to adhere to medication schedules if ketoacidosis occurs after a missed medication dose.

People with diabetes should monitor blood sugar levels regularly. If they have hyperglycemia, people with diabetes may take steps to lower their blood glucose level, such as exercising or increasing the dose of their medications. Exercise should be avoided if ketoacidosis is suspected, because exercise during ketoacidosis may actually increase blood sugar levels.

Hypoglycemia

Low blood sugar, or *hypoglycemia*, occurs when there is too little glucose and/or too much insulin in the blood. Many conditions may lead to hypoglycemia, including some types of cancer, critical illnesses (e.g., kidney, heart, or liver failure), anorexia nervosa and some medications. Pancreatic tumors may stimulate the pancreas to release too much insulin, leading to hypoglycemia. Otherwise healthy individuals may develop hypoglycemia if they do not consume adequate food, or if excessive amounts of alcohol are consumed without food.

Hypoglycemia is common in diabetic patients; it may be caused by taking too much insulin or other medications that lower glucose levels. Typical symptoms of hypoglycemia include confusion, abnormal behavior, impaired vision (such as blurred or double vision), irregular heartbeat, tremors, anxiety, sweating, and hunger. In rare cases, patients may develop seizures or lose consciousness. Short-term treatment may include increasing the patient's blood sugar level to relieve acute symptoms. Patients may take glucose tablets or eat foods high in carbohydrates to increase blood sugar levels. In severe cases, patients may require IV glucose or an injection of the glucagon hormone. Long-term treatment may involve identifying and treating the underlying cause of hypoglycemia.

Once initial symptoms of hypoglycemia are treated, health care providers work with the patient to determine the underlying cause, to prevent the recurrence of hypoglycemia. For example, if a pancreatic tumor is causing symptoms, it may be surgically removed. If a medication is causing the condition, an alternative dose or drug may be recommended.

Types of Diabetes

There are four main types of diabetes: type 1 diabetes, type 2 diabetes, and gestational diabetes. Other forms include metabolic syndrome (or syndrome X) and maturity-onset diabetes of the young.

Type 1 Diabetes

In type 1 diabetes the pancreas does not make enough insulin to facilitate the absorption of glucose into the cells. Although the exact cause of type 1 diabetes is unclear, genetics or other illnesses (such as viral infections) may be contributing factors. Type 1 diabetes is generally considered an *autoimmune* disease, in which the body's immune system attacks its own cells. In type 1 diabetes, the autoimmune reaction targets the pancreatic beta cells; as a result, these cells are often entirely nonfunctional and do not produce or secrete any insulin. Therefore, type 1 diabetes, previously called *insulin-dependent diabetes mellitus* (IDDM) requires insulin therapy. Oral glucose-lowering agents are not effective because their function depends on at least partially functioning beta cells. Because type 1 diabetes is more likely to occur in younger patients, it was previously known as juvenile-onset diabetes; however, it can also occur in older individuals. Glucose control is achieved by carefully monitoring the diet and regular insulin injections. Even if the individual takes insulin and eats on a rigid schedule, the amount of sugar in the blood can change unpredictably. Depending on what type of insulin therapy is prescribed, such as single-dose injections, multiple-dose injections, or an insulin pump, the individual may need to check and record blood sugar levels up to four or more times a day.

Type 2 Diabetes

Type 2 diabetes, previously called *non-insulin-dependent diabetes mellitus* (NIDDM) or adult-onset diabetes, occurs more frequently in older people, but also occurs in overweight young people. This type of diabetes is often discovered when the patient seeks medical care for related complications (e.g., eye problems). Patients with type 2 diabetes may have decreased insulin production from pancreatic beta cells, decreased sensitivity of cells to insulin, and decreased ability to transport glucose into cells. Although the initial treatment for type 2 diabetes was previously diet and exercise, current standards suggest that oral drug therapy (in addition to diet and exercise) should be initiated when type 2 diabetes is diagnosed. Stepwise pharmacological treatment of type 2 diabetes typically progresses from use of one oral agent to use of multiple oral agents. As beta-cell function continues to decline, many individuals with type 2 diabetes may eventually need insulin therapy.

Prediabetes

Type 2 diabetes is usually preceded by *prediabetes*, a condition characterized by blood glucose levels that are higher than normal but not high enough to be considered type 2 diabetes. Prediabetes typically involves impaired glucose tolerance or impaired fasting glucose. *Impaired glucose tolerance* (IGT) consists of decreased secretion of insulin from the pancreatic beta cells, as well as reduced sensitivity of the cells to the presence of insulin *(insulin resistance)*. In people with normal glucose tolerance, glucose levels return to normal within a few hours of consuming a meal. In those with prediabetes, glucose levels remain high because insulin does not function properly. High glucose levels further damage the pancreatic beta cells, which worsens the disease over time. When fasting, those with IGT tend to have normal or slightly elevated blood glucose levels.

Impaired fasting glucose (IFG) may overlap with IGT. In IFG, increased blood glucose levels cause further damage to the pancreatic beta cells, thereby decreasing their function. When the brain senses inadequate glucose supply to the cells, glucagon stimulates the conversion of glycogen into glucose for use by the cells and stimulates the liver to produce glucose through gluconeogenesis. As a result high levels of glucose circulate in the blood, even when the individual has not eaten.

Although diet and exercise can improve IGT and IFG, most people with these conditions go on to develop type 2 diabetes.

Gestational Diabetes

Gestational diabetes is a type of diabetes that occurs during pregnancy; it is caused when hormones secreted by the placenta cause insulin resistance. Women who are overweight before pregnancy, are older than age 25, or have a family history of type 2 diabetes are at increased risk of developing gestational diabetes. Symptoms of gestational diabetes are the same as for other types of diabetes (polydipsia, polyuria, polyphagia) but may not be apparent. A diagnosis of gestational diabetes does not mean that the patient will have chronic diabetes, but it does increase the risk of developing type 2 diabetes in the future. Gestational diabetes is treated with insulin therapy rather than oral medications because of the risks to the fetus.

Metabolic Syndrome

Metabolic syndrome (or *syndrome X*) is a combination of metabolic risk factors that include insulin resistance or glucose intolerance, abdominal obesity, dyslipidemia, hypertension, prothrombotic state (e.g., high fibrinogen), and proinflammatory state (e.g., elevated C-reactive protein). Aggressive lifestyle modifications and conventional or nonconventional medications may help reduce this collection of unhealthy measurements and abnormal laboratory tests.

Maturity-Onset Diabetes of the Young

Maturity-onset diabetes of the young (MODY) is a type of diabetes that is caused by genetic mutations. MODY may occur during childhood or adolescence; however, it is often misdiagnosed as type 1 or type 2 diabetes, or it may be unidentified until the patient is an adult. Research indicates that the genetic mutations responsible for MODY interfere with normal pancreatic secretion of insulin. Currently, six gene mutations (*MODY1* to *MODY6*) have been associated with MODY; these genes are involved with normal pancreatic function, and the MODY mutations interfere with insulin secretion. Each type of MODY has different signs and symptoms, clinical manifestations, complications, and treatments.

Diagnosis

Diabetes is diagnosed by measuring the amount of glucose in the blood, which may be done when the individual has been fasting, after ingesting glucose, or at random times throughout the day. Women who are pregnant are routinely screened for gestational diabetes between 24 and 28 weeks gestation (or earlier if at high risk).

Diabetes tests require a blood sample. Depending on the test used, the level of blood glucose can be affected by many factors, including eating or drinking (water is acceptable); taking medications known to elevate or reduce blood sugar levels, such as oral contraceptives, some diuretics ("water pills"), and corticosteroids; or a recent injury, physical illness, or surgery that may temporarily alter blood sugar levels.

Fasting Blood Glucose Test

Fasting blood glucose tests are performed after fasting for 12 to 14 hours. The individual can drink water during this time but should strictly avoid any other beverage. Individuals with diabetes may be asked to delay their diabetes medication or insulin dose until the test is completed. This test can be used to diagnose diabetes or prediabetes. The fasting plasma glucose (FPG) test is the preferred test for diagnosing diabetes because it is convenient and most reliable when done on an empty stomach in the morning (so that food and natural biorhythms do not cause fluctuations in blood sugar levels). If the FPG level is 100 to 125 mg/dL, the individual has a form of prediabetes called impaired fasting glucose, meaning that the individual is more likely to develop type 2 diabetes but does not yet have the condition. A blood glucose level equal to or greater than 126 mg/dL indicates the individual has diabetes. These results are confirmed by repeating the test on a different day.

Oral Glucose Tolerance Test

In the oral glucose tolerance test (OGTT), the subject must be in the fasting state. An initial blood glucose level is determined by a blood test. The subject then drinks a liquid containing 75 g of glucose. Blood glucose levels are then measured 30 minutes, 1 hour, 2 hours, and 3 hours after drinking the liquid. An OGTT can be used to diagnose diabetes or prediabetes.

Random Blood Glucose Test

A random (or "casual") blood glucose test checks blood glucose levels at various times during the day, regardless of when the individual last ate. Blood glucose levels tend to stay constant in those without diabetes. This test, along with an assessment of symptoms, may be used to indicate whether additional diabetes testing should be performed.

Metabolic Syndrome

Metabolic syndrome may be identified by the presence of three or more of the following traits: elevated waist circumference (men ≥40 inches, women ≥35 inches); elevated triglycerides (≥150 mg/dL); reduced HDL cholesterol (men <40 mg/dL, women <50 mg/dL); elevated blood pressure (≥130/85 mm Hg); or elevated fasting glucose (≥100 mg/dL).

Gestational Diabetes

Pregnant women are screened for gestational diabetes using the OGTT in a fasting state. Because of increased blood volume during pregnancy, glucose levels tend to be lower. Therefore the cutoff levels considered "normal" during pregnancy are lower than those in the general population. An initial blood glucose level is determined by a blood test; the woman then drinks a solution containing 100 g of glucose. Blood glucose levels are measured 30 minutes, 1 hour, 2 hours, and 3 hours after drinking the liquid. Gestational diabetes is diagnosed if blood glucose levels are at least 95 mg/dL fasting, 180 mg/dL within 1 hour of the OGTT, 155 mg/dL after 2 hours, or 140 mg/dL after 3 hours.

Alternatively, a simplified test known as the 2-hour postglucose test measures glucose only at baseline and 2 hours after drinking the liquid. If the second value is elevated, the OGTT may be performed.

Maturity-Onset Diabetes of the Young

Genetic testing can diagnose a predisposition for MODY in a patient's children before symptoms develop.

Monitoring Blood Glucose

For any type of diabetes, treatment aims to maintain glucose levels within the normal range. Patients with diabetes can measure their blood glucose by performing *self-monitoring of blood glucose* (SMBG) with a handheld finger-stick monitor that uses a small sample of blood. Target glucose levels are 90 to 130 mg/dL before meals *(preprandial)* and less than 180 mg/dL after meals *(postprandial)*.

The glycosylated hemoglobin A (HbA$_{1c}$) level may also be useful in diabetes monitoring. HbA$_{1c}$ level indicates an individual's average blood sugar control over the past 3 months. Glucose in the bloodstream can adhere to the *hemoglobin*, the part of the red blood cells (RBCs) that carries oxygen. This process is called *glycosylation*. Once the sugar is attached, it remains for the life of the RBC, which is about 120 days. Increased blood glucose levels are accompanied by increased amounts of glucose adhering to the RBCs. The HbA$_{1c}$ test measures the amount of glucose adhering to the hemoglobin in the RBCs. HbA$_{1c}$ values are not subject to the fluctuations that are seen with daily blood glucose monitoring. Results are given in percentages. The American Diabetes Association (ADA) states that the HbA$_{1c}$ is the best test to determine an individual's blood sugar control over time.[3] The test should be performed every 3 months for insulin-treated patients, during treatment changes, or when blood glucose is consistently elevated. The ADA currently recommends an HbA$_{1c}$ goal of less than 7.0%. Studies have reported that there is a 10% decrease in relative risk of microvascular complications, such as diabetic nephropathy (kidney damage) or diabetic neuropathy (nerve damage), for every 1% reduction in HbA$_{1c}$.[3]

SELECTED HERBAL THERAPIES

Note

To help make this educational resource more interactive, all pharmacokinetics, adverse effects, and interactions data have been compiled in Appendix A. Safety data specifically related to pregnancy and lactation are listed in Appendix B. Please refer to these appendices when working through the case studies and answering the review questions.

Alfalfa *(Medicago sativa)*

Grade C: *Unclear or conflicting scientific evidence (diabetes)*

Mechanism of Action

The hypoglycemic actions of alfalfa have been postulated to result from the potentiation (enhancement) of insulin secretion and improvement of insulin action,[1,4] however, clinical evidence is limited.[1,5]

Scientific Evidence of Effectiveness

Alfalfa has been associated with reductions in serum glucose levels in rat studies[5,6] and in a 1962 human case report.[7] After being unresponsive to conventional hypoglycemic agents, a diabetic man's blood glucose reached 648 mg/dL. Physicians allowed the patient to prepare an alfalfa extract he had used in the past. Two hours after the patient consumed the extract, he exhibited clinical signs of hypoglycemia, with a blood sugar level of 68 mg/dL. After consuming the extract 12 additional times, the patient had blood glucose levels ranging between 190 and 580 mg/dL, each time resulting in a reduction of blood glucose concentrations. Despite these positive findings, clinical trials evaluating the use of alfalfa for diabetes are currently lacking.

Dose

The dose of alfalfa for diabetes has not been determined.

Adverse Effects, Interactions, Pharmacokinetics. See Appendix A.

Aloe *(Aloe vera)*

Grade C: *Unclear or conflicting scientific evidence (diabetes)*

Mechanism of Action

The hypoglycemic action of aloe has not been extensively studied. Research conducted in mice suggests that aloe may exert antidiabetic effects by stimulating beta cell function.[8]

Scientific Evidence of Effectiveness

As a treatment for type 2 diabetes, aloe gel is supported by somewhat weak clinical evidence. When aloe gel was used in combination with glibenclamide (a sulfonylurea), it was found to decrease fasting blood glucose effectively compared with glibenclamide alone.[9,10] A small study of 16 patients, however, found no hypoglycemic effects associated with aloe juice ingestion.[11]

Dose

Standardized products are not widely available. One tablespoon of oral aloe gel in combination with 5 mg of glibenclamide twice daily was found to reduce fasting blood sugar.[10] One study found no hypoglycemic effects in patients taking 15 mL aloe juice twice daily.[11]

Adverse Effects, Interactions, Pharmacokinetics. See Appendix A.

Ashwagandha (Withania somnifera)

Grade C: *Unclear or conflicting scientific evidence (type 2 diabetes)*

Mechanism of Action

The mechanism of ashwagandha in diabetes is not well understood. It may improve insulin sensitivity.[12] Ashwagandha may also inhibit glycosylation ("glycation"), a nonenzymatic reaction as a protein molecule binds to a glucose molecule,[13] which may be beneficial for diabetes-related complications.

Scientific Evidence of Effectiveness

In a small case series, it was reported that powdered ashwagandha roots led to reductions in blood glucose levels that were comparable to those with an oral hypoglycemic drug; however, study details are unclear.[14]

Dose

In a case series, six patients with mild type 2 diabetes and six patients with mild hypercholesterolemia were administered powdered roots of ashwagandha (exact amount unspecified) for 30 days by mouth.[14]

Adverse Effects, Interactions, Pharmacokinetics. See Appendix A.

Astragalus (Astragalus membranaceus)

Grade C: *Unclear or conflicting scientific evidence (diabetes)*

Mechanism of Action

Based on laboratory and animal studies, polysaccharide fractions of astragalus have demonstrated hypoglycemic action.[15-18] It increases cellular uptake of glucose and protein synthesis in adipocytes.[19,20] Astragalus has also been shown to affect flux of glucose metabolism and insulin sensitivity by altering the activity of protein tyrosine phosphorylase and other regulatory enzymes.[21]

Scientific Evidence of Effectiveness

Although experimental evidence shows that astragalus alone and in combination with hypoglycemic medication has significant hypoglycemic properties, clinical evidence is weak. The clinical data suggest that combination products containing astragalus may help lower glucose levels in patients with type 2 diabetes.[22-27] Although the findings are suggestive, the validity of the data is confounded by methodological limitations and is therefore inconclusive.

Dose

The dose of astragalus for diabetes has not been determined.

Adverse Effects, Interactions, Pharmacokinetics. See Appendix A.

Banaba (Lagerstroemia speciosa)

Grade C: *Unclear or conflicting scientific evidence (diabetes)*

Mechanism of Action

Active constituents of banaba include corosolic acid and the ellagitannins: lagerstroemin, flosin B, and reginin A.[28-30] In vitro studies suggest that ellagitannins have an insulin-like effect.[28] Lagerstroemin may activate insulin receptors.[31]

Scientific Evidence of Effectiveness

Banaba has been used for thousands of years in the Philippines, as a folk remedy by American Indians, and more recently by Japanese populations as a tea preparation. Because of purported hypoglycemic effects, banaba leaves are popularly used for sugar control and weight loss.[32] Animal evidence supports this historical use.[33] Preliminary clinical evidence is promising. Type 2 diabetic patients who received banaba for 15 days reported a reduction in blood glucose.

Dose

Banaba has been standardized to 1% corosolic acid (Glucosol) in available clinical research. Soft-gel and dry-powder-filled hard-gelatin formulations of Glucosol showed a drop in blood glucose level in type 2 diabetic patients over a dose range of 16 to 48 mg daily (0.16-0.48 mg corosolic acid).[30]

Adverse Effects, Interactions, Pharmacokinetics. See Appendix A.

Barley (Hordeum vulgare)

Grade C: *Unclear or conflicting scientific evidence (hyperglycemia)*

Mechanism of Action

Barley contains more fermentable carbohydrates than other cereals such as rice. Fermentation of undigested carbohydrates produces short-chain fatty acids, some of which may reduce hepatic glucose production and affect postprandial glycemia. Because of viscous properties of beta-glucans, boiled flours appear to produce higher glucose and insulin responses compared with milled kernels.[34]

Scientific Evidence of Effectiveness

Barley and barley products enriched with beta-glucan have been shown to have positive effects on blood glucose and insulin parameters in various clinical trials.[35-38] Barley products enriched with beta-glucan (18 g/100 g dry weight) significantly lowered postprandial rises in blood glucose levels and serum insulin responses compared with white bread in healthy subjects.[35] Improved glucose tolerance is believed to result from fermentation of undigested carbohydrates in barley, which decreases hepatic glucose production by up to 30%. Barley products have been shown to have lower glycemic indices than wheat or rice.[36]

Dose

For glucose-lowering effects, 90 g of carbohydrates from barley grain with meals has been used.[36] Higher amounts of barley products enriched with beta-glucan may result in greater effect.[36-38]

Adverse Effects, Interactions, Pharmacokinetics. See Appendix A.

Beet (Beta vulgaris)

Grade C: *Unclear or conflicting scientific evidence (hyperglycemia; type 2 diabetes)*

Mechanism of Action

Dietary fibers such as beet fiber may improve glucose control through various mechanisms, including a decrease in glucose absorption, increase in hepatic extraction of insulin, increase in insulin sensitivity at the cellular level, and binding of bile acids. Beet fiber may also increase the secretion of motilin, which may be useful for disturbed gastric emptying.[39]

Scientific Evidence of Effectiveness

Dietary fiber has been shown to help improve glycemic control in type 2 diabetic patients.[40] Clinical trials evaluating the effects of beet fiber supplementation on glucose metabolism and glycemic control in subjects with abnormal glucose metabolism or in healthy volunteers have reported mixed results.[39,41-44] Some studies have shown a clinical benefit, whereas others have found no measurable effect. One available study found beet fiber to increase motilin secretion, which may be beneficial in diabetic gastroparesis (impaired gastric emptying).[39]

Dose

There is no well-known standardization for any part of the beet plant. Diets supplemented with 7 to 27 g of beet fiber daily may improve glucose control and lower insulin levels after meals.[39,42,43]

Adverse Effects, Interactions, Pharmacokinetics. See Appendix A.

Berberine

Grade C: *Unclear or conflicting scientific evidence (type 2 diabetes)*

Mechanism of Action

Berberine is the active constituent of goldenseal (*Hydrastis canadensis*) and coptis or goldenthread (*Coptis chinensis*), as well as plants in the genus *Berberis* such as barberry (*B. vulgaris*), Oregon grape (*B. aquifolium*), and tree turmeric *B. aristata*).[45] Berberine has been shown to influence glucose absorption and may act as an alpha-glucosidase inhibitor.[46] Berberine has also improved insulin resistance and liver glycogen levels similar to metformin when given to rats fed a high-fat diet.[47]

Scientific Evidence of Effectiveness

Historically, berberine has been suggested to aid in glycemic regulation. When berberine was being studied for diarrhea, a potential glucose-lowering effect was noted. In human studies designed to evaluate the efficacy of berberine for diabetes, researchers found positive results.[48,49] Fasting and postprandial glucose was reduced by 1.4 and 3.1 mmol/L, respectively, after 3 months and HbA$_{1c}$ by 0.9% from initial levels of 7.5%.[49] This decline is comparable to that of existing pharmacological products used for type 2 diabetes, such as metformin. Reductions in serum cholesterol, low-density lipoprotein (LDL) cholesterol, and triglycerides have also been noted.[48,49]

Dose

For glucose-lowering effects, 0.5 g of berberine was administered two to three times daily for 3 months.[48,49] A dose reduction to 0.25 g twice daily has been suggested when constipation occurs and lasts longer than 2 weeks.[49]

Adverse Effects, Interactions, Pharmacokinetics. See Appendix A.

Beta-Glucan (β-Glucan)

Grade B: *Good scientific evidence (diabetes)*

Mechanism of Action

Beta-glucan is a soluble fiber found in the cell walls of algae, bacteria, fungi, yeast, and plants. Dietary fibers may improve glucose control through various mechanisms, including decreased glucose absorption, increased hepatic extraction of insulin, increased insulin sensitivity at the cellular level, and binding of bile acids. Fermentation of undigested carbohydrate, especially from beta-glucan, produces short-chain fatty acids and may reduce hepatic glucose production and affect postprandial glycemia.[36]

Scientific Evidence of Effectiveness

Beta-glucan is popularly used to reduce cholesterol levels, but results from several studies suggest it may also be beneficial for glycemic control.[50-56] Beta-glucan–containing products appear to have positive effects on postprandial blood glucose and insulin parameters.[50] The long-term effects of beta-glucan on postprandial blood sugar have not been well established. Additionally, a beta-glucan–enriched snack in children did not result in reductions in nocturnal blood glucose levels.[52]

Dose

For diabetes, 50 to 90 g of carbohydrate portions of barley grain with meals have been studied.[56] Higher amounts of fiber and beta-glucan may result in a stronger effect.

Adverse Effects, Interactions, Pharmacokinetics. See Appendix A.

Bitter Melon (Momordica charantia)

Grade C: *Unclear or conflicting scientific evidence (diabetes)*

Mechanism of Action

Multiple mechanisms have been proposed as the source of bitter melon's hypoglycemic properties.[57] Components of bitter melon extract appear to have structural similarities to animal insulin, as measured by electrophoresis and infrared spectrum analysis.[58] Preliminary investigation has reported some insulin-like properties of bitter melon.[59-61] Other evidence suggests that bitter melon may decrease hepatic gluconeogenesis, increase hepatic glycogen synthesis, and increase peripheral glucose oxidation in erythrocytes and adipocytes.[62] There is limited evidence that bitter melon increases pancreatic insulin secretion,[63] but this was not confirmed by subsequent studies.[64,65] Although several constituents of bitter melon have been found to possess hypoglycemic properties,[66-70] most interest has focused on a polypeptide isolated from the seeds called *polypeptide P* and a mixture of two steroid glycosides named *charantin*.[71]

Scientific Evidence of Effectiveness

In the Ayurvedic tradition, bitter melon has been used to treat diabetes.[72] Bitter melon has been shown to decrease serum glucose levels in animal experiments and in a small number of methodologically limited human studies that were not randomized or controlled.[58-70, 73-77] Systematic studies on dosage, toxicity, and adverse effects are currently lacking. Preparation techniques have varied in the literature, and potency and chemical constituents may have varied accordingly. Nonetheless, the human, animal, and in vitro evidence collectively suggest a moderate hypoglycemic effect of bitter melon and some of its crude extracts. Reduction in serum blood sugar may occur as soon as 30 minutes after dosing, peak at 4 hours, and persist for at least 12 hours.[1,4] Properly designed randomized controlled trials (RCTs) are warranted to establish the clinical role of bitter melon for diabetes.

Dose

Because of the wide variation in preparation techniques for bitter melon, the proper dosing for diabetes cannot be determined at present. In the available studies, bitter melon has been administered as a fruit juice in doses of 50 mL[73] or 100 mL.[75] Juice formulations have been reported to have more potent effects on blood sugar and HbA_{1c} than the powder of the sun-dried fruit. A dose of 5 g of dried bitter melon fruit powder has also been used three times daily for 3 weeks.[81] However, safety and efficacy have not been established for any specific dose of bitter melon.

Adverse Effects, Interactions, Pharmacokinetics. See Appendix A.

Burdock (Arctium lappa)

Grade C: *Unclear or conflicting scientific evidence (diabetes)*

Mechanism of Action

The mechanism of burdock's effects on serum glucose is not clear.[78]

Scientific Evidence of Effectiveness

Burdock has been used traditionally to treat diabetes. Preliminary animal data and poor-quality human data suggest possible hypoglycemic effects of burdock root or fruit, although reliable data are lacking.[79,80] In a 1930s human case series evaluating the effects of the dried root in diabetic patients, burdock inhibited the expected hyperglycemia caused by administration of common polysaccharides at the measured intervals. In "mild diabetic" subjects, normal blood sugar levels were maintained by the administration of burdock in the form of crackers.[79]

Dose

The dose of burdock for diabetes has not been determined.

Adverse Effects, Interactions, Pharmacokinetics. See Appendix A.

Chrysanthemum (Chrysanthemum spp.)

Grade C: *Unclear or conflicting scientific evidence (diabetes)*

Mechanism of Action

According to limited clinical research, a product of chrysanthemum called *jiangtangkang* may improve insulin sensitivity and decrease blood viscosity.[81]

Scientific Evidence of Effectiveness

The chrysanthemum product jiangtangkang may improve fasting and postprandial blood glucose levels and increase sensitivity to insulin in patients with type 2 diabetes (NIDDM).[81] However, the effects do not appear to be similar to glibenclazide. In vitro, chrysanthemum extracts did not have the same activity.[82]

Dose

The dose of *Chrysanthemum* for diabetes has not been determined.

Adverse Effects, Interactions, Pharmacokinetics. See Appendix A.

Cinnamon (*Cinnamomum* spp.)

Grade C: *Unclear or conflicting scientific evidence (type 2 diabetes)*

Mechanism of Action

Cinnamon has been used in folkloric medicine to control blood sugar.[83] Recent pharmacological studies have shown that cinnamon may play a role in improving glucose and insulin metabolism.[84] The insulin-sensitizing effect of cinnamon has been established with in vitro cell line studies using adipocytes as well as with in vivo animal studies.[84-91] Bioactive compounds extracted from cinnamon may potentiate insulin activity.[85,87,89] Cinnamon was highly active in the insulin-dependent utilization of glucose using a rat epididymal adipocyte assay.[86] A hydroxychalcone from cinnamon functioned as an insulin mimetic in 3T3-LI adipocytes.[88] Cinnamaldehyde exhibited strong inhibition against aldose reductase,[91] an enzyme in carbohydrate metabolism that converts glucose into its sugar-alcohol form, *sorbitol*, using NADPH as the reducing agent. Aqueous extracts of cinnamon significantly lowered the absorption of alanine, an important amino acid for gluconeogenesis, from the rat intestine.[90]

Scientific Evidence of Effectiveness

Ingestion of cinnamon daily for 40 days reduced fasting serum glucose as well as triglycerides, serum cholesterol, and LDL cholesterol in type 2 diabetic patients.[92] Decreases for fasting glucose ranged from 18% to 29%. However, a study in postmenopausal women could not substantiate these effects; cinnamon supplementation did not improve whole-body insulin sensitivity or oral glucose tolerance and did not modulate blood lipid profiles.[93]

Dose

For type 2 diabetes, 1, 3, or 6 g of cinnamon daily for 40 days was shown to have beneficial effects.[92] A dose of 1500 mg of cinnamon daily for 6 weeks did not improve glucose in postmenopausal women with type 2 diabetes.[93]

Adverse Effects, Interactions, Pharmacokinetics. See Appendix A.

Dandelion (*Taraxacum officinale*)

Grade C: *Unclear or conflicting scientific evidence (diabetes)*

Mechanism of Action

The antidiabetic mechanisms of dandelion are not well understood. *Inulin,* a soluble fiber in dandelion, may act as a glucose modulator.[94]

Scientific Evidence of Effectiveness

Dandelion has been reported to decrease glucose levels in nondiabetic rabbits,[95] whereas no changes in mice were observed.[78] Effects in humans are unclear.

Dose

The dose of dandelion for diabetes has not been determined.

Adverse Effects, Interactions, Pharmacokinetics. See Appendix A.

Devil's Club (*Oplopanax horridus*)

Grade C: *Unclear or conflicting scientific evidence (diabetes)*

Mechanism of Action

Devil's club has purported hypoglycemic effects, though the mechanisms of action for these effects are unclear.

Scientific Evidence of Effectiveness

The hypoglycemic effect is one of many reported uses for devil's club, traditionally and currently used for diabetes. Several animal studies and limited human anecdotal evidence resulted after ethnobotanical research reported the hypoglycemic effect of devil's club.[96-100] However, patients given devil's club in conjunction with OGTT found no hypoglycemic effects that could be attributed to the product.[104] Animal trials have yielded conflicting results and clinical evidence is limited to case studies.

Dose

The dose of devil's club for diabetes has not been determined.

Adverse Effects, Interactions, Pharmacokinetics. See Appendix A.

Evening Primrose (*Oenothera biennis*)

Grade C: *Unclear or conflicting scientific evidence (diabetes; diabetic peripheral neuropathy)*

Mechanism of Action

The principal active ingredient in evening primrose oil (EPO) is thought to be gamma-linolenic acid (GLA), an omega-6 essential fatty acid. The mechanism of evening primrose or GLA in diabetes or diabetic neuropathy is not well understood. GLA may promote the production of vasodilator prostaglandin E1, which is capable of modulating blood flow to peripheral nerves.[101,102]

Scientific Evidence of Effectiveness

Animal studies[103-105] and small controlled human trials[106-108] have demonstrated beneficial effects of EPO on serum markers in diabetes mellitus, including prostaglandin levels and serum fatty acids. Changes have not been observed in HbA_{1c}. Notably, GLA has demonstrated beneficial effects for diabetic neuropathy. Significant improvements in neurophysiological parameters, thermal thresholds, and clinical sensory evaluations in human trials have been noted.[101,102]

Dose

For diabetic neuropathy, 480 mg of EPO was administered daily.[101,102] The dose of EPO for diabetes has not been determined.

Adverse Effects and Interactions, Pharmacokinetics. See Appendix A.

Fenugreek (Trigonella foenum-graecum)

Grade C: *Unclear or conflicting scientific evidence (types 1 and 2 diabetes)*

Mechanism of Action

The hypoglycemic effects of fenugreek observed in animal studies have been associated with the "A" subfraction that contains the testa and endosperm of the defatted seeds. These effects have not been observed with lipid extracts.[109,110] Hypoglycemic effects have been attributed to several mechanisms. The amino acid 4-hydroxyisoleucine in fenugreek seed has been shown to increase glucose-induced insulin release in vitro in human and rat pancreatic islet cells.[111] This amino acid appeared to act only on pancreatic beta cells, because somatostatin and glucagon were not altered in the study. However, another in vitro study indicated that fenugreek seed extract phosphorylates a number of proteins.[112] These results suggest that fenugreek's effects may be caused by activation of the insulin-signaling pathway in adipocytes and liver cells. Fenugreek seeds have also been postulated to exert hypoglycemic effects by stimulating glucose-dependent insulin release by beta cells,[113] or through inhibition of α-amylase and sucrase activity.[114] Another study further characterized 4-hydroxyisoleucine as one of the active ingredients for blood glucose control.[115]

Scientific Evidence of Effectiveness

Preliminary human trials suggest that oral fenugreek seed powder may be efficacious in diabetes.[71,116-123] Various fenugreek preparations have been found to reduce 24-hour urine glucose, fasting glucose, and OGTT in patients with type 1 or 2 diabetes. Improvement in beta-cell secretion and insulin resistance has also been reported.[119] It has been suggested that fenugreek seed extract and diet/exercise may be equally effective strategies for attaining glycemic control in type 2 diabetes.

Significant decreases in total cholesterol, LDL cholesterol, and triglyceride levels and increases in high-density lipoprotein (HDL) cholesterol were also noted.[124,125]

Dose

Different clinical trials have used different doses of fenugreek preparations. The active ingredients of fenugreek have yet to be identified, so it is difficult to relate these preparations to a standard dose.

For type 1 diabetes, 100 g of debitterized powdered fenugreek seeds divided in two equal doses added to meals has been used.[117]

For type 2 diabetes, 2.5 g of fenugreek seed powder in capsule form, twice daily for 3 months;[115] and 25 g of seed powder divided in two equal doses have been used.[120,126,127]

Adverse Effects, Interactions, Pharmacokinetics. See Appendix A.

Fig (Ficus carica)

Grade C: *Unclear or conflicting scientific evidence (type 1 diabetes)*

Mechanism of Action

The mechanism of action of fig in diabetes is not well understood. The antioxidants in fig leaf extracts have shown benefits in animal models of diabetes.[128]

Scientific Evidence of Effectiveness

In animals *Ficus carica* extraction normalized fatty acid and plasma vitamin E values in diabetic animals.[132] Clinical research examining fig as diabetic therapy has produced equivocal results, largely due to methodological limitations and small sample size.[129] Ten subjects (six men, four women) with type 1 diabetes were randomly assigned to drink 1 cup daily of a 13-g fig leaf decoction or a nonhypoglycemic tea (placebo). After 1 month and an unspecified washout period, the groups crossed over for 1 more month. All patients were maintained on two daily insulin injections. The average insulin dose was 12% lower during the fig tea phase in the experimental group. There was also a significant decline in postprandial blood glucose measurements during tea phases compared with placebo. No changes in lipid profile, glycosylated hemoglobin (HbA_{1c}) levels, or other measures of glycemic control were detected.

Dose

The exact dose of fig for diabetes has not been determined. However, preliminary evidence from human study noted positive results when subjects consumed 1 cup daily of a 13-g fig leaf decoction for 1 month.[129]

Adverse Effects, Interactions, Pharmacokinetics. See Appendix A.

Galega (Galega Officinalis)

Galega officinalis (commonly known as goat's rue, French lilac, Italian fitch, or professor-weed) has been traditionally used as an herbal remedy for diabetes.[138-140] Galega extracts contain guanidine, a chemical precursor to the class of drugs known as biguanides, which are standard treatments for type 2 diabetes mellitus.[141] The biguanide drug metformin (marketed under the brand names Glucophage, Riomet, Fortamet, Glumetza, Diabex, or Diaformin) inhibits gluconeogenesis in the liver,[142] and is one of two oral antidiabetic medications listed in the World Health Organization Model List of Essential Medicines.[143]

The general structure of guanidines.

The structure of Metformin.

Clinical studies using galega as a treatment for diabetes are lacking. However, there is convincing evidence from animal and basic science studies (as well as traditional use) to support its hypoglycemic effects. Furthermore, clinical evidence supports the efficacy of metformin, a synthetic derivative of galega, which is commonly used to type 2 diabetes. In 2007, nearly 37 million prescriptions for metformin were filled, making it the single most popular antidiabetic drug in the United States; moreover, of all generic medicines, metformin was the 11th most commonly prescribed.[144] Because metformin is has significantly lower toxicity than guanidine or its derivatives,[141] galega should not be used as a replacement for metformin or other conventional therapies.

Flax (Linum usitatissimum)

Grade C: *Unclear or conflicting scientific evidence (hyperglycemia/diabetes)*

Mechanism of Action
The mechanism of flaxseed in diabetes is not well understood but may be related to its antioxidant effects.[130-133]

Scientific Evidence of Effectiveness
There is equivocal evidence from several human studies, which have reported mixed effects of oral flaxseed on serum glucose levels.[133-136] Reductions in fasting blood glucose and postprandial glucose levels have been noted.[135,136] However, a case series found flaxseed to diminish insulin sensitivity.[137]

Dose
The dose of flaxseed for diabetes has not been determined.

Adverse Effects, Interactions, Pharmacokinetics. See Appendix A.

Ginseng (Panax spp.)

Grade B: *Good scientific evidence (type 2 diabetes; hyperglycemia)*

Grade C: *Unclear or conflicting scientific evidence (diabetic nephropathy)*

Mechanism of Action
Ginseng appears to have an insulin-mimetic,[145] hypoglycemic effect in type 2 diabetes, possibly accelerating glucose-utilization by the liver.[146,147] This hypoglycemic effect has also been seen in nondiabetic human subjects taking American ginseng, although one study found no such effect, perhaps because of variable ginsenoside concentrations in the *ginseng preparatic* used.[148,149] Several types of ginseng (Canadian white, American red, Korean red, Sanchi ginseng) decrease plasma glucose levels,[150] possibly from their sulfonylurea-like activity.[151]

Furthermore, ginseng seems to accelerate hepatic lipogenesis, stimulate glucose transport, enhance glycogen storage, inhibit lipolysis, and inhibit lipid peroxidation.[145,152-154] Ginseng may elicit an elevation in plasma insulin levels by increased insulin secretion from beta islet cells, through a different mechanism than glucose.[155] At least five glycans have been isolated from *Panax ginseng*[156] and three from *Panax quinquefolium*.[157] Although a hypoglycemic effect of ginseng was also found on postprandial glucose levels in healthy subjects, no hypoglycemia was observed.[146] A small study found that 50 g of ginseng extract had no effect on insulin after a standardized weight-training workout.[158] Some clinicians still believe that evidence is lacking to attribute a glycemic effect to ginseng[159] because of the methodological limitations in studies.[160] Ingestion of 3 g of American ginseng daily for 8 weeks significantly lowered fasting plasma plasminogen activator inhibitor-1

(PAI-1).[161] A strong relationship exists between glycemic control and the PAI-1.

Scientific Evidence of Effectiveness

TYPE 2 DIABETES. American ginseng has been found to reduce postprandial glucose levels in healthy patients and in patients with type 2 diabetes.[162] It decreased postprandial glycemic response to a 25-g oral glucose challenge in 12 healthy (nondiabetic) subjects.[163] American ginseng with a depressed ginsenoside profile did not affect postprandial glycemia in healthy subjects after OGTT.[148] Overall, however, results are promising, especially because ginseng does not seem to cause dangerous hypoglycemia. Future research needs to evaluate the long-term efficacy of American ginseng in treating type 2 diabetes compared with standard oral hypoglycemic drugs.

DIABETIC NEPHROPATHY. There is preliminary evidence that *Panax notoginseng* may have beneficial effects in patients with diabetic nephropathy. One study found equivalence between a *P. notoginseng* preparation and ticlopidine (Ticlid); however, no placebo was used in this study, and conclusions are limited. Additional studies are warranted. *P. notoginseng* is not commonly used or available in the United States.[164]

Dose

Ginseng extracts may be standardized to 4% to 7% total ginsenosides content[165] (e.g., in G115). Some sources indicate that ginsenosides constitute an average of 3% of the dried whole root[166] and that the usual concentration of ginsenosides may actually be 1% to 3%. Standardized extracts of *Panax quinquefolius* (CNT-2000) are also available. The German Federal Pharmacopeia standardizes a minimum ginsenoside content of 1.5%, calculated in terms of the ginsenoside Rg1.[167]

In clinical study of American ginseng (*P. quinquefolius*) for diabetes, 3 g was used daily.[146] *Panax ginseng*, 100 to 200 mg daily for 8 weeks, has also been found to improve glucose levels.[152]

Adverse Effects, Interactions, Pharmacokinetics. See Appendix A.

Gotu Kola (Centella asiatica)

Grade C: *Unclear or conflicting scientific evidence (diabetic microangiopathy)*

Mechanism of Action

The triterpenoid saponins found in gotu kola (asiatic acid, madecassic acid, and asiaticoside) appear to increase wound healing and decrease venous pressure.[168,169] Gotu kola may improve blood circulation in the lower legs by stimulating collagen synthesis in the vein wall. This results in greater vein tonicity and decreased vein distention.[170,171]

Scientific Evidence of Effectiveness

Studies suggest beneficial effects from the total triterpenoid fraction of *Centella asiatica* (TTFCA) on subjective and objective parameters of venous insufficiency of the lower extremities.[172-182] Based on these observations, gotu kola may be somewhat effective in the treatment of vascular disease associated with diabetes. However, diabetic patients often experience vascular disease with different etiology than venous insufficiency. Nonetheless, preliminary controlled trials of short duration have found that oral gotu kola (TTFCA, 60 mg twice daily) has statistically significant beneficial effects on microcirculatory parameters in patients with diabetic microangiopathy.[183-185]

Dose

For diabetic microangiopathy, 60 mg of TTFCA was administered twice daily.[183,184]

Adverse Effects, Interactions, Pharmacokinetics. See Appendix A.

Gymnema (Gymnema sylvestre)

Grade B: *Good scientific evidence (diabetes)*

Mechanism of Action

Few studies have closely evaluated the constituents of *Gymnema sylvestre* leaf. Proposed active components include gurmarin, conduritol A, and triterpene glycosides.[186-188] Gymnemoside b and gymnemic acids V and VII appear to be the key saponin constituents.[189]

Gymnema may act by enhancing insulin secretion through increased pancreatic beta-cell number and through improved cell function. Other proposed mechanisms include stimulation of the release of endogenous insulin[190,191] through interactions with insulinotropic enteric hormones or increased glucose utilization.[192] Such activities may explain the observed hypoglycemic effects in type 2 diabetic patients. Gymnema has also been reported to restore levels of glycoproteins in diabetic rats to normal, thereby potentially preventing diabetic microangiopathy and other pathological organ changes.[193]

Scientific Evidence of Effectiveness

Multiple animal studies report that gymnema lowers serum glucose levels.[186-189,192,194-201] There is some clinical evidence supporting the use of gymnema as an adjunct to insulin or oral hypoglycemic drugs; hypoglycemic effects of chronic oral gymnema were observed when used in patients with type 1 or type 2 diabetes. The onset of effect has not been clearly described, although one study noted that oral administration of gymnema did not have acute effects on fasting serum glucose levels (after 45 minutes).[190] The effects of gymnema were assessed after 10 days, for up to 20 months.

Although gymnema may lower serum glucose levels, further studies of dosing, safety, and efficacy are warranted. Multiple drugs are available to establish good long-term control of blood glucose levels, and gymnema has not been thoroughly evaluated as a safe or effective alternative or adjunct to these agents.

Dose

Gymnema may be standardized to 25% gymnemic acid. An ethanolic acid–precipitated extract from gymnema, labeled GS4, has been used in human trials.[190,202] GS4 has since been patented as the product Proβeta. This preparation is purportedly standardized to possess specific "pancreotropic" effects, as measured by a proprietary test.

For type 1 diabetes, a dose of 200 mg GS4 extract was administered orally twice daily[202] under careful continuation of insulin.

For type 2 diabetes, a dose of 200 mg GS4 extract was administered orally twice daily.[190] Also for type 2 diabetes, 2 mL of an aqueous decoction (containing 10 g shade-dried powdered leaves per dL) was administered three times daily.[203]

Doses of insulin or other concomitant hypoglycemic drugs may need to be adjusted or discontinued, under the supervision of a healthcare professional.

Adverse Effects, Interactions, Pharmacokinetics. See Appendix A.

Holy Basil *(Ocimum sanctum)*

Grade C: *Unclear or conflicting scientific evidence (diabetes)*

Mechanism of Action

The mechanism of action of holy basil in diabetes is not understood. Research on holy basil suggests that it contains powerful antioxidants that may be beneficial in diabetes.[204-208]

Scientific Evidence of Effectiveness

The two primary types of basil are closely related: *Ocimum basilicum* (sweet basil), which is prominent in Italian and Asian cooking, and *Ocimum sanctum* (holy basil), which is a sacred plant in the Hindu religion. Experiments in animal models indicate that holy basil may have a hypoglycemic effect.[209] Limited clinical evidence indicates a significant decrease in fasting and postprandial blood glucose levels during treatment with holy basil leaves compared with placebo.[210] These findings suggest that basil leaves may be useful as an adjunct to dietary therapy and drug treatment in mild to moderate diabetes mellitus. It is unclear whether common culinary basil (*O. basilicum*) would have similar effects.

Dose

The chemical content of basil oil varies widely because of numerous factors, such as plant variety and the time of harvest. This may account for some of the variability in medicinal efficacy demonstrated in studies.

For diabetes, 2.5 g of dried holy basil leaf powder was taken by mouth every morning; additionally, 1 tsp of dried herb brewed in 1 cup of water has been administered three times daily.[1,210]

Adverse Effects, Interactions, Pharmacokinetics. See Appendix A.

Jackfruit *(Artocarpus heterophyllus)*

Grade C: *Unclear or conflicting scientific evidence (high blood sugar/glucose intolerance)*

Mechanism of Action. Insufficient available evidence.

Scientific Evidence of Effectiveness

Preliminary clinical research has assessed the effects of jackfruit leaves and whole-plant material on gluclose tolerance. Improvements were noted in glucose tolerance in healthy subjects and diabetic patients.[211]

Dose

Jackfruit leaves and whole-plant material have been administered in oral doses equivalent to 20 g/kg).[211]

Adverse Effects, Interactions, Pharmacokinetics. See Appendix A.

Kudzu *(Pueraria lobata)*

Grade C: *Unclear or conflicting scientific evidence (diabetes/insulin resistance; diabetic retinopathy)*

Mechanism of Action

Based on animal studies, kudzu and its constituents may have hypoglycemic effects.[212-214] *Puerarin*, an isoflavone, in kudzu, has increased glucose utilization to lower plasma glucose.[215] It has also activated α_1-adrenoceptors on the adrenal gland to enhance the secretion of β-endorphin, resulting in decreased plasma glucose.[216,217]

Compounds that target the peroxisome proliferator-activated receptors PPAR-α and PPAR-γ are used to correct dyslipidemia and to restore glycemic balance, respectively.[218] Because diabetic patients often have atherogenic lipid abnormalities in addition to insulin resistance, molecules are required to activate both PPAR-α and PPAR-γ. *Pueraria thomsonii* and isolated daidzein were found to activate both PPARs. However, daidzein was not as potent as other common isoflavones, such as formononetin and calycosin from *Astragalus*.

Scientific Evidence of Effectiveness

Type 2 diabetes is typically preceded by insulin resistance; therefore, reversing insulin resistance can decrease the risk of developing type 2 diabetes. Preliminary evidence suggests that puerarin may improve insulin resistance and related lipid or fibrinolytic abnormality, particularly in patients with coronary heart disease (CHD).[219] Preliminary evidence also suggests that puerarin injections may reduce blood viscosity, improve microcirculation, and play a beneficial role in diabetic retinopathy.[220]

Dose

A specific kudzu extract (NPI-031, Natural Pharmacia) has been used in rats. This extract is standardized to contain 19% puerarin, 4% daidzin, and 2% daidzein.[221]

Puerarin in a 500-mg dose given by adding 250 mL of normal saline for IV drip once daily for 3 weeks has been shown to improve insulin resistance.[219]

Puerarin at 400 mg daily by IV drip for 3 weeks has been shown to improve diabetic retinopathy.[220]

Adverse Effects, Interactions, Pharmacokinetics. See Appendix A.

Maitake Mushroom *(Grifola frondosa)*

Grade C: *Unclear or conflicting scientific evidence (diabetes)*

Mechanism of Action

The mechanism of maitake mushroom in diabetes is not well understood but may be related to the enhancement of peripheral insulin sensitivity.[222]

Scientific Evidence of Effectiveness

Multiple animal studies have demonstrated hypoglycemic effects of maitake mushroom extracts. In insulin-resistant mice a water-soluble maitake extract was associated with enhanced peripheral insulin sensitivity.[222] Decreased blood glucose levels and glucosuria and elevated serum insulin levels have been found with dietary maitake extract in diabetic mice.[223,224] Human evidence is limited in this area.[225]

Dose

The dose of maitake mushroom for diabetes has not been determined.

Adverse Effects, Interactions, Pharmacokinetics. See Appendix A.

Milk Thistle *(Silybum marianum)*

Grade C: *Unclear or conflicting scientific evidence (diabetes)*

Mechanism of Action

The antidiabetic mechanisms of milk thistle are not well understood. *Silymarin*, the biologically active component of milk thistle, was observed to help protect the pancreas from damage in rats with experimentally induced diabetes mellitus.[226]

Scientific Evidence of Effectiveness

Preliminary evidence from animal studies has suggested a possible role of silymarin in the management of diabetes. Limited human data are available, and existing studies have focused on the treatment of type 2 diabetes associated with alcoholic cirrhosis. In rats pretreated with cyclosporin, silybin did not affect glucose levels; however, silybin and cyclosporin had an additive inhibitory effect on insulin secretion.[227] According to limited clinical research, silymarin taken for 1 year may decrease fasting plasma glucose, HbA$_{1c}$, and fasting insulin levels in patients with type 1 diabetes mellitus (IDDM) associated with cirrhosis.[228]

Dose

Milk thistle capsules, tincture, and powder are often standardized to contain 70% to 80% silymarin. As a treatment for type 1 diabetes associated with cirrhosis, silymarin (Legalon) has shown positive results when used daily (for up to 1 year) in 230- to 600-mg doses.[228-230]

Adverse Effects, Interactions, Pharmacokinetics. See Appendix A.

Myrcia *(Myrcia* spp.*)*

Grade C: *Unclear or conflicting scientific evidence (type 2 diabetes)*

Mechanism of Action

Myrcia has been found to reduce intestinal glucose absorption.[231] Additionally, portions of the leaves of one species, *Myrcia multiflora* DC, was found to inhibit aldose reductase and alpha-glucosidase.[232]

Scientific Evidence of Effectiveness

Myrcia has been used traditionally by indigenous tribes in the Brazilian rainforest to treat diabetes, and *Myrcia uniflora* has exhibited antidiabetic properties in animal studies.[231,232] Limited clinical study has investigated the hypoglycemic effects of *Myrcia uniflora* in normal subjects and type 2 diabetic patients, but found no clinical differences. More research is warranted to confirm this finding.

Dose

Traditionally, 1 cup of *Myrcia* leaf infusion two or three times daily with meals, or 1 to 2 g of leaf powder in tablets or capsules with meals, has been taken to treat diabetes. Infusion of 3 g of *Myrcia* leaves daily for 56 days was used in human study, but no clinical benefits were observed for diabetes.[233]

Adverse Effects, Interactions, Pharmacokinetics. See Appendix A.

Nopal *(Opuntia* spp.*)*

Grade C: *Unclear or conflicting scientific evidence (diabetes)*

Mechanism of Action

The antidiabetic mechanisms of nopal are not well understood. It appears to slow carbohydrate absorption and thus reduce the postprandial rise in blood glucose and serum insulin.[234]

Scientific Evidence of Effectiveness

Animal and clinical studies have suggested that nopal may reduce blood glucose levels in diabetes.[235-238] Preliminary clinical research has shown that prickly pear cactus may decrease blood glucose levels in patients with type 2 diabetes.[239-244] Single doses may decrease blood glucose levels by 17% to 46%

in some patients. Thus far only the species *Opuntia streptacantha* seems to be beneficial.[242,245] It is currently unclear if extended daily use may consistently lower blood glucose levels and decrease HbA_{1c} levels. The quality of available studies is low. The same author has conducted most of the available studies; in the absence of well-designed independent studies, conclusive evidence is lacking.

Dose

For diabetes, broiled *Opuntia streptacantha* stems (up to 500 g) have been used as in acute doses.[239,241-244] A dose of 10.1 g of nopal stem extract has also been used as an acute dose after a glucose load.[240]

Adverse Effects, Interactions, Pharmacokinetics. See Appendix A.

Onion (Allium cepa)

Grade C: *Unclear or conflicting scientific evidence (diabetes)*

Mechanism of Action

The antidiabetic action of onion is not well understood but may result from the inactivation of the thiol group, which may be involved in insulin breakdown.[246] Onion may have stimulating effects on glucose utilization and the antioxidant enzymes superoxide dismutase and catalase.[247]

Scientific Evidence of Effectiveness

Onion has been experimentally documented to possess antidiabetic potential.[248] A crossover comparative study in 20 diabetic outpatients was performed to assess the effects of a diet including onions or green beans on diabetic symptoms (hypercholesterolemia, serum glucose levels).[249] Ten patients consumed a specific diet (68% cal carbohydrate, 20% cal fat, 12% cal protein) plus either 20 g of fresh onion three times daily or 200 g of green beans three times daily in the first week, then the diet alone in the second week. The other 10 patients received diet alone the first week, then onion or green beans the second week. The onion group had a significant decrease in blood sugar level; however, no changes in blood lipid level occurred with these diets.

Dose

Fresh onion (20 g) was consumed three times daily by diabetic patients in a clinical study; significant decreases in blood sugar were observed.[249]

Adverse Effects, Interactions, Pharmacokinetics. See Appendix A.

Psyllium (Plantago spp.)

Grade C: *Unclear or conflicting scientific evidence (hyperglycemia)*

Mechanism of Action

The soluble fiber found in psyllium may help regulate blood glucose levels by slowing the access of glucose to the small intestine, delaying gastric emptying, or slowing carbohydrate digestion and absorption.[250-254]

Scientific Evidence of Effectiveness

Psyllium has been studied for its effect in acutely or chronically affecting glucose levels. Several studies have examined the administration of psyllium before, during, or after meals.[250-262] Psyllium fiber reduced the rise in postprandial glucose and insulin concentrations in type 2 diabetic patients. Postprandial glucose was lowered by 14% after breakfast and 20% after dinner doses.[251] Psyllium appears to have a dose-dependent blood-glucose-lowering effect, which is similar in normal and diabetic subjects; however, this effect seems only to be apparent when psyllium is mixed with food.[262] Psyllium may also lower blood sugar levels in patients with type 2 diabetes and hypercholesterolemia.[250,255,257,259] In addition to lowering glucose levels in this population, psyllium therapy revealed reductions in total cholesterol of 9%, LDL cholesterol of 16%, and triglycerides of 24%.[259]

Dose

Psyllium products may contain husks of *Plantago ovata* seeds or the seeds themselves, with the husks used more often. Amounts of psyllium in products are generally reported as total grams. Seed preparations contain approximately 47% soluble fiber by weight, and husk preparations generally contain 67% to 71% soluble fiber and 85% total fiber by weight.[263,264]

For hyperglycemia, 2.2 to 45 g has been used daily in divided doses for 6 to 8 weeks, often administered just before meals in experimental studies.[250,251,255-259,262]

Adverse Effects, Interactions, Pharmacokinetics. See Appendix A.

Pycnogenol (Pinus pinaster subsp. atlantica)

Grade C: *Unclear or conflicting scientific evidence (type 2 diabetes; diabetic microangiopathy)*

Note: Pycnogenol contains oligomeric proanthocyanidins (OPCs) as well as several other bioflavonoids. There has been some confusion in the U.S. market regarding OPC products containing Pycnogenol or grape seed extract (GSE) because one of the generic terms for chemical constituents ("pycnogenols") is the same as the patented trade name (Pycnogenol). Some GSE products were formerly erroneously labeled and marketed in the United States as containing "pycnogenols." Although GSE and Pycnogenol do contain similar chemical constituents, primarily in the OPC fraction, the chemical, pharmacological, and clinical literature on the two products is distinct. The term *Pycnogenol* should therefore be used only when referring to this specific proprietary pine bark extract. Scientific literature regarding this product should not be referenced as a basis for the safety or effectiveness of GSE.

Mechanism of Action

The mechanism of action of Pycnogenol in diabetes and diabetic microangiopathy is not well understood but may be related to its antioxidant effects.[265,266] Decreased retinal gamma-glutamyltransferase (GGT) activity in diabetic rats was normalized by administration of Pycnogenol alone or in combination with beta-carotene.[266] Treatment with Pycnogenol and alpha-lipoic acid alone or in combination decreased the activity of glutathione peroxidase. Elevated activity of superoxide dismutase in diabetic retina was normalized by treatment with Pycnogenol and beta-carotene in combination.

Scientific Evidence of Effectiveness

TYPE 2 DIABETES. Preliminary human data suggest that Pycnogenol as an adjunct to conventional treatment, may lower glucose levels and HbA_{1c} and may improve endothelial function in patients with type 2 diabetes.[267,268] A dose-dependent blood glucose–lowering effect has been noted.[268]

DIABETIC MICROANGIOPATHY. Preliminary human data suggest that supplementation with Pycnogenol may improve symptoms associated with diabetic microangiopathy in patients with type 2 diabetes.[269] After 4 weeks, microcirculatory and clinical evaluations showed a progressive decrease in skin flux at rest in the foot (indicating improvement in level of microangiopathy), significant decrease in capillary filtration, and significant improvement in the venoarteriolar response in all treated subjects. It was also suggested that Pycnogenol treatment may help to prevent diabetic ulcerations by controlling the level of microangiopathy.[269]

Dose

Pycnogenol at 50 to 200 mg daily for 3 to 12 weeks has been shown to decrease blood glucose and HbA_{1c} levels modestly in type 2 diabetic patients.[267,268]

For diabetic microangiopathy, 50 mg of Pycnogenol was administered three times daily for 4 weeks.[269]

Adverse Effects, Interactions, Pharmacokinetics. See Appendix A.

Red Clover *(Trifolium pratense)*

Grade C: *Unclear or conflicting scientific evidence (diabetes)*

Mechanism of Action

Red clover, like soy, is a legume and contains *phytoestrogens*, which are plant-based compounds structurally similar to estradiol. Phytoestrogens are capable of binding to estrogen receptors as an agonist or antagonist.[1] The exact mechanism of red clover isoflavones in diabetes is not well understood. In vitro studies have shown isoflavones to inhibit intestinal brush border uptake of glucose, alpha-glucosidase actions, and tyrosine kinase properties.[270-272]

Scientific Evidence of Effectiveness

Clinical research is limited on the use of red clover in diabetes; however, evidence suggests that a combination of soybean protein and isoflavones from red clover may have a positive effect on diabetes control. The available studies used different isoflavone preparations and focused on postmenopausal diabetic women alone.[273-275] Results have been inconsistent, possibly due to differences in isoflavones from different sources. One study reported a reduction in fasting insulin, and insulin resistance, HbA_{1c} using 30 g of soybean protein plus 132 mg of isoflavone,[273] while another showed no change in overall glycemic control using 50 mg of red clover isoflavone alone,[274] A soybean-based meal replacement was associated with reduced plasma glucose and HbA_{1c} at 3 and 6 months, an effect that diminished at 12 months.[275] Although both red clover and soy contain isoflavones, soy may have greater beneficial effects on diabetic parameters.

Dose

For diabetes, various isoflavone preparations have been used;[273-275] 30 g of soybean protein plus 132 mg of isoflavones resulted in a reduction in fasting insulin, insulin resistance and HbA_{1c}.[277]

Adverse Effects, Interactions, Pharmacokinetics. See Appendix A.

Red Yeast Rice *(Monascus purpureus)*

Grade C: *Unclear or conflicting scientific evidence (diabetes)*

Note: Red yeast rice is a form of the yeast *Monascus purpureus,* which is typically grown on rice and is a dietary staple in some Asian countries. *Monascus purpureus* produces several compounds collectively known as *monacolins,* substances known to inhibit cholesterol synthesis. One of these, *monacolin K,* is a potent inhibitor of hydroxymethylglutaryl coenzyme A (HMG-CoA) reductase (HMG is the liver enzyme responsible for producing cholesterol and the target of pharmaceutical intervention). This active ingredient is also known as the prescription drug lovastatin (Mevacor), approved for marketing in the United States for high cholesterol. Of note, lovastatin can cause severe muscle problems that could result in kidney damage. In 2007 the U.S. Food and Drug Administration (FDA) issued a warning to consumers to avoid red yeast rice products promoted on the Internet because these products were found to contain lovastatin. Although red yeast rice is still available in the United States, it is fermented using a different process, and the active ingredient has been removed. Its pharmacological effects are now questionable.

Mechanism of Action

The mechanism of action of red yeast rice in diabetes is not well understood, but may involve decreasing hepatic gluconeogenesis, resulting in lower plasma glucose levels.[276]

Scientific Evidence of Effectiveness

In animal studies, oral consumption of red yeast rice has been shown to decrease plasma glucose and increase plasma insulin.[277,278] Preliminary clinical evidence also suggests benefits in diabetic patients.[279] Results included a reduction in glycemia and insulinemia on an empty stomach (39.5% and 33.7%, respectively) and 20 hours after a meal (49.2% and 55.76%). Reductions in total cholesterol (27.1%) and triacylglycerol (42.3%) were also reported.

Dose

To lower glucose, two 300-mg capsules of *Monascus* extract was administered daily for 8 weeks.[279]

Adverse Effects, Interactions, Pharmacokinetics. See Appendix A.

Reishi Mushroom (Ganoderma lucidum)

Grade C: *Unclear or conflicting scientific evidence (type 2 diabetes)*

Mechanism of Action

The mechanism of action of reishi in diabetes is not well understood but may be caused by polysaccharides found in reishi products.[280]

Scientific Evidence of Effectiveness

Based on animal models of diabetes that demonstrated the hypoglycemic and lipid-lowering activities of *Ganoderma lucidum*, a clinical study was conducted to evaluate the effect of Ganopoly (reishi mushroom product) versus placebo in diabetic patients.[281] Treatment with Ganopoly slightly decreased the levels of plasma glucose and HbA_{1c} and improved other markers for diabetes. Because this research was conducted in collaboration with the manufacturer of Ganopoly, efficacy is uncertain in the absence of independent studies.

Dose

Standardization of extracts may not be clinically relevant in predicting effectiveness because the active ingredient in *G. lucidum* has not been fully determined. However, the dose of *G. lucidum* is often based on its content of polysaccharide peptide and triterpene. These doses can be extracted from spores or the whole–fruiting body preparation. The New Zealand product Ganopoly contains 600 mg of *G. lucidum* extract per capsule, with 25% (w/w) crude polysaccharides, equivalent to 30 g fruiting body of *G. lucidum*.[282]

To lower blood sugar, 1800 mg reishi mushroom extract was administered three times daily.[281]

Adverse Effects, Interactions, Pharmacokinetics. See Appendix A.

Seaweed

Grade C: *Unclear or conflicting scientific evidence (hyperglycemia, diabetes)*

Mechanism of Action

The antidiabetic mechanism of seaweed is not well understood, but may involve polysaccharide constituents such as those found in bladderwrack.[283]

Scientific Evidence of Effectiveness

Polysaccharides from bladderwrack lowered blood glucose in normoglycemic rabbits.[283,284] Effects appear to be dose dependent.[283] Clinical evidence is lacking.

Dose

Some bladderwrack products list iodine content, although there is no widely accepted standardization. The effective dose of bladderwrack for diabetes has not been determined.

Adverse Effects, Interactions, Pharmacokinetics. See Appendix A.

Soy (Glycine max)

Grade C: *Unclear or conflicting scientific evidence (type 2 diabetes)*

Mechanism of Action

Soy contains isoflavones, which are considered *phytoestrogens*, and have been used for various health conditions.[1,5] The antidiabetic mechanisms of soy isoflavones are not well understood, but they have been shown in vitro to have inhibitory effects on glucose uptake, alpha-glucosidase activity, and tyrosine kinase properties.[270,271]

Scientific Evidence of Effectiveness

There is limited clinical research using soy as a treatment for diabetes. Available studies used different isoflavone preparations and focused on postmenopausal diabetic women alone.[273-275] In one study, there was no change in overall glycemic control using 50 mg of red clover isoflavone alone.[274] Another study reported a reduction in fasting insulin, HbA_{1c}, and insulin resistance using 30 g of soybean protein plus 132 mg of isoflavone. In a study using a soybean-based meal replacement, there was a reduction in plasma glucose and HbA_{1c} at 3 and 6 months, an effect that diminished at 12 months.[275]

Dose

For diabetes, various isoflavone preparations have been used.[273-275] 30 g of soybean protein plus 132 mg of isoflavones resulted in a reduction in fasting insulin, HbA_{1c}, and insulin resistance.[273]

Adverse Effects, Interactions, Pharmacokinetics. See Appendix A.

Spirulina (Arthrospira spp.)

Grade C: Unclear or conflicting scientific evidence (diabetes)

Mechanism of Action

Hypoglycemic effect of spirulina may be caused by the downregulation of nicotinamide adenine dinucleotide phosphate-oxidase (NADPH) and nicotinamide adenine dinucleotide (NADH), which are involved in fat metabolism.[285] Enhanced activity in spirulina-treated rats suggests a greater uptake of glucose from the blood by liver cells.

Scientific Evidence of Effectiveness

In type 2 diabetic patients, oral spirulina treatment demonstrated beneficial effects on fasting blood sugar.[286,287] Patients were supplemented with 2 g of spirulina daily, one spirulina tablet (1 g) with lunch and dinner, for 2 months. The subjects were told not to change their lifestyle during this time (e.g., diet, exercise, medications). Reductions were noted in fasting blood sugar and HbA$_{1c}$ after 2 months of spirulina. With regard to lipids, the total cholesterol, LDL cholesterol, and triglycerides were lowered, and HDL cholesterol was increased.

Dose

A dose of 2 g of spirulina (Multinal), taken daily for 2 months, reduced fasting blood sugar in patients with type 2 diabetes.[286,287]

Adverse Effects, Interactions, Pharmacokinetics. See Appendix A.

Stevia (Stevia rebaudiana)

Grade B: Good scientific evidence (hyperglycemia)

Mechanism of Action

Stevia rebaudiana standardized extracts are used as natural sweeteners or dietary supplements in different countries for their content of stevioside or rebaudioside A. These compounds possess up to 250 times the sweetness intensity of sucrose and are noncaloric and noncariogenic.[288] *Stevioside*, a natural plant glycoside isolated from *S. rebaudiana*, has been commercialized as a noncaloric sweetener in Japan for more than 20 years. Stevia-based sweeteners recently gained FDA approval for use in foods and beverages.[1]

Stevia has also been shown to have beneficial effects in diabetes.[289-295] Various mechanisms have been described. Stevioside has been shown to regulate blood glucose levels by enhancing not only insulin secretion, but also insulin utilization; the latter effect has been attributed to the ability of stevia to slow down gluconeogenesis.[295] Stevioside has been found to act directly on pancreatic beta cells in vitro to secrete insulin, with actions independent of cyclic adenosine monophosphate (cAMP)– and adenosine triphosphate (ATP)–sensitive potassium channel activity.[296] Stevioside also exerts a stimulatory action on hepatic glycogen synthesis under gluconeogenic conditions. Steviol, isosteviol, and glucosilsteviol (constituents of stevia) have also been found to decrease glucose production and inhibit oxygen uptake.[279]

Scientific Evidence of Effectiveness

Stevia has been widely used for diabetes in South America, and animal studies have produced mixed results. There is some evidence that stevioside increases plasma glucose in animals.[298] Nonetheless, preliminary human studies report significant reductions in blood glucose.[289,290] Stevia has been studied in normal volunteers, and significant decreases were found in plasma glucose levels during tests and after overnight fasting.[290] Stevioside has also been shown to lower postprandial glucose levels by 18% in type 2 diabetic patients.[289]

Dose

Stevioside (1 g taken with meals) showed antihyperglycemic effects in patients with type 2 diabetes.[289] Aqueous extracts of stevia leaves (5 g) administered at 6-hour intervals for 3 days increased glucose tolerance and significantly decreased plasma glucose levels during the test and after overnight fasting in all healthy volunteers.[290]

Adverse Effects, Interactions, Pharmacokinetics. See Appendix A.

Tea (Camellia sinensis)

Grade C: Unclear or conflicting scientific evidence (diabetes)

Mechanism of Action

Antioxidant substances in tea, such as epigallocatechin gallate (EGCG) from green tea, may have beneficial effects in reducing diabetes risk by affecting insulin resistance and glucose metabolism.[299-301]

Scientific Evidence of Effectiveness

There is conflicting evidence regarding the use of tea in diabetes particularly regarding caffeine (present in both tea and coffee).[302-304] An increase in blood glucose may occur after low caffeine ingestion (200 mg).[302] Based on Finland's highest incidence of insulin dependent diabetes mellitus and high coffee consumption, a hypothesis of coffee as a trigger for insulin dependent diabetes mellitus has been proposed.[303] However, other research from Japan suggests that adults who consume 6 or more cups of green tea daily have a 33% reduced risk for developing diabetes compared with those who drink less than 1 cup per week. This effect appears to be more pronounced in women and in overweight men.[304]

Dose

The dose of tea for treating diabetes has not been determined.

Adverse Effects, Interactions, Pharmacokinetics. See Appendix A.

White Horehound (Marrubium vulgare)

Grade C: *Unclear or conflicting scientific evidence (diabetes)*

Mechanism of Action. Insufficient available evidence.

Scientific Evidence of Effectiveness
White horehound has been used traditionally in Mexico to manage diabetes mellitus. However, there is a lack of clinical evidence to support the safety or efficacy of this use. In animals, white horehound was found to decrease hyperglycemia induced in rabbits by dextrose solution compared with water and did not differ statistically in magnitude from tolbutamide.[305]

Dose
The maximum average concentration of white horehound in candy has been reported as 0.073%. Crude white horehound was formerly official in the *United States Pharmacopeia* (USP). Strengths of extracts have been expressed in terms of flavor intensities or weight-to-weight (w/w) ratios. Black horehound (*Ballota nigra*) may be found as an adulterant in compounds reported to contain only white horehound.

Adverse Effects, Interactions, Pharmacokinetics. See Appendix A.

HERBAL THERAPIES WITH NEGATIVE EVIDENCE

Garlic (Allium sativum)

Grade D: *Fair negative scientific evidence (type 2 diabetes)*
Animal studies have reported that garlic or its constituents may decrease glucose concentrations and increase insulin secretion.[306,307] However, multiple human trials have failed to demonstrate significant effects of oral garlic preparation on measures of glycemic control in diabetic or nondiabetic patients.[308,309] Trials have studied oral garlic in patients with type 2 diabetes as primary outcomes and found no significant effects. Several other trials have measured glucose levels as a secondary outcome (mainly in nondiabetic individuals) and found no significant effects, with the exception of a small yet statistically significant reduction in blood glucose (from mean of 89 mg/dL to 79 mg/dL) in a methodologically limited 4-week study.[310] Overall, it appears that garlic does not exert clinically relevant effects on glucose levels and is probably not a viable therapy for type 2 diabetes.

Safflower (Carthamus tinctorius)

Grade D: *Fair negative scientific evidence (glucose metabolism)*
Safflower oil is thought to be beneficial in diabetes, possibly because of antioxidant effects.[311-313] However, clinical studies suggest that safflower oil may actually affect glucose metabolism negatively. Fasting blood glucose increased by 11% during safflower oil supplementation compared with baseline; however, body weight, fasting serum insulin levels, and insulin sensitivity were unchanged.[314,315]

HERBAL THERAPIES WITH LIMITED EVIDENCE

African Wild Potato (Hypoxis hemerocallidea)
An aqueous extract of African wild potato was found to lower blood glucose in rats.[316] The exact mechanism is unclear; the effect may be caused by its phytosterol content.

Agrimony (Agrimonia spp.)
According to research conducted in animals agrimony may have insulin-like effects and may help to reduce symptoms of hyperglycemia.[5,317] Treatment with agrimony reduced the level of hyperglycemia in mice and was associated with reduced polydipsia, but it did not help to reduce the rate of body weight loss.[5]

Andrographis (Andrographis paniculata)
Animal studies suggest that a water extract of *Andrographis paniculata* may prevent hyperglycemia induced by oral glucose administration, probably through an effect on glucose absorption from the gut.[318] Increased glucose metabolism has also been reported with andrographis.[319] Further research is warranted.

Bilberry (Vaccinium myrtillus)
Bilberry is a traditional therapy for diabetes, often as tea made from bilberry leaves. Limited animal evidence suggests that bilberry leaf extract possesses hypoglycemic properties that may be beneficial in diabetes.[320-323] Clinical evidence is lacking.

Juniper (Juniperus communis)
An orally administered decoction of juniper showed significant hypoglycemic activity in normal rats after single doses. The effects may be attributed to an increase in peripheral absorption of glucose, independent of plasma insulin levels.[324]

Sage (Salvia officinalis)
Sage is among many plants with purported benefits in diabetes.[325-327] Animal research suggests that the effects of sage resemble those of metformin, an inhibitor of gluconeogenisis.[327] Sage may be useful for the prevention and treatment of type 2 diabetes, but more research is warranted.

ADJUNCT THERAPIES

1. The damaging effects of hyperglycemia are separated into *macrovascular* complications (coronary artery disease, peripheral arterial disease, stroke) and *microvascular* complications (diabetic nephropathy, neuropathy, retinopathy). Treatment goals focus on reducing symptoms of hyperglycemia and reducing these related complications. Keeping blood sugar levels close to normal most of the time can dramatically reduce the risk of these complications. Adjunct natural products and integrative therapies may also provide benefit.

2. Chronic high blood sugar levels may damage sensitive blood vessels in the eye, resulting in *diabetic retinopathy*, a disease of the small blood vessels in the retina. Preliminary research using oligomeric proanthocyanidins (the purported active ingredient in grape seed) and the brand-name product Endotelon has shown beneficial effects in stopping disease progression.[328] Preliminary evidence also suggests puerarin injections may reduce blood viscosity, improve microcirculation, and play a beneficial role in diabetic retinopathy.

3. *Diabetic nephropathy* causes kidney damage and is another complication of diabetes caused by uncontrolled

Herbs with Potential Hypoglycemic or Hyperglycemic Properties*

HERB	SPECIFIC THERAPEUTIC USE(S)†	HERB	SPECIFIC THERAPEUTIC USE(S)†
Abuta	Diabetes	Chia	Diabetes
Acacia	Diabetes	Chicory	Diabetes
Acerola	Diabetes	Chlorella	Diabetes, diabetic microangiopathy
Aconite	Diabetes		
Agave	Diabetes	Clove	Diabetes
Agrimony	Diabetes	Codonopsis	Diabetes
Algin	Diabetes	Coleus	Diabetes
Alpinia	Diabetes	Cordyceps	Diabetes
Andiroba	Diabetes	Couch grass	Diabetes
Annatto	Diabetes, hyperglycemia	Cowhage	Diabetes
Arnica	Diabetes	Damiana	Diabetes
Asparagus	Diabetes	Danshen	Diabetes
Astaxanthin	Diabetes	Devil's claw	Diabetes
Bael fruit	Diabetes	Dogwood	Diabetes, diabetic microangiopathy
Bamboo	Diabetes		
Barberry	Diabetes	Dong quai	Diabetes
Barley	Diabetes	Elder	Diabetes
Bay leaf	Diabetes	Elecampane	Diabetes
Betony	Hyperglycemia	Essiac	Diabetes
Bitter orange	Diabetes	Eucalyptus	Diabetes
Buchu	Diabetes	Euphorbia	Diabetes
Bugleweed	Hyperglycemia	Fo-ti	Diabetes
Bupleurum	Diabetes	Garcinia	Diabetes
Cajeput oil	Diabetes	Germanium	Diabetes
Calamus	Diabetes	Ginger	Hypoglycemia
Capers	Diabetes	Ginkgo	Diabetes
Carob	Diabetes	Goji	Diabetes, hyperglycemia
Carqueja	Diabetes	Goldenrod	Diabetes
Carrot	Diabetes	Goldenseal	Diabetes, hypoglycemia
Cat's claw	Diabetes	Grape seed	Diabetes
Chamomile	Hypoglycemia	Grapefruit	Diabetes
Chaparral	Diabetes	Greater celandine	Diabetes

Continued

Herbs with Potential Hypoglycemic or Hyperglycemic Properties—cont'd

HERB	SPECIFIC THERAPEUTIC USE(S)†	HERB	SPECIFIC THERAPEUTIC USE(S)†
Guggul	Diabetes	Neem	Diabetes
Hawthorn	Diabetes insipidus, diabetes mellitus	Noni	Diabetes
		Perilla	Diabetes
Hops	Diabetes	Rehmannia	Diabetes (type 2)
Horsetail	Diabetes	Rhodiola	Diabetes
Hydrangea	Hyperglycemia	Rose hip	Diabetes
Hydrazine sulfate	Impaired glucose tolerance	Rosemary	Hyperglycemia
Hyssop	Diabetes (type 1)	Sarsaparilla	Diabetes
Jequirity	Diabetes	Saw palmetto	Diabetes
Jiaogulan	Diabetes	Shiitake muskroom	Diabetes
Juniper	Hypoglycemia	Stinging nettle	Diabetes
Katuka	Diabetes	Tamarind	Diabetes
Ladies mantle	Diabetes	Turmeric	Diabetes, hyperglycemia
Lavender	Diabetes	Uva ursi	Diabetes
Lemongrass	Diabetes	Wheatgrass	Diabetes
Licorice	Diabetes	White oak	Diabetes
Mangosteen	Diabetes	Wild yam	Hypoglycemia
Meadowsweet	Diabetes	Willow	Diabetes
Morus nigra	Diabetes	Yarrow	Diabetes
Mugwort	Diabetes		

*This is not an all-inclusive or comprehensive list of agents that may affect serum glucose. A qualified health care provider should be consulted with specific questions or concerns regarding potential effects on blood sugar levels or interactions.
†Based on expert opinion, anecdote, case reports, and/or preliminary trial evidence.

high blood sugar. Herbs used in *traditional Chinese medicine* (TCM) and *acupuncture* may augment conventional Western medicine for better outcomes in diabetic nephropathy.

4. *Diabetic neuropathy*, or nerve damage, is another complication of diabetes that occurs when excess blood sugar levels injure the walls of capillaries that nourish the nerves, especially in the legs. A few clinical trials have administered gamma-linolenic acid (GLA) to diabetic patients with neuropathy symptoms.[101,102] Results suggest that GLA may be a viable treatment. Ginkgo may also be an option for diabetic retinopathy based on its antioxidant effects.[329]

5. Diabetes can also dramatically increase the risk of various cardiovascular problems, including coronary artery disease with angina, myocardial infarction, stroke, atherosclerosis, and hypertension. According to the American Heart Association, approximately 75% of diabetic individuals die of some type of heart or blood vessel disease. *Diabetic microangiopathy* is the damage to small blood vessels caused by high blood sugar levels. Microangiopathy causes the walls of capillaries to become so thick and weak that they bleed, leak protein, and slow the flow of blood. Diabetic patients may develop microangiopathy in many areas, including the eyes, feet, legs, and kidneys. Preliminary studies have suggested beneficial effects of the total triterpenoid fraction of gotu kola *(Centella asiatica)* (TTFCA) on subjective and objective parameters of venous insufficiency of the lower extremities. Supplementation with Pycnogenol may also improve symptoms associated with diabetic microangiopathy.

6. Lipid abnormalities are frequently associated with diabetes, as are complications of atherosclerotic disease. Therefore, defining the connection between lipids and diabetes may elucidate ways to reduce the morbidity and mortality of this disease. Beta-glucan, beta-sitosterol, niacin, omega-3 fatty acids, policosanol, psyllium, and soy all have strong scientific evidence to support their use in lipid abnormalities.

7. *Psychotherapy* may be useful as an adjunct to blood sugar control in adolescents and adults with poorly controlled type 1 diabetes, especially if blood sugar problems are related to depression. Also, cognitive behavioral therapy may reduce depression and improve blood sugar level control in patients with type 2 diabetes. Therapy may be less effective in people with diabetes complications or poorly controlled blood sugar levels.

8. Certain supplements may also provide benefit to patients with diabetes. *Chromium* has been studied for sugar abnormalities in patients with types 1 and 2 diabetes, as

well as at-risk populations. Some studies suggest that oral chromium may lower blood sugar levels, whereas other studies show no effects. Some research reports that chromium may improve symptoms of hypoglycemia.

INTEGRATIVE CARE PLAN

- Appropriate care of patients with diabetes mellitus involves setting goals for blood sugar, blood pressure, and lipid levels; monitoring for complications; dietary and exercise modifications; self-monitoring of blood glucose; and laboratory assessment.
- Blood sugar levels should be checked frequently, at least before meals and at bedtime. Even if the individual takes insulin and adheres to a rigid diet the amount of sugar in the blood can change unpredictably. Careful monitoring is the only way to make sure that the blood sugar level remains within the target range, usually 90 to 130 mg/dL before meals and less than 180 mg/dL after meals. A daily blood sugar logbook or diary may be valuable to see how the individual is responding to medications, diet, and exercise in the treatment of their diabetes.
- The glycosylated hemoglobin (HbA_{1c}) test should be performed every 3 months for insulin-treated patients, during treatment changes, or when blood glucose is elevated. For stable patients taking oral agents, health care professionals recommended testing HbA_{1c} at least twice yearly. The American Diabetes Association (ADA) currently recommends an HbA_{1c} goal of less than 7.0%. Studies have reported that there is a 10% decrease in relative risk of microvascular complications (e.g., diabetic nephropathy or neuropathy) for every 1% reduction in HbA_{1c}.
- Treatment goals for lipids include LDL cholesterol less than 100 mg/dL, triglycerides less than 150 mg/dL, and HDL cholesterol greater than 45 mg/dL for men and greater than 55 mg/dL for women.
- Treatment goals for blood pressure include levels less than 130/85 mm Hg.
- Trials evaluating natural products for diabetes have used a diversity of preparations, dosing regimens, and outcome measures. Good scientific evidence supports the use of beta-glucan, gymnema, and stevia for glycemic control. These agents have been mostly studied in type 2 diabetic patients. Beneficial results have been reported with gymnema in type 1 diabetes.
- Teach patients the diabetes ABCs: A_{1c} (blood glucose), B (blood pressure), and C (cholesterol). The goal A_{1c} is less than 7%; blood pressure for diabetic patients should be less than 130/80 mm Hg; and LDL cholesterol should be less than 100 mg/dL and HDL cholesterol greater than 45 mg/dL.
- Counsel the patient regarding healthy lifestyle choices, including diet and exercise. These healthy choices will help to improve glycemic control and prevent or minimize complications of diabetes.
- Recommend that the patient follow a low-fat diet enriched with fresh fruits, vegetables, and whole grains. Refined carbohydrates (sugars and white flour) and hydrogenated oils should be eliminated from the patient's diet.
- Thirty minutes of moderate physical activity for 5 or more days is recommended to all patients with diabetes.[330]
- Inform patients that alcohol consumption should be limited to no more than one drink per day for women, two per day for men, and none if there is difficulty controlling alcohol intake (addiction) or blood sugar levels.
- Promote smoking cessation to patients who smoke. Smoking cigarettes or use of any other form of tobacco raises the risks for developing complications from diabetes, such as heart attack, stroke, nerve damage, and kidney disease. Smoking damages blood vessels and contributes to heart disease, stroke, and poor circulation in the limbs. Smokers who have diabetes are three times more likely to die of cardiovascular disease than nonsmokers who have diabetes, according to the ADA.
- Inform the patient that regular health checkups are important. Regular diabetes checkups are not meant to replace yearly physical or routine eye examinations. Physicians will look for any diabetes-related complications, such as neuropathy, as well as screen for other medical problems. An eye specialist will check for signs of retinal damage, cataracts, and glaucoma. Annual foot exams should be performed on all patients with diabetes.
- Advise the patient to check the feet every day for blisters, cuts, sores, redness, or swelling. A physician should be contacted if a sore or other foot problem does not heal within a few days.
- Recommend that the patient brush the teeth at least twice daily, floss the teeth once a day, and schedule dental examinations at least twice a year.

Case Studies

CASE STUDY 18-1

UM is a 65-year-old male patient with a 14-year history of type 2 diabetes. Current diabetes medications include metformin (1000 mg twice daily) and pioglitazone (30 mg once daily). Average SMBG value is about 200 mg/dL. His most recent HbA_{1c} measurement was 8.0%, up from 6.8% 6 months ago. His fasting total cholesterol was 240 mg/dL, LDL 166 mg/dL and HDL 35 mg/dL. He does not follow any specific diet and does not exercise besides walking his dog. Although height and weight are not available for UM, visual inspection reveals he is overweight with abdominal obesity and a high waist circumference. UM was diagnosed with benign prostatic hyperplasia (BPH) 2 years ago, for which he takes tamsulosin (0.8 mg daily). At that time, he also started taking saw palmetto. UM states his prostate problem has dramatically improved since starting tamsulosin and saw palmetto. However, since he started using the herb at the same time as the prescription drug, he is uncertain whether one or both are responsible for the improvement. He also regularly takes *Ginkgo biloba* to improve his memory. He expresses concern about his poor blood sugar control and asks whether there are natural remedies for type 2 diabetes. How do you advise him?

Answer: It appears that UM has metabolic syndrome, as evidenced by elevated glucose levels, abdominal obesity, high LDL cholesterol, and low HDL cholesterol. Lifestyle change is key in the management of metabolic syndrome. UM should follow a low-fat diet enriched with fresh fruits, vegetables, and whole grains. Refined carbohydrates (sugars and white flour) and hydrogenated oils should be eliminated. He should also engage in 30 minutes of moderate physical activity for 5 or more days per week. Beta-glucan may be a reasonable choice for UM to help reduce cholesterol levels and improve blood sugar control. It is a soluble fiber typically used for its cholesterol-lowering effects but also used for diabetes. Beta-glucan may be added as a part of a healthy diet and appears to be well tolerated. Recommend that UM take his other medications 2 hours before or 2 hours after beta-glucan. Blood sugar levels should be checked more frequently when initiating beta-glucan. Notably, ginkgo may also reduce blood sugar levels. With the saw palmetto, UM is successfully treating his BPH, so this regimen currently does not need to be altered.

CASE STUDY 18-2

MM is a 42-year-old accountant who seeks advice regarding natural remedies because of frequent high blood sugar readings on self-monitoring. Four years ago, MM was diagnosed with type 2 diabetes after 6 months of polyuria, blurred vision, and weight loss. He lost 30 pounds, from 218 to 188 pounds (height: 5 feet, 9 inches). He was treated with oral metformin (1000 mg twice daily), and his blood sugar values improved. In the past year, however, he has been stressed during tax season and has regained 20 pounds. MM eats three meals daily and occasionally has a snack or two throughout the day. He consulted a dietician, who counseled him regarding an ADA diet; however, MM admits not using it consistently. His HbA_{1c} was 8.8% 1 month ago; his weight is 210 pounds. MM also has hypertension, treated with enalapril (10 mg every morning), and hypercholesterolemia, treated with atorvastatin (10 mg every evening). His blood pressure reading is 130/80 mm Hg, and his most recent lipid panel reveals a marginally elevated LDL cholesterol level. According to his most recent blood pressure reading and lipid panel, both are controlled. MM said he also started taking valerian and chamomile to help relieve stress. He asks you if there is an herbal product he can try to help reduce his glucose levels. How do you advise him?

Answer: Currently, MM's blood sugar is not well controlled based on an elevated HbA_{1c}. Gymnema may be a reasonable herbal product for MM. Evidence suggests that gymnema may reduce blood glucose levels when used with other diabetes agents. It may also help to lower MM's slightly elevated LDL cholesterol level. Interactions among gymnema, chamomile, and valerian are not well understood. MM should monitor his blood sugar levels when adding any agent to his current regimen.

MM should be counseled regarding the importance of a healthy diet that includes fiber, low saturated fat, and low refined sugars. Thirty minutes of physical exercise a day should also be recommended. The stress MM experiences during tax season may also lead to blood sugar regulation problems.

CASE STUDY 18-3

NS is a 55-year-old woman with a 7-year history of type 2 diabetes. She currently takes 5 mg of glyburide once daily. She performs SMBG; her fasting glucose values range from 100 to 115 mg/dL, with postprandial values of 130 to 150 mg/dL. At her regular follow-up examination 3 months ago, her HbA_{1c} was 5.8%. NS is also overweight and has high cholesterol. She is 5 feet, 5 inches tall and weighs 150 pounds (same as last visit). This indicates a body mass index (BMI, kg/m²) of 25 (BMI >25 considered overweight, BMI >30 considered obese). NS follows a low-fat diet that is high in fruits and vegetables. She rarely eats meat. NS has maintained a walking program since she was first diagnosed with type 2 diabetes and has recently increased her walking distance from 2 miles to 3 miles a day. Most recent cholesterol levels (recorded 6 months ago) are total 188 mg/dL, LDL 98 mg/dL, HDL 60 mg/dL, and triglycerides 145 mg/dL. She takes Lipitor (40 mg at bedtime) and a garlic supplement every morning. NS has no known drug allergies.

During your consultation with NS as a clinical pharmacist in the diabetes clinic, she expresses concern about a funny taste in her mouth and feeling unusually sluggish after her evening walk. When asked, NS replies she is taking her medication as prescribed. You then ask her if she is taking any dietary supplements in addition to garlic. NS indicates she started taking gymnema 2 weeks earlier. How should you advise and counsel?

Answer: NS is currently meeting her diabetes and cholesterol goals. No medication changes were made during this visit. However, she is concerned about the funny taste in her mouth and unusual sluggishness after her evening walk. After additional questions, you learn that NS generally performs SMBG before meals but does not tend to measure blood glucose after dinner or after her walk. You suggest that NS's evening sluggishness may result from hypoglycemia or low blood sugar, which may be caused by both her exercise and the addition of gymnema. There is good scientific evidence for the effect of gymnema used as adjunctive therapy in type 2 diabetes. Gymnema tends to be well tolerated and has few drug interactions. However, gymnema may cause an alteration in taste and is known as a "sugar destroyer." Gymnema may also add to the effects of her current hypoglycemic and cholesterol-lowering drugs.

NS should be counseled on the dangers of hypoglycemia and the importance of performing SMBG during or after her evening walk to prevent hypoglycemia. She should also carry a ready source of glucose in case her blood glucose levels drop to a dangerous range. Sources of easily absorbed glucose include sugar candies, 4 fluid ounces of orange juice, and Glucotabs. If her unusual sluggishness continues, NS should be urged to return to the clinic for follow-up.

Good scientific evidence supports the effect of garlic in the treatment of high cholesterol. However, the evidence for the effect of garlic on type 2 diabetes is fairly negative. In addition, garlic may cause bad breath and may be contributing to NS's altered taste.

In summary, NS's dietary supplement use may be contributing to her altered taste (gymnema and garlic) and unusual sluggishness (gymnema). NS should be counseled on the effects and side effects of gymnema and garlic as well as the tendency to develop tolerance with continued use. Nevertheless, if the altered taste becomes intolerable, NS may choose to discontinue one agent at a time, on consultation with her primary care provider or pharmacist.

References for Chapter 18 can be found on the Evolve website at http://evolve.elsevier.com/Ulbricht/herbalpharmacotherapy/

Review Questions

1. Which of the following constituents of bitter melon has been found to possess hypoglycemic properties?
   a. Polypeptide P
   b. Balsambirne
   c. Charantin
   d. Both a and c

2. True or false: Preliminary human evidence suggests that garlic may be efficacious for the management of serum glucose levels in type 1 and type 2 diabetes, as an adjunct to conventional drug therapy, for up to 20 months.

3. Which of the following agents is used as a natural sweetener?
   a. Stevia
   b. Gymnema
   c. Gotu kola
   d. Myrcia

4. Which of the following triterpenoids is found in gotu kola and appears to be responsible for its beneficial effects in diabetic microangiopathy?
   a. Asiatic acid
   b. Madecassic acid
   c. Asiaticoside
   d. All the above

5. Patients with lupus should avoid which of the following?
   a. Ashwagandha
   b. Aloe
   c. Alfalfa
   d. Astragalus

6. What constituent of dandelion may contribute to its hypoglycemic activity?
   a. Glycogen
   b. Inulin
   c. Rutin
   d. Tannins

7. Which of the following may be caused by chronic ingestion of devil's club?
   a. Headache
   b. Impotence
   c. Seizures
   d. Weight gain

8. True or false: The broiled stems of nopal (*Opuntia* spp.) seem to be beneficial in lowering blood glucose levels and decreasing HbA_{1c} levels.

9. Bladderwrack should be used cautiously in patients taking which of the following medications?
   a. Propylthiouracil
   b. Lithium
   c. Warfarin
   d. All the above

10. Puerarin, which has shown promise in the treatment of diabetic retinopathy, is derived from which plant?
    a. Ginseng
    b. Kudzu
    c. Maitake mushroom
    d. Milk thistle

Answers are found in the Answers to Review Questions section in the back of the text.

19 Pituitary and Thyroid Disorders

Outline

OVERVIEW
  Pituitary Disorders
    Growth Hormone Disorders
    Thyroid-Stimulating Hormone Disorders
    Adrenocorticotropic Hormone and Corticotropin-Releasing Hormone Disorders
    Antidiuretic Hormone Disorders
    Prolactin Disorders
    Luteinizing Hormone and Follicle-Stimulating Hormone Disorders
    Diagnosis
  Thyroid and Parathyroid Disorders
    Hyperthyroidism
    Hypothyroidism
    Thyroid Nodules
    Thyroid Tumors and Thyroid Cancer
    Hyperparathyroidism
    Hypoparathyroidism
    Diagnosis
SELECTED HERBAL THERAPIES
  Chasteberry *(Vitex agnus-castus)*
  Rehmannia *(Rehmannia glutinosa)*
  Seaweed
HERBAL THERAPIES WITH LIMITED EVIDENCE
ADJUNCT THERAPIES
INTEGRATIVE THERAPY PLAN
CASE STUDIES
REVIEW QUESTIONS

Learning Objectives

- Know the herbs that affect pituitary, thyroid, and parathyroid hormone levels.
- Describe how herbal agents may affect the levels of pituitary, thyroid, and parathyroid hormones in the blood, and how they affect laboratory evaluation of these hormones.
- Counsel a patient regarding herbs that affect pituitary, thyroid, and parathyroid disorders.

OVERVIEW[1-4]

Pituitary Disorders

The pituitary gland, also called the *hypophysis,* is a pea-sized gland located at the base of the brain. It is just one of many glands involved in the endocrine system. The pituitary gland is often called the "master" gland because it produces and secretes hormones that regulate the functions of many other endocrine glands (Figures 19-1 and 19-2). Because of this, patients with pituitary disorders may experience a disruption in many different body functions.

The pituitary gland is composed of three sections: anterior lobe, intermediate lobe, and posterior lobe. The anterior lobe produces *growth hormone* (GH), *prolactin, corticotropin* (also called adrenocorticotropin or *adrenocorticotropic hormone* [ACTH]), *thyroid-stimulating hormone* (TSH), *follicle-stimulating hormone* (FSH), and *luteinizing hormone* (LH). GH regulates bone and tissue growth and helps maintain a healthy balance between muscle and fat tissue. Prolactin stimulates milk production in women after they give birth. Corticotropin stimulates the adrenal glands to produce corticosteroids such as *cortisol* and androgens such as *dehydroepiandrosterone* (DHEA). TSH, also called *thyrotropin,* signals the thyroid gland to secrete *triiodothyronine* (T_3) and *thyroxine* (T_4), hormones that regulate the body's metabolism. Although T_4 is the major product released from the thyroid, T_3 is the active form. FSH signals sperm production in men and egg development and ovulation in women. LH regulates testosterone production in men and estrogen production in women.

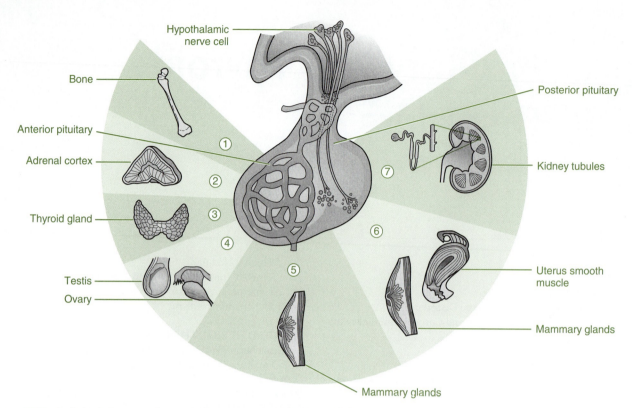

Figure 19-1 The hypothalamus and pituitary hormones. (Modified from Thibodeau GA, Patton KT: *Anatomy and physiology*, ed 5, St Louis, 2003, Mosby.)

The intermediate pituitary lobe produces *melanocyte-stimulating hormone* (MSH), which controls skin pigmentation. The posterior lobe produces *antidiuretic hormone* (ADH), also known as *vasopressin* and arginine vasopressin (AVP), which helps control urine production and manages the water balance in the body. ADH also produces *oxytocin,* which allows the uterus to contract during childbirth and stimulates milk production during breastfeeding.

Pituitary disorders may be inherited, but most cases are acquired. They may be caused by tumors within or near the pituitary gland, severe hemorrhage that decreases blood supply to the pituitary, chronic inflammation, or infection. Pituitary disorders most often result from the development of a noncancerous (benign) tumor, called *pituitary adenoma*. The tumors may result in hormone overproduction and serious endocrine disturbances. They may also press against optic nerves and lead to visual disturbances and headaches.

Growth Hormone Disorders

Deficiency of GH results in short stature in children. When GH disorders occur in adulthood, after full height has been reached, other effects are observed, including increased fat mass and decreased lean body mass, decreased bone mineral density, and worsening of cardiac function.

Excess GH during childhood or adolescence, before the bones have fully matured, is called *gigantism*. Children with gigantism show rapidly increased height disproportionate with normal age-related changes. In adults, excess GH does not affect height because the bones have already ceased to grow in length. Instead, a condition called *acromegaly* develops, which causes the bones to thicken. As a result, the hands, feet, and jaw are enlarged, and surrounding structures may become compressed. Other complications of acromegaly include type 2 diabetes, hypertension, arthritis, enlarged heart muscle (cardiomegaly), enlarged tongue (macroglossia), thickened skin, colon polyps, carpal tunnel syndrome, sleep apnea, uterine fibroids, and vision abnormalities. Although acromegaly can result from excess GH production by the pituitary, it can also be secondary to a tumor in the *hypothalamus*, another structure in the brain. The hypothalamus secretes GH-releasing hormone (GHRH) on the pituitary to increase the production and release of GH into the bloodstream.[1-4]

Thyroid-Stimulating Hormone Disorders[1-3,5]

Deficient TSH production by the pituitary gland results in a lack of thyroid hormone production, or *hypothyroidism*. Symptoms associated with hypothyroidism include weight gain, fatigue, menstrual irregularities, intolerance of cold climates, decreased mental function, depression, and changes in the texture of skin and hair. Excess TSH results in overactive thyroid hormone production, or *hyperthyroidism*. Symptoms of hyperthyroidism include elevated energy levels, palpitations, excessive sweating, intolerance of warm climates, increased appetite, weight loss, menstrual irregularities, tremors, and anxiety.

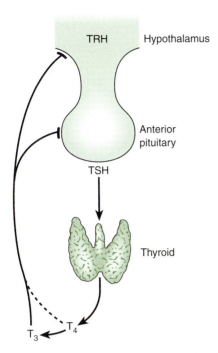

Figure 19-2 An endocrine axis and negative feedback. The axis shown is the hypothalamo-pituitary-thyroid axis. Thyrotropin releasing hormone (TRH), from the hypothalamus, stimulates the release of thyroid stimulating hormone (TSH) from the anterior pituitary. The TSH stimulates the thyroid gland to release T_4 and T_3, which exert a negative feedback inhibitory effect on the hypothalamus and pituitary glands. (From Hinson J, Raven P, Chew SL: *The endocrine system: systems of the body series*. Edinburgh, 2007, Churchill Livingstone.)

Graves' disease is characterized by hyperthyroidism. Some patients may experience Graves' ophthalmopathy, in which the eyeballs protrude from the sockets, and which may lead to dry, red, and swollen eyes; excessive tearing or eye discomfort; photosensitivity; blurry or distorted vision; and limited eye movement.

Adrenocorticotropic Hormone and Corticotropin-Releasing Hormone Disorders

When the pituitary gland produces insufficient corticotropin-releasing hormone (CRH), the adrenal glands are not stimulated. As a result, there is a deficiency in adrenal hormone production, called *secondary adrenal insufficiency*. Symptoms are predominantly caused by a lack of glucocorticoid hormones (e.g., cortisol) and include weakness, fatigue, muscle pain (myalgia), joint pain (arthralgia), and hypoglycemia.

Excess production of corticotropin, also known as adrenocorticotropic hormone (ACTH, results in *Cushing's syndrome*) also called hyperadrenocorticism or hypercortisolism. This condition is caused by hyperstimulation of the adrenal gland. A form of Cushing's syndrome called *Cushing's disease* is caused by a benign pituitary tumor that induces excessive ACTH secretion, which in turn stimulates the adrenal glands to produce more cortisol. Cushing's disease occurs five times more often in women than in men, and it is the most common form of endogenous Cushing's syndrome.[1-3] In rare cases, Cushing's syndrome may be caused by tumors in organs that do not normally produce ACTH, which subsequently may begin to secrete high levels of ACTH. This condition is called *ectopic ACTH syndrome*. These tumors, which can be benign or malignant, are most often found in the lung, thyroid, pancreas, or thymus gland. Lung tumors cause over half of all ectopic ACTH syndrome cases.

Excess cortisol causes various physical abnormalities, such as "buffalo hump" or a "fatty" hump between the shoulders, a rounded or "moon" face, and stretch marks on the skin. Other manifestations include hypertension, hyperglycemia, decreased lean body mass, increased fat mass, decreased bone mineral density, thinning of the skin, and menstrual irregularities in women. Because ACTH also controls the release of androgens from the adrenal gland, women with Cushing's disease may show male-pattern hair growth (hirsutism), increased acne, and increased libido.[1-4]

Antidiuretic Hormone Disorders

Antidiuretic hormone acts on the kidneys to increase water retention. Decreased ADH production results in excessive loss of fluid in the urine. Patients with low ADH may have *diabetes insipidus,* characterized by high urine output (polyuria) despite decreased water intake. Symptoms may also include excessive thirst (polydypsia).

Excess production of ADH is called the *syndrome of inappropriate antidiuretic hormone secretion* (SIADH). Low sodium levels in the blood, from too much water retention, cause symptoms in patients with SIADH. Patients may have central nervous system (CNS) symptoms such as headache, blurred vision, disorientation, and agitation. They may also experience nausea, vomiting, and muscle cramps. SIADH can occur with CNS infections or head trauma, for unknown reasons.[1-4]

Prolactin Disorders

Prolactin deficiency is a rare disorder resulting from partial or generalized anterior pituitary failure. Patients are usually asymptomatic unless they are breastfeeding because prolactin deficiency leads to decreased milk production.

Excess prolactin results in abnormal menstrual cycles and infertility in premenopausal women. It has also been linked to infertility in males. Patients may also have abnormal increases in breast fluid production (galactorrhea). Postmenopausal females are generally asymptomatic. Men with hyperprolactinemia experience decreased libido, impotence, infertility, and increased breast tissue (gynecomastia). Rarely, men also experience galactorrhea.

Luteinizing Hormone and Follicle-Stimulating Hormone Disorders[1-4]

Also referred to as *gonadotropins,* LH and FSH are responsible for stimulating the gonads in male testes and in female ovaries. These hormones are essential for reproduction but not for life.

Deficiencies in LH and FSH usually occur together because they are secreted by the same cell population. Low LH and FSH levels may result in infertility, lack of secondary sexual characteristics (e.g., breast development, pubic hair), amenorrhea (lack of menstrual bleeding), or irregular menstrual cycles.

Excessive production of LH and FSH usually reflects negative steroid feedback and results from gonadal failure or pituitary tumors. People with elevated gonadotropin levels are generally asymptomatic.

Diagnosis

To diagnose pituitary disorders, the levels of pituitary hormones, as well as hormones that stimulate the pituitary gland, are evaluated. Laboratory tests measure prolactin, LH, FSH, TSH, thyroxine (T_4), human chorionic gonadotropin (hCG, to detect pregnancy), corticotropin (ACTH), cortisol, glucose, GH, and insulin-like growth factor-1 (IGF-1). Other, nonlaboratory tests that may be ordered include computed tomography (CT), magnetic resonance imaging (MRI), and water deprivation tests to diagnose diabetes insipidus.[1-4]

Thyroid and Parathyroid Disorders[1,3,5]

The thyroid gland is one of the larger glands in the body (~2 in or 5 cm in length) and is located in the front of the neck below the larynx. It consists of two lobes, one on each side of the trachea (windpipe). The lobes are connected by the thyroid isthmus, which consists of follicular and parafollicular cells. The thyroid needs *iodine* to produce hormones. Follicular cells secrete the iodine-containing hormones thyroxine (T_4) and triiodothyronine (T_3), which stimulate all body tissues to produce proteins and increase the amount of oxygen used by cells. Thyroid hormones are also produced in response to thyroid-stimulating hormone (TSH, thyrotropin) secreted by the pituitary gland. Parafollicular cells secrete the hormone *calcitonin*, which works along with *parathyroid hormone* (PTH, parathormone) to regulate calcium levels in the body. The pituitary gland produces TSH, which controls synthesis of T_3 and T_4. The thyroid cells combine iodine and the amino acid *tyrosine* to make the thyroid hormones.

The parathyroid glands are four small glands located adjacent to the thyroid gland lobes in the neck. They produce PTH, the most important endocrine regulator of calcium. PTH stimulates the mobilization of calcium from bone, enhances absorption of food and calcium from the small intestines, and suppresses calcium loss in urine.

Thyroid disorders affect about 4.5 million Americans, with an estimated 600,000 yet to be diagnosed. Although thyroid disorders can affect anyone, women are about five times more likely to develop thyroid disorders than men.

Hyperthyroidism

Hyperthyroidism occurs when the thyroid gland produces excessive T_4. Several conditions may lead to hyperthyroidism, including a toxic diffuse goiter *(Graves' disease)*, toxic adenoma, toxic multinodular goiter *(Plummer's disease)*, painful subacute thyroiditis (inflamed thyroid gland), silent thyroiditis (includes lymphocytic and postpartum variations), iodine-induced hyperthyroidism (related to amiodarone therapy), excessive pituitary TSH or trophoblastic disease, and excessive ingestion of thyroid hormonal agents.

Signs and Symptoms

Signs and symptoms of hyperthyroidism may include nervousness, irritability, palpitations, tachycardia, heat intolerance or increased sweating, tremors, weight loss or gain, alterations in appetite, frequent bowel movements or diarrhea, dependent lower-extremity edema, sudden paralysis, exertional intolerance and dyspnea, menstrual disturbances (decreased flow), infertility, mental disturbances, sleep disturbances (insomnia), changes in vision, photophobia, eye irritation, diplopia, exophthalmos, fatigue, muscle weakness, thyroid enlargement, and pretibial myxedema (in Graves' disease).

Hypothyroidism

Hypothyroidism occurs when the thyroid gland does not produce enough thyroid hormone. *Hashimoto's thyroiditis* is the most common cause of hypothyroidism in the United States; it is an *autoimmune disorder* that attacks the thyroid gland, resulting in low levels of thyroid hormone. Many factors are involved in this disorder, including age, heredity, and gender. Hashimoto's thyroiditis is most common among middle-aged women and is often found among biological family members. A less common type of hypothyroidism is *de Quervain's thyroiditis*, in which the thyroid gland swells rapidly and is very painful and tender.

Hypothyroidism may also occur if the individual does not consume enough iodine in the diet. Iodine is an essential element that helps the thyroid gland produce hormones. Inadequate iodine consumption is most common in countries where malnutrition is also common.

Goiter is hypertrophy of the thyroid gland that is typical in hypothyroidism; the gland enlarges as it tries to make more thyroid hormone in the absence of iodine. Goiter may also occur as a result of hyperthyroidism. Although goiters generally do not cause pain, a large goiter may interfere with swallowing or breathing and may affect the individual's appearance and self-esteem. Goiters are more common in women and older adults. The most common cause of goiter is a lack of iodine in the diet in areas where the soil is deficient in iodine. However goiters may occur in both hyperthyroid and hypothyroid patients. In many cases, goiters are cured once hormone replacement therapy is started. However, some individuals may need to have their goiter surgically removed.

Signs and Symptoms

Common symptoms of hypothyroidism include sensitivity to cold temperatures, weight gain, fatigue, constipation, small thyroid gland or goiter, dry skin, hair loss, muscle cramps, heavy and irregular menstruation, and difficulty thinking or concentrating. Less common symptoms include facial swelling and joint stiffness.

Thyroid Nodules

Thyroid nodules are lumps that usually arise within an otherwise normal thyroid gland. Often, these abnormal growths of thyroid tissue are located at the edge of the thyroid gland, so they can be felt as a lump in the throat. If they are large or occur in very thin individuals, they may even be seen as a lump in the front of the neck. One in 12 to 15 young women and 1 in 40 young men has a thyroid nodule. More than 95% of all thyroid nodules are benign. Some nodules are actually cysts filled with fluid rather than thyroid tissue. The incidence of thyroid nodules increases with age; at least one thyroid nodule will occur in 50% of 50-year-olds, 60% of 60-year-olds, and 70% of 70-year-olds. Individuals with nodules of the thyroid gland may have normal thyroid function.

Signs and Symptoms

Thyroid nodules are generally asymptomatic. They may produce a visible or palpable mass in the neck. If they become extremely large, thyroid nodules may compress adjacent structures, such as the larynx or nearby vessels and nerves, although this is rare. Laryngeal obstruction may cause difficulty in swallowing and breathing. Compression of vessels or nerves results in numbness or tingling of the face, head, or neck.

Thyroid Tumors and Thyroid Cancer

Many types of tumors can develop in the thyroid gland. Most of these tumors are benign. Anyone can develop cancer of the thyroid gland, but certain factors may increase the risk, including gender (women are three times more likely than men), low-iodine diets, exposure to radiation (e.g., treatment for acne), family history (e.g., parent with medullary thyroid cancer), inherited conditions (e.g., Gardner's syndrome), race (e.g., white), age (20-60), and reproductive history (women who were pregnant at age 30 or later).

Signs and Symptoms

Thyroid tumors usually do not produce symptoms other than a mass in the neck. As with thyroid nodules, tumors may grow large enough to compress adjacent structures and produce difficult breathing, numbness, and tingling. Some tumors may secrete excessive amounts of thyroid hormone, resulting in hyperthyroidism.

Hyperparathyroidism

The parathyroid glands are small organs located on the thyroid. Most people have four parathyroid glands, but some may have more or less. The parathyroid glands regulate serum calcium and phosphorus levels through PTH secretion. PTH acts directly on bone cells called *osteoclasts*, which function to break down bone (a process called *resorption*). PTH thus stimulates the release of calcium from the bones, which in turn raises serum calcium and lowers serum phosphorus concentration. The regulation of PTH secretion occurs through a negative feedback loop in which calcium-sensing receptors on the membranes of parathyroid cells trigger decreased PTH production as serum calcium concentrations increase.

Primary hyperparathyroidism, which accounts for most cases of hyperparathyroidism, results from excessive release of PTH and manifests as *hypercalcemia* (high blood levels of calcium). In 80% of patients with hyperparathyroidism, the symptoms of hypercalcemia are mild or absent. Both hypercalcemia and hypocalcemia are associated with *end-stage renal disease* (ESRD), also known as chronic kidney failure or chronic renal failure.

Signs and Symptoms

Many patients with hyperparathyroidism are asymptomatic and are diagnosed based on abnormally high calcium levels on routine laboratory screening. When symptoms do occur, they may include malaise, bone pain, abdominal pain, headache, heartburn, kidney stones, and psychiatric symptoms, including depression, anxiety, irritability, and memory problems. Additional symptoms may include thinning hair, decreased libido, stomach ulcers, hypertension, and palpitations. As calcium levels increase in the bloodstream, the bones may lose calcium, placing patients at increased risk for fractures.

Hypoparathyroidism

Hypoparathyroidism is the secretion of insufficient PTH. The symptoms of hypoparathyroidism are the same as for *hypocalcemia* (low blood calcium level). Symptoms range from mild tingling in the hands/fingers and around the mouth, to more severe forms of muscle cramping that lead to *tetany* (strong muscular spasms) and rarely convulsions.

Signs and Symptoms

Hypoparathyroidism results in low serum calcium levels, and the person may be asymptomatic. When symptoms occur, they usually include tingling or numbness of the lips, fingers, and toes; muscle cramps; and abdominal pain. Other symptoms include dry hair and nails, weakened fingernails, and painful menstruation. Very low calcium levels may produce convulsions or tetany, which can result in death if the larynx is involved.

Diagnosis

Thyroid Disorders

Various tests and procedures are used to diagnose thyroid disorders, including blood and imaging studies.

Thyroid disorders are diagnosed based on blood tests for thyroid hormones (TSH, T_3, T_4). Low T_3 and T_4 levels in combination with high TSH levels generally lead to a diagnosis of hypothyroidism. High T_3 and T_4 levels combined with low TSH levels usually indicate hyperthyroidism.

If an autoimmune disease is suspected as causing hypothyroidism or hyperthyroidism, the patient's serum is tested for abnormal antibodies called *autoantibodies*. The autoantibodies bind to components of an individual's cells and cause the immune system to attack the body. In Graves' disease, patients usually have the *thyrotropin receptor–stimulating antibody* (TRS-Ab). *Antinuclear antibodies* (ANAs) may be detected in patients with Graves' disease or autoimmune hypothyroidism.

A nuclear scan/radioactive iodine uptake (RAI-U) may be ordered to look for thyroid gland abnormalities and to evaluate thyroid function in different areas of the thyroid. Thyroid ultrasound may be performed to evaluate nodules, lumps, or enlargement of the gland. It can also help determine whether a nodule is a fluid-filled cyst or a solid tissue mass. A biopsy may be performed to determine the cause of a thyroid nodule or a goiter.

Parathyroid Disorders

To diagnose parathyroid disorders, blood levels of PTH and calcium are measured. Normal PTH level is 10 to 55 picograms per milliliter (pg/mL), and normal serum calcium is 8.5 to 10.2 milligrams per deciliter (mg/dL). Abnormally low levels of PTH are indicative of hypoparathyroidism, whereas high levels indicate hyperparathyroidism. In both cases, serum calcium levels may be either higher or lower than normal values.

SELECTED HERBAL THERAPIES

Note
To help make this educational resource more interactive, all pharmacokinetics, adverse effects, and interactions data have been compiled in Appendix A. Safety data specifically related to pregnancy and lactation are listed in Appendix B. Please refer to these appendices when working through the case studies and answering the review questions.

Chasteberry *(Vitex agnus-castus)*

Grade B: *Good scientific evidence (Hyperprolactinemia)*

Mechanism of Action

In vitro, constituents in chasteberry bind selectively to estrogen receptor beta.[6-8] The flavonoid *apigenin* has been identified as an active phytoestrogen in chasteberry. It has been debated whether chasteberry alters the secretion of FSH or LH. Most clinical trials have found that levels remain unaffected.[9,10] The reported effects of chasteberry on prolactin levels in humans are variable and not well characterized. In vitro and animal studies report that constituents of chasteberry bind to dopamine-2 receptors in the pituitary, thereby inhibiting prolactin secretion.[9,11] Haloperidol (Haldol), a dopamine agonist, was able to counteract the prolactin-lowering effect of chasteberry.[12] Animal study suggests that chasteberry possesses antiandrogenic effects.[13] A flavonoid-rich fraction of chasteberry administered to male dogs resulted in disruption of the latter stages of spermatogenesis. Reduced androgen production was reflected in low levels of sialic acid in the testes.

Scientific Evidence of Effectiveness

Several controlled trials and preclinical studies report that chasteberry inhibited prolactin secretion.[9-12,14] Doses of 480 mg produced a 10% drop in prolactin.[15]

Three months of therapy with supplementation standardized to 10 mg of chasteberry reduced prolactin release in response to thyrotropin-releasing hormone (TRH)–normalized luteal phase and eliminated deficits in progesterone synthesis.[16] Long-term use of chasteberry has not been systematically investigated.

Dose

Although there is no universal standardization for chasteberry products, many extracts are standardized to contain 0.5% agnuside or 0.6% aucubin and may be standardized to casticin content.

For hyperprolactinemia, standard dosing recommendations are currently lacking. Studies have used Strotan capsules (each standardized to 20 mg of chasteberry), one capsule daily in women for 3 months.[16] In men, doses of 40 to 160 mg of a chasteberry extract up to three times daily for 6 weeks has been used.[15]

Adverse Effects, Interactions, Pharmacokinetics. See Appendix A.

Rehmannia *(Rehmannia glutinosa)*

Grade C: *Unclear or conflicting scientific evidence (Hypopituitarism; Sheehan's syndrome)*

Mechanism of Action

A study in hyperthyroid rats compared the effects of T_4 and traditional Chinese medicine (TCM) herbs (*Ophiopogon japonicus, Pseudostellaria heterophylla,* and *Rehmannia glutinosa*).[17] The results suggest that these herbs may have an effect in lowering receptor affinity and the peripheral conversion of T_4 to T_3. In another study evaluating the effects on *Rehmannia glutinosa* on hyperthyroid rats, rehmannia significantly reduced the binding capacity of the beta-adrenergic receptors of kidney in rats ($p < 0.01$).[18]

Scientific Evidence of Effectiveness

In a case series conducted to evaluate the effects of *R. glutinosa* in the treatment of Sheehan's syndrome (postpartum hypopituitarism), subjects showed marked improvement in clinical symptoms after 2 to 5 months of treatment.[19]

Dose

A preparation of rehmannia standardized to contain 1% glutannic acid per dose has been used. The crude or dried root or steamed root of *R. glutinosa* showed different pharmacological activities, and the quality of rehmannia root preparations may vary with concentration changes in its constituents.[20]

For Sheehan's syndrome, 90 g of cleaned and finely chopped *R. glutinosa* root, added to 900 mL of water and boiled down to 200 mL, has been used three times daily with an intermission of 3, 6, and 14 days. After a cessation period of 1 month, daily doses of 45 to 50 g of *R. glutinosa* in 5-day courses, with an intermission of 5 days each time, for 2 to 5 months were then used in the second treatment phase.[19]

Adverse Effects, Interactions, Pharmacokinetics. See Appendix A.

Seaweed

Grade B: *Good scientific evidence (goiter/thyroid disease)*

Mechanism of Action

Kelp or bladderwrack products have been used traditionally for thyroid diseases. The high iodine content of these products may be effective in preventing hypothyroidism and goiter; however, trace amounts of iodine (such as the levels found in iodized salt) are generally sufficient for this purpose. In human case reports, transient hyperthyroidism resulted from bladderwrack ingestion.[21,22] Bladderwrack products contain up to 600 micrograms per gram (mcg/g) of iodine, whereas normal human iodine intake is 100 to 200 mcg daily. Individuals ingesting bladderwrack or kelp products as food or supplements may exceed the maximum recommended daily dose of iodine (about 1 mg); chronic iodine toxicity may result in hypothyroidism, hyperthyroidism, goiter, or myxedema, although many individuals continue to have normal thyroid function.[23] In terms of iodine content, there is no widely accepted standardization of iodine content in bladderwrack, although some products may list iodine content on the label.

Scientific Evidence of Effectiveness

Bladderwrack contains variable levels of iodine, up to 600 mcg/g. There have been case reports of hyperthyroidism resulting from sea kelp ingestion,[21,22] but systematic studies of dosing, safety, or efficacy are currently lacking. There is no widely accepted standardization of iodine content for these products. Although evidence suggests thyroid activity, there are inadequate studies to strongly support this use of bladderwrack.

Dose

Some bladderwrack products list iodine content, although there is no widely accepted standard at this time.

The dose of seaweed for thyroid disease has not been determined.

Adverse Effects, Interactions, Pharmacokinetics. See Appendix A.

HERBAL THERAPIES WITH LIMITED EVIDENCE

Aconite (Aconitum napellus)

Radix aconiti praeparata, or prepared aconite root, is a Chinese herbal therapy shown to decrease T_3 levels in animal models.[24] There is a current lack of clinical evidence of efficacy in treating thyroid disease.

Cassia (Cortex cinnamomi)

Cortex cinnamomi is a Chinese herbal therapy that has been shown to decrease T_3 levels in animals.[24] There is a current lack of clinical evidence of efficacy in treating thyroid disease.

Maca (Lepidium meyenii)

Traditionally, maca has been used in Peru to enhance fertility and to boost sexual desire. However, according to clinical study in healthy men, maca (1.5 and 3 g) had no effect on reproductive hormone levels, including LH, FSH, prolactin, 17α-hydroxyprogesterone, testosterone, and 17β-estradiol.[25]

Herbs with Potential Pituitary and/or Thyroid Gland Effects*

HERB	SPECIFIC THERAPEUTIC USE(S)†
Astragalus	Hyperthyroidism
Babassu	Hyperthyroidism
Bael fruit	Thyroid disorders
Bamboo	Hyperthyroidism
Blue flag	Goiter
Bugleweed	Graves' disease, hyperthyroidism, thyroid disorders
Cinnamon	Hyperthyroidism
Codonopsis	Thyroid disorders
Coleus	Hypothyroidism
Comfrey	Thyroid disorders
Cowhage	Hyperprolactinemia
Essiac	Thyroid disorders
Fenugreek	Hyperthyroidism
Ginseng	Endocrine disorders
Horny goat weed	Thyroid disorders
Horsetail	Hypothyroidism, thyroiditis
Lemon balm	Graves' disease
Myrcia	Goiter, hyperthyroidism
Rhodiola	Thyroid disorders
Stinging nettle	Goiter
Watercress	Goiter

*This is not an all-inclusive or comprehensive list of herbs with potential pituitary and/or thyroid effects; other herbs and supplements may possess these qualities. A qualified health care provider should be consulted with specific questions or concerns regarding potential effects of agents or interactions.
†Based on expert opinion, anecdote, case reports, and/or preliminary trial evidence.

ADJUNCT THERAPIES

1. *Calcium* is the most abundant mineral in the body and is responsible for many cellular functions, as well as maintenance of bone health. In patients with hypoparathyroidism, calcium supplementation may be beneficial.[26]
2. Some individuals may develop secondary hyperparathyroidism from low vitamin D levels; initial treatment is vitamin D.[27] For patients with primary or refractory hyperparathyroidism, health care professionals usually recommend surgical removal of the parathyroid glands. Postoperative hypoparathyroidism, though rare, may develop after this procedure.[28] High doses of dihydrotachysterol, calcitriol, or ergocalciferol taken orally can assist in increasing serum calcium concentrations in patients with hypoparathyroidism or pseudohypoparathyroidism. Vitamin D is also found in numerous dietary sources, such as fish, eggs, fortified milk, and cod liver oil. The sun is also a significant contributor to the body's daily production of vitamin D, and 10 minutes of exposure may be sufficient to prevent deficiencies.[1]
3. *Gamma oryzanol* is a mixture of ferulic acid esters of sterol and triterpene alcohols; it is found in rice bran oil at a level of 1% to 2% and has been extracted from corn and barley oils as well.[29] Preliminary evidence indicates that gamma oryzanol affects several parts of the endocrine system and may reduce TSH level in patients with hypothyroidism.[30] More studies are needed in this and other areas of endocrinology to establish these effects. Gamma oryzanol has been shown to inhibit platelet aggregation in animals fed high-cholesterol diets;[31] it may increase bleeding in some individuals, particularly those taking blood-thinning medications, such as aspirin and warfarin (Coumadin).
4. *Iodine* is an element that is required by humans for the synthesis of thyroid hormones (triiodothyronine and thyroxine). Iodine deficiency is one of the causes of goiter and generally occurs in individuals with poor diets, usually in the developing world. Iodine supplementation is warranted in cases of proven iodine deficiency.[32] Only trace levels of iodine (such as those supplied by iodized salt) are generally sufficient to prevent iodine deficiency.
5. *L-Arginine* helps maintain the body's fluid balance, resulting in normalization of serum urea and creatinine levels. Arginine also aids in wound healing, hair growth, spermatogenesis, vasodilation, and infection. Intravenous arginine can be used to evaluate growth hormone reserve in people with suspected GH deficiencies. One study showed that IV arginine increased serum GH levels in acromegaly patients treated with corticosteroids.[33] More research is needed to clarify the effect of long-term arginine supplementation in patients with GH deficiency.
6. *L-Carnitine,* also known as acetyl-L-carnitine or carnitine, plays a role in energy metabolism. In hyperthyroidism, carnitine may be depleted from the body. Supplementing with L-carnitine may be beneficial in reversing and preventing symptoms of this disorder by inhibiting thyroid hormone entry into the nucleus fibroblasts, hepatocytes, and neurons.[34]
7. *Selenium* is a trace mineral found in soil, water, and some foods, such as brewer's yeast, wheat germ, butter, garlic, grains, sunflower seeds, Brazil nuts, walnuts, raisins, liver, kidney, shellfish (lobster, oyster, shrimp, scallops), and freshwater and saltwater fish (red snapper, salmon, swordfish, tuna, mackerel, halibut, flounder, herring, smelts). Selenium is also found in alfalfa, burdock root, catnip, fennel seed, ginseng, raspberry leaf, radish, horseradish, onion, chives, medicinal mushrooms (reishi, shiitake), and yarrow. In patients with autoimmune thyroiditis, such as Hashimoto's thyroiditis, selenium supplementation decreased the concentration of thyroid peroxidase autoantibodies.[35] Selenium may be beneficial in areas of the world where the population has mild iodine deficiency.

INTEGRATIVE THERAPY PLAN

- Interview patient to determine the presence of symptoms associated with a specific pituitary, thyroid, or parathyroid hormone disorder. Pituitary diseases may involve multiple hormones and therefore may cause a wide array of symptoms. Patients may also complain of nonspecific symptoms associated with a pituitary mass, such as visual changes and headache.
- Physical examination may reveal signs of excess or deficient hormones. A thorough evaluation by a physician is required of all patients suspected of having endocrine disorders.
- Based on the patient's signs and symptoms, appropriate laboratory tests are ordered, including blood tests to determine levels of the hormone in question. Skull or thyroid radiography and provocative tests are designed to elicit certain laboratory findings associated with a disorder.
- Thyroid disorders may require nuclear medicine testing or thyroid biopsy if a tumor is suspected. If an autoimmune disease is suspected, laboratory evaluation of specific antibodies should be performed.
- Parathyroid disorders are diagnosed based on blood tests of PTH and calcium levels.
- Pituitary deficiency that causes clinical symptoms is treated with hormone replacement. Hypersecretion of pituitary hormones may be treated with medications or surgery. Pituitary tumors may require surgical removal if they are growing in size, compressing adjacent structures, or not responding to medical treatment.
- Thyroid disorders may be treated with hormone replacement (for deficiency) or medical/radioactive ablation of the thyroid (for excess). Benign tumors may require no treatment or may be removed if they are causing symptoms.
- No herbal or alternative therapy currently available has been shown to be effective in the treatment of pituitary, thyroid,

or parathyroid disorders. Physicians should ask their patients if they are taking any herbs or supplements, because some agents may affect endocrine function or laboratory test results.

- Iodine deficiency is the most common cause of hypothyroidism worldwide, although it is uncommon in the United States. Iodine is found in seawater and thus in foods from the sea, particularly seaweed (e.g., kelp, bladderwrack, dulce). Although it comes from the ocean, sea salt is not a good source of iodine. Iodized salt may be the most common source of iodine in the Western diet and can generally provide enough iodine to prevent iodine deficiency. An adult requires only about 1 tsp of iodine over a lifetime, so eating fish once a week fulfills the average iodine requirement. The value of dietary iodine can be reduced by cruciferous vegetables from the Brassica family, which includes cabbage, Brussels sprouts, raw turnip, broccoli, and cauliflower. In circumstances in which large quantities of these foods are eaten and dietary iodine levels are low, goiter could develop.

Case Studies

CASE STUDY 19-1

CS is a 42-year-old woman who comes to you with questions regarding herbal supplements. She was recently diagnosed with mild prolactinemia. CS has undergone a complete workup, including brain MRI, and no abnormalities were noted. Her physician recommends prolactin level monitoring but no other therapy. CS mentions that her menses are somewhat irregular and her sex drive has decreased. She is interested in a hormonal remedy to resolve her prolactinemia. CS reports a history of schizophrenia, which is well controlled with risperidone (Risperdal). She also takes soy extract to prevent osteoporosis.

Answer: Antipsychotic therapy is capable of elevating prolactin levels. Mild prolactinemia is frequently treated with observation only. Bromocriptine (Parlodel) is often used to lower prolactin levels in patients who develop symptomatic disease, such as infertility or galactorrhea. If CS's only symptom is an elevated prolactin level, medical or herbal treatment is merely treating a laboratory test and not a symptomatic disease. However, her irregular menses and decreased libido may be caused by hyperprolactinemia.

Chasteberry *(Vitex agnus-castus)* has been shown to lower prolactin levels. Furthermore, the herb appears to be generally well tolerated, with few significant side effects. A 3-month course of chasteberry accompanied by prolactin monitoring could be instituted. However, CS should be warned of potential interactions with her current medications. Chasteberry has dopaminergic effects and may inhibit the effects of risperidone on her schizophrenia symptoms. If CS decides to initiate chasteberry supplementation, she should be carefully monitored by her physician for exacerbation of schizophrenia. Chasteberry also increases plasma levels of estrogen, which may negate the effects of soy supplementation.

CASE STUDY 19-2

MT is a 35-year-old woman who comes to the pharmacy and tells you she has been trying to get pregnant for the past year. She is in good health except for occasional blood pressure elevation, as noted inconsistently at the medical office. A friend told MT that she took maca for 2 months and promptly became pregnant. MT currently takes St. John's wort for depression, dandelion for her blood pressure, and licorice for gastritis. How do you consult?

Answer: Human studies have failed to demonstrate that maca *(hepidium meyenii)* induces changes in LH, FSH, prolactin, testosterone, or estradiol. In addition, maca has been reported to cause hypertension in some patients. MT's inability to achieve a pregnancy for 1 year may indicate an underlying fertility problem; therefore, she should visit a gynecologist and a fertility specialist.

MT is also taking *St. John's wort,* which has been reported to cause hypertension; she should be warned of this potential effect. St. John's wort has also been associated with anorgasmia, or the inability to achieve an orgasm during sexual activities, which may exacerbate MT's infertility problems.

Dandelion has been shown to increase the expression of estrogen, progesterone, and FSH receptors and decrease the level of serum androgens. The effect of dandelion on fertility is unknown; it may alter laboratory evaluation of estrogens and androgens.

Licorice has been reported to cause high levels of prolactin and estrogen in women, which may lead to infertility. MT should be counseled to discuss each of these herbs with her physician before a workup for infertility, because they may interfere with testing or may exacerbate the underlying problem.

CASE STUDY 19-3

RG is a 42-year-old man recently diagnosed with mild hypothyroidism who comes to you for advice. His family practitioner recommended thyroid replacement with levothyroxine (Synthroid). RG states that he is generally distrustful of hormones and has heard that bladderwrack can cure his hypothyroidism. He currently takes policosanol and licorice for heart disease. How do you counsel this patient?

Answer: Although rare in the United States, hypothyroidism may be caused by iodine deficiency. Bladderwrack *(Fucus vesiculosus)*, with its high iodine content, is excessive for iodine deficiency. Ingestion of iodine-containing foods such as iodized salt, sea vegetables, dairy products, strawberries, and seafood (to varying degrees) is generally sufficient. Because value of dietary iodine can be reduced by cruciferous vegetables from the Brassica family (cabbage, Brussels sprouts, raw turnip, broccoli, cauliflower), large quantities of these foods should be avoided if the levels of dietary iodine are low. RG should be reassured that levothyroxine is an appropriate therapy for his condition and that this replacement hormone is common and generally very safe; the only significant danger is excess intake, and RG could develop hyperthyroidism. Before instituting thyroid therapy, RG should undergo a thorough endocrine workup to detect any medical problems contributing to or causing his hypothyroidism.

RG should also be warned of the potentially additive antiplatelet effects of bladderwrack combined with policosanol. He should also be counseled that licorice may interfere with the absorption of some drugs. He should take any other medications several hours before or after taking licorice. Notably, licorice may cause increased blood pressure; caution is warranted because RG has a history of heart disease.

References for Chapter 19 can be found on the Evolve website at http://evolve.elsevier.com/Ulbricht/herbalpharmacotherapy/

Review Questions

1. Which of the following best describes apigenin, a constituent of chasteberry?
   a. It is a soluble fiber.
   b. It is an insoluble fiber.
   c. It is a phytoestrogen.
   d. It is a potent CNS stimulant.

2. Which of the following is true regarding chasteberry?
   a. It may be standardized to agnuside, aucubin, or casticin content.
   b. It is only standardized to agnuside or aucubin.
   c. It has not shown any effect in the treatment of hyperprolactinemia.
   d. All the above are true.

3. Which of the following adverse effects is *not* known to occur with maca ingestion?
   a. Stomach pain
   b. Urticaria
   c. Flatulence
   d. Leukocytosis

4. Which of the following best describes maca?
   a. It has been used in traditional medicine to enhance fertility and libido.
   b. It has been shown to increase levels of luteinizing hormone (LH).
   c. It has been shown to increase testosterone levels.
   d. It has been shown to inhibit follicle-stimulating hormone (FSH).

5. Rehmannia preparations have been standardized to what percentage of glutannic acid content?
   a. 0.1%
   b. 0.3%
   c. 1%
   d. 3%

6. True or false: Rehmannia may increase the toxicity of aminoglycosides if administered concomitantly.

7. Bladderwrack has been associated with which of the following adverse events?
   a. Heavy metal poisoning
   b. Anticoagulant effects
   c. a and b
   d. None of the above

8. Which of the following conditions has been traditionally treated with bladderwrack?
   a. Hyperthyroidism
   b. Hypothyroidism
   c. Goiter
   d. Gout

9. Which of the following herbs has clinical evidence supporting its use for treating Sheehan's Syndrome, also known as postpartum hypopituitarism?
   a. Chasteberry *(Vitex agnus-castus)*
   b. Cassia bark *(Cortex cinnamomi)*
   c. Maca *(Lepidium meyenii)*
   d. Rehmannia *(Rehmannia glutinosa)*

Answers are found in the Answers to Review Questions section in the back of the text.

20 Obesity

Outline

OVERVIEW
  Signs and Symptoms
  Diagnosis
SELECTED HERBAL THERAPIES
  Bitter Orange (*Citrus aurantium*)
  Capsicum (*Capsicum* spp.)
  Cinnamon (*Cinnamomum* spp.)
  Coleus (*Coleus forskohlii*)
  Damiana (*Turnera diffusa*)
  Ephedra (*Ephedra sinica*)
  Evening Primrose (*Oenothera biennis*)
  Garcinia (*Garcinia cambogia*)
  Ginger (*Zingiber officinale*)
  Guarana (*Paullinia cupana*)
  Guggul (*Commiphora mukul*)
  Licorice (*Glycyrrhiza glabra*)
  Psyllium (*Plantago* spp.)
  Rhubarb (*Rheum* spp.)
  Soy (*Glycine max*)
  Spirulina (*Arthrospira platensis*)
  Tea (*Camellia sinensis*)
HERBAL THERAPIES WITH NEGATIVE EVIDENCE
HERBAL THERAPIES WITH LIMITED EVIDENCE
ADJUNCT THERAPIES
INTEGRATIVE THERAPY PLAN
CASE STUDIES
REVIEW QUESTIONS

Learning Objectives

- Define obesity, morbid obesity, abdominal obesity, body mass index (BMI), and metabolic syndrome (syndrome X).
- Identify natural products used for obesity and understand their mechanism for weight management.
- Recognize dose, side effects, and interactions of natural products used for obesity.
- Assess and counsel a patient for integrative therapy treatment.
- Identify and implement clinical monitoring to assess for tolerance of natural products and weight loss outcomes.

OVERVIEW

Obesity is typically defined as 20% to 30% above normal body weight for a person of a certain age, gender, and height.[1] *Morbid obesity* (also called "clinically severe obesity") is defined as 50% to 100% above normal body weight. If more than 100 lb (45 kg) above ideal weight, an individual may also be classified as "morbidly obese."

Many factors, including an individual's age, gender, and height, are considered when determining whether a person is overweight. Normally, people gain weight until they are fully grown. Women gain about 16 lb (7.2 kg) between ages 25 and 54. In contrast, men tend to gain about 10 lb (4.5 kg) between ages 25 and 45. The body weights of both men and women tend to decline after age 55. Women are more likely to become obese than men because they typically have more body fat and less muscle mass than men. Furthermore, women burn fewer calories at rest than men.

Obesity is a chronic condition that may persist for many years. Researchers believe that numerous factors contribute to obesity, including poor diet, overeating, decreased physical activity, pregnancy, medications, medical conditions, genetics, gender, and age.[1] Calorie intake and physical activity are major determinants of body weight. Basal metabolism (which controls the rate at which the body breaks down, stores, and uses food for energy) also plays a role in regulating body weight. Metabolism can be altered by physical activity or by stimulating the sympathetic nervous system with drugs such as caffeine. To a certain degree, diet may also influence metabolism. For example, dietary fats are easier for the body to convert and store than carbohydrates and proteins, so a diet high in fats may lead to weight gain.

Food intake is largely controlled by appetite, which in turn is controlled by hormones such as *cholecystokinin*, *leptin*, and *ghrelin*. An increase or decrease in the activity of these hormones, depending on their effects, may lead to increased appetite or overeating. Obesity can have serious long-term effects on health. Individuals who are overweight are at an increased risk of developing many life-threatening illnesses, including heart disease, high blood pressure, stroke, diabetes, osteoporosis, and cancer.[2] Approximately 280,000 adult deaths are attributed to obesity each year in the United States,[3] where obesity is considered an epidemic. More than half of all Americans are considered overweight, and almost 33% are considered obese.[4] According to the American Heart Association (AHA), 140 million Americans were considered overweight or obese in 2005.[5] About 20% of children are currently overweight, so the number of obese adults will likely continue to increase.

Signs and Symptoms

Besides having excess body fat and body weight, obese individuals may have shortness of breath, difficulty walking, and may become easily tired. Conditions often associated with obesity include hypercholesterolemia, diabetes mellitus (type 2 and gestational), and hypertension.[2] These increased risk factors, along with insulin resistance, are among the factors that define *metabolic syndrome* (or syndrome X). Because excess weight places more stress on the joints, obesity is also commonly associated with osteoarthritis, joint pain, and limited mobility. Other symptoms include sleep apnea, gallstones, stress incontinence, polycystic ovarian syndrome, and depression.

Diagnosis

Health care professionals often use the *body mass index* (BMI, kg/m²) to determine if a person is obese. The BMI may be calculated as weight in kilograms divided by height in meters squared (kg/m²), or as weight in pounds divided by height in inches squared, multiplied by 703 ([lb/in²] × 703).[6] Individuals with a BMI between 25 and 29.9 are considered overweight, and those with a BMI of 30 and above are obese.[2] There are three classes of obesity: class I (BMI 30-34.9), class II (BMI 35-39.9), and class III (BMI ≥40). Table 20-1 lists the standard weight categories associated with BMI ranges for adults.

Although BMI is considered to be the standard by which obesity is measured, it has its limitations. First, BMI only considers weight and height, which do not always correlate with body fat. Second, BMI ranges are not necessarily accurate for children or teenagers, because the BMI ranges are based on adult measures. Third, BMI does not take into account frame size. Athletes and bodybuilders may have skewed results because of lower body fat and heavier muscle mass.

Central obesity, or *abdominal obesity,* is excess fat in the trunk or abdomen and a specific risk factor for cardiovascular and other diseases. Abdominal obesity is independent of general obesity and may affect individuals of normal weight or BMI. Clinicians may use the waist circumference as a measure of abdominal obesity. Men with waist circumferences greater than 40 inches (102 cm) and women with waist circumferences greater than 35 inches (88 cm) are defined as "abdominally obese." However, waist circumference thresholds are not reliable for patients with a BMI greater than 35.[6]

SELECTED HERBAL THERAPIES

Note

To help make this educational resource more interactive, all pharmacokinetics, adverse effects, and interactions data have been compiled in Appendix A. Safety data specifically related to pregnancy and lactation are listed in Appendix B. Please refer to these appendices when working through the case studies and answering the review questions.

Bitter Orange *(Citrus aurantium)*

Grade C: *Unclear or conflicting scientific evidence (weight loss)*

Mechanism of Action

Bitter orange extract comes from the *Citrus aurantium* plant. Products containing bitter orange typically have the active ingredients synephrine alkaloids and para-octopamine.[7-10] Similar to those found in ephedra, *C. aurantium* alkaloids have adrenergic agonist effects and are often incorporated into supplements claimed to aid in weight loss.[11] Para-synephrine, often called simply *synephrine* or *oxedrine,* is thought to be the primary ingredient in *C. aurantium* that promotes weight loss. It has been shown to be an alpha-adrenergic agonist[12] that may also have beta-adrenergic properties.[13] *C. aurantium* has also been reported to aid in weight loss by increasing thermogenesis, especially in women.[14]

Scientific Evidence of Effectiveness

Since the U.S. Food and Drug Administration (FDA) banned the sale of ephedrine-containing dietary supplements, some products previously containing ephedrine have been reformulated to include *Citrus aurantium*. It is marketed to be a "safe" alternative to ephedra.

A systematic review identified one randomized controlled trial (RCT) that assessed a bitter orange preparation for weight loss.[15] One study reported that subjects who received

TABLE 20-1	Body Mass Index (BMI) and Weight Categories
BMI	WEIGHT STATUS
<18.5	Underweight
18.5-24.9	Normal
25.0-29.9	Overweight
≥30.0	Obese

From Centers for Disease Control and Prevention. www.cdc.gov.

a combination of *C. aurantium*, caffeine, and St John's wort in correlation with strict diet and exercise regimen lost significant amounts of body fat (average fat loss of 3.1 kg).[16] Those in the placebo and control groups, who followed the same diet and exercise regimen, did not show significant fat loss. However, intergroup analysis did not reveal statistical significance between the weight changes in the three groups.

At present, *C. aurantium* may be the best thermogenic substitute for ephedra. However, more studies are needed to establish efficacy as well as safety. Because bitter orange has not been studied as monotherapy, it is difficult to determine if the effects were caused by bitter orange or the combination therapy.

Dose

Bitter orange extract has been standardized to 4% to 6% synephrine for thermogenic action.[17] A dose of 975 mg of bitter orange extract in combination with 900 mg of St. John's wort and 528 mg of caffeine daily for 6 weeks has been reported to promote weight loss.[16] All subjects followed an exercise and diet program.

Adverse Effects, Interactions, Pharmacokinetics. See Appendix A.

Capsicum (*Capsicum* spp.)

Capsaicin is the major component that imparts pungency to chili peppers and other fruits of the genus *Capsicum*. The capsaicin content in *Capsicum* ranges from 37.6 to 497.0 mg/100 g in ripe fruits and 27.8 to 404.5 mg/100 g in green fruit.[18] Topical capsaicin is widely used for pain relief. It acts as an agonist for the receptors of the transient receptor potential vanilloid subfamily member 1 (TRPV1) type, and by saturating pain receptors it may reduce sensations of pain and burning. TRPV1 also appears to play a role in regulating body weight.[19] Numerous animal studies have revealed a role for capsaicin, capsaicin analogues, and TRPV1 in body weight regulation.[20-25] Capsaicin-induced thermogenesis is likely mediated by beta-adrenergic stimulation.[26]

Several clinical studies have demonstrated weight loss when capsaicin is administered with other thermogenic agents (such as green tea) and/or stimulants (such as caffeine), suggesting possible synergistic effects. Capsaicin supplementation was shown to stimulate energy metabolism in men during aerobic exercise[27] and after meals.[28] Similar effects have also been demonstrated with capsinoids (capsaicin analogues with low pungency). In a randomized controlled trial, capsinoid intake was correlated with increased energy expenditure and fat oxidation, particularly in subjects with high BMI (≥25).[29] However, in another study, an acute capsaicin dose stimulated a thermogenic response in women of normal weight but not in obese women.[30] This suggested that resistance to physiological stimulants may be a factor in obesity. After modest weight loss, capsaicin treatment was also shown clinically to sustain fat oxidation during weight maintenance, but did not affect 3-month weight regain.[31] Taken together, the clinical evidence suggests that capsaicin may be effective in increasing energy expenditure, an effect that may be altered by other physiological factors. The effect of capsaicin supplementation on long-term weight loss remains unclear.

Cinnamon (*Cinnamomum* spp.)

Grade C: *Unclear or conflicting scientific evidence (increase lean body mass)*

Mechanism of Action

In vitro evidence shows that cinnamon may modulate energy utilization in adipocytes by stimulating glucose uptake and glycogen synthesis.[32-34] Doubly linked polyphenol type A polymers are thought to be the bioactive component.[35]

Scientific Evidence of Effectiveness

Preliminary clinical research found that a daily dose of 500 mg of a specific aqueous extract of cinnamon (Cinnulin PF) improved body composition in patients with prediabetes and metabolic syndrome.[35] Subjects maintained their normal diets and levels of physical activity.

Dose

To increase lean body mass, 500 mg daily of a specific aqueous extract of cinnamon (Cinnulin PF) has been used; this dose is equivalent to approximately 10 g of whole-cinnamon powder (20:1 extract) and contains at least 1% doubly linked polyphenol type A polymers. Subjects were advised to take two capsules (250 mg) twice daily (with breakfast and dinner) for 12 weeks.[35]

Adverse Effects, Interactions, Pharmacokinetics. See Appendix A.

Coleus (*Coleus forskohlii*)

Grade C: *Unclear or conflicting scientific evidence (increase lean body mass)*

Mechanism of Action

Forskolin, isolated from plants of the genus *Coleus*, is thought to aid in weight management by stimulating the cellular production of cyclic adenosine monophosphate (cAMP), an important component in energy production and utilization; this was demonstrated in animals.[36,37] In humans, forskolin was also shown to stimulate the production of hormone-sensitive lipase, a key enzyme involved in the mobilization of fatty acids from adipose tissues.[38]

Scientific Evidence of Effectiveness

In clinical studies, forskolin decreased body fat percentage and fat mass compared with placebo treatment.[38,39] Men taking coleus showed a significant 11% decrease in body fat percentage, an almost 6% increase in lean mass, and a 17% increase in total testosterone.[38] *Coleus forskohlii* supplementation has also been shown to help prevent weight gain, particularly in women.[40]

Dose

A dose of 250 mg of 10% standardized forskolin extract has been taken twice daily by mouth for 12 weeks to promote weight loss and prevent weight gain.[38-40]

Adverse Effects, Interactions, Pharmacokinetics. See Appendix A.

Damiana *(Turnera diffusa)*

Grade C: *Unclear or conflicting scientific evidence (weight loss in obese patients)*

Mechanism of Action

Although damiana is promoted as a stimulant, its mechanism of action is not well understood.[7]

Scientific Evidence of Effectiveness

Damiana, a plant that grows in the Americas and Africa, has been widely used in traditional medicine for cough, diuresis, and as an aphrodisiac. A preparation called "YGD" is frequently used for weight loss, and contains yerba mate (leaves of *Ilex paraguayensis*), guarana (seeds of *Paullinia cupana*), and damiana (leaves of *Turnera diffusa* var. *aphrodisiaca*). There is some evidence that YGD delays gastric fullness and induces weight loss over 45 days in overweight patients.[41]

Dose

The dose of damiana for weight loss has not been determined.

Adverse Effects, Interactions, Pharmacokinetics. See Appendix A.

Ephedra *(Ephedra sinica)*

Grade A: *Strong scientific evidence (weight loss)*

Note: All dietary supplements that contain a source of ephedrine alkaloids such as ephedra have been banned by the FDA. However, products regulated as drugs that contain chemically synthesized ephedrine are not dietary supplements and not covered by this rule. These include drugs used for the short-term treatment of respiratory problems, and allergic reactions.[42]

Mechanism of Action

Ephedrine and *pseudoephedrine* are found in the leaves and stems of ephedra (also commonly known as *ma huang*) and are structurally related to amphetamines. They increase the availability and action of the endogenous neurotransmitters *norepinephrine* and *epinephrine* and directly and indirectly stimulate catecholamine receptors in the brain, heart, and blood vessels. Both ephedrine and pseudoephedrine elicit central nervous system (CNS) stimulation, bronchodilation, hypertension, and chronotropic/inotropic effects.[43] The synthetic form of pseudoephedrine is widely used in nonprescription decongestants. Pseudoephedrine may also have diuretic properties more potent than ephedrine.

Based on in vitro and animal studies, ephedrine stimulates thermogenesis in adipocytes, an effect that appears to be enhanced by chronic administration.[44] This effect has been associated with significant weight loss.[45-49] Ephedrine has inhibited gastric emptying, which may cause a feeling of satiety and thus assist in weight loss.[50]

Scientific Evidence of Effectiveness

In 1998, up to 7% of the U.S. population was using nonprescription weight loss products, and 14% of those taking such products used an ephedra- or ephedrine-containing formulation.[51] Scientific evidence from several trials lasting 1 to 12 months suggests that the ephedra constituent ephedrine can elicit a modest short-term weight loss when combined with caffeine.[52-58] This combination, however, may cause adverse cardiovascular effects.

Studies of ephedra or ephedrine monotherapy have been equivocal. Overall, the available trials have been small with methodological inadequacies, including incomplete reporting of blinding or randomization; furthermore, treatment-related adverse effects led to high dropout rates.[59-62] Because of the variable concentrations of ephedrine found in commercial preparations and numerous reports of serious adverse effects (particularly when combined with caffeine), ephedra may not be a safe therapy for weight loss.

Dose

The alkaloid content of different preparations of ephedra varies widely. One study examined the pseudoephedrine and ephedrine content of nine nutritional supplements containing *Ephedra sinica* and found significant variations in content for pseudoephedrine, ranging from 0.52 to 9.46 mg, and for ephedrine, from 1.08 to 13.54 mg, per recommended dose.[63] A study of 22 different ephedra products collected from herbal shops throughout Taiwan found a fourfold difference in the amounts of the various alkaloids, ranging from 0.536% to 2.308%.[64] Average ephedra supplement content is 1% of the crude plant. Different *Ephedra* species, yielding greatly different quantities of active alkaloids, are all sold as Ma huang in China, which makes finding standardized products difficult for consumers. *Ephedra sinica* plants grown in northern China often have a different morphology and alkaloid content than the same species grown in southern China.[65]

There is a lack of consistent evidence regarding the optimal form and dose of ephedra. Traditionally, herbalists have recommended a wide range of doses, which are typically higher than former FDA recommendations. The FDA formerly recommended a maximum of 8 mg every 6 hours (total daily dose of 24 mg) for up to 7 days. However, some experts recommend doses up to 25 mg of total ephedra alkaloids four times daily, and some studies have used doses as high as 50 to 100 mg of ephedra three times daily. Over-the-counter (OTC) drugs containing ephedra generally contain warning labels advising adults to take 12.5 to 25 mg every 4 to 6 hours and not to exceed 150 mg in 24 hours.

Although ephedra has been shown to help reduce weight, it is unsafe in humans for this indication, especially when combined with caffeine. The FDA has banned sales of ephedra dietary supplements because of adverse cardiovascular effects.

Adverse Effects, Interactions, Pharmacokinetics. See Appendix A.

Evening Primrose *(Oenothera biennis)*

Grade C: *Unclear or conflicting scientific evidence (obesity/weight loss)*

Mechanism of Action

The active ingredient in evening primrose oil (EPO) is thought to be gamma-linolenic acid (GLA), one of the omega-6 essential fatty acids (EFAs). The exact mechanism of EPO in reducing weight is not well understood. However, EFAs may alter lipogenesis and adipocyte differentiation as well as enhance insulin sensitivity.[66-68]

Scientific Evidence of Effectiveness

In humans, the use of GLA (a major component of EPO) has resulted in weight loss.[69] However, the use of EPO as a part of a weight loss regimen has not been linked to any benefit.[69,70] One study of 100 obese women found no anorectic effect of EPO.[70] Subjects were randomly assigned to receive either EPO, two 600-mL capsules four times daily, or placebo in combination with a 1000-kcal dietary regimen for 12 weeks. No difference in weight loss was observed between treatment groups.

Dose

The effective dose of EPO for weight loss has not been determined. In one study, two 600-mL capsules four times daily did not appear to promote weight loss.

Adverse Effects, Interactions, Pharmacokinetics. See Appendix A.

Garcinia *(Garcinia cambogia)*

Grade C: *Unclear or conflicting scientific evidence (weight loss)*

Mechanism of Action

Hydroxycitric acid (HCA), the active ingredient in garcinia, has been found to be a competitive inhibitor of the enzyme adenosine triphosphate (ATP) citrate-lyase and an inhibitor of lipogenesis.[71-73] HCA appears to increase fat metabolism and decrease glycogen utilization.[73] HCA may also promote weight loss by suppressing appetite, although the mechanism is not well understood.[74]

Scientific Evidence of Effectiveness

Garcinia's active constituent, HCA, may promote weight loss. However, clinical studies have demonstrated mixed results.[71,74-76] No significant weight loss or fat mass loss was noted in obese patients receiving garcinia compared with patients receiving placebo.[71] HCA, and to a greater degree the combination of HCA with niacin-bound chromium, facilitates a reduction in excess body weight, BMI, and cholesterol levels. Theoretically, HCA may be a good choice for weight loss in patients with dyslipidemias caused by effects on lipogenesis.[75] Other studies have reported reductions in weight loss and abdominal visceral fat in overweight patients;[74,76] however, no beneficial effects on appetite variables and dietary compliance have been noted.[74]

Dose

No well known standardization exists for garcinia. A total of 4.7 g of HCA in three divided daily doses 30 to 60 minutes before meals for 8 weeks reduced body weight index and BMI by 5% to 6% in one RCT.[75] Smaller daily garcinia doses of 2.4 g (1.2 g daily HCA) reduced body weight but had no effect on appetite variables and dietary compliance.[74]

Adverse Effects, Interactions, Pharmacokinetics. See Appendix A.

Ginger *(Zingiber officinale)*

Grade C: *Unclear or conflicting scientific evidence (weight loss)*

Mechanism of Action

The "pungent principles" or nonvolatile constituents of ginger are responsible for its flavor, aromatic properties, and proposed pharmacological activity. Spiced foods or herbal drinks, such as those that contain ginger, have the potential to produce significant effects on metabolic targets, such as satiety, thermogenesis, and fat oxidation.[77] Significant clinical outcomes may seem straightforward in some cases, but results are strongly dependent on the full compliance of subjects. Thermogenic ingredients such as ginger may be considered as functional agents that could help regulate body weight and prevent obesity.

Scientific Evidence of Effectiveness

In one clinical trial an herbal combination product containing ginger (as well as rhubarb, astragalus, red sage, turmeric, and gallic acid) was found to be ineffective in healthy adults.[78] Because ginger was combined with other herbs, the effects cannot be attributed to ginger alone. It remains unclear if ginger can effectively promote weight loss.

Dose

The dose of ginger for weight loss has not been determined.

Adverse Effects, Interactions, Pharmacokinetics. See Appendix A.

Guarana (Paullinia cupana)

Grade C: *Unclear or conflicting scientific evidence (weight loss)*

Mechanism of Action

The mechanism of action of guarana is related to its significant caffeine content. As with green tea, caffeine, which is a methylxanthine, appears to elevate free fatty acid mobilization and enhance weight loss.[79] Based on animal study, methylxanthines contained in guarana were reported to induce a thermogenic response and increase daily energy expenditure when combined with ephedrine.[80] Trials have been carried out with caffeine, however, so their outcomes cannot be directly related to guarana.

Scientific Evidence of Effectiveness

In the available studies, guarana alone has not been studied for its ability to induce weight loss. Instead, it has been studied in combination products that contain other potentially active substances. Preliminary research suggests that the combination product "YGD" (yerba mate, guarana, and damiana) delays gastric emptying, reduces the time to perceived gastric fullness, and induces weight loss.[27] Because this study used a combination product, the true effect of guarana alone on weight management cannot be clearly identified.

Scientific evidence supports the use of caffeine, the active ingredient of guarana, in combination with ephedra for weight loss.[41,81-83] These study results are of limited value because the FDA has removed dietary supplements containing ephedrine from the market. The FDA banned these products after determining that ephedra posed an unreasonable health risk to those who used it.

Dose

Guarana is generally standardized in terms of caffeine content, which is the active ingredient.[43] The amount of caffeine varies among products and manufacturers.[84,85]

The dose of guarana for weight loss has not been determined.

Adverse Effects, Interactions, Pharmacokinetics. See Appendix A.

Guggul (Commiphora mukul)

Grade C: *Unclear or conflicting scientific evidence (obesity)*

Mechanism of Action

The mechanism if action of guggul in weight loss is not well understood. Guggul has been found to stimulate thyroid activity, which may contribute to its effects in weight loss.[86]

Scientific Evidence of Effectiveness

Guggul is used in Ayurvedic medicine to treat obesity.[87] Modest weight loss has been reported in several RCTs in overweight patients who used guggul.[87-91] Nonsignificant weight reduction compared with placebo was reported in an open comparative trial.[88] In this study, patients weighing more than 90 kg received either exercise and diet or instruction on exercise and diet plus guggul. More evidence is needed to support the use of guggul or its derivatives for the management of obesity.

Dose

Guggulipid, a standardized guggul extract from the resin of the mukul myrrh tree native to India, is often standardized to contain 2.5% to 5% of guggulsterones (thought to be the active constituents).

Guggul (1.5-3 g daily) plus diet and exercise for 30 days resulted in a nonsignificant trend toward weight loss.[92]

Adverse Effects, Interactions, Pharmacokinetics. See Appendix A.

Licorice (Glycyrrhiza glabra)

Grade C: *Unclear or conflicting scientific evidence (reducing body fat mass)*

Mechanism of Action

According to animal study, licorice flavonoids have been found to suppress abdominal fat accumulation and decrease blood glucose levels.[93,94] This mechanism may be mediated through activation of peroxisome proliferator-activated receptor gamma (PPAR-γ).[94,95]

Scientific Evidence of Effectiveness

Preliminary evidence suggests that daily supplementation of licorice may reduce body fat in healthy subjects 21 to 26 years of age.[96] Endpoints included body fat mass, which was reduced, and extracellular water, which significantly increased after licorice consumption. BMI remained unchanged. Notably, because licorice may cause sodium retention and hypertension, obese patients should be discouraged from consuming large amounts of licorice.

Dose

Consuming 3.5 g of licorice daily for 2 months may help reduce body fat.[96]

Adverse Effects, Interactions, Pharmacokinetics. See Appendix A.

Psyllium (Plantago spp.)

Grade C: *Unclear or conflicting scientific evidence (obesity)*

Mechanism of Action. Insufficient available evidence.

Scientific Evidence of Effectiveness

Early research shows that supplementation with dietary psyllium and chitosan (see Adjunct Therapies) may help to increase the excretion of fat in the stool.[97] Although the administration of mucilage was shown to result in a weight loss greater than that obtained with diet alone,[98] the available evidence suggests that body weight reduction has not been proven to be associated with psyllium use in adults.[99,100]

Dose

The exact dose of psyllium for obesity has not been determined.

Adverse Effects, Interactions, Pharmacokinetics. See Appendix A.

Rhubarb (*Rheum* spp.)

Grade C: Unclear or conflicting scientific evidence (obesity)

Mechanism of Action

The mechanisms that underlie rhubarb's purported antiobesity effects are not well understood. In animals, a combination product containing refined rhubarb was shown to reduce food intake, prolong stomach emptying, and accelerate intestinal movement.[101]

Scientific Evidence of Effectiveness.

Preliminary study suggests that rhubarb may reduce weight in obese children and adults.[102] According to available study, rhubarb appears to be more effective at reducing weight than fenfluramine (a weight loss agent sold under the brand name Pondimin that was withdrawn from the U.S. market in 1997). More high-quality studies are needed to confirm these results.

Dose

Active ingredients of rhubarb vary by species.

For obesity in adults, five tablets containing 0.25 g of refined rhubarb extract (1.0 g crude drug) has been taken two or three times daily 30 minutes before meals for 12 weeks.[102]

For obesity in children, five tablets of 2.5 to 3.75 g containing refined rhubarb extract every night for 1 week has been used.[102]

Adverse Effects, Interactions, Pharmacokinetics. See Appendix A.

Soy (*Glycine max*)

Grade C: Unclear or conflicting scientific evidence (obesity, weight reduction)

Mechanism of Action

Soy protein appears to affect the upregulation of genes involved in lipid and glucose metabolism, enhance insulin sensitivity, regulate hepatic fatty acid oxidation, and promote loss of adipose tissue.[103-106]

Scientific Evidence of Effectiveness

Soy-based diets have been shown to reduce body fat and weight in overweight and obese patients more than calorie restriction alone.[107,108] Additionally, consuming soy milk appears to be as effective in reducing weight, fat, and abdominal circumference as consuming skim milk.[109,110]

Dose

The exact dose of soy for weight loss has not been determined. A high–soy protein, low-fat diet with or without physical exercise has been shown to reduce weight and fat mass in obese subjects.[107]

Adverse Effects, Interactions, Pharmacokinetics. See Appendix A.

Spirulina (*Arthrospira* spp.)

Grade C: Unclear or conflicting scientific evidence (weight loss)

Mechanism of Action. Insufficient available evidence.

Scientific Evidence of Effectiveness

Spirulina is a popular supplement for weight loss, sometimes marketed as a "vitamin-enriched" appetite suppressant. Preliminary research has been conducted in animals, with limited human data. A small, methodologically flawed study found no benefit of spirulina compared with placebo.[111] At this time the evidence does not support a recommendation either for or against the use of spirulina for weight loss.

Dose

The dose of spirulina for weight loss has not been determined.

Adverse Effects, Interactions, Pharmacokinetics. See Appendix A.

Tea (*Camellia sinensis*)

Grade C: Unclear or conflicting scientific evidence (weight loss)

Mechanism of Action

The chemical composition of tea varies with climate, season, horticultural practices, age of the leaf (position of leaf on the harvest shoot) and the degree of oxidation (depending on how the leaves are processed). Tea leaves contain various polyphenols, including catechins, epicatechin, epicatechin gallate, epigallocatechin gallate (EGCG), and proenthocyanidins.[112] EGCG accounts for 40% of the total polyphenol mixture, and catechins constitute about 30% of the dry weight of green tea (vs. 9% of dry weight of black tea).[113] Both EGCG and catechins have been implicated as the most significant antioxidants. The bud leaf and the first leaves are richest in EGCG.[114]

The catechins found in green tea may increase energy expenditure and fat oxidation for weight loss.[80,115,116-118] Green tea extract inhibits gastric and pancreatic lipases and stimulates thermogenesis.[119] It also inhibits the digestion and absorption of carbohydrates.[120,121] There is evidence that EGCG may suppress appetite by modulating the endocrine system.[122] Green tea is also a source of caffeine, which appears to elevate free fatty acid mobilization and enhance weight loss[80].

Scientific Evidence of Effectiveness

Several clinical studies have assessed the use of green tea in weight loss or weight maintenance.[119,123-126] Study results have been mixed, with most studies showing results similar to that of placebo.[119,123,124,126] Decaffeinated green tea products may offer the similar weight loss–enhancing effects as their caffeinated counterparts because these properties appear related to the catechin and polyphenol content. Decaffeinated products may also be associated with reduced risks of cardiovascular adverse effects. One study found that habitual consumption of green tea does not appear to affect weight loss management.[123] However, others found that obese patients who consumed green tea had weight loss after 12 weeks.[118,125]

Dose

Two capsules of a green tea extract (AR25; Exolise) standardized to 25% EGCG (taken twice daily for 12 weeks) reduced weight in obese patients.[118]

Adverse Effects, Interactions, Pharmacokinetics. See Appendix A.

HERBAL THERAPIES WITH NEGATIVE EVIDENCE

Beta-Glucan (β-Glucan)

Evidence suggests that different types of fiber may affect satiety and energy intake. A pilot study examined whether a fermentable fiber, such as beta-glucan, decreases hunger and energy intake and promotes weight loss more than nonfermentable fiber.[127] However, the results do not support a role for short-term use of fermentable fiber and nonfermentable fiber supplements in promoting weight loss.

HERBAL THERAPIES WITH LIMITED EVIDENCE

Barley (Hordeum vulgare)

In a study evaluating the effects of barley versus wheat in mildly overweight individuals, 60 subjects received muffins with barley endosperm (containing 7 g of beta-glucan) in an easily absorbed form, barley (5 g beta-glucan) in a less easily absorbed form, or refined wheat flour.[128] All groups followed the National Cholesterol Education Program's Step 1 diet. Subjects were asked to rank their feelings of fullness, hunger, and satiety throughout the study. Results showed that those who ate barley muffins felt "fuller" and "more satisfied" throughout the study than those who ate wheat muffins. Other results revealed an average weight loss of 0.5 lb weekly in those who ate barley, versus a weight gain of 0.5 lb in those who ate wheat muffins. The barley groups demonstrated significant reductions in total (11%) and low-density lipoprotein (LDL; 12%) cholesterol. These results suggest beneficial weight loss effects with barley but are unpublished and cannot be analyzed in detail.

Galega (Galega officinalis)

Galega has been traditionally used to increase lactation and treat diabetes mellitus (see Chapter 18). Galega's hypoglycemic effects have been attributed to guanidine and its derivative galegine. These compounds are chemical precursors to the drug *metformin,* a biguanide that inhibits gluconeogenesis in the liver. Metformin (Glucophage, Riomet, Fortamet, Glumetza, Diabex, Diaformin) is the single most popular antidiabetic drug in the United States. In obese patients with type 2 diabetes, beneficial effects of metformin on body weight were observed.[129,130] This prompted clinical research to test its ability to promote weight loss in nondiabetic subjects, and multiple human trials have shown efficacy.[131] Galega has demonstrated weight-reducing effects in animals;[132,133] however, studies examining galega for weight loss are lacking.

Ginseng (Panax spp.)

Despite the widespread use of ginseng for its stimulant effects, there is a lack of clinical evidence regarding its role in weight reduction. According to preliminary animal research, an extract from the ginseng berry decreased weight by reducing appetite and increasing activity levels in mice.[134-137]

Gymnema (Gymnema sylvestre)

Preliminary research suggests that gymnema may be beneficial in patients with type 1 or type 2 diabetes mellitus. However, though gymnema has been used historically to treat obesity, clinical evidence is lacking. Gymnema's effects may be linked to its ability to delay glucose absorption in the blood.[138]

Hoodia (Hoodia gordonii)

Although hoodia was introduced to the West in early 2004, the Bushmen of the Kalahari Desert in southern Africa have long used it to suppress hunger and thirst during long trips in the desert. Unlike ephedra, hoodia does not act as a stimulant. The pharmaceutical company Phytopharm found promising evidence from an isolated appetite-suppressing molecule, P57 (P57AS3), which is an oxypregnane steroidal glycoside. According to animal study, hoodia reduced food intake.[139] The P57 molecule was once licensed to Pfizer for development, but was discontinued in 2003.

Noni (Morinda citrifolia)

It is unclear whether noni can affect energy expenditure or fat metabolism. Of two recent laboratory studies, one reported that noni had energy-enhancing effects,[140] while the other reported noni had sedative and anxiolytic effects.[141] Currently, clinical research is lacking on the effects of noni on body weight, body composition, or fat metabolism.

Nopal (Opuntia spp.)

Nopal, or prickly pear, is high in fiber. Nopal has been suggested as a weight loss aid based on its purported ability to absorb water and provide a feeling of satiety. Nopal has been used traditionally to treat diabetes, and has demonstrated hypoglycemic effects (see Chapter 18). However, there is a lack of research using nopal in body weight regulation.

Seaweed

Bladderwrack and other seaweed products are often marketed for weight loss. However, their anorectic properties and safety for this purpose have not been adequately evaluated in humans. Theoretically, the thyroid-stimulating properties of seaweed (see Chapter 19) may be responsible for its effects on body weight.

Herbs with Appetite Suppressant or Weight Loss Properties*

HERB	SPECIFIC THERAPEUTIC USE(S)†	HERB	SPECIFIC THERAPEUTIC USE(S)†
Annatto	Obesity	Hoodia	Appetite suppressant, weight reduction, obesity
Aristolochia spp.	Weight loss	Jojoba	Appetite suppressant, weight loss
Arrowroot	Weight loss	Kava	Weight reduction, appetite suppressant
Astragalus	Weight loss		
Babassu	Obesity	Khat	Obesity
Barley	Appetite suppressant	Lemongrass	Body fat reducer (cellulite)
Betel nut	Appetite suppressant	Maitake mushroom	Weight loss
Black currant	Weight loss	Massage	Body fat reducer (cellulite)
Black pepper	Obesity	Nopal	Obesity, weight loss
Black tea	Obesity	Oleander	Weight gain
Cardamom	Weight loss	Onion	Obesity
Carob	Obesity	Perilla	Obesity
Carqueja	Weight loss	Pycnogenol	Fat burning, prevention of fat formation
Chia	Obesity		
Chicory	Obesity, weight loss	Raspberry	Obesity, weight loss
Chitosan	Appetite suppressant	Red clover	Appetite suppressant
Codonopsis	Obesity, weight gain	Red yeast rice	Obesity, weight loss
Coleus	Obesity	Rhodiola	Obesity
Dandelion	Obesity, weight loss	Safflower	Appetite suppressant
Desert parsley	Weight gain	Sarsaparilla	Weight reduction
Devil's club	Weight loss	St. John's wort	Weight loss
Garlic	Obesity	Stevia	Obesity
Ginseng	Weight loss	Thyme	Obesity
Goldenseal	Obesity	Turmeric	Weight reduction
Grape seed	Body fat reducer (cellulite), weight loss (maintenance)	Usnea	Weight loss
		Uva ursi	Weight loss
Grapefruit	Weight loss	Wheatgrass	Weight loss aid
Gymnema	Obesity	Yohimbe bark extract	Obesity
Hibiscus	Weight loss		

*This is not an all-inclusive or comprehensive list of herbs with appetite suppressant or weight loss properties; other herbs and supplements may possess these qualities. A qualified health care provider should be consulted with specific questions or concerns regarding potential weight loss effects or interactions of agents.
†Based on expert opinion, anecdote, case reports, and/or preliminary trial evidence.

ADJUNCT THERAPIES

1. Obesity is a disease that may precipitate or exacerbate co-morbid conditions such as metabolic syndrome, which includes diabetes, hypertension, and hyperlipidemia. Loss of weight typically results in improvement or normalization of physical signs and symptoms of these other conditions. A balanced *diet*, decreased *portion sizes*, and regular *exercise* are essential first-line therapies for obesity and any concomitant cardiovascular conditions. Obesity should be evaluated with any comorbid conditions. Subsequently, therapy with herbal remedies and dietary supplements may be used to target obesity and other underlying conditions. The following adjunct therapies may be beneficial to select populations of obese patients.

2. *Chitosan* is derived from the shells of crustaceans and has been found to have some efficacy in reducing weight when used as an adjunct to diet and exercise. A meta-analysis of RCTs evaluating chitosan as a weight loss therapy shows some positive results overall.[142] However, other available evidence suggests that chitosan is ineffective as a monotherapeutic weight loss agent. Some studies using chitosan in combination with other active ingredients (e.g., garcinia, guar meal, ascorbic acid) report some effect, but it is not clear whether these effects are caused by chitosan or the combination of chitosan with other active compounds.

3. Serotonergic agents such as *tryptophan*, or 5-hydroxy-tryptamine (5-HTP), the precursor for serotonin, may augment serotonin levels in the brain. Serotonin is the brain chemical associated with sleep, mood, movement, feeding, and nervousness. 5-HTP and other serotonergic agents such as selective serotonin reuptake inhibitors (SSRIs) may reduce carbohydrate cravings, elevate mood, and promote weight loss in obese individuals.[143-146] Such agents may be most effective for weight loss in patients with a history of depression and in patients with salty carbohydrate cravings.

4. *Dehydroepiandrosterone* (DHEA) is a hormone produced by the adrenal glands. Despite some negative results, most human studies investigating the effects of DHEA on weight or fat loss support its use for this purpose.[147-154] DHEA may be a useful adjunct in obese individuals with underlying endocrine abnormalities, such as hypothyroidism.

5. *Taurine* is an amino acid that the human body may synthesize from cysteine and pyridoxine. Taurine is found in high levels in meats and fish. In the human body, taurine is found in highest concentrations in the brain. Taurine acts as an inhibitory neurotransmitter in the body and has been studied for the treatment of epilepsy, hypertension, and abnormal heart rhythms. Taurine is currently a component of several energy drinks (e.g., Monster, Red Bull, Rockstar, Full Throttle). The role of taurine supplementation in weight loss requires further study; however, it may act as an energy and protein source that may be substituted for other caloric sources to increase catabolism.[155] Taurine may be an effective adjunctive therapy for weight loss in individuals with low serum concentrations of taurine.[156]

6. *Chromium* is a mineral associated with regulation of blood glucose and insulin function. Deficiencies in chromium may predispose individuals to hyperglycemia, hyperinsulinemia, hypertriglyceridemia, and low levels of high-density lipoprotein (HDL) cholesterol. Chromium may play an integral role in carbohydrate and lipid metabolism and may influence body mass and composition. Several small RCTs of short duration revealed equivocal results with respect to weight loss. Special populations with chromium deficiency may benefit from chromium supplementation and, through correction of an underlying deficiency, may lose weight; however, concrete evidence is currently insufficient.[157]

7. Diets with higher *calcium* density (high levels of calcium per total calories) have been associated with a reduced incidence of overweight or obesity in several studies. Although more research is needed to understand the relationship between calcium intake and body fat, these findings emphasize the importance of maintaining adequate calcium intake while attempting to diet or lose weight. One possible mechanism relates to calcium's role in proper insulin functioning. Low dietary calcium may impede insulin activity. This may lead to metabolic disturbances and weight gain.[158]

8. The Atkins Diet is an eating style that radically departs from the FDA's Food Pyramid. The Atkins Diet advocates increased consumption of fats as the primary source of energy and simultaneous restriction of carbohydrates. Carbohydrate restriction is based on the premise that eating carbohydrates (e.g., bread, cereal, potatoes, pasta) causes excessive secretion of insulin, which may increase fat storage. A carbohydrate-restricted diet has been shown to cause weight loss in obese and nonobese individuals. Effects at 1 year may be lower, and dropout rates are high. Overall, studies suggest that the Atkins Diet does result in long-term weight loss.[159] However, patients should consult with qualified health care professionals before beginning any new diet to discuss possible adverse effects and negative health consequences. The Atkins Diet should be avoided in patients with kidney disorders and diabetic patients (adequate protein/carbohydrate ratio required). The AHA dietary recommendations are preferred to "quick weight loss" diets. Adherence to a balanced diet produces better long-term outcomes and maintenance of weight loss.

9. The *macrobiotic diet* stresses vegetarianism and the consumption of whole, healthy foods. Proponents of macrobiotics advocate a flexible approach that allows supplementation with dairy, fish, or other supplements as needed on an individual basis. Evidence suggests that a macrobiotic diet may lead to reduced body size and

increased leanness in preschool children compared with children consuming normal diets.[160-161]

10. *Psychotherapy* is an interactive process between a person and a qualified mental health professional. The patient explores thoughts, feelings, and behaviors to help with problem solving. Several studies indicate that people who are overweight or obese may benefit from behavioral and cognitive-behavioral psychotherapy in combination with diet and exercise to lose weight.[162]

11. *Acupuncture* is used worldwide. According to traditional Chinese medicine (TCM) theory, the human body contains a network of energy pathways through which vital energy, *chi*, circulates. These pathways contain specific "points" that function as gates, allowing chi to flow through the body. Needles are inserted into these points to regulate the flow of chi. Studies have produced inconclusive evidence on whether acupuncture might contribute to weight loss, and the exact mechanism is unknown. Some studies show modest benefit, but others show none.[163] Currently, available evidence is insufficient to recommend either for or against acupuncture for weight loss.

12. *Moxibustion* is a therapeutic method in TCM, classical (five-element) acupuncture, and Japanese acupuncture. An herb (usually mugwort) is burned above the skin or on acupuncture points to introduce heat into a point to alleviate symptoms. The herb may be applied in the form of a cone, stick, or loose herb or may be placed on the head of an acupuncture needle to manipulate its temperature gradient. Evidence does not support moxibustion to aid in weight loss at this time, although it may contribute to increased psychological well-being and improved eating behaviors in obese patients.[164]

13. *Hypnosis* induces a trancelike state in which a person becomes more aware and open to suggestion. Hypnotherapy has been used to treat health conditions or to change behaviors. Research suggests that hypnosis may be valuable as an adjunct to cognitive-behavioral therapy for weight loss.[165]

14. *Yoga* is an ancient practice of relaxation, exercise, and healing with origins in Indian philosophy. Yoga has been described as "the union of mind, body, and spirit," which addresses physical, mental, intellectual, emotional, and spiritual dimensions toward an overall harmonious state of being. Yoga, in addition to healthy eating habits, may reduce weight. Better studies are necessary to form conclusions about the potential benefits of yoga alone. Yoga and other forms of meditation have been shown to lower blood pressure, heart rate, and stress and improve motivation. A meditative technique called the *relaxation response* has been studied extensively for benefits in patients with excessive stress and other disease states that improve with lifestyle modification.[166]

INTEGRATIVE THERAPY PLAN

- Perform a comprehensive medical history, and ask questions about lifestyle habits (e.g., smoking, alcohol consumption, exercise routine, dietary intake), history of comorbid conditions (particularly cardiovascular conditions), family history of obesity, and psychosocial history.
- Discuss weight history, eating, and activity behaviors.
- Identify potential causes of obesity, including poor diet, overeating, alcohol intake, inactivity, and stress level.
- Rule out secondary causes of obesity, such as hypothyroidism, eating disorders (e.g., binge-eating disorder), growth hormone deficiency, hypogonadism, medications (usually involving certain classes of agents, such as antidepressants, anticonvulsants, glucocorticoids, antipsychotics, and oral contraceptives), and polycystic ovarian syndrome.
- Measure weight and height, and calculate body mass index (BMI) and waist-to-hip ratio (WHR).
- The BMI is a measurement of weight (in pounds) for height (in inches) in adults older than 20 years. BMI falls into one of these categories: below 18.5 units is underweight, 18.5 to 24.9 is normal, 25.0 to 29.9 is overweight, and 30.0 and above is obese. For adults the accepted formula is BMI = $703 \times [\text{weight in pounds}/(\text{height in inches})^2]$.
- The WHR is the circumference of the waist divided by the circumference of the hips. For women a healthy ratio is 0.8 or lower. For men a healthy ratio is 1.0 or lower. A high ratio means that the patient is overweight or obese. A low ratio means that the patient is underweight.
- Obtain baseline metabolic panel, complete blood count with differential, liver function tests, thyroid function tests, and lipid profile.
- Perform baseline blood pressure and pulse measurements. A baseline electrocardiogram (ECG) is warranted in patients with a history of cardiovascular problems.
- Patients diagnosed with obesity and/or with preexisting comorbid cardiovascular risks (hypertension, diabetes, dyslipidemias, history of heart disease) should be referred to a comprehensive clinic that includes support groups, diet, and exercise counseling, psychosocial interventions, and diagnostic and pharmacotherapeutic evaluation.
- Ask if the patient uses any prescription or nonprescription agents for weight loss, including orlistat (alli, Xenical), sibutramine (Meridia), or diethylpropion (Tenuate).
- Determine the patient's readiness to lose weight, and discuss goals and expectations.
- Urge patients to try to lose weight gradually to reduce the risk of nutritional deficiencies and increase the likelihood of long-term success. Overweight patients should aim to lose about 0.5 to 2 pounds per week.
- Counsel patients on the importance of exercise and diet. In general, overweight patients should participate in 45 to 60 minutes of moderate exercise (e.g., brisk walking or jogging) daily to prevent obesity or to lose weight. Individuals

should eat well-balanced meals containing sensible portions. Recommend that the patient visit a registered dietitian (RD) to create an individualized eating plan.
- Encourage the patient to increase fiber intake and water consumption (6-8 glasses of water daily). Adding psyllium to the diet is an effective means of increasing dietary nonabsorbable fiber intake that may improve gastrointestinal motility and help eliminate waste in the body. Psyllium is also a useful adjunct therapy in patients with concomitant dyslipidemia or diabetes.
- Adding green tea (caffeinated or decaffeinated) without added sugars may provide beneficial antioxidants and catechins. In addition, the polyphenols in green tea will augment thermogenesis. Patients with contraindications may elect to drink decaffeinated green tea.
- Classes of herbal weight loss agents containing ephedra or ephedra-like constituents are not recommended for patients taking antiarrhythmic drugs or with histories of hypertension or cardiovascular disease.
- Guggulipid may be an appropriate herbal weight loss supplement as an adjunct to diet and exercise in patients with history of diabetes and/or dyslipidemias.
- People considering the use of herbs and supplements with potential for QT-interval prolongation require baseline ECG and QT measurement. Subsequent QT-interval calculation is recommended at 1 week, 2 weeks, and every 4 to 6 weeks thereafter, as well as with addition of agents affecting the ECG. Discontinue the herb or supplement if QT widening is greater than 25% to 35% over baseline, because this places patients at increased risk of life-threatening arrhythmias, such as torsades de pointes. Routine monitoring of potassium and magnesium levels is recommended to ensure normal values for cardioprotection and prevention of arrhythmias.
- Discourage "quick weight loss" diets, such as the Atkins Diet, because of the inherent health risks and high incidences of rebound weight gain.
- Patients and clinicians should record average weight loss weekly. Clinicians should provide positive feedback and encouragement and acknowledge weight loss.

Case Studies

CASE STUDY 20-1

NR is a 50-year-old man with a 10-year history of type 2 diabetes with high LDL cholesterol and blood pressure. His current medications include metformin (Glucophage, 1000 mg) twice daily, glargine (Lantus, 60 U insulin) at bedtime, rosuvastatin (Crestor, 5 mg), and lisinopril (Zestril). He presents to the diabetes clinic where you are the clinical pharmacist complaining of excessive fatigue, difficulty losing weight, and lack of motivation. He reports no polyphagia, polydipsia, polyuria, or blurred vision.

NR states he has gained about 30 pounds since he started using insulin therapy about 3 years ago, although he acknowledges that insulin therapy has helped him better manage his blood sugar. He is 6 feet tall and currently weighs 225 pounds. He performs self-monitoring of blood glucose (SMBG) four times daily. His fasting glucose usually ranges from 100 to 120 mg/dL. Postprandial glucose generally ranges from 140 to 160 mg/dL. Most recent glycosylated hemoglobin (HbA_{1c}) was 6.6%. His blood pressure was 132/80 mm Hg. He has no known allergies. NR's mother died 2 months ago. Since then, he has started taking St. John's wort for depression, which he believes is helping. NR inquires about his BMI and about herbal supplements to help with weight loss.

Answer: Currently, NR has BMI (kg/m^2) of 30.5 (>30 considered obese) and high LDL cholesterol. It is imperative for NR to lose weight to better control his diabetes and reduce the risk of macrovascular complications of diabetes (cardiovascular disease, stroke, peripheral vascular disease). A gradual weight loss plan should be employed for NR, with a goal of losing about ½ to 2 pounds per week.

Soy may play a beneficial role in obesity, diabetes, high cholesterol, and hypertension. The dose of soy for weight loss is unknown; however, scientific studies show that consumption of 25 g of soy protein daily may lower cholesterol levels. Advise NR to incorporate soy beverages, tofu, tempeh, and soy-based meat alternatives into his diet. Along with soy, the addition of psyllium, fiber, and plenty of water (6-8 glasses daily) will help improve gastrointestinal motility and help eliminate waste. Decaffeinated green tea, a healthful diet, exercise (45-60 minutes of moderate exercise, including brisk walking or jogging), depression counseling, and group support for diet and exercise would bring greatest success for this patient.

Currently, NR's diabetes and depression appear to be well controlled, and there is no need at this time to change these agents. Additionally, although St. John's wort appears to be an inducer of cytochrome P450, rosuvastatin has not been shown to be subject to oxidative biotransformation by the cytochrome P450 3A4 isoenzyme. Reduced effectiveness of this agent by St. John's wort is unlikely.

Low-dose aspirin should also be recommended to help prevent heart and blood vessel disease. However, caution is warranted because concurrent use of St. John's wort with aspirin may increase the risk of bleeding.

NR should routinely monitor his blood glucose and blood pressure and report any changes to his physician. Eye and foot examinations should be performed regularly by a clinician. A lipid profile should also be obtained to assess the effectiveness of rosuvastatin.

CASE STUDY 20-2

KA is a 27-year-old woman of normal weight who uses a free blood pressure test near the pharmacy counter. After completing the test, she approaches the counter and says her blood pressure is 160/100 mm Hg. KA adds that she came to the pharmacy for an herbal remedy that would help "calm her nerves." For the past few months she has noted that her "heart was racing," and she had occasional palpations. She also has insomnia. She switched to decaffeinated coffee but did not notice any improvement. You inquire about any medicines or herbs she is taking. KA replies that she is taking only an herbal product that she found on the Internet for weight loss. You ask to see the product and find that it contains ephedra, guarana, and evening primrose oil (EPO). How do you counsel?

Answer: Although strong scientific evidence indicates that ephedra *(Ephedra sinica)* can promote weight loss, the FDA has taken action to ensure that all ephedra-containing weight-loss products are no longer marketed and sold. However, some ephedra-containing products can still be obtained. Ephedra is a CNS stimulant, bronchodilator, and vasoconstrictor. These effects are exacerbated when combined with other ingredients, such as caffeine and guarana *(Paullina cupana)*, which contains caffeine. Use of ephedra-containing products can result in hypertension, tachycardia, CNS stimulation, cardiac arrhythmia, myocardial infarction, and stroke. EPO *(Oenothera biennis)* may have some efficacy for weight control and may have a hypotensive effect; however, EPO may increase the risk of seizures. You should advise KA to immediately cease taking the weight loss product; most likely her symptoms will disappear once the substances are no longer present in her system. Because she appears to be of normal weight, KA should also be assessed for potential eating disorders; thus you should suggest that she make an appointment to see a physician.

CASE STUDY 20-3

RR is a 46-year-old man who presents at your pharmacy and asks for refills of metformin (Gluchophage) for his type 2 diabetes and atenolol (Tenormin) for control of hypertension. He is 5 feet, 10 inches tall and weighs 390 pounds. He asks if you can recommend an herbal remedy to help him lose weight. He adds that he has tried bitter orange and damiana and found them to be ineffective. How do you counsel?

Answer: RR is more than 100 pounds over his ideal weight and is therefore considered to be morbidly obese. While none of the herbal remedies currently available in the United States has proved effective, several may be useful in moderately obese individuals when combined with a diet and exercise program. RR should enroll in an intensive, medically supervised weight loss program. If he is unsuccessful, he might consider bariatric surgery, in which the stomach is greatly reduced in size and intestinal realignment is performed. Bariatric surgery is associated with significant risk, but successful outcomes have included achievement of goal body weight, resolution of type 2 diabetes, and normalization of blood pressure.

Bitter orange *(Citrus aurantium)* is *not* recommended for RR. Animal and clinical studies have reported increases in systolic and diastolic blood pressure with use of *C. aurantium*. Damiana *(Turnera diffusa)* is also not recommended for RR. Animal studies have reported conflicting results on the effect of damiana on blood glucose levels, and it might interfere with RR's metformin therapy.

Together with an intense weight loss program, other herbal remedies might have a supplemental benefit. Cinnamon *(Cinnamomum* spp.) might be beneficial for RR. In vitro evidence suggests that cinnamon may modulate energy utilization in adipocytes by stimulating glucose uptake, glycogen synthesis, and activated glycogen synthase. One study reported a significant decrease in blood glucose and blood pressure with use of cinnamon, as well as an increase in lean body mass. Coleus *(Coleus forskohlii)* has been reported to stimulate the cellular production of cAMP, an important component in energy production and utilization. It also has been reported to lower blood pressure through vasodilation. Colenol is a compound isolated from coleus that stimulates insulin release; however, it may increase insulin levels.

Ensure that RR's blood pressure, HbA_{1c}, and blood glucose are appropriately monitored periodically to assess drug effectiveness.

References for Chapter 20 can be found on the Evolve website at http://evolve.elsevier.com/Ulbricht/herbalpharmacotherapy/

Review Questions

1. True or false: Patients with a BMI of 35 are considered obese.

2. All the following statements are true *except*:
   a. Bitter orange is marketed as a safe alternative to ephedra.
   b. Hydroxycitric acid (HCA), the active ingredient in *Garcinia cambogia,* has been shown to facilitate a reduction in body weight.
   c. Hoodia acts as a stimulant, similar to ephedra, to aid in weight loss.
   d. Theoretically, the thyroid-stimulating properties of bladderwrack may cause hypermetabolic weight loss.

3. Which component of guarana contributes to its weight loss effects?
   a. Flavonoids
   b. Methylxanthines
   c. Saponins
   d. Terpenoids

4. All the following statements are true *except*:
   a. "YGD," which contains yerba mate, guarana, and damiana, is an herbal preparation used for weight loss.
   b. Bitter orange extract (975 mg) in combination with St. John's wort (900 mg) and caffeine (528 mg) daily has been reported to aid in weight loss.
   c. The FDA banned ephedra products after reports of serious adverse effects, including toxicity and death.
   d. There is strong evidence to support the use of spirulina as an appetite suppressant.

5. What dose of HCA contained in garcinia has been shown to reduce BMI?
   a. 4.7 g daily
   b. 475 mg daily
   c. 47 mcg daily
   d. 0.47 g daily

6. True or false: Consuming soy milk appears to be as effective in reducing weight, fat, and abdominal circumference as consuming skim milk.

Answers are found in the Answers to Review Questions section in the back of the text.

21 Menopause

Outline

OVERVIEW
- Perimenopause
- Postmenopause
- Surgical Menopause
- Signs and Symptoms
- Diagnosis
- Hormone Replacement Therapy Controversy

SELECTED HERBAL THERAPIES
- Alfalfa (*Medicago sativa*)
- Belladonna (*Atropa* spp.)
- Black Cohosh (*Actaea racemosa*, formerly *Cimicifuga racemosa*)
- Dong Quai (*Angelica sinensis*)
- Flax (*Linum usitatissimum*)
- Ginseng (*Panax* spp.)
- Hop (*Humulus lupulus*)
- Kudzu (*Pueraria lobata*)
- Red Clover (*Trifolium pratense*)
- Rhubarb (*Rheum* spp.)
- Sage (*Salvia officinalis*)
- Soy (*Glycine max*)
- St. John's Wort (*Hypericum perforatum*)
- Wild Yam (*Dioscorea villosa*)

HERBAL THERAPIES WITH NEGATIVE EVIDENCE
HERBAL THERAPIES WITH LIMITED EVIDENCE
ADJUNCT THERAPIES
INTEGRATIVE THERAPY PLAN
CASE STUDIES
REVIEW QUESTIONS

Learning Objectives

- Assess for physical and psychological signs and symptoms of menopause.
- Describe the mechanism of action, side effects, and drug interactions associated with herbs used in menopause.
- Provide evidence-based information, adjunct therapies, and an integrative care plan for menopause and associated symptoms.

OVERVIEW

According to the World Health Organization (WHO), menopause is the permanent cessation of menstrual periods, or *menses*, following the loss of ovarian follicular activity.[1] From the Greek *mens* ("monthly") and *pausis* ("cessation"), menopause can be diagnosed after 12 consecutive months of *amenorrhea* (absence of menstrual bleeding). The age at which menopause occurs (also known as the *climacteric*) is genetically determined; the mean age in the United States is approximately 51 years (range, 45-55 years). Cessation of menses before age 40 is known as *premature ovarian failure*. The endometrium is the uterine lining that sloughs at menstruation, then regenerates for another cycle. Woman who menstruate past age 55 are at increased risk for endometrial hyperplasia or endometrial carcinoma.[1-4]

A woman is born with a finite reserve of primordial *follicles* (primary oocytes with one layer of follicular cells) in her ovaries. At menopause, few to no mature follicles remain in the ovaries. The gradual loss of *oocytes* (immature eggs) and follicles results in a series of changes in endocrine function involving gonadotropins and estrogen.[1-4]

Follicular maturation is induced by pituitary release of *follicle-stimulating hormone* (FSH). As a woman ages, her oocytes become increasingly resistant to FSH. These changes are more pronounced in the 40s, as are changes in menstrual patterns. As a woman ages, the ovary requires high amounts of FSH to stimulate estrogen.[1-4]

The hypothalamic-pituitary-ovarian (HPO) axis, a network of hormonal relationships that regulate reproductive status, becomes less stable with age. The ovaries become less predictable because of the hormonal fluctuations, and the oocytes cease to respond predictably to the hormones.[5]

Researchers once thought that menopause was caused exclusively by a lack of estrogen production by the ovaries, which resulted in higher levels of FSH and the cessation of menses. More recently, however, it was found that *inhibin B*, a glycoprotein synthesized by ovarian granulosa cells, plays a role in triggering the menopause transition.[6,7] As the number of ovarian follicles diminishes, inhibin B declines and stimulates a rise in FSH by a negative feedback loop.[8] Around age 45, FSH stimulation triggers the remaining follicles to increase estradiol level during the late reproductive years. However, 6 to 12 months before menopause, higher FSH levels fail to increase estradiol production, and these reduced levels can result in menopause-related symptoms, such as hot flashes and vaginal dryness.[2-4]

A woman's menses may become longer or shorter, heavier or lighter, and more or less frequent. Eventually, the ovaries cease to function, and there are no more menses. Rarely, a woman may menstruate every month until the last egg is released; however, a gradual tapering off is more common. Signs and symptoms depend on the amount of hormone loss in the body. Therefore, replacement of these hormones or hormonelike compounds may play a role in the treatment of menopausal symptoms.[2-4]

Perimenopause[2-4]

Perimenopause is the transition period before menopause, marked by great instability and upredictability of reproductive hormone secretion. It usually begins between ages 45 and 55, but some women experience perimenopause earlier, even in their 30s. The body undergoes various endocrine and biological changes. The ovaries' production of estrogen is erratic. Estradiol levels are unpredictable and can fluctuate among normal, high, and low.

During perimenopause the woman may begin to experience menopausal physical and emotional signs and symptoms, even though she still menstruates. The average length of perimenopause is 4 years, but for some women this stage may last only a few months or continue for 10 years.

Postmenopause

Postmenopause represents the time after menopause. A woman is considered to be postmenopausal after her menses have ceased for an entire year. Symptoms of menopause may be milder or less frequent, and energy, emotional, and hormonal levels may have stabilized. As estrogen levels decline, bone mass and lipid profiles may also change, thereby increasing a woman's risk of osteoporosis and cardiovascular disease.[2-4]

Surgical Menopause

A *hysterectomy* generally refers to the surgical removal of the uterus. A *total hysterectomy* is the removal of the uterus, fallopian tubes, ovaries, and cervix. Hysterectomies are used to treat fibroids, endometriosis, uterine prolapse, cancer, persistent vaginal bleeding, and chronic pelvic pain. This procedure usually does not cause menopause. Although women no longer have menses, their ovaries still release eggs and produce estrogen and progesterone. However, surgery that removes the uterus and the ovaries (total hysterectomy or bilateral oophorectomy) does cause menopause, without any perimenopausal phase. Instead, menses stop immediately, and hot flashes and other menopausal signs and symptoms appear.[2-4]

Signs and Symptoms

Symptoms that may indicate menopause include changes in menstrual patterns; *vasomotor* (referring to nerves and muscles that cause blood vessels to constrict or dilate) symptoms; psychological, emotional, and mental disturbances; sexual dysfunction; and somatic symptoms (e.g., back pain, fatigue, joint pain).

Many women experience changes in menstrual patterns because of their changing hormone levels and decreased frequency of ovulation. The changes may be subtle at first, then gradually become more noticeable. Common changes include irregular cycles (shorter or longer), unusual bleeding (heavier or lighter), and missed menses.

Hot flashes (or hot flushes) are vasomotor responses that cause sensations of warmth or heat, usually beginning in the head and face and then radiating down the neck to other parts of the body. There may be red blotches on the skin. Each hot flash averages 2.7 minutes and is characterized by a sudden increase in heart rate; an increase in peripheral blood flow, which leads to a rise in skin temperature; and a sudden onset of sweating, particularly on the upper body. Flashes can begin when a woman's cycles are still regular or, more often, as menopause approaches and her cycles become irregular (e.g., less frequent). Hot flashes usually continue for less than 1 year after the last menstrual period (LMP), although some women still experience flashes 5 to 10 years after menopause. They can occur once a month, once a week, or several times an hour and at any time of day or night. When occurring at night (e.g., night sweats), hot flashes can interrupt sleep and drench clothing and sheets. Loss of sleep can eventually lead to irritability and fatigue.

Psychological and mental disturbances are common problems of menopause. Depression, anxiety, irritability, mood swings, and loss of concentration may result from hormonal imbalances and life circumstances surrounding middle age (e.g., aging parents, children going to college).

Sexual dysfunction, which includes desire, arousal, orgasmic, and sex pain disorders (e.g., pain during intercourse caused by vaginal dryness), may occur during menopause. The problem may be caused by several factors, including vaginal changes. In particular, the tissues of the vagina and vulva may become thin and dry *(vaginal atrophy)*, which may lead to itching and discomfort during sexual intercourse. In some women, vaginal dryness is the first sign of menopause.

Somatic symptoms are increased during menopause. These complaints include nausea, dizziness, backache, headaches, tiredness, and clumsiness. Other changes include urinary incontinence (leaking urine when coughing, sneezing, laughing, or exercising), breast enlargement or tenderness, thinning hair, "electric shock" sensation under the skin, tingling in extremities, hair growth on face, and gum problems.[2-4]

Diagnosis

A careful medical history should be performed along with a physical examination, including a pelvic examination (Figure 21-1). During the pelvic exam, reproductive organs should be screened for abnormalities or indication of infection. Many clinicians advise women to keep diaries of menstrual cycles and the physical and psychological changes they experience over the course of several months. The menstrual diary provides clues to the physician and helps the woman understand and cope with the changes.

The signs and symptoms of menopause, such as hot flashes and mood swings, are an indication to women that they have begun the transition. Laboratory tests, such as FSH and estradiol tests, may be performed to confirm menopause or perimenopause. Tests to determine the level of thyroid function may be conducted, because hypothyroidism may cause symptoms similar to those of menopause.[9]

Hormone Replacement Therapy Controversy

Some women take hormone replacement therapy (HRT) to relieve the symptoms associated with menopause. HRT is medication containing one or more female hormones, usually estrogen plus progestin (synthetic progesterone). HRT may also protect against osteoporosis. However, HRT also has risks. In 2002 the National Institutes of Health (NIH) halted a large study that was evaluating a widely used HRT medication, Prempro (combination product of estrogen and progestin).[10] This study was one of five major studies in the Women's Health Initiative (WHI). Of the five major arms of the WHI, the HRT was the only study terminated. This study found that HRT was associated with an increased risk of breast cancer, heart disease, blood clots, and stroke. This abrupt cessation of the study was widely publicized in the media. Clinicians should consider the unique needs of their patients and weigh the risks and benefits of HRT on an individual basis. Certain types of HRT carry a higher risk, and each woman's own risks can vary depending on her health history and lifestyle.

SELECTED HERBAL THERAPIES

Note

To help make this educational resource more interactive, all pharmacokinetics, adverse effects, and interactions data have been compiled in Appendix A. Safety data specifically related to pregnancy and lactation are listed in Appendix B. Please refer to these appendices when working through the case studies and answering the review questions.

Alfalfa (*Medicago sativa*)

Grade C: *Unclear or conflicting scientific evidence (menopausal symptoms)*

Mechanism of Action

Alfalfa isoflavonoid constituents—coumestrol, genistein, biochanin A, and daidzein—appear to have estrogenic effects. However, the exact mechanism of alfalfa in menopause is not well understood.[11]

Scientific Evidence of Effectiveness

Alfalfa, when used in combination with sage, reduced menopausal symptoms, including hot flushes and night sweating, in limited available clinical study. Levels of estradiol, luteinizing hormone (LH), FSH, prolactin, and thyroid-stimulating hormone (TSH, thyrotropin) were unchanged in women who received the sage-alfalfa extract treatment.[12]

Dose

To alleviate menopausal symptoms, tablets containing 120 mg of sage extract and 60 mg of alfalfa extract (*Medicago sativa*) have been used daily for up to 3 months.[12]

Adverse Effects, Interactions, Pharmacokinetics. See Appendix A.

Belladonna (*Atropa* spp.)

Grade C: *Unclear or conflicting evidence (menopausal symptoms)*

Mechanism of Action. Insufficient available evidence.

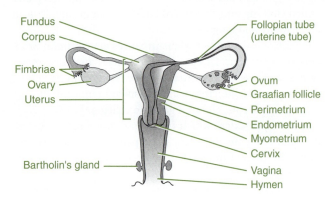

Figure 21-1 Anterior view of female reproductive organs. (Modified from LaFleur Brooks M: *Exploring medical language: a student-directed approach,* St Louis, 2002, Mosby.)

Scientific Evidence of Effectiveness

There are anecdotal reports that Bellergal, a proprietary combination formula containing 40 mg phenobarbital, 0.6 mg ergotamine tartrate, and 0.2 mg levorotatory alkaloids of belladonna (not available in the United States), may reduce the incidence of hot flashes. One randomized control trial (RCT) noted a trend toward improved symptoms with Bellergal.[13]

Dose

The dose of belladonna for menopause has not been determined. However, one Bellergal tablet (see combination and doses above) three times daily for 8 weeks has been used in clinical study.[13]

Adverse Effects, Interactions, Pharmacokinetics. See Appendix A.

Black Cohosh (Actaea racemosa, formerly Cimicifuga racemosa)

Grade C: *Unclear or conflicting scientific evidence (menopausal symptoms)*

Mechanism of Action

The mechanism of action of black cohosh remains unclear, and its effects on estrogen receptors (ERs) or hormonal levels (if any) have not been fully elucidated. Recent studies suggest no direct effects of black cohosh on ERs, although this area is controversial.[14-21] In animals and in vitro studies, initial reports of ER-binding activity[22] contrast with more recent data suggesting no significant ER-binding or estrogenic activities.[23-26] Available in vitro studies found no effects of black cohosh alone on ERs, but that black cohosh antagonized proliferative effects on cells induced by estradiol.[27] A similar in vitro study on estrogen-sensitive breast cancer cells (MCF-7) reported isopropanolic black cohosh extract did not stimulate MCF-7 growth and exerted inhibitory effects on cellular proliferation, indicating strong estrogen-antagonist effects.[28]

Scientific Evidence of Effectiveness

Black cohosh is popularly used as an alternative to prescription hormonal therapy in the treatment of climacteric symptoms such as hot flashes, mood disturbances, diaphoresis, palpitations, and vaginal dryness.[27,29-33] The German Commission E approved it for perimenopausal symptoms. Between 2002 and 2003, sales of black cohosh rose 26% in the United States.[34] However, in recent years, negative publicity and reports of liver damage have been associated with black cohosh.

Several controlled trials and case series reported improved menopausal symptoms for up to 6 months with black cohosh treatment.[35] A combination of black cohosh and St. John's wort appears to be beneficial for climacteric complaints, including the related psychological component.[36] Although promising, initial studies have been small in number with methodological weaknesses. Most recent, more definitive trials indicate that black cohosh has little or no effect on menopausal symptoms.[37-39] When used with other botanicals, the combination had no effects on vaginal dryness, menstrual cyclicity, vaginal epithelium, endometrium, or reproductive hormones.[39]

Most trials have used a standardized measurement scale to assess menopausal symptoms, the Kupperman Index, which does not measure vaginal dryness/atrophy, but does measure paresthesias and vertigo (not traditionally associated with menopause). Because of the conflicting studies in this area, it remains unclear whether black cohosh has any effect on menopausal symptoms.

Dose

The dosage of black cohosh is often based on its content of triterpenes, calculated as 27-deoxyactein. The German product Remifemin, used in most clinical studies, contains an alcoholic extract of black cohosh rhizoma standardized to contain 1 mg of 27-deoxyactein per 20-mg tablet.[40] The manufacturing process and dosing recommendations for Remifemin have changed over the past 20 years, and doses used in different studies may not be comparable. A standardized liquid formulation of Remifemin has been used in some studies.

For perimenopausal symptoms, studies have used 20-mg to 40-mg Remifemin tablets (corresponding to 1-2 mg of 27-deoxyactein) twice daily, or 40 drops of a liquid ethanolic extract. The dosing regimen currently recommended is 20 mg twice daily. Other preparations of black cohosh have been used as well, with mixed results. A study of 40 mg/day versus 127 mg/day of an isopropanolic extract of black cohosh for 6 months reported similar effects on menopausal symptoms.[41] However, black cohosh at 160 mg/day has been used for up to 1 year to treat vasomotor symptoms associated with menopause, although this preparation was not found beneficial.[37] Also, 40 mg of *Actaea* or *Cimicifuga racemosa* extract (CR BNO 1055) has also been studied in postmenopausal women with symptoms related to estrogen deficiency for 1 year; it was safe and greatly decreased hot flushes.[42] However, one 20-mg capsule of *C. racemosa* twice daily for 4 weeks to reduce hot flashes was not found effective.[38] The combination of ethanolic St. John's wort extract and isopropanolic black cohosh extract taken for 16 weeks has been found beneficial for climacteric complaints with psychological symptoms in women.[36] In another study, 40 mg of isopropanolic black cohosh daily for 12 weeks was beneficial.[43]

Adverse Effects, Interactions, Pharmacokinetics. See Appendix A.

Dong Quai (Angelica sinensis)

Grade C: *Unclear or conflicting scientific evidence (menopausal symptoms)*

Mechanism of Action. Insufficient available evidence.

Scientific Evidence of Effectiveness

Dong quai is used in traditional Chinese formulas for menopausal symptoms.[2,11] It has been proposed that dong quai may contain *phytoestrogens*, or chemical structures resembling endogenous estrogens that exert hormonal effects, which may benefit conditions such as menopause. A survey revealed that dong quai was among remedies used to treat menopausal symptoms.[44] However, clinical studies are limited. A well-designed clinical trial that evaluated the effects of dong quai on menopausal symptoms found no significant estrogenic effects in 71 women with menopausal symptoms who received either dong quai (4.5 g) or placebo for 6 months.[45] The study also showed no difference in endometrial thickness, maturation of vaginal cells, serum estradiol, or estrone levels. This study evaluated dong quai alone, but it is traditionally used in combination with several other herbs. The synergistic activity of dong quai with other herbs appears to account for its beneficial effects. In addition, the extract used may not be manufactured in the same way as other products and may have different effects.

No specific recommendations for menopausal symptoms can be made because of the lack of high-quality studies and the variety of products and doses evaluated.

Dose

The dose of dong quai for menopause has not been determined.

Adverse Effects, Interactions, Pharmacokinetics. See Appendix A.

Flax (Linum usitatissimum)

Grade C: Unclear or conflicting scientific evidence (menopausal symptoms)

Mechanism of Action

The plant lignans found in flaxseed (*not* flaxseed oil) are considered to be phytoestrogens.[46,47] Because phytoestrogens have a chemical structure similar to that of 17β-estradiol, they may possess estrogen receptor agonist or antagonist properties.[48] Flaxseed is a concentrated food source of the lignan secoisolariciresinol diglycoside, which is metabolized to the mammalian lignans enterodiol and enterolactone (ENL) by colonic bacteria.[49,50] Flaxseed also appears to exert more favorable effects on modulation of estrogens than does soy, indicated by changes in urinary estrogen metabolite excretion.[51]

Scientific Evidence of Effectiveness

Preliminary research has examined the effects of flaxseed on menopausal symptoms and cholesterol levels in menopausal women.[52] A dose of 40 g of flaxseed was as effective as an oral estrogen-progesterone replacement (0.625 mg of conjugated equine estrogens and 100 mg of micronized progesterone) in improving the presence and severity of menopausal symptoms after 2 months of treatment, as measured by the Kupperman Index. High-density lipoprotein (HDL) cholesterol levels were reported to increase, but low-density lipoprotein (LDL) cholesterol remained unchanged.[52]

Dose

To treat mild menopausal symptoms, 40 g of flaxseed has been given daily in divided doses.[52]

Adverse Effects, Interactions, Pharmacokinetics. See Appendix A.

Ginseng (Panax spp.)

Grade C: Unclear or conflicting scientific evidence (menopausal symptoms)

Mechanism of Action

The exact effects of ginseng in menopause are not well understood; its purported estrogenic effects have not been definitively established in studies. Some in vitro studies indicate an estrogenic effect in human breast cancer cells, possibly by binding and activating the estrogen receptor.[25,53-57] Other in vitro data did not show this effect.[58] This discrepancy may be caused by the type of ginseng extract used, because methanol extract has demonstrated estrogenic properties in vitro in breast cancer cells, but water extracts have not.[59] The traditional Japanese herbal medicine *unkei-to*, which contains *Panax ginseng* and other herbs, stimulated the secretions of 17β-estradiol and progesterone from highly luteinized granulosa cells.[60]

Scientific Evidence of Effectiveness

Results from two trials suggest that *P. ginseng* may be moderately effective in relieving postmenopausal symptoms, including fatigue, insomnia, and depression.[61,62] Efficacy was assessed by a number of validated symptom indices, including the Women's Health Questionnaire, Psychological General Well-Being Index, visual analog scales, and Cornell Medical Index (CMI). The beneficial effects of ginseng do not appear to be mediated by hormone replacement effects, because FSH and estradiol levels, endometrial thickness, maturity index, and vaginal pH were not affected by treatment.[61]

Dose

For symptomatic relief of postmenopausal symptoms, two capsules of standardized ginseng extract (Ginsana, containing 100 mg of standardized ginseng extract G115) have been taken daily for 16 weeks.[61]

Adverse Effects, Interactions, Pharmacokinetics. See Appendix A.

Hop (Humulus lupulus)

Grade C: Unclear or conflicting scientific evidence (menopausal symptoms)

Mechanism of Action

Hop is an essential ingredient in beer; it is also a source of prenylflavonoids, including 8-prenylnaringenin (8-PN), one of the most potent phytoestrogens.[63-65] A high level of estrogenic activity has also been reported in the beta-bitter acids of the hop plant.[66] Furthermore, this bitter fraction has been shown to bind competitively to estrogen receptor alpha and beta in vitro[67] and to intracellular receptors for estradiol in human breast cancer cells.[68]

Scientific Evidence of Effectiveness

Hop is popularly used to treat sleeping disorders and may help alleviate menopausal symptoms, such as hot flashes.[69-71] According to preliminary research, the phytoestrogen flavone 8-PN found in hop has been shown to help alleviate hot flushes, as measured by a modified Kupperman Index.[71] A vaginal gel containing hop, hyaluronic acid, liposomes, and vitamin E may help relieve vaginal dryness, as well as burning, itching, inflammation, rash, and dyspareunia.[69]

Dose

A hop extract similar to the standardized food supplement, MenoHop (corresponding to 100 and 250 mcg 8-PN), for 12 weeks has been shown to alleviate menopausal symptoms.[71]

Adverse Effects, Interactions, Pharmacokinetics. See Appendix A.

Kudzu (Pueraria lobata)

Grade C: *Unclear or conflicting scientific evidence (menopausal symptoms)*

Mechanism of Action

Kudzu contains several constituents that display estrogenic effects, including puerarin, genistein, glycetein, daidzin, and daidzein.[72-74] These phytoestrogens may be synergistic with each other.[56,72,73,75-84]

Scientific Evidence of Effectiveness

There is conflicting evidence regarding the effects of kudzu on menopausal symptoms. Preliminary study found that kudzu supplementation (both 50 mg and 100 mg daily) for 6 months improved hot flashes and night sweats in perimenopausal women.[85] Another study found that kudzu reduces vaginal dryness and dyspareunia (painful sexual intercourse), improves signs of vaginal atrophy, and restores the atrophic vaginal epithelium in healthy postmenopausal women.[86] Contrary to these findings, a separate clinical trial found that 3 months of kudzu supplementation had no effect on menopausal symptoms, lipid profiles, sex hormone levels, or bone turnover markers. Beneficial effects were noted only in cognitive function in postmenopausal women.[76]

Dose

A specific kudzu extract (NPI-031, Natural Pharmacia) has been used in rats. This extract is standardized to contain 19% puerarin, 4% daidzin, and 2% daidzein.[87]

Doses of 50 mg and 100 mg of a related plant, *Pueraria mirifica*, have been used once daily for 6 months to treat menopausal symptoms.[85]

Adverse Effects, Interactions, Pharmacokinetics. See Appendix A.

Red Clover (Trifolium pratense)

Grade C: *Unclear or conflicting scientific evidence (menopausal signs and symptoms)*

Mechanism of Action

Isoflavones, such as those in red clover, are believed to reduce signs and symptoms of menopause. In vitro estrogenic responses have been observed with the isoflavones genistein and daidzein and their respective precursors, biochanin A and formononetin, as well as with the steroidlike phytochemical coumestrol. These isoflavones possess varying affinity for estradiol receptors and are capable of acting as both agonists and antagonists.[88] Isoflavones may affect levels of gonadotropin-releasing hormone, FSH, and LH through hormonal feedback mechanisms.[89]

Scientific Evidence of Effectiveness

Red clover is a legume and, as with soy, is a source of isoflavones, which act as phytoestrogens. Although the isoflavones present in red clover have demonstrated estrogenic properties in preclinical studies, clinical evidence is currently insufficient to support the efficacy for climacteric vasomotor symptoms and as an alternative to conventional HRT. Some small studies have reported reductions in frequency and severity of hot flashes as well as improvements in vaginal cytology.[90-92] Other studies report that red clover supplementation is no more effective than placebo.[93,94] Trials have been methodologically weak and short in duration,[93-95] which may not be sufficient to assess efficacy for menopausal symptoms because symptoms tend to wax and wane over longer periods. Nonetheless, red clover products remain popular.

The specific doses of red clover isoflavone extract that would be equivalent to ethinyl estradiol or conjugated equine estrogens have not been established.[96] It has not been definitively demonstrated that isoflavones possess similar benefits to those purported for estrogens (reduction of cardiovascular disease, positive effects on lipid profiles, vascular benefits) and this remains controversial for estrogens in general.[97-99]

Dose

The brand of red clover isoflavone extract used in most trials and most available commercially is Promensil (Novogen). Each tablet is standardized to contain 40 mg of total isoflavones: 4 mg genistein, 3.5 mg daidzein, 24.5 mg biochanin A, and 8.0 mg of formononetin (present as hydrolyzed aglycons).

Doses of 40, 80, or 160 mg of red clover isoflavones (Promensil) have been taken daily for 12 weeks to treat menopausal symptoms.[93,94]

Adverse Effects, Interactions, Pharmacokinetics. See Appendix A.

Rhubarb (*Rheum* spp.)

Grade C: *Unclear or conflicting scientific evidence (menopausal symptoms)*

Mechanism of Action

The exact mechanism of rhubarb in menopause is not well understood. Sibiric rhubarb *(Rheum rhaponticum)* does not appear to contain anthraquinones, estrogens, or any activators of estrogen receptor alpha, suggesting that it likely has a decreased risk of adverse estrogenic effects.[2,11]

Scientific Evidence of Effectiveness

A special extract from the roots of Sibiric rhubarb *(Rheum rhaponticum)*, ERr 731 (Phytoestrol N, Chemisch-Pharmazeutische Fabrik Goeppingen), has been used in Germany to treat women with climacteric complaints in perimenopause and postmenopause for many years. In clinical study, ERr 731 reduced climacteric complaints, including frequency and severity of hot flashes, and improved general well-being in perimenopausal women.[100,101] ERr 731 also reduced the Hamilton Anxiety Scale (HAM-A) scores for somatic and anxiety symptoms, from "moderate" or "severe" to "slight."[101] When comparing this extract to placebo, no differences in gynecological findings, including endometrial biopsies, bleeding, weight, blood pressure, pulse, and laboratory safety parameters, were noted.[100]

Dose

The standardized extract from the roots of Sibiric rhubarb *(Rheum rhaponticum)*, ERr 731, consists of rhaponticin, desoxyrhaponticin, and their aglycons rhapontigenin and desoxyrhapontigenin. To treat hot flashes in perimenopausal women, one ERr 731 tablet has been taken daily for 12 weeks.[100]

Adverse Effects, Interactions, Pharmacokinetics. See Appendix A.

Sage (*Salvia officinalis*)

Grade B: *Good scientific evidence (menopausal symptoms)*

Mechanism of Action

The sage constituent *geraniol* appears to exert estrogenic activity.[102,103] It has also been hypothesized that reduced menopausal symptoms may result from central antidopaminergic actions.[12]

Scientific Evidence of Effectiveness

Sage may contain compounds with mild estrogenic activity,[102,103] which may in theory decrease the symptoms of menopause. Sage in combination with alfalfa reduced menopausal symptoms, including hot flushes and night sweating, in limited available clinical research.[12] Levels of estradiol, LH, FSH, prolactin, and TSH were unchanged in sage-alfalfa extract treated women.

Dose

Tablets containing 120 mg of sage extract and 60 mg of alfalfa extract *(Medicago sativa)* have been used daily for up to 3 months to alleviate symptoms of menopause.[12]

Adverse Effects, Interactions, Pharmacokinetics. See Appendix A.

Soy (*Glycine max*)

Grade B: *Good scientific evidence (menopausal hot flashes)*

Mechanism of Action

Isoflavones (e.g., genistein) from soy are believed to have estrogen-like effects in the body and to be structurally related to estradiol-17β (Figure 21-2). As a result, these isoflavones are referred to as "phytoestrogens." In laboratory studies, it is not clear if isoflavones stimulate or block the effects of estrogen, or both (acting as "mixed receptor agonists/antagonists").[2,11]

Scientific Evidence of Effectiveness

A lifelong diet rich in soy foods may be related to a lower incidence of menopausal hot flashes. Asian women, who traditionally consume more soy than women from Western countries, reportedly experience a lower incidence of menopausal hot flashes. Various clinical trials have examined the effects of soy on menopausal symptoms.[104-120]

Most studies have found that soy minimally reduces, but does not eliminate, night sweats and the number of hot flashes.[106,111,113] Improvements in other menopausal symptoms, including sleep disorders, depression, vaginal dryness, anxiety, and loss of libido have also been reported.[107] However, no beneficial effects have been found on cognitive function, bone mineral density, or plasma lipids when postmenopausal women took soy supplements for 1 year.[121] Published evidence is variable and results are conflicting. Soy has not been shown to be more effective than conventional HRT.

Dose

Isolated soy protein such as Supro (60 g), soy flour (45 g), and a range of isoflavone products have been studied for menopausal symptoms. Doses of 20 to 60 g of soy protein, providing 40 to 80 mg of isoflavones, for up to 1 year have been used in research.[108,119,120]

Adverse Effects, Interactions, Pharmacokinetics. See Appendix A.

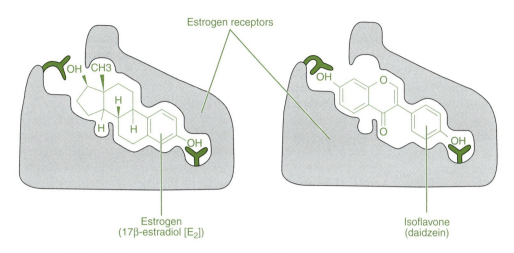

Figure 21-2 Estrogen and soy isoflavones. (From www.womentowomen.com.)

St. John's Wort *(Hypericum perforatum)*

Grade C: *Unclear or conflicting scientific evidence (perimenopausal symptoms)*

Mechanism of Action

The apparent broad-spectrum mechanisms of St. John's wort (SJW) are not fully understood, but biologically active constituents may include hyperforin and adhyperforin (phloroglucinols), hypericin and pseudohypericin (naphthodianthrones), flavonoids, xanthones, oligomeric procyanidins, and amino acids.[122,123] SJW's antidepressant activity may be mediated by serotonergic (5-hydroxytryptamine), noradrenergic, and dopaminergic systems,[124-129] as well as by gamma-aminobutyric acid (GABA) and glutamate amino acid neurotransmitters.[130-133] This activity may explain SJW in the management of symptoms of depressed mood in perimenopausal women.

Scientific Evidence of Effectiveness

St. John's wort may help treat psychological and psychosomatic symptoms associated with perimenopause or menopause, including depression.[134,135] After 12 weeks of SJW use, improvement was also noted in climacteric complaints, as measured by self-rating and physician rating.[134]

Dose

St. John's wort products are often standardized to 0.3% hypericin extract, although the manufacturing industry encourages standardization to hyperforin (usually 2%-5%). Standardization of extracts may not be clinically relevant in predicting effectiveness, because the active ingredients in SJW have not been definitively determined.

St. John's wort standardized extract (Kira) at 900 mg orally three times daily has been used to manage psychological symptoms, including depressed mood associated with perimenopause or menopause.[134]

Adverse Effects, Interactions, Pharmacokinetics. See Appendix.

Wild Yam *(Dioscorea villosa)*

Grade C: *Unclear or conflicting scientific evidence (menopausal symptoms)*

Grade D: *Fair negative scientific evidence (hormonal effects)*

Mechanism of Action

Diosgenin, a constituent of wild yam (*Dioscorea villosa* and other species of the genus *Dioscorea*), is thought to possess dehydroepiandrosterone (DHEA)–like properties, and may likewise act as a precursor to human sex hormones such as estrogen and progesterone. Based on this proposed mechanism, extracts of the plant have been used to treat hot flashes and headaches associated with menopause.[2] However, it is a misconception that wild yam contains hormones or hormonal precursors; this is largely based on the historical fact that progesterone, androgens, and cortisone were chemically manufactured from Mexican wild yam in the 1960s. It is unlikely that this chemical conversion to progesterone actually occurs in the human body.

Scientific Evidence of Effectiveness

Wild yam preparations are traditionally used to treat hot flashes and headaches associated with menopause. Manufacturers of a vaginal cream containing *Dioscorea* have claimed that the cream possesses progesterone-like effects and is a source of "natural hormones," although this is not supported by animal or human studies. Steroidal effects may be attributable to the presence of synthetic progesterone, which is sometimes added to commercial wild yam products. Some marketers also promote wild yam as a natural precursor of DHEA, a claim that is not supported by scientific evidence. Available studies have noted no direct effect of wild yam extract on the estrogen or progesterone receptors and no increases in DHEA levels.[136,137] At this time, evidence is inconclusive regarding the use of wild yam for menopausal symptoms.

Dose

Typically, wild yam products are standardized to 10% diosgenin per dose. Diosgenin levels vary greatly among different wild yam species.[138,139] Unless a product is standardized, consumers can expect a considerable range of diosgenin-related effects based on the source species, as well as growing, harvesting, processing, and storage conditions. Synthetic progesterone has reportedly been added to some wild yam products.

The dose of wild yam for menopausal symptoms has not been determined.

Adverse Effects, Interactions, Pharmacokinetics. See Appendix A.

 Traditional Chinese Medicine: MF101

> Medical systems such as Traditional Chinese Medicine (TCM) involve complete systems of theory and practice that have developed independently from or parallel to conventional medicine. TCM practitioners typically use herbs, acupuncture, and massage to unblock *qi* (or vital energy) and maintain "balanced energy." The evidence regarding TCM for menopause is mixed, although promising. The oral drug MF101 (BioNovo) is an estrogen receptor beta–selective agonist found to stimulate endometrium and breast tissue. It is based on mixed botanicals of 22 TCM herbs. MF101 is being designed for perimenopausal and menopausal women. In Phase 1 clinical study, MF101 was found to be safe and well tolerated. Phase 2 study found potential efficacy at reducing frequency and severity of menopausal symptoms with two doses of MF101.[140]

HERBAL THERAPIES WITH NEGATIVE EVIDENCE

Evening Primrose *(Oenothera biennis)*

Grade D: *Fair negative scientific evidence (menopausal symptoms)*

Literature review reveals a lack of available evidence that evening primrose oil (EPO) is useful in the management of menopausal symptoms. Small trials investigating its effects on flushing as well as bone mineral density have been negative overall.[141-143]

HERBAL THERAPIES WITH LIMITED EVIDENCE

Chasteberry *(Vitex agnus-castus)*

In vitro, constituents in chasteberry bind selectively to estrogen receptor beta.[144,145] Apigenin (a flavonoid) has been identified as an active phytoestrogen in chasteberry and may alter FSH and LH. Chasteberry has been found to bind to dopamine-2 receptors in the pituitary, thereby inhibiting prolactin secretion.[146,147] Historically, chasteberry has been used to reduce libido. Despite its demonstrated mechanisms of action, clinical evidence evaluating the effects of chasteberry on menopausal symptoms is currently lacking.

Maca *(Lepidium meyenii)*

Maca has been used for centuries in Peru to improve hormonal function. According to anecdotal evidence, female patients experienced reduced menopausal symptoms, including hot flashes and vaginal dryness. Improvements in mood swings, libido, hair/bone loss, and sleep have also been noted.

Tea *(Camellia sinensis)*

Constituents of green tea such as beta-sitosterol (a phytoestrogen) may contribute to its beneficial effects in menopause. A study conducted in healthy postmenopausal women showed that a morning/evening menopausal formula containing green tea was effective in relieving menopausal symptoms, including hot flashes and sleep disturbance.[148] However, these formulas also contained popularly used botanicals for menopause, including soy and black cohosh. The exact effects of green tea are not well understood.

ADJUNCT THERAPIES

1. The onset of menopause triggers profound changes in bone strength and cardiovascular health, which can greatly increase a woman's risk for developing osteoporosis and heart disease. Various lifestyle modifications and integrative treatments can prevent these long-term health risks.
2. During the first few years after menopause, women may lose bone density at a rapid rate, increasing their risk of osteoporosis. *Osteoporosis* ("porous bone") causes bones to become brittle and weak, leading to an increased risk of fractures (see Chapter 22). Until about age 30, people normally build more bone than they lose. After age 35, bone breaks down faster than it builds up and results in gradual loss of bone mass. At this point, the person has begun to develop osteoporosis.
3. Postmenopausal women are especially susceptible to fractures of the hip, wrist, and spine. It is important for women to start building stronger bones early to help protect against osteoporosis and fractures (see Chapter 22).
4. Women also tend to gain weight during the menopausal transition. Individuals may need to eat less, perhaps 200 to 400 fewer calories a day, and exercise more just to maintain their current weight. However, although menopausal women tend to require fewer calories to maintain or lose weight, they have equal or greater nutrient needs that may be difficult to meet. Health care professionals generally recommend a balanced diet that includes a variety of fruits, vegetables, and whole grains and that limits saturated fats, oils, and sugars. Eating smaller, more frequent meals each day may reduce bloating and the

Herbs with Potential Progestogenic or Estrogenic Activity*

HERB	SPECIFIC THERAPEUTIC USE(S)†	HERB	SPECIFIC THERAPEUTIC USE(S)†
Aconite	Menopausal symptoms	Deer velvet	Hormonal disorders
Anise	Estrogenic effects, menopausal symptoms	Dill	Estrogenic effects
Asarum	Menstrual stimulation	Echinacea	Menopausal symptoms
Ashwagandha	Menstrual stimulation, menstrual disorders	Eucalyptol	Menopausal symptoms
		Fenugreek	Menopausal symptoms
Astragalus	Menstrual disorders	Feverfew	Menstrual stimulation
Avocado	Menstrual stimulation	Fo-ti	Hormonal effects
Bay leaf	Menstrual stimulation	Garlic	Menstrual stimulation, hormonal effects
Betony	Menstrual stimulation	Ginger	Menstrual stimulation
Black currant	Menopausal symptoms	Ginkgo biloba	Estrogenic effects
Black haw	Menstrual stimulation, menopausal symptoms	Goji	Gynecological disorders (ovulation)
		Gotu kola	Menstrual stimulation, menopausal symptoms (hot flashes)
Black horehound	Menstrual stimulation, menopausal symptoms	Ground ivy	Menstrual disorders
		Guggul	Menstrual disorders
Blessed thistle	Dysmenorrhea, menstrual stimulation	Hawthorn	Menstrual stimulation
Bloodroot	Menstrual stimulation	Hop	Estrogenic effects
Blue cohosh	Menstrual stimulation, hormonal imbalances, menstrual disorders	Horny goat weed	Menstrual stimulation, menopausal symptoms, gynecological disorders (ovulation)
Blue flag	Menstrual stimulation		
Boneset	Menstrual stimulation	Hyssop	Menstrual stimulation
Borage seed oil	Menopausal symptoms	Jointed flatsedge	Menstrual disorders
Boswellia	Menstrual stimulation	Kava	Menopausal symptoms
Bugleweed	Hormonal regulation	Ladies mantle	Hormonal imbalances, menopausal symptoms
Bupleurum	Menstrual stimulation, hot flashes, menstrual disorders	Lavender	Menstrual stimulation, menopausal symptoms, menstrual disorders
Burdock	Hormonal effects		
Calabar bean	Menopausal symptoms	Lemongrass	Menstrual stimulation
Calendula	Menstrual disorders	Licorice	Hormonal regulation, hot flashes, menopausal symptoms
Camphor	Menopausal symptoms		
Cannabis indica	Menopausal symptoms	Maca	Hormonal imbalances (female), menstrual disorders
Carrot	Menopausal symptoms		
Cat's claw	Menstrual disorders	Milk thistle	Menstrual disorders
Chamomile	Menstrual disorders, menopausal symptoms	Mistletoe	Menstrual stimulation
		Mugwort	Menstrual stimulation
Chasteberry	Menstrual stimulation, menopausal symptoms	Muira puama	Menstrual disorders
		Mullein	Estrogenic effects
Cherry	Gynecological disorders	Neem	Estrogenic effects
Chia	Hormonal disorders	Noni	Menstrual disorders
Chicory	Menstrual stimulation	Nux vomica	Menopausal symptoms, menstrual disorders
Cinnamon	Menstrual stimulation, gynecological disorders		
		Oleander	Menstrual stimulation
Cleavers	Menopausal symptoms	Oregano	Menstrual disorders, menstrual stimulation
Comfrey	Gynecological disorders		
Cordyceps	Menstrual disorders	Ovaraden	Menopausal symptoms
Cornflower	Menstrual stimulation	Ovariin	Menopausal symptoms
Dandelion	Hormonal disorders, menopausal symptoms, menstrual stimulation	Passion flower	Menopausal symptoms (hot flashes)
		Physostigma	Menopausal symptoms
Danshen	Menstrual disorders		

Continued

Herbs with Potential Progestogenic or Estrogenic Activity—cont'd

HERB	SPECIFIC THERAPEUTIC USE(S)†	HERB	SPECIFIC THERAPEUTIC USE(S)†
Pleurisy root	Estrogenic effects	Stinging nettle	Menstrual stimulation
Quassia	Menstrual stimulation	Sweet almond	Estrogenic effects
Raspberry	Menstrual irregularities	Tansy	Menstrual stimulation
Rehmannia	Menstrual stimulation	Thyme	Dysmenorrhea
Rhodiola	Menstrual stimulation, menopausal symptoms	Tribulus	Menopausal symptoms
		Turmeric	Dysmenorrhea, menstrual stimulation
Rose hip	Menstrual disorders	Uva ursi	Menopausal symptoms
Safflower	Menstrual stimulation, vaginal dryness	Valerian	Menstrual stimulation, hot flashes, menopausal symptoms
Sarsaparilla	Estrogenic effects		
Saw palmetto	Hormonal imbalances	Verbena	Estrogenic effects
Scullcap	Menopausal symptoms	White water lily	Menstrual disorders
Shepherd's purse	Menstrual disorders, menstrual stimulation	Yarrow	Menstrual stimulation
		Yellow dock	Menopausal symptoms
Star anise	Menstrual stimulation	Yew	Menstrual stimulation

*This is not an all-inclusive or comprehensive list of herbs with progestational or estrogenic properties; other herbs and supplements may possess these qualities. A qualified health care provider should be consulted with specific questions or concerns regarding potential progestational or estrogenic effects of agents or interactions.
†Based on expert opinion, anecdote, case reports, and/or preliminary trial evidence.

sensation of fullness. A high-protein diet or high coffee consumption increases calcium excretion and may increase the body's calcium needs. Fiber, oxalates (found in rhubarb, spinach, beets, celery, greens, berries, nuts, tea, cocoa), and high-zinc foods (e.g., oysters, red meats) decrease calcium absorption, requiring more calcium supplementation. It is also recommended that patients limit salt intake to reduce bloating and fluid retention. A multivitamin should be recommended in menopausal women.

5. A regular exercise program of at least 30 minutes 5 days a week that includes various activities to improve aerobic, strength, and flexibility performance should also be established. Low-impact weight-bearing exercises such as walking, jogging, tennis, and dancing are helpful. Strength training with free weights, weight machines, and resistance bands will help strengthen muscles and bones. Flexibility exercises, including yoga, may help to increase mobility of joints and are considered important in overall fitness.

6. Nutritional supplements along with diet will also help build healthy bones. Calcium and vitamin D supplements are essential for menopausal women. Daily calcium intake for postmenopausal women should be about 1200 mg. Women should eat foods rich in calcium (e.g., dairy products, leafy green vegetables, tofu, calcium-fortified foods), as well as foods that promote calcium absorption. A glass of milk provides about 300 mg of calcium. Intake of foods that deplete the bones of calcium, such as animal protein and salt, should be limited. Vitamin D helps the body absorb calcium. Fifteen minutes of sun exposure daily provides sufficient vitamin D. Foods such as fortified milk, liver, and tuna also contain vitamin D. Women should ask their health care providers or nutritionists if they should take a vitamin D supplement; some calcium supplements include vitamin D. Supplements such as shark and bovine cartilage are sometimes used for their high amounts of calcium.

7. When estrogen levels decline, the woman is also at greater risk for cardiovascular disease, the leading cause of death in women as well as men. Risk reduction steps for heart disease include smoking cessation, reducing high blood pressure, regular aerobic exercise, and eating a diet low in saturated fats and plentiful in whole grains, fruits, and vegetables. Natural agents such as beta-glucan, psyllium, and soy may protect menopausal women from this disease through cholesterol-lowering effects. Consuming higher amounts of vitamins C, E, and beta-carotene have also been linked to a lower incidence of heart disease.

8. As the tissues of the vagina and urethra lose their elasticity, postmenopausal women may experience a frequent, sudden, strong urge to urinate, followed by an involuntary loss of urine (called *urge incontinence*), or the loss of urine with coughing, laughing, or lifting (called *stress incontinence*). Exercise involving the muscles of the pelvic floor, called *Kegel exercises,* can improve some forms of urinary incontinence. These exercises consist of the regular clenching and unclenching of the "sex muscles" that form part of the pelvic floor (sometimes called the "Kegel muscles").

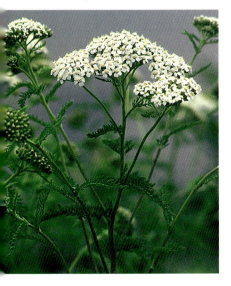
Achillea millefolium (yarrow)

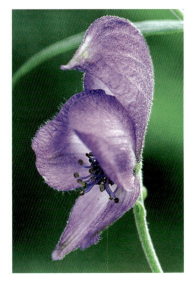
Aconitum napellus (aconite)

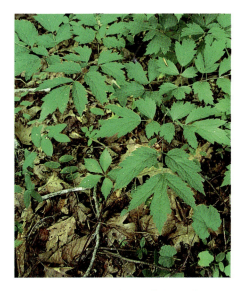
Actaea racemosa, formerly *Cimicifuga racemosa* (black cohosh)

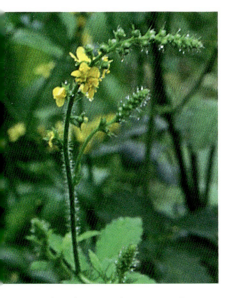
Agrimonia eupatoria (agrimony)

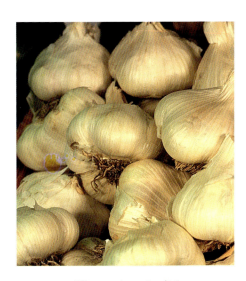
Allium sativum (garlic)

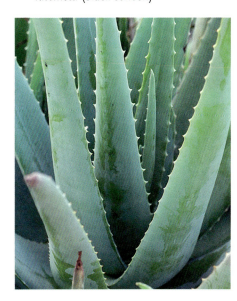
Aloe vera (aloe)

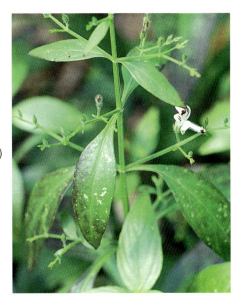
Andrographis paniculata (andrographis)

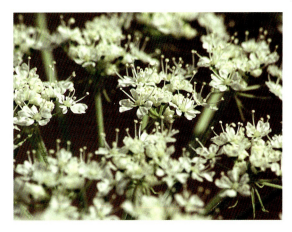
Angelica sinensis (dong quai, Chinese angelica)

All photographs from Martin Wall Botanical Services.

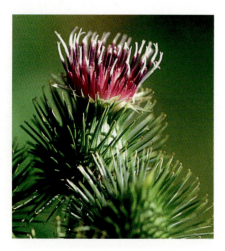
Arctium lappa (burdock)

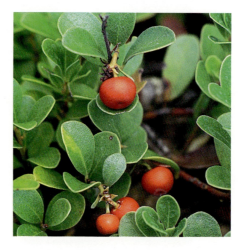
Arctostaphylos uva-ursi (uva ursi)

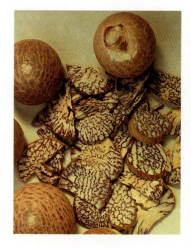
Areca catechu (betel nut)

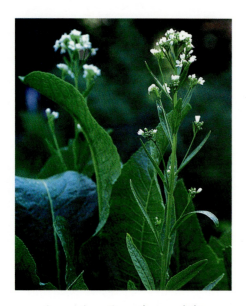
Armoracia rusticana (horseradish)

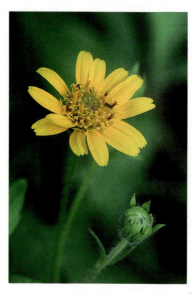
Arnica chamissonis spp. (arnica)

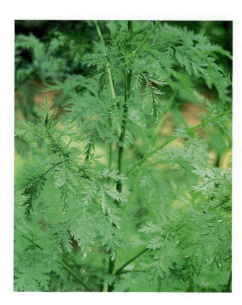
Artemisia annua (sweet Annie)

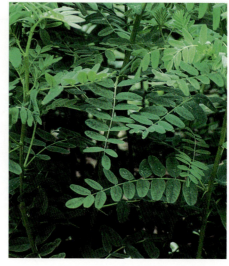
Astragalus membranaceus (astragalus)

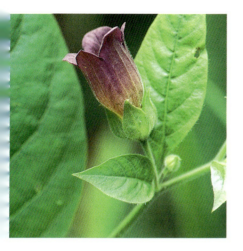

Atropa belladonna (belladonna, deadly nightshade)

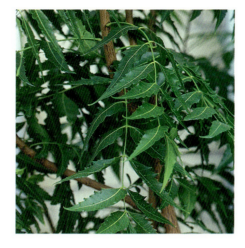

Azadirachta indica (neem)

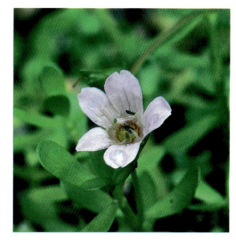

Bacopa monnieri (bacopa)

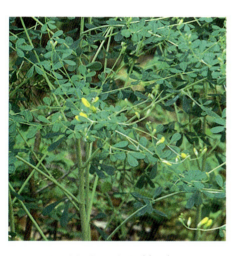

Baptisia tinctoria (wild indigo)

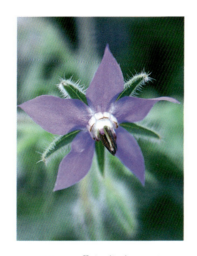

Borago officinalis (borage)

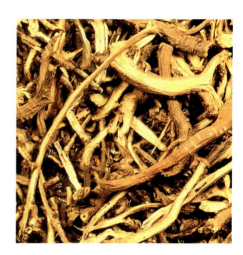

Bupleurum chinense (bupleurum)

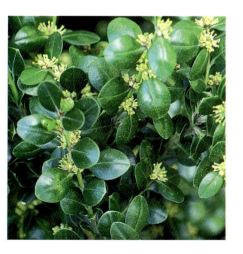

Buxus sempervirens (boxwood)

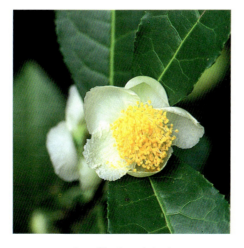

Camellia sinensis (tea)

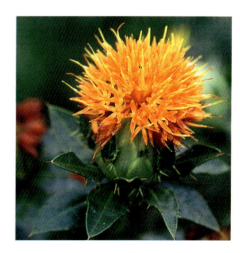

Carthamus tinctorius (safflower)

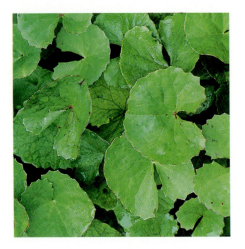
Centella asiatica (gotu kola)

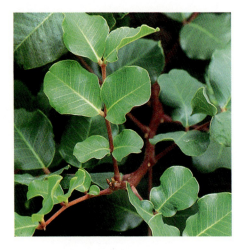
Ceratonia siliqua (carob)

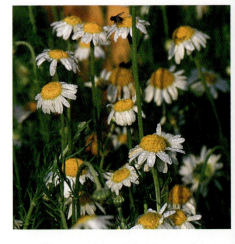
Chamaemelum nobile (chamomile)

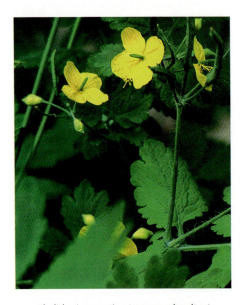
Chelidonium majus (grater celandine)

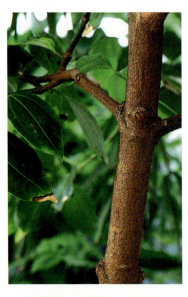
Cinnamomum verum (cinnamon)

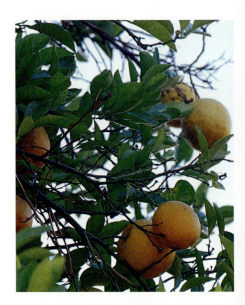
Citrus aurantium (bitter orange)

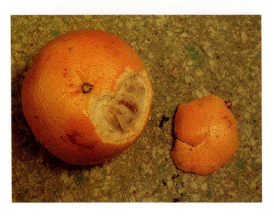
Citrus x *paradisi* (grapefruit)

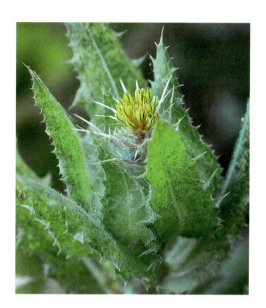
Cnicus benedictus (blessed thistle)

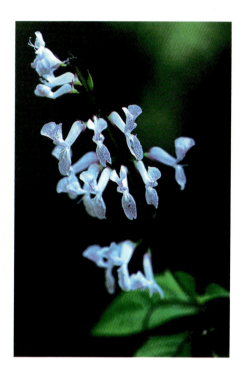
Coleus forskohlii (coleus)

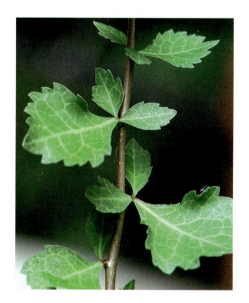
Commiphora wightii (guggul)

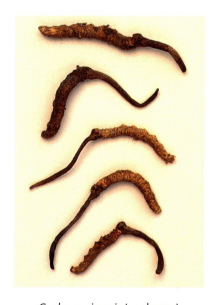
Cordyceps sinensis (cordyceps)

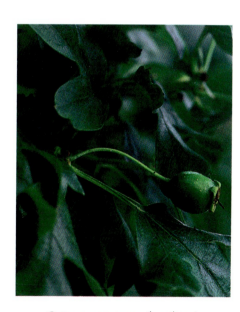
Crataegus monogyna (hawthorn)

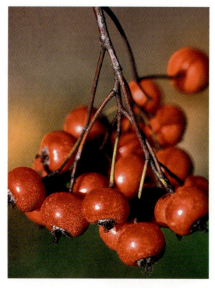
Crataegus phaenopyrum (Washington hawthorn)

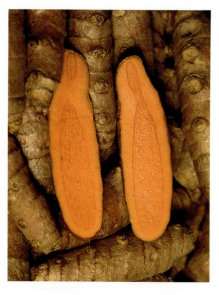
Curcuma longa (turmeric)

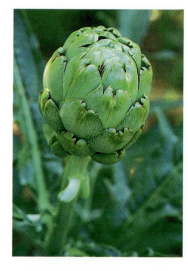
Cynara scolymus (globe artichoke)

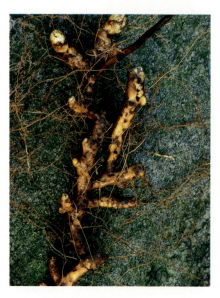
Dioscorea villosa (wild yam)

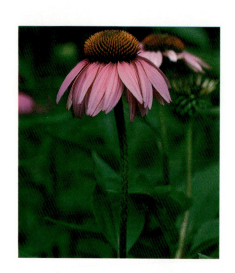
Echinacea purpurea (echinacea)

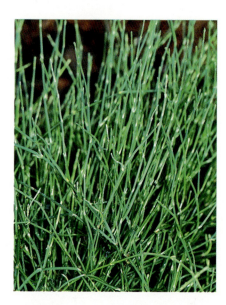
Ephedra sinica (ephedra, ma huang)

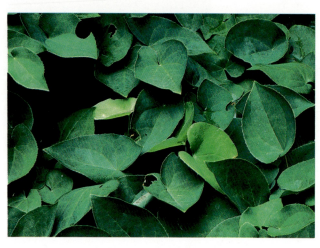
Epimedium spp. (horny goat weed)

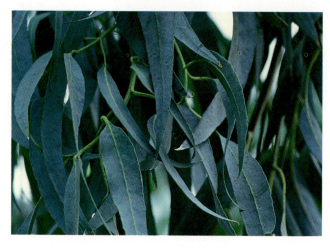
Eucalyptus globulus (eucalyptus)

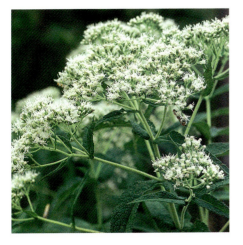
Eupatorium perfoliatum (boneset)

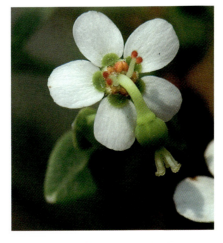
Euphorbia corollata (euphorbia, flowering spurge)

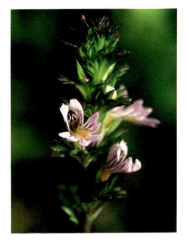
Euphrasia nemorosa (eyebright)

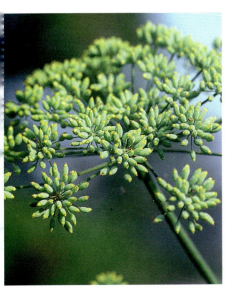
Foeniculum vulgare (fennel)

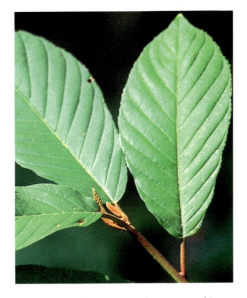
Frangula purshiana, syn. *Rhamnus purshiana* (cascara)

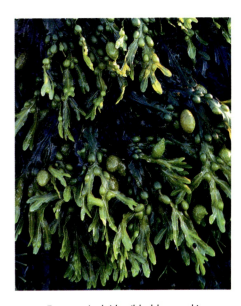
Fucus vesiculoides (bladderwrack)

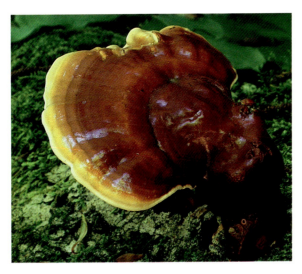
Ganoderma lucidum (reishi mushroom)

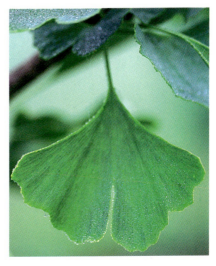
Ginkgo biloba (ginkgo)

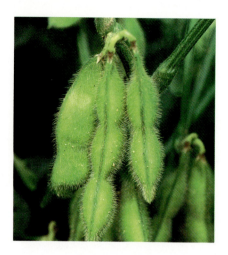
Glycine max (soy)

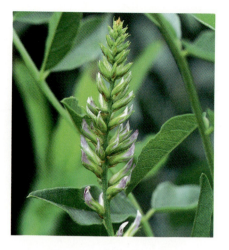
Glycyrrhiza glabra (licorice)

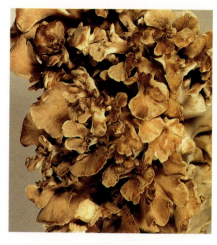
Grifola frondosa (maitake mushroom)

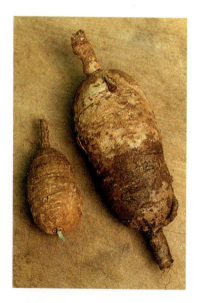
Harpagophytum procumbens (devil's claw)

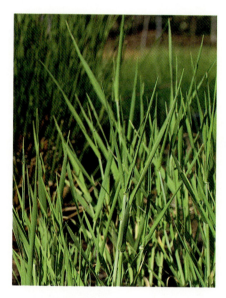
Hordeum vulgare (barley)

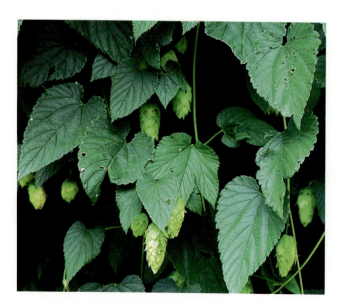
Humulus lupulus (hop)

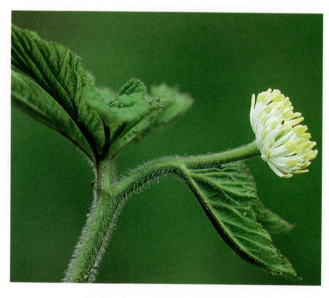
Hydrastis canadensis (goldenseal)

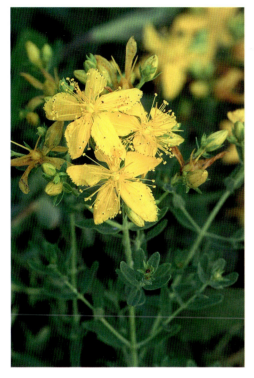
Hypericum perforatum (St. John's wort)

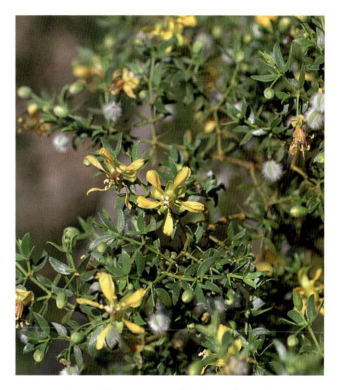
Larrea tridentate, Larrea divaricata (chaparral)

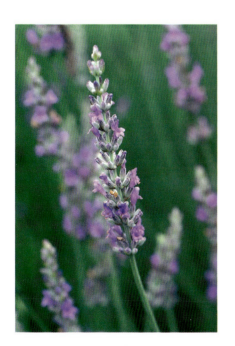
Lavandula angustifolia (lavender)

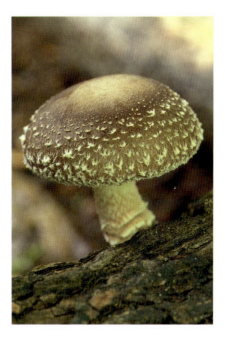
Lentinus edodes (shiitake mushroom)

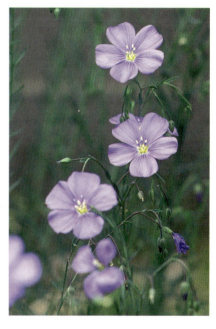
Linum usitatissimum (flax)

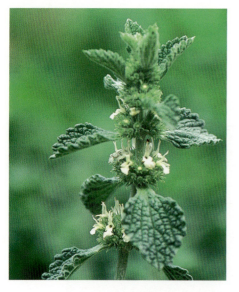
Marrubium vulgare (white horehound)

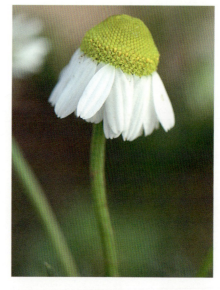
Matricaria recutita (German chamomile)

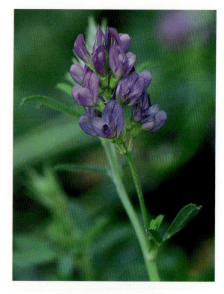
Medicago sativa (alfalfa)

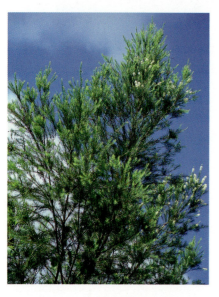
Melaleuca alternifolia (tea tree)

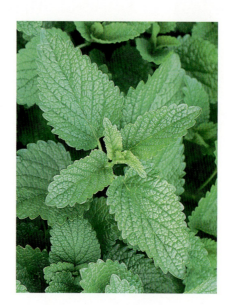
Melissa officinalis (lemon balm)

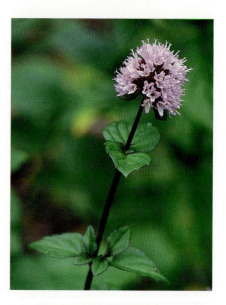
Mentha x *piperita* (peppermint)

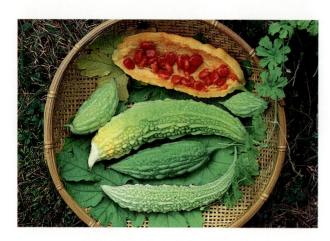
Momordica charantia (bitter melon)

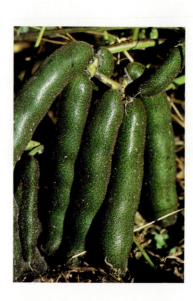
Mucuna pruriens (cowhage)

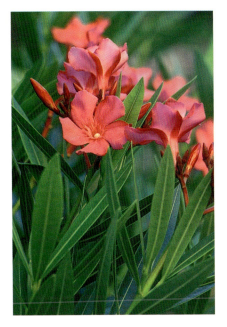
Nerium oleander, Thevetia peruviana (oleander)

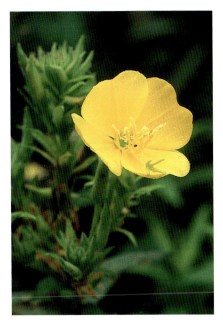
Oenothera biennis (evening primrose)

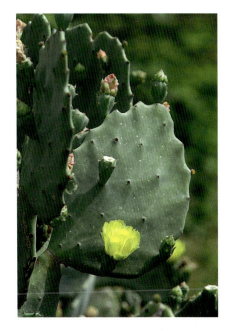
Opunita spp. (nopal)

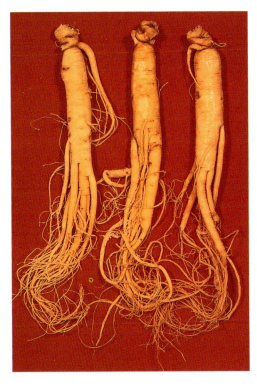
Panax ginseng (ginseng)

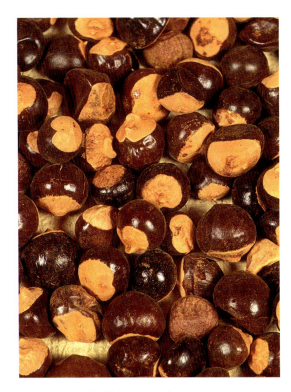
Paullinia cupana (guarana)

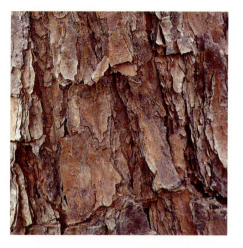
Pinus spp. (pine)

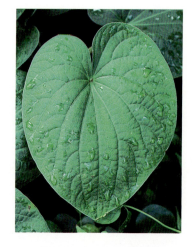
Piper methysticum (kava)

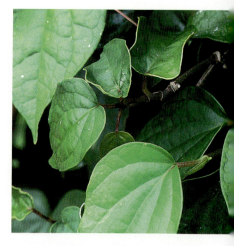
Piper nigrum (black pepper)

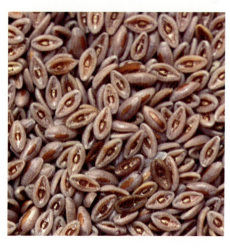
Plantago ovata (desert Indian wheat, blond psyllium)

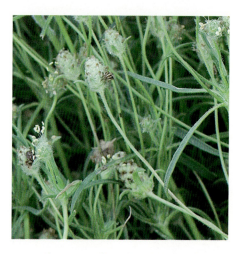
Plantago psyllium (sand plantain)

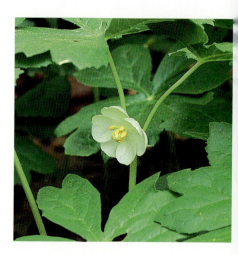
Podophyllum peltatum (mayapple)

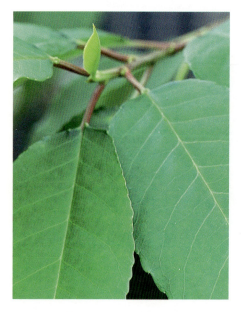
Prunus africana, syn. *Pygeum africanum* (pygeum)

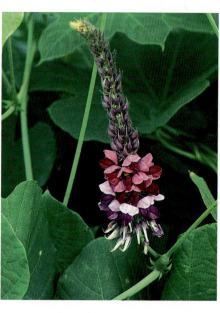
Pueraria lobata, syn. *Pueraria montana* (kudzu)

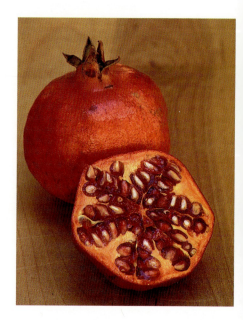
Punica granatum (pomegranate)

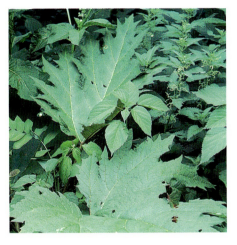
Rheum palmatum (rhubarb)

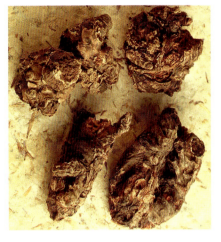
Rhodiola rosea (rhodiola)

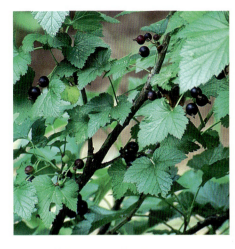
Ribes nigrum (black currant)

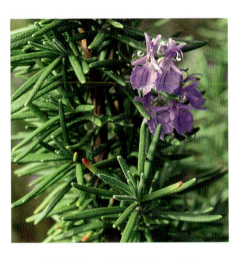
Rosmarinus officinalis (rosemary)

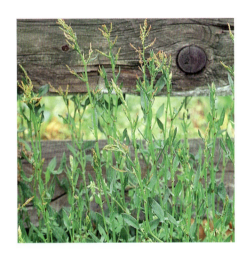
Rumex acetosella (sheep's sorrel)

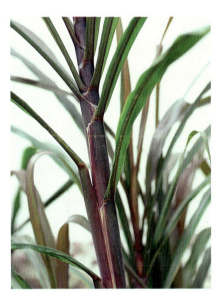
Saccharum officinarum (sugar cane)

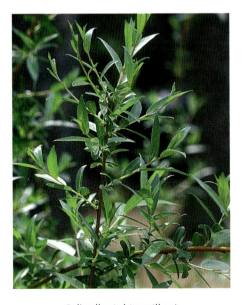
Salix alba (white willow)

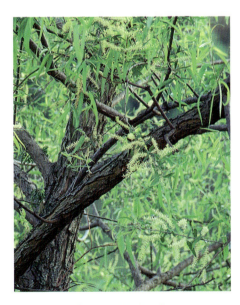
Salix nigra (black willow)

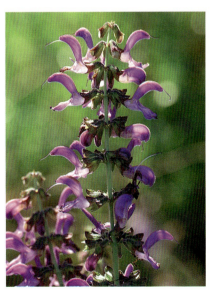
Salvia miltiorrhiza (danshen)

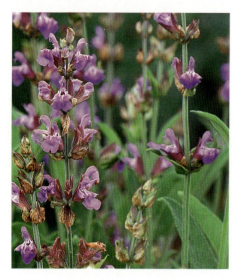

Salvia officinalis (sage)

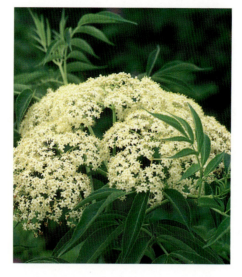

Sambucus nigra subsp *canadensis* (elderberry, American black elderberry)

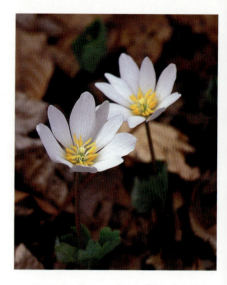

Sanguinaria canadensis (bloodroot)

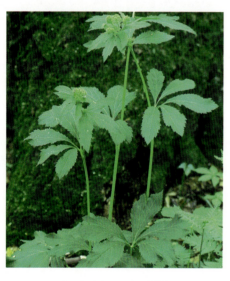

Sanicula spp. (sanicle)

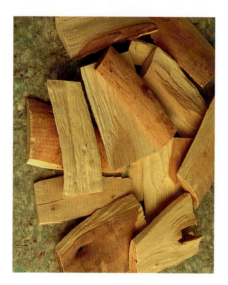

Santalum album (sandalwood)

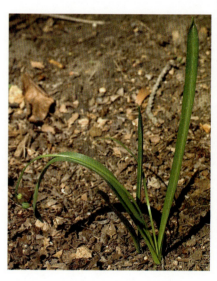

Scilla siberica (Siberian squill)

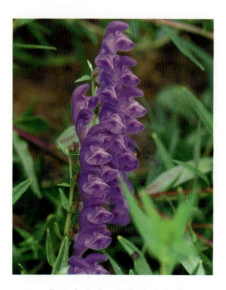

Scutellaria baicalensis (baikal skullcap)

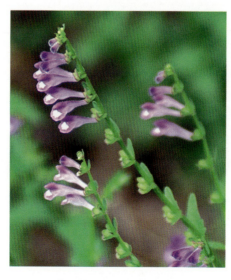

Scutellaria barbata (barbat skullcap)

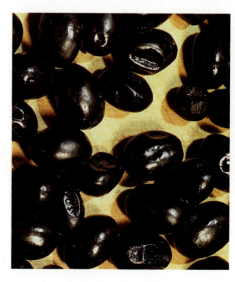

Serenoa repens (saw palmetto)

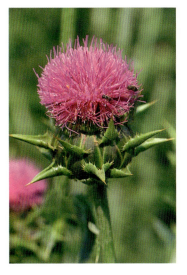
Silybum marianum (milk thistle)

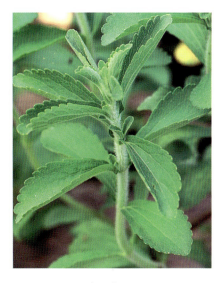
Stevia rebaudiana (stevia)

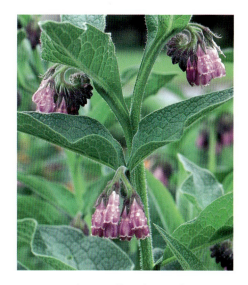
Symphytum officinale (comfrey)

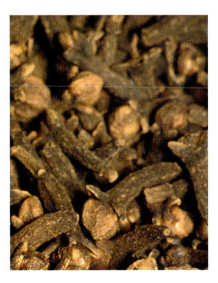
Syzygium aromaticum, syn. *Eugenia aromaticum* (clove)

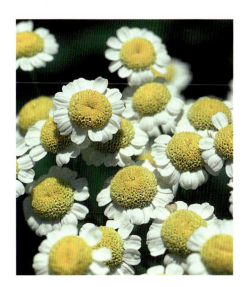
Tanacetum parthenium (feverfew)

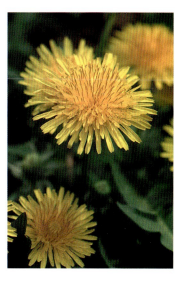
Taraxacum officinale (dandelion)

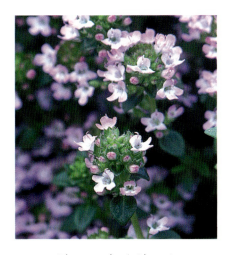
Thymus vulgaris (thyme)

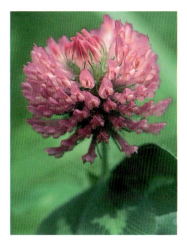
Trifolium pratense (red clover)

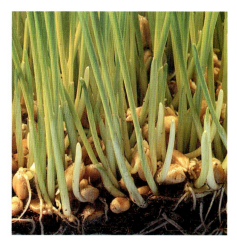
Triticum spp. (wheatgrass)

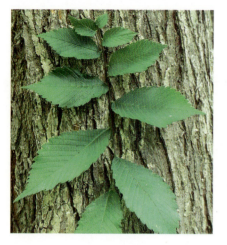
Ulmus rubra, syn. *Ulma fulva* (slippery elm)

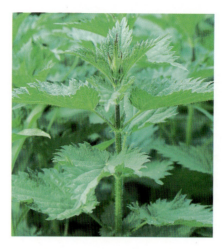
Urtica dioica (stinging nettle)

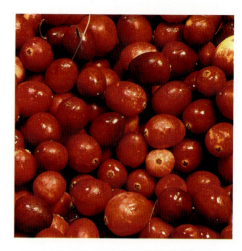
Vaccinium macrocarpon (cranberry)

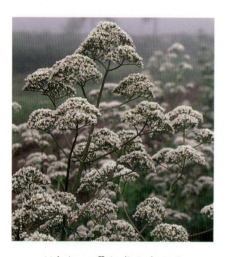
Valeriana officinalis (valerian)

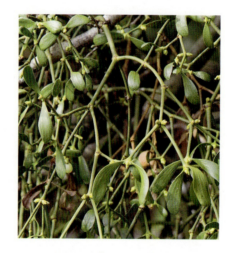
Viscum album (mistletoe)

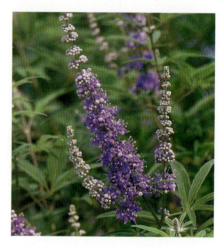
Vitex agnus-castus (chasteberry)

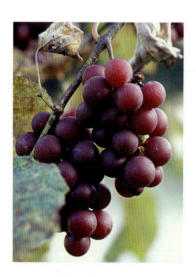
Vitis vinifera (grape)

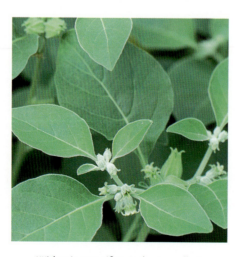
Withania somnifera (ashwagandha)

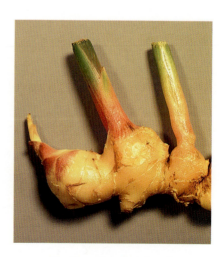
Zingiber officinale (ginger)

9. Menopausal women may experience a variety of psychological symptoms, such as depression, anxiety, stress, and insomnia. Depression may occur after or during the transition to menopause. During midlife and perimenopause, women may be more vulnerable to depression. *St. John's wort* may be beneficial in treating this psychological component of menopausal symptoms. *Cognitive-behavioral psychotherapy* may be used alone or with antidepressant agents to help women identify and change pessimistic thoughts and beliefs associated with depression. Many women also experience anxiety during perimenopause and menopause caused by hormonal imbalances, the condition itself, and life stresses. *Kava* may effectively treat symptoms of anxiety. Depression and anxiety disorders may lead to chronic insomnia. *Melatonin, lavender, chamomile,* and *valerian* are popular dietary supplements used for sleep. These products may help the individual to relax and may promote healthy sleep patterns.

INTEGRATIVE THERAPY PLAN

- Discuss the patient's medical, family, and social history. Inquire about the age of the patient's mother when she began menopause and what types of symptoms she experienced.
- Ensure that the patient has had a complete physical examination and appropriate laboratory testing, including lipid panel, glucose, bone density, mammogram, cancer screening, thyroid test, urine screens, and hormone levels.
- Ask detailed questions about the patient's menopausal symptoms, including hot flashes, night sweats, vaginal dryness, depression, anxiety, difficulty sleeping, joint pain, and weight gain.
- Review the patient's current medication use, including prescription and nonprescription drugs, herbs, and supplements, as well as alternative or complementary therapies. Ask about the patient's current or past use of hormone replacement therapy (HRT) and oral contraceptives.
- Discuss the benefits and short-term and long-term side effects of HRT.
- Weigh the potential benefits and risks, preferences, and needs before the patient begins HRT or natural therapy. Menopausal symptoms and therapeutic benefits and side effects vary greatly among women.
- Menopause is a popular reason for using herbal medicine. Several natural therapies show promise in reducing hot flashes. In general, studies evaluating phytoestrogens, including isoflavones, lignans, and coumestans, which are found in a variety of edible plants, may display both estrogenic and antiestrogenic effects. However, studies have been highly variable.
- Soy and red clover are sources of isoflavones. A reduction in menopausal symptoms, including hot flashes and vaginal dryness, has been reported with these isoflavones, but research is inconclusive. Data suggest that phytoestrogens are well tolerated. It is important to caution women that these herbs may have similar effects in the body as estrogen and therefore may carry some of the same potentially serious risks as HRT. There is some concern regarding cancer risk with isoflavones from soy and red clover. Patients who have or have had breast cancer should consult with their physician before supplementation. Soy allergy is a fairly common food allergy. Patients who have peanut allergies or asthma should avoid soy products.
- Black cohosh (*Actaea racemosa*, formerly known as *Cimicifuga racemosa*) is a popular alternative to hormonal therapy in the treatment of menopausal symptoms, such as hot flashes, mood disturbances, diaphoresis, palpitations, and vaginal dryness. Studies report that black cohosh improves menopausal symptoms for up to 6 months. Black cohosh is generally well tolerated, but liver damage has been reported with its use. Patients with liver disease should consult with their physician before using black cohosh.
- Recommend techniques to help women deal with hot flashes, such as wearing loose clothing and dressing in layers for removal during a hot flash; wearing fabrics that absorb moisture and dry quickly; avoiding foods (e.g., hot drinks, spicy foods) that may trigger hot flashes; splashing the face with cool water at the start of a hot flash; and avoiding stress.
- Advise the patient to use over-the-counter (OTC) water-based vaginal lubricants (Astroglide, K-Y) or moisturizers (Replens, Vagisil) to help relieve vaginal dryness associated with low estrogen levels such as in menopause.
- Discuss with the patient other changes that may occur, including urinary incontinence (leaking urine when coughing, sneezing, laughing, or exercise), breast enlargement or tenderness, thinning hair, electric shock sensation under the skin, tingling in extremities, and gum problems.
- Suggest that the patient keep a diary to record symptoms (frequency, duration, character, intensity, triggers).
- Monitor for response to therapy, as demonstrated by alleviation of symptoms and improvement in quality of life.
- Discuss lifestyle modifications with all menopausal women, including weight management, regular exercise, and smoking cessation.
- Emphasize the importance of eating a balanced diet that includes a variety of fruits, vegetables, and whole grains and that limits saturated fats, oils, and sugars.
- Urge the patient to establish a regular exercise program. Thirty minutes of moderate-intensity weight-bearing exercise on most days will help protect against cardiovascular disease, diabetes, osteoporosis, and other conditions associated with aging in women. Walking, jogging, and tennis are all examples of weight-bearing exercises.
- Postmenopausal women are especially susceptible to fractures of the hip, wrist, and spine. It is important for all women to intake adequate amounts of calcium and vitamin D.
- Postmenopausal women should ingest 1200 to 1500 mg of elemental calcium and 800 IU of vitamin D daily. Dietary

sources of calcium, including dairy products, salmon, and dark-green leafy vegetables, are also important to include as part of a healthy lifestyle.

Case Studies

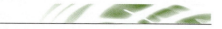

CASE STUDY 21-1

JR is a thin, 49-year-old female mail carrier who comes to the clinic with complaints of premenstrual discomfort and hot flashes once or twice daily lasting about a minute. She was recently prescribed gabapentin for migraines and has not had a migraine since starting therapy. However, gabapentin has not helped with the hot flashes. She drinks an herbal tea every night that contains peppermint, chamomile, and fennel to help with digestion. She recently had a hipbone mineral density test, which revealed a T-score of –0.8 (mild bone thinning). How should you counsel?

Answer: JR is currently perimenopausal and undergoing various menopausal symptoms. Hot flashes, premenstrual discomfort, and migraine headache can be related to hormonal imbalances and fluctuations. The isoflavones in soy and red clover are phytoestrogens and may act similar to estrogens. Studies suggest that these products may help relieve hot flashes, and they may be a reasonable option for JR. Soy products include tofu and soy milk. Phytoestrogen supplements are also available. Doses of 20 to 60 g of soy protein, providing 40 to 80 mg of isoflavones, have been used in research. Ensure that JR is not allergic to soy or peanuts.

The dose of gabapentin, prescribed for the migraines likely related to menopause, does not currently need to be altered because JR appears to be responding well to treatment.

JR is also at risk of developing osteoporosis, as evidenced by a less-than-ideal bone mineral density test. Menopause dramatically speeds up bone loss, and women who are risk should try to minimize and treat this loss. Successful treatment of osteoporosis usually involves a combination of lifestyle changes and supplements. Women such as JR should begin taking 1200 to 1500 mg of calcium daily. To receive enough calcium, JR should eat a well-balanced diet that includes dairy and other calcium-rich products and should take a daily calcium supplement. JR also needs to take vitamin D; her daily intake should be 400 to 800 IU/day. Bones may remain stronger if they are used in exercise, especially weight-bearing activities. Exercise may also help with menopausal hot flashes.

Interactions among these various agents, including the peppermint, chamomile, and fennel in her herbal tea, are not well understood. JR should be aware of any unusual symptoms or side effects.

CASE STUDY 21-2

TH is a 55-year-old woman with a history of hypothyroidism and hyperlipidemia who takes levothyroxine (Synthroid, 100 mcg) and atorvastatin (Lipitor, 10 mg) daily. She presents to the clinic where you are the clinical pharmacist, complaining of hot flashes and depression. On her daughter's recommendation, TH recently began taking valerian root for her sleep problems caused by the hot flashes, but she uses this herb inconsistently. TH asks you if there are any natural remedies for menopausal symptoms and depression. She has been considering trying St. John's wort (SJW) for the depression. How do you counsel TH?

Answer: Women experience menopause differently, and it is not always clear which symptoms are caused by the condition. Hot flashes are common in women undergoing menopause and are usually accompanied by night sweats. TH is currently taking valerian to treat her sleep difficulties. Several studies have shown that valerian improves sleep quality and reduces time to fall asleep, but there is a lack of evidence in the population of menopausal women. Several studies, however, report a benefit in menopausal symptoms with the use of black cohosh, which may be a reasonable option for TH.

TH is also experiencing symptoms of depression during midlife, which may or may not be caused by menopause itself. At this time of life, it is common for women to feel symptoms of depression because of life stressors and role changes. SJW is a natural product used for depression. Notably, the combination of black cohosh and SJW may improve various menopausal symptoms, including hot flashes and psychological symptoms.

Many symptoms of menopause overlap with symptoms of depression, including difficulty sleeping and physical symptoms such as fatigue and anxiety. TH may want to try black cohosh before SJW to see if any depressive symptoms improve by taking one product. If her depressive symptoms continue, she may consider adding SJW to her medication regimen. Liver function tests should be performed because of the potential black cohosh–atorvastatin interaction. Black cohosh has been associated with hepatotoxicity and may inhibit cytochrome P450 3A4. Inhibition of cytochrome P3A4 by black cohosh could elevate levels of atorvastatin, increasing liver enzymes.

TH is also taking levothyroxine. Although evidence of an interaction between black cohosh or SJW and levothyroxine is not clear, thyroid function should be monitored when adding a new agent. Liver function should also be assessed during treatment with black cohosh, which has been linked to cases of liver damage. Remind TH to have her thyroid function monitored regularly.

Photosensitivity is a rare reaction that may occur with SJW. Advise TH to use sunscreen when taking this herb. Also, ensure that TH is having her lipid profiles monitored, and emphasize the importance of a healthy diet and regular exercise.

CASE STUDY 21-3

RW is a 48-year-old, slightly overweight woman who comes to the clinic complaining of feeling sweaty and overheated at bedtime. The symptoms began 6 months ago, and she tried taking black cohosh. After 3 months, her symptoms did not improve, so RW tried taking phytoestrogens, but she is still experiencing night sweats. She is frustrated and asks for your advice. She does not take any other medication; however, she smokes a pack of cigarettes a day. How should you counsel?

Answer: Black cohosh and phytoestrogens have been credited for reducing the frequency of hot flashes. Another option may be dong quai, which has been used in China for menopausal symptoms. Although studies evaluating dong quai alone have not shown a significant benefit, it may have a synergistic effect when used with other natural remedies such as soy.

It is also important to discuss lifestyle measures with RW to help minimize hot flashes, including weight management and regular exercise. Emphasize the importance of eating a balanced diet that includes a variety of fruits, vegetables, and whole grains and that limits saturated fats, oils, and sugars. Advise RW to take a multivitamin and get at least 30 minutes of moderate-intensity physical activity daily. Smoking cessation is also an important step to enhancing health. These lifestyle measures may reduce menopausal symptoms and can help reduce the risk of cardiovascular disease, osteoporosis, and cancer.

References for Chapter 21 can be found on the Evolve website at http://evolve.elsevier.com/Ulbricht/herbalpharmacotherapy/

Review Questions

1. All the following statements regarding black cohosh are true *except*:
   a. Studies on the effects of black cohosh on estrogen receptors remain controversial.
   b. The German Commission E has approved black cohosh for perimenopausal symptoms.
   c. Clinical research shows that black cohosh combined with kava improves climacteric complaints as well as psychological disorders.
   d. Cases of liver damage have been reported with black cohosh use.

2. What is the recommended dose of Remifemin (black cohosh) for perimenopausal symptoms?
   a. 20 to 40 mcg once daily
   b. 20 to 40 mg twice daily
   c. 2 to 4 g twice daily
   d. 200 to 400 mg twice daily

3. True or false: Phytoestrogens are chemical structures resembling endogenous estrogens that exert estrogenic and antiestrogenic effects.

4. According to available research, what dose of soy isoflavones may be effective in relieving menopausal symptoms?
   a. 20 to 60 g of soy protein providing 40 to 80 mg of isoflavones
   b. 2 to 6 g of soy protein providing 4 to 8 mg of isoflavones
   c. 20 to 60 mg of soy protein providing 40 to 80 mg of isoflavones
   d. 40 to 80 mg of soy protein providing 20 to 60 mcg of isoflavones

5. True or false: A vaginal cream containing red clover has been used to treat dysmenorrhea, hot flashes, and headaches associated with menopause.

6. All the following statements are true *except*:
   a. Dong quai may increase sun sensitivity and risk of severe skin reactions.
   b. The brand of soy isoflavone extract used in most trials and most available commercially is Promensil.
   c. A dose of 40 g of flaxseed was shown to be as effective as oral estrogen-progesterone replacement to improve mild menopausal symptoms.
   d. Literature review reveals no evidence that evening primrose oil is useful in the management of symptoms associated with menopause.

7. Sage has been used with which of the following agents to reduce symptoms of menopause?
   a. Black cohosh
   b. Alfalfa
   c. Red clover
   d. Soy

8. Black cohosh may interact with which of the following?
   a. Fluoxetine
   b. Enalapril
   c. Ketoconazole
   d. All the above

9. What is the recommended daily elemental calcium and vitamin D intake for postmenopausal women?
   a. 12 mg calcium and 800 IU vitamin D
   b. 1200 mg calcium and 800 IU vitamin D
   c. 1200 mcg calcium and 800 mg vitamin D
   d. None of the above

10. True or false: St. John's wort may reduce psychological and psychosomatic symptoms, including depression, associated with perimenopause or menopause.

Answers are found in the Answers to Review Questions section in the back of the text.

22 Osteoporosis

Outline

OVERVIEW
 Signs and Symptoms
 Diagnosis
SELECTED HERBAL THERAPIES
 Horny Goat Weed (*Epimedium grandiflorum*)
 Horsetail (*Equisetum* spp.)
 Red Clover (*Trifolium pratense*)
 Soy (*Glycine max*)
 Tea (*Camellia sinensis*)

HERBAL THERAPIES WITH LIMITED EVIDENCE
ADJUNCT THERAPIES
INTEGRATIVE THERAPY PLAN
CASE STUDIES
REVIEW QUESTIONS

Learning Objectives

- Recognize the signs and symptoms of osteoporosis, and cite current diagnostic strategies.
- Discuss the herbal products used to reduce fracture risk and bone loss, and the evidence supporting their use.
- Describe the mechanisms of action, adverse effects, and interactions associated with herbs used to treat and prevent osteoporosis.
- Provide an integrative care plan for patients with osteoporosis, or those seeking to prevent osteoporosis.

OVERVIEW

Osteoporosis is a condition in which bones have decreased density and altered structure, which weakens them such that they are prone to fractures (Figure 22-1). Osteoporosis is considered a "silent" disease because bone loss itself is gradual and painless; symptoms may not become apparent until the bones weaken to the point of fracture.[1-5]

In the United States about 8 million women and 2 million men have osteoporosis.[3-5] Those over age 50 are at greatest risk of osteoporosis and related fractures. In this age group, 1 in 2 women and 1 in 6 men will have an osteoporosis-related fracture at some point in their lives.[1-5]

Osteoporosis can occur at any age, in all ethnic groups, and in both sexes, although it is much more common in women. The incidence of osteoporosis increases with age and is more common among individuals with slender frames, such as Asians and Scandinavians. Africans and African Americans are genetically endowed with denser bones; thus it takes longer for their bone mass to decrease to the level of osteoporosis.[1-5] Calcium is generally considered the most important dietary component in osteoporosis prevention (Table 22-1). Because vitamin D and calcium are essential for healthy bones, malnourished individuals, including those with eating disorders, may also develop osteoporosis.[6] Prevention of osteoporosis includes various areas of treatment (Figure 22-2).

Three main cell types make up bone: osteoblasts, osteocytes, and osteoclasts. *Osteoblasts* are the cells primarily responsible for new bone formation and its mineralization. They are balanced by the activity of *osteoclasts*, which are responsible for breaking down old bone in a process called *resorption*. *Osteocytes* are calcified osteoblasts that make up the hard part of the bone structure. In normal bones there is a regulated balance between the activity of cells that create bone and those that break it down, a process called *bone remodeling*.

Healthy bone remains stable because osteoblasts and osteoclasts are working at a similar rate, allowing bone to remodel continuously and heal when damaged. If osteoclast activity outpaces osteoblast activity, however, bones become weakened. In other words, if bone resorption is greater than bone formation, bone loss occurs.

By their mid-30s, most men and women gradually begin to lose bone strength. When bones become less dense and

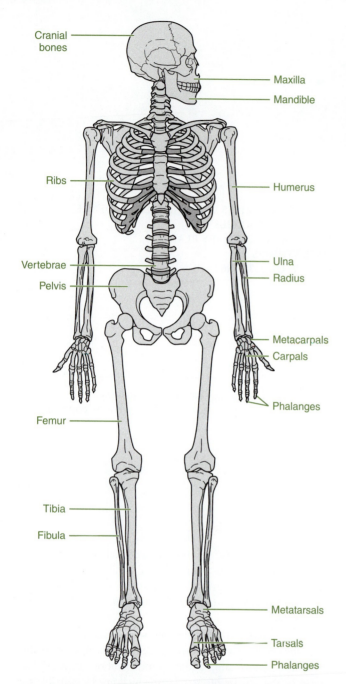

Figure 22-1 The human skeleton. (Modified from Damjanov I: *Pathology for the health professions*, ed 3, St Louis, 2006, Saunders-Elsevier.)

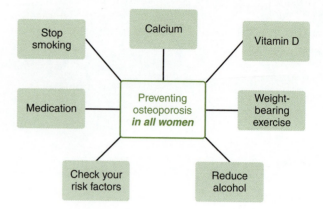

Figure 22-2 Osteoporosis prevention chart. (From www.womenshealthcareforum.com.)

TABLE 22-1	Daily Calcium Requirements
AGE (YEARS)	DAILY CALCIUM REQUIREMENT
4 to 8	800 mg
9 to 18	1300 mg
19 to 50	1000 mg
50+	1500 mg
Pregnant or lactating women 18+	1000 mg

From Osteoporosis Canada, www.osteoporosis.ca

structurally weaker, the condition is known as *osteopenia*. Osteopenia refers to mild bone loss that is not as severe as osteoporosis. Individuals with osteopenia are at increased risk of developing osteoporosis. As the condition progresses, bones lose calcium, phosphorus, boron, and other minerals, and bones become lighter, less dense, and more porous. If untreated, osteopenia can progress painlessly to osteoporosis, increasing the likelihood of fracture. Although any bone is susceptible to fracture, the most common fractures in osteoporosis occur at the spine, wrists, and hips. Spine and hip fractures in particular may lead to chronic pain, long-term disability, and even death.[1-5]

Extracellular levels of calcium, vitamin D, and certain hormones are key factors in bone remodeling. *Parathyroid hormone* (PTH, parathormone) enhances the release of calcium and stimulates bone resorption and formation. *Estrogen* is thought to have a direct effect on bone cells; it enhances bone formation by stimulating the estrogen receptors, which are located on the osteoblasts. A direct link exists between the estrogen loss after menopause and the development of osteoporosis. Low hormone levels that occur in early menopause can significantly increase the risk of osteoporosis. Using antiinflammatory corticosteroids may also significantly impact bone health. These drugs are often taken by women over 55 for conditions such as arthritis, and are known to directly lead to bone loss.[1-5] An estimated 20% of all osteoporosis cases may be attributed to corticosteroid use.[3-5]

Although often regarded as a condition of older individuals, osteoporosis can occur at any age. In rare cases, osteoporosis can affect children (a condition known as *juvenile osteoporosis*); it is usually secondary to other medical conditions, including thyroid abnormalities and Cushing's disease (a rare condition involving insufficient adrenal hormone output). Use of certain medications, such as corticosteroids, can also contribute to juvenile osteoporosis. Because the bone loss occurs during the prime bone-building years, juvenile osteoporosis may lead to severe consequences later in life.[1-5]

Signs and Symptoms

Once bones have been weakened by osteoporosis, signs and symptoms may include fractures (usually wrists, hips, or vertebrae) and back pain, which can be severe if a vertebra has fractured or collapsed. Some fractures are obvious, as in the wrist or hip, but fractures in the spinal cord can be more difficult to diagnose. Spinal fractures may be painless, and even if pain occurs from a vertebral fracture, it might be attributed to another cause. More obvious signs of spinal fractures are reduced height and *kyphosis* (curved upper spine, sometimes called "dowager's hump").

Diagnosis[1-5,7]

The diagnosis of osteoporosis involves an initial physical examination, various x-rays to detect skeletal problems, laboratory studies on metabolic process of bone breakdown and formation, and a bone density test.

Laboratory tests may include serum calcium and vitamin D levels, which are good indicators of bone resorption. Because hormones play major roles in the regulation of bone remodeling, tests may also be performed to measure thyroid function, PTH levels, estradiol levels (in women), follicle-stimulating hormone (FSH), luteinizing hormone (LH) to establish menopause status, testosterone levels (in men), and osteocalcin levels. Urine tests include a 24-hour collection to measure calcium metabolism.

Bone mineral density (BMD) testing measures the amount of calcium in the bones and is one of the best predictors of fracture risk (Table 22-2). Dual-energy x-ray absorptiometry (DEXA) is the "gold standard" for osteoporosis diagnosis. Physicians generally do not recommend osteoporosis screening for men because it is much less common than in women; however, BMD testing may be performed in men if other underlying conditions are present that may promote bone loss. The National Osteoporosis Foundation recommends a BMD test in women if they are not taking estrogen and if they are taking medications such as corticosteroids (e.g., prednisone) that can cause osteoporosis; have type 1 diabetes, liver disease, kidney disease, or family history of osteoporosis; experience early menopause; are postmenopausal (older than 50) and have at least one risk factor for osteoporosis; or older than 65 and have never had a BMD test.[5]

The DEXA measurements are compared to the BMD of young, healthy individuals, resulting in a measurement called a *T-score*. If the T-score is −2.5 or lower, the individual is considered to have osteoporosis and therefore is at high risk for fracture. Individuals with T-scores between −1.0 and −2.5 are generally considered to have osteopenia. The risk of fractures is generally lower in patients with osteopenia than in those with osteoporosis, but if bone loss continues, the fracture risk increases.

TABLE 22-2 Bone Mineral Density (BMD) Results and Treatment

T-SCORES		BMD CATEGORY	WHEN TO CONSIDER TREATMENT WITH OSTEOPOROSIS MEDICATION
POSSIBLE SCORES	SCORE RANGE		
+1.0 +0.5 0 −0.5 −1.0	−1 and higher	Normal BMD	Most individuals with T-scores of −1 or higher do not need to consider medication.
−1.1* −1.5 −2.0 −2.4*	−1.1 to −2.4	Low BMD (osteopenia)	Individuals with T-scores between −1.0 and −2.5 should consider a medication when certain risk factors are present.
−2.5 −3.0 −3.5 −4.0	−2.5 and lower	Osteoporosis	All individuals with osteoporosis should consider medication.

Data from The National Osteoporosis Foundation (NOF) and The World Health Organization.
*To help understand osteopenia, NOF has presented the T-scores differently than in its clinical guidelines.

Radiographic studies may be performed to show the alignment of the spine and to detect degenerative joint disease or fractures. However, x-rays cannot accurately determine BMD. Radiographs are also appropriate if a person has experienced a loss of height or change in posture.

SELECTED HERBAL THERAPIES

Note

To help make this educational resource more interactive, all pharmacokinetics, adverse effects, and interactions data have been compiled in Appendix A. Safety data specifically related to pregnancy and lactation are listed in Appendix B. Please refer to these appendices when working through the case studies and answering the review questions.

Horny Goat Weed *(Epimedium grandiflourm)*

Grade C: *Unclear or conflicting scientific evidence (osteoporosis prevention)*

Mechanism of Action

The mechanism of horny goat weed in osteoporosis is not well understood. However, flavonoids in horny goat weed, such as icariin, appear to stimulate osteoblasts, which are the principal cells involved in bone formation.[8]

Scientific Evidence of Effectiveness

According to animal research, flavonoid extracts of horny goat weed may protect against osteoporosis.[9] Preliminary clinical evidence suggests flavonoids derived from *Epimedium brevicornum* may prevent bone loss in late postmenopausal women and may have benefits against osteoporosis.[10] After 2 years of supplementation, BMD at the hip (femoral neck) and lower spine (lumbar) increased by 1.6% and 1.3%, respectively, for the *E. brevicornum* group and decreased by 1.8% and 2.4% for the placebo group. The study also reported that supplementation with *E. brevicornum* significantly decreased levels of deoxypyridinoline (a marker of bone resorption) by 39% after 2 years. Changes to the uterus were not observed despite concerns.

Dose

In one clinical study, late postmenopausal women received a daily dose of *Epimedium brevicornum* consisting of 60 mg icariin, 15 mg daidzein, and 3 mg genistein for 24 months. Patients also received 300 mg elemental calcium daily.[10] The dose of horny goat weed as a monotherapy is unclear.

Adverse Effects, Interactions, Pharmacokinetics. See Appendix A.

Horsetail (*Equisetum* spp.)

Grade C: *Unclear or conflicting scientific evidence (osteoporosis)*

Mechanism of Action

Animal and in vitro studies suggest that *silicon* plays a role in bone development[1,11] and may increase the rate of bone mineralization and enhance calcium deposition in bone. Because it contains silicon, horsetail has been hypothesized to be an effective natural treatment for osteoporosis.

Scientific Evidence of Effectiveness

In a randomized controlled trial (RCT), 122 women received placebo, no treatment, horsetail dry extract (a horsetail-calcium combination used in Italy for osteoporosis and fractures; dose not specified), or calcium (270 mg) twice daily (a horsetail-calcium combination used in Italy for osteoporosis and fractures).[12] After 40, 80, and 365 days, a statistically significant improvement in bone density was reported in both the horsetail and the calcium group, with an average improvement of 2.3% in vertebral BMD in the calcium group. Although effects of horsetail on BMD were equivalent to the effects of calcium, well-designed clinical trials are needed before a recommendation can be made.

Dose

The dose of horsetail as a monotherapy for osteoporosis has not been determined.

Adverse Effects, Interactions, Pharmacokinetics. See Appendix A.

Red Clover (*Trifolium pratense*)

Grade C: *Unclear or conflicting scientific evidence (osteoporosis)*

Mechanism of Action

Isoflavones such as those found in red clover are considered to be *phytoestrogens,* plant compounds structurally similar to estradiol and capable of binding to estradiol receptors. Isoflavones have a varying affinity for the estradiol receptors alpha and beta and are capable of acting as both agonists and antagonists.[13] Some evidence suggests a preferential binding to estrogen receptor beta (found in bone) as opposed to estrogen receptor alpha (found in the ovaries, breast, uterus, and adrenal glands). Red clover may slow bone loss and protect against osteoporosis because of its estrogen-like properties.

Scientific Evidence of Effectiveness

It is unclear to what extent bone loss is affected by dietary isoflavones, such as those in red clover. Most studies investigating isoflavones and bone metabolism have used soy products,[14-16] which have a higher concentration of the isoflavones genistein and daidzein than red clover. Soy also contains other potentially active ingredients, such as saponins, pectins, and essential fatty acids.

Red clover supplementation has been shown to increase BMD by 4.1% over 6 months in subjects taking 57 mg daily. Subjects taking 85.5 mg had a 3% increase in BMD.[14] Additionally, loss of lumbar spine BMD was reduced in women after 12 months of treatment with red clover isoflavone supplement.[16]

Dose

Doses of 57 and 85.5 mg of red clover isoflavones daily (Rimostil, containing genistein, daidzein, formonetin, and biochanin) for 6 months increased BMD in postmenopausal women.[16]

Adverse Effects, Interactions, Phamacokinetics. See Appendix A.

Soy (*Glycine max*)

Grade C: *Unclear or conflicting scientific evidence (osteoporosis/postmenopausal bone loss)*

Mechanism of Action

The main isoflavones in soy are genistein and daidzein and their respective beta glycosides, genistin and daidzin. The structure and function of isoflavones are similar to 17β-estradiol. Laboratory and animal studies have shown that isoflavones affect bone health in various ways, acting on both osteoblasts and osteoclasts through genomic and nongenomic mechanisms.[17-25] In vitro, in vivo, and clinical studies suggest that genistein and daidzein suppress osteoclast activity by induction of apoptosis, cytokine inhibition, protein tyrosine phosphate activation, and changes in calcium and membrane depolarization.[19,20,22,24,25] Osteoblasts secrete bone-forming proteins, including osteocalcin and alkaline phosphatase, and are capable of synthesizing cytokines such as interleukin-6 and osteoprotegrin.[18,25]

Scientific Evidence of Effectiveness

Results are mixed regarding the effects of soy on postmenopausal bone loss. Soy isoflavones appear to have beneficial effects on BMD, bone turnover markers, and bone mechanical strength in postmenopausal women in some,[26-33] but not all, available studies.[34-36] There are differences in study design and in estrogen status, isoflavone metabolism, and other dietary factors among women.[26,32,37] Also, BMD changes occur slowly over time. It is therefore difficult to draw a conclusion from studies lasting less than 1 year.

Dose

For osteoporosis prevention, oral doses of 60 to 126 mg of soy isoflavones have been used daily. Soy isoflavone supplementation has been found to be beneficial after 6 months of use and has been used safely up to 2 years.[31,34]

Adverse Effects, Interactions, Phamacokinetics. See Appendix A.

Tea (Camellia sinensis)

Grade C: *Unclear or conflicting scientific evidence (osteoporosis prevention)*

Mechanism of Action

Black tea may slow bone loss and protect against osteoporosis because of its estrogen-like properties. Black tea appears to increase serum estradiol level, reduce bone turnover, and increase bone mineral density.[38] The antioxidant effects of green and black tea may also help protect bone.

Scientific Evidence of Effectiveness

Preliminary research showed that elderly women who drank tea (green or black tea) had higher BMD in their hips and less bone loss than women who did not drink tea. Researchers surveyed 275 women between ages 70 and 85 participating in a cross-sectional 5-year study of calcium supplements and osteoporosis. BMD was measured in the trochanter, a bony prominence on the upper femur, which is a common site of hip fracture. Measurements were taken at the start and the end of the 5-year study. Women who were regular tea drinkers (75% of women in the study) had higher total bone density and higher trochanter density of the hip compared with non–tea drinkers. However, a relationship between the number of cups of tea consumed per day and BMD was not found.[39]

Notably, high amounts of caffeine have been associated with bone loss and increased urinary calcium excretion[40,41] and have been considered a risk factor for fractures.[42] Calcium supplementation has been suggested to counteract the effects of high caffeine consumption.[43-45]

Dose

The dose of black or green tea to reduce bone loss has not been determined.

Adverse Effects, Interactions, Phamacokinetics. See Appendix A.

HERBAL THERAPIES WITH LIMITED EVIDENCE

Black Cohosh (Actaea racemosa, formerly Cimicifuga racemosa)

Black cohosh is one of the top-selling herbs in the United States and is popular as an alternative to hormonal therapy in the treatment of menopausal (climacteric) symptoms. Isopropanolic extract of black cohosh has been shown to diminish significantly the urinary content of pyridinoline and deoxypyridinoline, specific markers for bone loss, in animal study. The triterpenoid glycoside 25-acetylcimigenol xylopyranoside (ACCX), found in black cohosh, has been shown to block osteoclastogenesis induced by tumor necrosis factor alpha (TNF-α) both in vitro and in vivo.[46]

Onion (Allium cepa)

Onion is used worldwide for food and also for medicinal applications. Animal research has found that gamma-L-glutamyl-*trans*-S-1-propenyl-L-cysteine sulfoxide from the onion family inhibits bone resorption in a dose-dependent manner.[47] Clinical studies are lacking.

Sage (Salvia officinalis)

Sage has been used in Europe for centuries as a spice and as medicine.[48] There are many different species of sage, with some reports describing more than 500 species. It is popularly used for cognitive and mood improvement. In animals, sage was found to inhibit bone resorption when added to food.[49] The mechanism for this effect has not been thoroughly elucidated, and clinical studies are lacking.

ADJUNCT THERAPIES

1. *Calcium* is consistently found to be the most important nutrient for attaining and maintaining peak bone mass and preventing osteoporosis.[1-7] However, adequate *vitamin D* intake is also important because it is required for optimal calcium absorption. Adequate consumption of both calcium and vitamin D is essential for the prevention of bone loss in general, including postmenopausal osteoporosis. Calcium intake of 1200 mg daily is recommended for adults older than 50; 600 to 800 IU of vitamin D daily is

Herbs That May Help Prevent or Reduce Bone Loss*

HERB	SPECIFIC THERAPEUTIC USE(S)†	HERB	SPECIFIC THERAPEUTIC USE(S)†
Anise	Osteoporosis prevention	Maca	Osteoporosis (postmenopausal)
Barberry	Osteoporosis	Mistletoe	Osteoporosis
Chamomile	Osteoporosis	Papain	Osteochondrosis, osteoporosis
Chicory	Osteoporosis	Perilla	Osteoporosis
Dong quai	Osteoporosis	Policosanol	Postmenopausal osteoporosis
Fennel	Bone loss (inhibition of bone resorption)	Pycnogenol	Osteoporosis
Folate	Osteoporosis	Raspberry	Osteoporosis prevention
Goji	Osteoporosis	Rosemary	Osteoporosis
Goldenseal, berberine	Osteoporosis	Shiitake	Osteoporosis
Hop	Osteoporosis	Wasabi	Osteoporosis
Kudzu	Osteoporosis	Wild yam	Osteoporosis

*This is not an all-inclusive or comprehensive list of herbs that may help prevent or reduce bone loss; other herbs and supplements may possess these qualities. A qualified health care provider should be consulted with specific questions or concerns regarding the potential adverse effects of agents or interactions with other therapies.
†Based on expert opinion, anecdote, case reports, and/or preliminary trial evidence.

recommended for those over age 60. Approximately 73% of calcium in the food supply comes from dairy products, with 9% from fruits and vegetables, 5% from grain products, and 12% from other sources, including dietary supplements. Milk and milk products are calcium-rich foods that provide about 300 mg of calcium per serving. These foods also contain other nutrients important to bone health, such as vitamin D (if fortified), phosphorus, and magnesium. Sun exposure of 15 minutes a day to hands and face also helps the body make vitamin D.

2. The recommended dietary allowance (RDA) for calcium is 1000 mg daily for adults younger than 50 (except pregnant or lactating women) and children older than 4 years. Adequate intake (AI) recommendations published in August 1997 were set at 1000 mg for men and women age 19 to 50 years and 1200 mg for adults older than 50.
3. Exercise can help prevent osteoporosis and maintain bone strength. Weight-bearing aerobic activities (in which the bones support body weight) have been shown to help maintain and increase bone mass and prevent osteoporosis. These activities include weightlifting, walking, jogging, hiking, stair climbing, step aerobics, dancing, racquet sports, and other activities that require muscles to work against gravity. Swimming, cycling, and water aerobics, although good for cardiovascular fitness, are not the best exercises for building bone because they are not considered weight-bearing activities. Individuals who live a sedentary lifestyle have weaker bones and are at higher risk of sustaining fractures. Physical activities, including tai chi and yoga, may also be included in a patient's exercise program. Supervised or home-based physical therapy, used in combination with resistance and endurance training, may help improve bone density.
4. *Estrogen therapy*, either alone or in combination with *progestin*, has been reported to decrease the risk of osteoporosis and osteoporotic fractures in women. However, the combination of estrogen with progestin has been shown to increase the risk for breast and ovarian cancer, strokes, heart attacks, and blood clots (see Chapter 21). Health care professionals recommend weighing all options before choosing hormone replacement therapy (HRT) as part of osteoporosis prevention or treatment.

INTEGRATIVE THERAPY PLAN

- Identify the patient's risk factors for osteoporosis, including age, gender (more common in women than men), family history of osteoporosis, body weight (low body weight and small bones), race and ethnicity (Caucasian, Asian, and Latino people are at higher risk), history of broken bones, menopause status, diet, activity level, smoking, and alcohol use (Figure 22-3).
- Discuss the patient's past medical history, including diseases that may increase the risk of osteoporosis, including thyroid disease, diabetes mellitus, cystic fibrosis, cancer, and renal disease.
- Ask what medications the patient is taking. Drugs that may affect bone strength include steroids, anticonvulsants, antipsychotics, furosemide, and heparin.
- Recommend bone mineral density (BMD) testing for women age 65 and older and men 70 and older. Women and men age 50 to 70 who are at risk for developing osteoporosis should undergo BMD testing to establish a baseline T-score. BMD testing is usually performed about every 2 years.

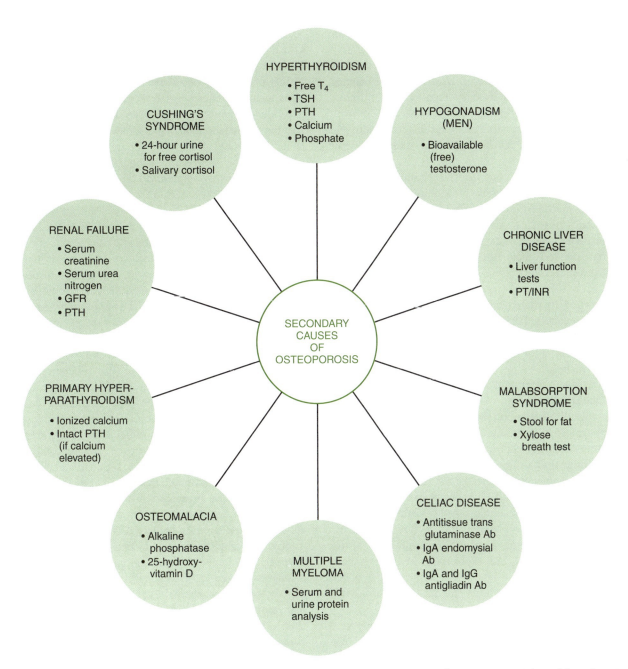

Figure 22-3 Recommended tests in selected patients for the evaluation of secondary causes of osteoporosis. (Adapted from American Medical Directors Association, *Osteoporosis and fracture prevention in the long-term care setting clinical practice guideline*, Columbia, MD, 2009, AMDA.)

- Osteoporosis treatment should be initiated in postmenopausal women and in men 50 years and older who have low bone mass or osteopenia; a T-score of −1.0 to −2.5 at the femoral neck, total hip, or spine; and a 10-year hip fracture probability of 3% or more or a 10-year all major osteoporosis–related fracture probability of 20% or more based on the United States–adapted World Health Organization (WHO) Absolute Fracture Risk model.
- Pharmacological options currently approved by the U.S. Food and Drug Administration (FDA) include the bisphosphonates, such as alendronate (Fosamax), ibandronate (Boniva), risedronate (Actonel), and zoledronate (Zometa).
- Hormone-related treatments include calcitonin, estrogens or hormone therapy, raloxifene (Evista), and parathyroid hormone (PTH 1-34).
- Implement preventive measures, including discontinuing tobacco, avoiding excessive alcohol intake, engaging in weight-bearing activities, maintaining a healthy weight, adequate calcium and vitamin D intake, and herbal therapies.
- Smokers lose bone more rapidly than nonsmokers. Eighty-year-old smokers have up to 10% lower BMD, which translates into twice the risk of spinal fractures and a 50% increase in risk of hip fracture. Fractures heal slower in smokers and are more likely to heal improperly.
- Excessive alcohol intake has been associated with osteoporosis because of the degenerative metabolic effects of alcohol. Alcohol abuse may inhibit calcium absorption and bone formation.
- Exercise is an important treatment for osteoporosis to maintain healthy bones. Weight-bearing aerobic activities involve the bones supporting body weight and have a positive effect in maintaining and increasing bone mass and preventing osteoporosis. These activities include weightlifting, walking, jogging, hiking, stair climbing, step aerobics, dancing, and racquet sports. A sedentary lifestyle leads to weaker bones and a higher risk of fractures.
- Advise patients on sufficient intake of calcium (at least 1200 mg daily, including supplements if necessary) and vitamin D (800-1000 IU daily of vitamin D_3 for individuals at risk for inadequate intake). Sun exposure of 15 minutes daily to hands and face helps the body make vitamin D, which helps the body absorb calcium. Patients should be advised to avoid overexposure to the sun.
- Strong evidence is lacking to support the use of any herb for the treatment and prevention of osteoporosis. However, soy and red clover isoflavones may increase BMD in postmenopausal women and, in combination with diet and exercise, may help to reduce the risk of fractures.
- Emphasize good practices to prevent falls. Recommend eliminating hazards that can increase the risk of falling, such as removing loose wires or throw rugs, installing grab bars in the bathroom and nonskid mats near sinks and in the tub, and not walking in slick shoes or socks; using caution when carrying or lifting items because of the risk for spinal fracture; wearing sturdy shoes; and using a cane or walker if the individual has balance problems or other difficulties walking. Hip protectors or pads may also be worn to help prevent hip fractures.

Case Studies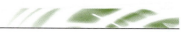

CASE STUDY 22-1

TP is a 70-year-old African-American woman with a medical history of type 2 diabetes and hypertension. Current medications include metformin (Glucophage, 1000 mg) twice daily, glipizide (Glucotrol, 10 mg) twice daily, atenolol (Tenormin, 100 mg) daily, and clopidogrel (Plavix, 75 mg) daily. At a recent checkup, her glycosylated hemoglobin (HbA_{1c}) was 5.9%, which is below the recommended threshold of 7% (values above 7% indicate poor control), and her blood pressure was 135/85 mm Hg. At that visit, a DEXA scan was performed. Her T-score was −2.0, and TP was diagnosed with osteopenia. She was given a prescription for ibandronate (Boniva). She heard that estrogen will make her bones stronger, but she is concerned about adverse effects; however, she asks if there is an herbal remedy that would work as well. She asks specifically about red clover to prevent bone loss. She leads a healthy lifestyle, walks her dog 2 miles a day, attends an exercise program at a local senior center 5 days a week, and takes a multivitamin. How do you counsel?

Answer: Red clover contains phytoestrogens called isoflavones. Phytoestrogens are estrogen-like substances that are similar to 17β-estradiol. They promote bone health by inhibiting the activity of osteoclasts (bone-decreasing cells) and promoting the activity of osteoblasts (bone-increasing cells). However, using this herbal product with TP's current drug regimen poses a few risks. Red clover contains coumarin and coumarin-like compounds, which may potentiate the anticoagulation effect of clopidogrel. In addition, it might lower serum glucose levels. The increased risk of bleeding and the possibility of lowering her serum glucose outweigh the possible benefit of using red clover to reduce bone loss for TP.

Soy, an agent similar to red clover that also contains isoflavones, may benefit her postmenopausal bone loss without the same interactions. Traditionally, soy is found in foods such as tofu, bean curd, tempeh, soy milk, miso, and soy sauce. A growing number of soy-based products are also available, including soy burgers (veggie burgers), soy hot dogs, soy-based cheese, soy ice cream, and soy yogurts. Soy supplements also may provide benefit.

Although TP's African-American heritage puts her at a reduced risk for osteoporosis, her diagnosis of osteopenia underscores the need to prevent further bone loss. All women over age 50, regardless of race, should take calcium and vitamin D supplements (1200 mg calcium and 600-800 IU vitamin D daily). Milk and milk products also contain calcium (~300 mg/serving). These products also contain other nutrients important to bone health, such as vitamin D (if fortified), phosphorus, and magnesium. Sun exposure of 15 minutes a day also provides vitamin D.

TP should continue exercising regularly and taking daily multivitamins.

CASE STUDY 22-2

GH is the daughter of the frail-looking man she wheels into your pharmacy. She places him in the waiting area to view videos on health care topics. GH has a new prescription for alendronate (Fosamax) and atorvastatin (Lipitor). She states that her 67-year-old father, WD, was recently released from the hospital after being treated for a hip fracture sustained during a fall. She states that WD had a DEXA scan that revealed a T-score of −2.5, which denotes osteoporosis.

GH says she thought that osteoporosis was much more common in women, but she thinks she knows the reason why her father developed it: "He drinks like a fish, smokes like a chimney, and sits on the couch watching TV all day. When he is not drinking alcohol, he is drinking coffee." She explains that her father is a widower and lost his job 2 years ago because of alcohol-related issues. After his discharge from the hospital, she has taken him into her home to convalesce. She adds that his presence has put a real strain on herself, her husband, and their three children. She tells you that he is averse to taking prescriptions and only takes aspirin (81 mg/day) for cardiovascular health and red yeast rice for hyperlipidemia. GH states, however, that "his cholesterol is sky high." In the past he has thrown away prescriptions because he "has no faith in doctors or their medicines." She is worried about his lack of compliance with the new prescriptions and asks if there is "a hormone shot or something to give him for his osteoporosis." How do you counsel?

Answer: As GH stated, WD's osteoporosis is most likely caused by the combined effects of alcohol abuse, cigarette smoking, and inactivity. Furthermore, alcoholics often do not eat proper diets. Testosterone can promote bone growth but can cause liver damage. WD most likely has liver damage from his alcohol intake, so testosterone would not be recommended. Additionally, high amounts of caffeine in coffee may contribute to bone loss and increased urinary calcium excretion.

Strong efforts should be made to counsel WD on the benefit of smoking cessation and reduced alcohol intake. He also must consume a healthy diet, ingest 1200 mg of calcium daily, and take a multivitamin that includes vitamin D. He should also begin weight-bearing exercises, such as walking, after his hip heals.

The alendronate will promote bone growth, but compliance may be a problem. WD must sit upright for 30 minutes after taking his weekly dose, and he may experience abdominal discomfort and nausea.

Although supportive evidence suggests that red yeast rice lowers blood cholesterol, there are potential risks. Red yeast rice may have an anticoagulant effect and, combined with WD's aspirin and (current) alcohol intake, may cause gastrointestinal bleeding. You may suggest discontinuing the red yeast rice and trying atorvastatin. This agent may be beneficial for high cholesterol levels if WD is compliant.

CASE STUDY 22-3

GT is a 32-year-old Vietnamese woman who presents at your pharmacy to refill her oral contraceptive (OC) prescription (Ortho-Novum 7/7/7). She is accompanied by her mother, who has an obvious dowager's hump and walks with a cane. The older woman hobbles off to the gift card section, and GT whispers that her 52-year-old mother was recently diagnosed with osteoporosis; "I don't want to be all humped over like that when I'm my mom's age." She asks you if there is anything she can do or take to prevent osteoporosis. GT also takes St. John's wort for mild depression and valerian for sleep. She drinks about 3 to 4 glasses of wine daily, smokes about one pack of cigarettes per day, and rarely exercises. How do you counsel?

Answer: GT has several risk factors for developing osteoporosis, and she should take precaution now. Asians are at higher risk for osteoporosis because they tend to have slender frames and less bone mass. Her mother's development of osteoporosis at a relatively young age is further indication of GT's increased risk.

Preventive measures that GT should implement include avoiding excess alcohol intake and engaging in exercise, including weight-bearing activities. Most importantly, GT must stop smoking. OC use may potentiate harmful effects of smoking on the cardiovascular system and increase her risk of developing a blood clot. Additionally, smokers lose bone more rapidly than nonsmokers.

The OC's estrogen content will help prevent bone loss, which is an added benefit for GT. At some time in the future, GT will discontinue her OC and lose its osteoporosis-preventing effect. At that point or when she becomes perimenopausal, GT may consider low-dose estrogen replacement therapy.

GT should also be counseled regarding possible interactions between her medication and herbal treatments. St. John's wort induces cytochrome P450 3A4 enzymes and may reduce the efficacy of OCs. Advise GT to consider adding a barrier method of contraception if using St. John's wort with OCs, or switching OCs, or implementing methods of coping with depression.

References for Chapter 22 can be found on the Evolve website at http://evolve.elsevier.com/Ulbricht/herbalpharmacotherapy/

Review Questions

1. What component of horsetail may contribute to its role in bone health?
   a. Oxygen
   b. Magnesium
   c. Nitrogen
   d. Silicon

2. True or false: If the T-score is −2.5 or lower, the individual is considered to have osteoporosis and therefore at high risk for fracture.

3. Which of the following doses of red clover has been studied in osteoporosis?
   a. 57 mg red clover isoflavones daily
   b. 5.7 g red clover isoflavones daily
   c. 85.5 mg red clover isoflavones daily
   d. Both a and c

4. All the following statements are true *except*:
   a. Soy isoflavones suppress osteoclast activity by induction of apoptosis.
   b. Soy isoflavones act only on osteoblasts, not osteoclasts.
   c. The structure and function of isoflavones are similar to 17β-estradiol.
   d. Osteoblasts secrete bone formation proteins, including osteocalcin and alkaline phosphatase.

5. True or false: Soy isoflavones have demonstrated beneficial effects on BMD, bone turnover markers, and bone mechanical strength.

Answers are found in the Answers to Review Questions section in the back of the text.

23 Arthritis

Outline

OVERVIEW
  Osteoarthritis
    Signs and Symptoms
    Diagnosis
  Rheumatoid Arthritis
    Signs and Symptoms
    Diagnosis
  Periarthritis
    Signs and Symptoms
    Diagnosis
  Juvenile Rheumatoid Arthritis
    Signs and Symptoms
    Diagnosis
  Infectious Arthritis
    Signs and Symptoms
    Diagnosis
  Reiter's Syndrome (Reactive Arthritis)
    Signs and Symptoms
    Diagnosis
  Gout
    Signs and Symptoms
    Diagnosis
SELECTED HERBAL THERAPIES
  Arnica (*Arnica* spp.)
  Ash (*Fraxinus* spp.)
  Ashwagandha (*Withania somnifera*)
  Avocado (*Persea americana*)
  Black Cohosh (*Actaea racemosa,* formerly *Cimicifuga racemosa*)
  Black Currant (*Ribes nigrum*)
  Borage (*Borago officinalis*)
  Boswellia (*Boswellia serrata*)
  Bromelain (Bromeliaceae)
  Cat's Claw (*Uncaria* spp.)
  Cherry (*Prunus avium, Prunus cerasus,* and various *Prunus* spp.)
  Devil's Claw (*Harpagophytum procumbens*)
  Evening Primrose (*Oenothera biennis*)
  Feverfew (*Tanacetum parthenium*)
  Ginger (*Zingiber officinale*)
  Guggul (*Commiphora mukul*)
  Hop (*Humulus lupulus*)
  Mistletoe (*Viscum album*)
  Papaya (*Carica papaya*)
  Podophyllum (*Podophyllum* spp.)
  Rose Hip (*Rosa* spp.)
  Stinging Nettle (*Urtica dioica*)
  Turmeric (*Curcuma longa*)
  Willow (*Salix* spp.)
HERBAL THERAPIES WITH NEGATIVE EVIDENCE
HERBAL THERAPIES WITH LIMITED EVIDENCE
ADJUNCT THERAPIES
INTEGRATIVE THERAPY PLAN
CASE STUDIES
REVIEW QUESTIONS

Learning Objectives

- List at least 10 herbs that are used for arthritis.
- Understand the mechanism of action and evidence supporting the use of herbs in arthritis.
- Describe the adverse effects and drug interactions associated with herbs used for arthritis.
- Create a specific integrative treatment plan for a patient with arthritis.

OVERVIEW

The term *arthritis* is derived from the Greek word roots for "joint" *(arthro)* and "inflammation" *(itis)*. More than 100 different diseases fall under the general category of "arthritis," which affects not only the joints but also the tissues surrounding joints and other connective tissues. Arthritis may be caused by autoimmune (rheumatic) disease, overuse of drugs, infection, metabolic conditions (gout), or a reaction to infection (reactive arthritis).[1] Common forms of arthritis include rheumatoid arthritis, osteoarthritis, and periarthritis. Other types of arthritis and related conditions include juvenile rheumatoid arthritis, infectious arthritis, Reiter's syndrome (reactive arthritis), and gout.

The symptoms associated with arthritis are variable, but most patients experience some degree of pain, swelling, and difficulty moving the affected joint. The type of arthritis has significant impact on the exact symptomatology and the extent of involvement of other organ systems.

Osteoarthritis

Osteoarthritis (OA), also called *degenerative joint disease* (DJD), is marked by the breakdown of cartilage that lines the ends of most limb bone. This type of cartilage, known as *articular* cartilage, serves to cushion the bones and allow painless joint movement; its breakdown causes patients to experience pain and reduced mobility in their joints (Figure 23-1). OA may affect any joint in the body but occurs most often in fingers, spine, and weight-bearing joints. Patients with OA often experience inflammation around the affected joint, caused by bits of cartilage that break off and aggravate the synovial tissue lining the joints (Figure 23-2).

Besides cartilage loss, OA is characterized by irregular thickening and remodeling of bone. The synovial tissue may bulge out of joints to form cysts *(Baker cysts)* or may become hardened with fibrous tissue overgrowth *(sclerosis)*. Bony protrusions called *osteophytes* (also known as "bone spurs") may also form. These pathological changes result in increased blood flow and joint inflammation.

Osteoarthritis occurs most often in individuals older than 45 years, but OA may develop at any age.[2] The exact cause of OA remains unclear. Most researchers believe that several factors contribute to its development, including obesity, age, joint injury or stress, genetics, and muscle weakness.[3] Regardless of the specific cause, the end result is pain and destruction of the joint from a breakdown of cartilage and bone.

Signs and Symptoms

Osteoarthritis may affect any joint in the body. Because OA develops slowly, however, many patients do not experience symptoms initially. The pain and inflammation in OA is typically less severe and more localized than that of rheumatoid arthritis, which is more systemic. Common symptoms of OA include joint pain (arthralgia), swelling and stiffness in a joint (especially after movement), joint discomfort before or during a change in the weather (e.g., conditions of low pressure and high humidity), bony lumps on the fingers, and loss of joint flexibility.

When individuals have OA, the cells that form cartilage *(chondrocytes)* cannot efficiently repair the damaged cartilage. Thus, OA represents a failure of the chondrocytes to maintain a proper balance between cartilage formation and destruction. Instead, new bone grows alongside the existing bone, causing small lumps to form. Although these lumps cause minimal pain, they may be disfiguring and limit joint mobility. The joints most often affected by OA include the fingers, spine, and weight-bearing joints (such as the hips, ankles, feet, and knees). If patients overuse the affected joints without proper treatment, the cartilage in the joints may wear down completely. When this happens, bone may rub against bone and may cause severe pain.

Diagnosis

The diagnosis of OA is largely based on medical history and physical examinations that reveal tenderness and joint enlargement. Laboratory tests may reveal mildly elevated white blood cell (WBC) counts, but other tests used to diagnose rheumatic disease, such as erythrocyte sedimentation rate (ESR) and *rheumatoid factor* (RF), are generally negative. Nonetheless, these tests are often performed to distinguish patients with OA from those with other connective tissue diseases, especially rheumatoid arthritis. Radiographs can provide objective evidence of the disease. Findings consistent with OA include asymmetrical joint space narrowing, subchondral sclerosis (fibrous growth under cartilage), osteophyte formation, and joint misalignment (subluxation).

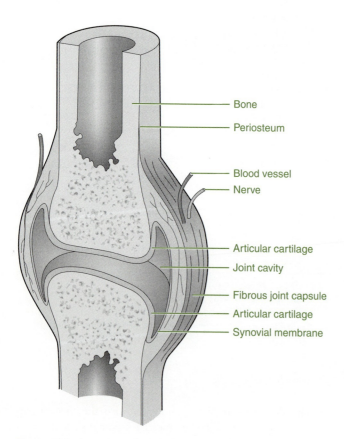

Figure 23-1 Structure of a typical synovial joint. (Modified from Thibodeau GA, Patton KT: *Anatomy & physiology*, ed 5, St Louis, 2003, Mosby.)

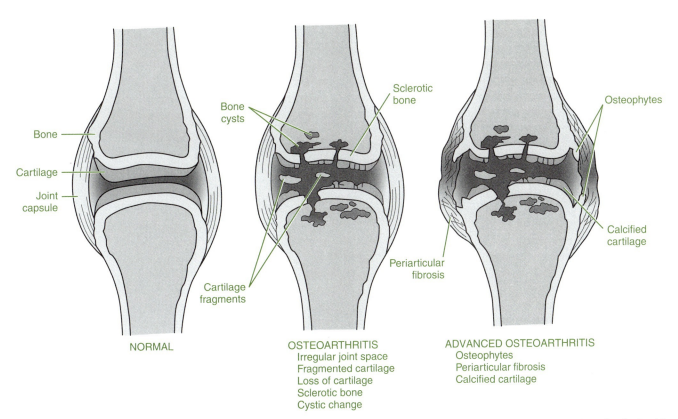

Figure 23-2 Schematic presentation of the pathologic changes in osteoarthritis. (Modified from Damjanov I: *Pathology for the health professions*, ed 3, St Louis, 2006, Saunders-Elsevier.)

Rheumatoid Arthritis

Rheumatoid arthritis (RA) is a systemic inflammatory disease that affects the peripheral joints in a symmetrical pattern. Although the exact cause is unclear, RA is thought to be an autoimmune phenomena, characterized by abnormal immune responses against healthy host tissue. In RA, autoimmune reactions can cause joint inflammation and degeneration[4,5] (Figure 23-3).

Because RA is a type of autoimmune disorder, most patients have antibodies called *rheumatoid factors*. The presence of these antibodies in the blood confirms a diagnosis of RA,[6] but does not necessarily indicate the severity. Proinflammatory factors such as tumor necrosis factor (TNF) interleukin, T cells, prostaglandins, and histamine may also be elevated. Blocking these proinflammatory substances is the major target of most RA therapies. The presence of chronic inflammation in the joints eventually leads to breakdown of synovial tissue, cartilage, and bone.

Women are two to three times more likely than men to develop RA. Most cases of RA occur in individuals 20 to 50 years old. Some researchers believe that during certain infections or inflammatory responses, the immune system may inadvertently produce antibodies that attack "self" tissues. Thus, autoimmunity often develops after an illness. Genetics may also play a role in the development of RA.[3]

Signs and Symptoms

Rheumatoid arthritis is marked by pain and swelling in the joints. Unlike osteoarthritis, which affects only bones, cartilage, and synovial tissue, RA may also cause swelling in other areas, including the tear ducts, salivary glands, lining of the heart, lungs, and occasionally the blood vessels. Furthermore, whereas OA tends to be localized to a few joints, RA often affects many joints at the same time.

The severity of symptoms varies among patients. Early nonspecific symptoms of RA include fatigue, weakness, low-grade fever, loss of appetite, and joint pain. Generalized aching or stiffness of the muscles (myalgias) may precede pain and swelling in the joints (synovitis). Joint pain is usually symmetrical and transitory. Some studies indicate that symptoms may worsen with changes in the weather, such as conditions of low atmospheric pressure and high humidity.

Diagnosis

Diagnosing RA begins with a medical history and physical examination. The clinical presentation of RA varies, but the most frequent finding is pain with symmetrical swelling of the joints in the hands, feet, and cervical spine over several weeks to months. In clinical practice the classification criteria from 1987 American College of Rheumatology (formerly the American Rheumatism Association) are often used.[6]

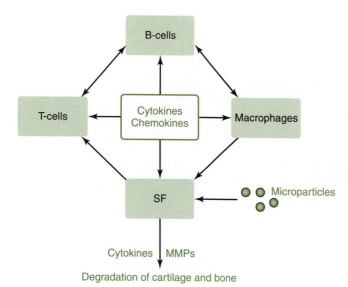

Figure 23-3 Interactions in the pathophysiology of joint destruction in rheumatoid arthritis. *SF*, Synovial fibroblasts; *MMPs*, matrix metalloproteinases. (From Knedla A, Neumann E, Müller-Ladner U: Developments in the synovial biology field, 2006, *Arthritis Res Ther* 9(2): 209, 2007.)

A patient is considered to have RA if she has satisfied at least four of the following seven criteria:
1. *Morning stiffness.* Morning stiffness felt in and around the joints, lasting at least 1 hour before maximal improvement.
2. *Arthritis of three or more joint areas.* At least three joint areas simultaneously have had soft tissue swelling or fluid (not bony overgrowth alone) observed by a physician; the 14 possible joint areas are right or left proximal interphalangeal (PIP) joints, metacarpophalangeal (MCP) joints, wrist, elbow, knee, ankle, and metatarsophalangeal (MTP) joints.
3. *Arthritis of hand joints.* At least one area swollen (as defined above) in a wrist, MCP joint, or PIP joint.
4. *Symmetrical arthritis.* Simultaneous involvement of the same joint areas (see 2 above) on both sides of the body (bilateral involvement of PIPs, MCPs, or MTPs is acceptable without absolute symmetry).
5. *Rheumatoid nodules.* Subcutaneous nodules, over bony prominences, or extensor surfaces, or in juxtaarticular regions, observed by a physician.
6. *Serum rheumatoid factor.* Demonstration of abnormal amounts of serum RF, an autoantibody, by any method for which the result has been positive in less than 5% of normal control subjects.
7. *Radiographic changes.* Radiographic changes typical of RA on posteroanterior hand and wrist radiographs, which must include erosions or unequivocal bony decalcification localized to, or most marked adjacent to, the involved joints (osteoarthritis changes alone do not qualify).

Rheumatoid arthritis is diagnosed if at least 4 of these criteria are met. Criteria 1 through 4 must have been present for at least 6 weeks.

Most patients with RA will have a positive test for RF. However, a positive result may take many years to manifest because the test has low sensitivity in the early stages of RA. Recent research has focused on anticitrullinated protein/peptide antibodies (anti-CCP), which are highly specific and sensitive markers for RA that may be positive early in the course of disease.

Standard blood tests may be obtained to evaluate for anemia, which is inversely related to inflammatory disease activity. Other test results may show increased number of WBCs or platelets or abnormal liver function. ESR and levels of C-reactive protein (CRP) are nonspecific markers of inflammation that are also evaluated. Plain film radiography is the standard investigation to assess the extent of anatomical changes in RA patients. The radiographic features of the hand joints early in the disease are characterized by soft tissue swelling and mild juxtaarticular osteoporosis. Other imaging techniques, such as magnetic resonance imaging (MRI), computed tomography (CT), and scintigraphy, may also be used to monitor the progression of RA.

Periarthritis

Periarthritis is used as an umbrella term to refer to chronic inflammation that results in stiffness over time.[7] Periarthritis is a chronic inflammatory disease of the tissues surrounding a joint, and typically occurs after injuries that cause scarring, thickening, or shrinkage of the joint. It may also occur after exposure to cold temperatures. Periarthritis most often affects the shoulder, and may involve tendons, ligaments, synovial tissue, or other soft tissues. Periarthritis of the shoulder is also called *adhesive capsulitis* or "frozen shoulder."

Individuals with other types of chronic arthritis affecting the shoulders have an increased risk of developing periarthritis of the shoulder. Periarthritis primarily affects patients over 50 years of age and is more common in patients with diabetes mellitus. It has been suggested that complications of diabetes, including protein glycosylation and blood vessel damage, may cause connective tissue disorders such as periarthritis in patients with diabetes. Periarthritis is also often associated with calcified deposits within the joint,[8] and it is reported to be more common in patients with chronic renal disease because they are more prone to calcium deposits.

Signs and Symptoms

Periarthritis causes swelling, pain, and restricted motion in the joint; it most commonly affects the shoulder. If not treated early, the pain and restricted motion may become permanent.

Diagnosis

Periarthritis is usually diagnosed after a detailed medical history is obtained and physical examination is performed. The affected joint will have very limited mobility. In some cases a radiograph may be needed to confirm a diagnosis; a contrast dye is injected into the affected joint and x-rays are taken. If the patient has periarthritis, the joint will appear shrunken and scarred. Periarthritis may also show swelling of the soft tissue or calcified deposits on radiographs.

Juvenile Rheumatoid Arthritis

Juvenile rheumatoid arthritis (JRA), also referred to as *juvenile idiopathic arthritis* (JIA), occurs in children 6 months to 16 years of age. It is estimated that JRA occurs in approximately 1 in 1000 children in the United States. Research suggests that JRA may be an autoimmune disease, but the exact cause is unclear. The different types of JRA are based on the particular joints affected and include *systemic* JRA (affecting the whole body), *polyarticular* JRA (affecting five or more joints), and *pauciarticular* JRA (affecting four or fewer joints).

Signs and Symptoms

Symptoms of JRA may not always be obvious and unlike other severe joint diseases, it may not worsen. Signs and symptoms may include sore, painful, or stiff joints (fingers, hands, knees), spiking fever, limping, weak muscles, unexplained rash, and a feeling of tiredness or lack of energy. Some children may have infrequent or temporary symptoms, whereas others may have persistent symptoms.

Diagnosis

The diagnosis of JRA typically begins with complete physical examination and medical history. Blood tests, including a complete blood count (CBC), ESR, antinuclear antibody (ANA), and RF test, may also be performed. Radiographs of the patient's joints may be taken to help rule out other complications, such as fractures or infections. In some cases, joint fluid may be removed and analyzed.

Infectious Arthritis

Infectious arthritis, also referred to as *septic arthritis* or *bacterial arthritis*, is an acute process caused by bacterial, fungal, or viral invasion of the joint space (the area located between components of a joint). *Staphylococcus, Streptococcus, Haemophilus, Salmonella, Pseudomonas,* and gonococci are the most common infectious agents. Bacteria may enter a joint through the blood or may enter directly during surgery, by injection, or through an injury. Infectious arthritis may occur after trauma near the joint, infection in the blood, or in patients predisposed to infection (e.g., with diabetes, immune deficiency, HIV/AIDS, some forms of cancer, existing arthritis) or in people who use intravenous (IV) drugs. Infectious arthritis develops rapidly in a single joint, with severe pain, swelling, redness, and restricted movement.

Because it may cause fatal septic shock, bacterial infectious arthritis is considered a medical emergency and requires urgent drainage and antibiotic therapy.[9] Viral infectious arthritis is usually less severe in intensity, has a slower onset, does not cause a fever, and generally resolves without treatment. In rare cases, joint infections may be caused by a fungus. Fungal infections may be treated with the antifungal amphotericin B. An infection-related type of arthritis known as *reactive arthritis* may cause joint pain in response to an infection in another part of the body, even though the infection does not actually occur in the joint (see Reiter's syndrome).

Signs and Symptoms

Infectious arthritis develops rapidly in a single joint with severe pain, warmth in the affected area, restricted movement, and redness and swelling in the affected joint (especially when moved). Patients may also have fever, chills, and swollen lymph nodes.

Diagnosis

A combination of physical examination and laboratory tests are used to diagnose infectious arthritis. Specific questions may be asked to determine coexisting medical conditions, past or present infections, recent travel, and potential contact with infectious individuals. Radiography may show increased fluid within the joint space, which usually indicates significant inflammation. Blood cultures are then taken if infectious arthritis is suspected. A joint fluid sample is also usually taken to identify the presence of bacteria or other infectious organisms. Other tests (sputum, spinal fluid, urine) may also be performed to confirm the diagnosis.

Reiter's Syndrome (Reactive Arthritis)

Reiter's syndrome, or reactive arthritis, is a type of arthritis resulting from infection, but in joints that are not actually infected. *Chlamydia* is the genus of bacteria typically associated with Reiter's syndrome. Many types of bacteria known to cause infections in the gastrointestinal tract (e.g., *Salmonella, Shigella, Yersinia, Campylobacter*) have also been linked to Reiter's syndrome. It remains unclear why only some patients develop Reiter's syndrome after they are exposed to these bacteria. However, researchers have discovered a genetic (biological) factor that increases an individual's chance of developing the disorder. Reiter's syndrome has been associated with a mutated HLA-B27 gene that leads to the development of an abnormal human leukocyte antigen (HLA).[10] HLA-B27 has been linked with a number of inflammatory and autoimmune disorders; however, its role in these disorders remains unclear.

Patients with Reiter's syndrome develop pain and swelling in large joints (knee, ankle, and pelvic joints) and inflammation of the eyes (uvea, iris, conjunctiva) and the urethra. For unknown reasons, women rarely develop the disorder, and typically experience milder symptoms than men.

Signs and Symptoms

Reiter's syndrome causes three main symptoms: arthritis, redness of the eyes, and urinary tract symptoms, such as increased need to urinate (especially in men) and burning sensation during urination.[10] Symptoms usually develop within days or weeks of an infection.

Diagnosis
Specific tests to diagnose Reiter's syndrome are currently unavailable. Instead, the clinician will take a detailed medical history and perform a physical examination. A culture swab may be used to determine if *Chlamydia* is causing symptoms. Blood tests may be performed to diagnose a bacterial infection that may have caused Reiter's syndrome. A blood test may also be performed to determine if the patient has the HLA-B27 tissue type, although this does not necessarily mean that the patient has Reiter's syndrome; the HLA-B27 molecule has also been linked to other conditions, including rheumatic diseases. An eye examination may also be performed to determine if the patient has eye infections (conjunctivitis, uveitis, or iritis). However, a lack of eye problems does not rule out Reiter's syndrome, because only 50% of patients with Reiter's syndrome have conjunctivitis, and even fewer develop uveitis or iritis.

Gout
Gout, also referred to as *gouty arthritis,* is considered the most common metabolic disease associated with arthritis. Patients with gout have abnormally high levels of uric acid in the blood (hyperuricemia). This may be caused by a diet high in protein or alcohol, a genetic predisposition, hormonal changes, or certain medications (e.g., thiazide diuretics). The excess uric acid is deposited in the joint space as sharp crystals, which cause inflammation and pain. The joint most often affected in gout is the joint between the big toe and the foot. Gout is typically marked by the sudden onset of severe pain, restriction of movement, joint swelling, and redness caused by the sharp uric acid crystals. Patients with chronic gout may also develop deposits of uric acid crystals called *tophi* in the subcutaneous tissue.

Signs and Symptoms
Symptoms of gout include intense pain and redness of a single joint, most frequently the joint of the big toe. Gout attacks are precipitated when water is reabsorbed from the joint space at night, leaving behind a supersaturated solution of monosodium urate. For this reason, most patients experience attacks of gout at night. Patients often have recurrent attacks and, if they have chronic gout, may develop deposits within the joint that cause permanent deformity. The pain of gout may be so severe that a light touch (as with a bed sheet) will cause severe pain.

Diagnosis
If gout is suspected, the health care provider will take a sample of synovial fluid from the affected joint. This sample is analyzed for uric acid crystals in the WBCs. If crystals are present, a positive diagnosis is made. If gout is diagnosed, the health care provider may also take a urine sample to determine how much uric acid is being excreted.

Serum uric acid levels are often used to monitor the status of patients diagnosed with gout but are generally not used in the diagnosis of the disorder.[11]

SELECTED HERBAL THERAPIES

Note
To help make this educational resource more interactive, all pharmacokinetics, adverse effects, and interactions data have been compiled in Appendix A. Safety data specifically related to pregnancy and lactation are listed in Appendix B. Please refer to these appendices when working through the case studies and answering the review questions.

Arnica (*Arnica* spp.)

Grade C: *Unclear or conflicting scientific evidence (osteoarthritis)*

Mechanism of Action
Arnica has shown antiinflammatory effects in vitro and may act by preventing the action of histamine on blood vessels, thus preventing fluid from leaking into the surrounding tissue.[12,13] The sesquiterpene lactones (SLs) in arnica may also block molecules within inflammatory cells that activate the cells.[14-16]

Scientific Evidence of Effectiveness
Because of its purported antiinflammatory constituents, topical arnica gel has been used for osteoarthritis pain and stiffness. Although one clinical trial reported positive effects of topical arnica gel on pain, stiffness, and function,[17] common homeopathic arnica preparations contain negligible amounts of the purported active ingredients; thus, the scientific basis of efficacy remains unclear.

Dose
Note: Arnica is toxic if taken internally except when diluted into homeopathic preparations.

Topical application of fresh plant gel, applied twice daily, has been used for mild to moderate osteoarthritis of the knee for up to 6 weeks.[17] Homeopathic arnica that may be taken orally is created by taking the alcohol tincture of fresh arnica flowers and repeatedly diluting it to create an oral solution.[18]

Adverse Effects, Interactions, Pharmacokinetics. See Appendix A.

Ash (*Fraxinus* spp.)

Grade C: *Unclear or conflicting scientific evidence (gouty arthritis)*

Mechanism of Action

In clinical studies of RA and OA, the antiinflammatory properties of ash *(Fraxini excelsior)* have been demonstrated in combination with trembling poplar *(Populus tremula)*, and true goldenrod *(Solidago virgaurea)*.[19] The combination product is reported to be similar in efficacy to nonsteroidal antiinflammatory drugs (NSAIDs) but to have half as many adverse effects.[19] Antiinflammatory properties may result from the hydroxycoumarin in ash bark, which may directly inhibit the activity of inflammatory cells and to inhibit activation of inflammatory cytokines.[20]

Scientific Evidence of Effectiveness

Ash has been used historically for its antiinflammatory and analgesic properties in combination products for more than 40 years in Europe. One clinical trial evaluated the efficacy of a combination product, Rebixiao granule (RBXG), which contained ash bark and sarsaparilla *(Smilax glabra)* root, in the treatment of repeated gouty arthritis compared to the NSAID Futalin (diclofenac sodium).[21] A higher cure rate and lower serum uric acid levels were reported with RBXG.

Dose

The effective dose of ash for gouty arthritis is not clear. Currently, there is a lack of published research evaluating ash as a monotherapy for arthritis.

Adverse Effects, Interactions, Pharmacokinetics. See Appendix A.

Ashwagandha *(Withania somnifera)*

Grade C: *Unclear or conflicting scientific evidence (osteoarthritis)*

Mechanism of Action

The use of ashwagandha in OA has been suggested based on reported antiinflammatory[22-26] and antiarthritic[27] properties in rodents. Many of the beneficial properties have been attributed to the specific compound *withaferin A*,[28] which has been reported to have immunosuppressive properties[29] and to protect cells and DNA from the cytotoxic agent peroxide.[30] Prevention of granuloma formation, a type of inflammation, has been noted in rats.[31,32] Other studies also show antiinflammatory and immune-modulating effects in mice and rats,[23,25,26] including enhanced cytokine production.[33]

Scientific Evidence of Effectiveness

There is limited clinical evidence of efficacy for ashwagandha in arthritis. OA patients were treated with a formulation called Articulin-F, which contains roots of *Withania somnifera*, the stem of *Boswellia serrata*, rhizomes of *Curcuma longa*, and a zinc complex. Patients experienced significant improvement in pain and disability rating with the combination product compared with placebo, but no radiographic improvements were seen.[34] Currently, research evaluating ashwagandha alone for the treatment of arthritis is lacking.

Dose

The dose of ashwagandha monotherapy for osteoarthritis has not been determined.

Adverse Effects, Interactions, Pharmacokinetics. See Appendix A.

Avocado *(Persea americana)*

Grade B: *Good scientific evidence (osteoarthritis of the knee and hip)*

Mechanism of Action

The applicable parts of avocado are the fruit, leaves, and seed. Avocado oil is derived from the fruit pulp, which is a good source of potassium and vitamin D. Mexican avocado is reported to contain estragole and anethole, shown to be hepatotoxic in animals and structurally similar to safrole, a known carcinogen.

Avocado oil and soybean oil are mixed together in a preparation called *avocado/soybean unsaponifiables* (ASU). ASU has been shown to interfere with chondrocytes, reducing their ability to produce inflammatory molecules, including prostaglandin E_2 (PGE_2), metalloproteinase, and other cytokines.[35-36] There is also evidence that ASU can increase the synthesis of aggrecan, a key component of cartilage. These results suggest that ASU could prevent the breakdown of cartilage and promote cartilage repair.[37]

An in vivo model of cartilage destruction evaluated avocado, soy, and their combination (ASU). Both ASU and avocado oil alone protected cartilage from damage.[38] This protective effect may be caused by the free-radical scavengers tocopherol and beta-sitosterol in ASU. Free-radical scavengers are molecules that deactivate free radicals, which are unstable molecules that can damage tissue. ASU may also inhibit the inflammatory cytokine interleukin-1 (IL-1), which causes cartilage breakdown. IL-1 is released from mononuclear cells, and avocado and ASU both prevent mononuclear cells from entering inflamed tissue surrounding cartilage.[38] ASU increases the production of some molecules that may protect cartilage, including transforming growth factor beta ($TGF-\beta_1$, $TGF-\beta_2$), and plasminogen activator inhibitor 1 (PAI-1).[39]

Scientific Evidence of Effectiveness

Clinical trials have been done to assess the effect of avocado/soybean unsaponifiables (ASU) on OA.[40-43] One trial investigated OA in the knee, another investigated OA in the hip, and two assessed the effect on OA in both the knee and the hip. Three of four trials showed significant positive effects, including improved function, decreased pain, and decreased use of pain medication. The fourth trial reported positive radiographic evidence of benefit only in the most severe patients. Only one trial was longer than 90 days. Long-term trials are needed to evaluate properly the effect of ASU. It is unclear how much of the effect is caused by avocado versus soybean. Separate trials are needed to distinguish the relative effects of avocado and soybean.

Dose
When used as a fruit, avocado is not standardized. Clinical trials have used ASU doses of 300 to 600 mg for 3 months to 2 years.[40-43]

Adverse Effects, Interactions, Pharmacokinetics. See Appendix A.

Black Cohosh (Actaea racemosa, formerly Cimicifuga racemosa)

Grade C: Unclear or conflicting scientific evidence (rheumatoid arthritis, osteoarthritis)

Mechanism of Action
The mechanism of action of black cohosh in arthritis relief is unclear. It has been demonstrated to have bone-conserving effects, including stimulation of osteoblast and osteoclast products,[44,45] which may have beneficial effects in arthritis. Native black cohosh is reported to contain small amounts of salicylates, which may have analgesic effects, although it is not clear if salicylates are present in therapeutic amounts in commercial preparations.

Scientific Evidence of Effectiveness
There is a lack of definitive evidence that black cohosh monotherapy may effectively treat RA or OA. Native black cohosh does contain small amounts of salicylates, although it is unclear whether these are present in therapeutic amounts in commercial preparations. One study of a combination product (Reumalex) containing black cohosh and other salicylate-containing herbs (white willow bark, sarsaparilla, or poplar bark, containing 10-20 mg of salicylates per tablet) for RA or OA reported small improvements in pain scores, but no improvement in joint function or decrease in self-medication, with analgesics.[46]

Dose
The dose has not been determined for black cohosh monotherapy in treating arthritis.

Adverse Effects, Interactions, Pharmacokinetics. See Appendix A.

Black Currant (Ribes nigrum)

Grade C: Unclear or conflicting scientific evidence (rheumatoid arthritis)

Mechanism of Action
Black currant has shown antiinflammatory effects in vitro.[47] Black currant seed oil is a source of polyunsaturated fatty acids, which have been suggested as a treatment of inflammatory disease.[48] Black currant has been shown to be rich in phenolic compounds.[49] In one study, black currant seed oil was found to contain 14.5% alpha-linolenic acid (18:3n3), 12.6% gamma-linolenic acid (18:3n6), 47.5% linoleic acid (18:2n6), and 2.7% stearidonic acid (18:4n3).[50] Black currant seed oil has been shown to modulate membrane lipid composition and eicosanoid production.[51]

A study of inflammatory cells (monocytes) isolated from patients given black currant seed oil showed greatly altered PGE_2 production and production of the cytokines IL-1β, tumor necrosis factor alpha (TNF-α), and interleukin-6 (IL-6) from the cultured monocytes.[47] Results suggest antiinflammatory effects due to a reduction in IL-1β and TNF-α.

In vitro studies of the effect of black currant on cyclooxygenase (COX) enzymes indicated that black currant inhibited PGE_2 synthesis, but prodelphinidin did not affect COX in the whole-blood assay.[52] These results suggest that the prodelphinidin fractions in black currant may be a useful additive in OA prevention.

Scientific Evidence of Effectiveness
Treatment of RA patients with black currant seed oil reduced signs and symptoms, according to one double-blind, placebo-controlled study.[53] In another study, RA patients given black currant seed oil had marked changes in levels of the inflammatory cytokines IL-1β, TNF-α, IL-6, and PGE_2 compared with those given placebo.[47] The treatment group also showed improvement in morning stiffness. Additional research is needed before a firm conclusion can be made.

Dose
No well-known method of standardization exists for black currant.

For RA, doses of 10.5 g of black currant seed oil (subdivided in 15 capsules) have been taken daily for 24 weeks.[53]

Adverse Effects, Interactions, Pharmacokinetics. See Appendix A.

Borage (Borago officinalis)

Grade B: Good scientific evidence (rheumatoid arthritis)

Mechanism of Action
The main constituent of interest in borage seed oil is gamma-linolenic acid (GLA), which is responsible for most of the pharmacological effects.[54] It has been hypothesized that the antiinflammatory effects of borage may be caused by GLA.[55] GLA increases levels of PGE and cyclic adenosine monophosphate (cAMP), which suppress TNF-α synthesis.[55]

Scientific Evidence of Effectiveness

A clinical study of RA patients found a clinically important reduction in swelling and tenderness in patients treated with borage seed oil compared with placebo.[56] Another trial in patients with active RA found symptomatic improvement and significant reductions in the inflammatory markers PGE_2, leukotriene B_4 (LTB_4), and leukotriene C_4 (LTC_4) produced by stimulated monocytes after 12 weeks of GLA supplementation.[57]

A review of clinical studies assessed the overall effects of essential fatty acids on rheumatological conditions and reported that several clinical trials have found borage oil to improve arthritis symptoms.[58]

Dose

In a few clinical studies, borage oil has been standardized to 23% to 25% GLA.[59-61] Another clinical trial standardized 6 mL of borage oil to contain 1.17 g GLA.[62]

For RA, 1 to 3 g of GLA in borage seed oil has been taken orally daily for up to 24 weeks.[56,63] Nine capsules of borage seed oil (providing 1.1 g of GLA) have also been taken daily for 12 weeks.[57]

Adverse Effects, Interactions, Pharmacokinetics. See Appendix A.

Boswellia (Boswellia serrata)

Grade C: *Unclear or conflicting scientific evidence (osteoarthritis, rheumatoid arthritis)*

Mechanism of Action

Boswellia serrata is a branching tree found in India, North Africa, and the Middle East. A gummy oleo-resin is found under the bark. Oleogum resin from *Boswellia* species has been used in traditional medicine in India and Africa for the treatment of a variety of diseases.[64]

Boswellic acids have been identified as major antiinflammatory components of boswellia gum resin extract.[65-74] Doses of 50 to 200 mg/kg of boswellia extract orally inhibit inflammatory cell migration in rats, simulating the effect of the potent antiinflammatory indomethacin.[72] Boswellic acids also inhibit the activation and proliferation of acute inflammatory cells.[65,67,72] Rat models of arthritis have demonstrated that boswellia has antiinflammatory effects.[68] Results of studies suggest that boswellia extract may also inhibit the TNF-α–induced inflammatory response.[75,76] Boswellic acids also reduce enzymes that are elevated in inflammatory conditions such as arthritis, including glutamic-pyruvic transaminase (GPT; alanine transaminase), glycohydrolase, and β-glucuronidase.[77-79]

Scientific Evidence of Effectiveness

Animal and in vitro studies report that boswellia possesses antiinflammatory properties. Clinical studies have reported conflicting results for boswellia monotherapy.[80,81] In one study, boswellia had additive effects when used with some other therapies (e.g., NSAIDs). Positive studies of combination products containing boswellia (RA-1, Articulin-F) have not provided adequate data regarding the effects of boswellia alone.[82-84]

Dose

The dose of boswellia alone for arthritis has not been determined.

Adverse Effects, Interactions, Pharmacokinetics. See Appendix A.

Bromelain (Bromeliaceae)

Grade C: *Unclear or conflicting scientific evidence (rheumatoid arthritis)*

Mechanism of Action

The mechanism of the putative antiinflammatory activity of bromelain is not well understood. Bromelain may inhibit biosynthesis of proinflammatory prostaglandins by lowering kininogen and bradykinin levels in serum and tissues, and it may alter prostaglandin synthesis.[85] One animal study found a dose-dependent decrease in bradykinin and prekallikrein levels and in plasma exudation.[86]

Combined bromelain and trypsin decreased laboratory-induced edema in rabbits.[87] These results suggest that the inhibitory action of the bromelain-trypsin combination against edema formation may depend on these molecules' ability to prevent vascular leakage.

Scientific Evidence of Effectiveness

One preliminary study examined bromelain combined with corticosteroids such as prednisone.[88] Improvements in joint swelling and mobility were reported in more than 70% of patients. Additional research evaluating bromelain alone is needed before a recommendation can be made for or against the use of bromelain for RA.

Dose

Bromelain is standardized to milk-clotting unit (mcu; officially recognized by Food Chemistry Codex) or gelatin-digesting unit (gdu) activity. Bromelain at 240 mg (Ananase) has been used for 5 days to treat inflammation.[89] Bromelain has also been used in 20-mg to 40-mg doses with standard corticosteroid therapy.[88]

Adverse Effects, Interactions, Pharmacokinetics. See Appendix A.

Cat's Claw (Uncaria spp.)

Grade C: *Unclear or conflicting scientific evidence (osteoarthritis, rheumatoid arthritis)*

Mechanism of Action

Most commercial preparations of cat's claw contain the plant species *Uncaria tomentosa*. Both *U. tomentosa* and *Uncaria guianensis* showed effective antiinflammatory activity, although *U. guianensis* was shown to be more potent.[90] The antiinflammatory properties of *U. guianensis* and *U. tomentosa* may result from their ability to inhibit production of TNF-α and, to a lesser extent, PGE_2.[91-94] Additional studies have demonstrated the ability of cat's claw to inhibit COX-1 and COX-2.[95]

When tested, the isolated compounds from cat's claw had minimal antiinflammatory activity.[96,97] In preliminary pharmacological investigations by Senatore et al,[98] sterols (β-sitosterol, stigmasterol, campesterol) in *U. tomentosa* seemed to contribute to antiinflammatory activity. In animal research, alkaloids of *U. tomentosa* quinovic acid glycosides have also been found to reduce edema.[97]

Scientific Evidence of Effectiveness

Several studies have reported the ability of cat's claw to reduce inflammation.[90-94,96-99] A small preliminary study demonstrated relative safety and modest benefit of a highly purified cat's claw extract for RA patients taking prescription drugs.[100] Patients treated with cat's claw had significantly fewer painful and swollen joints than those who received placebo. Large, high-quality human studies are needed comparing the effects of cat's claw alone to placebo before a conclusion can be drawn.

Dose

Cat's claw is usually administered orally. Most experts recommend that cat's claw be standardized to contain 3% alkaloids and 15% total phenols per dose. In Europe an extract of cat's claw containing only pentacyclic oxindole alkaloids is available on the market. Saventaro root extract is standardized to contain at least 1.3% pentacyclic oxindole alkaloids.

For RA, 20-mg Krallendorn capsules (containing 20 mg of *uncaria tomentosa* with 14.7 mg/g pentacyclic oxindole alkaloids and no tetracyclic oxindole alkaloids) have been taken three times daily for 52 weeks.[100]

Adverse Effects, Interactions, Pharmacokinetics. See Appendix A.

Cherry (Prunus avium, Prunus cerasus, and various Prunus spp.)

Grade B: *Good scientific evidence (arthritis, gout)*

Mechanism of Action

Cherries have long been reputed to relieve the symptoms of arthritis, particularly gouty arthritis.[101] This effect may result from various phenolic compounds in cherries thought to have antiinflammatory effects, notably the hydroxycinnamates and anthocyanins. Further, although most fruits generally contain the reduced form of vitamin C (ascorbic acid), cherries appear to contain only the oxidized form, *dehydroascorbic acid* (DHA).[102] It is unclear whether DHA possesses antigout effects, but cherry consumption has been shown to lower plasma urate concentrations and increase plasma elimination in the urine.[102]

Scientific Evidence of Effectiveness

Cherries have long been popular remedies for relieving arthritis and gout, although the scientific literature is limited. Clinical case reports of a few patients have shown cherry consumption to reduce plasma urate and alleviate gout attacks.[101] Metabolic studies have demonstrated that cherry consumption lowers plasma urate concentrations in healthy women.[102]

Dose

In clinical case reports, reduced plasma urate was observed in gout patients after they consumed 227 g of cherry products daily for 3 days to 3 months.[101] In healthy women, plasma urate was lowered 5 hours after consuming an acute dose of 280 g of depitted cherries (about 45 cherries).[102]

Adverse Effects, Interactions, Pharmacokinetics. See Appendix A.

Devil's Claw (Harpagophytum procumbens)

Grade B: *Good scientific evidence (degenerative joint disease, osteoarthritis)*

Mechanism of Action

One molecule found in devil's claw, *aucubin*, has been shown to inhibit the release of leukotriene C_4 (LCT_4), whereas other molecules have been reported to inhibit the effects of thromboxane B_2 (TXB_2). However, these findings conflict with another study that found no effect of devil's claw on the 5-lipoxygenase pathway.[103]

Extracts of devil's claw have been reported to decrease the activity of inducible nitric oxide synthase (iNOS), TNF-α, COX-2 expression, and matrix-degrading enzymes.[104-108]

Devil's claw extracts have been reported to exert antiinflammatory properties,[109-112] although these results are not confirmed by other studies.[113,114] Antiinflammatory effects in acute and chronic treatment of laboratory-induced arthritis in rats have also been noted.[115] Administration of harpagosides extracted from devil's claw has been reported to produce an analgesic effect[109] and to reduce pain in rats.[116]

Scientific Evidence of Effectiveness

A growing body of scientific evidence suggests that devil's claw is safe and beneficial in the short-term management of pain related to DJD or OA; it was suggested that it may be equally as effective as drug therapies such as

NSAIDs, or may allow for dose reductions or cessation of these drugs in some patients.[117-122] However, many of the available studies have been small or methodologically limited. Additional trials lasting longer than 8 to 12 weeks are necessary.

Dose

Moderate evidence of effectiveness exists for *Harpagophytum* powder standardized to 60 mg harpagoside per day, but there is limited evidence for *Harpagophytum* extract containing less than 30 mg harpagoside.[122]

Adverse Effects, Interactions, Pharmacokinetics. See Appendix A.

Evening Primrose (Oenothera biennis)

Grade C: *Unclear or conflicting scientific evidence (rheumatoid arthritis)*

Mechanism of Action

The active ingredient in evening primrose oil (EPO) is thought to be gamma-linolenic acid (GLA), one of the omega-6 essential fatty acids (EFAs). The amount of GLA in EPO varies but is approximately 9%.[123] EPO also contains linoleic acid (LA), which may be found in a variety of other vegetable oils. LA is metabolized to GLA, which is further metabolized to dihomo-GLA and arachidonic acid.

A review of clinical studies assessing the effects of EFAs on rheumatological conditions[124] found that GLA in EPO improved arthritis symptoms. GLA in EPO promotes the production of prostaglandin E1 (PGE1), which has inhibitory effects on polymorphonuclear leukocytes[125] and lymphocytes.[126] GLA also appears to have an inhibitory effect on leukotriene production.[127] GLA has been shown to decrease leukocyte aggregation and to increase fibrinolysis.[124]

Scientific Evidence of Effectiveness

Evening primrose grows in Europe, North America, and the Southern Hemisphere. Traditionally, EPO has been used to treat eczema. More recently, it has become popular for RA treatment.[128] Clinical trials of EPO for arthritis began in the early 1980s and focused on patients with RA. Studies have been small with methodological limitations. Two clinical trials have found that GLA supplementation reduced the need for pain medication and improved joint pain, tenderness, and global functioning in RA patients.[129,130] Based on inconsistent results and poorly designed trials,[129,131-133] evidence is currently inadequate to recommend for or against this use of EPO for arthritis.

Dose

Evening primrose oil is generally taken orally. Standardized capsules of EPO contain approximately 320 mg LA, 40 mg GLA, and 10 IU vitamin E.[134] Preparations may also be identified according to percent content (70% LA, 9% GLA).[123] Dietary conversion of LA provides approximately 250 to 1000 mg/day of GLA.[135]

For arthritis, clinical trials have used 20 mL EPO and EPO standardized to 540 mg GLA for up to 15 months.[136]

Adverse Effects, Interactions, Pharmacokinetics. See Appendix A.

Feverfew (Tanacetum parthenium)

Grade C: *Unclear or conflicting scientific evidence (rheumatoid arthritis)*

Mechanism of Action

Feverfew's antiinflammatory actions may result from inhibition of prostaglandin synthesis[137,138] and inhibition of the cyclooxygenase and lipoxygenase pathways.[139,140] In vitro inhibition of prostaglandin synthetase activity has also been demonstrated.[141] Extracts of feverfew leaves and commercially available powdered leaves inhibit the generation of TXB_2 and LTB_4 by stimulated rat and human leukocytes.[142] Feverfew extract has also demonstrated inhibition of histamine release from stimulated rat peritoneal mast cells.[143]

Oral administration of feverfew extract has produced significant dose-dependent antiinflammatory and pain-relieving effects in rodents.[144] One experiment showed that parthenolide inhibits the proinflammatory protein I-κB kinase-β.[145] Compounds in feverfew may also affect the ability of inflammatory cells to bind and travel through target tissue, which may further decrease the inflammation response.[146]

Scientific Evidence of Effectiveness

There is limited clinical evidence that feverfew can effectively manage joint inflammation. The only significant finding in one study was an increase in grip strength in the feverfew group compared to baseline and to placebo at 6 weeks of treatment.[147]

Dose

In Great Britain and Canada, feverfew products are standardized to contain at least 0.2% parthenolide. In France, standardized products must contain at least 0.1% parthenolide.[148] One clinical trial of RA used capsules containing a mean dose of 76 mg of dried feverfew leaf, which corresponds to 2 to 3 μmol parthenolide.[147] Traditional doses include 70 to 86 mg of dried chopped feverfew leaves taken once daily.

Adverse Effects, Interactions, Pharmacokinetics. See Appendix A.

Ginger (Zingiber officinale)

Grade C: *Unclear or conflicting scientific evidence (osteoarthritis, rheumatoid arthritis)*

Mechanism of Action

Ginger has been found to inhibit prostaglandin biosynthesis[149] and to interfere with the inflammatory cascade and the vanilloid pain receptor.[150] Ginger demonstrated pain-relieving and antiinflammatory qualities in animal models.[151] Ginger shares pharmacological properties with NSAIDs because it suppresses prostaglandin synthesis through the inhibition of COX-1 and COX-2.[152] However, ginger can be distinguished from NSAIDs based on its ability to suppress leukotriene biosynthesis by inhibiting 5-lipoxygenase. Also, a ginger extract (EV.EXT. 77) derived from *Zingiber officinale* (and *Alpinia galanga*) inhibits the induction of several genes involved in the inflammatory response, including genes encoding cytokines, chemokines, iNOS,[153] and the inducible enzyme COX-2.[152] It has been shown that ginger inhibits T-cell proliferation, IL-1α production,[154] and the synthetic and functional activity of macrophages in vitro.[155,156]

Scientific Evidence of Effectiveness

A literature review that evaluated the efficacy of oral herbal medicines in the treatment of lower back or joint pain reported that the evidence of efficacy for ginger was "moderate."[157] Multiple clinical trials have evaluated ginger's effect on arthritis,[158-161] with some reporting benefit and others reporting no benefit. Based on these mixed results, more clinical trials are necessary before ginger's effect in OA can be confirmed.

It is not clear whether ginger is effective in treating RA. Studies have produced conflicting results, with one reporting improvement in pain and swelling[162] and another finding no benefit.[160] Additional randomized controlled trials (RCTs) are required to confirm whether ginger possesses analgesic properties in rheumatic patients. Currently, there is insufficient evidence to recommend for or against the use of ginger for RA or OA.

Dose

Common forms of ginger include fresh root, dried root, tablets, capsules, liquid extract, tincture, and tea. Many publications note that the maximum recommended daily dose of ginger is 4 grams (g). Some forms of ginger, such as ginger powder, have been reported to cause mild stomach upset; this effect may be reduced by taking ginger capsules rather than powder.

For OA, 200 mg of EV.EXT. 77, which contains the extract of two ginger species (*Zingiber officinale* and *Alpinia galanga*), was given twice daily for 6 weeks.[159]

For RA, a daily dose of 1 to 2 g of powdered ginger has been used.[162] In this study, patients who mistakenly took 2 to 4 g daily of ginger (number of patients not specified) reported faster and superior pain relief.

Adverse Effects, Interactions, Pharmacokinetics. See Appendix A.

Guggul (Commiphora mukul)

Grade C: Unclear or conflicting scientific evidence (rheumatoid arthritis, osteoarthritis)

Mechanism of Action

Resin from the guggul *(Commiphora mukul)* tree has been used in Ayurvedic medicine since around 600 BC. This thorny tree has little foliage and is indigenous to western India. Guggul (gum guggul) is a resin produced by the mukul mirth tree. *Guggulipid* is extracted from guggul and contains plant sterols (guggulsterones E and Z), which are believed to be its bioactive compounds.

The results of several studies suggest possible antiinflammatory and antiarthritic activities of guggul.[163-170] Guggul extract has been demonstrated to reduce edema, arthritis, and inflammatory cell count in rats.[166,168-170] On a per-mcg basis, guggulipid appears to be significantly less potent than indomethacin or hydrocortisone.[165] Possible effects on the inflammatory marker high-sensitivity C-reactive protein (hs-CRP) have recently been observed in a clinical trial.[171]

Scientific Evidence of Effectiveness

One clinical trial using guggul reported improvement in morning stiffness, fatigue, grip strength, writing, dressing, and walking times in RA patients.[172] Another trial reported improvement in RA symptoms in patients treated with a combination product that included guggul.[173]

Dose

The dose of guggul for arthritis is unclear.

Adverse Effects, Interactions, Pharmacokinetics. See Appendix A.

Hop (Humulus lupulus)

Grade C: Unclear or conflicting scientific evidence (rheumatic diseases)

Mechanism of Action

Humulon, one of the bitter constituents in the hop plant, has shown antiinflammatory activity in mice by inhibiting activity against 12-O-tetradecanopyphorbo-13-acetate (TPA)–induced inflammation and arachidonic acid–induced inflammation.[174]

Scientific Evidence of Effectiveness

The Cherokee Native Americans traditionally used hop to treat rheumatic disorders. Early clinical research suggests that Meta050, a proprietary standardized combination of reduced iso-alpha-acids from hop, rosemary extract, and oleanolic acid may help reduce pain in patients with rheumatic diseases (e.g., OA, RA, fibromyalgia).[175] However, well-designed human trials that use hop as monotherapy are needed to determine if these positive effects are specifically the result of hop.

Dose

Patients with rheumatic disease used 440 mg of Meta050 three times daily for 4 weeks.[175] In most subjects the dose was then increased to 880 mg twice daily for the subsequent 4 weeks of the trial.

Adverse Effects, Interactions, Pharmacokinetics. See Appendix A.

Mistletoe (Viscum album)

Grade C: *Unclear or conflicting scientific evidence (arthritis)*

Mechanism of Action

Mistletoe's beneficial results in arthritis may be related to its effects on the immune system. Mistletoe has been shown to increase the number and activity of various WBC types. Increased secretion of immune system–enhancing cytokines (e.g., TNF, IL-1, IL-6) by WBCs has been observed after exposure to mistletoe.[176-183]

Scientific Evidence of Effectiveness

Viscum album has a long history of use in European rituals, folklore, and folk medicine. This shrub has been regarded as a sacred medicinal plant and was called "all-healer" or "cure-all" by the Gauls and Celts. One retrospective case series of 319 patients documented reduced pain in arthritis patients treated with mistletoe extract injection.[184]

Dose

Mistletoe is usually taken orally; one clinical trial used joint injections. Extracts of mistletoe may be standardized based on the content of several different compounds.[185] Commercial preparations are available as aqueous extracts of *Viscum album* obtained from several host trees fermented with *Lactobacillus plantarum* (Iscador). Helixor is obtained similarly without fermentation. Eurixor extracts are said to be standardized to 50 to 70 ng/mL.

For arthritis, Plenosol injected with a tuberculin syringe has been given directly into the site at 0.1 to 0.7 mL (100-5000 NKE) twice weekly for several weeks.[184]

Adverse Effects, Interactions, Pharmacokinetics. See Appendix A.

Papaya (Carica papaya)

Grade C: *Unclear or conflicting scientific evidence (rheumatic disorders)*

Mechanism of Action

When aerial parts of the papaya plant *(C. papaya)* are damaged, the plant releases latex that contains enzymes, including cysteine proteinases, papain, chymopapain, caricain, and glycyl endopeptidase. These enzymes may be an important part of the plant's defense mechanism that cleans and seals the damaged areas of the plant.[186]

An in vitro study indicated that exposure of inflammatory cells (polymorphonuclear lymphocytes) to Wobenzym, which contains pancreatin, papain, bromelain, trypsin, and chymotrypsin, stimulated production of reactive oxygen species (ROS).[187] In a clinical trial of healthy subjects, Wobenzym significantly increased ROS production in a dose-dependent and time-dependent manner.[187] The mechanism of action in the relief of arthritis symptoms is unclear.

Scientific Evidence of Effectiveness

A review found inconsistent results from studies using proteolytic enzymes, including combinations of bromelain, papain, trypsin, and chymotrypsin, to treat rheumatic disorders.[188] Although often inconsistent, results of the reviewed studies do suggest that oral therapy with proteolytic enzymes produces certain analgesic and antiinflammatory effects. More research is needed before papain can be recommended for arthritis treatment.

Dose

The dose of papain for arthritis has not been determined.

Adverse Effects, Interactions, Pharmacokinetics. See Appendix A.

Podophyllum (Podophyllum spp.)

Grade C: *Unclear or conflicting scientific evidence (rheumatoid arthritis)*

Mechanism of Action

The applicable parts of podophyllum are the root, rhizome, and resin. Major active constituents are podophyllotoxins (including 4α- and 4β-podophyllotoxin-4-O-(D)-6-acetylglucopyranoside), quercetin, kampherol, alpha-peltatin, and beta-peltatin.[189-192]

According to an ex vivo study, *Podophyllum hexandrum* treatment of mouse peritoneal macrophages inhibited the production and release of several inflammatory molecules, including nitrites, interferon gamma (IFN-γ), IL-6, and TNF-α.[193]

Scientific Evidence of Effectiveness

One study evaluated the use of 300 mg of CPH 82, which is composed of two purified semisynthetic lignan glycosides of *Podophyllum emodi*. Patients treated with CPH 82 showed a statistically significant improvement in most clinical and immunological variables compared with patients given placebo.[194] Additional research is needed before a firm conclusion can be drawn.

Dose

Podophyllum dosing has not been rigorously tested in human trials. A dose of 300 mg of CPH 82, composed of two purified semisynthetic lignan glycosides of *Podophyllum emodi*, taken orally daily for 12 weeks has been used for treatment of RA.[194]

Adverse Effects, Interactions, Pharmacokinetics. See Appendix A.

Rose Hip (*Rosa* spp.)

Grade B: *Good scientific evidence (osteoarthritis)*

Mechanism of Action

Fresh rose hips contain 0.03% to 1.3% vitamin C.[195] They are also high in flavonoid and nonflavonoid polyphenols as well as major and minor carotenoids, all of which contribute to rose hips' antioxidant capacity.[196,197] Rose hip constituents have demonstrated antiinflammatory properties,[198] which may help to clarify their use in the treatment of arthritis.

Extracts or fractions obtained from *Rosa canina* roots have demonstrated in vitro inhibitory activity against one model of inflammation by inhibiting IL-1α, IL-1β, and TNF-α biosynthesis.[199] A standardized rose hip powder, Hyben Vital, has been shown to reduce serum CRP levels in humans.[200] This rose hips preparation has also reduced the rate of migration of polymorphonuclear leukocytes in vitro.[200,201] The galactolipid (2S)-1,2-di-*O*-[(9Z,12Z,15Z)-octadeca-9,12,15-trienoyl]-3-*O*-β-d-galactopyranosyl glycerol, isolated from dried and milled fruits of *R. canina*, has demonstrated antiinflammatory properties through its inhibitory effects on chemotaxis of human peripheral blood neutrophils in vitro.[198]

Scientific Evidence of Effectiveness

Two review articles have supported the use of rose hip extract for relief of joint pain, improvement in functioning, increased joint flexion, decreased use of pain medication,[202,203] and decreased CRP and creatinine levels.[202]

Several placebo-controlled trials evaluating the efficacy of rose hip extract on OA symptoms found that it decreased pain, stiffness, global disease severity, and use of pain medication.[200,201,204,205]

Dose

Rose hip concentrate is most often administered orally. Hyben Vital, a biologically standardized rose hip powder, has been studied in clinical trials.[200,201] Hyben Vital is composed of dried fruits, seeds, and husks of LiTo, a subtype of *Rosa canina*, and is standardized to contain at least 500 mg vitamin C per 100 g Hyben Vital powder, plus pectins 58.0 mg/g, beta-carotene 57.9 mg/kg, beta-sitosterol 0.5 mg/g, folic acid 1.6 mg/kg, vitamin E 4.6 mg/100 g, magnesium 170 mg/100 g, zinc 1.0 mg/100 g, and copper 10.9 mcg/100 g.

For osteoarthritis, 5 g (five 0.5-g capsules twice daily) of Hyben Vital has been taken for 3 months.[200,201,205] Twice-daily standardized rose hip powder at a dose of 0.5 g has also been used in clinical trials.[200]

Adverse Effects, Interactions, Pharmacokinetics. See Appendix A.

Stinging Nettle (*Urtica dioica*)

Grade C: *Unclear or conflicting scientific evidence (arthritis)*

Mechanism of Action

The proposed use of stinging nettle in the treatment of arthritis may be the result of antiinflammatory and immunomodulatory effects demonstrated in animals. Extracts of stinging nettle have a number of effects on the immune system. Stinging nettle extracts inhibit edema in rats and stimulate lymphocytes and the complement system.[206,207] They have been shown to inhibit the enzyme *human leukocyte elastase* (HLE). HLE is one of the most destructive enzymes released by neutrophils that migrate into tissues during the inflammatory process.[208] Stinging nettle extracts have also been found to inhibit the production of cytokines, prostaglandins, leukotrienes, and other mediators of the inflammatory response.[209-212]

Scientific Evidence of Effectiveness

A trial comparing stinging nettle combined with low-dose diclofenac (50 mg) to higher-dose diclofenac (200 mg) in acute arthritis attacks found a comparable decrease in pain and stiffness in the two groups,[213] suggesting that stinging nettle combined with low-dose diclofenac may be as effective as diclofenac at higher doses. Results also showed a comparable decrease in CRP in both groups. More research is necessary to determine if stinging nettle extract is effective on its own.

Dose

There is no well-known standardization for nettle.

For arthritis, 50 mg stewed nettle leaves in combination with 50 mg diclofenac daily for 14 days has been used.[213]

Adverse Effects, Interactions, Pharmacokinetics. See Appendix A.

Turmeric (*Curcuma longa*)

Grade C: *Unclear or conflicting scientific evidence (osteoarthritis, rheumatoid arthritis)*

Mechanism of Action

In vitro and animal studies have demonstrated antiinflammatory properties of turmeric and its constituent curcumin that may play a role in the symptomatic relief of OA and RA. Multiple mechanisms have been implicated, including effects on prostaglandins and cytokines.

Turmeric has been associated with the inhibition of TNF-α, interleukin-8 (IL-8), monocyte inflammatory protein-1, IL-1β, and monocyte chemotactic protein-1.[214] Turmeric and its constituent curcumin have been found to inhibit lipoxygenase and cyclooxygenase in rat tissues and in vitro,[215-217] as well as inhibit TXB_2 formation[218] and LTB_4 formation[217,219] in vitro. Based on animal studies, oral administration of curcumin may reduce expression of several cytokines, chemokines, and proteinases.[220] In rat macrophages, curcumin inhibited the incorporation of arachidonic acid into membrane lipids, as well as PGE_2, LTB_4, and LTC_4, but did not affect the release of arachidonic acid.[221]

Scientific Evidence of Effectiveness

Turmeric has been used historically to treat rheumatic conditions. Promising preliminary results were found in a clinical study in which 1200 mg of curcumin was given daily for two weeks in patients with rheumatoid arthritis.[222] Treatment with two capsules of Articulin-F (containing extracts of 50 mg turmeric root, 100 mg *Boswellia serrata*, 450 mg *Withania somnifera*, and 50 mg zinc complex) daily for 3 months significantly improved the mean pain severity score and mean disability score in OA patients.[34] Because Articulin-F is a combination product, further studies are needed to distinguish the effects of turmeric as a monotherapy.

Dose

Turmeric may be standardized to contain 95% curcuminoids per dose. The dried root of turmeric is reported to contain 3% to 5% curcumin.[223] Subjects with RA received 1200 mg of curcumin daily.[222] In other clinical study, subjects with OA received two capsules of Articulin-F (extracts of 50 mg turmeric root, 100 mg *Boswellia serrata*, 450 mg *Withania somnifera*, and 50 mg zinc complex) daily for 3 months.[34]

Adverse Effects, Interactions, Pharmacokinetics. See Appendix A.

Willow (*Salix* spp.)

Grade A: *Strong scientific evidence (osteoarthritis)*

Grade C: *Conflicting scientific evidence (rheumatoid arthritis)*

Mechanism of Action

The active constituent of willow bark is the salicylate *salicin*. Willow bark also contains other salicylates, glycosides, tannins, and flavonoids. Salicin is a chemical precursor to aspirin, and has some similar pharmacological effects. An ethanolic extract of willow bark extract inhibited COX-2–mediated prostaglandin release. In animal study in vivo, all doses of willow bark studied showed antiinflammatory activity, and only high doses of aspirin and acetylsalicylic acid showed the same effect.[224] Willow bark may also act as a weak inhibitor of proinflammatory cytokines (including TNF-α, IL-1β, and IL-6), all of which are inflammatory mediators.[225]

Scientific Evidence of Effectiveness

OSTEOARTHRITIS. The benefits of willow bark extract on patients with OA have been studied in several placebo-controlled trials.[226-228] All studies showed a significant difference between willow bark extract and placebo in the treatment of chronic pain. One trial comparing willow bark to diclofenac (100 mg) for both OA and RA found significant improvement in pain with diclofenac but not with willow bark.[229] Another trial found that the combination product Reumalex significantly improved pain compared with placebo.[226] The ingredients in Reumalex include 100 mg pulverized white willow bark, 40 mg pulverized guaiacum resin, 35 mg pulverized black cohosh, 25 mg pulverized extract of sarsaparilla 4:1, and 17 mg pulverized extract of poplar bark 7:1. Because Reumalex contains multiple active ingredients, the effect of willow bark extract is difficult to discern.

Larger clinical trials of longer duration are needed to determine the true efficacy of willow bark extract, and if the clinical improvement seen with willow bark treatment results only from the salicylate content or from additional active components as well.

RHEUMATOID ARTHRITIS. Although in vitro studies have demonstrated the ability of willow bark extract to inhibit the production and release of inflammatory mediators,[224,225,230,231] one available trial of 26 patients with RA found no improvement in pain comparing willow bark extract to placebo.[229] Based on these limited findings, willow bark does not appear to be effective in RA.

Dose

Willow bark extract may be taken orally as a tablet or tea or may be used in the form of an ointment or cream. In arthritis clinical trials, it has been used as a tablet. A dose of 2 g of willow bark has been reported to contain about 20 mg total salicin. European products are typically standardized to 1% salicin.[232] The proprietary preparation Assalix is standardized to 15.2% salicin, which corresponds to 240 mg of salicin per tablet.[233] Based on unsubstantiated reports, a typical 500-mg dose of aspirin may have equivalent therapeutic effects to 794 mg of salicin. If extraction was 100% effective, this amount of salicin could be derived from 80 to 150 g of dried willow bark. For OA pain, 1360 to 2160 mg of willow bark extract, containing 240 mg of salicin, has been taken daily for 2 weeks in clinical study.[227,228]

Adverse Effects, Interactions, Pharmacokinetics. See Appendix A.

Ayurveda

> Ayurveda uses a combination of dietary changes, herbal supplementation, and physical and spiritual exercises. An Ayurvedic formula containing roots of *Withania somnifera*, the stem of *Boswellia serrata*, rhizomes of *Curcuma longa*, and a zinc complex (Articulin-F) may contribute to significant improvement in the pain and disability caused by OA.[82]

HERBAL THERAPIES WITH NEGATIVE EVIDENCE

Willow (*Salix* spp.)

Grade D: *Fair negative scientific evidence (gout)*
Willow bark contains salicylic acid, a chemical precursor to aspirin. Because aspirin is known to increase uric acid retention and trigger gout attacks, especially at low doses,[234] willow bark is not recommended for use by gout patients.

HERBAL THERAPIES WITH LIMITED EVIDENCE

African Wild Potato (*Hypoxis hemerocallidea*)

The constituents responsible for the pharmacological activity of African wild potato and the mechanism of action are unclear. A study in rats compared the antiinflammatory activity of *Hypoxis hemerocallidea* extracts with aspirin, also known as acetylsalicylic acid (ASA).[235] The extract was found to be less potent than ASA as an antiinflammatory agent. Another study in rats found that the aqueous extract of African wild potato possesses antiinflammatory properties.[236]

Dandelion (*Taraxacum officinale*)

Dandelion's therapeutic effects have historically been attributed to the bitter constituents found in its roots and leaves.[237] Research in animals suggests that dandelion root may possess antiinflammatory properties.[238] Sesquiterpene lactones may contribute to dandelion's mild antiinflammatory activity.[238]

Dong Quai (*Angelica sinensis*)

Dong quai (*Angelica sinensis*), also known as Chinese angelica, has been used for thousands of years in traditional Chinese, Korean, and Japanese medicine. It remains one of the most popular plants in Chinese medicine and is used primarily for health conditions in women. In Chinese medicine, dong quai is most often used in combination with other herbs. It is traditionally used to treat arthritis. However, there is insufficient reliable human evidence to recommend the use of dong quai alone or in combination with other herbs for OA or RA.

Flax (*Linum usitatissimum*)

Flaxseed and flaxseed oil may possess antiinflammatory properties because of the fatty acids EPA and DHA, which inhibit the neutrophil inflammatory responses in humans.[239] These abilities may also result from the inhibition of LTB_4 formation and from the inhibition of LTB_4 and platelet-activating factor (PAF)–stimulated chemotaxis. Also, alpha-linolenic acid (ALA) was found to decrease the production of arachidonic acid, thereby causing a reduction in inflammation.[240] ALA may suppress cell-mediated immunity and T-cell function without affecting humoral immunity and B-cell function (shown in immunocompromised patients).[241]

Marijuana (*Cannabis sativa*)

Constituents of marijuana have been reported to have antiarthritic properties in mice.[242] A small clinical trial compared the use of the cannabis-based medicine Sativex to placebo in RA.[243] Patients treated with Sativex reported significantly less pain and global disease severity than those receiving placebo.

Pycnogenol (*Pinus pinaster* subsp. *atlantica*)

In vitro, Pycnogenol reduced the production of IL-1β and its messenger ribonucleic acid (mRNA) levels and reduced the expression of IL-2.[244] The activation of nuclear factor kappa B (NF-κB) and activator protein-1 (AP-1), two major transcription factors centrally involved in IL-1β gene expression, was also reduced. Pycnogenol inhibited TNF-α–stimulated release of superoxide anion and hydrogen peroxide from human umbilical vascular endothelial cells.[245] Blood samples from healthy volunteers who had been supplemented with 200 mg of Pycnogenol daily for 5 days showed significantly inhibited NF-κB activation.[246] These blood samples also inhibited COX-1 and COX-2 activities.[247]

Tea (*Camellia sinensis*)

The components of green tea include caffeine, polyphenols, trace elements, and vitamins. Green tea polyphenols mainly include catechins, anthocyanins, and phenolic acids.[248] The alkaloids (caffeine, theobromine, and theophylline) in tea are nervous system stimulants, while the polyphenols are antioxidant compounds.

Epigallocatechin-3-gallate (EGCG) is a compound found in green tea that inhibits the expression of matrix metalloproteinase-1 (MMP-1) and MMP-13 in human chondrocytes in vitro and inhibits the activation of the enzyme c-Jun N-terminal kinase.[249,250] Both these enzymes are involved in the inflammatory response. EGCG also inhibits the activity and expression of COX-2 and NOS-2 in human chondrocytes and the production of nitric oxide.[251,252] Further, catechins from green tea prevent the breakdown of cartilage in vitro.[253] In mice fed green tea polyphenols, there was a marked reduction in the expression of inflammatory mediators (e.g., COX 2, IFN-γ, TNF-α) in arthritic joints compared with control mice.[254]

Based on laboratory evidence of antiinflammatory and chondroprotective effects of green tea extracts, potential benefit exists for patients with arthritis. Clinical trials will be necessary before green tea can be recommended as a useful therapy in arthritis.

Thunder God Vine (Tripterygium wilfordii)

Thunder god vine (TGV) has been shown to inhibit T-cell autocrine stimulation[255] and inflammatory cytokine production.[256,257] Parts of the TGV plant are poisonous and can cause death.[128] In a placebo-controlled trial, patients treated with TGV showed significant improvement in RA symptoms.[258]

Herbs with Possible Antiarthritic Properties*

HERB	SPECIFIC THERAPEUTIC USE(S)†	HERB	SPECIFIC THERAPEUTIC USE(S)†
Abuta	Rheumatic disorders	Bupleurum	Rheumatoid arthritis, autoimmune disorders
Aconite	Arthritis, inflammation joint pain, rheumatoid arthritis	Burdock	Arthritis, rheumatoid arthritis
Agrimony	Rheumatic disorders	Calamus	Autoimmune disorders
Alfalfa	Rheumatoid arthritis	Capers	Inflammation, rheumatic disorders
Aloe	Osteoarthritis, rheumatoid arthritis, autoimmune disorders	Carqueja	Rheumatic disorders
Alpinia	Arthritis	Celery	Arthritis, inflammation
American pennyroyal	Joint disorders	Chamomile	Arthritis, inflammation, rheumatic disorders
Andiroba	Arthritis		
Angel's trumpet	Arthritis, rheumatic disorders	Chaparral	Arthritis, autoimmune disorders, rheumatic disorders
Anise	Rheumatic disorders	Chia	Joint disorders
Aristolochia spp.	Rheumatic disorders	Cinnamon	Arthritis, inflammation, rheumatic disorders
Asarum	Rheumatic disorders		
Astragalus	Joint disorders, autoimmune disorders	Codonopsis	Autoimmune disorders
		Coleus	Autoimmune disorders
Babassu	Rheumatic disorders	Comfrey	Arthritis, autoimmune disorders
Bacopa	Rheumatic disorders	Coral	Arthritis
Barberry	Arthritis, rheumatic disorders	Cordyceps	Autoimmune disorders
Bay leaf	Arthritis, rheumatic disorders	Couch grass	Rheumatic disorders
Belladonna	Arthritis	Cramp bark	Arthritis
Bellis perennis	Arthritis, joint disorders, rheumatic disorders	Cranberry	Rheumatoid arthritis
		Datura wrightii	Arthritis, rheumatic disorders
Betel nut	Rheumatic disorders, joint pain	Desert parsley	Rheumatic disorders
Betony	Rheumatic disorders	Devil's club	Arthritis
Bilberry	Arthritis	Eastern hemlock	Rheumatic disorders
Bitter melon	Rheumatoid arthritis	Echinacea	Rheumatic disorders
Bitter orange	Rheumatic disorders	English ivy	Arthritis, rheumatic disorders
Black horehound	Arthritis	Ephedra	Arthritis, joint disorders
Bloodroot	Rheumatic disorders	Essiac	Arthritis, autoimmune disorders
Blue cohosh	Arthritis, inflammation, rheumatic disorders	Eucalyptus	Rheumatic disorders
		Euphorbia	Arthritis, rheumatic disorders
Boldo	Rheumatic disorders	Fo-ti	Autoimmune disorders
Boneset	Arthritis, rheumatic disorders	Garcinia	Rheumatic disorders
Buchu	Rheumatic disorders		
Bulbous buttercup	Rheumatic disorders	Ginkgo	Rheumatic disorders

Continued

Herbs with Possible Antiarthritic Properties—cont'd

HERB	SPECIFIC THERAPEUTIC USE(S)†	HERB	SPECIFIC THERAPEUTIC USE(S)†
Ginseng	Autoimmune disorders, inflammation, rheumatic disorders	Onion	Arthritis
Globe artichoke	Arthritis, rheumatic disorders	Oregano	Arthritis, rheumatoid arthritis
Goji	Arthritis	Peppermint oil	Arthritis, rheumatic disorders
Goldenrod	Arthritis	Pokeweed	Arthritis, rheumatic disorders
Goldenseal	Arthritis, autoimmune disorders	*Polypodium leucotomos*	Autoimmune disorders, rheumatic disorders, joint disorders
Gotu kola	Rheumatic disorders, autoimmune disorders	Populus	Rheumatic disorders
Grape seed	Arthritis, joint disorders	Raspberry	Rheumatic disorders
Ground ivy	Arthritis, inflammation, rheumatic disorders	Red clover	Arthritis
Guarana	Rheumatic disorders	Rehmannia	Autoimmune disorders, rheumatoid arthritis
Gymnema	Rheumatoid arthritis	Reishi mushroom	Arthritis
Heartsease	Arthritis, autoimmune disorders, inflammation, rheumatic disorders	Rhubarb	Rheumatic disorders
Holy basil	Arthritis	Rosemary	Joint pain, rheumatic disorders
Horse chestnut	Rheumatic disorders, rheumatoid arthritis	Sarsaparilla	Arthritis
Horseradish	Arthritis, rheumatic disorders	Scotch broom	Rheumatic disorders
Horsetail	Reiter's syndrome, rheumatoid arthritis	Sea buckthorn	Arthritis, autoimmune disorders
Hyssop	Rheumatic disorders	Seaweed	Arthritis, rheumatic disorders
Jequirity	Rheumatic disorders	Shepherd's purse	Rheumatic disorders
Jewelweed	Rheumatic disorders	Shiitake mushroom	Arthritis
Juniper	Arthritis	Skunk cabbage	Rheumatic disorders
Katuka	Rheumatoid arthritis	Slippery elm	Rheumatic disorders
Kava	Arthritis, joint pain, rheumatic disorders	Soy	Autoimmune disorders, rheumatoid arthritis
Labrador tea	Arthritis	Spirulina	Autoimmune disorders
Ladies mantle	Rheumatic disorders	Squill	Arthritis
Lavender	Rheumatic disorders	St. John's wort	Joint pain, rheumatic disorders
Lemongrass	Arthritis, rheumatic disorders	Star anise	Arthritis, rheumatic disorders
Licorice	Rheumatoid arthritis	Tamanu	Rheumatic disorders
Lime	Arthritis, rheumatic disorders	Tamarind	Rheumatic disorders
Maitake mushroom	Arthritis	Tansy	Rheumatic disorders
Marshmallow	Arthritis	Thyme	Arthritis, inflammation, rheumatic disorders
Mastic	Arthritis, rheumatic disorders	Tribulus	Rheumatic disorders, joint disorders
Meadowsweet	Rheumatic disorders, rheumatoid arthritis	Tylophora	Joint pain
Morus nigra	Rheumatic disorders	Usnea	Autoimmune disorders
Mugwort	Rheumatic disorders	Uva ursi	Arthritis
Muira puama	Rheumatic disorders	Valerian	Arthritis, rheumatic disorders
Mullein	Rheumatic disorders	Verbena	Rheumatic disorders
Noni	Arthritis, inflammation, joint pain, rheumatic disorders	Watercress	Arthritis, rheumatoid arthritis
		Wheatgrass	Rheumatoid arthritis
		White oak	Rheumatic disorders
		Wild yam	Joint pain, rheumatic disorders
Nopal	Arthritis	Yellow dock	Arthritis
		Yerba santa	Arthritis
Nux vomica	Reiter's syndrome, rheumatic disorders	Yew	Arthritis, rheumatic disorders

*This is not an all-inclusive or comprehensive list of herbs with possible antiarthritic properties; other herbs and supplements may possess these qualities. A qualified health care provider should be consulted with specific questions or concerns regarding the potential effects of agents or interactions.
†Based on expert opinion, anecdote, case reports, and/or preliminary trial evidence.

ADJUNCT THERAPIES

1. Several other alternative therapies have been studied for the relief of arthritis symptoms and may be used in conjunction with herbal therapies. The most common may be glucosamine with or without chondroitin. Glucosamine, a molecule found in the joint fluid, and chondroitin, a component of healthy cartilage, have been used alone and in combination for the treatment of arthritis. *Glucosamine* increases synthesis of proteoglycans in cultures of normal human chondrocytes in vitro,[259,260] as well as in chondrocytes isolated from human osteoarthritic articular cartilage,[260,261] and may have clinical effects as well.[262] Glucosamine has a beneficial effect in animal models of experimental arthritis[263,264] and also appears to display mild antiinflammatory activity.[265-267]
2. *Chondroitin* is a building block of the proteoglycan molecules found in cartilaginous tissues of most mammals. Chondroitin is hydrophilic and can help attract water molecules into the cartilage matrix.[268] Chondroitin sulfates have been shown to influence the formation of new cartilage matrix by stimulating chondrocyte metabolism and synthesis of collagen and proteoglycan.[269]
3. Several systematic reviews and meta-analyses of glucosamine and chondroitin in osteoarthritis (OA) have been conducted.[269-273] Results are conflicting, with some reviews revealing moderate benefit and others finding none. Despite the relatively large number of trials performed, poor study design and variation in outcome measures prevent a conclusion as to the efficacy of glucosamine and chondroitin in OA.
4. The antiinflammatory properties of *fish oil* have also been studied as adjunctive therapies in arthritis. Fish oil contains high amounts of two omega-3 fatty acids: EPA (eicosapentaenoic acid) and DHA (docosahexaenoic acid). Fish oil, as the exclusive source of lipid, suppressed autoimmune disorders in mice by decreasing lymphoid hyperplasia and macrophage surface I_a expression and by delaying the onset of renal disease.[274] Another mouse model of lupus suggested that suppression of autoimmune disease by DHA and EPA was related to a decrease in IL-1β gene transcription.[275-277] Omega-3 fatty acids compete with omega-6 fatty acids to inhibit production of inflammatory products from arachidonic acid.[278-286] Several small clinical trials have shown improvements in pain, stiffness, strength, and functional status in rheumatoid arthritis (RA) patients.[287-302]
5. Physical activity may also be beneficial. A clinician such as a physical therapist may organize range-of-motion exercises and individualized exercise programs. These exercises may reduce stiffness, help maintain joint movement, increase muscle strength and flexibility, and help keep cartilage and bone healthy.
6. *Acupuncture* has been used for centuries to heal a variety of ailments, including arthritis. The precise mechanism of action of acupuncture remains unclear, particularly within the framework of Western medicine. There is conflicting evidence regarding the efficacy of acupuncture in the treatment of OA, with several randomized trials, primarily studying knee, cervical, and hip OA symptoms. Most studies have been methodologically flawed and have yielded mixed results. Differences in technique may account for this discrepancy, although descriptions of technique in the studies are not adequate to make this distinction. A recent randomized trial demonstrated a significant improvement in OA pain and disability,[303] but two prior well-designed small trials were negative.[304,305] Ezzo et al[306] conducted a small systematic review of randomized or quasirandomized trials using needle insertion for OA of the knee. Short-term results showed reductions in pain for four studies,[303,307-309] improvement in function for two studies,[303,307] and reduced cost of treatment for the only study that collected cost data.[307]
7. *Magnetic therapy* is a highly controversial and poorly understood therapy for numerous ailments, but claimed by proponents to aid in the relief of arthritis symptoms. Numerous theories exist on the possible medicinal value of static magnets or electromagnetic fields, although high-quality scientific research is lacking. There are many proposed mechanisms. Magnet therapy may affect blood vessels and improve blood circulation, relax blood vessels (from effects on cellular calcium channels), increase blood oxygen levels, and decrease toxic materials or plaques in blood vessel walls. Magnet therapy may also have effects on the nervous system and cause alterations in nerve impulses, block nerve-cell conduction, increase endorphins, and reduce edema. Magnet therapy may lead to the alkalinization of body fluids, increase oxygen in local tissues, relax muscles, or change cell membranes. In addition, magnet therapy may stimulate acupoints and thus may have activity similar to acupuncture.
8. Several studies have evaluated the use of magnetic field therapy applied to areas of OA or degenerative joint disease (DJD).[310-314] In particular, this research has focused on knee OA. However, most reported studies have been small or poorly designed or reported, and efficacy remains unclear. Notably, one promising small study in 2004 reported some benefits.[315] Another study evaluating magnet therapy in RA found no benefit.[316] Larger and better-quality studies are needed before a recommendation can be made in this area.
9. *Hydrotherapy* includes a variety of different methods that use water therapeutically, including heated baths, hot-spring or seawater baths, mineral baths,

and water-jet massages. Hydrotherapy is also called *balneotherapy*.[128] There are numerous proposed mechanisms of action for hydrotherapy, depending on the specific technique used. Hydrotherapy practitioners and texts propose that immersion treatments and wraps may serve to detoxify the blood. Alternating cold with hot temperatures is suggested to alter blood circulation, enhance the immune system, and improve digestion. Warmth also causes muscle relaxation. Some hydrotherapy techniques make use of these physiological changes, although correlation to long-term health benefits is not clear. Multiple studies have examined hydrotherapy in arthritis treatment and are largely based on therapy given at Dead Sea spa sites in Israel.[317-327] Most studies report benefits in pain, range of motion, or muscle strength but have design flaws. Therefore, insufficient reliable evidence exists on which to base recommendations.

10. *Mind-body techniques* are based on the concept that one's mental state can affect one's physical health. These techniques attempt to modify the interactions present among the mind, emotions, and body. Types of mind-body techniques include relaxation, meditation, tai chi, and spirituality.[128] A review of mind-body techniques in RA evaluated 25 trials and concluded that mind-body techniques may be effective additions to conventional RA therapy.[328] Mind-body practices were reported to improve pain, disability, and psychological state.[128]

11. Arthritic individuals who are overweight may benefit from losing weight, by putting less strain on the weight-bearing joints such as the ankles. It may also decrease uric acid levels in the body. However, weight loss should be gradual because sudden weight loss has been shown to temporarily increase uric acid levels and worsen symptoms.

12. Patients with gouty arthritis may benefit from eating a diet low in animal protein, including red meat, organ meat (e.g., kidneys, liver), and oily fish (e.g., salmon, sardines, mackerel, anchovies, herring). These foods contain high amounts of purine and may worsen gout symptoms. It is generally recommended that all individuals, including those who do not have gout, eat no more than 5 to 6 ounces of lean meat, poultry, or fish daily.

13. It is also recommended that gout patients limit alcohol intake. Consuming too much alcohol may prevent the body from excreting sufficient uric acid. Men with gout should limit their alcohol consumption to two drinks or less and women to one drink daily. Alcohol should not be consumed at all during a gout attack. Instead, patients should drink plenty of other fluids (especially water). Drinking sufficient water will help dilute uric acid in the blood and urine, reduce gout symptoms, and may even prevent future attacks.

INTEGRATIVE THERAPY PLAN

- Interview the patient to determine family history and the onset and duration of symptoms, type of symptoms, joints involved, and other nonarthritic symptoms. The most common symptoms include joint pain, stiffness, swelling, and decreased range of motion.
- Osteoarthritis (OA) typically produces pain in fingers and weight-bearing joints that feel worse with physical activity; swelling may be absent. OA may only affect one joint.
- Rheumatoid arthritis (RA) most often affects the hands, wrists, and knees, with swelling, stiffness, and pain that is worse in the morning. Joints are usually affected symmetrically.
- Periarthritis results in stiffness, swelling, pain, and restricted motion in joints and most often develops in the shoulder.
- Juvenile arthritis symptoms may be mild and may include fever, limping, sore, painful, or stiff joints, weak muscles, and a feeling of tiredness. Symptoms may be infrequent and temporary or may be persistent.
- Infectious arthritis develops rapidly in a single joint, with severe pain, swelling, redness, and restricted movement. Patients may also have fever. This type of arthritis is considered a medical emergency and requires immediate medical attention.
- Reactive arthritis (Reiter's syndrome) symptoms usually include pain with urination (dysuria), eye pain, and arthritis of the large joints. Patients may also have fever and fatigue.
- Gout symptoms include intense pain and redness of a single joint, most frequently the joint of the big toe. Symptoms usually begin at night and may resolve within several days or may be recurrent.
- Before treatment, a physician should evaluate all patients with arthritis symptoms to determine the type of arthritis and to rule out acute conditions such as infection and trauma.
- Determine if the patient has additional medical conditions such as liver disease, kidney disease, or immunosuppression.
- In addition to a thorough physical examination and medical history, additional studies that may be warranted include radiography, joint aspiration, arthroscopy, CT, MRI, and blood tests. A specific blood test for diagnosing RA called the anti-CCP antibody test may help to distinguish RA from other types of arthritis.
- Determine if the patient is taking prescription or over-the-counter drugs, herbs, or dietary supplements for the management of symptoms. Common medications for OA include aspirin, acetaminophen, ibuprofen, naproxen, COX-2 inhibitors (e.g., Celebrex), and corticosteroids (e.g., prednisone).
- Ask if the patient has any allergies to medications, including aspirin or nonsteroidal antiinflammatory drugs (NSAIDs).

- Common medications for RA include NSAIDs, corticosteroids, and disease-modifying antirheumatic drugs (DMARDs). DMARDs include methotrexate, sulfasalazine, leflunomide (Arava), etanercept (Enbrel), infliximab (Remicade), adalimumab (Humira), abatacept (Orencia), rituximab (Rituxan), anakinra (Kineret), antimalarials, gold salts, penicillamine, cyclosporin A, cyclophosphamide, and azathioprine (Imuran).
- Willow bark may be suggested to the patient with OA considering dietary supplements. The proprietary preparation Assalix is standardized to contain 15.2% salicin, which corresponds to 240 mg of salicin per tablet. Doses of 1360 to 2160 mg willow bark extract containing 240 mg of salicin can be taken daily. Willow bark should be avoided in patients with gastrointestinal ulcers, bleeding, or gastritis. It should be used cautiously in patients with liver disease or diabetes.
- Avocado oil, rose hip, and devil's claw may also be suggested for OA patients. The proprietary formula Piascledine 300 is standardized to 100 mg of one-third avocado oil and 200 mg of soybean oil. The topical cream Regividerm is standardized to contain 82.9 mg/kg avocado oil. A dose of 5 g of Hyben Vital, a proprietary rose hip extract, can be taken daily. Doses of 670 to 2460 mg of devil's claw have been used in clinical trials.
- Both rose hip and devil's claw should be avoided in patients on antiplatelet or anticoagulant medication. Devil's claw may potentiate the anticoagulant effect of other medications. Rose hip has platelet-aggregating activity in vitro and may inhibit the effects of anticoagulant or antiplatelet medications.
- Glucosamine with or without chondroitin may be effective for the treatment of OA and is a relatively safe supplement. Numerous studies have evaluated the concomitant use of glucosamine and chondroitin sulfate,[329-332] which suggests that they may work synergistically. There are also anecdotal reports of additive effects of glucosamine with concomitant use of supplements such as manganese or vitamin C.
- If the patient has RA, you might suggest borage oil. A dose of 1 to 3 g of gamma-linolenic acid in borage seed oil daily for up to 24 weeks has been used.[56,63] Nine capsules of borage seed oil daily for 12 weeks has also been used.[57] Borage oil may increase the risk of bleeding and may potentiate the effect of warfarin. Borage should be avoided in pregnant or immunosuppressed patients.
- Monitor patients for improvement in symptoms. Specifically, effective therapy should result in decreased joint pain and swelling, increased joint flexibility, and decreased use of pain medication. Duration of therapy, estimated duration for improvement of symptoms, and expected degree of symptomatic improvement should be determined and discussed with the patient.
- Osteoarthritis is a slowly progressive disorder that should be monitored symptomatically. Radiographs may be used periodically to demonstrate the degree of joint space narrowing and loss of articular cartilage. Patients who continue to experience pain and decreased joint function with medical therapy may be candidates for joint replacement surgery.
- Because RA can affect other body systems, patients should be monitored on a regular basis. In addition to joint pain and swelling, patients with poorly controlled disease may develop vasculitis, pleuritis, or anemia. High-dose antiinflammatory medications may be necessary in patients with these complications and with refractory arthritis symptoms. Regular laboratory monitoring of hemoglobin/hematocrit, ESR, and WBC count is recommended.
- Exercise benefits both OA and RA if the patient can tolerate physical activity. Weight loss may improve symptoms of OA in overweight patients. Patients can incorporate exercise into their lifestyle in many ways, including gardening, walking, and sports activities such as golfing, dancing, yoga, and swimming. Experts recommend that different types of exercises should be incorporated into the patient's exercise program, such as range-of-motion exercises (for increasing flexibility), strengthening exercises (for weight training), and aerobic or endurance exercises (for cardiovascular and overall health). Patients who are beginning an exercise program should choose activities that fit their level of strength and endurance. Exercise that causes extreme pain or discomfort may be unhealthy and may even cause permanent damage to the body.
- Maintaining a proper body weight will significantly reduce the amount of stress on joints. A healthy diet is recommended for all arthritis patients; in particular, a low-purine diet is strongly recommended for those with gout. Aspirin should be avoided; although high doses can promote uric acid excretion, low-dose aspirin regimens (which are more common) are known to increase uric acid retention and worsen gout symptoms.

Case Studies

CASE STUDY 23-1

KP is a 68-year-old woman in no acute distress, but has a history of hyperlipidemia, depression, and rheumatoid arthritis. Her prescription medications include simvastatin (20 mg/day), methotrexate (25 mg/week), and infliximab (3 mg/kg). Her most recent lipid profile was total cholesterol 220 mg/dL, low-density lipoprotein cholesterol (LDL-C) 120 mg/dL, high-density lipoprotein cholesterol (HDL-C) 35 mg/dL, and triglycerides 150 mg/dL. She occasionally takes 325 mg of aspirin for back pain. KP recently began taking St. John's wort for depression and guggul for hyperlipidemia, but she cannot remember the doses. She walks daily and has recently begun to eat a low-fat, low-cholesterol diet. She hopes to eliminate all prescription medications.

KP's rheumatoid arthritis is generally well controlled but becomes painful when gardening or playing the piano. The infliximab helps and allows her to resume these activities, but she is very afraid of needles; she says "I'm tired of my doctor treating me like a pin cushion." She wants to find a more natural alternative to the infliximab. Devise an integrative therapy plan for KP, keeping in mind her current medication and exercise regimens.

Answer: Because KP tolerates methotrexate and does not appear to have major problems without the infliximab, it may be useful to try an herbal product that also has anti-TNF activity. Cat's claw, podophyllum, and turmeric may be helpful. If patients are not taking other medications, cat's claw may be a better choice because it has slightly more data and fewer side effects than podophyllum. Because she occasionally takes aspirin, however, cat's claw may not be a good choice because it may interact with salicylates. You should determine how often she takes aspirin. If she takes aspirin daily or multiple times per week, podophyllum or turmeric may be more reasonable to try. Podophyllum may be beneficial, although research on safety and efficacy is limited. Turmeric may also have cholesterol-lowering effects, although this is unproven. Regardless of what she tries, KP should inform her physician of the new product so that her condition can be monitored and her infliximab can be temporarily discontinued to evaluate the efficacy of her herbal supplement(s).

The recent addition of St. John's wort and guggul should be discussed. Methotrexate has been reported to cause increased sensitivity to the sun, thereby increasing the risk of sunburn and skin rash. Because St. John's wort may cause a similar problem, taking this herbal agent with methotrexate may add to this risk. Advise KP to wear sunscreen and protective clothing during sun exposure.

St. John's wort has also been shown to reduce the effectiveness of simvastatin. KP should be monitored for continued lipid-lowering effectiveness. Encourage her to continue walking daily and eating a low-fat, low-cholesterol diet.

CASE STUDY 23-2

LP is a 52-year-old man who approaches you with questions about osteoarthritis in his knees. He was recently diagnosed and wants to try something to prevent his condition from worsening. Currently, his knees do not bother him enough to take pain medication, but he occasionally uses ibuprofen (400 mg daily). He strongly believes in herbal treatments and read that avocado might help his cartilage. His past medical history is significant for a recent deep vein thrombosis (DVT), for which he takes warfarin (5 mg/day), and hypertension, which is treated with atenolol (100 mg/day). LP takes 600 mg of valerian every night to help him sleep and 50 mg of *Ginkgo biloba* daily to help his memory. Advise LP regarding the integration of avocado into his current regimen.

Answer: Avocado and soybean extracts have been tested in several studies for relief of OA symptoms. It is important to ask LP about any known allergies before recommending dietary supplements. In this situation, banana, chestnut, and latex allergies are of most importance because cross-allergy to avocado may be possible.

If LP has no allergies or sensitivity to these substances, the potential benefits and limitations of avocado and soybean extracts can be discussed. Studies suggest that the antiinflammatory effects of these extracts may help prevent cartilage degeneration and may even help cartilage repair. Several clinical studies have shown a benefit for those using avocado/soybean unsaponifiables (ASU). It is important to note that there are no long-term trials showing beneficial effects or side effects and no evidence to show effects on cartilage repair or degradation in actual patients. If LP understands the lack of data showing long-term safety and the limitations on the benefits observed, he can make an educated decision whether to use ASU. Avocado can be ingested as a fruit, and ASU can be taken at doses of 300 to 600 mg daily.

LP should be counseled regarding the potential for avocado to decrease the effects of warfarin. It may be prudent to delay avocado therapy until his warfarin treatment is complete. International normalized ratio (INR) should be monitored if avocado and warfarin are used concomitantly.

LP should be asked whether he has had any problems with concentration. One small study found the combination of valerian and propranolol impaired concentration, and this interaction may be the underlying cause of the memory problems for which he takes ginkgo. Ginkgo has been shown to decrease blood pressure. It would be helpful to determine if his blood pressure has decreased since the addition of ginkgo to his treatment regimen. There have been numerous case reports of spontaneous hemorrhage in patients taking *Ginkgo biloba*. Because LP is also taking warfarin, he should be counseled about these risks and encouraged to stop ginkgo until his warfarin therapy is completed.

CASE STUDY 23-3

TN is a 65-year-old woman who brings a bottle of Krallendorn to the pharmacy counter as well as a prescription for mesalamine (Pentasa), 1000 mg four times daily. Examining her prescription history, you notice she has been regularly using mesalamine and has used azathioprine once or twice a year. TN also tells you that she takes horse chestnut for varicose veins and licorice for a past history of peptic ulcer disease. How would you counsel this patient?

Answer: Mesalamine is typically used for maintenance of inflammatory bowel disease (IBD), whereas azathioprine is often used to control flares. TN seems to have flares a few times a year, which suggests that her bowel problems are not under optimal control. This may indicate that she is sensitive to immune changes.

Determine TN's purpose for using Krallendorn, a standardized cat's claw extract used with some success to treat rheumatoid arthritis. Ask TN if she has been diagnosed with RA or another type of bone and joint disorder. If not, she should undergo an appropriate physical examination and laboratory tests. The side effects generally seem to be minimal; however, cat's claw is often associated with immunostimulant effects, and it is unclear how these will affect her IBD. Cat's claw causes gastrointestinal upset in some patients, which may further aggravate her IBD.

Because licorice may increase the absorption of some drugs, TN should be counseled to take other medications several hours before or after her licorice. Licorice also may cause electrolyte abnormalities and hypertension, and TN should be appropriately warned. Horse chestnut is generally safe and well tolerated, but it may cause hypoglycemia and should therefore be used carefully in patients with diabetes.

References for Chapter 23 can be found on the Evolve website at http://evolve.elsevier.com/Ulbricht/herbalpharmacotherapy/

Review Questions

1. Which component(s) of borage seed oil is(are) thought to exert antiinflammatory effects?
   a. Gamma-linolenic acid (GLA)
   b. Alpha-linolenic acid (ALA)
   c. Both a and b
   d. None of the above

2. Which constituent of devil's claw has been shown to inhibit the release of leukotriene C4, thereby reducing the inflammatory response?
   a. Curcumin
   b. Aucubin
   c. Procumben
   d. Rhynchophylline

3. Devil's claw has been shown to inhibit which of the following inflammatory mediators?
   a. Leukotriene B_4
   b. Cyclooxygenase-2 (COX-2)
   c. Both a and b
   d. None of the above

4. Avocado, combined with which of the following, may be effective in treating osteoarthritis?
   a. Borage seed oil
   b. Soybean
   c. Safflower oil
   d. Flaxseed oil

5. Willow bark is noted to contain which precursor to aspirin?
   a. Glucose
   b. Salicylate
   c. Cadmium
   d. Aromatic aldehydes

6. Bromelain is thought to reduce which of the following proinflammatory mediators?
   a. Kininogen
   b. Bradykinin
   c. Both a and b
   d. None of the above

7. All of the following are true concerning rose hips, *except*:
   a. It has been shown to inhibit TNF-alpha.
   b. It contains the antioxidants vitamin C, polyphenols, and carotenoids.
   c. The medicinal uses of *Rosa* spp. are confined to the fruits.
   d. Rose hip extract may reduce C-reactive protein (CRP) levels.

8. CPH 82, which has been used to treat rheumatoid arthritis, is composed of which constituent(s) derived from *Podophyllum emodi*?
   a. Two purified semisynthetic lignan glycosides
   b. Quercetin
   c. Kampherol
   d. All the above

9. What is the proposed mechanism of action for cherry in treating gouty arthritis?
   a. Reducing plasma urate
   b. Increasing plasma urate
   c. Reducing urinary oxalate
   d. Increasing urinary oxalate

10. What characteristic(s) of ginger differs from over-the-counter NSAIDs?
    a. Ginger may suppress prostaglandin synthesis through the inhibition of cyclooxygenase-1 and cyclooxygenase-2
    b. Ginger is a selective cyclooxygenase-2 inhibitor
    c. Ginger may suppress leukotriene biosynthesis by inhibiting 5-lipoxygenase
    d. None of the above

Answers are found in the Answers to Review Questions section in the back of the text.

24 Gastrointestinal Disorders

Outline

OVERVIEW
    Upper Gastrointestinal Disorders
        Dyspepsia
        Gastroesophageal Reflux Disease
        Peptic Ulcer Disease
        Nausea and Vomiting
    Lower Gastrointestinal Disorders
        Diarrhea
        Colic
        Constipation
        Inflammatory Bowel Disease
        Irritable Bowel Syndrome
SELECTED HERBAL THERAPIES
    Agrimony (*Agrimonia* spp.)
    Aloe (*Aloe vera*)
    Arnica (*Arnica* spp.)
    Arrowroot (*Maranta arundinacea*)
    Asparagus (*Asparagus officinalis*)
    Bacopa (*Bacopa monnieri*)
    Barley (*Hordeum vulgare*)
    Blessed Thistle (*Cnicus benedictus*)
    Boswellia (*Boswellia serrata*)
    Carob (*Ceratonia siliqua*)
    Cascara (*Rhamnus purshiana*)
    Chamomile (*Matricaria recutita*, syn. *Matricaria suaveolens*, *Matricaria chamomilla*, *Anthemis nobilis*, *Chamaemelum nobile*, *Chamomilla chamomilla*, *Chamomilla recutita*)
    Cinnamon (*Cinnamomum* spp.)
    Dandelion (*Taraxacum officinale*)
    Fennel (*Foeniculum vulgare*)
    Flax (*Linum usitatissimum*)
    Ginger (*Zingiber officinale*)
    Globe Artichoke (*Cynara scolymus*)
    Goldenseal (*Hydrastis canadensis*)
    Lemon Balm (*Melissa officinalis*)
    Licorice (*Glycyrrhiza glabra*)
    Mastic (*Pistacia lentiscus*)
    Neem (*Azadirachta indica*)
    Papaya (*Carica papaya*)
    Peppermint (*Mentha x piperita*)
    Psyllium (*Plantago* spp.)
    Rhubarb (*Rheum* spp.)
    Sea Buckthorn (*Hippophae rhamnoides*)
    Slippery Elm (*Ulmus rubra*, syn. *Ulmus fulva*)
    Soy (*Glycine max*)
    Turmeric (*Curcuma longa*)
    Wheatgrass (*Triticum aestivum*)
    White Horehound (*Marrubium vulgare*)
HERBAL THERAPIES WITH NEGATIVE EVIDENCE
HERBAL THERAPIES WITH LIMITED EVIDENCE
ADJUNCT THERAPIES
INTEGRATIVE THERAPY PLAN
CASE STUDIES
REVIEW QUESTIONS

Learning Objectives

- Describe the use, adverse effects, and drug interactions of herbs used to treat disorders of the gastrointestinal system, including upper gastrointestinal disorders, diarrhea, constipation, and nausea/vomiting.

- Develop an appropriate integrative care plan for the management of gastrointestinal disorders.

OVERVIEW

The gastrointestinal (GI) tract is an organ system involved in ingesting, digesting, absorbing, and excreting food. The upper GI tract includes the mouth, esophagus, and stomach; the lower GI tract includes the small intestine, large intestine (colon), rectum, and anus (Figures 24-1 and 24-2). Gastrointestinal disorders occur when any part of the digestive tract does not function properly. As a result, patients may have difficulty with food digestion, food absorption, and bowel movements (Figure 24-2).

The digestive process begins when food is broken down in the mouth, not only mechanically by chewing, but also chemically by salivary enzymes such as amylase.[1,2] After food is swallowed, it enters the esophagus, a muscular tube that carries food and liquids from the mouth to the stomach.

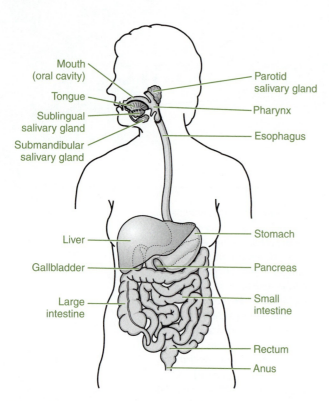

Figure 24-1 Digestive system (midsagittal section and frontal view). (Modified from Fehrenbach MJ, editor: *Dental anatomy coloring book*, St Louis, 2008, Saunders-Elsevier.)

The stomach contains strong enzymes such as pepsin and stomach acids such as hydrochloric acid (HCl), which further break down food. Food then enters the small intestine, which contains three parts: the duodenum, jejunum, and ileum. At this point the pancreas releases the peptide hormone insulin to aid in glucose absorption, as well as several other digestive enzymes. Bile is also secreted by the liver and facilitates the digestion and absorption of fats in the small intestine.

Most of the digestive process occurs in the small intestine because it is responsible for absorbing nutrients from food. The remaining food then enters the large intestine, which includes the colon, cecum, appendix, and rectum. The large intestine absorbs water from indigestible food matter; the stool is normally solid by the time it reaches the rectum because the body reabsorbs most of the water. Muscle contractions *(peristalsis)* in the colon then push the stool toward the rectum; the unusable food matter, or *feces*, is then excreted through the anus.[1-3]

There are many different types of gastrointestinal disorders; some affect multiple parts of the digestive tract, and others affect only a specific portion, such as the upper GI tract (e.g., esophagus, stomach) or the lower GI tract (e.g., small bowel, large bowel, anus/rectum). The severity of gastrointestinal disorders varies significantly, depending on the specific type of disease. Some disorders, such as indigestion, are mild; others, such as Crohn's disease, are lifelong and debilitating and may lead to serious complications.[1-3]

Upper Gastrointestinal Disorders[1-5]

Dyspepsia

Dyspepsia, also called *nonulcer dyspepsia* or simply *indigestion*, is a general term that describes discomfort in the upper abdomen. The pathophysiology of dyspepsia is not well understood, possible mechanisms include abnormal motility, delayed gastric emptying, altered visceral sensation (in stomach and duodenum), and psychosocial factors. Patients with indigestion typically have several symptoms, including heartburn (pyrosis), bloating, belching, and nausea. Indigestion affects almost everyone at some time and is not considered a serious health condition; it may occur if a person eats too much of a particular food (especially fatty or spicy foods) or eats too quickly. Alcohol, stress, and anxiety may also contribute to indigestion. Because it is such a common condition, indigestion generally does not require a diagnosis. However, those who frequently experience indigestion should visit their health care providers because it may be a symptom of an underlying medical condition, such as acid reflux disease.

Gastroesophageal Reflux Disease

Gastroesophageal reflux disease (GERD), also called *acid reflux disease,* occurs when liquid from the stomach regurgitates into the esophagus. This liquid may contain stomach acids and bile. In some cases the regurgitated stomach liquid (acid) can cause inflammation, irritation, and damage to the esophagus. The exact cause of GERD is not well understood; factors associated with GERD include hiatal hernia (stomach pushing up through weak spot in diaphragm), abnormally weak contractions of the lower esophageal sphincter (LES), and abnormal emptying of the stomach after a meal.

Common symptoms of GERD include a burning sensation in the chest that may spread to the throat; this condition is known as *pyrosis* or "heartburn." This chest pain commonly occurs after eating a large meal, or when lying down (especially soon after eating). GERD can also cause dysphagia (difficulty swallowing), regurgitating food or sour liquid, coughing, hoarseness, sore throat, and wheezing. Factors such as weight gain may worsen symptoms. Other exacerbating factors include spicy foods, fatty foods, chocolate, caffeine, tomato sauce, carbonated beverages, mint, alcoholic beverages, large meals, certain medications (e.g., sedatives, tranquilizers, blood pressure drugs, aspirin), and cigarette smoking.

Most cases of GERD can be diagnosed based on the patient's symptoms. GERD may be a lifelong condition because no cure exists; however, many drugs are approved for its treatment. Patients may also modify their dietary and daily habits (e.g., avoid spicy foods, stop smoking) to manage symptoms; some patients require long-term drug therapy. In intractable cases, patients may undergo a surgical procedure (Nissen fundoplication) to strengthen the pyloric sphincter and prevent acid reflux.

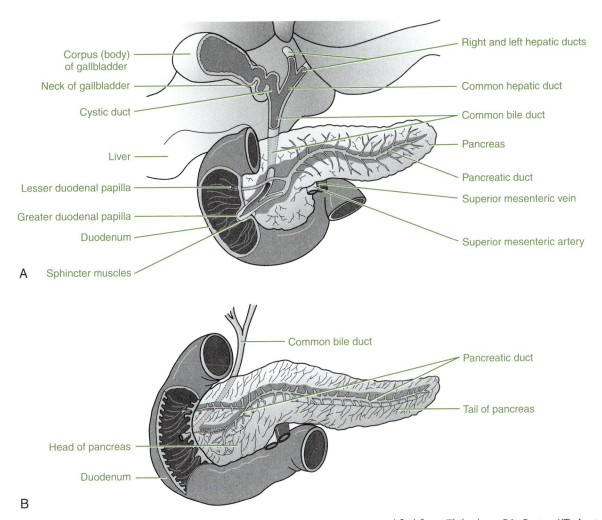

Figure 24-2 **A,** Accessory organs of the gastrointestinal system. **B,** Pancreas. (**A,** modified from Thibodeau GA, Patton KT: *Anatomy & physiology,* ed 5, St Louis, 2003, Mosby. **B,** modified from LaFleur Brooks M: *Exploring medical language: a student-directed approach,* St Louis, 2002, Mosby.)

Peptic Ulcer Disease

An ulcer is an open sore or break in a body tissue. Peptic ulcers may be caused by abnormalities in the secretion of gastric acid and pepsin or by bacterial infections. Peptic ulcers may develop on the inside lining of the stomach (*gastric* peptic ulcer), upper small intestine (*duodenal* peptic ulcer), or esophagus (*esophageal* peptic ulcer). Researchers have found that a bacterial infection with *Helicobacter pylori* is the most common cause of gastric and duodenal ulcers. Some medications, including aspirin and nonsteroidal antiinflammatory drugs (NSAIDS) such as ibuprofen (Motrin, Advil), can damage the stomach lining (mucosa) and thus may also cause gastric and duodenal ulcers. In addition, smoking tobacco increases a person's risk of developing ulcers. It remains unclear whether excessive alcohol consumption leads to an increased risk of ulcers.

Esophageal peptic ulcers are usually associated with acid reflux disease. Contrary to popular belief, diet and stress do *not* cause peptic ulcers. However, high levels of stress and acidic foods and beverages (e.g., coffee) may aggravate symptoms of peptic ulcers. Peptic ulcers generally cause pain that may be felt from the chest to the stomach. Pain may last a few minutes to several hours and can worsen on an empty stomach. The timing of symptoms in relation to meals help differentiate gastric from duodenal ulcers; gastric ulcers are relieved by food, whereas duodenal ulcers are worsened by food. Symptoms may also come and go for a few days to weeks. Less common symptoms include vomiting blood, dark blood in the stool, nausea, vomiting, and unexplained weight loss.

Most ulcers are diagnosed after radiography of the upper GI tract. An endoscopy may also be performed; a thin tube with a camera (endoscope) is inserted into the mouth and digestive tract so that the clinician can see if ulcers are present.

Nausea and Vomiting

Nausea is an unpleasant sensation in the stomach; it is often accompanied by an urge to vomit, which is a forceful expulsion of gastric contents through the mouth and sometimes the nose. The chemoreceptor trigger zone (CTZ) in the brain, the vestibular system, the visceral afferents from the GI tract, and the cerebral cortex are involved in nausea and vomiting. These areas can stimulate the vomiting center of the brain, which induces stimulation of the salivary and respiratory centers and the pharyngeal, gastrointestinal, and abdominal muscles. An activated CTZ invokes the release of various neurotransmittors, including serotonin (5-hydroxytryptamine type 3, $5-HT_3$), neurokinin-1 (NK_1), histamine, dopamine (D_2), and substance P receptors, which also stimulate vomiting.

Vomiting is intended to protect a person from harmful ingested substances; it can also be a symptom of many common conditions, including cough, motion sickness or seasickness, migraine headaches, overeating, and food sensitivities. Nausea and vomiting may also be symptoms of serious conditions, including heart attack, blocked intestines, concussion or brain injury, and appendicitis; it can also occur after surgery, as a side effect of certain medications, during infections (especially "food poisoning") or during pregnancy *(hyperemesis gravidarum* or "morning sickness").

A comprehensive history and physical examination can often reveal the cause of nausea and vomiting, making further evaluation unnecessary. The patient should be asked about medical history, surgeries, and medications, including a thorough history of recreational drug and alcohol use or abuse. A complete physical examination includes a neurological examination and brain function tests. Acute symptoms generally result from infectious, inflammatory, or unknown causes. Evaluation first focuses on detecting any emergencies or complications that require hospitalization, such as bowel obstruction, cancer, opiate addiction, or internal bleeding. Blood tests are performed to determine if the person is dehydrated and may include electrolyte levels (sodium, potassium, chloride). Tests for kidney function may also be performed, including blood urea nitrogen (BUN) and serum creatinine levels.

Lower Gastrointestinal Disorders[1-6]

Diarrhea

Diarrhea is an increase in the volume of stool fluidity or frequency of defecation. It is often caused by inflammation of the small intestine. Diarrhea is a symptom of an underlying health problem, such as an infection, that prevents the intestines from properly absorbing nutrients from food. *Acute* diarrhea lasts a few days and is experienced by virtually everyone at some point. *Chronic* diarrhea generally lasts longer than 4 weeks and may be a sign of a serious condition, such as inflammatory bowel disease or gastroenteritis.

Diarrhea can result from viral, bacterial, or parasitic infections. Diarrhea caused by an infection, often called *infectious diarrhea*, may be acquired through direct contact with the pathological microbes. For example, an infection may be transmitted if a person consumes contaminated food or water. Viruses such as the Norwalk virus, cytomegalovirus, viral hepatitis, herpes simplex virus, and rotavirus are likely causes of diarrhea. Infants and young children are most likely to develop diarrhea from a rotavirus infection (rotaviruses cause digestive problems and diarrhea in young children). If an individual consumes food or water contaminated with certain bacteria or parasites, the person may develop diarrhea. This type of diarrhea is often called *traveler's diarrhea* because it frequently occurs in people who are traveling to developing countries. Common bacterial causes of diarrhea include *Campylobacter, Salmonella, Escherichia coli, Shigella dysenteriae,* and *Clostridium difficile.* Common parasites known to cause diarrhea include *Giardia lamblia* and *Cryptosporidium.*

Diarrhea may also be caused by lactose intolerance; certain medications, especially antibiotics, chemotherapies, and anti-HIV medications; artificial sweeteners such as sorbitol and mannitol, often found in sugar-free products (e.g., chewing gum); sugary foods; and other gastrointestinal disorders (e.g., irritable bowel syndrome).

Symptoms of diarrhea include frequent and loose stools, abdominal pain or cramping, bloating, and fever. Excessive thirst and dehydration may occur because the body loses water and salts. Infants and young children are at risk of severe dehydration as a result of diarrhea. People with severe diarrhea may be unable to control the passage of stool, a condition known as *fecal incontinence.*

Adults should seek medical attention if diarrhea continues longer than 4 days, if blood is present in the stool, or if they have signs of dehydration (dry skin, thirst, less frequent urination, lightheadedness, dark-colored urine). Infants, young children, and older adults should receive medical attention if diarrhea lasts longer than 24 to 48 hours, if they have a high fever, or if they have signs of dehydration. The physician will perform a physical examination and take a detailed medical history. Patients should tell their physician if they are taking any prescription or over-the-counter drugs, herbs, or supplements because these agents may be causing diarrhea. A physician may take blood or stool samples to check for infection.

Colic

Colic is usually defined as "excessive crying," for more than 3 hours a day, 3 days a week, and longer than 3 weeks, in an otherwise healthy baby. Its underlying cause remains unclear. However, researchers suggest that colic may be caused by gastrointestinal problems (such as lactose intolerance or an immature digestive system) because sometimes a colic episode stops after a baby passes gas or has a bowel movement. Other possible causes include maternal anxiety, differences in the way an infant is fed or comforted, and allergies.

Currently, no treatment has been proved to be effective for the treatment of colic in babies. Colic typically goes away once the infant reaches 3 months of age.

Constipation

Constipation is the infrequent passage of small amounts of hard, dry bowel movements, usually fewer than three times a week. Some individuals who are constipated find it painful to have a bowel movement and often experience straining, bloating, and the sensation of a full bowel.

Constipation is a symptom, not a disease. Almost everyone experiences constipation at some point, and most periods of constipation are temporary, self-treatable, and not serious health issues. Common causes of constipation include prescription medications (e.g., narcotics, antidepressants), hormonal changes, bowel habits, diet, dehydration, lack of exercise, laxatives, diseases (e.g., colon cancer, irritable bowel syndrome), and stress. Bowel movements are different for each individual, depending on genetic makeup, types of food and drink, and amount of exercise. Bowel movements do not have to occur daily. Normal stool elimination may range from three times a day to three times a week.

An individual's medical history is very important in determining the cause of constipation. A medical history from a patient with constipation will determine dietary habits, physical activity level, medications, and existing diseases that can contribute to constipation. A physical examination may identify diseases that can cause constipation, such as *scleroderma* (excessive deposits of connective tissue in organs), *intestinal pseudo-obstruction* (decreased ability of intestines to move stool), *Hirschsprung's disease* (enlargement of colon that stops flow of stool), irritable bowel syndrome, *diverticulitis* (formation of pouches in the colon), and *Chagas disease* (tropical parasitic disease). A rectal examination may uncover a tight anal sphincter that may be making defecation difficult. Blood tests, abdominal radiograph, barium enema, and colonoscopy may be used to evaluate underlying conditions causing constipation.

Inflammatory Bowel Disease

Inflammatory bowel disease (IBD) refers to two chronic diseases that cause inflammation of the intestines: colitis (or ulcerative colitis) and Crohn's disease. The symptoms of these two illnesses are very similar, which often makes it difficult to distinguish them. In fact, about 10% of colitis (inflamed-colon) cases cannot be diagnosed as either ulcerative colitis or Crohn's disease. When physicians cannot diagnose the specific IBD, the condition is called *indeterminate colitis*. Researchers estimate that about 1 million Americans have IBD. Although it can develop at any age, IBD is most prevalent in persons between 15 and 30 years of age.

Inflammatory bowel disease causes chronic inflammation of the GI tract; it is not to be confused with *irritable bowel syndrome* (IBS, see below), though they share some of the same symptoms. Both cause discomfort and distress, but IBD may cause permanent damage to the intestines and may also lead to complications such as colon cancer.

The cause of IBD remains unclear; however, there is mounting evidence that it involves a complex interaction of factors, including heredity, the immune system, and antigens in the environment. Because IBD occurs more often among people who live in cities and industrialized nations, environmental and dietary factors (including a diet high in fat or refined foods) contribute to the disease. Individuals with a family history of the disease are more likely to develop IBD; therefore researchers believe that an individual's genetic makeup may also play a role. Some evidence suggests that a virus or bacterium may cause IBD; when the immune system attacks the invading substance, the GI tract may become inflamed. Other researchers speculate that the inflammation may stem from the virus or bacterium directly. *Mycobacterium avium* subsp. *paratuberculosis* (MAP) may be involved in the development of Crohn's disease and ulcerative colitis. This microorganism is known to cause intestinal diseases in cattle. In addition, researchers have found MAP in the blood and intestinal tissue of individuals diagnosed with Crohn's disease, but rarely in individuals with ulcerative colitis.

The symptoms of IBD vary in severity among patients and may develop gradually or occur suddenly. Some individuals experience long periods with no symptoms, whereas others experience chronic or recurrent symptoms.

The most common symptoms of both ulcerative colitis and Crohn's disease are diarrhea (ranging from mild to severe), abdominal pain, decreased appetite, and weight loss. If extreme, diarrhea may lead to dehydration, increased heart rate, and decreased blood pressure. As food moves through inflamed areas of the GI tract, it may cause bleeding. Continued loss of blood in the stool may result in anemia. In addition, Crohn's disease may also cause intestinal ulcers, fever, fatigue, arthritis, eye inflammation, skin disorders, and inflammation of the liver or bile ducts.

Irritable Bowel Syndrome

Irritable bowel syndrome (IBS), also called spastic colon, mucous colitis, spastic colitis, nervous stomach, or irritable colon, is a functional bowel disorder in which the bowel appears normal but does not function normally. The most common symptoms are lower abdominal pain and bloating associated with alteration in bowel habits (constipation, diarrhea) and abdominal discomfort relieved with defecation. In patients with IBS the contents inside their colon do not move properly. The pain is usually felt in one of the four quadrants of the abdomen, especially the lower left quadrant. Other symptoms may include headache and anxiety.

Although the exact cause is unclear, IBS may result from poor dietary choices, neurotransmitter imbalances, cigarette smoking, and infection.

The syndrome can be divided into four main types, depending on which symptom is reported. Symptoms include abdominal pain, diarrhea, constipation, and diarrhea alternating with constipation. The abdominal pain type is usually described in a patient as *diarrhea predominant* (IBS-D), *constipation predominant* (IBS-C), or IBS with *alternating stool pattern* (IBS-A). In some individuals, IBS may have a sudden onset and develop after an infectious illness, characterized by two or more of the following: fever, vomiting, acute diarrhea, and positive stool culture. This syndrome caused by an infection is termed *postinfectious* IBS (IBS-PI).

Typically, the diagnosis begins with a medical history, including questions about the duration, severity, and characteristics of symptoms. IBS is diagnosed by its signs and symptoms and by the absence of inflammatory bowel diseases such as Crohn's disease and ulcerative colitis. These diseases are inflammatory conditions and have been associated with cancer. In contrast, the colon is not inflamed in IBS, and the condition does not seem to harm the intestines or lead to cancer.

SELECTED HERBAL THERAPIES

Note
To help make this educational resource more interactive, all pharmacokinetics, adverse effects, and interactions data have been compiled in Appendix A. Safety data specifically related to pregnancy and lactation are listed in Appendix B. Please refer to these appendices when working through the case studies and answering the review questions.

Agrimony (*Agrimonia* spp.)

Grade C: *Unclear or conflicting scientific evidence (gastrointestinal disorders)*

Mechanism of Action
The applicable parts of agrimony are the dried, aboveground parts. The aerial plant parts contain 4% to 10% condensed tannins, which may account for its astringent properties. Because of its tannin content and astringent properties, agrimony is thought to be helpful for gastrointestinal conditions such as diarrhea. The antidiarrheal effect of tannins occurs by increasing colonic water and electrolyte reabsorption.[7,8]

Scientific Evidence of Effectiveness
Traditionally, agrimony has been used for many gastrointestinal conditions, including appendicitis, mild diarrhea, lack of appetite, and ulcers. Clinical data are lacking for these uses. Agrimony has been used in a combination product also containing St. John's wort (*Hypericum perforatum*), plantain (*Plantago major*), peppermint (*Mentha x piperita*), and German chamomile (*Matricaria chamomile*). In gastroduodenitis patients, after 25 days of therapy, 75% of patients claimed to be pain free, 95% free of dyspeptic symptoms, and 76% free from palpitation pains.[9] Gastroscopy indicated that previous erosion and hemorrhagic mucous changes had healed.

Dose
The dose of agrimony for gastrointestinal disorders has not been determined.

Adverse Effects, Interactions, Pharmacokinetics. See Appendix A.

Aloe (*Aloe vera*)

Grade B: *Good scientific evidence (constipation)*

Grade C: *Unclear or conflicting scientific evidence (inflammatory bowel disease)*

Mechanism of Action
Aloe latex contains anthraquinone glycosides (aloin, aloe-emodin, and barbaloin) that act as potent colonic-specific stimulant laxatives.[10-16] These water-soluble glycosides increase the rate of colonic motility and enhance colonic transit. Anthraquinones are split by intestinal bacteria into aglycons. One of these compounds, aloe-emodin-9-anthrone, has been shown to increase the water content in rat large intestine.[17] This effect appeared to be a more important cathartic mechanism than increased intestinal motility (also proposed).[12,13]

Scientific Evidence of Effectiveness
CONSTIPATION. Few clinical studies have been conducted to evaluate the laxative effect of aloe latex in humans.[18,19] However, the laxative effect of anthraquinone glycosides found in aloe, such as aloin, aloe-emodin, and barbaloin, is well established scientifically.[10-16] A combination product containing celandine, aloe, and psyllium (6:3:1 ratio) produced more frequent bowel movements, softer stools, and less laxative dependence than placebo in patients with chronic constipation.[20] Pain scores (related to constipation) remained unchanged in both groups. Further study is warranted to establish dosing and compare efficacy and safety with common laxative agents.

INFLAMMATORY BOWEL DISEASE (ULCERATIVE COLITIS). Preliminary evidence from a small, randomized placebo-controlled trial (RCT) in 44 individuals suggests that oral *Aloe vera* gel (100 mL twice daily for 4 weeks) is beneficial in the management of ulcerative colitis.[21,22] Clinical improvement ("remission") was seen in 30% of aloe patients versus 7% of placebo patients, although no sigmoidoscopic improvements were seen in either group. The small study population limits the interpretation of this data.

Dose
Standardized aloe products are not widely available. Most experts recommend that the minimum dose needed to maintain a soft stool is usually 0.04 to 0.17 g of dried juice (corresponds to 10-30 mg hydroxyanthraquinones). A combination product of celandine (300 mg) plus aloe (150 mg) plus psyllium (50 mg), starting with one capsule daily and increasing up to three times daily for 28 days, has benefited patients with chronic constipation.[20]

The dose of aloe for ulcerative colitis has not been determined.

Adverse Effects, Interactions, Pharmacokinetics. See Appendix A.

Arnica (*Arnica* spp.)

Grade C: *Unclear or conflicting scientific evidence (acute diarrhea in children)*

Mechanism of Action. Insufficient available evidence.

Scientific Evidence of Effectiveness

Arnica has not been well studied for its effects on diarrhea. One study suggests a decrease in the duration of diarrhea in children with homeopathic doses of arnica.[23] Because homeopathic remedies contain little (if any) of the purported active ingredients, the scientific basis for this observation remains unclear.

Dose

Note: Arnica is toxic if taken internally, except when highly diluted into homeopathic preparations. The homeopathic dose of arnica for children with acute diarrhea has not been determined.

Adverse Effects, Interactions, Pharmacokinetics. See Appendix A.

Arrowroot (*Maranta arundinacea*)

Grade C: *Unclear or conflicting scientific evidence (diarrhea; irritable bowel syndrome)*

Mechanism of Action

Arrowroot is an edible starch with proposed demulcent (soothing) effects.[1]

Scientific Evidence of Effectiveness

Arrowroot is a well-known traditional remedy for diarrhea and gastrointestinal complaints. One small pilot study investigated powdered arrowroot as a treatment for diarrhea in IBS patients and found a small, potentially lasting benefit.[24] Most patients who completed the study reported slight to moderate improvements. These patients experienced a decrease in diarrhea episodes during treatment and lessened pain after 1 month of arrowroot use. Bowel habits, however, did not appear to be more regular, and arrowroot had no effect on the odor of stools or on mucus production. Constipation was reported with long-term use.

Dose

For IBS-D (diarrhea predominant), two 5-mL spoonfuls of powdered arrowroot (Thornton & Ross UK Pharmaceutical) were taken three times daily with, or as part of, meals for 1 month.[24]

Adverse Effects, Interactions, Pharmacokinetics. See Appendix A.

Asparagus (*Asparagus officinalis*)

Grade C: *Unclear or conflicting scientific evidence (dyspepsia)*

Mechanism of Action

The exact mechanism of asparagus in dyspepsia is not clear, but researchers have suggested that it may be a mild dopamine antagonist.[25]

Scientific Evidence of Effectiveness

Asparagus racemosus (Shatavari) is used in Ayurveda for dyspepsia. In a preliminary study, asparagus was compared with metoclopramide (Reglan).[25] The results showed asparagus to be equivalent to metoclopramide in reducing gastric-emptying time. Notably, a pungent odor is produced with asparagus consumption by some individuals, making placebo-controlled trials difficult to conduct.

Dose

The effective dose of asparagus in dyspepsia has not been determined. A small study used 2 g of powdered asparagus root in the morning for 2 days.[25]

Adverse Effects, Interactions, Pharmacokinetics. See Appendix A.

Bacopa (*Bacopa monnieri*)

Grade C: *Unclear or conflicting scientific evidence (irritable bowel syndrome)*

Mechanism of Action

Bacopa may have direct antispasmodic effects on intestinal smooth muscle by inhibiting calcium influx across cell membrane channels.[26,27] This effect may be beneficial in patients with IBS who experience intestinal spasm.

Scientific Evidence of Effectiveness

Bacopa and bael fruit have been used in combination to treat IBS. A clinical trial compared treatment with an Ayurvedic compound preparation (2 g bacopa and 3 g *Aegle marmelos correa* fruit powder) to standard therapy (2.5 mg clidinium bromide, 5 mg chlordiazepoxide [Librax], and 5 g isaphaghulla) and placebo (5 g cornstarch with 1 g excipient).[28] The compound preparation treatment containing bacopa was found effective and particularly beneficial in patients with IBS-D. The beneficial effects cannot be isolated to bacopa because *A. marmelos* is a common antidiarrheal in India. Long-term use (>6 months) of bacopa and bael fruit was found to be no better than a placebo in reducing the chance of relapse.

Dose

The dose of bacopa for IBS has not been determined.

Adverse Effects, Interactions, Pharmacokinetics. See Appendix A.

Barley (Hordeum vulgare)

Grade C: *Unclear or conflicting scientific evidence (constipation; inflammatory bowel disease)*

Mechanism of Action

Germinated barley foodstuff (GBF) is derived from the aleurone and scutellum fractions of germinated barley. GBF appears to induce proliferation of intestinal epithelial cells and facilitate defecation through bacterial production of short-chain fatty acids, especially butyrate.[29] GBF is believed to facilitate epithelial repair and suppress epithelial nuclear factor kappa B (NF-κB)–DNA binding activity through butyrate (by the microflora *Bifidobacterium* and *Eubacterium*). GBF has been associated with increased growth of microflora in the intestinal tract, which is considered beneficial.[30]

Scientific Evidence of Effectiveness

CONSTIPATION. GBF appears to induce proliferation of intestinal epithelial cells and facilitate defecation through bacterial production of short-chain fatty acids, especially butyrate.[30] Butyrate, a key substrate for colonic cell and mucosal barrier function, modulates water and electrolyte absorption ability.[30,31]

INFLAMMATORY BOWEL DISEASE (ULCERATIVE COLITIS). GBF has been shown to improve clinical symptoms of ulcerative colitis when added to baseline antiinflammatory treatment.[32-33] A decrease in clinical activity index compared with baseline, particularly in the degree of visible blood in stools and nocturnal diarrhea, has been noted.[33] Ulcerative colitis patients who were unresponsive or intolerant to standard therapy also showed clinical and endoscopic improvements after taking 30 grams daily for 4 weeks.[34]

Dose

For constipation, 9 g of GBF daily for up to 20 days may be used. For IBD (ulcerative colitis), 20-30 g GBF was taken daily in divided doses for 4 weeks.[32-34]

Adverse Effects, Interactions, Pharmacokinetics. See Appendix A.

Blessed Thistle (Cnicus benedictus)

Grade C: *Unclear or conflicting scientific evidence (dyspepsia, indigestion, flatulence)*

Mechanism of Action

Blessed thistle is recommended for the treatment of dyspepsia and indigestion; it has historically been known to stimulate gastric acid secretion. However, evidence is currently lacking.[1,29]

Scientific Evidence of Effectiveness

Blessed thistle leaves, stems, and flowers have traditionally been used in "bitter" tonic drinks and in other oral preparations to enhance appetite and digestion. Although blessed

Belladonna (*Atropa* spp.)

Belladonna alkaloids are competitive inhibitors of the muscarinic actions of acetylcholine. Belladonna induces smooth muscle relaxation and reduces spasm in the GI tract. Belladonna may also act as an antiemetic, inhibiting acetylcholine directly at the area postrema, the vomiting center of the brain.[1,29] The belladonna constituent *hyoscine* (scopolamine) is approved by the FDA for preventing motion sickness.

Anticholinergic medications have been used for years as standard therapies for IBS patients. IBS is thought to have abnormal colonic motility, and symptoms may be replicated with a cholinergic agonist. The anticholinergic action of belladonna provides a compelling case for its use for treating IBS, and controlled trials have used FDA-approved belladonna-phenobarbital combination products in heterogeneous samples.[35,36] One study showed a trend toward improved symptoms in patients treated with the scopolamine.[37] Evidence is currently insufficient to recommend belladonna as a monotherapy for IBS treatment.

Placebo-controlled trials during the 1960s and 1970s examined several doses and preparations of belladonna for irritable bowel, including hyoscine butylbromide, 10 mg four times daily, or a combination preparation containing 0.25 mg levorotatory alkaloids of belladonna plus 50 mg phenobarbital.[36,37]

Belladonna products (available by prescription) should be adjusted to meet the needs of the individual patient to ensure control of symptoms with limited adverse reactions.

The usual dose of Donnatal Extentabs is one tablet every 12 hours. When indicated, one tablet every 8 hours may be given. Each Donnatal Extentabs tablet contains 48.6 mg phenobarbital, 0.3111 mg hyoscyamine sulfate, 0.0582 mg atropine sulfate, and 0.0195 mg scopolamine hydrobromide.[38]

The usual dosage for Donnatal Elixir is 1 or 2 tsp three or four times daily, according to conditions and severity of symptoms. Each 5-mL (teaspoonful) of elixir contains 16.2 mg phenobarbital, 0.1037 mg hyoscyamine sulfate, 0.0194 mg atropine sulfate, and 0.0065 mg scopolamine hydrobromide.[39]

thistle is sometimes recommended for dyspepsia, indigestion, and flatulence, the evidence is lacking and unclear.

Dose

No universally accepted standardization exists for blessed thistle, although assays are available to determine the presence of the bitter constituent *cnicin*, a sesquiterpene lactone. Pharmacopeial-grade blessed thistle herb is reported to require a "bitterness value" that is 800 or higher. Blessed thistle herbal preparations are often obtained from the leaves and flowers of the plant.

The dose of blessed thistle for dyspepsia and flatulence has not been determined.

Adverse Effects, Interactions, Pharmacokinetics. See Appendix A.

Boswellia (Boswellia serrata)

Grade C: *Unclear or conflicting scientific evidence (inflammatory bowel disease)*

Mechanism of Action

Boswellia's beneficial effects in gastrointestinal disorders may be related to its antiinflammatory effects. Multiple pentacyclic triterpenic acids, referred to as *boswellic acids*, have been isolated from resins of *Boswellia* species and identified as major antiinflammatory components of boswellia gum resin extract.[40-49]

Scientific Evidence of Effectiveness

Preparations from the gum resin of *Boswellia serrata* have been used as a traditional remedy in Ayurvedic medicine to treat inflammatory diseases.[50] Boswellia has been noted in animal and in vitro studies to possess antiinflammatory properties.[40-49] Based on these observations, boswellia has been suggested as a potential treatment for Crohn's disease and ulcerative colitis, both inflammatory bowel diseases. A survey of German patients with IBD (246 with Crohn's disease; 164 with ulcerative colitis) found that 38% had tried *B. serrata* extracts, and some reported positive therapeutic effects.[50] However, limited high-quality clinical data exist, and evidence is inadequate for or against this use for boswellia.

Dose

For Crohn's disease, 1200 mg of standardized *Boswellia serrata* gum resin H15 has been taken three times daily for up to 8 weeks.[51] For ulcerative colitis, 350 to 400 mg (extract standardized to 37.5% boswellic acids per dose) has been taken three times daily for 6 weeks.[52] Another study used *B. serrata* gum resin (S compound manufactured in India), 900 mg daily in three divided doses for 6 weeks, although details of benefit are unclear.[53]

Adverse Effects, Interactions, Pharmacokinetics. See Appendix A.

Carob (Ceratonia siliqua)

Grade C: *Unclear or conflicting scientific evidence (vomiting in infants, diarrhea in children; gastroesophageal reflux disease in infants)*

Mechanism of Action

Carob bean gum has been shown to alter food structure, texture, and viscosity, and thus the rate of starch degradation during digestion.[54] The effect of carob bean gum on bowel transit time is uncertain. In a clinical study, bowel transit time was not significantly affected by the carob bean gum; however, total dry fecal weight was significantly increased after the refined fibers compared with the basal diet.[55] This finding was supported by a clinical study in infants.[56] In another clinical trial, however, addition of locust bean gum to a nutrient semisolid meal strongly delayed the emptying rate in healthy subjects.[57] This result is supported by a animal research, in which the addition of carob bean gum to test diets reduced the rate of gastric emptying and thus slowed the passage of food from the stomach into the upper small intestine.[58] Although carob bean gum has uncertain effects on gastric emptying, it does affect mineral absorption, fecal weight, and urinary nitrogen. In animal study a 10% carob bean gum diet significantly decreased urinary nitrogen and significantly increased fecal dry matter and fecal nitrogen loss, resulting in a marked reduction in apparent protein digestibility.[59]

Scientific Evidence of Effectiveness

VOMITING IN INFANTS. Literature on gastroesophageal reflux in infants can be divided into studies addressing clinically apparent reflux (vomiting or regurgitation) and reflux as measured by pH probe or other methods. Carob bean gum used as a formula thickener decreases reflux, as measured by intraluminal impedance, but not by pH probe.[60] Minimal evidence or expert opinion is available on breastfed infants, particularly with regard to preservation of breastfeeding during therapy.[61-63] Although thickened formulas do not appear to reduce measurable reflux, they may reduce vomiting.[64]

DIARRHEA IN CHILDREN. Traditionally, carob has been used for the treatment of gastrointestinal conditions, especially diarrhea. Clinical trials have used different types of carob products (carob bean juice and carob pod powder) as an adjunct to oral rehydrating solution and showed promising results.[65,66] Duration of diarrhea was shortened, stool output was reduced, and oral rehydration requirement was decreased. However, the studies do not show carob's efficacy as a monotherapy for diarrhea.

GASTROESOPHAGEAL REFLUX DISEASE IN INFANTS. Pediatricians are familiar with infants complaining of regurgitation and emesis from gastroesophageal reflux. These subjects, usually growing satisfactorily and healthy, are affected by "functional" or "symptomatic" gastroesophageal reflux and are treated with posture changes and thickened feedings. Locust bean gum is a common food thickener, and studies have shown that it may be helpful in infantile gastroesophageal reflux.[60,67-69] Because locust bean gum may increase feces, studies should examine safety concern for potentially underweight infants. In addition, locust bean gum's efficacy should be compared with other forms of food thickeners.

Dose

Carob pod powder at 1.5 g/kg/day to a maximum of 15 g for up to 6 days has been used in infants (3-21 months) with acute diarrhea.[66]

The dose of carob for GERD has not been determined.

Adverse Effects, Interactions, Pharmacokinetics. See Appendix A.

Cascara (Rhamnus purshiana)

Grade C: *Unclear or conflicting scientific evidence (constipation; bowel cleansing)*

Mechanism of Action

The active constituents of cascara are the anthraquinones. Free anthraquinone and hydroxyanthracene derivative (HAD) give cascara its laxative action. These compounds promote more peristalsis in the large intestine and trigger a nerve center, which facilitates bowel movements. The active constituents of cascara are absorbed through the small intestine, then enter the circulatory system and stimulate the autonomic nervous system to create peristalsis. Cascara also contains small amounts of bitter anthracene and aloin compounds, which account for the cathartic action.

Scientific Evidence of Effectiveness

CONSTIPATION. Cascara is widely accepted and used as a mild laxative and effective short-term treatment for chronic constipation; however, limited data are available.[70-73]

BOWEL CLEANSING. Evidence from a methodologically weak study found that using a combination of cascara, bisacodyl, and sodium picosulfate along with a tap-water enema 1 hour before colon examination yielded 96% adequate bowel cleansing.[74] Evidence is insufficient to suggest efficacy over conventional treatments for this indication.

Dose

Traditionally, 4 to 6 mL of aromatic fluid extract has been administered at bedtime for constipation. As a tea, cascara can be given for constipation in a dose of 1 cup of tea, made by steeping 2 g of finely chopped bark in 150 mL of boiling water for 5 to 10 minutes, and then straining. The appropriate amount of cascara is the smallest dose necessary to maintain soft stools.

Adverse Effects, Interactions, Pharmacokinetics. See Appendix A.

Chamomile (Matricaria recutita, syn. Matricaria suaveolens, Matricaria chamomilla, Anthemis nobilis, Chamaemelum nobile, Chamomilla chamomilla, Chamomilla recutita)

Grade C: *Unclear or conflicting scientific evidence (diarrhea in children; gastrointestinal conditions; infantile colic)*

Mechanism of Action

The mechanism of action of chamomile for diarrhea is not well understood. However, it may benefit other gastrointestinal conditions. Constituents of chamomile, alpha-bisabolol and apigenin, are considered antispasmodics.[29,75-77] Other constituents, including coumarins and flavonoids, have been found to possess minor smooth muscle relaxant activity.

Scientific Evidence of Effectiveness

DIARRHEA IN CHILDREN. There is some preliminary evidence that chamomile with apple pectin (Diarrhoesan, a liquid preparation containing apple pectin and chamomile fluid extract standardized to 2.5 g/100 g of chamazulen) may reduce the length of time that children experience diarrhea.[78] This combination product revealed superior efficacy over placebo, with a significantly reduced stool frequency in the treatment group compared with the control group.

GASTROINTESTINAL CONDITIONS. Chamomile is a popular home remedy for gastrointestinal complaints. The German Commission E has approved internal use of chamomile for GI complaints. However, scant evidence exists to support its use in this area. Chamomile appears to be of some benefit when used in the combination product Diarrhoesan, which resulted in 85% relief of symptoms when taken for 3 days.[79] Studies using chamomile monotherapies are lacking.

INFANTILE COLIC. The herbal combination preparation Iberogast containing chamomile (*Matricaria recutita*) plus lemon balm (*Melissa officinalis*), iber (*Iberis amara*), garden angelica (*Angelica archangelica*), caraway (*Carum carvi*), milk thistle (*Silybum marianum*), greater celandine (*Chelidonium majus*), licorice (*Glycyrrhiza glabra*), and peppermint (*Mentha x piperita*) has been found to reduce symptoms of dyspepsia (see Lemon Balm). Studies evaluating chamomile monotherapy for dyspepsia are currently lacking.

Dose

As a common remedy for unspecified gastrointestinal complaints, chamomile tea (2-3 g chamomile steeped in 150 mL hot water) has been used three or four times daily between meals. Doses of 5 mL of 15 chamomile tincture three times daily and 12 g of German chamomile flowers daily have also been used.

Based on unsubstantiated sources, 3 g of dried flowers in 5 oz of hot water three to four times daily has been used for IBS.

Adverse Effects, Interactions, Pharmacokinetics. See Appendix A.

Cinnamon (Cinnamomum spp.)

Grade C: *Unclear or conflicting scientific evidence (Helicobacter pylori infection)*

Mechanism of Action
Cinnamon extracts have shown inhibitory activity against *Helicobacter pylori* in vitro, although the exact mechanism of action is not well understood.[80]

Scientific Evidence of Effectiveness
Based on positive effects of cinnamon on *H. pylori*, a pilot study was conducted to test the activity of an alcoholic extract of cinnamon in a group of patients infected with *H. pylori*.[81] The cinnamon extract, 40 mg taken twice daily, was ineffective in eradicating *H. pylori*. However, the combination of cinnamon with other antimicrobials, or cinnamon extract at a higher concentration, may prove useful. Further studies are warranted.

Dose
In a pilot study, patients infected with *Helicobacter pylori* took 40 mg cinnamon extract twice daily for four weeks.[81]

Adverse Effects, Interactions, Pharmacokinetics. See Appendix A.

Dandelion (Taraxacum Officinale)

Grade C: *Unclear or conflicting scientific evidence (colitis)*

Mechanism of Action
Dandelion's therapeutic effects have historically been attributed to the bitter constituents found in roots and leaves.[82] Research in laboratory animals suggests that dandelion root may possess antiinflammatory properties.[83] Sesquiterpene lactones are responsible for diuretic effects and may contribute to dandelion's mild antiinflammatory activity.[83] This effect may be beneficial in patients with colitis.

Dandelion has also been shown to be *cholertic,* or to increase bile production and flow to the gallbladder. It may also have a direct *cholagogic* effect on the gallbladder, causing contraction and release of stored bile.[84]

Scientific Evidence of Effectiveness
A combination herbal preparation containing dandelion, St. John's wort (*Hypericum perforatum*), lemon balm (*Melissa officinalis*), calendula (*Calendula officinalis*), and fennel (*Foeniculum vulgare*) reportedly improved chronic pain associated with colitis.[85] The contribution of dandelion to this effect is unclear.

Dose
The dose of dandelion as a monotherapy for colitis has not been determined.

Adverse Effects, Interactions, Pharmacokinetics. See Appendix A.

Fennel (Foeniculum vulgare)

Grade B: *Good scientific evidence (infantile colic)*

Grade C: *Unclear or conflicting scientific evidence (colitis)*

Mechanism of Action
Fennel seed appears to increase gastrointestinal motility and acts as an antispasmodic at high doses (dose not given). Fennel extracts produce a reduction in acetylcholine-induced contraction and decrease maximum possible contractility.[86]

Scientific Evidence of Effectiveness
INFANTILE COLIC. Fennel grows in the Mediterranean region. For centuries, fennel fruits have been used as herbal medicines in Europe and China. An emulsion of fennel seed oil and a combination herbal tea containing fennel (along with chamomile, vervain, licorice, balm-mint) have reduced infantile colic in RCTs.[86,87] The use of the fennel oil emulsion eliminated colic, according to the Wessel criteria, in 65% (40/62) of infants. It was also found to decrease the intensity of colic.

COLITIS. Patients with nonspecific colitis who took a combination herbal product containing fennel plus dandelion (*Taraxacum officinale*), St. John's wort (*Hypericum perforatum*), calendula (*Calendula officinalis*), and lemon balm (*Melissa officinalis*) demonstrated cessation of spontaneous and palpable pains along the large intestine.[85] Studies evaluating lemon balm monotherapy for colitis are currently lacking.

Dose
For infantile colic (age 2-12 weeks), 0.1% fennel seed oil in a water emulsion and 0.4% polysorbate-80 was used for 1 week.[87]

The dose of fennel as a monotherapy for colitis has not been determined.

Adverse Effects, Interactions, Pharmacokinetics. See Appendix A.

Flax (Linum usitatissimum)

Grade B: *Good scientific evidence (constipation/laxative [flaxseed, not flaxseed oil])*

Mechanism of Action
Flaxseed (not flaxseed oil) may produce laxative effects by increasing volume and stimulating peristalsis from stretch reflexes. Flaxseed does not appear to be affected by gastric acid or intestinal alkaline conditions. Also, flaxseed has been suggested to coat and protect intestinal mucosa.[1,29]

Scientific Evidence of Effectiveness
It has been proposed that flaxseed (not flaxseed oil) produces laxative effects. Loose stools have been observed in patients

participating in studies of flaxseed for other indications.[88,89] These effects were noted at doses of 45 g/day.[90] Additional evidence available from a small trial suggests that flaxseed is a more effective treatment for constipation than the popular laxative agent psyllium.[91] Preliminary clinical evidence plus a plausible mechanism suggest that flaxseed does possess laxative properties.[1,29,91,92] Notably, in large doses, or when taken with inadequate water, flaxseed may precipitate bowel obstruction through a mass effect.[90]

Dose

Flaxseed products are not standardized based on specific chemical components, but rather are evaluated with identity and quality tests, including microscopic/macroscopic inspection and organoleptic evaluation. Flaxseed is approximately 35% oil, of which 55% is alpha-linolenic acid (ALA). From 58% to 60% of flaxseed is omega-3 fatty acids, with 18% to 20% omega-6 fatty acids. Flaxseed and linseed oil contain 30% to 45% unsaturated fatty acids, and approximately 8% of the plant contains soluble fiber mucilage. The plant also contains 20% protein. Flaxseed oil is composed of 73% polyunsaturated fatty acids, 18% monounsaturated fatty acids, and 9% saturated fatty acids.

As a laxative, the dose of flaxseed used commonly is 2 to 3 tbsp of bulk seed mixed in 10 times the amount of water, although 45 g/day has had laxative effects in clinical studies.

Adverse Effects, Interactions, Pharmacokinetics. See Appendix A.

Ginger (Zingiber officinale)

Grade B: *Good scientific evidence (hyperemesis gravidarum [morning sickness])*

Grade C: *Unclear or conflicting scientific evidence (motion sickness; chemotherapy-induced nausea and vomiting; postoperative nausea and vomiting; Heliobacter pylori infections)*

Mechanism of Action

The "pungent principles" or nonvolatile constituents of ginger are considered responsible for its flavor, aromatic properties, and pharmacological activity. These include gingerols such as 6-gingerol (usually <1% of the root's weight), 6-shagaol (dehyroxylated analog of 6-gingerol), 6- and 6-dehyrogingerdione, 6-gingerdion and (10)-gingerdione, 6-paradol, vallinoids, galanals A and B, and zingerone. Other compounds include carbohydrates, fats, minerals, oleoresins, vitamins, waxes, and *zingibain* (a proteolytic enzyme). The rhizome of ginger contains pungent vanillyl ketones, including 6-gingerol and 6-paradol, and has been reported to possess strong antiinflammatory activity as well as anti–tumor-promoting properties.[93]

Mechanisms have been proposed for ginger's effects on nausea and vomiting. The components in ginger responsible for its antiemetic effect are thought to be the gingerols, shogaols, and galanolactone, a diterpenoid of ginger.[94-96] Animal and in vitro studies have shown ginger to have antiserotoninergic and $5-HT_3$ receptor antagonism effects, which play an important role in the etiology of postoperative nausea and vomiting.[95-99] In a randomized, placebo-controlled, crossover trial of 16 healthy volunteers, ginger (1 g orally) had no effect on gastric emptying.[100] It appears unlikely that ginger's antiemetic or antinausea effects are mediated through increased gastroduodenal motility or through increased gastric emptying.[101]

It has been suggested that ginger rhizome (root) increases stomach acid production. However, other in vitro and animal studies report gastroprotective properties.[102,103] In addition, the ginger constituent 6-shogaol (generally more potent than 6-gingerol) has inhibited intestinal motility in intravenous preparations and facilitated gastrointestinal motility in oral preparations. Ginger extract has also been reported to inhibit the growth of *Helicobacter pylori* in vitro.[104]

Scientific Evidence of Effectiveness

HYPEREMESIS GRAVIDARUM (MORNING SICKNESS). Because many conventional antiemetics have the potential of teratogenic effects during pregnancy, researchers have begun studying herbal remedies as possible alternatives.[105] A limited number of RCTs suggest that 1 g/day of ginger may be safe and effective for pregnancy-associated nausea and vomiting when used for short periods (≤4 days). Significant improvements in nausea, retching, and vomiting episodes have been observed.[106,107] Follow-up of pregnancies and deliveries revealed normal ranges of birth weights, gestational ages, Apgar scores (to determine if neonates require urgent medical care), and frequencies of congenital abnormalities when ginger group infants were compared to the general population of infants.[106]

Studies have shown ginger to be superior to vitamin B_6 for treating morning sickness.[108] Two 325-mg capsules of ginger three times daily for 4 days has been found more effective than vitamin B_6, based on an equivalence study.[108] Another equivalence study showed that one capsule of ginger (350 mg) was equivalent to 25 mg of vitamin B_6 when taken three times daily for 3 weeks.[109]

Doses of 500 to 1500 mg (0.5-1.5 g) have been evaluated in studies using ginger to treat morning sickness.[106,107,110-112] However, some advise women not to consume ginger in amounts greater than typically found in food (>1 g dry weight daily) during pregnancy because of purported emmenagogic (menstrual discharge–promoting) effects, as well as abortifacient, mutagenic, and antiplatelet effects.[113] However, others have reported no scientific or medical evidence for a pregnancy contraindication.[113,114] Additional research is warranted regarding the safety and efficacy of ginger during pregnancy before it can be routinely recommended to patients for extended courses.

MOTION SICKNESS. Results evaluating the effects of ginger in motion sickness have been inconsistent. Several studies have found ginger to have no effect on motion sickness.[115-119] However, a study of naval cadets found that powdered ginger root (1 g) significantly reduced vomiting (but not nausea or vertigo) throughout a 4-hour test period.[120] In an RCT comparing the effects of ginger (100 mg total given as two divided doses, 4 hours apart) with six other medications (combination of 20 mg cinnarizine and 15 mg domperidone twice daily, 4 hours apart; 50 mg cyclizine; combination of 50 mg dimenhydrinate and 50 mg caffeine; combination of 12.3 mg meclizine and 10 mg caffeine; 25 mg cinnarizine; and 0.5 mg scopolamine), found ginger to be equivalent in tolerability and efficacy.[116]

CHEMOTHERAPY-INDUCED NAUSEA AND VOMITING. Supportive evidence from one RCT and an open-label study indicates that ginger reduces the severity and duration of self-reported nausea (but not vomiting) during chemotherapy.[121,122] Effects appear to be additive to prochlorperazine (Compazine).[122] However, another study failed to find any significant effects of ginger on cisplatin-induced emesis.[123]

POSTOPERATIVE NAUSEA AND VOMITING. A limited number of RCTs have found a significant decrease in postoperative nausea and/or vomiting after prophylactic administration of ginger before surgery,[124,125] whereas other research shows perioperative ginger to be no more efficacious than placebo.[126-129] Powdered ginger root (1 g) and metoclopramide (10 mg) orally were similarly effective in prevention of postoperative nausea and vomiting in an RCT of 120 female patients having gynecological surgery.[124]

Use of ginger in the perioperative period should be approached cautiously; ginger may inhibit platelet aggregation, decrease platelet thromboxane production, and thus theoretically increase perioperative bleeding risk. Increased prothrombin time (PT) and international normalized ratio (INR) were reported in a woman taking both warfarin and ginger, suggesting an interaction between ginger and anticoagulants.[130]

Dose

Most experts, including the European Scientific Cooperative on Phytotherapy (ESCOP), and the German Commission E, recommend a dose of 1 to 4 g daily of powder, tablets, or fresh-cut ginger in divided doses. Many publications note that the maximum recommended daily dose of ginger is 4 g.

For hyperemesis gravidarum (nausea/vomiting of pregnancy), 1 to 2 g of powdered ginger orally has been taken daily in divided doses for up to 3 weeks.[107,109,112]

For motion sickness, 1 to 2 g of ginger has been taken daily in divided doses.[131]

For chemotherapy-induced nausea and vomiting, the optimal dose remains unclear, as does the effectiveness.[121]

According to the results of a meta-analysis, a fixed dose of at least 1 g of ginger is more effective than placebo for the prevention of postoperative nausea and vomiting.[132]

Adverse Effects, Interactions, Pharmacokinetics. See Appendix A.

Globe Artichoke (Cynara scolymus)

Grade C: *Unclear or conflicting scientific evidence (dyspepsia; irritable bowel syndrome)*

Mechanism of Action

One proposed etiology of nonulcer dyspepsia is bile duct dyskinesia.[133] Because globe artichoke extract has been studied as a choloretic, artichoke has been suggested to function as an antidyspeptic agent.[134]

Scientific Evidence of Effectiveness

DYSPEPSIA; IRRITABLE BOWEL SYNDROME. Globe artichoke is authorized for use in dyspeptic complaints by the German Commission E. An available RCT found a standardized artichoke extract (LI 220 Hepar SL forte) to be more effective than placebo in relieving symptoms of functional dyspepsia.[135] Symptoms that improved more with artichoke were fullness, early satiety, and flatulence; however, nausea, vomiting, and pain were not affected by artichoke treatment. In subset analysis, artichoke leaf extract reduced symptoms and incidence of IBS and improved quality of life in otherwise healthy volunteers with concomitant dyspepsia.[136]

A recommendation for the use of artichoke in the management of nonulcer dyspepsia cannot be made in the absence of better-designed, adequately powered RCTs. Also, patients with chronic or recurrent dyspepsia might require medical evaluation to rule out ulcer or neoplasm; nonulcer dyspepsia is a diagnosis of exclusion.

Dose

It is recommended that artichoke dietary supplements be standardized to 15% chlorogenic acid, 2% to 5% cynarin per dose, or 1% caffeoyl acid derivatives.[133]

For dyspepsia, 640 mg of standardized artichoke extract three times daily for 6 weeks has been used.[135] Patients with concomitant dyspepsia and IBS have taken 320 to 1920 mg of extract daily for 6 to 8 weeks.[135,137,138]

Adverse Effects, Interactions, Pharmacokinetics. See Appendix A.

Goldenseal (Hydrastis canadensis)

Grade C: *Unclear or conflicting scientific evidence* (Helicobacter pylori *infection; infectious diarrhea*)

Mechanism of Action

Berberine, the active constituent in goldenseal, appears to have a broad spectrum of antibiotic activity against *Helicobacter pylori*, *Escherichia coli*, and cholera.[139-147] Berberine has been found to inhibit cholera toxin and to have an antisecretory effect in the intestines of animals induced by *E. coli* enterotoxin or *Vibrio cholerae*.[147-153]

Scientific Evidence of Effectiveness

Helicobacter pylori infection. Berberine has been used as an antidiarrheal medication in Ayurvedic medicine and traditional Chinese medicine (TCM) for thousands of years. In several animal and preliminary clinical studies, berberine has been evaluated as a treatment for infectious diarrhea (including choleric diarrhea).[154,155] One review suggests the efficacy of berberine sulfate in treating diarrhea caused by a number of etiologies.[156] Berberine appears to be more effective in *Escherichia coli*–related diarrhea than in cholera. However, human studies have produced equivocal and conflicting results. The efficacy of berberine remains uncertain in the management of infectious diarrhea.

Infectious diarrhea. Berberine has been compared with antibacterial drugs (gentamicin, terramycin) and ranitidine in stimulation of ulcer healing and *H. pylori* clearance.[157] Berberine was suggested to be less effective at ulcer healing than ranitidine, but potentially more effective at *H. pylori* clearance.

Dose

The dose of berberine for *Helicobacter pylori* infection has not been determined.

For infectious diarrhea, a single dose of 400 mg of berberine sulfate has been studied over a 24-hour period.[158]

Adverse Effects, Interactions, Pharmacokinetics. See Appendix A.

Lemon Balm (Melissa officinalis)

Grade C: *Unclear or conflicting scientific evidence (dyspepsia; colitis)*

Mechanism of Action

Currently, there is a lack of clinical evidence using lemon balm alone for the treatment of gastrointestinal disorders.[159,160] The mechanism of action is not clear.

Scientific Evidence of Effectiveness

Dyspepsia. The herbal combination preparation Iberogast, containing lemon balm (*Melissa officinalis*) plus chamomile (*Matricaria recutita*), iber (*Iberis amara*), garden angelica (*Angelica archangelica*), caraway (*Carum carvi*), milk thistle (*Silybum marianum*), greater celandine (*Chelidonium majus*), licorice (*Glycyrrhiza glabra*), and peppermint (*Mentha x piperita*), has been found to reduce symptoms of dyspepsia.[161-163] Studies evaluating lemon balm monotherapy for dyspepsia are currently lacking.

Colitis. Patients with nonspecific colitis who took a combination herbal product containing lemon balm plus dandelion (*Taraxacum officinale*), St. John's wort (*Hypericum perforatum*), calendula (*Calendula officinalis*), and fennel (*Foeniculum vulgare*) demonstrated cessation of spontaneous and palpable pains along the large intestine.[85] Studies evaluating lemon balm monotherapy for colitis are currently lacking.

Dose

The percentage of essential oil that can be obtained from lemon balm leaves can range from 0.08 to 0.25 mL/100 g and 0.06 to 0.167 mL/100 g from the herb.[164] The content and quality of essential oils from lemon balm may also differ depending on the height and location of the harvest cut of a particular plant, the vegetation period of the plant, and between different populations of the plant. For example, the oil content in lemon balm appears to be highest in the top third of the plant, and the percentage of the constituents may be highest when the plant is cut in the basipetal direction (from top to base).[164-171] Clinical trial data suggest that different preparations of lemon balm may result in products that exhibit different properties depending on the process used for the sample preparation.[172]

For dyspepsia, the combination product Iberogast, 20 drops three times daily for a minimum of 4 weeks, may be recommended.[161-163] The dose of lemon balm as a monotherapy for colitis has not been determined.

Adverse Effects, Interactions, Pharmacokinetics. See Appendix A.

Licorice (Glycyrrhiza glabra)

Grade C: *Unclear or conflicting scientific evidence (dyspepsia; bleeding stomach ulcers caused by aspirin; peptic ulcer disease)*

Mechanism of Action

The exact mechanism of licorice in dyspepsia is not well understood. For peptic ulcers, licorice may accelerate healing by interfering with prostanoid synthesis and increasing blood flow and stimulating mucus secretion.[173] It may also inhibit *Helicobacter pylori* in the intestine.

Scientific Evidence of Effectiveness

Dyspepsia. The herbal combination preparation Iberogast, containing licorice (*Glycyrrhiza glabra*) plus lemon balm (*Melissa officinalis*), chamomile (*Matricaria recutita*), iber (*Iberis amara*), garden angelica (*Angelica archangelica*), caraway (*Carum carvi*), milk thistle (*Silybum marianum*), greater celandine (*Chelidonium majus*), and peppermint (*Mentha x piperita*), has been found to reduce symptoms of dyspepsia.[161-163]

Bleeding stomach ulcers caused by aspirin. Human fecal blood loss induced by 975 mg aspirin orally three times daily was demonstrated to be less when 350 mg deglycyrrhizinated licorice (DGL) was given with each dose of aspirin.[174]

Peptic ulcer disease. A peptic ulcer may occur in the lining of the stomach (gastric ulcer), duodenum (duodenal ulcer), or esophagus (esophageal ulcer). The use of licorice extracts, DGL and carbenoxolone, for duodenal and gastric ulcers has demonstrated some benefit, primarily for duodenal ulcers.[175-182]

Both DGL and cimetidine (Tagament) have demonstrated a healing effect on gastric and duodenal ulcers.[179] For duodenal ulcers, however, cimetidine appears to be more effective than DGL.[177]

It is not clear whether DGL or the synthetic derivative carbenoxolone is more effective in the treatment of peptic ulcers. Some studies show that DGL is similar to carbenoxolone, whereas in other research, carbenoxolone appeared more effective at healing gastric ulcers than DGL.[1,29,182] Ulcer size and percentage of radiological healing appeared slightly greater with the use of carbenoxolone.[181]

Dose

For dyspepsia, the combination product Iberogast (20 drops three times daily for a minimum of 4 weeks) may be recommended.[161-163]

To reduce gastric mucosal damage caused by aspirin, 350 mg of DGL was given with each dose of aspirin (975 mg) for an unspecified duration.[174] For peptic ulcers, DGL has been used at 760 mg orally three to five times daily for up to 2 years.[178,179]

Adverse Effects, Interactions, Pharmacokinetics. See Appendix A.

Mastic (Pistacia lentiscus)

Grade C: *Unclear or conflicting scientific evidence (gastric and duodenal ulcers)*

Mechanism of Action

The exact mechanism of action of mastic in the healing of gastric and duodenal ulcers has not yet been identified. Through animal and in vitro studies, investigators hypothesize that mastic exhibits antisecretory and cytoprotective effects on the gastric and duodenal mucosa.[183,184] Also, mastic has shown antibacterial action against *Helicobacter pylori* in vitro, which may help to explain its ulcer-healing properties.[1]

Scientific Evidence of Effectiveness

Mastic has been used by traditional Mediterranean healers to treat peptic ulcers since the thirteenth century. The results of one study showed the efficacy of mastic versus placebo to heal duodenal ulcers.[185] An RCT showed mastic to be superior to placebo in both relieving the symptoms of and healing duodenal ulcers, with no reported adverse effects. These results led to an observational study to determine mastic's efficacy in healing gastric ulcers as well.[186] Six patients, all with endoscopically diagnosed gastric ulcer, were followed over 4 weeks to assess the healing capabilities of twice-daily mastic ingestion. Mastic healed gastric ulcers in five of the six subjects, with no reported adverse effects. Additional research is needed to determine mastic's mechanism of action and efficacy in treating duodenal or gastric ulcer and compare it to current medical treatment.

Dose

For duodenal ulcers, 1 g of mastic powder has been ingested orally, once daily before breakfast, for 2 weeks.[185]

For gastric ulcers, 1 g of mastic powder has been ingested orally, twice daily before breakfast and at bedtime, for 4 weeks.[186]

Adverse Effects, Interactions, Pharmacokinetics. See Appendix A.

Neem (Azadirachta indica)

Grade C: *Unclear or conflicting scientific evidence (gastroduodenal ulcers)*

Mechanism of Action

Neem appears to have antisecretory and antiulcer effects. According to animal research, neem dose-dependently blocked gastric ulcer.[187] Compared to ranitidine, neem was equipotent, and more potent than omeprazole (Prilosec) in inhibiting pylorus ligation–induced acid secretion. Neem appeared to offer gastroprotection against stress ulcers by preventing adhered mucus and endogenous glutathione depletion. Furthermore, neem prevented oxidative damage of the gastric mucosa by significantly blocking lipid peroxidation and scavenging of hydroxyl radical.

Scientific Evidence of Effectiveness

Protective and healing effects of neem on gastroduodenal ulcers have been reported in a preliminary clinical study.[188] Neem bark extract resulted in a 63% reduction in total volume of gastric section and a 77% inhibition of total amount of acid secretion. Comparisons to other agents used for this purpose, such as proton pump inhibitors or H_2-receptor antagonists, are lacking.

Dose

The bark extract, 30 to 60 mg twice daily for 10 weeks, has been used to treat gastroduodenal ulcers.[188]

Adverse Effects, Interactions, Pharmacokinetics. See Appendix A.

Papaya (Carica papaya)

Grade C: *Unclear or conflicting scientific evidence (gastrointestinal disorders [phytobezoar])*

Mechanism of Action

Papain is a proteolytic enzyme that is thought to break up protein linkages within enteric stones called *bezoars*,[189] specifically, *phytobezoars*, composed of nondigestible food particles found in fruits and vegetables.

Scientific Evidence of Effectiveness

Nonsurgical methods, including the use of natural enzymes such as papain, have been used to disintegrate bezoars, which collect in the stomach and cannot pass through intestines. Papase tablets (no longer available in the United States) have successfully treated phytobezoars (bezoars caused by plants) in various case reports.[190-192] Papain successfully treated 87% of patients with phytobezoars; however, papain appeared to be less effective and less well tolerated than cellulose.[193]

Dose

The dose of papain for phytobezoars is unclear.

Adverse Effects, Interactions, Pharmacokinetics. See Appendix A.

Peppermint (Mentha x piperita)

Grade B: *Good scientific evidence (colonic spasm; dyspepsia; gastric spasm; irritable bowel syndrome)*

Grade C: *Unclear or conflicting scientific evidence (abdominal distention; esophageal spasm; postoperative nausea)*

Mechanism of Action

The principal effect of peppermint oil relevant to the GI tract is a dose-related antispasmodic effect on the smooth musculature caused by menthol, which interfers with calcium movement across the cell membrane. The choleretic and antifoaming effects of peppermint oil may play an additional role in medicinal use.[194] Carminative properties of peppermint are believed to result from relaxation of the esophageal sphincter.[195-199] Peppermint oil appears to inhibit enterocyte glucose uptake by directly acting on the brush border membrane of the intestine in animals.[200] Increased bile secretion, attributable to the flavonoid, terpene, and menthol content of peppermint oil, and improvements in the solubility of bile have been noted in animal studies.[201,202] In 12 healthy volunteers, 90 mg of peppermint oil in a non-enteric-coated gelatin capsule inhibited gallbladder contraction, as demonstrated by ultrasound, and slowed intestinal transit time, as determined by a lactulose H_2 breath test.[203] When combined with caraway oil, peppermint oil reduces the visceral hyperalgesia in rats exposed to colonic inflammatory agents.[204]

Scientific Evidence of Effectiveness

COLONIC SPASM. Based on purported smooth muscle relaxant properties, peppermint oil has been proposed to help reduce colonic spasm during and after endoscopic procedures.[199,205] Peppermint may be added as an ingredient in barium enema preparations for rectal use. Because definitive evidence is still lacking, however, it remains unclear if peppermint oil is beneficial in the treatment of colonic spasm during barium enemas or colonoscopies.

DYSPEPSIA. Preliminary evidence from a small number of controlled trials indicates that a combination of peppermint oil and caraway oil may help alleviate moderate to severe pain from nonulcerative dyspepsia.[206-211] However, most studies had methodological limitations, which complicates data interpretation. It is unclear which constituent(s) may be beneficial. Nonetheless, the existing evidence does suggest efficacy for the peppermint-caraway combination.

Dyspepsia can actually be a side effect of oral peppermint oil and has been reported by patients in several controlled trials.[195-198,212] This may be caused by relaxation of the lower esophageal sphincter by peppermint oil. Therefore, patients with underlying GERD should use peppermint oil cautiously. Patients with chronic heartburn should be evaluated by qualified health care providers and may be advised to undergo a diagnostic endoscopy before initiating any treatment for heartburn.

GASTRIC SPASM. Preliminary research suggests that peppermint oil may effectively reduce colonic spasm during endoscopy. One RCT compared intraluminal peppermint solution to hyoscine (antimuscarinic alkaloid).[213] The contraction ratio of peppermint oil was lower than that of hyoscine, and the time required for disappearance of the antral contraction ring(s) was shorter in the peppermint oil group than the hyoscine group. Fewer side effects were noted with peppermint oil.

IRRITABLE BOWEL SYNDROME. Multiple RCTs using peppermint to treat IBS suggest significant improvements in symptoms of IBS.[195,197,212,214-222] The smooth muscle–relaxing properties of peppermint and calcium antagonism may play a role. Enteric-coated peppermint preparations are generally recommended. Average response rates in terms of "overall success" are 58% (range, 39%-79%) for peppermint oil and 29% (range, 10%-52%) for placebo.[223] Studies of peppermint versus smooth muscle relaxants showed no differences between treatments, suggesting therapeutic equivalence. Overall, studies have been brief, with small sample sizes and methodological weaknesses (unclear diagnostic criteria, lack of validated measurement scales, unclear blinding and randomization procedures). Well-designed large trials are necessary before a strong recommendation can be made. Future studies should use standardized symptom scales and established diagnostic criteria to classify patients before enrollment (e.g., Rome II Diagnostic Criteria), uniform dosing and standardization, and longer duration.

ABDOMINAL DISTENTION. Preliminary evidence suggests peppermint hot compress may help relieve abdominal distention and pain as well as shorten duration of first gas passage after surgery.[1,29]

ESOPHAGEAL SPASM. Preliminary evidence suggests intraluminal peppermint oil will help decrease spasm in the esophagus, lower stomach, and duodenal bulb in patients undergoing double-contrast barium meal examination.[224]

POSTOPERATIVE NAUSEA (AROMATHERAPY). Research is insufficient to determine if peppermint oil aromatherapy is beneficial in the treatment of postoperative nausea. Peppermint aromatherapy effectively reduced the perceived severity of postoperative nausea.[225] However, it was compared to saline "placebo," which was also effective. Beneficial effect may be related more to controlled breathing patterns than to the actual aroma inhaled.

Dose

For decreasing colonic spasms during barium enema, 8 mL of peppermint oil was added to 100 mL water with Tween 80 (surfactant and emulsifier). The insoluble fraction was removed, then 30 mL of the remaining peppermint solution was added to 300 mL of barium solution (dose and duration unspecified).[205]

For gastric spasm (endoscopy), 16 mL of peppermint oil dissolved in hot water and infused intraluminally has been used during upper endoscopy.[213]

For dyspepsia, enteric-coated capsules containing a fixed combination of 90 mg peppermint oil and 50 mg caraway oil two to three times daily for up to 4 weeks have been used.[206,226]

For IBS, one or two enteric-coated capsules of Colpermin (0.2- 0.4 mL peppermint oil or 187-374 mg peppermint oil in thixotropic gel) has been used three times daily 15 to 30 minutes before meals for up to 1 month.[195] Also, patients have taken 180 to 200-mg peppermint oil in enteric-coated capsules.[223]

For abdominal distention, the dose of peppermint oil monotherapy has not been determined.

For esophageal spasm, patients ingested a solution containing 5 drops of peppermint oil in 10 mL of water (duration unspecified).[227]

For other digestive disorders, 0.2 to 0.4 mL of peppermint oil may be used three times daily in dilute preparations or suspension.[228]

Adverse Effects, Interactions, Pharmacokinetics. See Appendix A.

Psyllium (*Plantago* spp.)

Grade B: *Good scientific evidence (constipation; diarrhea)*

Grade C: *Unclear or conflicting scientific evidence (anal fissures; hemorrhoids; inflammatory bowel disease; irritable bowel disease)*

Mechanism of Action

The laxative properties of psyllium result from the soluble fiber component of the husk, which swells when it comes in contact with water. The polysaccharides in psyllium form a gel in the intestine and lubricate stool contents, easing defecation.[229] The resulting bulk stimulates a reflex contraction of the walls of the bowel, followed by emptying.[230] Studies exploring the mechanism of the laxative effects of psyllium are conflicting but generally reveal an increase in bowel movements daily, an increase in wet and dry stool weight, and a decrease in total gut transit time with psyllium administration.[231-235] In persons with diarrhea, the mucilage may increase the water-holding capacity and viscosity of stools, which delays gastric emptying and improves stool consistency.[229,236-238] Psyllium maintains remission in ulcerative colitis because fermentation of blond psyllium in the colon yields butyrate, a short-chain fatty acid known to inhibit cytokine production and have an antiinflammatory effect.[239] With IBS, blond psyllium (*plantago ovata*) may normalize bowel function and relieve symptom severity by reducing rectosigmoidal pressure.[240] Psyllium fiber has also been shown to delay intestinal gas transit by decreasing bolus propulsion to the rectum and promote gas retention.[241]

Scientific Evidence of Effectiveness

CONSTIPATION. Psyllium has long been used as the chief ingredient in "bulk laxatives." Studies show that psyllium decreases constipation, increases weekly stool frequency, decreases the number of incomplete evacuations, reduces straining, and produces softer stools.[20,232,233,242-250] Psyllium appears to be superior to docusate sodium for softening stools by increasing water content, with greater overall laxative effect. Psyllium plus senna improved objective symptoms of stool frequency and weight greater than with psyllium alone.[247]

DIARRHEA. Several trials studied psyllium as treatment for diarrhea, particularly in patients undergoing tube feeding.[251-254] As an adjunct to orlistat (alli) therapy, psyllium was used to decrease the gastrointestinal manifestations of the weight loss drug.[255] Compared with loperamide (Imodium), psyllium in combination with calcium appeared to be as effective in reducing urgency and improving stool consistency.[256]

ANAL FISSURES. Results from a preliminary clinical trail suggested that psyllium reduced the number of surgeries necessary to heal anal fissures.[257] Recurrence rate was also reduced.

HEMORRHOIDS. Hemorrhoids are caused by the straining and hardness of stools associated with constipation. Two clinical studies reported that psyllium-containing products reduced the symptoms of hemorrhoids.[258,259] Fewer bleeding episodes and less pain on defecation have been reported with psyllium use.[258-260]

INFLAMMATORY BOWEL DISEASE. Minimal evidence addresses IBD remission with psyllium preparations. Results from available human study evaluating patients with ulcerative colitis in remission found that psyllium was helpful in the management of gastrointestinal symptoms.[261-263] A higher rate of improvement was noted with psyllium than with placebo.

IRRITABLE BOWEL SYNDROME. Studies have shown that treatment with psyllium improved constipation, abdominal pain, and bloating in IBS patients.[264-267] Diarrhea and overall well-being also improved.[264,265] According to clinical study, a combination approach with lorazepam, hyoscine butylbromide, and psyllium may provide added benefit.[268]

Dose

Psyllium products may contain husks of *Plantago ovata* seeds or the seeds themselves. Amounts of psyllium in products are generally reported as total grams. Seed preparations contain approximately 47% soluble fiber by weight; husk preparations generally contain 67% to 71% soluble fiber and 85% total fiber by weight.[234,235]

For colonoscopy preparation, 1 tbsp of sugar-free Metamucil has been combined with 8 oz of water for 4 days before a colonoscopy.[269]

For constipation, single or divided doses of 7 to 30 g of psyllium have been taken daily for 2 to 16 weeks.*

For diarrhea, single or divided doses of 7.5 to 30 g of psyllium have been taken daily for 3 to 7 days.[238,252,253]

For anal fissures, the dose of psyllium has not been determined.

For hemorrhoids, patients received 7 g of psyllium daily for 6 weeks and reported improvement in symptoms.[271]

For IBD, 7 to 20 g of psyllium has been taken daily in divided doses.[239,261,262] Patients in one study received up to 12 months of therapy.[262]

For IBS, doses of 6 to 30 g of psyllium have been taken daily for 2 to 8 weeks.[245,262,264-267,272,273]

Adverse Effects, Interactions, Pharmacokinetics. See Appendix A.

Rhubarb (*Rheum* spp.)

Grade B: *Good scientific evidence (upper gastrointestinal bleeding)*

Grade C: *Unclear or conflicting scientific evidence (chronic constipation; gastrointestinal disorders; diarrhea)*

Mechanism of Action

Rhubarb contains tannins, anthraquinones, and pectin. At high doses, anthraquinone effects predominate and produce a stimulant-laxative effect. These constituents exert action on the colon wall and increase motility.[274] Because of its ability to increase peristalsis, rhubarb may be able to eliminate blood in cases of gastrointestinal (GI) bleeding. At low doses the tannin activity in rhubarb supersedes the anthraquinone activity, thus leading to a constipating effect and decreasing the number of stools. The pectin in rhubarb also tends to be antidiarrheal. In conjunction with tannins, pectin's effect may supersede the effect of anthraquinones when rhubarb is given in small doses (exact dose not given).[275]

Scientific Evidence of Effectiveness

UPPER GASTROINTESTINAL BLEEDING. Rhubarb has been used in TCM for many gastrointestinal disorders, including upper GI bleeding. Relatively low-quality studies suggest that rhubarb may be beneficial in reducing upper GI bleeding.[276-281] Rhubarb has displayed a higher effective rate and a shorter hemostatic time than Western medicine (e.g., oral magnesium-aluminium compound, intramuscular norepinephrine, intravenous PAMBA).[277] Disappearance of occult blood occurred 5 days earlier than in those treated with Western medicine.

CHRONIC CONSTIPATION. Historically, rhubarb has been widely used as a laxative, but it frequently causes intestinal griping and colic. One RCT studied the effects of a rhubarb–Glauber's salt mixture on chronic constipation.[282] Effects with this combination product were noted in 7 to 12 hours. Although this study indicates that the combination has positive effects, the contribution of rhubarb is difficult to distinguish.

GASTROINTESTINAL DISORDERS. One double-blind controlled trial examined the herbal extract "Amaro Medicinale Giuliani," which contains rhubarb, gentian, cascara, and boldo, for its effect on mild gastrointestinal disturbances.[283] Significant improvements were noted in asthenia, loss of appetite, coated tongue (whitish layer on upper surface of tongue), postprandial bloating, difficult digestion, constipation, flatulence, and abdominal fullness. Although the herbal extract and a combination of rhubarb and gentian seem promising, more studies using rhubarb as a monotherapy are needed to discern rhubarb's effect on gastrointestinal disturbances.

DIARRHEA. Rhubarb contains tannin constituents and may be beneficial for the treatment of diarrhea when consumed in low doses. However, evidence is lacking.

Dose

Various doses for constipation have been used: 1 tsp (5-6 g) of powdered root boiled in 1 cup of water for 10 minutes and ingested 1 tbsp (15 mL) at a time, up to 1 cup daily; ½ to 1 tsp or 1 to 4 g of dried root daily to produce a mild laxative effect; and 1 tsp daily of tincture or 1 to 2 tsp daily of decoction.

For upper GI bleeding, 3 g alcoholic extract tablets or powder or 6 mL of rhubarb syrup two to four times daily for up to 2 weeks has been used.[276,277,280]

Various doses for diarrhea have been traditionally used: powdered rhubarb root (1 g) boiled in 1 cup of water and taken 1 tbsp (15 mL) at a time up to 1 cup daily, 100 to 300 mg of the dried root daily, and 1 tsp of tincture or decoction once daily.

For gastritis and dyspepsia, 100 to 300 mg of rhubarb has been used.

Adverse Effects, Interactions, Pharmacokinetics. See Appendix A.

Sea Buckthorn (*Hippophae rhamnoides*)

Grade C: *Unclear or conflicting scientific evidence (gastric ulcers)*

---

*References 232, 234, 244, 245, 247, 248, 269, 270.

Mechanism of Action

In animals, sea buckthorn seed and fruit oil reduced ulcer formation, likely from inhibition of gastric acid and pepsin secretion and increased gastric mucus.[284] Also, sea buckthorn has inhibited various strains of *Helicobacter pylori*.[285]

Scientific Evidence of Effectiveness

When sea buckthorn oil was added to therapeutic endoscopy to treat gastroduodenal ulcers, patients underwent 1.5 to 2 times fewer treatments.[286] Results were positive in 93.7% of cases.

Dose

The dose of sea buckthorn for gastric ulcers has not been determined.

Adverse Effects, Interactions, Pharmacokinetics. See Appendix A.

Slippery Elm (*Ulmus rubra*, syn. *Ulmus fulva*)

Grade C: *Unclear or conflicting scientific evidence (diarrhea; gastrointestinal disorders)*

Mechanism of Action

The inner bark of slippery elm is rich in mucilage, consisting of insoluble polysaccharides (hexose, pentose, methylpentose), which form a viscous material after oral or topical administration.[287] After hydrolysis, these polysaccharides break down to produce galactose with traces of glucose and fructose. The fiber content is thought to reduce gastrointestinal transit time and to act as a bulk-forming laxative.

Scientific Evidence of Effectiveness

DIARRHEA. Slippery elm has been used traditionally to treat diarrhea. Although the tannins found in the herb may theoretically decrease water content of stool, and mucilage may act as a soothing agent to inflamed mucous membranes, reliable scientific evidence is lacking to support this indication.

GASTROINTESTINAL DISORDERS. Slippery elm is also traditionally used to treat inflammatory conditions of the digestive tract, such as gastritis, peptic ulcer disease, and enteritis. It may be taken alone or in combination with other herbs. Although anecdotally reported to be effective, supporting evidence is largely based on traditional evidence and the soothing properties attributed to mucilage in the herb. Clinical evidence is lacking.

Dose

Traditionally, for gastrointestinal upset, 7 g of slippery elm powder in 20 oz (1 pint) of boiling water has been used as a hot or cold infusion. Also, 1 tsp of slippery elm powder in 1 cup of boiling water has been taken multiple times during the day.

Adverse Effects, Interactions, Pharmacokinetics. See Appendix A.

Soy (*Glycine max*)

Grade B: *Good scientific evidence (acute diarrhea in infants and young children; diarrhea in adults)*

Mechanism of Action

Soy fiber may improve gastrointestinal function by regulating transit time and absorbing fluid from the intestinal lumen.[288,289]

Scientific Evidence of Effectiveness

ACUTE DIARRHEA IN INFANTS AND YOUNG CHILDREN. Numerous studies report that infants and young children (2-36 months old) with diarrhea who are fed soy formulas experience fewer daily bowel movements and fewer days of diarrhea.[290-296] Soy has been shown to be effective in reducing the duration of diarrhea as well as producing weight gain and reducing stool frequency.[291,293,296] This research suggests that soy has benefits over other types of formula, including cow's milk–based solutions.[292,294] The addition of soy fiber to soy formula may increase the effectiveness.[1] Parents should be advised to speak with qualified health care providers if their infants experience prolonged diarrhea, become dehydrated, develop signs of infections (e.g., fever), or have blood in the stool.

DIARRHEA IN ADULTS. Preliminary RCT results on the effect of tube feeding with soy-polysaccharide fiber suggest that it may not be effective for adult diarrhea in an acute setting.[297] Limited evidence makes soy difficult to recommend in the treatment of diarrhea.

Dose

Because of potential safety concerns, a qualified physician should be consulted regarding the choice of infant formula. The dose of soy for diarrhea in adults has not been determined.

Adverse Effects, Interactions, Pharmacokinetics. See Appendix A.

Turmeric (*Curcuma longa*)

Grade C: *Unclear or conflicting scientific evidence (dyspepsia; irritable bowel syndrome; peptic ulcer disease)*

Mechanism of Action

Curcuminoids (including curcumin), the compounds responsible for the bright-yellow color of turmeric, are also the principal pharmacological agents in turmeric. Curcuminoids are believed to stimulate bile secretion, which may contribute to its beneficial effects for dyspepsia.[298]

Oral administration of turmeric to rats (500 mg/kg) significantly reduced the incidence of chemically induced duodenal ulcers and is associated with an increase in intestinal wall mucus and nonprotein sulfhydryl content.[299] However, preliminary research in guinea pigs reported that various constituents of turmeric do not protect against histamine-induced gastric ulcerations.[300]

Scientific Evidence of Effectiveness

DYSPEPSIA. Turmeric has been used traditionally to treat a variety of gastrointestinal disorders, particularly indigestion associated with fatty meals. Data are limited in the area of dyspepsia therapy, although preliminary evidence suggests that turmeric may provide some benefit. In an RCT of 116 patients, 71% of patients receiving turmeric experienced symptom relief.[301] Notably, turmeric may cause GI irritation or upset, particularly in high or prolonged doses.

IRRITABLE BOWEL SYNDROME. A randomized, double-blind, placebo-controlled trial investigated the effect of *Curcuma xanthorriza* on IBS-related symptoms.[302] *C. xanthorriza* is related to *Curcuma longa*, and it is unclear whether its effects are the same as turmeric (*C. longa*). IBS-related distention decreased in the patients given *C. xanthorriza*. However, the global assessment of changes in IBS symptoms and psychological stress from IBS did not differ significantly among the treatment groups. It was concluded that *C. xanthorriza* showed no therapeutic benefit over placebo in patients with IBS.

PEPTIC ULCER DISEASE. Turmeric has also been used historically to treat gastric and duodenal ulcers, and it was approved for the treatment of benign gastric ulcers in Thailand in 1986. In rats, oral turmeric reduces the incidence of duodenal ulcers and is associated with an increase in intestinal wall mucus.[299] However, the mixed clinical findings in this area make an evidence-based recommendation difficult.[303-305] In a comparison trial of turmeric to an antacid, an improvement of gastric ulcers, presumably based on reduction in size, was observed in an additional 51.9% of the turmeric group and 34.8% of the antacid group. Beneficial results have not been noted in patients with duodenal ulcers.[305]

With the discovery of the role of *Helicobacter pylori* in duodenal and some gastric ulcers, and the demonstrated efficacy of antibiotics and proton pump inhibitors (PPIs), turmeric may not be an appropriate first-line therapy. Comparisons of turmeric with PPIs or H_2 blockers have not been conducted.

Dose

Turmeric may be standardized to contain 95% curcuminoids per dose. The dried root of turmeric is reported to contain 3% to 5% curcumin.[306] The effective dose of turmeric for dyspepsia has not been determined. Traditional doses range from 1.5 to 3 g of turmeric root daily in divided doses. Studies have used 750 mg to 1.5 g of turmeric daily in three or four divided doses,[301,307] Doses up to 8 g daily have been used for duodenal ulcer.[305] As a tea, 1 to 1.5 g of dried root may be steeped in 150 mL of water for 15 minutes and taken twice daily.

For IBS, patients have received 60 mg of *Curcuma xanthorriza* three times daily for 18 weeks.[302]

For gastric ulcers, clinical studies have used 250-mg powdered turmeric root capsules four times daily.[303]

Adverse Effects, Interactions, Pharmacokinetics. See Appendix A.

Wheatgrass (Triticum aestivum)

Grade C: *Unclear or conflicting scientific evidence (inflammatory bowel disease)*

Mechanism of Action

The mechanism of action of wheatgrass in IBD (ulcerative colitis) is not well understood but may be attributed to antioxidative properties.[308]

Scientific Evidence of Effectiveness

Wheatgrass juice appears to be effective as a single or adjuvant treatment of active distal ulcerative colitis.[308] Treatment with wheatgrass juice was associated with significant reductions in the overall disease activity index and in the severity of rectal bleeding.

Dose

Wheatgrass is not consistently standardized; however, advocates claim that wheatgrass has nutritional benefits similar to dark, leafy greens, such that seven 500-mg tablets (for a total dose of 3500 mg) or 1 tsp of wheatgrass powder may be equivalent to about 1 cup dark, leafy green salad. As a single or adjunct therapy for ulcerative colitis, a daily dose of 100 mL of wheatgrass juice has been used for 1 month.[308]

Adverse Effects, Interactions, Pharmacokinetics. See Appendix A.

White Horehound (Marrubium vulgare)

Grade C: *Unclear or conflicting scientific evidence (dyspepsia, bile flow stimulant)*

Mechanism of Action

A hydroalcoholic extract of *Marrubium vulgare* has exhibited antispasmodic and antinociceptive effects in animals.[309] The exact mechanisms remain to be determined but do not appear to involve the inhibition of cyclooxygenase or opioid receptors. In vitro study of white horehound demonstrated noncompetitive antagonism and a concentration-dependent manner of muscle contractions induced by several agonists of smooth muscle tissue.[310] White horehound may also stimulate bile secretion.

Scientific Evidence of Effectiveness

White horehound has been used traditionally as an antispasmodic to treat gastrointestinal disorders. The German Commission E has approved white horehound as a choleretic for the treatment of dyspepsia and lack of appetite. The evidence supporting this use is largely anecdotal and based on historical use. A 1959 study reported that the white horehound constituent marrubin acid and its sodium salt transiently stimulated bile flow, but the constituent marrubiin did not.[311]

Dose

For choleretic (bile-stimulating) effects, dyspepsia, and appetite stimulation, the German Commission E recommends 4.5 g/day of cut herb, 2 to 6 tbsp fresh plant juice, or equivalent of white horehound. Other traditional dosing suggestions are 1 to 2 g of dried herb or infusion three times daily.

Adverse Effects, Interactions, Pharmacokinetics. See Appendix A.

HERBAL THERAPIES WITH NEGATIVE EVIDENCE

Garlic (Allium sativum)

Grade D: *Fair negative scientific evidence* (Helicobacter pylori *infection*)

Garlic has a long history of use in the treatment of various infectious agents, including bacteria, fungi, and viruses. Garlic has been effective in vitro against numerous gram-negative and gram-positive bacteria, including resistant strains,[312-317] mycobacteria,[318-320] and *Helicobacter* spp.[321-323] Several human case studies have examined the effects of garlic on *Helicobacter pylori* infection and found a lack of benefit. This preliminary negative evidence may merit follow-up with more rigorous trials.

HERBAL THERAPIES WITH LIMITED EVIDENCE

Betel Nut (Areca catechu)

Betel nut may have some type of protective effect in IBD (ulcerative colitis), but its mechanism of action is not well understood. Both smoking and chewing betel nut appear to reduce the risk of developing ulcerative colitis, and the effects may be linked.[324] Based on the known toxicities associated with acute or chronic betel use, the risks probably outweigh any potential benefits. Despite widespread recreational use, because of documented toxicity associated with acute or chronic chewing or oral consumption, betel nut cannot be recommended for human use, particularly when used chronically or in high doses.

Bilberry (Vaccinium myrtillus)

The specific anthocyanidin from bilberry (IdB 1027) has been shown to possess antiulcer activity, possibly by potentiating defensive barriers in gastrointestinal mucosa and antiinflammatory effects.[325,326] IdB 1027 has been shown to antagonize chronic gastric ulcers induced by acetic acid,[325] as well as increase gastric mucosal release of prostaglandin E_2, which may also explain its antiulcer and gastroprotective properties.[327] Bilberry may also be more potent when given intraperitoneally than orally.[325]

Berry extracts have been shown to inhibit *Helicobacter pylori* in vitro and enhance susceptibility to clarithromycin (Biaxin).[328]

At this time, however, clinical evidence is inadequate to recommend for or against this use of bilberry. *H. pylori* has been implicated in many cases of gastric and duodenal ulcers, and testing or treatment for *H. pylori* should be considered in patients with known or suspected peptic ulcer disease.

Bilberry products are popularly used to treat diarrhea. However, literature review reveals that laboratory, animal, and clinical studies investigating this role for bilberry products are lacking.

Cinchona (Cinchona officinalis)

The alkaloid constituent of cinchona, quinine, has been found to induce gastrointestinal transit in animal study.[329] Traditionally, cinchona has been used for stimulating appetite. Currently, clinical reports are lacking.

Cranberry (Vaccinium macrocarpon)

The antiadhesion properties of cranberry, shown in *Escherichia coli*, have also been studied in *Helicobacter pylori*.[330] A high-molecular-weight compound in cranberry juice with antibacterial properties was incubated with three strains of *H. pylori*. In vitro, this compound inhibited the sialic acid–specific adhesion of *H. pylori* to human gastric mucus and to human erythrocytes. Consumption of cranberry may be beneficial in prevention or treatment of *H. pylori*, but this has yet to be studied in vivo.

False Hellebore (Veratrum spp.)

False hellebore has historically been used for profuse and painful diarrhea. However, this plant is considered toxic when used orally.

Guar (Cyamopsis tetragonoloba)

Guar gum is a thickening agent that is used in various gastrointestinal disorders, including constipation, diarrhea, and IBS. It may work by slowing gastric emptying and intestinal transit, thereby producing a feeling of satiety.[331]

Podophyllum (Podophyllum spp.)

Podophyllum has been historically used by North American Indians as an intestinal purgative and emetic. In large amounts, however, the herb may be fatal.

ADJUNCT THERAPIES

1. The use of natural remedies for gastrointestinal (GI) disorders is widespread both currently and throughout history. Probiotics and certain vitamins and minerals may provide additional benefit when used with drug therapy or natural remedies in the management of GI

Herbs with Potential Gastrointestinal Effects*

HERB	SPECIFIC THERAPEUTIC USE(S)†
Abuta	Colic, stomach ache, dyspepsia
Acacia	Dyspepsia
Ackee	Ulcers
Aconite	Esophagitis
African wild potato	Abdominal pain, vomiting
Agave	Dyspepsia
Alfalfa	Gastrointestinal disorders, dyspepsia, peptic ulcers
Allspice	Dyspepsia, vomiting
Alpinia	Antispasmodic, gastrointestinal disorders, dyspepsia, *Helicobacter pylori* infections, ulcers, nausea and vomiting, motion sickness
American pawpaw	Emetic
Andiroba	Esophagitis, ulcers
Andrographis paniculata	Dyspepsia, ulcers
Angel's trumpet	Antispasmodic
Anise	Antispasmodic, colic, dyspepsia, *H. pylori* infection
Annatto	Colic, stomach ache, stomach disorders, antacid, heartburn, emetic, nausea, vomiting
Apricot	Antispasmodic, enteritis, gastritis, gastrointestinal disorders
Aristolochia spp.	Antispasmodic
Asafoetida	Antispasmodic
Asarum	Gastrointestinal disorders, emetic, nausea
Asparagus	Gastric ulcers
Astragalus	Gastrointestinal disorders, gastric ulcers
Bael fruit	Antispasmodic, stomach ache, ulcers, nausea
Banaba	Dyspepsia
Barberry	Abdominal cramps, heartburn, *H. pylori* infection, dyspepsia
Bay leaf	Gastric ulcers, emetic
Bellis perennis	Antispasmodic
Betony	Antispasmodic, heartburn, *H. pylori* infection
Bilberry	Dyspepsia, infantile dyspepsia
Bitter almond	Antispasmodic
Bitter melon	Gastrointestinal cramps, diabetic gastropathy
Bitter orange	Gastrointestinal disorders, duodenal ulcers, dyspepsia, nausea
Black cohosh	Antispasmodic
Black currant	Colic
Black haw	Colic, gastrointestinal cramps
Black horehound	Antispasmodic, stomach disorders, motion sickness, nausea and vomiting
Black pepper	*H. pylori* infection
Black tea	Stomach disorders, vomiting
Bloodroot	Gastrointestinal conditions, dyspepsia, emetic
Blue cohosh	Antispasmodic, colic, gastric disorders
Blue flag	Enteritis, gastritis, heartburn, ulcers, emetic, morning sickness, vomiting
Boldo	Gastrointestinal disorders, dyspepsia, nausea
Boneset	Antispasmodic, gastrointestinal distress, dyspepsia, emetic
Borage seed oil	*H. pylori* infection
Bromelain	Phytobezoar, leaky gut syndrome, malabsorption, gastric ulcers, dyspepsia, ulcer (prevention)
Buchu	Antispasmodic, stomach ache
Bulbous buttercup	Stomach ailments
Bupleurum	Gastric ulcer, dyspepsia, ulcers, nausea, vomiting
Burdock	Ulcers
Butterbur	Antispasmodic, gastric ulcers, dyspepsia
Cajeput oil	*H. pylori* gastric infection
Calamus	Antispasmodic, colic, dyspepsia, ulcers
Calendula	Bowel irritation, gastrointestinal disorders, gastritis, dyspepsia, peptic ulcers, gastric ulcers, ulcerative colitis, nausea
California jimson weed	Antispasmodic, bloating
Cardamom	Gastrointestinal disorders, irritable bowel syndrome (IBS), stomach aches, antacid, dyspepsia, nausea
Carqueja	Stomach ailments
Carrot	Gastrointestinal disorders
Cascara sagrada	Abdominal pain, dyspepsia, emetic
Cat's claw	Bowel diseases, diverticulitis, gastrointestinal disorders, leaky gut syndrome, stomach pain, gastritis, ulcers
Chaparral	Bowel cramps, gastrointestinal cramps, gastrointestinal disorders, dyspepsia, heartburn, peptic ulcers, emesis
Chia	Celiac disease
Chicory	Gastrointestinal disorders
Cleavers	Stomach ailments

Herbs with Potential Gastrointestinal Effects—cont'd

HERB	SPECIFIC THERAPEUTIC USE(S)†	HERB	SPECIFIC THERAPEUTIC USE(S)†
Clove	Abdominal pain, antispasmodic, colic, dyspepsia, ulcers, nausea, vomiting	Grape seed	Gastrointestinal disorders, ulcers (gastroduodenal), nausea
Codonopsis	Gastrointestinal motility disorders, gastric ulcers, vomiting	Greater celandine	Antispasmodic, IBS, dyspepsia, ulcers
		Ground ivy	Antispasmodic, gastritis, ulcers
Coleus	Abdominal colic, bloating, IBS, malabsorption, peptic ulcers	Hawthorn	Abdominal colic, abdominal distention, abdominal pain, dyspepsia
Comfrey	Gastritis, ulcers	Heartsease	Antispasmodic, ulcers (throat), emetic
Corn poppy	Gastric ulcers	Holy basil	Antispasmodic, stomach ailments, enteritis, dyspepsia, ulcers, vomiting
Cramp bark	Antispasmodic, colic, gastric ulcers		
Damiana	Gastrointestinal disorders, gastrointestinal motility disorders, ulcers	Hop	Antispasmodic, IBS, dyspepsia
		Horse chestnut	Ulcers
Danshen	Gastric ulcers	Horseradish	Colic, emetic
Datura wrightii	Antispasmodic, bloating, stomach ache	Horsetail	Stomach upset, dyspepsia
Desert parsley	Gastrointestinal disorders	Hyssop	Antispasmodic, dyspepsia
Devil's claw	Gastrointestinal disorders, dyspepsia, heartburn	Jequirity	Abdominal pain, colic, gastritis, emetic
		Jewelweed	Abdominal cramps
Devil's club	Gastric ulcers, emetic	Jointed flatsedge	Abdominal pain, colic, nausea, vomiting
Dong quai	Abdominal pain, antispasmodic, IBS, gastric ulcers, heartburn	Juniper	Bloating, dyspepsia, heartburn
		Katuka	Dyspepsia
Eastern hemlock	Gastrointestinal distress	Kava	Antispasmodic, stomach upset, dyspepsia
Echinacea	Stomach upset, dyspepsia		
Elder	Antispasmodic, colic, gastrointestinal disorders, vomiting	Khat	Gastric ulcers
		Khella	Urinary colic
Elecampane	Antispasmodic, IBS	Kudzu	Gastritis, gastroenteritis
English ivy	Ulcers (gastroduodenal)	Labrador tea	Stomach ache, heartburn
Eucalyptus oil	Antispasmodic	Ladies mantle	Stomach ailments
Euphorbia	Bloating, emetic	Lady's slipper	Antispasmodic
Evening primrose oil	IBS, gastrointestinal disorders, ulcerative colitis	Lavender	Colic, heartburn, dyspepsia, motion sickness, nausea, vomiting
Eyebright	Gastric acid stimulation	Lemongrass	Abdominal pain, antispasmodic, gastrointestinal disorders, gastroenteritis, nausea, vomiting
False hellebore	Emetic		
Fenugreek	Colic, gastrointestinal disorders, stomach upset, dyspepsia, gastric ulcers, gastritis, peptic ulcers	Lesser celandine	Heartburn/poor appetite, ulcers
		Lime	Stomach ailments, dyspepsia, ulcers, nausea
Feverfew	Abdominal pain, gastrointestinal distress	Lotus	Enteritis, gastric ulcers (bleeding), dyspepsia
Fo-ti	Stomach ailments	Mangosteen	Abdominal pain, ulcers
Garcinia	Intestinal disorders, gastric ulcer prophylaxis, gastrointestinal motility disorders	Marshmallow	Diverticulitis, functional gastrointestinal disorders, ileitis, IBS, duodenal ulcer, enteritis, gastroenteritis, dyspepsia, peptic ulcer disease, ulcerative colitis, vomiting
Garlic	Antispasmodic, stomach ache, peptic ulcer disease		
Ginseng	Gastrointestinal motility disorders, gastritis, *H. pylori* infection, peptic ulcers, emesis, nausea, vomiting	Meadowsweet	Antispasmodic, intestinal disorders, stomach disorders, antacid, dyspepsia, heartburn, peptic ulcer disease, ulcers
Goldenrod	Antispasmodic		
Gotu kola	Gastric ulcers (treatment and prevention), gastritis	Milk thistle	Dyspepsia, ulcers
Grapefruit	Gastric ulcers	Mistletoe	Gastrointestinal disorders, dyspepsia, ulcers

Continued

Herbs with Potential Gastrointestinal Effects—cont'd

HERB	SPECIFIC THERAPEUTIC USE(S)†	HERB	SPECIFIC THERAPEUTIC USE(S)†
Mugwort	Antispasmodic, gastric ulcers	Sarsaparilla	Gastrointestinal disorders
Muira puama	Asthenia, dyspepsia, gastric ulcers	Saw palmetto	Antispasmodic, dyspepsia
Mullein	Antispasmodic, ulcers	Scotch broom	Emetic, nausea
Myrcia	Enteritis, ulcers (mouth)	Seaweed	Stomach upset, dyspepsia, heartburn, ulcers
Noni	Stomach ache, ulcers	Shepherd's purse	Colic, cramping, ulcers
Nopal	Ulcers	Shiitake mushroom	Ulcers
Nux vomica	Gastrointestinal disorders, IBS, dyspepsia	Skunk cabbage	Antispasmodic, emetic
Oleander	Dyspepsia, emetic	Sorrel	Gastrointestinal disorders
Onion	Gastrointestinal disorders	Spirulina	Bowel health, stomach acid excess, ulcers
Oregano	Bloating, gastrointestinal disorders, dyspepsia, ulcers	Squill	Emetic
Passion flower	Antispasmodic, gastrointestinal discomfort (nervous stomach), *H. pylori* infection	St. John's wort	Heartburn, ulcers
		Star anise	Gastrointestinal distress, dyspepsia
Pennyroyal	Antispasmodic, colic, gastrointestinal disorders, stomach ache, dyspepsia	Stinging nettle	Stomach ache, gastric secretory inhibition
		Sweet woodruff	Antispasmodic, stomach ache
Peony	Antispasmodic, gastrointestinal disorders, stomach pain, chronic gastritis, emetic	Tamarind	Colic, gastrointestinal disorders, dyspepsia, morning sickness
		Tangerine	Gastrointestinal disorders, *H. pylori* infection
Perilla	Gastrointestinal disorders, nausea, vomiting	Tansy	Antispasmodic, dyspepsia, ulcers (stomach or duodenal), nausea
Podophyllum	Emetic	Tea	Stomach disorders, vomiting, gastritis, *H. pylori* infection
Pokeweed	Emetic		
Pomegranate	Colic, ulcers (mouth and genitals)	Thyme	Colic, stomach cramps, gastritis, *H. pylori* infection, heartburn, dyspepsia
Pycnogenol	Motion sickness		
Pygeum	Stomach upset		
Quassia	Dyspepsia, ulcers	Tribulus	Colic
Quinoa	Celiac disease	Tylophora	Antispasmodic
Raspberry	Constipation, colic, gastrointestinal bleeding, stomach ache, *H. pylori* infection, nausea, morning sickness, vomiting	Usnea	Gastric ulcers
		Valerian	Bloating, abdominal cramping, IBS, viral gastroenteritis, heartburn, gastric ulcers, nausea
Red clover	Antispasmodic, dyspepsia	Wasabi	Gastric ulcers
Red yeast rice	Colic, gastrointestinal disorders, dyspepsia	Watercress	Gastrointestinal disorders
		White oak	Gastrointestinal disorders, ulcers
Reishi mushroom	Ulcers	White water lily	Gastrointestinal inflammation, ulcers (mouth and throat)
Rooibos	Colic		
Rose hip	Ulcer	Wild indigo	Emetic
Rosemary	Antispasmodic, colic, dyspepsia, peptic ulcers	Wild yam	Diverticulitis, IBS, emesis, morning sickness, vomiting
Sage	Abdominal pain, bloating, dyspepsia, *H. pylori* infection	Yarrow	Dyspepsia, ulcers
		Yew	Antispasmodic, intestinal disorders
Salvia divinorum	Gastrointestinal motility disorders		

*This is not an all-inclusive or comprehensive list of herbs with possible gastrointestinal properties; other herbs and supplements may possess these qualities. A qualified health care provider should be consulted with specific questions or concerns regarding potential gastrointestinal effects or interactions.

†Based on expert opinion, anecdote, case reports, and/or preliminary trial evidence.

disorders. Other potential therapies to use with natural remedies or conventional medicines include hypnotherapy, massage, and acupuncture. Although not conclusively shown to be effective, these therapies may offer some benefit.

2. Certain strains of bacteria can colonize the GI tract, and some beneficial strains are taken as *probiotics* to help establish favorable microflora in the colon. Some intestinal bacteria are necessary for producing essential nutrients such as vitamin B_{12}. Most probiotics come from food sources, especially cultured milk products. Probiotics are thought to be beneficial for a number of GI problems, including inflammatory bowel disease (IBD), antibiotic-related diarrhea, *Clostridium difficile* toxin-induced colitis, infectious diarrhea, hepatic encephalopathy, irritable bowel syndrome (IBS), constipation, diarrhea, and food allergies. Probiotics may be used as part of a healthy diet or used in combination with other conventional medications. The most common probiotics taken as supplements are from the genera *Lactobacillus* and *Bifidobacterium*.

3. Vitamin and mineral deficiencies are potential complications of many GI disorders, especially diarrhea. Malnutrition is especially dangerous in infants and young children. Diarrheal diseases kill more young children worldwide than any other condition. Symptoms of overall poor nutrition may include weight loss, diarrhea, abdominal cramps, gas, bloating, fatigue, foul-smelling or grayish stools that may be oily (steatorrhea), stunted growth in children, and osteoporosis. The body needs 13 essential vitamins: vitamins A, C, D, E, and K, and the B vitamins (thiamine, riboflavin, niacin, pantothenic acid, biotin, vitamin B_6, vitamin B_{12}, and folate). Essential minerals include calcium, chromium, copper, fluorine, iodine, iron, magnesium, manganese, molybdenum, phosphorus, potassium, selenium, sodium, and zinc. Supplementation with some or all of these vitamins and minerals may be recommended if a patient is malnourished from diarrhea.

4. *Saccharomyces boulardii* is a nonpathogenic, probiotic yeast strain that has been used to treat and prevent diarrhea resulting from multiple etiologies. *S. boulardii* has been isolated from the skins of tropical fruits found in Indochina, where the indigenous population has long used these fruit skins to prevent and treat diarrhea.[332] There is strong evidence that concurrent use of *S. boulardii* with antibiotic therapy reduces the incidence of developing antibiotic-associated diarrhea (AAD).[333]

5. *Hypnotherapy* has been shown to lower sensory and motor component of the gastrocolonic response in patients with IBS; however, systematic review of the evidence suggests that more evidence is needed to establish efficacy.[334]

6. *Abdominal massage* may be useful in patients with constipation. According to systematic review, the available evidence (though weak overall) suggests possible benefits for massage in treating constipation.[335]

7. *Acupressure* or *acupuncture* may be useful as adjunct therapy for nausea and vomiting as well as IBS. Specifically, stimulation of the P6 acupuncture point may benefit chemotherapy patients with nausea and vomiting.[336]

INTEGRATIVE THERAPY PLAN

- Ask about the patient's medical history, including any herbs, supplements, or medications that the patient is taking, as well as any changes in bowel function. It is also important to ask about lifestyle choices, such as diet, stress, exercise, and if and how much the patient smokes or drinks alcohol.
- Inquire about the patient's symptoms, including frequency, duration, and severity.
- Recommend appropriate diagnostic tests, including blood, urine and fecal occult tests; endoscopy; and colonoscopy.
- Treatment with conventional medications may be used in conjunction with various natural products. Conventional medications that may be used in gastrointestinal disorders include proton pump inhibitors (e.g., omeprazole [Prilosec]) and H_2-receptor antagonists (ranitidine [Zantac]) for dyspepsia; loperamide (Imodium) for diarrhea; and polyethylene glycol (MiraLax) for constipation.
- Psyllium contains a high level of soluble dietary fiber and is the main ingredient in many common laxatives, such as Metamucil and Serutan. Psyllium has long been used as a chief ingredient in bulk laxatives. Generally, an increase in stool weight, an increase in bowel movements per day, and a decrease in total gut transit time has been observed in most studies. Psyllium has been studied for the treatment of diarrhea, particularly in patients undergoing tube feeding. It has also been studied in addition to orlistat (Alli, Xenical) therapy in hopes of decreasing GI effects (diarrhea and oily discharge) of this weight loss agent.
- Globe artichoke is authorized for use in dyspeptic complaints by the German Commission E. It may also be used for relieving symptoms of IBS, including fullness, early satiety, and flatulence.
- Fennel tea is often used to treat infants with digestive disorders. It has a mild flavor and seems to be well tolerated. An emulsion of fennel seed oil and an herbal tea containing fennel have reduced infantile colic.
- Nutritional and lifestyle choices may help prevent or relieve symptoms of various GI disorders.
- Advise the patient to reduce the consumption of alcohol, caffeine, dairy products, refined sugar, and fatty foods.
- Advise the patient not to smoke because it may worsen symptoms of various GI disorders.
- Eating sufficient amounts of fiber may alleviate constipation, relieve diarrhea, and prevent muscle spasms. Soluble and insoluble fiber can be found in foods such as whole-grain cereals and breads, fruits, vegetables, and legumes (dried peas and beans). Fiber should be introduced gradually into the diet to avoid adverse gastrointestinal effects, such as flatulence and bloating.

- Regular exercise (especially abdominal muscle exercises) and brisk walking are recommended according to the patient's age and physical condition. Regular exercise may help reduce stress, decrease constipation, and improve physical performance.
- Stress may be decreased through relaxation and meditation methods.
- Recommend immediate medical care to all individuals who have experienced vomiting for longer than 24 hours; blood in the vomit; severe abdominal pain; headache and stiff neck; or signs of dehydration, such as dry mouth, infrequent urination, or dark urine.
- Patients with diarrhea should drink plenty of water to prevent dehydration. They may also benefit from drinks that contain electrolytes, including Pediatric Electrolyte, Pedialyte, or Enfalyte. Patients should avoid diuretics such as caffeine, because they worsen symptoms of dehydration. Certain foods, especially those in the BRAT diet (bananas, rice, applesauce, and toast), may help reduce symptoms of diarrhea.

Case Studies

CASE STUDY 24-1

WP is a 53-year-old woman who takes spironolactone (Aldactone, 50 mg twice daily) to control her hypertension and ibuprofen (400 mg three times daily) for arthritis of her hips, knees, and fingers. She takes licorice to reduce the chance of developing an ulcer with her aspirin therapy. She also takes aloe daily because she tends to be constipated.

At a recent physical examination, WP's blood pressure was 140/90 mm Hg and serum potassium 3.5 milliequivalents per liter (mEq/L), the lower limits of normal. Six months earlier her blood pressure was 116/78 mm Hg and serum potassium 4.5 mEq/L. Her physician increased her spironolactone to 100 mg twice daily, prescribed a potassium supplement, and asked WP to return for follow-up in 2 weeks.

WP consults you in regard to an herbal supplement that might "naturally" lower her blood pressure and raise her serum potassium. When asked, she says she did not inform her physician about the licorice and aloe because he inquires about any "medicines" she is taking, not herbs. She is mystified that her potassium level dropped because she was told that spironolactone was a potassium-sparing agent. Based on WP's test results, medications, and dietary supplements, what advice would you give?

Answer: Licorice root (*Glycyrrhiza glabra*) may reduce the incidence of gastric ulcers and help promote healing. It is thought to accelerate healing by interfering with prostanoid synthesis, increasing gastric blood flow, and stimulating mucus secretion. However, licorice may deplete serum potassium and elevate blood pressure. Strong scientific evidence exists that aloe *(Aloe vera)* can resolve constipation. Aloe latex contains anthraquinone glycosides (aloin, aloe-emodin, barbaloin), which act as potent colonic-specific stimulant laxatives. These are water-soluble glycosides, which increase the rate of colonic motility and enhance colonic transit. However, aloe may lower serum potassium. Furthermore, the combined use of aloe and licorice might result in a synergistic effect to lower serum potassium. WP should immediately discontinue the use of aloe and licorice.

Other potentially beneficial herbs may be safer choices for WP. Sea buckthorn (*Hippophae rhamnoides*) may provide benefit in preventing ulcer formation, possibly as a result of inhibition of gastric acid and pepsin secretion plus increased gastric mucus secretion. Furthermore, sea buckthorn has been reported to inhibit various strains of *Helicobacter pylori*, the bacterium implicated in peptic ulcer disease. Another benefit for WP is the possibility that sea buckthorn may lower her blood pressure.

An alternative laxative for WP is flaxseed (*Linum usitatissimum*), which may increase stool volume and stimulate peristalsis. Flaxseed also may coat and protect intestinal mucosa.

The most appropriate recommendations for WP currently are (1) discontinue licorice and aloe; (2) visit her physician at the scheduled follow-up (if she experiences any symptoms of dizziness or lightheadedness, which may be symptoms of hypotension, she should immediately have her blood pressure checked); and (3) consider addition of other herbs at a future date when her condition stabilizes. Consult with the physician to determine if WP can return to the lower dose of spironolactone and discontinue the potassium supplement, without a return of her hypertension or hypokalemia.

Remind WP to monitor her blood pressure regularly; readings should be below 140/90 mm Hg. Lifestyle changes can help control and prevent high blood pressure as well as help constipation. Emphasize the importance of eating fruits, vegetables, and whole grains. Regular physical activity of 30 minutes a day will also provide benefit for her conditions.

CASE STUDY 24-2

PW is a 50-year-old man who presents at your pharmacy to refill his prescription for diazepam (Valium, 5 mg three times daily). He also takes hydrochlorthiazide (Hydrodiuril, 50 mg daily) and a potassium supplement for hypertension. You note that PW has an enlarged, bulbous, and coarsely thickened nose characteristic of rhinophyma. You also notice a strong odor of tobacco and alcohol. When asked about his cigarette smoking and alcohol consumption, he replies that he "smokes about a pack a day" and "drinks an occasional beer." He tells you that he takes the diazepam for his "nerves" and finds it helpful. He adds that he had hoped it would help his irritable bowel syndrome (IBS), but it hasn't helped. He is plagued by intermittent cramping and bouts of diarrhea. He is often fearful of traveling outside his home because he might "have the urge to go." On the advice of a friend, he began taking bacopa, but it did not benefit his IBS and made him feel dizzy. He asked if another herb might help his IBS. How do you counsel?

Answer: PW's dizziness may be caused by his combined use of diazepam and bacopa *(Bacopa monnieri)*, as a synergistic effect may occur when the herb is used with an antianxiety medication. Bacopa may exert a direct antispasmodic effect on intestinal smooth muscle through inhibition of calcium influx across cell membrane channels. However, because bacopa has a possible synergistic effect with diazepam and PW has derived no apparent benefit, it should be discontinued.

Multiple RCTs have found that peppermint oil *(Mentha x piperita)* can significantly improve IBS symptoms. It has a dose-related antispasmodic effect on intestinal smooth musculature because menthol interferes with calcium passage across the cell membrane. It might also lower PW's blood pressure.

In a study evaluating arrowroot *(Maranta arundinacea)* for IBS, a number of participants reported a slight to moderate improvement in their condition. Constipation has been reported with long-term use of arrowroot.

Globe artichoke *(Cynara scolymus)* has been reported to improve IBS symptoms. Side effects are minimal.

Cigarette smoking and alcohol use can both aggravate IBS. PW's IBS might dramatically improve if he discontinued smoking and drinking. Tobacco also injures blood vessel walls and speeds up the process of hardening of the arteries. Advise PW to quit smoking, and discuss the available products that aid in smoking cessation.

Also, ensure that PW is monitoring his blood pressure regularly. Counsel him on the benefits of healthy diet and exercise.

CASE STUDY 24-3

BL is a 47-year-old woman who presents to the pharmacy with a prescription for a scopolamine (Transderm-Scop) patch and a refill of insulin. She and her husband are taking a 2-week ocean cruise to celebrate their 25th wedding anniversary. Her physician gave her the prescription for scopolamine because she is prone to seasickness; "I can get seasick in my bathtub." After discussing the cruise and her scopolamine prescription with a neighbor, BL became concerned about the medication. Her friend told BL that when she took scopolamine, she did not recall getting seasick, but did not recall much else about the trip either. Her friend attributed the amnesia to the patch plus "a bit of partying." BL asks for advice regarding an herbal remedy instead of the prescription. Her diabetes is in good control; however, her blood pressure is slightly elevated, 136/84 mm Hg at her last checkup. Based on BL's medical history and her current plans, help her determine an appropriate integrative therapy plan to adopt for her trip.

Answer: Scopolamine, derived from belladonna *(Atropa* spp.) can indeed cause amnesia, particularly when mixed with alcohol. It also has a number of other side effects, such as blurred vision, drowsiness, confusion, and hallucinations. Ginger *(Zingiber officinale)* has been reported to be beneficial in reducing nausea and vomiting associated with motion sickness. The components in ginger responsible for the antiemetic effect are reportedly the gingerols, shogaols, and galanolactone. Ginger may have a hypoglycemic affect, so BL should closely monitor her blood glucose levels and adjust her insulin dosage if necessary. Ginger might also have a mild hypotensive effect, which would improve BL's blood pressure elevation. Peppermint oil *(Mentha x piperita)* might also decrease the symptoms of motion sickness and slightly lower BL's blood pressure. It has no known effect on serum glucose levels. BL should be advised to take a supply of ginger and peppermint to try. She could have the scopolamine patch on hand in case the herbal remedies were ineffective. If she uses the patch, she should avoid alcohol.

References for Chapter 24 can be found on the Evolve website at http://evolve.elsevier.com/Ulbricht/herbalpharmacotherapy/

Review Questions

1. Which of the following constituents in psyllium has laxative effects?
   a. Magnesium
   b. Soluble fiber
   c. Omega-3 fatty acid
   d. Omega-6 fatty acid

2. Which of the following chemicals is responsible for aloe's stimulant-laxative effects?
   a. Tannins
   b. Pentacyclic triterpenic acids
   c. Anthocyanidins
   d. Anthraquinone glycosides

3. True or false: Arrowroot has been reported to be equivalent to metoclopramide in reducing gastric emptying time.

4. Peppermint has been used for which of the following gastrointestinal disorders?
   a. Postoperative nausea
   b. Irritable bowel syndrome
   c. Abdominal distention
   d. All the above

5. Globe artichoke may interact with which of the following agents?
   a. Warfarin
   b. Metformin
   c. Methyldopa
   d. Ciprofloxacin

6. True or false: Bacopa may have direct antispasmodic effects on intestinal smooth muscle by inhibiting calcium influx across cell membrane channels.

7. Psyllium has been used for which of the following gastrointestinal conditions?
   a. Constipation
   b. Diarrhea
   c. Irritable bowel syndrome
   d. All the above

8. Fennel may interact with which of the following agents?
   a. Synthroid
   b. Cipro
   c. Lasix
   d. Avandia

9. All the following statements are true regarding flaxseed *except*:
   a. Flaxseed may be more effective than psyllium.
   b. Flaxseed may produce laxative effects at doses of 45 g daily.
   c. Flaxseed oil produces laxative effects.
   d. Flaxseed may precipitate bowel obstruction.

10. True or false: Soy-containing infant formula may have beneficial effects over milk-based formulas when used in infants with diarrhea.

Answers are found in the Answers to Review Questions section in the back of the text.

25 Liver Disorders

Outline

OVERVIEW
    Stages of Liver Disease
        Fatty Liver
        Liver Fibrosis
        Cirrhosis
        Liver Failure
    Types of Liver Disorders
        Hepatitis
        Drug-Induced Liver Disease
        Wilson's Disease
    Diagnosis
SELECTED HERBAL THERAPIES
    Astragalus (*Astragalus membranaceus*)
    Bupleurum (*Bupleurum* spp.)
    Caper (*Capparis spinosa*)
    Chicory (*Cichorium intybus*)
    Cordyceps (*Cordyceps sinensis*)
    Dandelion (*Taraxacum officinale*)
    Danshen (*Salvia miltiorrhiza*)
    Ginseng (*Panax* spp.)
    Licorice (*Glycyrrhiza glabra*)
    Milk Thistle (*Silybum marianum*)
    Mistletoe (*Viscum album*)
    Peony (*Paeonia* spp.)
    Reishi Mushroom (*Ganoderma lucidum*)
    Rhubarb (*Rheum* spp.)
    Safflower (*Carthamus tinctorius*)
    Sea Buckthorn (*Hippophae rhamnoides*)
HERBAL THERAPIES WITH NEGATIVE EVIDENCE
HERBAL THERAPIES WITH LIMITED EVIDENCE
ADJUNCT THERAPIES
INTEGRATIVE THERAPY PLAN
CASE STUDIES
REVIEW QUESTIONS

Learning Objectives

- Recognize and evaluate signs and symptoms associated with liver disease.
- Discuss herbal products that may be used for liver disorders.
- Review data currently available to support herbal therapies for liver disorders.
- Explain the mechanisms of action, adverse effects, and interactions associated with herbs used for liver disorders.
- Develop an integrative pharmacotherapy plan for patients with liver disorders.

OVERVIEW

The liver is the second largest organ in the body (after the skin) and is located in the upper right-hand side of the abdomen. Its important bodily functions include processing nutrients, manufacturing bile to help digest fats, synthesizing proteins, producing glucose (gluconeogenesis), regulating blood clotting, and filtering toxins from the blood. Liver disorders may interfere with these processes and allow potentially toxic substances to accumulate. Inflammation can occur while the liver is performing normal functions, such as drug metabolism. The liver is able to regenerate, or repair, up to two thirds of injured tissue, including hepatocytes, biliary epithelial cells, and endothelial cells.[1-4]

Liver disorders are categorized by the cause, such as infection, exposure to certain drugs or toxins, an autoimmune process, or a genetic defect (e.g., hemochromatosis). These causes may lead to fatty liver disease, cirrhosis, or hepatitis.[1-3]

Stages of Liver Disease[1-3]

Fatty Liver

Fatty liver, also known as steatorrheic hepatosis or *steatohepatitis*, is the accumulation of triglycerides and other fats in liver cells. It is normal for the liver to contain some fat; however, excess fat can be pathological. If the liver contains more than 10% fat by weight, it is considered a fatty liver. Alcohol abuse is a common cause of fatty liver (*alcoholic steatohepatitis*). Other causes can lead to *nonalcoholic steatohepatitis* (NASH). Certain drugs, such as amiodarone (Cordarone, Pacerone) and methotrexate (Rheumatrex, Trexall), are known to increase the risks of steatohepatitis. Fatty liver may also be caused by metabolic syndrome, nutrition problems (severe malnutrition), or it may be a symptom of other conditions (e.g., Wilson's disease). NASH is very common in overweight persons over age 30. The liver is invaded by an excessive amount of fat, which replaces normal healthy liver tissue. The liver cells and the spaces in the liver are filled with fat, so the liver becomes enlarged.

It is not entirely clear how fatty liver develops, but proposed mechanisms include mitochondrial abnormalities, enhanced delivery of fatty acids to the liver, and defects in lipid uptake and metabolism. Inflammation is implicated in the pathological progression of fatty liver.

Liver Fibrosis

If severe, hepatic inflammation may cause necrosis (tissue death) and the formation of fibrous scar tissue. Fibrosis occurs as the scar tissue grows and builds up faster than it can be broken down and removed. If excessive, the scar tissue may obstruct liver blood flow and impair metabolic functions of the liver. The liver is able to regenerate up to 60% of injured tissue and can recover function after fibrosis; however, if fibrosis progresses it may lead to cirrhosis.

Cirrhosis

Cirrhosis is the endpoint of many chronic liver diseases; it occurs when the liver is seriously damaged and normal tissue is replaced with nonfunctional scar tissue. Cirrhosis can lead to further complications, and may even lead to liver cancer. In some patients the symptoms of cirrhosis may be the first signs of liver disease. For this reason, liver diseases are often considered "silent" diseases, and many patients are asymptomatic until the liver damage becomes severe. Symptoms of cirrhosis often affect the skin and result in easy bruising, edema, jaundice (yellowing of the skin), and intense itching. Other symptoms include esophageal varices, hepatomegaly, portal hypertension, liver obstruction and rupture, decreased drug metabolism, insulin resistance, and type-2 diabetes. The accumulation of toxins in the liver may lead to hepatic encephalopathy (resulting in impaired cognition or memory), difficulty sleeping, and mental status changes.

Liver Failure

Liver failure is the loss of liver function beyond repair. Many conditions besides cirrhosis may lead to liver failure, including hepatitis B, hepatitis C, hemochromatosis, and malnutrition. Alcohol abuse is a leading cause of liver failure; excessive intake of hepatotoxic medications such as acetaminophen (Tylenol) can also contribute to liver failure. Poisons and toxins may also cause the liver to fail.

The first symptoms of liver failure often include nausea, loss of appetite, fatigue, and diarrhea. Because these symptoms are nonspecific, it may be difficult to diagnose liver failure in the early stages. As liver failure progresses, the symptoms become more serious. The individual may become confused, disoriented, and somnolent (sleepy) and is at risk for coma and death; immediate medical attention is required. If liver failure is severe, a liver transplant may be needed.

Types of Liver Disorders

Hepatitis[1-5]

Hepatitis is inflammation of the liver that is caused by viruses (e.g., hepatitis B virus), chemicals, drugs, alcohol, inherited diseases, or autoimmune disorders. Hepatitis can be *acute* (flaring, then resolving in a few weeks to months) or *chronic* (lasting many years). Chronic hepatitis can result in liver cirrhosis or cancer and may lead to death.

Viruses cause most cases of acute and chronic hepatitis. There are five identifiable forms of viral hepatitis: A, B, C, D, and E. The liver is the primary site of replication and cellular damage. All hepatitis viruses can cause an acute infection; however, the viruses that cause hepatitis A and E are usually cleared from the body within 6 months and do not cause persistent infections. On the other hand, hepatitis B, C, and D may lead to chronic infections, cirrhosis, and increased risk of liver cancer.

Classic symptoms of acute hepatitis last for several weeks and include jaundice, dark urine, extreme fatigue, nausea, vomiting, abdominal pain, and decreased appetite. Some patients are asymptomatic or present with flulike illness. Patients with chronic hepatitis B or C usually report fatigue among their chief complaints.

Hepatitis A is transmitted primarily through the fecal-oral route. In rare cases it may spread via infected blood. Hepatitis A may resolve without treatment after several weeks. It may also be prevented with gamma globulin (which provides short-term protection against acute exposure) or vaccination for long-term protection. Hepatitis A may be diagnosed with the hepatitis A viral antibody immunoglobulin test (HAV-AB-M).

Hepatitis B virus (HBV) causes a serious liver infection. The infection can become chronic in some people, possibly leading to liver failure, liver cancer, cirrhosis, or death. HBV is transmitted through contact with bodily fluids, such as the blood and semen of an infected person. There is no cure for HBV; however, the hepatitis B vaccine can prevent the disease. Also, potentially infected individuals can take precautions to help prevent the spread of HBV by being tested for the virus, abstaining from sex, using protection during sexual contact, and not sharing intravenous (IV) needles. HBV is diagnosed on the basis of serology (blood analysis), which reveals detectable hepatitis B surface antigen (HBsAg) in almost all HBV-infected patients. It is produced in excess during viral replication. Other serological and molecular markers include hepatitis B anticore antibody (HBcAb), hepatitis B "e" antigen and hepatitis B "e" antibody (HBeAg and HBeAb), and hepatitis B surface antibody (HBsAb). Tests such as polymerase chain reaction (PCR) may also be performed to detect HBV genetic material.

Hepatitis C is primarily spread via blood. In rare cases, it may also be transmitted through sexual contact and childbirth. Currently, there is no vaccine for hepatitis C. The only way to prevent hepatitis C is to reduce the risk of exposure to the hepatitis C virus (HCV). Individuals can minimize exposure to HCV by using only sterilized needles and razors. Avoiding unprotected sex will also minimize the risk of acquiring HCV. According to the U.S. Centers for Disease Control and Prevention (CDC), individuals who underwent hemodialysis or received blood-clotting factors before 1987 are at a high risk of developing chronic hepatitis C because blood products were not tested for hepatitis C before then.[4] Hepatitis C is usually diagnosed through enzyme-linked immunosorbent assay (ELISA), which detects the presence of antibody to two HCV regions. Although rare, a false-positive reaction may occur. To confirm a true-positive reaction, the recombinant immunoblot assay (RIBA) is performed.

Hepatitis D virus primarily infects those with hepatitis B because it can replicate only by attaching to HBV. Injection (IV) drug users with hepatitis B have the greatest risk of acquiring hepatitis D. Individuals who are infected with both HBV and hepatitis D are more likely to develop cirrhosis or liver cancer than patients who only have HBV. As with hepatitis C, hepatitis D is also diagnosed by ELISA.

Hepatitis E is rare in the United States and occurs mainly in tropical and subtropical areas, especially South Asia and North Africa.[4] This disease is transmitted by fecal-oral route. No vaccine exists for hepatitis E; the only way to prevent the disease is to reduce the risk of exposure to the virus. Hepatitis E is self-limiting and usually resolves without treatment, within several weeks to months. To diagnose hepatitis E, blood tests are performed to detect elevated levels of specific antibodies to hepatitis E.

Drug-Induced Liver Disease[1-3]

The liver is responsible for the metabolism of alcohol, drugs, and environmental toxins. It breaks them down into substances that can be used or excreted by the body. Many prescription and nonprescription drugs, including anesthetics, antibiotics, anabolic steroids, and antiepileptic drugs, are metabolized in the liver, and overuse may cause liver damage.

Natural remedies can also have hepatotoxic potential, including kava *(Piper methysticum)*, chaparral *(Larrea taridentata)*, comfrey *(Symphytum officinale)*, germander *(Teucrium chamaedrys)*, mistletoe *(Viscum album)*, pennyroyal *(Mentha pulegium)*, and skullcap *(Scutellaria lateriflora)*. Fat-soluble vitamins, including vitamins A, D, E, and K, may accumulate in the liver if taken in excess and are potentially hepatotoxic. However, the two most common causes of drug-induced liver disease are alcohol and acetaminophen (Tylenol).

Chronic alcoholism, the excessive and habitual consumption of alcohol, is harmful to the liver and is one of the most common causes of chemical hepatitis. The liver can metabolize only limited amount of alcohol in a given time, irrespective of the quantity ingested. Alcohol intake causes the body to overproduce liver transaminases. Long-term alcohol abuse may lead to cirrhosis, pancreatitis, anemia, upper gastrointestinal bleeding, nerve damage, impotence, and brain damage. Heavy drinkers may also develop severe malnutrition if alcohol is consumed in place of food.

Acetaminophen (Tylenol) is potentially toxic to the liver in high doses, or even in regular doses when combined with alcohol. Although manufacturers set a maximum dose of 4 g of acetaminophen daily, equivalent to eight 500-mg ("extra-strength") tablets or capsules; health care professionals recommend that patients who take other prescription medications or drink alcohol daily should only take a maximum of 2 to 3 g per 24 hours.

Mild drug-induced liver disease may be asymptomatic. As the disease progresses, it may manifest as fatigue, abdominal pain, loss of appetite, weight loss, jaundice, or easy bruising. To diagnose drug-induced liver disease, a careful history should be obtained, particularly drug and alcohol use, along with blood and liver tests.

Wilson's Disease

Wilson's disease (or hepatolenticular degeneration) is a rare inherited disorder in which copper is not eliminated properly and accumulates in the liver and other vital organs (e.g., brain, eyes, kidneys), possibly to a life-threatening level. If left untreated, Wilson's disease is fatal. When diagnosed early, Wilson's disease is easily treated by removing excess copper with chelators (such as penicillamine) or zinc (which prevents copper absorption), and many patients live normal lives.

In patients with Wilson's disease, copper begins accumulating in the liver immediately after birth, but signs and symptoms rarely occur before 5 years of age. Symptoms may not appear until age 40 to 50 years. The most common characteristic of Wilson's disease is the Kayser-Fleisher ring, a rusty-brown ring around the cornea of the eye, which can be viewed using an ophthalmologist's slit lamp. Blood and genetic tests can help screen and diagnose Wilson's disease.[1-3,6]

Diagnosis

The diagnosis of liver disease depends on patient history, physical examination, laboratory testing, and in some cases, radiological studies and biopsy. Patient history should include an assessment of signs and symptoms and risk factors, including alcohol abuse, risk of viral hepatitis, and obesity.[1-3]

In general, when a liver abnormality is suspected, a liver function test (LFT) or "liver panel" is performed. The term "panel" refers to a battery of routine chemistry tests, including *alanine transaminase* (ALT; or glutamic-pyruvic transaminase [GPT]), *aspartate transaminase* (AST; or glutamic-oxaloacetic transaminase [GOT]), *alkaline phosphatase* (ALP), *gamma-glutamyl transferase* (GGT), *lactic dehydrogenase* (LDH), bilirubin, albumin, and total protein. Other tests that may be ordered include complete blood count (CBC) with platelets and prothrombin time (PT) to measure the liver's capacity to synthesize clotting factors. Serological studies may be pursued if LFTs are persistently abnormal.[1-6]

SELECTED HERBAL THERAPIES

 Note

To help make this educational resource more interactive, all pharmacokinetics, adverse effects, and interactions data have been compiled in Appendix A. Safety data specifically related to pregnancy and lactation are listed in Appendix B. Please refer to these appendices when working through the case studies and answering the review questions.

Astragalus (*Astragalus membranaceus*)

Grade C: *Unclear or conflicting scientific evidence (hepatoprotection, antiviral activity)*

Mechanism of Action

Active constituents of astragalus root have been identified and characterized, including polysaccharide cycloartane glycoside fractions (astragalosides I-IV, trigonosides I-III), four major isoflavonoids (formononetin, ononin, calycosin, and calycosin glycoside), several minor isoflavonoids, gamma-aminobutyric acid (GABA), and other biogenic amines.[7-12]

Astragalus constituents, particularly the flavonoids, exert significant cellular antioxidant effects, which appear to be protective against hepatic changes.[13,14] Astragalus polysaccharide and flavonoid extracts have been shown to preserve liver function in response to hepatotoxins.[15-21] The polysaccharides have also been found to induce endogenous interferon (IFN) production in animals and humans and to potentiate IFN actions in viral infections.[22-25]

Scientific Evidence of Effectiveness

HEPATOPROTECTION. Preliminary evidence suggests that combination products containing astragalus may offer benefit in the treatment of liver fibrosis.[26,27] LFTs and blood flow in the portal vein were improved with these astragalus-containing products. However, because astragalus was used in combination with other products, the effects cannot be isolated to astragalus alone.

ANTIVIRAL ACTIVITY. Evidence indicates that astragalus induces endogenous IFN production in vitro and in vivo and is an effective treatment for several viral illnesses. The available clinical data tentatively support this hypothesis, particularly in immunocompromised patients with hepatitis C.[26,28] In contrast, clinical data to date do not support the efficacy of astragalus in treating hepatitis B or viral myocarditis.[29,30]

Dose

The dose of astragalus for liver protection has not been clearly established. Astragalus is typically taken in combination formulas with other herbs, such as ginseng, angelica, and licorice, and has not been thoroughly studied as a monotherapy.

Adverse Effects, Interactions, Pharmacokinetics. See Appendix A.

Bupleurum (*Bupleurum* spp.)

Grade C: *Unclear or conflicting scientific evidence (hepatitis)*

Mechanism of Action

The root is believed to be the most biologically active part of bupleurum because of the presence of triterpene saponins (saikosaponins a, b, d, e, f, and h; related compounds, saikogenins a-g),[31] polysaccharides, and polyacetylenes.[32]

In animal studies, bupleurum showed marked hepatoprotective effects in fatty liver degeneration and cell necrosis, which manifested in a relative decrease in transaminase levels and in pathological changes.[33-36] The effect was much more pronounced for *Bupleurum falcatum* and *Bupleurum kaoi* than for *Bupleurum chinense*.[34]

Bupleurum is a key ingredient in the formula *sho-saiko-to* (also known as "Xiao Chai Hu Tang") with active constituents known as saikosaponins. Other ingredients include jujube, ginger, and licorice. *Sho-saiko-to* is often used in Asia to treat liver disorders. In vitro studies indicate that *sho-saiko-to* may modulate both cellular and humoral immune responses specific for HBV-associated antigens.[37] Extracts of bupleurum have been found to stimulate B-lymphocyte proliferation in mice, by an unclear mechanism.[38,39]

Scientific Evidence of Effectiveness

Bupleurum belongs to the Apiaceae family, which includes dill and fennel plants; however, unlike the characteristic lacey leaves of dill and fennel, bupleurum has lanceolate (lance-shaped) leaves. It has been used in Chinese medicine for more than 2000 years as a "liver tonic." Traditional use from China, as well as at least one rigorous clinical trial and several small clinical reports, suggest that bupleurum and the herbal combination formula *sho-saiko-to* (which contains bupleurum) may help treat chronic hepatitis B.[40,41] After 12 weeks of bupleurum treatment, AST and ALT decreased significantly in patients with chronic hepatitis B.[40] A nonsignificant trend toward decreased HBeAg and increased Anti-HBe has also been noted.[40] Although studies to date are small and some not well controlled, they do suggest that further research into this question is warranted.

Prospective clinical evidence suggests that *sho-saiko-to* may be hepatoprotective in hepatocellular carcinoma.[42] Phase II clinical studies are currently investigating *sho-saiko-to* in hepatitis C patients who cannot tolerate IFN therapy.[43]

Dose

Bupleurum is typically taken in combination formulas with other herbs and has not been thoroughly researched as a monotherapy. For hepatitis, a combination therapy, *sho-saiko-to*, at doses of 5.4 g daily for 12 weeks, has been used in clinical study.[40]

Adverse Effects, Interactions, Pharmacokinetics. See Appendix A.

Caper (Capparis spinosa)

Grade C: *Unclear or conflicting scientific evidence (cirrhosis)*

Mechanism of Action

A constituent of caper, *p*-methoxybenzoic acid, appears to have hepatoprotective effects.[44] It also contains significant amounts of the antioxidant flavonoid *rutin*, which may also have liver-protecting effects.

Lyophilized extracts of *Capparis spinosa* have been shown to counter the effects of oxidative inflammatory stress in human chondrocyte cultures stimulated with proinflammatory cytokine interleukin-1 beta (IL-1β).[45] The extracts are thought to offset three key pathogenetic mechanisms of degenerative joint disease: oxidative stress, inflammation, and chondrodegeneration. This is done by reducing the production of nitric oxide, reactive oxygen species, and prostaglandins induced by IL-1β and by increasing the synthesis of glycosaminoglycans in a dose-dependent manner. It is hypothesized that the action of *C. spinosa* extracts may be partially caused by the scavenger action of its polyphenolic active constituents, in particular flavonoids, such as quercetin, kampferol glycosides, and hydroxycinnamic acids (caffeic acid, ferulic acid, *p*-coumaric acid, and cinnamic acid). These flavonoid extracts, once introduced into the lipid bilayer of cell membranes, perform an antiapoptotic or cytoprotective action, preventing cell death caused by reactive oxidative substances. The flavonoids also inhibit enzymes involved in the production of these oxidative substances, protecting DNA against their toxic effects. The antioxidant effect of *C. spinosa* extract is also associated with an antiinflammatory action based on the control of the degranulation of some hyperactive cells, such as mast cells, basophils, and neutrophils, and on the inhibition of the inflammatory cytokines.

Scientific Evidence of Effectiveness

In humans, the combination therapy Liv-52 (Himalayan Co., India), containing ferric oxide and *Capparis spinosa* as one of seven herbal ingredients, was shown to be a potentially effective treatment for cirrhosis.[46] However, the efficacy of *C. spinosa* as sole treatment for cirrhosis or other conditions remains unproved, but worthy of further investigation.

Dose

Each tablet of Liv-52 reportedly contains "Mandur bhasma," 33 mg (prepared from ferric oxide), and extracts of *Capparis spinosa* (65 mg), *Cichorium intybus* (65 mg), *Solanum nigrum* (32 mg), *Cassia occidentalis* (16 mg), *Terminalia arjuna* (32 mg), *Achillea millefolium* (16 mg), and *Tamarix gallica* (16 mg). Patients with cirrhosis have taken three tablets of Liv-52 daily for 6 months.[46]

Adverse Effects, Interactions, Pharmacokinetics. See Appendix A.

Chicory (Cichorium intybus)

Grade C: *Unclear or conflicting scientific evidence (chronic hepatitis)*

Mechanism of Action

The exact hepatoprotective mechanism of chicory is not fully understood. The active compounds in chicory are inulin, sesquiterpene lactones, vitamins, minerals, fat, mannitol, and latex. The root callus extracts and seeds of chicory, specifically compound AB-IV, have liver-protective effects, as measured by reductions in AST, ALT, ALP, and total protein.[47,48] In animals, chicory seed consumption led to an almost complete normalization of liver tissues, with effects comparable to milk thistle *(Silybum marianum)*.[47]

Scientific Evidence of Effectiveness

The seed of the chicory plant is one of the main ingredients of Jigrine, a commercial product of India used to treat liver disease. Preliminary research suggests that chicory alone may provide some benefit to patients with chronic hepatitis;[49] however, the strength of this evidence is unclear.

Dose

The dose of chicory for chronic hepatitis has not been clearly established.

Adverse Effects, Interactions, Pharmacokinetics. See Appendix A.

Cordyceps (Cordyceps sinensis)

Grade B: *Good scientific evidence (hepatitis B)*

Grade C: *Unclear or conflicting scientific evidence (liver disease [hepatic cirrhosis])*

Mechanism of Action

Constituents found in cordyceps with pharmacological activity include adenosine, alkenoic acids, cordycepin, ergosterol, galactomannan, linoleic acid, oleic acid, d-mannitol, nucleosides, polysaccharides, sterols, and tryptophan.[50-54]

Cordyceps appears to inhibit hepatic fibrogenesis from liver injury, slow the development of cirrhosis, and restore liver function. Possible mechanisms appear to involve the inhibition of transforming growth factor beta (TGF-β), thereby downregulating platelet-derived growth factor (PDGF) and reducing deposition of procollagens I and III.[55]

Scientific Evidence of Effectiveness

HEPATITIS B. In traditional Chinese medicine (TCM), cordyceps has been used to support and improve liver function. Human studies indicate that cordyceps may stimulate the immune system and improve serum gamma globulin levels in hepatitis B patients.[56-58] Although studies have provided somewhat weak evidence supporting cordyceps as a treatment for chronic hepatitis B, the results are promising.

LIVER DISEASE (HEPATIC CIRRHOSIS). Preliminary studies evaluating the use of herbal combinations containing cordyceps found that these products improve liver and immune function, as evidenced by cellular immune function modulation and inhibition of humoral immune hyperfunction.[59,60] Because these studies used combination treatments, however, the effect of cordyceps alone is difficult to discern.

Dose

The dose of cordyceps for liver disorders has not been clearly established.

Adverse Effects, Interactions, Pharmacokinetics. See Appendix A.

Dandelion (Taraxacum officinale)

Grade C: *Unclear or conflicting scientific evidence (hepatitis B)*

Mechanism of Action. Insufficient available evidence.

Scientific Evidence of Effectiveness

Modern naturopathic physicians believe that dandelion has the ability to detoxify the liver and gallbladder, reduce the side effects of medications processed by the liver, and relieve symptoms of diseases in which impaired liver function plays a role. However, in vitro data and human studies are lacking.[1]

There is limited clinical evidence that dandelion improves liver function in hepatitis B patients; after taking a combination herbal preparation containing dandelion root, called Jiedu Yanggan Gao, symptoms improved after up to 5 months of treatment. However, the product also contained *Artemisia capillaris, Taraxacum mongolicum, Plantago* seed, *Cephalanoplos segetum, Hedyotis diffusa,* flos chrysanthemi indici, *Smilax glabra, Astragalus membranaceus, Salvia miltiorrhiza,* fructus polygonii orientalis, Radix paeoniae alba, and *Polygonatum sibiricum*.[61] Therefore the contribution of dandelion is unclear.

Dose

The dose of dandelion for hepatitis B has not been clearly established.

Adverse Effects, Interactions, Pharmacokinetics. See Appendix A.

Danshen (Salvia miltiorrhiza)

Grade C: *Unclear or conflicting scientific evidence (hepatitis B)*

Mechanism of Action

The exact mechanism of danshen in liver disease is not well understood. In a human study, injection with danshen reduced ALT, AST, and liver fibrosis indices (procollagen type III and collagen type IV).[62] In animals, danshen reduced carbon tetrachloride–induced hepatic fibrosis in rats.[63] Treated animals had reduced levels of TGF-β1 and procollagens I and II. In vitro study showed that salvianolic acid A offered protection for hepatocyte biomembranes.[64]

Scientific Evidence of Effectiveness

Danshen, in combination with other herbs, has been used traditionally for liver disorders. Human and animal studies suggest hepatoprotective effects as well as possible benefits for treating hepatitis B.[62,63,65,66] It is unclear whether there are any clinically significant effects of danshen in patients with hepatitis B, because of inadequately powered studies.

Dose

Danshen is often used in combination with other therapeutic extracts (e.g., *Salvia miltiorrhiza, Panax notoginseng, Cinnamomum camphora*). Standardization and dosing of danshen alone or in combination are not well established.

Adverse Effects, Interactions, Pharmacokinetics. See Appendix A.

Ginseng (Panax spp.)

Grade C: *Unclear or conflicting scientific evidence (hepatoprotection)*

Mechanism of Action

The metabolite of oral ginsenosides, 20-*O*-beta-D-glucopyranosyl-20(S)-protopanaxadiol, protected mouse liver cells from cytotoxicity induced by tert-butylhydroperoxide and significantly inhibited the increment of ALT and AST induced by tert-butylhydroperoxide in mice.[50,67] The metabolite of this compound also stabilized cell membranes.

Scientific Evidence of Effectiveness

Preliminary evidence suggests that *Panax ginseng* may have hepatoprotective properties, as evidenced by improved biochemical parameters associated with liver function, particularly in elderly patients.[68,69] One laboratory study investigated compound K, a ginseng metabolite that shows promise in protecting against liver injury.[67]

Dose

Two capsules of Pharmaton Capsules (Pharmaton Natural Health Products, Boehringer Ingelheim Pharmaceuticals) containing 40 mg of G115 (ginseng extract standardized to

4% to 7% ginsenosides as well as dimethylaminoethanol bitartrate, vitamins, minerals, and trace elements; phospholipids; and linolenic acid), daily for 12 weeks, improved liver function in elderly patients with chronic liver disease.[68]

Adverse Effects, Interactions, Pharmacokinetics. See Appendix A.

Licorice (Glycyrrhiza glabra)

Grade C: *Unclear or conflicting scientific evidence (hepatitis C)*

Mechanism of Action

The protective mechanism of licorice may involve antiinflammatory action that helps protect the hepatic cellular membrane.[70,71] Protection likely results from the induction of heme oxygenase-1 and the downregulation of proinflammatory mediators.[71] *Glycyrrhizin,* a constituent of licorice, may enhance interferon production and the immunogenicity of HBsAg at the *trans*-Golgi area after *O*-linked glycosylation and before its sialylation.[72,73]

Glycyrrhizin may also exhibit antiviral activity against the hepatitis A virus.[74,75] It is unlikely to induce viral clearance of chronic hepatitis C because transaminase levels increase after stopping treatment. This effect indicates that the inflammation may still be present.[76]

Scientific Evidence of Effectiveness

Note: The licorice constituent glycyrrhizin may worsen *ascites,* or the accumulation of fluid in the abdomen. In some cases, ascites can be caused by cirrhosis.[77]

The Japanese IV solution Stronger Neo-Minophagen C (SNMC), which contains 0.2% glycyrrhizin, 0.1% cysteine, and 2.0% glycine, has been evaluated for use in hepatitis C.[70,76,78-83] Studies have reported improvements in ALT in patients with chronic hepatitis C.[76,78,80,82,83] After discontinuing SNMC, serum transaminases returned to baseline elevated values; however, low-dose maintenance therapy could have prevented this effect.[76] Long-term use among patients with chronic hepatitis C has resulted in significantly lower rates of hepatocellular carcinoma.[79,84]

Dose

The standardized licorice root extract SNMC has been used in various clinical trials for hepatitis C. SNMC is made up of aqueous extract of licorice root containing 0.2% glycyrrhizin, 0.1% cysteine, and 2.0% glycine dissolved in saline. Hepatitis C patients taking IV glycyrrhizin at 80 to 240 mg (40-100 mL) three times weekly for 4 to 12 weeks showed improvement in liver transaminases.[76,80-82] In evaluations of long-term administration of SNMC, the average duration of use was 10 years.[70,83]

Adverse Effects, Interactions, Pharmacokinetics. See Appendix A.

Milk Thistle (Silybum marianum)

Grade B: *Good scientific evidence (cirrhosis; chronic hepatitis)*

Grade C: *Unclear or conflicting scientific evidence (acute viral hepatitis;* Amanita phalloides *mushroom poisoning; liver damage from drugs or toxins)*

Mechanism of Action

Silymarin, a flavonoid complex that can be extracted from the seeds of milk thistle, is composed of three isomers. Silymarin is typically extracted with 95% ethanol, yielding a bright-yellow fluid. A frequently studied and used milk thistle product, Legalon (Madeus, Gemany), is prepared by extraction with ethyl acetate. A standard milk thistle extract contains 70% silymarin, a mixture of the flavonolignans silydianin and silychristin, and silibinin (the most biologically active constituent, according to in vitro assays). Other constituents, including dehydrosilybin, desoxysilydianin, and silybinomer, have also been isolated.

Antioxidant activity, or free-radical antagonism, has been cited as the likely mechanism of action of milk thistle. Other suggested effects include increased protein synthesis, decreased tumor-promoter activity, stabilized immunological response, protection against cellular radiation damage, and alteration and increased stability of cellular membranes. Hepatoprotective qualities of milk thistle have been attributed to antioxidant properties. Flavonoids present in milk thistle, such as silymarin and silybin, have been shown to act as antioxidants and free-radical scavengers.[85-93] Silymarin abolished hepatotoxicity of microcystin-LR (toxin from the alga *Microcystis aeruginosa*) in rats and mice, possibly by preventing oxidation of protein-thiol groups.[94] Silymarin may also exert an antioxidant effect on human platelets, and it provides antioxidant protection against liver toxicity in iron-overloaded rats.[95] In human subjects with alcoholic cirrhosis, levels of erythrocyte/lymphocyte superoxide dismutase are raised in the presence of silymarin.[96]

Numerous other hepatoprotective mechanisms of milk thistle have been proposed. In vitro and animal studies have demonstrated protective effects of silymarin, particularly silybin, against hepatotoxins as diverse as acetaminophen, alcohol, carbon tetrachloride, tetrachloromethane, thallium, toluene, and xylene.[97-105] The protective effects of silymarin against *Amanita phalloides,* as observed in preliminary clinical and animal studies,[106-111] have been attributed to inhibition of toxin binding and uptake in hepatocytes. A membrane-stabilizing effect of silymarin has been demonstrated in rat hepatocytes.[112] The protection of silymarin on rat livers from D-galactosamine toxicity has been attributed to an activation of enzymes involved in the UDP–glucuronic acid biosynthesis pathways in detoxification of phenols and other toxic substances.[113] Silibinin also had a regenerating effect on the livers of hepatectomized rats, increasing DNA synthesis by 23% to 25%.[114-116] A similar effect was observed in cells exposed to various nephrotoxic agents.[117] Silybin stimulated DNA polymerase, increasing the synthesis of ribosomal RNA and stimulating liver cell regeneration; it also stabilized cellular membranes and increased the glutathione content of the liver.[118-121] Malignant cell lines, specifically HeLa and Burkitt lymphoma cells, were not stimulated by this compound.[114,115]

Scientific Evidence of Effectiveness

CIRRHOSIS. Milk thistle products are popular in Europe and the United States for the management of various types of liver disease, including hepatitis, cirrhosis, gallstones, jaundice, and toxin-induced liver damage. Multiple randomized, double-blind, placebo-controlled trials have been conducted in Europe to evaluate the effects of milk thistle on alcoholic and nonalcoholic cirrhosis.[122-129] Studies have examined both short-term and longer-term (4-5 years) outcomes, including mortality. Overall, this research has reported milk thistle to lower serum transaminase levels, improve liver histology, and improve survival. However, methodological weaknesses in study design and reporting limit interpretation and clinical applicability. Confounding factors (e.g., alcohol consumption) have not been well controlled, and inclusion criteria (e.g., diagnostic criteria for liver diseases) have not been well defined. A high-quality systematic review and meta-analysis prepared for the Agency for Healthcare Research and Quality (AHRQ) concluded that the clinical efficacy of milk thistle for liver disease has not been clearly established.[122] Although the existing evidence does suggest benefits of milk thistle, most effect sizes are small or not statistically significant when data are pooled. Rigorous controlled trials using serological, histological, and survival outcomes are necessary before a strong recommendation can be made.

CHRONIC HEPATITIS (VIRAL AND ALCOHOLIC). Several trials have examined milk thistle as a treatment for chronic hepatitis of viral or alcoholic origin. Most studies have produced statistically significant results showing that milk thistle improves transaminase, bilirubin, and PT values,[130] with consistently positive results for viral hepatitis.[131,132] Significant histological improvements were noted in the silymarin-treated patients with chronic hepatitis.[132] However, a systematic review and a meta-analysis both concluded that the clinical efficacy of milk thistle for liver disease, as for hepatitis, has not been clearly established.[122,123]

ACUTE VIRAL HEPATITIS. Several low-quality studies have examined the use of milk thistle for acute viral hepatitis.[133-137] Beneficial serological outcomes have been reported, but because of methodological weaknesses, these results are not conclusive. There is insufficient evidence to recommend for or against milk thistle for the treatment of acute viral hepatitis.

AMANITA PHALLOIDES MUSHROOM POISONING. For several decades, milk thistle has been reported anecdotally to be beneficial in the management of Amanita phalloides mushroom poisoning. Amatoxins, the main toxins in A. phalloides, are taken up by hepatocytes and interfere with messenger RNA synthesis, thereby suppressing protein synthesis and leading to acute hepatitis and potential liver failure. Most research consists of animal studies, human case reports, case series, and retrospective analyses.[109,110,138] The quality of reports has been limited by confounding factors and lack of controls or prospective design. However, several authoritative natural medicine texts support the use of milk thistle in the treatment of A. phalloides mushroom poisoning based on traditional precedent and expert opinion. At this time, insufficient evidence is available to recommend for or against milk thistle for the treatment of A. phalloides mushroom toxicity.

LIVER DAMAGE FROM DRUGS OR TOXINS. Milk thistle has been used as a hepatoprotective agent against drug- and toxin-induced liver damage.[139-148] Numerous studies have reported improvements in serum transaminase levels (improved AST, ALT, and platelet counts), histology, and symptoms (pruritus, nausea) in patients with toxin or drug-induced liver damage after treatment with oral milk thistle. Although these results are promising, they are confounded by weaknesses in study design and reporting.

Dose

Milk thistle capsules, tinctures, and powders are often standardized to contain 70% to 80% silymarin.

For cirrhosis, 280 to 420 mg of silymarin (Legalon) has been taken daily in two or three divided doses.[124-128] Up to 450 mg daily in three divided doses has been studied for 2 years, although silymarin had no effect on survival or the clinical course in alcoholics with liver cirrhosis.[129]

For chronic hepatitis, 160 to 480 mg of Silipide (IdB 1016) has been taken daily in silybin equivalents,[131,149,150] or silymarin (Legalon), 420 mg daily in three divided doses.[132] Silipide is a complex of silybin and phosphatidylcholine designed to improve oral absorption of silymarin, with demonstrated greater bioavailability.

For acute viral hepatitis, 420 mg of silymarin has been taken daily in three divided doses.[134,136,137,151] However, the efficacy of this dose is unclear.

For Amanita phalloides mushroom poisoning, silibinin at 20 to 50 mg/kg in 500 mL 5% dextrose solution, given intravenously every 6 hours over 24 hours, has been used in clinical trials.[109,110,138]

For drug/toxin-induced hepatotoxicity, 280 to 420 mg of silymarin (Legalon) has been taken orally daily in three divided doses.[140-142,152,153] Up to 800 mg daily has been studied for 90 days;[144] however, nonsignificant improvements in transaminases were observed in both the milk thistle and the no-drug groups. It is not clear if this study was adequately powered to detect between-group differences, and the results may not be clinically relevant.

Adverse Effects, Interactions, Pharmacokinetics. See Appendix A.

Mistletoe (Viscum album)

Grade C: Unclear or conflicting scientific evidence (hepatitis)

Mechanism of Action

Mistletoe extracts contain carbohydrate-binding proteins (lectins) and thionins (viscotoxins), which may be responsible for immunomodulating effects. Mistletoe appears to increase its production of immune cells, including T lymphocytes and natural killer (NK) cells.[154-157] Mistletoe has also been shown to enhance tumor necrosis factor alpha (TNF-α), interleukin-1 (IL-1), interleukin-6 (IL-6), and endogenous interferon (IFN).[158-161]

Scientific Evidence of Effectiveness

Note: Mistletoe has the potential to be hepatotoxic and should be used cautiously in patients with liver disorders.

Mistletoe is popularly used as an alternative cancer treatment. Preliminary evidence suggests that mistletoe may reduce liver transaminase levels, viral load, and inflammation as well as the signs and symptoms associated with hepatitis C (tiredness, musculoskeletal pain, abdominal discomfort).[154,162,163] Complete elimination of the virus after treatment with mistletoe has been noted.[154,163] It has been suggested that mistletoe may improve inflammation and reduce long-term complications associated with liver damage.[163]

Dose

Extracts of mistletoe may be standardized based on the content of several different compounds.[164] Commercial preparations such as Iscador are available as aqueous extracts of *Viscum album* obtained from several host trees fermented with *Lactobacillus plantarum*. Iscador is an unlicensed, experimental drug produced by Weleda in Switzerland. The U.S. trade name of Iscador is Iscar.

For hepatitis C, 5 mg of Iscador Qu Special (composed of 380 ng/mL lectins and 14 ng/mL viscotoxins) has been used subcutaneously three times weekly for 12 months.[162]

Adverse Effects, Interactions, Pharmacokinetics. See Appendix A.

Peony (Paeonia spp.)

Grade C: Unclear or conflicting scientific evidence (chronic hepatitis/liver cirrhosis)

Mechanism of Action

The gallate structure, 1,2,3,4,6-penta-O-galloyl-β-D-glucose, of peony may play a role in its activity against viral hepatitis.[165] Peony appears to prevent the process of virus attachment and penetration.[166] The aqueous extract of peony inhibited the virus from attaching to the cell surface.[166]

Scientific Evidence of Effectiveness

Peony has been used in TCM to treat liver disease.[167] In preliminary research, *Paeonia rubra* root was given to patients with chronic active hepatitis or chronic active hepatitis with liver cirrhosis.[168] "Heavy doses" (unspecified) of *P. rubra* were effective in promoting the reabsorption of collagen fibers and arresting the development of liver fibrosis.[168] The positive results of this small case series warrant further rigorous studies.

Dose

The dose of peony for chronic hepatitis and liver cirrhosis has not been established.

Adverse Effects, Interactions, Pharmacokinetics. See Appendix A.

Reishi Mushroom (Ganoderma lucidum)

Grade C: Unclear or conflicting scientific evidence (chronic hepatitis B)

Mechanism of Action

Constituents of *Ganoderma lucidum* with proposed or demonstrated pharmacological activity include lanostanoids,[169] lectins,[170] steryl esters and steroids,[171] polysaccharides, and triterpenes.[172-174] The major active constituents found in reishi are polysaccharides and triterpenoids, which contain ganoderic acids.

Ganoderma lucidum appears to stimulate cytokine (TNF-α), IL-1, and IL-6.[175,176] Polysaccharides isolated from reishi yielded a decrease in serum AST, ALT, ALP, and total bilirubin and reduced collagen content in the liver. The implications of collagen inhibition are not fully understood.[177] Another study performed in rats showed that extracts from reishi reduced free radicals that potentially harm the liver.[178] Chloroform toxicity was dramatically decreased with the administration of a reishi water extract. Serum AST and LDH levels decreased in rats given reishi.

Scientific Evidence of Effectiveness

Preliminary clinical evidence suggests that Ganopoly, a reishi product from New Zealand, may be beneficial for the treatment of hepatitis B virus (HBV).[179] Within a 6-month study period, 33% of Ganopoly-treated patients had normal transaminase values, and 13% had cleared HBsAg from serum, whereas none of the controls had normal transaminase values or had lost HBsAg. This study had a small sample size and short duration of treatment and follow-up, reducing its validity. Chronic hepatitis B must be studied for a longer period. HBV is also notoriously difficult to clear from the body, and recurrence after treatment is common. Additionally, the authors' affiliation with the drug's manufacturer may represent a conflict of interests.

Dose

Standardization of extracts may not be clinically relevant in predicting effectiveness because the active ingredient in *Ganoderma lucidum* has not been fully determined. However, the dose of *G. lucidum* is often based on its content of polysaccharide peptide and triterpene. These doses can be extracted from spores or the whole–fruiting body preparation. The New Zealand product Ganopoly contains 600 mg, which equals 30 g fruiting body of *G. lucidum*. For chronic hepatitis B, patients received oral Ganopoly capsules (1800 mg) three times daily.[179]

Adverse Effects, Interactions, Pharmacokinetics. See Appendix A.

Rhubarb (*Rheum* spp.)

Grade C: *Unclear or conflicting scientific evidence (hepatitis; nonalcoholic fatty liver disease)*

Mechanism of Action

The mechanism of action of rhubarb for liver disorders is not well understood. However, rhubarb's antioxidant effects may play a potential role.[180]

Scientific Evidence of Effectiveness

Note: Chronic ingestion of rhubarb may cause liver damage.

HEPATITIS. Preliminary study suggests that rhubarb may reduce symptoms and serum transaminase levels associated with hepatitis.[181,182] However, more rigorous studies are needed to establish rhubarb's effect.

NONALCOHOLIC FATTY LIVER DISEASE. Preliminary evidence from a large clinical trial found that a rhubarb-containing therapy reduced ALT levels, blood lipids, and fatty liver in patients with nonalcoholic fatty liver disease.[183] Because the therapy involved multiple herbs and other treatments, rhubarb's effects on nonalcoholic fatty liver disease are difficult to discern.

Dose

Active ingredients of rhubarb vary by species. Different species are frequently substituted for one another in commercially available, medicinal rhubarb products. There is marked variation in the anthraquinone content of commercial preparations, as well as the potential for contamination with related species and heavy metals in imported products. The British and some European pharmacopeias specify that products must contain not less than 2.2% of hydroxyanthracene derivatives, calculated as rhein. The German Pharmacopeia describes rhubarb root extract as 70% alcohol and adjusted with lactose as needed to obtain 4% to 6% anthranoid content.

For hepatitis, adults ingested 50 g of *Rheum officinale* decocted in 200 mL of liquid (unknown) once daily for 16 days.[181] The subjects had a 1-day break after every six treatments, and elderly patients had a 1-day break after every 2 days of treatment.[181]

The dose of rhubarb for nonalcoholic fatty liver has not been established.

Adverse Effects, Interactions, Pharmacokinetics. See Appendix A.

Safflower (*Carthamus tinctorius*)

Grade C: *Unclear or conflicting scientific evidence (chronic hepatitis C)*

Mechanism of Action

The mechanism of action of safflower in hepatitis is not well understood; however, immunomodulatory effects may play a role. According to in vitro study, N-(p-coumaroyl) serotonin and its derivatives in safflower seeds have a suppressive effect on proinflammatory cytokine production from monocytes.[184,185]

Scientific Evidence of Effectiveness

The traditional Japanese Kampo formula EH0202 contains safflower seed extract and is used for immunostimulation. According to preliminary study, EH0202 significantly decreased HCV-RNA levels in patients with high viral titers.[186] More studies with safflower as a monotherapy are needed to define safflower's effect on hepatitis C.

Dose

Although some trials have standardized safflower oil to 74% linoleic acid, standardization is not consistent for safflower or safflower oil.[187,188] The dose of safflower monotherapy for hepatitis C has not been established.

Adverse Effects, Interactions, Pharmacokinetics. See Appendix A.

Sea Buckthorn (*Hippophae rhamnoides*)

Grade C: *Unclear or conflicting scientific evidence (cirrhosis)*

Mechanism of Action

The mechanism of sea buckthorn for cirrhosis is not well understood. Sea buckthorn may have antioxidant and immunomodulatory activity.[189] It has been shown to protect the liver from damage from carbon tetrachloride (CCl_4), a hepatotoxic agent.[189,190]

Scientific Evidence of Effectiveness

Preliminary evidence indicates that sea buckthorn extract may improve hepatic markers for cirrhotic patients.[191] Those treated with sea buckthorn had higher serum levels of TNF-α, IL-6, laminin, and type IV collagen. Also, the sea buckthorn treatment notably shortened the duration for normalization of transaminases.

Dose

The dose of sea buckthorn for cirrhosis has not been determined.

Adverse Effects, Interactions, Pharmacokinetics. See Appendix A.

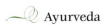 Ayurveda

> Katuka *(Picrorhiza kurroa)* is an herbal preparation used in the Ayurvedic system. Kutkin is the principal constituent of katuka and is composed of kutkoside and the iridoid glycoside picrosides I, II, and III. In animal study, katuka stimulated liver regeneration by increasing nucleic acid and protein synthesis.[192] In experimental study, *Picrorhiza kurroa* improved levels of bilirubin, AST (GOT), and ALT (GPT) in patients with viral hepatitis.[193]
>
> A different Ayurvedic preparation, Kamalahar, has been reported to reduce clinical signs and indicators of liver damage in acute viral hepatitis.[194] Kamalahar is a fixed combination of *Tecoma undulate, Phyllanthus urinaria, Embelia ribes, Taraxacum officinale, Nyctanthes arbortistis,* and *Terminalia arjuna.*

HERBAL THERAPIES WITH NEGATIVE EVIDENCE

St. John's Wort *(Hypericum perforatum)*

Grade D: *Fair negative scientific evidence (chronic hepatitis C)*

Hypericin from St. John's wort does not appear to be effective for treating chronic hepatitis C, as it has shown no detectable antiviral activity against the virus in patients with chronic HCV infection.[195]

Spirulina *(Arthrospira* spp.)

Grade D: *Fair negative scientific evidence (chronic viral hepatitis)*

The hepatoprotective properties of spirulina are attributed to its antiinflammatory, antioxidant, membrane-stabilizing, and immunocorrecting actions.[196] Preliminary animal study reported that oral *Spirulina fusiformis* significantly reduced the extent of lipid peroxidation with concomitant increases in the liver enzymatic (GPx, GST, SOD, CAT) and nonenzymatic antioxidants.[197] It has also been proposed that carotenoids found in *Spirulina* are responsible for its hepatoprotective effects.[198] Despite positive preliminary findings, subsequent clinical research showed spirulina to be ineffective for chronic viral hepatitis.[199]

HERBAL THERAPIES WITH LIMITED EVIDENCE

Eyebright *(Euphrasia officinalis)*

Eyebright contains iridoid glycosides (e.g., aucubin),[200,201] flavonoids (e.g., quercetin, apigenin), and tannins. The most studied constituent of eyebright is *aucubin* and its aglycon, aucubigenin. Limited evidence from animal studies suggests that aucubin may inhibit hepatic RNA and protein synthesis in vivo. These properties have been associated with protective effects in CCl4-induced and alpha-amanitin–induced hepatotoxicity in mice. Conversion of aucubin to its algycon appears to be a prerequisite step for these hepatic effects to occur.[202-204] It is unclear if animal study results are clinically significant to humans.

Schisandra *(Schisandra chinensis)*

Schisandra is a fruit traditionally used to improve liver function in patients with hepatitis. Schisandra appears to have immunomodulatory properties and has been found to reduce circulating monocyte count.[205] It has also been shown to inhibit secretion of HbsAg and HBeAg in hepatocellular carcinoma.[206]

Turmeric *(Curcuma longa)*

In traditional Indian Ayurvedic medicine, turmeric has been used to "tone the liver." In animals, turmeric reversed hepatonecrosis and fatty changes in the liver, with reversal of aflatoxin-induced liver damage.[207] However, the turmeric constituent *curcumin* has been reported to induce abnormalities in liver function tests in rats and may be mildly hepatotoxic in high doses.[208]

Yellow Dock *(Rumex crispus)*

Yellow dock is an herbal product used as a general health tonic. Purportedly, it may strengthen the blood and protect the liver; however, scientific evidence is lacking in this area.

ADJUNCT THERAPIES

1. An integrative approach to liver disorders may involve dietary changes, dietary supplements, and healing techniques. These techniques may be used to improve the immune system and relieve symptoms associated with various liver conditions.
2. Low-protein and low-fat diets are sometimes recommended to patients with liver damage. The liver's workload may be reduced by decreasing the amount of consumed protein. Iron and fat-soluble vitamin intake may need to be monitored; these can accumulate in the liver, with negative effects. Patients may benefit from certain vitamin

Herbs with Possible Hepatoprotective Properties*

HERB	SPECIFIC THERAPEUTIC USE(S)†	HERB	SPECIFIC THERAPEUTIC USE(S)†
Abuta	Jaundice	Cranberry	Liver disorders
Acacia	Hepatitis	Desert parsley	Hepatitis C
Acerola	Liver disorders	Devil's claw	Hepatoprotection
Aconite	Hepatitis	Dong quai	Hepatitis, cirrhosis, hepatoprotection
Agave	Jaundice	Elder	Liver disorders
Agrimony	Jaundice, liver disorders	English ivy	Liver disorders
Alfalfa	Jaundice	Eucalyptus	Hepatoprotection
Alkanna	Jaundice	Evening primrose	Hepatitis B
Aloe	Hepatitis	Eyebright	Jaundice, liver disorders
Andrographis	Hepatoprotection, jaundice	Fenugreek	Liver disorders, hepatoprotection
Annatto	Hepatitis, hepatoprotection, jaundice, liver disorders	Flax	Hepatoprotection
		Fo-ti	Liver disorders
Arnica	Hepatitis, liver disorders	Garcinia	Hepatoprotection
Ashwagandha	Liver disorders	Garlic	Liver toxicity
Asparagus	Hepatoprotection, liver disorders	Ginger	Hepatitis, liver disorders, liver toxicity
Barberry	Hepatoprotection, liver toxicity (acetaminophen-induced), jaundice, cirrhosis (hypertyraminemia)	Ginkgo	Hepatitis B
		Globe artichoke	Hepatoprotection, jaundice
		Goji	Hepatoprotection, liver toxicity
Bellis perennis	Liver disorders	Goldenseal	Alcoholic liver disease, hepatitis, jaundice, liver disorders
Betony	Hepatitis, hepatoprotection		
Bilberry	Liver disorders	Gotu kola	Alcoholic liver disease, liver disorders, hepatitis, jaundice
Black cohosh	Liver disorders		
Black currant	Hepatitis, liver disorders	Grape seed	Hepatoprotection, cirrhosis
Black haw	Jaundice	Grapefruit	Liver disorders
Blessed thistle	Liver disorders, jaundice	Greater celandine	Jaundice, liver disorders
Bloodroot	Hepatoprotection	Ground ivy	Jaundice
Blue cohosh	Liver cancer	Gymnema	Hepatoprotection, liver disorders
Blue flag	Jaundice, liver cleanser, liver disorders	Hibiscus	Liver disorders, hepatoprotection
		Holy basil	Liver disorders
Boldo	Liver disorders, hepatoprotection	Horny goat weed	Hepatitis, hepatoprotection
Boneset	Jaundice, liver disorders	Horse chestnut	Liver congestion
Boswellia	Hepatitis C, liver toxicity	Horsetail	Hepatitis, hepatoprotection
Burdock	Hepatoprotection, liver disorders	Hyssop	Liver disorders
Calendula	Jaundice, liver cancer, liver disorders	Jequirity	Jaundice
Cardamom	Liver disorders	Jewelweed	Jaundice
Carqueja	Liver disorders, hepatoprotection	Jiaogulan	Hepatoprotection
Cascara	Liver disorders	Katuka	Hepatitis, liver disorders, hepatoprotection
Cat's claw	Cirrhosis, liver disorders, hepatoprotection		
		Khella	Liver disorders
Chamomile	Liver disorders	Kudzu	Cirrhosis
Chaparral	Liver toxicity, liver metabolic function	Lesser celandine	Hepatoprotection
Chia	Liver disorders	Lime	Jaundice, liver disorders
Chickweed	Hepatitis B	Maca	Hepatoprotection
Cinnamon	Liver disorders	Maitake mushroom	Hepatitis
Club moss	Liver disorders	Mangosteen	Hepatoprotection (hydrocholeretic)
Codonopsis	Hepatoprotection	Morus nigra	Liver disorders
Coleus	Liver disorders	Mugwort	Hepatoprotection, liver disorders
Couch grass	Liver disorders	Neem	Hepatoprotection

Herbs with Possible Hepatoprotective Properties—cont'd

HERB	SPECIFIC THERAPEUTIC USE(S)†	HERB	SPECIFIC THERAPEUTIC USE(S)†
Noni	Jaundice	Shiitake mushroom	Hepatitis B, hepatoprotection
Nopal	Hepatoprotection	Skullcap	Hepatitis, liver disorders, hepatoprotection
Nux vomica	Liver cancer	Sorrel	Jaundice
Pennyroyal	Liver disorders	Soy	Hepatitis
Peppermint	Liver disorders	Sweet woodruff	Hepatitis, jaundice, liver disorders
Podophyllum	Hepatitis, jaundice, liver disorders	Tamarind	Jaundice, liver disorders
Psyllium	Liver disorders	Tansy	Jaundice, liver disorders (increasing appetite and alleviating pain)
Quassia	Hepatoprotection		
Red yeast rice	Liver toxicity (acetaminophen-induced), liver disorders	Tea	Liver cancer
Rehmannia	Hepatoprotection	Tribulus	Hepatitis
Rhodiola	Hepatoprotection	Valerian	Liver disorders
Rooibos	Hepatoprotection	Verbena	Liver metabolic function
Rose hip	Liver disorders	White horehound	Jaundice, liver disorders
Rosemary	Hepatoprotection, cirrhosis	White water lily	Hepatoprotection
Sage	Liver disorders	Wild yam	Hepatoprotection
Sarsaparilla	Hepatitis B, hepatoprotection	Yellow dock	Hepatitis
Scotch broom	Jaundice, liver disorders	Yew	Liver disorders

*This is not an all-inclusive or comprehensive list of herbs with hepatoprotective (liver-protecting) properties; other herbs and supplements may possess these qualities. A qualified health care provider should be consulted with specific questions or concerns regarding potential effects of agents or interactions.
†Based on expert opinion, anecdote, case reports, and/or preliminary trial evidence.

Herbs with Possible Hepatotoxic Properties*

Ackee	Lobelia
Birch oil	Mate
Blessed thistle	Mistletoe
Borage	Paraguay tea
Bush tea	Pennyroyal
Butterbur	Periwinkle
Chaparral	Rue
Coltsfoot	Sassafras
Comfrey	Scullcap
Echinacea	*Senecio* spp./groundsel
Echium spp.	Sorrel
English plantain	Tansy
Germander	Tea
Greater celandine	Turmeric
Heliotrope	Uva ursi
Horse chestnut	Valerian
Kava	White chameleon

*This is not an all-inclusive list of herbs with hepatotoxic properties; other herbs and supplements may possess these qualities.

supplements, especially B-complex vitamins. Because patients with chronic liver disease are at increased risk for developing osteoporosis, foods rich in calcium and/or supplements should be added to their diets. Increasing fiber intake may help bind toxins and detoxify the body.

3. *Probiotics* are beneficial bacteria (sometimes referred to as "friendly germs") that are believed to help the body maintain a healthy intestinal tract and assist with digestion. They are also thought to help inhibit potentially harmful organisms (e.g., bacteria, yeasts) in the gut. Most probiotics come from food sources, especially cultured milk products. Probiotics such as *Lactobacillus acidophilus*, *L. casei*, and *Saccharomyces boulardii* can be consumed as capsules, tablets, beverages, powders, yogurts, and other foods. Liver cirrhosis may be accompanied by an imbalance of intestinal bacteria flora. Probiotic supplementation in cirrhosis patients has been found to reduce the level of fecal acidity (pH) and fecal and blood ammonia, which are beneficial changes.
4. Various healing techniques, including acupuncture, massage, and physical therapy, may be used with conventional and nonconventional treatments to help boost the immune system in patients with hepatitis. However, there is currently a lack of clinical evidence supporting the therapeutic efficacy of these techniques.

INTEGRATIVE THERAPY PLAN

- Assess the patient's medical, family, and sexual history. Identify the possible cause of liver disease (e.g., alcohol abuse, cirrhosis).
- Discuss the patient's social history, including recreational drug use and alcohol use.

- Determine if the patient has been exposed to environmental hepatic toxins, including arsenic, carbon tetrachloride, copper, toluene, or flourine.
- Inquire about the patient's use of potentially hepatotoxic drugs, including acetaminophen (Tylenol).
- Assess the patient's nutritional status, including malnourishment because of alcohol abuse or a diet heavy in charcoal-grilled meats and vegetables.
- Determine if the patient is taking any herbal remedies that may be associated with a high risk of hepatotoxicity, including kava *(Piper methysticum)*, chaparral *(Larrea taridentata)*, comfrey *(Symphytum officinale)*, germander *(Teucrium chamaedrys)*, kombucha tea, mistletoe *(Viscum album)*, pennyroyal *(Mentha pulegium)*, and skullcap *(Scutellaria laterifolia)*. Fat-soluble vitamins, including vitamins A, D, E, and K, may also be potentially toxic to the liver; intake of these vitamins should be monitored.
- Evaluate the patient for signs and symptoms of liver disease, including jaundice, abdominal pain and swelling, chronic itchy skin, dark urine, pale or tar-colored stools, joint pain, nausea, and loss of appetite.
- Determine if the patient has liver panel abnormalities, including elevated ALT or AST, or has serologic markers of liver disease.
- An important measure in the treatment of alcoholic liver disease is to ensure that the patient immediately and totally abstains from alcohol.
- Milk thistle *(Silybum marianum)* has been used medicinally for more than 2000 years, most often for the treatment of liver disorders. Several studies of oral milk thistle for hepatitis caused by viruses or alcohol report improvements in liver tests. Multiple studies from Europe suggest benefits of oral milk thistle for cirrhosis. In studies lasting up to 5 years, milk thistle has improved liver function and decreased the number of deaths that occur in cirrhotic patients. Milk thistle may cause loose stools in higher dosages.
- The active compound in licorice is glycyrrhizin. This constituent may improve liver tissues damaged by hepatitis and may prevent liver cancer. However, glycyrrhizin may worsen *ascites*, or the accumulation of fluid in the abdomen, which may be a symptom of cirrhosis.[77]
- In traditional Chinese medicine, cordyceps *(Cordyceps sinensis)* has been used to support and improve liver function. In studies using herbal combinations that included cordyceps, liver and immune function improved. Studies also indicate that cordyceps may stimulate the immune system and improve serum gamma globulin levels in hepatitis B patients.
- Stress the importance of a healthy diet that includes five or more daily servings of fruits and vegetables, foods rich in soluble fiber (e.g., oatmeal, beans), foods rich in calcium (e.g., dairy products, spinach), soy products (e.g., tempeh, miso, tofu, soy milk), and foods rich in omega-3 fatty acids, including cold-water fish (e.g., salmon, mackerel, tuna).
- Regular exercise, at least 30 minutes a day, should also be encouraged. Even if an individual does not drink alcohol, obesity may contribute to nonalcoholic fatty liver disease.
- Advise patients with liver damage to avoid alcohol consumption and certain drugs, such as acetaminophen (Tylenol). The maximum daily dose of acetaminophen is 4 g.
- Counsel alcoholic patients on decreasing alcohol consumption and considering a referral to Alcoholics Anonymous to seek additional counseling on habitual routines.
- Patients at increased risk for hepatitis, or who have had past infections with any hepatitis virus, should receive the hepatitis B vaccine. Individuals should not engage in unprotected sex, especially if they do not know the health status of their partners. Individuals who use needles to inject drugs should use sterile needles and avoid sharing used needles with other people.
- Protective measures should be used when spraying insecticides, fungicides, paint, and other toxic chemicals.

Case Studies

CASE STUDY 25-1

JK is a 54-year-old man with a 25-year history of heavy alcohol consumption. Recently, his wife noticed that he had "turned yellow," and she convinced him to seek medical help. The physician informed JK that he had cirrhosis and would soon die if he did not stop drinking. Physical examination and laboratory studies revealed that JK had hypertension (150/114 mm Hg), was 50 pounds overweight, and had type 2 diabetes. The physician prescribed glipizide (Glucotrol) for JK's diabetes and spironolactone (Aldactone) for his hypertension and also recommended that he lose 50 pounds with diet and exercise.

On his return home, JK promised his wife that he would quit drinking but was not that interested in diet, exercise, or taking the prescribed medications. He consulted a co-worker who told him that he had little faith in doctors or the medication they prescribed. The co-worker suggested that instead of the medication, JK should take astragalus root, licorice, and silymarin. What kind of advice could you give to JK?

Answer: Astragalus *(Astragalus membranaceus)*, licorice *(Glycyrrhiza glabra)*, and silymarin, a milk thistle *(Silybum marianum)* extract, may improve his cirrhosis, but these herbs only supplement prescribed medications and other recommendations. Most importantly, JK must avoid all alcohol, including that contained in medications such as cough syrup. Glipizide will help him to maintain normal glucose (blood sugar) levels, and the diuretic ("water pill"), spironolactone, will reduce the fluid load in his cardiovascular system, reducing his blood pressure. Diet and exercise are also extremely important. If he loses the recommended 50 pounds, his type 2 diabetes will likely improve, and he might even be able to discontinue the glipizide. Diet and exercise may also improve his blood pressure, and JK might be able to discontinue the spironolactone.

The liver is one of the few internal organs that can regenerate up to two thirds of its tissue. This ability, plus a regimen of prescribed medication, herbal remedies, diet, and exercise, could lead to a resolution of JK's cirrhosis. Astragalus appears to be protective against cardiovascular, hepatic, pulmonary, and renal pathological changes and reportedly reduces the risk of diabetes-induced myocardial hypertrophy (enlarged heart). Astragalus also may improve congestive heart failure, diabetes, and hypertension and may have additive effects with glipizide and spironolactone.

Licorice contains glycyrrhizic acid, which has been implicated in many of the side effects reported with licorice intake (see Appendix A). Adverse effects from glycyrrhizin are primarily a result of hormonal and electrolyte disturbances. Possible effects include hypokalemia, hypernatremia, and metabolic alkalosis. Numerous cases of hypokalemia, hypotension, and hypertension have been associated with licorice use. Licorice has also been documented to exhibit diuretic effects, and may potentially interact with certain drugs; thus, with JK's current medication schedule, licorice supplementation is not recommended.

Evidence exists that silymarin is beneficial for cirrhosis and chronic hepatitis. It has been reported to decrease fasting plasma glucose, glycosylated hemoglobin (HbA_{1c}), and fasting insulin levels in diabetic patients; therefore an adjustment of JK's glipizide dosage might be necessary.

CASE STUDY 25-2

AJ is a 45-year-old Caucasian man with a liver disease secondary to hepatitis C and alcohol abuse. He has a history of IV drug use since adolescence. AJ states that for the past 10 years he has consumed "a few beers" each weekday and a "six-pack" on weekends. AJ recently began taking lorazepam (Ativan), 2 mg orally at bedtime for insomnia, which he attributes to stress. AJ also has hypertension, which is under control; his blood pressure was 130/88 mm Hg on his last visit to the family practitioner 6 months ago. His current prescription medications include lactulose (Enulose), 2 g (30 mL) orally four times daily as needed; spironolactone (Aldactone), 100 mg daily; furosemide (Lasix), 40 mg twice daily; nadolol (Corgard), 40 mg daily; and lisinopril (Prinivil), 20 mg daily.

AJ presents at your ambulatory care clinic and requests information on herbal remedies for hepatitis and hepatic cirrhosis. After reading a newspaper article on herbal options a few months ago, he began taking fermented cordyceps (3 g daily) and dried aqueous extract of mistletoe (2 mL daily) with the goal of improving his overall health. AJ states that since adding the herbs to his daily medication regimen, he feels lightheaded when arising in the morning. This sensation persists throughout the day; it is relieved if he lies down but returns when he arises. He adds that the lightheaded feeling was worse today, prompting his visit. How would you counsel?

Answer: The herbal therapies cordyceps (*Cordyceps sinensis*) and mistletoe (*Viscum album*) are natural treatment options for liver disease; however, in view of AJ's past medical history and current medications, these agents are not ideal. AJ's lightheadedness when arising is most likely caused by orthostatic hypotension secondary to a combination of adverse effects from his prescription medications and new herbal treatments. Both of his diuretic/antihypertensive medications, spironolactone and furosemide, can interact with the mistletoe preparation, resulting in bradycardia, hypotension, and dehydration. Mistletoe in combination with other antihypertensive medications, such as AJ's nadolol, could result in cardiotoxic and negative effects on heart contractility, induce reflex bradycardia, lower blood pressure, depolarize cardiac muscle, and cause severe dehydration. This could lead to hypovolemic shock and cardiovascular collapse. AJ's angiotensin-converting enzyme (ACE) inhibitor, lisinopril, also may have enhanced effect when used concomitantly with mistletoe. Furthermore, high doses of mistletoe can produce an increase in liver enzymes (AST, ALT). Moreover, the hypotensive adverse effects could be attributed to an interaction between both herbal agents, cordyceps and mistletoe, which may result in enhanced hypotensive effects.

Although AJ did not experience increased sedation, he should be aware that concomitant use of lorazepam and mistletoe can have additive sedative effects. This patient should also be counseled on decreasing his alcohol consumption and given a referral to Alcoholics Anonymous to seek counseling on habitual routines. AJ should be advised to discontinue all current herbal preparations (cordyceps and mistletoe) because of drug-herb and herb-herb interactions. However, AJ could be informed about another herbal preparation, milk thistle (*Silybum marianum*), which might benefit him and not interact with his other prescribed medications. The recommended dose for chronic hepatitis is 420 mg of silymarin (Legalon) daily in three divided doses. Conversely, a positive interaction has been noted with milk thistle and concomitant alcohol consumption, resulting in reduced hepatotoxicity associated with ethanol ingestion. If AJ decides to try silymarin, he must inform his physician before initiating treatment.

CASE STUDY 25-3

RM, a 47-year-old man with hepatitis C, is interested in herbal remedies for his condition. For the past 6 months he has been taking St. John's wort for depression. He was recently diagnosed with thrombophlebitis (inflammation and clotting in veins) in both lower legs and began a course of warfarin (Coumadin) therapy. He has heard that milk thistle can improve his liver disease. When asked, RM says he did not inform his physician that he was taking St. John's wort because it is "just an herb, not a drug." How do you counsel?

Answer: You inform RM that herbal remedies must be included in a medication list and that a number of prescription medications are derived from plant products. You add that he must immediately inform his physician that he is taking St. John's wort because the substance interacts with a number of drugs, herbs, and supplements (through induction of cytochrome P450 enzyme CYP3A4, as well as CYP2C9), enhancing or inhibiting the way the body processes these agents. In fact, St. John's wort has been shown to affect warfarin, which RM is currently taking.

Some individuals claim that St. John's wort improves depression; others do not. It has been studied for liver disorders but has not been shown to be effective. RM should discuss his use of this herb and whether or not it is improving his depression.

Although current evidence regarding the benefits of silymarin, an extract from milk thistle *(Silybum marianum)*, for viral hepatitis is unclear or conflicting, it has no known interactions with warfarin, so RM may add silymarin to his drug regimen.

References for Chapter 25 can be found on the Evolve website at http://evolve.elsevier.com/Ulbricht/herbalpharmacotherapy/

Review Questions

1. All the following statements are true regarding milk thistle *except:*
   a. Milk thistle protects liver cells against oxidation damage.
   b. High-quality studies have concluded strong evidence supports the use of milk thistle for all liver disorders.
   c. Studies of milk thistle up to 5 years have reported improved transaminase levels and survival in patients with cirrhosis.
   d. Milk thistle has been reported as generally well tolerated for up to 6 years.

2. True or false: Neo-Minophagen C (SNMC) is a product containing deglycyrrhizinated licorice extracts, and is used to treat hepatitis C.

3. Which of the following herbs is hepatotoxic?
   a. Comfrey
   b. Germander
   c. Kava
   d. All the above

4. All the following statements are true regarding mistletoe *except:*
   a. Lectins and thionins are constituents in mistletoe likely responsible for its immunomodulating effects.
   b. Mistletoe may reduce liver transaminase levels, viral load, and inflammation.
   c. Mistletoe is a key herb in *sho-saiko-to* for hepatitis C.
   d. Mistletoe has the potential to be hepatotoxic.

5. True or false: Cirrhosis is often considered a "silent" disease, and many patients are asymptomatic until decompensation occurs.

6. Which of the following doses of milk thistle has been studied in patients with chronic hepatitis?
   a. 42 mg silymarin daily in three divided doses
   b. 420 mg silymarin daily in three divided doses
   c. 4 g silymarin daily in three divided doses
   d. 420 mcg silymarin daily in three divided doses

7. The mechanism of cordyceps' action to help restore liver function may involve which of the following?
   a. Inhibition of hepatic fibrogenesis
   b. Inhibition of TGF-β
   c. Interference with viral replication
   d. Both a and b

8. Which of the following mechanisms may lead to inflammation of the liver?
   a. Defects in metabolism of lipids
   b. Increased delivery of fatty acids to liver
   c. Mitochondrial abnormalities
   d. All the above

9. True or false: Compound K, a constituent of caper, appears to have hepatoprotective effects.

10. Which test is usually performed to diagnose hepatitis C?
    a. ELISA
    b. HBsAg
    c. HAVAB-M
    d. None of the above

Answers are found in the Answers to Review Questions section in the back of the text.

26 Genitourinary Disorders

Outline

OVERVIEW
    Benign Prostatic Hyperplasia
        Signs and Symptoms
        Diagnosis
    Erectile Dysfunction
        Signs and Symptoms
        Diagnosis
    Urinary Incontinence
        Signs and Symptoms
        Diagnosis
    Interstitial Cystitis
        Signs and Symptoms
        Diagnosis
    Neurogenic Bladder
        Signs and Symptoms
        Diagnosis
    Prolapsed Uterus
        Signs and Symptoms
        Diagnosis
    Prostatitis
        Signs and Symptoms
        Diagnosis
    Kidney Stones (Renal Calculi)
        Signs and Symptoms
        Diagnosis
    Lupus Nephritis
        Signs and Symptoms
        Diagnosis
    Pelvic Inflammatory Disease
        Signs and Symptoms
        Diagnosis
SELECTED HERBAL THERAPIES
    African Wild Potato *(Hypoxis hemerocallidea)*
    Beta-Sitosterol (β-Sitosterol), Sitosterol (22,23-Dihydrostigmasterol, 24-Ethylcholesterol)
    Chamomile *(Matricaria recutita,* syn. *Matricaria suaveolens, Matricaria chamomilla, Anthemis nobilis, Chamaemelum nobile, Chamomilla chamomilla, Chamomilla recutita)*
    Coleus *(Coleus forskohlii)*
    Cranberry *(Vaccinium macrocarpon)*
    Damiana *(Turnera diffusa)*
    Danshen *(Salvia miltiorrhiza)*
    Ephedra *(Ephedra sinica)*
    Flax *(Linum usitatissimum)*
    Ginkgo *(Ginkgo biloba)*
    Ginseng *(Panax* spp.)
    Grapefruit *(Citrus x paradisi)*
    Horny Goat Weed *(Epimedium grandiflorum)*
    Maca *(Lepidium meyenii)*
    Muira Puama *(Ptychopetalum olacoides)*
    Nopal *(Opuntia* spp.)
    Pycnogenol *(Pinus pinaster* subsp. *atlantica)*
    Pygeum *(Prunus africanum,* syn. *Pygeum africanum)*
    Red Clover *(Trifolium pratense)*
    Rye *(Secale cereale)*
    Saw Palmetto *(Serenoa repens)*
    Soy *(Glycine max)*
    Stinging Nettle *(Urtica dioica)*
    Yohimbe *(Pausinystalia yohimbe)*
HERBAL THERAPIES WITH LIMITED EVIDENCE
ADJUNCT THERAPIES
INTEGRATIVE THERAPY PLANS
    Benign Prostatic Hyperplasia
    Erectile Dysfunction
CASE STUDIES
REVIEW QUESTIONS

Learning Objectives

- Assess various genitourinary conditions.
- Recognize herbal treatment options for genitourinary conditions.
- Describe the mechanism of action, adverse effects, and drug interactions of herbal products used for genitourinary conditions.
- Provide the patient with an integrative care plan for genitourinary conditions.

OVERVIEW

Genitourinary disorders are illnesses that affect the urinary organs or genital organs and may result from aging, illnesses, or injuries. The urinary organs include the kidneys, ureters, bladder, sphincter muscles, and the urethra (Figure 26-1). The female genital (or reproductive) organs include the uterus, cervix, fallopian tubes, and vagina. The male reproductive organs include the testicles, epididymis (tubular organ where sperm collect after leaving the testes), prostate gland, and penis. Examples of genitourinary disorders include benign prostatic hyperplasia, erectile dysfunction, urinary incontinence, prostatitis, kidney stones, lupus nephritis, pelvic inflammatory disease, interstitial cystitis, neurogenic bladder, and prolapsed uterus. In addition to causing urinary problems, many of these conditions may also affect the reproductive organs. Treatment of genitourinary disorders depends on the specific type and the severity of the disorder. *Urinary tract infections* (UTIs), caused by pathogenic microorganisms, are discussed in Chapter 27.

Benign Prostatic Hyperplasia

As men age, their testosterone levels drop, and their relative levels of estrogen increase. These hormonal changes may trigger prostate growth. Benign prostatic hyperplasia (BPH), often called *benign enlargement of the prostate* (BEP) or (inaccurately) *benign prostatic hypertrophy*, is a normal, gradual enlargement of the prostate caused by hormonal fluctuations, such as decreases in testosterone and increases in dihydrotestosterone (DHT) and estrogen. It affects about half of men older than 60 and 80% of men 80 or older.[2] Almost every man over age 45 years has some prostate enlargement, but symptoms are rarely apparent until age 60. In addition to hormonal fluctuations and age, BPH may be influenced by cell-growth factors and possibly by genetic makeup.

Although it generally does not cause pain, BPH may cause an uncomfortable feeling of pressure in the groin. As the prostate enlarges, it presses against the urethra and interferes with urination. At the same time, the bladder wall becomes thicker and irritated. The bladder may contract even when it contains small amounts of urine, which results in more frequent urination. As the bladder continues to weaken, it may not empty completely during urination.

Signs and Symptoms
Common symptoms of BPH include difficulty initiating urine flow, poor urinary flow and a variable flow rate, frequent urination, dribbling of urine at the end of urination, and nocturia (frequent urination at night). Blockage of the urethra and partial emptying of the bladder cause many of the problems associated with BPH, including UTIs, bladder stones, and kidney damage.

Diagnosis
Patients who experience BPH symptoms should undergo a detailed medical history, evaluation of symptoms, and a digital rectal examination (DRE). Various tests may be performed when evaluating the patient for BPH. Laboratory tests may include urinalysis to screen for kidney disorders, urine culture to detect signs of UTI, and blood urea nitrogen and creatinine to evaluate kidney function. A blood test that detects *prostate specific antigen* (PSA), along with DRE, may be performed to screen for prostate cancer.

Erectile Dysfunction

Erectile dysfunction (ED), sometimes called *impotence*, is the failure to achieve a penile erection suitable for intercourse. Impotence may also be used to describe other problems that interfere with sexual intercourse, such as infertility, lack of libido, and ejaculatory disorders. The pathophysiology of these disorders is distinct and treated with different agents.

Although ED is more common in men older than 65, it can occur at any age.[3] Occasional ED episodes happen to most men and are normal. As men age, it is also normal to experience changes in erectile function. Erections may take longer to develop, may not be as rigid, or may require more direct stimulation to be achieved. Men may also notice that orgasms are less intense, the volume of ejaculate is reduced, and recovery time increases between erections.

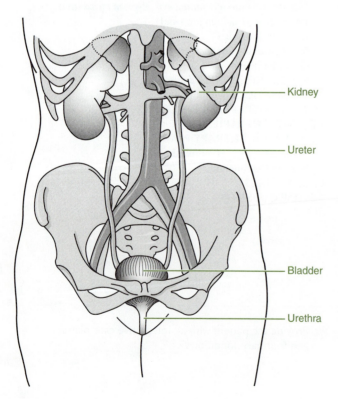

Figure 26-1 Urinary system (frontal view). (Modified from Fehrenbach MJ, editor: *Dental anatomy coloring book*, St Louis, 2008, Saunders-Elsevier.)

Signs and Symptoms
Symptoms associated with ED include inability to obtain a full erection and inability to maintain an erection throughout intercourse. Lack of morning erections are also noted along with a decreased libido.

Diagnosis
If ED occurs for more than 2 months or is a recurring problem, a physical examination is recommended. A medical history should include the frequency and duration of symptoms, the presence or absence of morning erections, and the quality of the relationship with the sexual partner. A psychosocial examination, using an interview and questionnaire, may reveal possible psychological factors (e.g., stress, anxiety, depression). A man's sexual partner may also be interviewed to determine expectations and perceptions during sexual intercourse. Questions about how and when the condition developed, medications taken, and other physical or emotional conditions are included. Diseases that predispose patients to ED include arteriosclerosis, diabetes mellitus, hypertension, and concurrent use of certain medications (e.g., antidepressants, diuretics, antihypertensives).

A physical examination should include a check for signs of *hypogonadism* (lack of male hormone production), which include *gynecomastia* (increase in breast size) or loss of axillary (underarm) and pubic hair. A genital examination should be performed to evaluate the size and consistency of the testes. The penis should be examined for any fibrosis (scar tissue) indicative of *Peyronie disease,* an inflammatory condition causing scar tissue formation in the penis.

Laboratory tests may be performed to test for underlying conditions that may cause ED. Tests should include thyroid function tests, blood glucose levels, lipid profile, and testosterone levels.

Urinary Incontinence
Urinary incontinence describes the inability to control the bladder. The bladder spontaneously empties all or some of the urine.

Most children, especially those younger than 7 years old, experience nighttime incontinence, also called bed-wetting or *nocturnal enuresis.* This may occur because the child's bladder is still developing, and it cannot hold all the urine produced during sleep. Children may be unable to recognize when they have full bladders; the nerves that control the bladder take a long time to develop.

Urinary incontinence may also occur in adults, usually as a symptom of an underlying medical condition. For example, pregnant women may experience incontinence because their bodies are going through hormonal and weight changes. Vaginal childbirth may damage the pelvic nerves and supportive tissues and muscles involved in bladder control. Aging is also associated with urinary incontinence because the bladder muscles become weaker over time. When incontinence is caused by weak pelvic floor muscles, it is called *stress incontinence.* Also, elderly women produce less estrogen, a hormone that helps keep the lining of the bladder and urethra healthy. Other medical conditions, including an inflamed prostate gland (prostatitis), enlarged prostate, prostate cancer, bladder stones, neurological disorders (e.g., Parkinson's disease, multiple sclerosis), and tumors that block the urinary tract may lead to urinary incontinence. In addition, alcohol, caffeine, dehydration, overhydration, bladder irritation, medications (e.g., sleeping pills, antidepressants, diuretics), UTIs, sleep apnea (pauses in breathing during sleep), diabetes, and constipation may lead to temporary urinary incontinence.

Urge incontinence occurs when the bladder muscles contract inappropriately, causing urine to leak involuntarily from the bladder. These contractions can occur regardless of how much urine is present in the bladder. Common causes of urge incontinence include neurological diseases or injuries, bladder cancer, infection, bladder stones, bladder inflammation, and bladder obstruction.

Signs and Symptoms
Patients with urinary incontinence are unable to control urine release. Urine may leak out when the patient laughs, coughs, exercises, or lifts heavy weights. Small amounts of urine may leak out periodically throughout the day or night. Some patients may experience a sudden urge to urinate followed by an uncontrolled emptying of the bladder. Some patients may be unable to empty their bladder completely. As a result, urine may build up in the bladder until it cannot hold any more fluid. When this occurs, the bladder may spontaneously release the urine.

Diagnosis
A complete medical history, including assessment of symptoms, and physical and neurological examination are essential in diagnosing the patient with urinary incontinence. Physical examinations should include an abdominal exam to rule out a distended bladder, a neurological exam to assess reflexes and sensory or motor deficiencies, a pelvic exam in women, and a genital and prostate exam in men. Several diagnostic tests may be performed, including a urine test to check for infection. *Postvoid residual* (PVR) measurement may be performed to determine if the patient is able to empty the bladder. In this test, patients urinate into a container, the clinician measures the amount of urine, and then a soft, thin tube (catheter) is inserted into the urethra and bladder to drain any remaining urine. If a large amount of urine remains in the bladder, it may indicate an obstruction (e.g., tumor) or a muscle or nerve problem.

Interstitial Cystitis
Interstitial cystitis (also called "painful bladder syndrome" or "frequency-urgency-dysuria syndrome") is a long-term inflammatory condition that causes frequent urination and bladder pain. In healthy individuals the bladder expands until it is full.

Once this happens, the brain receives a message from the pelvic nerves, which induces the urge to urinate. Patients with interstitial cystitis feel the urge to urinate more often than normal.

Although interstitial cystitis can affect anyone at any age, it is most common among women age 30 to 70 years,[4] with a median age of 43 years.[5] The exact cause of interstitial cystitis remains unknown. Most experts believe that patients are born with a leaky epithelium, which is the protective lining of the bladder. If toxic or harmful substances enter the bladder through the epithelium, this may cause irritation and lead to cystitis. Other possible causes of interstitial cystitis that are being investigated include heredity, infections, allergic reactions, or *autoimmunity*, when the immune system mistakenly attacks the body's own tissues.

Signs and Symptoms
Symptoms of interstitial cystitis vary among patients. Individual patients may also experience changes in the severity of symptoms over time. Stress, menstruation, allergies, and sexual activity may worsen symptoms. Common symptoms include a frequent urge to urinate and frequently passing small amounts of urine. Patients with severe interstitial cystitis may urinate more than 50 times daily. Patients may experience pain in the pelvis or perineum (area between the anus and external genitalia). Some patients may experience pain during sexual intercourse.

Diagnosis
A *potassium sensitivity test* is the standard diagnostic test for interstitial cystitis. A flexible tube (catheter) is used to fill the bladder with distilled water, and then the bladder is filled with a potassium solution. After each solution is instilled into the bladder, the patient assesses pain and urgency to urinate. Healthy patients notice no difference between the two solutions. If the potassium solution induces more pain and urgency than distilled water, the patient is diagnosed with interstitial cystitis. Although patients with interstitial cystitis are almost always sensitive to the potassium solution, researchers are unsure whether this indicates increased bladder permeability or hypersensitive nerves.

Neurogenic Bladder
Neurogenic bladder occurs when the pelvic nerves do not function properly. This may lead to either an overactive or an underactive bladder. Common causes of neurogenic bladder include diabetes, infections, tumors, heavy metal poisoning, vaginal childbirth, stroke, multiple sclerosis, and brain or spinal cord injuries. Some patients are born with genetic nerve problems that cause the condition.

Signs and Symptoms
Damaged or defective nerves may send signals to the bladder at the wrong time, causing the muscles to contract spontaneously. This causes the bladder to become *overactive*. Symptoms of an overactive bladder may include frequent urination, a persistent urge to urinate, and incontinence. Occasional urine leakage is common.

In patients who have an *underactive* bladder, the nerves do not receive the message that the bladder is full, or the message is too weak for the bladder to be completely emptied. When the nerves do not function properly, urine builds up in the bladder (urinary retention). An overfull bladder may empty without warning. If the bladder is too full, it may back up and put pressure on the kidneys. Urinary retention may also lead to bladder infections or *pyelonephritis* (kidney infections).

Diagnosis
If a patient is suspected of having a neurogenic bladder, the bladder and nervous system should be evaluated. Tests may be performed to determine how much water the bladder can hold and whether it is able to empty completely and efficiently. Imaging studies, including radiography, computed tomography (CT), and magnetic resonance imaging (MRI), may be performed to visualize the urinary tract and nervous system. The images may show abnormalities that indicate nerve damage.

Prolapsed Uterus
A prolapsed uterus occurs when the uterus collapses into the vaginal canal. Various conditions may cause prolapse, such as weakened pelvic muscles from aging. Vaginal childbirth and medical conditions, such as chronic cough, straining from constipation, pelvic tumors, or accumulation of fluid in the abdomen, may also put extra strain on the pelvic muscles and result in a prolapsed uterus.

Signs and Symptoms
Symptoms of a prolapsed uterus vary depending on the severity of the condition. Mild cases may be asymptomatic. Common symptoms include a feeling of fullness or pressure in the pelvis, lower back pain, a sensation that something is falling out of the vagina, difficulty urinating or moving the bowels, and difficulty walking.

Diagnosis
Among prolapsed uterus patients, a common complaint is the sensation that something is falling out of the vagina. Diagnosis is made after a pelvic examination, which readily determines the degree of prolapse. Imaging studies are generally not needed.

Prostatitis
Infections may cause inflammation of the prostate, a condition known as prostatitis. Blocked or irritated prostatic ducts may lead to the infection. The most common causal organisms for bacterial prostatitis are gram-negative members of the Enterobacteriaceae family and include *Escherichia coli, Proteus mirabilis, Klebsiella* spp., *Enterobacter* spp., *Pseudomonas aeruginosa,* and *Serratia* spp. *Staphylococcus aureus* infections

may occur from prolonged catheterization. With treatment, prostatitis generally resolves within several days to 2 weeks. Treatment of chronic bacterial prostatitis usually involves antimicrobial medication for 4 to 12 weeks. Chronic prostatitis is difficult to treat, and recurrence is possible.

There are four types of prostatitis: *acute bacterial prostatitis* (least common type, but most common in men under 35), *chronic bacterial prostatitis* (uncommon, but affects mostly men age 40-70), *asymptomatic inflammatory prostatitis* (no outward symptoms and occurs mainly in men ≥60), and *chronic nonbacterial prostatitis* (most common type). Prostadynia, also known as *chronic pelvic pain syndrome*, is associated with symptoms that are similar to chronic non-bacterial prostatitis but does not involve actual bacteria or prostate inflammation (Table 26-1).[6]

Signs and Symptoms
Symptoms of prostatitis may include painful, burning, or frequent urination; weak urine flow; and incomplete emptying. Other symptoms may include fever and chills, lower abdominal pain or pressure, painful ejaculation, impotence, and low back pain.

Diagnosis
A diagnosis may be based on clinical signs and symptoms. Urinary cultures should be obtained before antimicrobial treatment. Often this test reveals *Escherichia coli* as the most prevalent pathogen. A blood test should measure white blood cells (WBCs) because elevated WBC count may indicate an infection. DRE may be performed to visualize the prostate and aid in diagnosis. If the gland seems enlarged and tender, this may indicate prostatitis.

Chronic prostatitis is diagnosed after other possible causes are ruled out, such as infections and kidney stones. Because the differential diagnosis includes many possible conditions, several tests may be performed, including MRI, ultrasound, blood tests, and biopsy. If chronic prostatitis/chronic pelvic pain syndrome is diagnosed, the physician may use the National Institutes of Health (NIH)-Chronic Prostatitis Symptom Index, a standard questionnaire, to help understand the symptoms and measure the effects of treatment.[7]

Kidney Stones (Renal Calculi)
Kidney stones (also called renal calculi, urolithiasis, or nephrolithiasis) often develop when there are excessive levels of minerals and salts in the urine. These substances in the urine form crystals, which may combine over time to form hard masses or stones. Kidney stones may contain various combinations of chemicals, including calcium in combination with either oxalate or phosphate. Other types of stones are made up of struvite, uric acid, or cystine. A *struvite stone* or "infection" stone may form after UTI. These stones contain magnesium ammonium phosphate (struvite) and calcium carbonate apatite. A *uric acid stone* may form when the urine contains too much urate. *Cystine stones* are rare and result from an inherited genetic disorder called cystinuria; these calculi result from a buildup of cystine (a dimer of two cysteine amino acids) in the urine.

TABLE 26-1 Clinical Characteristics of Major Types of Prostatitis

TYPICAL PRESENTATION	PROSTATE EXAMINATION	PROSTATIC FLUID WBCs*	BACTERIAL CULTURES	ANTIBIOTIC RESPONSE	PERCENTAGE OF ALL CASES
ACUTE BACTERIAL PROSTATITIS					
Acute illness Age 40-60 years	Tender, warm	Contra-indicated†	Positive	Predictable and prompt	1%-5%
CHRONIC BACTERIAL PROSTATITIS					
Recurrent urinary tract infections Age 50-80 years	Enlarged, "boggy"	Always	Positive 4-cup test (prostatic specimens)	Usual, but slow	5%-10%
CHRONIC NONBACTERIAL (INFLAMMATORY) PROSTATITIS					
Genitourinary and voiding discomfort Age 30-50 years	Highly variable	Always	Negative	Occasional	40%-65%
CHRONIC PELVIC PAIN SYNDROME					
Pain, voiding problems Age 30-40 years	Usually normal	Rarely	Negative	None	20%-40%

From Lipsky BA: Prostatitis and urinary tract infection in men: what's new; what's true?, *Am J Med* 106(3):327-334, 1999.
*At least 10 white blood cells per high-power field (WBCs/hpf).
†Prostatic massage is contraindicated; examination and culture of urine are sufficient.

Signs and Symptoms

If the kidney stone is small, patients may not experience any symptoms of the condition. However, if the stone is large enough to block the ureters, patients may experience intermittent intense pain. Pain usually begins in the lower back and may last 5 to 15 minutes. As the stone moves from the kidney toward the bladder, the patient may feel pain near the abdomen, groin, or genitals. Additional symptoms may include blood in the urine, cloudy or foul-smelling urine, nausea, vomiting, and constant urge to urinate. In some patients the renal calculus may cause infection.

Diagnosis

Imaging studies (e.g., CT, MRI) may be performed if kidney stones are suspected. These scans allow health care providers to detect kidney stones.

Lupus Nephritis

Lupus nephritis is inflammation of the kidney caused by *systemic lupus erythematosus* (SLE), an autoimmune disease. The disease affects both males and females. Lupus nephritis occurs in approximately 50% of patients during the first year following a diagnosis of SLE.[8] It is a rare disease but a strong predictor of poor outcome in patients with SLE.

Signs and Symptoms

Some patients with SLE have no evidence of kidney disease. Others may experience weight gain, hypertension, dark urine, or swelling around the eyes, legs, ankles, or fingers.

Diagnosis

The diagnosis of lupus nephritis involves urine and blood tests and possibly kidney biopsy. Urinalysis will determine if there is blood or protein in the urine. Blood tests may be performed to evaluate antinuclear antibodies (ANAs), blood urea nitrogen (BUN), and creatinine. A kidney biopsy will confirm the diagnosis as well as the progression of the disease.

Pelvic Inflammatory Disease

Pelvic inflammatory disease (PID) is an infection of the female reproductive organs that causes pain and swelling. PID usually develops when a sexually transmitted bacterium enters the uterus and reproduces in the upper genital tract. The most common bacteria causing PID also cause the sexually transmitted diseases (STDs) gonorrhea and chlamydia. If left untreated, PID may lead to long-term pelvic pain. It may also result in infertility if the fallopian tubes are partially blocked or damaged. Complications during pregnancy may also occur, such as ectopic pregnancy.

Signs and Symptoms

Common symptoms of PID include pain in the lower abdomen and pelvis, irregular menstrual bleeding, foul-smelling vaginal discharge, lower back pain, fever, fatigue, diarrhea, vomiting, pain during intercourse, and difficulty or pain during urination.

Diagnosis

A diagnosis of PID is made after pelvic examination, cervical culture, and analysis of the vaginal discharge. During a pelvic exam, a small instrument called a speculum is inserted into the vagina, and the clinician is able to examine the vagina, cervix, and uterus. The reproductive organs, including the uterus, will appear inflamed during a pelvic exam. Cervical cultures and analyses of vaginal discharge are performed to detect bacteria known to cause PID. If bacteria are present, a positive diagnosis is made.

SELECTED HERBAL THERAPIES

 Note

To help make this educational resource more interactive, all pharmacokinetics, adverse effects, and interactions data have been compiled in Appendix A. Safety data specifically related to pregnancy and lactation are listed in Appendix B. Please refer to these appendices when working through the case studies and answering the review questions.

African Wild Potato (*Hypoxis hemerocallidea*)

Grade C: *Unclear or conflicting scientific evidence (benign prostatic hyperplasia)*

Mechanism of Action

Major components of the African wild potato are phytosterols such as beta-sitosterol,[9,10] beta-sitosterin,[11] and sitosterin[12] and lectinlike proteins such as agglutinins.[13] The rhizomes of some species contain glycosides of uncommon aglucons, which may be considered *norlignans*.[14]

Beta-sitosterol is thought to decrease prostate proliferation and to improve the symptoms of BPH. Animal and human studies report the African wild potato to be useful in prostate cancer and BPH.[10,12,15-21]

Scientific Evidence of Effectiveness

Clinical evidence indicates that African wild potato is a potentially effective treatment option for BPH. The mechanism of action is unclear; the effect may be attributed to β-sitosterol.

A literature review and meta-analysis was performed with the following inclusion criteria: men with symptomatic BPH treated for at least 30 days with a phytotherapeutic preparation (alone or combined) and compared with placebo controls.[17] A total of 18 trials involving 2939 men were reviewed (4 studies with 519 men for African potato). *Hypoxis rooperi* was demonstrated to be effective in improving symptom scores and flow measures compared with placebo. However, review of the literature found inadequate reporting of outcomes, which currently limits the determination of safety and efficacy. Adverse events caused by phytotherapies were generally mild and infrequent. Randomized studies of *Serenoa repens*, alone or in combination with other plant extracts, have provided the strongest evidence for efficacy and tolerability in treatment of BPH compared with other phytotherapies. *H. rooperi* and *Secale cereale* also appear to improve BPH symptoms, although the evidence is weaker for these products. The authors concluded that overall, phytotherapies are inexpensive and well tolerated, generally with mild and infrequent adverse effects.

A multicenter, randomized, double-blind, placebo-controlled clinical trial was conducted to assess the efficacy and safety of 130 mg free beta-sitosterol (phytosterol) daily, using the International Prostate Symptom Score (IPSS) as the primary outcome variable.[10] In total, 177 patients with BPH were recruited for 6 months of treatment. The drug used in the trial consisted of a chemically defined extract of phytosterols, derived from species of *Pinus*, *Picea*, or *Hypoxis*, with β-sitosterol as the main component. Those treated with β-sitosterol showed significant ($p <0.01$) improvement over placebo; the mean difference in the IPSS between placebo and β-sitosterol, adjusted for the initial values, was 5.4, and in the quality-of-life index was 0.9. Significant improvements were also seen in the secondary outcome variables, with an increase in maximum urinary flow rate (Qmax, 4.5 mL/sec) and decrease in PVR (33.5 mL) in favor of β-sitosterol.

Dose

For BPH, treatment doses have included 60 to 130 mg daily of beta-sitosterol, in two or three divided doses.[10]

Adverse Effects, Interactions, Pharmacokinetics. See Appendix A.

Beta-Sitosterol (β-Sitosterol), Sitosterol (22,23-dihydrostigmasterol, 24-ethylcholesterol)

Grade B: *Good scientific evidence (benign prostatic hyperplasia)*

Mechanism of Action

Beta-sitosterol appears to inhibit 5α-reductase,[22,23] which metabolizes testosterone into DHT. Agents that inhibit this enzyme appear to reduce the size of the prostate gland and consequently reduce the symptoms of BPH. Beta-sitosterol has also been found to have antiproliferative effects and to inhibit growth factors on prostate tissue, which may contribute to its beneficial effects.[24]

Scientific Evidence of Effectiveness

Beta-sitosterol and β-sitosterol glucoside have been used to treat symptoms of BPH. Several studies have analyzed the effects of phytosterols on BPH.[25-38] Both subjective and objective symptom improvements (e.g., IPSS, Q_{max}, PVR) have been inconsistently demonstrated.[23,28,37-39] Beta-sitosterol has been associated with reducing urinary symptoms associated with BPH and prostatitis, including increased urine flow and reduced PVR;[10,38] however, a reduction in prostate size has not been noted.[25,26,30,38]

Dose

For BPH, 60 to 130 mg of beta-sitosterol divided into two or three daily doses has been used.

Adverse Effects, Interactions, Pharmacokinetics. See Appendix A.

Chamomile (*Matricaria recutita*, syn. *Matricaria suaveolens*, *Matricaria chamomilla*, *Anthemis nobilis*, *Chamaemelum nobile*, *Chamomilla chamomilla*, *Chamomilla recutita*)

Grade C: *Unclear or conflicting scientific evidence (hemorrhagic cystitis, vaginitis)*

Mechanism of Action

The exact mechanism by which chamomile may affect hemorrhagic cystitis and vaginitis is not well understood; however, this agent appears to exhibit antiinflammatory and antibacterial effects.[40-44]

Several constituents of chamomile have been studied for their antiinflammatory activity, including apigenin-7-glucoside, luteoline, terpene compounds, herniarine, matricin, chamazulene, (–)-alpha-bisabololoxides A and B, (–)-alpha-bisabolol, patuletin, umbelliferone, quercetin, myricetin, rutin, and spiroethers. However, most studies have found that the whole extracts were more active than their individual constituents. *Chamazulene, alpha-bisabolol,* and *apigenin* have the highest antiinflammatory actions against proinflammatory agents. *Matricin*, the precursor of chamazulene, demonstrates antiinflammatory activity that is superior to chamazulene. In vitro, chamomile extract has been found to inhibit both cyclooxygenase (COX) and lipoxygenase and therefore prostaglandins and leukotrienes.[45] Chamazulene inhibits leukotriene B_4 (LTB_4).[41] Both bisabolol and bisabolol oxide have been shown to inhibit 5-lipoxygenase. Apigenin inhibits histamine and serotonin release.

Antibacterial activity of chamomile has been studied in vitro, with encouraging results. It was most effective against *Staphylococcus aureus*, *Streptococcus mutans*, and *Streptococcus salivarius*, but it also had bactericidal activity against *Bacillus megatherium*, *Leptospira icterohaemorrhagiae*, and *Trichomonas*.[44]

Scientific Evidence of Effectiveness

HEMORRHAGIC CYSTITIS (BLADDER IRRITATION WITH BLEEDING). Preliminary evidence suggests that the combination of chamomile baths plus chamomile bladder washes and antibiotics is superior to antibiotics alone for hemorrhagic cystitis.[46]

VAGINITIS. A before-and-after study was conducted to evaluate the treatment of vaginitis with a chamomile-extract vaginal douche.[48] Thirty symptomatic female subjects of fertile age were given 20 mL of diluted chamomile twice daily for 15 days (including during menstruation). Outcome measures included microscopic evaluation of vaginal secretions, bacteriology, odor, and edema. All patients showed improvement and tolerated treatment.

Dose

The dose of chamomile for hemorrhagic cystitis has not been determined. For vaginitis, a douche of 30 mL diluted chamomile has been used twice daily for 15 days.[47]

Adverse Effects, Interactions, Pharmacokinetics. See Appendix A.

Coleus (Coleus forskohlii)

Grade C: *Unclear or conflicting scientific evidence (erectile dysfunction)*

Mechanism of Action

Forskolin, a component of coleus classified as a diterpene derivative, is a potent activator of the enzyme adenylate cyclase, which activates cyclic adenosine monophosphate (cAMP) in the cell. It may act as an intracavernosal vasoactive agent in the management of vasculogenic impotence caused by vascular dysfunction.[48]

Scientific Evidence of Effectiveness

Promising evidence supporting coleus as an ED treatment was obtained from a series of in vitro and in vivo studies,[49] which demonstrated synergistic effects of forskolin with prostaglandin E_1 (PGE_1), which resulted in augmented cAMP synthesis and enhanced corporeal smooth muscle relaxation. An open case series found preliminary evidence of efficacy and safety of forskolin in combination with other vasoactive agents in patients with vasculogenic impotence resistant to standard three-agent pharmacotherapy (papaverine, phentolamine, PGE_1).[48] Improved rigidity and erection duration was experienced by 61% of patients using intracavernosal forskolin (98 mcg/mL), papaverine (29 mg/mL), phentolamine (0.98 mg/mL), and PGE_1 (9.8 mcg/mL) at 11 to 18 months of follow-up.

Dose

The dose of coleus alone for ED has not been determined; however, forskolin at 98 mcg/mL has been used in a combination product.[48]

Adverse Effects, Interactions, Pharmacokinetics. See Appendix A.

Cranberry (Vaccinium macrocarpon)

Grade C: *Unclear or conflicting scientific evidence (kidney stones)*

Mechanism of Action

Although cranberry contains small amounts of oxalate, which may potentially promote calcium oxalate stone formation, it also increases magnesium and potassium excretion, which can decrease the rate of stone formation.[50,51]

Scientific Evidence of Effectiveness

The effect of cranberry on kidney stone formation is unclear. According to preliminary research, cranberry juice of unspecified amounts decreased urinary calcium by 50% in patients with renal stones.[52] However, it has also been found to increase urine levels of oxalate. It currently remains unclear whether cranberry will increase or decrease the risk of kidney stones.

Dose

Cranberry products are not widely standardized, though some preparations are standardized to 11% to 12% quinic acid per dose. In general, cranberry juice contains glucose, fructose, ascorbic acid, benzoic acid, citric acid, quinic acid, malic acid, proanthocyanidins, triterpenoids, catechins, lectins, and 90% water. The dose of cranberry for nephrolithiasis (kidney stones) has not been determined.

Adverse Effects, Interactions, Pharmacokinetics. See Appendix A.

Damiana (Turnera diffusa)

Grade C: *Unclear or conflicting scientific evidence (sexual dysfunction)*

Mechanism of Action

According to animal evidence, damiana may increase performance and achievement of ejaculation.[53] However, the exact mechanism of action is not well understood.

Scientific Evidence of Effectiveness

Damiana has been traditionally used as an aphrodisiac. Two clinical studies found that ArginMax (combination of damiana, *Ginkgo biloba*, *Panax ginseng*, L-arginine, and multivitamin/minerals) improved sexual function in menopausal women and those with *hyposexual disorder* (low sexual desire).[54,55] The studies were well conducted with large sample sizes. However, the studies were performed with a multiherb/vitamin combination product, so the effect of damiana alone as a supplement for sexual function in women is difficult to interpret.

Dose

Because there is a lack of research using damiana monotherapy to treat sexual dysfunction, the dose of damiana alone for sexual dysfunction has not been established.

Adverse Effects, Interactions, Pharmacokinetics. See Appendix A.

Danshen (Salvia miltiorrhiza)

Grade C: *Unclear or conflicting scientific evidence (kidney disease; prostatitis)*

Mechanism of Action

Danshen may improve blood circulation and increase the rate of urinary clearance, which may help slow the progression of renal failure after renal transplantation.[56] However, the exact mechanism of action of danshen in prostatitis and renal failure is not clear.

Scientific Evidence of Effectiveness

KIDNEY DISEASE. In an RCT, patients were injected with danshen in the early stages after renal transplantation.[56] Use of danshen in addition to conventional medications resulted in a significant increase in urine volume and endogenous creatinine clearance rate and a significant decrease in serum creatine, incidence of renal function recovery impairment, blood viscosity, platelet aggregation, and blood flow resistance in the graft.

PROSTATITIS. There is somewhat unclear evidence from a clinical trial, which found danshen plus Western medicine to be less effective than Western medicine plus warming needle moxibustion (burning an herb close to the skin to facilitate healing).[57]

Dose

Danshen is often used in combination with other therapeutic agents, and standardized preparations are not widely used in the available literature. The dose of danshen for kidney disease or prostatitis has not been determined.

Adverse Effects, Interactions, Pharmacokinetics. See Appendix A.

Ephedra (Ephedra sinica)

Grade C: *Unclear or conflicting scientific evidence (aphrodisiac)*

Mechanism of Action

Ephedra contains the alkaloids ephedrine and pseudoephedrine.[58] Ephedrine stimulates alpha-adrenergic and beta-adrenergic receptors. Sexual arousal by ephedrine may be caused by increased sympathetic (adrenaline-dependent) nervous system reaction.[59]

Scientific Evidence of Effectiveness

According to preliminary research, epinephrine enhances plethysmographic (VPA and vaginal blood volume) measures of sexual arousal in women.[59] Ephedrine had no significant influence on subjective measures of sexual arousal, suggesting that physiological sexual arousal noted with ephedrine administration probably is not caused by changes in cognitive factors, such as mood. This study only examined the effects of ephedrine on sexual response in women, which limits generalizability.

Dose

The dose of ephedra for sexual arousal has not been determined.

Adverse Effects, Interactions, Pharmacokinetics. See Appendix A.

Flax (Linum usitatissimum)

Grade C: *Unclear or conflicting scientific evidence (lupus nephritis)*

Mechanism of Action

Flaxseed and flaxseed oil (also known as linseed oil) are rich sources of the essential fatty acid alpha-linolenic acid (ALA), which is a biological precursor to omega-3 fatty acids such as eicosapentaenoic acid. ALA has a variety of antiinflammatory, antioxidant, and lipid-lowering properties, potentially reducing the progression of nephritis and vascular disease associated with lupus.[69,70]

Scientific Evidence of Effectiveness

Flaxseed fed to rats with polycystic kidneys has reportedly increased citrate excretion and reduced histological damage.[71] In animal models of nephritis, mice fed diets supplemented with flaxseed or its constituent (secoisolariresinol diglucoside) had a delay in the development of proteinuria, better preservation of glomerular filtration rate, and significantly reduced mortality compared with controls.[72-75]

Several human studies have been conducted by the same research group, suggesting possible improvements in glomerular filtration rate (GFR) and serum creatinine levels in lupus nephritis patients treated with flaxseed.[73,76,77] However, stronger evidence is warranted in this area before a recommendation can be made.

Dose

Flaxseed (30 g daily) has been used to improve GFR and serum creatinine levels.

Adverse Effects, Interactions, Pharmacokinetics. See Appendix A.

Ginkgo (Ginkgo biloba)

Grade C: *Unclear or conflicting scientific evidence (decreased libido, sexual dysfunction, and erectile dysfunction [impotence])*

Mechanism of Action

Based on its vasodilatory effects (possibly related to the inhibition of nitric oxide), *Ginkgo biloba* may effectively treat ED.[78] According to animal and human studies, ginkgo possesses vascular smooth muscle relaxant properties, which may act on corpus cavernosum tissue[79] and has been reported to improve penile blood flow in patients with ED.[80]

Scientific Evidence of Effectiveness

Ginkgo has been used traditionally to treat sexual dysfunction in both men and women. Ginkgo reportedly is beneficial in antidepressant-induced sexual dysfunction, including the reduction of fluoxetine-induced "genital anesthesia."[81-83] In an open study, ginkgo has been shown to improve ED in men unresponsive to the vasodilator papaverine.[80] Similar results were noted in a subsequent published case series by the same research group.[84] Notably, these subjects had responded to intracavernous injections of papaverine before the study. Improved blood flow was noted in all subjects on ultrasonography compared to baseline, although statistical analysis was not documented.

Two clinical studies found that ArginMax (combination of Ginkgo biloba, damiana, Panax ginseng, L-arginine, and multivitamin/minerals) improved sexual function in menopausal and hyposexual females.[54,55] The studies were well conducted with large sample sizes. However, the studies were performed with a multiherb/vitamin combination product, so the effectiveness of Panax ginseng as a monotherapy for sexual function in women is unclear.

Dose
For decreased libido and ED, 240 mg of Ginkgo biloba has been taken daily for 12 weeks.[82]

Adverse Effects, Interactions, Pharmacokinetics. See Appendix A.

Ginseng (Panax spp.)

Grade C: *Unclear or conflicting scientific evidence (erectile dysfunction, premature ejaculation, sexual function in women)*

Mechanism of Action
Ginsenosides, the active constituents of ginseng, enhance nitric-oxide release from nitrergic nerves in tissue samples of rabbit corpus cavernosum[85,86] and cause relaxation of the smooth muscle.[87] In a clinical trial of 90 patients with erectile dysfunction, ginseng saponins changed early detumescence and penile rigidity, penile girth, and libido.[88]

Scientific Evidence of Effectiveness
ERECTILE DYSFUNCTION. Preliminary evidence suggests that Panax ginseng may effectively improve the signs and symptoms of erectile dysfunction. Studies have found Panax ginseng to be superior to placebo and trazodone in the treatment of erectile dysfunction.[88,89] Rigidity, swelling, libido, and patient satisfaction were improved in the ginseng group.

PREMATURE EJACULATION. Clinical research has assessed the efficacy of a topical cream containing ginseng as well as nine other agents (clove, angelica root, Cistanche deserticola, zanthoxyl species, torlidis seed, clove flower, asiasari root, cinnamon bark, and toad venom) in the treatment of premature ejaculation.[90] Despite the fact that the contribution of ginseng to this effect was not evaluated, this finding deserves further scientific attention.

SEXUAL FUNCTION IN WOMEN. Two clinical studies found that ArginMax (a combination of Panax ginseng, L-arginine, Ginkgo biloba, damiana, and multivitamin/minerals) improved sexual function in menopausal and hyposexual women.[54,55] The studies were well conducted with large sample sizes. However, the studies were performed with a multi-herb/vitamin combination product, so the effectiveness of P. ginseng as a monotherapy for sexual function in women is unclear.

Dose
Because it has been used in combination with other agents (L-arginine, ginkgo, damiana, vitamins, minerals), the dose of ginseng alone for premature ejaculation and sexual dysfunction is unclear.

Adverse Effects, Interactions, Pharmacokinetics. See Appendix A.

Grapefruit (Citrus x paradisi)

Grade C: *Unclear or conflicting scientific evidence (kidney stones)*

Mechanism of Action
The effects of grapefruit in the prevention of kidney stones are not clear. In seven healthy subjects with no history of kidney stones, ingestion of a soft drink containing grapefruit juice diluted to 10% in mineral water increased urinary excretion of citrate, calcium, and magnesium compared to subjects who consumed mineral water.[91]

Grapefruit has also been associated with an increased risk of kidney stones,[92,93] although the mechanism is not clear. Naringin, a flavone found in grapefruit, apparently is excreted in the urine[94] and binds to calcium, which is delivered to the renal system. Stone formation may be caused by high renal concentrations of calcium and probably unrelated to alteration in urinary pH or absorption of oxalate.[92]

Scientific Evidence of Effectiveness
Research on the use of grapefruit for kidney stones is limited and conflicting.[91-93] One small study found that a soft drink containing 10% grapefruit juice may have a beneficial effect in the prevention of calcium renal stones.[91] However, two large epidemiological studies linked drinking grapefruit juice to an increased risk of kidney stones.[92,93] Further research is needed to clarify the effect of grapefruit on kidney stone formation.

Dose
The dose of grapefruit for kidney stones has not been determined.

Adverse Effects, Interactions, Pharmacokinetics. See Appendix A.

Horny Goat Weed (Epimedium grandiflorum)

Grade C: *Unclear or conflicting scientific evidence (sexual dysfunction in renal failure patients)*

Mechanism of Action

Animal studies indicate that horny goat weed may increase nitric oxide (NO) levels, which relax smooth muscle and allow more blood to flow to the penis or clitoris.[95] Horny goat weed also appears to inhibit phosphodiesterase type 5 enzyme inhibitor (PDE-5), resulting in vasodilation in the corpus cavernosum of the penis and increasing testosterone production, which may increase libido.[9,96-100]

Scientific Evidence of Effectiveness

Horny goat weed is traditionally used to increase fertility and enhance sexual desire. According to folklore, it was discovered when a Chinese goat herder noticed enhanced sexual activity in his flock after they consumed the weed. One controlled trial suggests that *Epimedium* might improve sexual performance and quality of life in patients with renal failure undergoing chronic hemodialysis.[101]

Dose

Dosing regimen for horny goat weed is based on traditional health practice patterns and expert opinion. Reliable human trials demonstrating safety or efficacy for a particular dose are lacking.

For sexual dysfunction, 6 to 15 g daily has been used. A decoction (5 g horny goat weed simmered in 250 mL water for 10-15 minutes) three times daily also has been used; duration was not noted. A similar amount of horny goat weed in the form of granules (freeze-dried grains from decocted herb) or powdered herb in capsules has been used for sexual dysfunction (duration not specified).

Adverse Effects, Interactions, Pharmacokinetics. See Appendix A.

Maca (Lepidium meyenii)

Grade C: *Unclear or conflicting scientific evidence (aphrodisiac in men; increased sperm count)*

Mechanism of Action

Maca is rich in plant sterols such as beta-sitosterol.[102] Its effects on sexual function may be caused by these compounds, as well as benzyl- and *p*-methoxygenzyl glucosinolates.[103-106] Maca may improve penile endothelial L-arginine–NO activity.[107] Testosterone levels increased significantly in mice that received maca, which may explain its ability to stimulate sexual desire.[108,109]

Based on animal studies, maca appears to stimulate spermatogenesis by acting on the initial stages of sperm development (IX-XIV).[110,111] Treatment with maca has also resulted in increased seminal volume, sperm count, motile sperm count, and sperm motility.[109,110,112]

Scientific Evidence of Effectiveness

APHRODISIAC IN MEN. In Peru, maca has been used as an aphrodisiac for centuries. Preliminary evidence indicates that maca could improve sexual desire, according to self-perception of healthy men.[113] However, the use of an unvalidated tool to assess the primary outcome of subjective sexual desire and the lack of description of blinding techniques are significant shortcomings. Higher-quality studies are needed in this area, in both men and women.

INCREASED SPERM COUNT. Maca has also been used to enhance fertility and spermatogenesis in both humans and animals. A small, uncontrolled study provides some preliminary evidence that maca may improve semen quality, which was not associated with changes in hormone levels.[112]

Dose

To increase spermatogenesis, 1500 to 3000 mg has been taken daily for 8 to 12 weeks.[113]

Adverse Effects, Interactions, Pharmacokinetics. See Appendix A.

Muira Puama (Ptychopetalum olacoides)

Grade C: *Unclear or conflicting scientific evidence (erectile dysfunction; sexual dysfunction in women)*

Mechanism of Action

The lipophilic constituent *lupeol* was identified in the bark of muira puama bark. Lupeol content is much higher in the bark of *Ptychopetalum olacoides* than in *Ptychopetalum uncinatum*.[114] Muira puama is proposed to have testosterone-like properties, which may contribute to its ability to stimulate sexual desire.[115] Relaxation of the corpus cavernosum can be related to penile erection; in rabbits, the extract showed dose-dependent relaxation effects.[116]

Scientific Evidence of Effectiveness

ERECTILE DYSFUNCTION. Muira puama has long been used by Brazilian indigenous people as a treatment for impotence. Three preliminary case series suggest efficacy, but overall evidence is weak; furthermore, all were published by the same research group.[117-119] Significant improvements were seen in patients with low libido, reduced coital frequency, absent morning erections, latent time to achieve maximal erection, instability of erection during coitus, excessive feelings of postcoital fatigue, and global inadequacy described as "erectile dysfunction."

SEXUAL DYSFUNCTION IN WOMEN. Muira puama has also historically been recommended to enhance libido. Recent clinical data suggest that muira puama in combination with *Ginkgo biloba* (Herbal vY) may enhance libido.[120] A study in women showed improvements in intensity of sexual desires, ability to reach orgasm, intensity of orgasm, and excitement of sexual fantasies based on a nine-point Likert scale. Well-designed, adequately powered human trials of the single agent versus placebo or standard of care, as well as safety data, are necessary before a conclusion can be made in this area. The same authors who conducted the ED studies also conducted the available study for sexual dysfunction in women.

Dose
For ED, subjects received six tablets, each containing 430 mg of muira puama (HV 430), daily for 10 days.[117] From 10 to 16 drops of a muira puama tincture has been mixed with a small amount of water and used topically three times daily on genitalia for 1 month and repeated every 3 months.[121]

Adverse Effects, Interactions, Pharmacokinetics. See Appendix A.

Nopal (*Opuntia* spp.)

Grade C: *Unclear or conflicting evidence (benign prostatic hyperplasia)*

Mechanism of Action
Nopal, also called "prickly pear," appears to inhibit aromatase and 5α-reductase activity.[122] It may also interfere with free-radical processes. These mechanisms may explain the benefits of nopal for BPH.

Scientific Evidence of Effectiveness
Preliminary evidence suggests that prickly pear flowers may help reduce symptoms of BPH, which include urinary urgency, emergency urination, and the feeling of bladder fullness.[123]

Dose
Prickly pear flowers were dried, ground, and packed into 250-mg gelatin capsules. Subjects took two capsules three times daily for 2 to 6 months.[123]

Adverse Effects, Interactions, Pharmacokinetics. See Appendix A.

Pycnogenol (*Pinus pinaster* subsp. *atlantica*)

Grade C: *Unclear or conflicting scientific evidence (erectile dysfunction)*

Note: Pycnogenol contains oligomeric proanthocyanidins (OPCs) as well as several other bioflavonoids. There has been some confusion in the U.S. market regarding OPC products containing Pycnogenol or grape seed extract (GSE) because one of the generic terms for chemical constituents ("pycnogenols") is the same as the patented trade name (Pycnogenol).

Some GSE products formerly were erroneously labeled and marketed in the United States as containing "pycnogenols." Although GSE and Pycnogenol do contain similar chemical constituents (primarily in OPC fraction), the chemical, pharmacological, and clinical literature on the two products is distinct. The term *Pycnogenol* should therefore be used only when referring to this specific proprietary pine bark extract. Scientific literature regarding this product should not be referenced as a basis for the safety or effectiveness of GSE.

Mechanism of Action
The proposed mechanism of Pycnogenol for erectile dysfunction involves increasing the production of nitric oxide (NO) by NO synthase.[124] NO causes the arteries to dilate, increasing blood flow into the penile tissues.

Scientific Evidence of Effectiveness
Pycnogenol, alone or in combination with L-arginine, may improve ED.[124,125] Men reported improvement from "moderate" to "mild" ED, as determined with the International Index of Erectile Function (IIEF-5).[125]

Dose
Men using Pycnogenol (120 mg) daily for 3 months had improved measures of erectile function.[125] Improvements were also noted when Pycnogenol was combined with 1.7 g of L-arginine daily.[124]

Adverse Effects, Interactions, Pharmacokinetics. See Appendix A.

Pygeum (*Prunus africanum*, syn. *Pygeum africanum*)

Grade B: *Good scientific evidence (benign prostatic hyperplasia)*

Mechanism of Action
Pygeum contains ferulic acid esters of fatty acids, phytoesterols, and triterpenes. Preliminary research reported reductions in urethral obstruction and improved bladder function.[126-130] Laboratory studies report inhibition of enzymes, including 5-lipoxygenase[131] and 5α-reductase,[132] a mechanism similar to the prescription drug finasteride. Stimulation of secretory activity of the prostate and seminal vesicles has been reported in rats and humans.[133,134]

Scientific Evidence of Effectiveness
Extracts of *Prunus africanum* bark may moderately improve urinary symptoms associated with enlarged prostate gland or prostate inflammation. Numerous controlled trials in humans[135-157] and meta-analyses[135,158,159] report significant reductions in the number of nighttime urinary episodes (nocturia), urinary hesitancy, urinary frequency, and pain with urination (dysuria) in men who experience mild to moderate

symptoms. However, pygeum does not appear to reduce the size of the prostate gland or reverse the process of BPH. It is unclear how pygeum compares to the effectiveness or safety of other medical therapies, such as prescription drugs (e.g., α-adrenergic blockers, 5α-reductase inhibitors), surgical approaches, or other herbs or supplements (e.g., saw palmetto).

Overall, the scientific evidence supports the benefits of pygeum. Better research would strengthen the scientific support for this therapy, and research is ongoing. It is recommended that patients with BPH seek medical advice about the various available treatment options.

Dose

The active components of *Prunus africanum* bark extract have not been identified. Tadenan (Laboratoires DEBAT, Garches, France), the most popular and most frequently studied brand in Europe, is a lipophilic extract of *P. africanum* standardized to 13% total sterols. Other guidelines specify standardization to 14% triterpenes with 0.5% *n*-docosanol.[137] One capsule of Tadenan contains 50 mg of standardized extract. Other studied brands include Pigenil (Inverni della Beffa, Milan, Italy), Harzol (Hoyer, Germany), and Prostatonin (Pharmaton SA, Lugano, Switzerland). Some brands may contain other herbs in addition to pygeum.

Capsules of standardized pygeum extract (75-200 mg), taken daily as a single dose or two equal doses, have been studied.[141,143] Pygeum (25 mg) has also used in combination with stinging nettle (*Urtica dioica*, 300 g), which showed some efficacy in treating BPH and its symptoms.[160]

Adverse Effects, Interactions, Pharmacokinetics. See Appendix A.

Red Clover *(Trifolium pratense)*

Grade C: *Unclear or conflicting scientific evidence (benign prostatic hyperplasia)*

Mechanism of Action

The mechanism of red clover in BPH is not well understood. In animal study, red clover constituents (biochanin A, formononetin, genistein, daidzein) displayed antiandrogenic properties, which may explain effects on prostate growth.[161]

Scientific Evidence of Effectiveness

A study presented at the Endocrine Society's 82nd annual meeting in 2000 outlined a case series of red clover isoflavones (Trinovin) used for BPH symptomatology.[162] Three months of treatment decreased mean nocturia frequency, increased urine flow rates, improved quality-of-life score, and decreased IPSS. PSA values, blood biochemistry, and hematology were not altered from baseline, and prostate size remained unchanged. The abstract did not disclose the estimated prostate volumes for the study participants on enrollment, an important variable in the assessment of disease severity and projected response to therapy. Although these results are suggestive, BPH is a chronic condition meriting a long-term study of outcomes, comparison to standard of care, and adequate reporting of methodology. Notably, this study was funded by an unrestricted educational grant from Novogen, the manufacturer of Trinovin.

Dose

A dose used for BPH was one or two 500-mg tablets Trinovin (standardized to 40 mg of red clover isoflavones per tablet) taken daily by mouth.[162]

Adverse Effects, Interactions, Pharmacokinetics. See Appendix A.

Rye *(Secale cereale)*

Grade B: *Good scientific evidence (benign prostatic hyperplasia)*

Grade C: *Unclear or conflicting scientific evidence (prostatitis)*

Mechanism of Action

The mechanism of rye grass for BPH is unclear; however, evidence suggests that rye grass may act on α-adrenergic receptors and may relax the internal and external sphincter muscles.[163,164]

Scientific Evidence of Effectiveness

BENIGN PROSTATIC HYPERPLASIA. Cernilton, prepared from the rye grass pollen *Secale cereale,* is a popular phytotherapeutic agent for mild to moderate BPH and has been used in various clinical trials.[164-168] Cernilton improved self-rated urinary symptoms compared with placebo.[168] Rye grass reportedly improved symptoms of frequent urination, nocturia, urinary urgency, urinary incontinence, and painful urination.[165,166] Results are mixed on whether rye grass reduces prostate size or improves residual volume.[164,165,167,168] Studies have been generally of short duration with unknown standardization of preparations.

PROSTATITIS. Preliminary evidence suggests that 6 months of rye grass pollen extract (Cernilton N) may improve symptoms of prostatitis in people without complicating factors (urethral strictures, prostatic calculi, bladder neck sclerosis).[169]

Dose

Cernilton is a registered pharmaceutical throughout Western Europe, Japan, Korea, and Argentina.[168] One dose of Cernilton contains 60 mg of a water-soluble pollen extract fraction (Cernitin T60) and 3 mg of an acetone-soluble pollen extract fraction (Cernitin GBX).

Trials evaluating Cernilton for BPH have ranged from 12 to 24 weeks in duration, and used capsules of Cernilton two or three times daily.[165,167,168]

One tablet of Cernilton N, taken three times daily for 6 months, has been used for chronic prostatitis syndrome.[169]

Adverse Effects, Interactions, Pharmacokinetics. See Appendix A.

Saw Palmetto (Serenoa repens)

Grade A: *Strong scientific evidence (benign prostatic hyperplasia)*

Grade C: *Unclear or conflicting scientific evidence (hypotonic neurogenic bladder, prostatitis/chronic pelvic pain syndrome)*

Mechanism of Action

Active constituents within saw palmetto (*Serenoa repens, Sabal serrulata*) may be sterols and fatty acids, such as myristoleic acid.[170] The exact mechanism of action is unknown. Saw palmetto may increase the metabolism and excretion of dihydrotestosterone (DHT) through inhibition of cellular and nuclear receptor binding. Saw palmetto extract has demonstrated inhibition of androgen activity through competition with DHT at the androgen receptor in several animal and human tissue culture studies.[171-174] It has been shown to inhibit 5α-reductase activity on testosterone in vitro, thereby preventing the conversion of testosterone to DHT. However, evidence of 5α-reductase inhibition from RCTs is conflicting.[175-180]

The possible estrogenic effects of saw palmetto may come from β-sitosterol,[181] although subsequent evaluation reports possible competitive inhibitory effects on estrogen receptor binding.[182]

Scientific Evidence of Effectiveness

BENIGN PROSTATIC HYPERPLASIA. Saw palmetto has a long history of use as a treatment for BPH.[183] A 2006 report noted that more than 2 million men in the United States used saw palmetto as a treatment for BPH, and it is often recommended as an alternative to conventional drugs approved by the U.S. Food and Drug Administration (FDA).[184] Numerous RCTs have reported that saw palmetto is superior to placebo and may be equivalent to the antiandrogenic agent finasteride (Proscar) (with fewer adverse effects) in the alleviation of nocturia, improvement of urine flow, reduction in PVR bladder volume, and improvement of quality of life (but possibly not measurable reduction in prostate size). However, the majority of studies have been brief (1-6 months), included small sample sizes, and have not employed standardized outcomes measurements (e.g., IPSS). Furthermore, more recent, well-designed trials failed to find any significant benefit of saw palmetto for BPH treatment. Nonetheless, the weight of available evidence favors the efficacy of saw palmetto for this indication. Despite the heterogeneity of study designs and results reporting, two pooled analyses have suggested modest benefits of saw palmetto.[185-187] One trial reported superiority of a European α-adrenergic agent (alfuzosin) over saw palmetto, although methodological weaknesses limit the clinical significance of this result.[188] Most available studies have used the standardized saw palmetto product Permixon.

HYPOTONIC NEUROGENIC BLADDER. There is currently insufficient evidence regarding the use of saw palmetto for the management of hypotonic neurogenic bladder (also known as underactive or flaccid neurogenic bladder). One available study reported improvement in bladder capacity and PVR volume in patients taking saw palmetto (Urgenin) with neurogenic bladder.[189]

PROSTATITIS/CHRONIC PELVIC PAIN SYNDROME. The available scientific evidence of saw palmetto as a prostatitis treatment is conflicting, with many studies evaluating saw palmetto as part of combination therapies, making it difficult to isolate the effects of saw palmetto.[190-193]

Dose

Standardized extracts of saw palmetto containing 80% to 95% sterols and fatty acids (liposterolic content) are often recommended.

For BPH, 320 mg daily in one dose or two divided doses (80%-90% liposterolic content) has been used in multiple clinical trials[184-195] and is recommended by the German Commission E. A dosing evaluation reports that taking two 160-mg tablets once daily may be as effective as 160 mg twice daily, although the lack of a placebo group limits the clinical significance of this finding.[196] Rectal administration of saw palmetto (640 mg once daily) extract was reported as clinically equivalent to oral administration (160 mg four times daily) in a 30-day controlled trial in 40 men; however, it is unclear whether this sample size was large enough to assess equivalence.[197]

For prostatitis/chronic pelvic pain syndrome, 320 mg daily of prostamol (saw palmetto plant extract) has been used.[191]

Soy (Glycine max)

Grade C: *Unclear or conflicting scientific evidence (kidney disease [chronic renal failure, nephrotic syndrome, proteinuria])*

Mechanism of Action

Although the exact mechanism of soy in renal disease has not been identified, beneficial effects may be attributed to nicotinamide-N, N-(3-amino-3-carboxypropyl)-azetidine-2-carboxylic acid (an angiotensin-converting enzyme inhibitor) and phytic acid (an antiinflammatory).[198]

Scientific Evidence of Effectiveness

Dietary soy has been suggested to reduce or ameliorate proteinuria in patients with nephrotic syndrome. Soy diets produced lower GFR, renal plasma flow, BUN, and 24-hour urine creatinine/phosphate than animal-based diets.[199,202,203]

Dose

A diet of 700 to 800 mg/kg soy protein daily for 4 months has displayed beneficial effects on proteinuria in nephrotic patients.[202]

Adverse Effects, Interactions, Pharmacokinetics. See Appendix A.

Stinging Nettle *(Urtica dioica)*

Grade C: *Unclear or conflicting scientific evidence (benign prostatic hyperplasia)*

Mechanism of Action

The mechanism of action of stinging nettle in BPH is not clear but may involve aromatase inhibition, sex hormone–binding globulin (SHBG), and epidermal growth factor (EGF). It appears to be less likely that 5α-reductase is involved. High doses of a methanolic extract have been found to inhibit 5α-reductase.[204]

Aromatase is a key enzyme in steroid (sex) hormone metabolism. It is responsible for the conversion of androgens into estrogens. Estrogens appear to be involved in the etiology of BPH. Therefore, inhibition of aromatase could improve prostatic disorders.[205] Some constituents of the methanol extract of stinging nettle root demonstrated weak to moderate aromatase inhibition (concentration dependent), including the secondary fatty alcohol 14-octacosanol, two pentacyclic triterpenes (oleanolic acid, ursolic acid), and the fatty 13-hydroxy-9,11-octadecadienoic acid.[204,206-208]

It seems that SHBG plays a role in the regulation of prostate cells. A hydroethanolic and a methanolic root extract interfered with DHT binding with SHBG.[206,209,210] An aqueous extract was able to inhibit SHBG binding to receptors on the membrane of human prostate cells.[206,211]

Stinging nettle directly inhibited cell proliferation and the binding of EGF to its receptor in a tumor cell line.[206,212] Subfractions of an aqueous ethanolic stinging nettle root extract inhibited growth of BPH tissue in vitro; a methanolic extract suppressed proliferation of BPH tissue ex vivo.[213-215] This activity may contribute to antiinflammatory and antiprostatic activity of the extracts.[206] The polysaccharide fraction of the 20% methanolic extract of stinging nettle roots decreased the induced growth of prostate gland by 33.8% in mice.[215] Chronic intraperitoneal administration of Bazoton solution at 20 mg/kg daily in male rats for 10 days induced a reduction in prostate weight.[216] A reduction in biological activity in prostate cells was noted on fluorescent microscopy, under the effect of extract of stinging nettle root in patients with BPH.[217]

Different organic-solvent extracts of nettle root have demonstrated inhibition of the Na^+,K^+-ATPases from human prostatic hyperplastic tissue.[206,218] Steroidal components in stinging nettle roots (e.g., stigmasterol, campesterol) showed inhibitory activity on BPH-enzyme activity. Consequently, prostate cell metabolism and growth were suppressed.

Scientific Evidence of Effectiveness

Stinging nettle is used frequently in Europe to treat symptoms associated with BPH. Several case studies and RCTs have demonstrated an improvement in symptoms and quality of life as a result of nettle therapy.[219-225] Improvements were noted in urinary frequency, nocturia, quality of urine flow, and dripping.[219-223] Stinging nettle may be used alone or in combination with other herbal products such as saw palmetto or pygeum.[226-230] Nettle appears to be an appropriate treatment for the alleviation of lower urinary tract symptoms associated with stage I or II BPH.

Dose

Nettle products are not consistently standardized. Various types of nettle, including capsules and extract, have been used in clinical trials for the treatment of BPH. Doses have included one or two Bazoton capsules (300 mg ERU) twice daily for up to 6 months.[219,221,222,225] Bazoton Liquidum has been used at 3 mL twice daily for 3 months.[220]

Adverse Effects, Interactions, Pharmacokinetics. See Appendix A.

Yohimbe *(Pausinystalia yohimbe)*

Grade C: *Unclear or conflicting scientific evidence (erectile dysfunction, sexual side effects of SSRIs, libido [women])*

Mechanism of Action

Yohimbe bark extract contains approximately 6% indole alkaloids, of which 10% to 15% is the active constituent yohimbine. A 1995 chemical analysis of 26 commercial yohimbe products reported that most contained virtually no yohimbine.[231] The pharmacological activity of yohimbine has been well characterized in studies, although these effects may or may not apply to yohimbe, depending on the concentration of yohimbine present.

Yohimbine acts as an α_2-adrenoceptor antagonist and is significantly more active at presynaptic adrenoceptors than postsynaptic receptors. This action blocks the decrease in both central noradrenergic response and peripheral sympathetic activity.[232-238] Yohimbine has also demonstrated dopamine antagonist and serotonin-like properties.[239]

The purported aphrodisiac effects of yohimbine may be caused by genital blood vessel dilation, nerve impulse transmission to genital tissue, and increased reflex excitability in the sacral spinal cord. Yohimbine is thought to be most effective for impotence in men with organic vascular dysfunction. The effects of yohimbe on ED are said to be mediated through increased penile blood flow and increased central excitatory impulses to the genital tissue.[240,241]

Scientific Evidence of Effectiveness

ERECTILE DYSFUNCTION. Yohimbine is an active indole alkaloid constituent found in the bark of the *Pausinystalia yohimbe* tree. Yohimbine hydrochloride (HCl), a standardized form of yohimbine available as a prescription drug in the United States, has been demonstrated in multiple clinical trials to be efficacious in the management of male impotence.[242-245] Although yohimbine alkaloid isolated from yohimbe bark has been used traditionally to reduce ED, clinical evidence specifically studying these effects of yohimbe bark extract are lacking. Notably, yohimbe bark extract generally contains low concentrations of yohimbine (6% indole alkaloids, of which only 10%-15% is yohimbine), and commercial preparations may or may not share the pharmacological and clinical effects of yohimbine HCl.[231] Therefore, although strong evidence supports the efficacy of yohimbine HCl in the management of certain types of ED, evidence is insufficient to support the use of yohimbe bark extract for this indication. It should be noted that currently, yohimbine HCl is less frequently used in the United States than other drug therapies such as sildenafil (Viagra). Additionally, the German Commission E does not recommend yohimbe bark for sexual disorders because of a high risk/benefit ratio.

SEXUAL SIDE EFFECTS OF SSRIs. Yohimbine HCl has been suggested as a potential agent to improve impaired sexual function resulting from the use of selective serotonin reuptake inhibitor (SSRI) antidepressants. However, there is currently limited human evidence in this area from methodologically weak studies (case series and single-blind study).[246-249] Therefore, insufficient scientific data exist to recommend for or against the use of yohimbine or yohimbe bark extract for SSRI effects.

LIBIDO (WOMEN). Yohimbine is primarily used in men to boost sexual desire. It has been shown to increase the number of erections and orgasms in impotent males.[250] Evidence of this effect is lacking in women. Preliminary evidence suggests that yohimbine may increase the female libido;[251] however, there is currently insufficient evidence demonstrating beneficial effects of yohimbine or over-the-counter (OTC) yohimbe preparations in this area.

Dose

Standardization has not been widely established to regulate the production of yohimbe bark extract products. A gas chromatographic chemical analysis of 26 commercial yohimbe products concluded that most contain virtually no yohimbine. Concentrations ranging from less than 0.1 up to 489 parts per million (ppm) of yohimbine were found in the products. Nine of the 26 had no yohimbine, and seven contained trace amounts (0.1-1 ppm) of yohimbine. This was compared to a standard product that contained 7089 ppm.[231] Yohimbine tablets are typically standardized to contain 5.4 mg of yohimbine HCl.

Recommended doses are based on those most often used in available trials for pharmaceutical standardized yohimbine HCl. Clinical trials are lacking regarding the administration of OTC yohimbe.

For ED, 15 to 30 mg yohimbine HCl daily in three divided doses (e.g., 5.4-10 mg three times daily) has been used.[242,244,245,252-256] More adverse effects may occur with higher doses.[257-259]

Adverse Effects, Interactions, Pharmacokinetics. See Appendix A.

HERBAL THERAPIES WITH LIMITED EVIDENCE

Clove (Syzygium aromaticum, syn. Eugenia aromaticum)

A topical cream containing clove and eight other herbal agents (*Panax ginseng* root, angelica root, *Cistanche deserticola*, zanthoxyl species, torlidis seed, asiasari root, cinnamon bark, toad venom) was used clinically to treat premature ejaculation.[90] Although results were promising, well-designed clinical trials assessing clove monotherapy are needed before recommending for or against the use of clove for premature ejaculation.

Cornflower (Centaurea cyanus)

Cornflower has been used in clinical study to examine its effects on urolithiasis recurrence; however, the results were unclear.[260]

Maitake Mushroom (Grifola frondosa), Shiitake Mushroom (Lentinus edodes)

Maitake and shiitake mushrooms have been suggested to help the body fight infections and cancer. Evidence is lacking regarding their effects in preventing or treating prostate conditions.

Milk Thistle (Silybum marianum)

Milk thistle has been used traditionally to "detoxify" the liver and as an antioxidant. Recent studies have reported that milk thistle may be effective against prostate cancer cells in vitro.[261] Caution is advised when taking milk thistle; adverse effects (e.g., drug interactions) are possible.

Quercetin

Some evidence suggests that quercetin, a bioflavonoid and antioxidant, may be useful for the treatment of chronic prostatitis. Further research is needed to confirm these results. Quercetin is reported to be safe in recommended dosages.

Herbs with Possible Genitourinary Effects*

HERB	SPECIFIC THERAPEUTIC USE(S)†	HERB	SPECIFIC THERAPEUTIC USE(S)†
Aconite	Urinary retention	Holy basil	Genitourinary disorders
Annatto	Urinary retention	Horsetail	Urinary tract inflammation, enuresis, (bed wetting), urinary incontinence
Asparagus	Urinary tract inflammation		
Barberry	Urinary tract disorders	Hydrangea	Urinary tract disorders
Belladonna	Urinary tract disorders, enuresis (bed-wetting)	Kava	Urinary tract disorders, urinary incontinence
Blue cohosh	Genitourinary disorders	Lime	Genitourinary tract disorders
Boldo	Urinary tract inflammation	Marshmallow	Urinary irritation
Buchu	Urinary tract disorders, incontinence	Meadowsweet	Urinary retention (from prostate enlargement)
Butterbur	Urinary tract disorders		
Calendula	Urinary retention	Morus nigra	Urinary incontinence
Cat's claw	Urinary tract inflammation	Mullein	Urinary tract disorders
Chaparral	Genitourinary infections	Noni	Urinary tract disorders
Cordyceps	Urinary incontinence (nocturia)	Psyllium	Incontinence
Dandelion	Urinary tract inflammation, frequent urination	Raspberry	Urinary tract disorders
		Rose hip	Urinary irritation
Garcinia	Urinary tract disorders	St. John's wort	Enuresis (bed-wetting)
Goldenrod	Urinary tract disorders	Shepherd's purse	Urinary retention
Goldenseal	Urinary tract disorders	Thyme	Enuresis (bed-wetting)
Gotu kola	Urinary retention	Valerian	Urinary tract disorders
Ground ivy	Urinary tract inflammation (chronic)	White water lily	Enuresis (bed-wetting)
Heartsease	Urinary tract inflammation, enuresis (bed-wetting)	Wild yam	Urinary tract disorders

*This is not an all-inclusive or comprehensive list of herbs with possible genitourinary effects; other herbs and supplements may possess these qualities. A qualified health care provider should be consulted with specific questions or concerns regarding potential genitourinary effects of agents or interactions.
†Based on expert opinion, anecdote, case reports, and/or preliminary trial evidence.

ADJUNCT THERAPIES

1. Common disorders of the genitourinary system include benign prostatic hyperplasia (BPH), erectile dysfunction (ED, impotence), and urinary incontinence. *Lifestyle choices,* including a low-fat diet, at least 30 minutes of daily exercise five times a week, and smoking cessation, may help to reduce symptoms of these conditions. Other integrative approaches, including psychological counseling and physical therapy, may provide additional benefit to conventional and nonconventional therapies for various genitourinary conditions.
2. *Psychological counseling* can help with ED caused by stress, anxiety, or depression. ED can also cause these issues. The individual and his partner may be instructed to visit a sex therapist, psychologist, or psychiatrist with experience in treating sexual problems. Qualified therapists work with couples to reduce tension, improve sexual communication, and create realistic expectations for sex, all of which may improve symptoms of ED. Therapists also help individuals work through issues such as sexual abuse as a child. Psychological therapy may be effective along with medical or surgical treatment. However, medicosurgical treatment may not help the man with ED from psychological causes.
3. A variety of techniques have been used to improve urinary incontinence, such as pelvic floor neuromuscular *electrostimulation* combined with exercises, or pelvic floor muscle exercises alone *(Kegel exercises)*. *Vaginal cones* and *vaginal balls* may also be used to increase the pelvic wall muscles. Vaginal cones or balls are inserted into the vagina and stimulate the pelvic floor muscles to contract and anchor them. Outcome measures include bladder volume, vaginal palpation, and perceptions of improvement. Overall, short-term improvements have been seen with pelvic floor exercises and vaginal balls.[262]
4. Genitourinary disorders such as BPH may increase the risk of developing urinary tract infections (UTIs). *Cranberry* may be useful in preventing UTIs; preliminary evidence

suggests that cranberry may prevent *Escherichia coli* from attaching to the bladder wall, thus preventing infection.[263-267] The acidity of cranberry and the reduction in urinary pH may prevent the malodor of fermenting urine from incontinent patients.[9]

5. *Acupuncture* may provide relief for a variety of conditions. It may be an effective treatment option in patients with genitourinary conditions caused by psychological factors, including stress, anxiety, and depression.

INTEGRATIVE THERAPY PLANS

Benign Prostatic Hyperplasia

- Gather a careful medical history, including a list of symptoms and other disorders that may contribute to voiding symptoms.
- Obtain a thorough medication history, including prescription and nonprescription medications and dietary supplements.
- Identify any drugs that may cause voiding symptoms, including ipratropium, albuterol, and epinephrine.
- Perform laboratory tests, and be aware of elevated serum BUN, creatinine values, and abnormal urinalysis.
- Prostate-specific antigen (PSA) and digital rectal examination (DRE) should be performed to screen for prostate cancer.
- Numerous human trials report that saw palmetto improves BPH symptoms such as nocturia, urine flow, and overall quality of life, although it may not greatly reduce prostate size. Evidence is lacking that saw palmetto is beneficial in the treatment of prostate cancer, and theoretically it may lower PSA values, making it more difficult to determine when a cancer is growing.
- Pygeum (*Prunus africanum*, syn. *Pygeum africanum*) has moderately improved urinary symptoms associated with prostate enlargement or prostate inflammation. Numerous human studies report that pygeum significantly reduces nocturia episodes, urinary hesitancy, urinary frequency, and pain with urination in men who experience mild to moderate symptoms. However, pygeum does not appear to reduce prostate size. It is unclear how pygeum's effectiveness or safety compares to that of other medical therapies, such as prescription drugs (e.g., alpha blockers, 5α-reductase inhibitors), surgical approaches, or other herbs/supplements (e.g., saw palmetto).
- Recommend that patients with BPH have annual PSA tests starting at age 50, or at age 40 if they are in high-risk groups, such as African-American men or those with male relatives with BPH.
- Advise the patient to record the amount of fluid intake, trips to the bathroom, and episodes of urine leakage every day over the course of several days to weeks. This record may have a pattern, and patients may be able to avoid accidents by planning to use the bathroom at certain times of the day. Once patients gain control over their bladders, they may be able to increase the time between urination.

Erectile Dysfunction

- Obtain a full medical history, including the frequency and duration of ED symptoms, presence or absence of morning erections, and quality of the relationship with sexual partner.
- Determine if the patient has any condition that may predispose him to ED, including arteriosclerosis, diabetes mellitus, hypertension, or concurrent medications.
- Recommend a psychosocial examination in an interview and questionnaire format to reveal psychological factors.
- Identify any drugs that may cause ED, including antidepressants, antihistamines, and antihypertensives.
- Obtain laboratory tests to check for underlying conditions that may cause ED. Tests should include thyroid function, blood glucose, lipid profile, and testosterone level.
- Yohimbine hydrochloride, a standardized form of yohimbine available as a prescription drug in the United States, is efficacious in the management of male impotence, as demonstrated in multiple clinical trials. It may also be used for sexual side effects caused by some antidepressants (SSRIs), female hyposexual disorder, low blood pressure, and xerostomia. Yohimbine HCl improves erections for 10% to 20% of men. It stimulates the parasympathetic nervous system, which is linked to erection, and may increase libido. For ED, 16 to 30 mg yohimbine HCl daily in three divided doses for 6 to 8 weeks may be recommended. Yohimbine HCl has a stimulatory effect, and side effects include elevated heart rate and blood pressure, mild dizziness, nervousness, and irritability.
- Yohimbe bark extract contains low concentrations of yohimbine (6% indole alkaloids, of which only 10%-15% is yohimbine), and commercial preparations may or may not share the pharmacological and clinical effects of yohimbine HCl.[231] Although strong evidence suggests the efficacy of yohimbine HCl in the management of certain types of ED, evidence is insufficient to support the use of yohimbe bark extract for ED.
- Offer some preventive tips: ingest alcohol in moderation or not at all; discontinue use of tobacco and use of all recreational drugs (e.g., marijuana); exercise regularly (at least 30 minutes daily); reduce stress; get enough sleep (8 hours a night); and deal with anxiety or depression (through counseling, healthy lifestyle, and medication).

Case Studies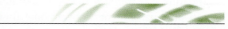

CASE STUDY 26-1

Over the past 2 years, DW, a 68-year-old man, has been experiencing an increase in BPH symptoms. He was getting up three times a night to urinate, had difficulty initiating urination, and often had urinary urgency. His wife, exasperated by having her sleep disturbed, insisted that he see their family physician. DW underwent a complete physical examination, including laboratory work. His PSA test was 2 ng/mL, well below the 4-ng/mL threshold that indicates increased risk of prostate cancer. He was given a prescription for tamsulosin (Flomax) and was advised to take one 0.4-mg capsule daily. DW is currently taking warfarin (Coumadin, 5 mg/day) for chronic atrial fibrillation and yohimbine (10 mg three times daily) for ED. He prefers an herbal remedy for his BPH and has heard that African wild potato and red clover may be beneficial.

Answer: DW may not be aware that yohimbine (yohimbe; *Pausinystalia yohimbe*) may exacerbate the symptoms of BPH. Merely discontinuing yohimbine may reduce DW's symptoms.

Both African wild potato (*Hypoxis hemerocallidea*) and red clover (*Trifolium pratense*) have been used to treat BPH; to date, however, their efficacy has not been clearly established.

The literature contains strong scientific evidence that saw palmetto (*Serenoa repens*) can improve BPH, and it is often recommended as an alternative to prescription medications. Saw palmetto is well tolerated, and side effects are usually mild; however, hemorrhage has been reported in patients using saw palmetto. DW's prothrombin time should be closely monitored if he begins taking saw palmetto. DW should watch for signs of bleeding, including bleeding nose or gums, unusual bruising, purplish spots on skin, and excessive or prolonged bleeding from cuts. If a significant change or side effect occurs, either the saw palmetto should be discontinued or his warfarin dosage adjusted.

Although current evidence is not as strong as that for saw palmetto, pygeum (*Prunus africanum*, syn. *Pygeum africanum*) has been used to treat BPH. According to most studies, the herb is well tolerated with few adverse effects; to date, however, the safety of pygeum has not been well documented. Ingestion of pygeum and saw palmetto may have a synergistic effect on the prostate. Combination products that contain pygeum and stinging nettle (*Urtica dioica*) are available for the treatment of BPH. The evidence for the efficacy of stinging nettle for the treatment of BPH is currently unclear or conflicting.

CASE STUDY 26-2

MJ is a 65-year-old woman who presents at the pharmacy with a prescription for sulfanilamide vaginal cream (AVC Cream) for bacterial vaginitis. She asks if an herbal remedy is available because she "has had it with drugs, doctors, and hospitals." She was recently hospitalized for ureterolithiasis (kidney stone lodged in ureter), and she likened the pain to that of childbirth. She asks if a natural remedy is available for her vaginitis instead of the sulfanilamide cream. She is also interested in an herbal remedy that will reduce the risk of recurrence of her kidney stones. She is currently taking no medications. Based on MJ's medical history, devise an intergrative therapy plan to help her manage vaginitis.

Answer: Douching with chamomile (*Matricaria recutita*, syn. *Matricaria suaveolens*, *Matricaria chamomilla*, *Anthemis nobilis*, *Chamaemelum nobile*, *Chamomilla chamomilla*, *Chamomilla recutita*) might improve MJ's vaginitis and has minimal side effects. MJ is in her menopausal years and is not taking a hormone replacement. Vaginitis is often associated with estrogen deficiency. Systemic or topical estrogen therapy would be beneficial; however, its use is controversial, particularly in postmenopausal patients. Topical estrogen is systemically absorbed. Estrogen replacement therapy should be discussed with her physician.

Once an individual has had a kidney stone, the person is more prone to a recurrence than the average population. Adequate fluid intake (2-3 L of water daily) and avoidance of excess calcium (calcium tablets, calcium-rich foods) should be stressed for MJ. A number of herbal remedies have been proposed to reduce the risk of developing nephrolithiasis and ureterolithiasis; however, currently available evidence is unclear or conflicting. Cornflower (*Centaurea cyanus*) flowers may help prevent the recurrence of kidney stones. Grapefruit (*Citrus x paradisi*) and cranberry (*Vaccinium macrocarpon*) might be beneficial. Cranberry juice may increase urinary excretion of oxalate, possibly increasing the risk of calcium oxalate stone formation; however, it also stimulates potassium and magnesium, which can decrease the rate of stone formation. Cranberry juice (amount unspecified) has been reported to decrease urinary calcium by 50% in patients with kidney stones.[52] One or two glasses of cranberry or grapefruit juice daily can be added to MJ's diet with extremely minimal risks of harmful side effects. Due to the high sugar content of cranberry juice "cocktails" that only partially contain cranberry juice, recommend that MJ try unsweetened cranberry juice.

CASE STUDY 26-3

DK is a 57-year-old man who presents at the pharmacy with a prescription for sildenafil (Viagra). One year ago, he was noted to be mildly hypertensive, with blood pressure of 146/94 mm Hg. He also was found to have a mildly elevated fasting blood sugar (108 mg/dL). He restricted his sodium intake and lost 35 pounds; his blood pressure returned to the normal range (120/80 mm Hg) and his fasting blood sugar dropped to 80 mg/dL. Although his health had improved, he was experiencing increasing difficulty obtaining and maintaining an erection. When informed of the price of Viagra, he asked if something cheaper, perhaps an herbal remedy, was available. What recommendations could you offer DK?

Answer: Sildenafil and similar medications, such as vardenafil (Levitra) and tadalafil (Cialis), are effective in the treatment of ED. Herbal remedies are available for ED treatment, but none has currently been proved effective. Anecdotal responses of individuals to the efficacy of an herbal remedy range from very effective to totally ineffective. A common effect of most herbal remedies for ED is vasodilation (penile vessels and elsewhere), so these herbs can lower blood pressure; DK's increased blood pressure in the past reduces this concern.

Grapefruit (*Citrus x paradisi*) has been shown to increase the absorption of sildenafil; however, some individuals report an increase of efficacy with grapefruit, whereas others report a decrease. Theoretically, grapefruit may alter the efficacy of other drugs and herbs used to treat ED.

Ginseng (*Panax* spp.) is a popular herbal remedy for ED. Ginseng enhances NO release, which facilitates smooth muscle relaxation of veins. In a clinical trial of 90 ED patients, ginseng increased penile rigidity, penile girth, and libido.[88] Ginseng has been shown to lower blood glucose; DK has a history of an elevated fasting blood sugar, so this effect does not negate his use of ginseng.

Ginkgo (*Ginkgo biloba*) is another popular herbal remedy for ED and can also stimulate NO release. L-Arginine is an amino acid that stimulates NO release. ArginMax (combination of L-arginine, *Panax*, *Ginkgo biloba*, damiana, and multivitamin/minerals) is a commercially available product designed to treat ED.

Coleus (*Coleus forskohlii*) is another herb used to treat ED. It is generally regarded to be safe, with few reports of adverse effects. Coleus stimulates insulin release, but this is not a negative effect for DK.

Yohimbe (*Pausinystalia yohimbe*) bark extract contains yohimbine, which has been used to treat ED. The concentration of yohimbine in yohimbe is quite low; thus it is unlikely that yohimbe bark extract will benefit ED. Yohimbine may exacerbate the symptoms of BPH.

DK should be aware that many factors can lead to sexual dysfunction, including tobacco and alcohol use, other medications, or emotional state. Refer DK to a primary care physician to determinate whether his sexual dysfunction is related to substance use, psychological state, or an underlying physiological problem.

References for Chapter 26 can be found on the Evolve website at http://evolve.elsevier.com/Ulbricht/herbalpharmacotherapy/

Review Questions

1. Which of the following statements is true?
   a. Yohimbine is safe for over-the-counter sale.
   b. Yohimbe is an active indole alkaloid constituent found in the bark of the yohimbine tree.
   c. Commercial preparations of yohimbe may or may not share the pharmacological and clinical effects of yohimbine hydrochloride.
   d. Most commercial yohimbe products contain a significant amount of yohimbine.

2. True or false: Cernilton, prepared from rye grass pollen, is a registered pharmaceutical throughout Western Europe, Japan, Korea, and Argentina, and is most popularly used for the treatment of erectile dysfunction.

3. Pygeum has been reported to reduce which of the following?
   a. Urinary frequency
   b. Size of the prostate gland
   c. Dysuria
   d. Both a and c

4. All the following statements are true *except:*
   a. Stinging nettle may be used alone or in combination with saw palmetto for BPH.
   b. Nettle does not appear to be well tolerated.
   c. The mechanism of action of stinging nettle in BPH is not clear but may involve aromatase inhibition, SHBG, and epidermal growth.
   d. Nettle appears to be an appropriate treatment for the alleviation of lower urinary tract symptoms associated with stage I or II BPH.

5. Which of the following appears to inhibit aromatase activity?
   a. Stinging nettle
   b. Nopal
   c. Clove
   d. Both a and b

6. True or false: *Panax* has been shown to be superior to placebo and trazodone in the treatment of erectile dysfunction.

7. The effects of ginkgo in ED treatment may be related to:
   a. Inhibition of nitric oxide
   b. Testosterone-like properties
   c. Alpha-2 antagonist effects
   d. None of the above

8. Which of the following doses for saw palmetto may be recommended for BPH?
   a. 320 mcg daily in one or two divided doses
   b. 3.2 g daily in one or two divided doses
   c. 320 mg daily in one or two divided doses
   d. None of the above

9. All the following are true about maca *except:*
   a. Maca is rich in isoflavones.
   b. Maca may increase testosterone levels.
   c. Maca may improve penile endothelial l-arginine–NO activity.
   d. Maca has been traditionally used as an aphrodisiac.

10. True or false: Saw palmetto may be superior to the finasteride (Proscar) in improving symptoms of BPH.

Answers are found in the Answers to Review Questions section in the back of the text.

27 Bacterial Infections

Outline

OVERVIEW
  Gram-Positive Bacteria
  Gram-Negative Bacteria
  Mycobacteria
  Oxygen Dependence
  Types of Infections
    Bacterial Conjunctivitis
    Bacterial Meningitis
    Cholera
    Foodborne Illness
    Leprosy
    Methicillin-Resistant *Staphylococcus aureus*
    Mycobacterium avium Complex
    Otitis Media
    Periodontal Disease
    Trachoma (*Chlamydia* Eye Infection)
    Tuberculosis
    Upper Respiratory Tract Infection (Bacterial)
    Urinary Tract Infection
SELECTED HERBAL THERAPIES
  Acacia (*Acacia* spp.)
  Andrographis (*Andrographis paniculata*)
  Astragalus (*Astragalus membranaceus*)
  Betel Nut (*Areca catechu*)
  Bloodroot (*Sanguinaria canadensis*)
  Bromelain (Bromeliaceae)
  Cranberry (*Vaccinium macrocarpon*)
  Eucalyptus (*Eucalyptus* spp.)
  Eyebright (*Euphrasia officinalis*)
  Ginseng (*Panax* spp.)
  Goldenseal (*Hydrastis canadensis*)
  Horseradish (*Armoracia rusticana*, syn. *Cochlearia armoracia*)
  Lime (*Citrus aurantifolia*)
  Lingonberry (*Vaccinium vitis-idaea*)
  Mastic (*Pistacia lentiscus*)
  Neem (*Azadirachta indica*)
  Pycnogenol (*Pinus pinaster* subsp. *atlantica*)
  Rhubarb (*Rheum* spp.)
  Tea (*Camellia sinensis*)
  Tea Tree (*Melaleuca alternifolia*)
  Thyme (*Thymus vulgaris*)
  Uva Ursi (*Arctostaphylos uva-ursi*)
HERBAL THERAPIES WITH NEGATIVE EVIDENCE
HERBAL THERAPIES WITH LIMITED EVIDENCE
ADJUNCT THERAPIES
INTEGRATIVE THERAPY PLAN
CASE STUDIES
REVIEW QUESTIONS

Learning Objectives

- Identify natural products used for bacterial infections and understand their mechanisms of action.
- Recognize dose, side effects, and interactions of natural products used for bacterial infections.
- Assess the patient and create an integrative therapy plan for a bacterial infection.

OVERVIEW

Bacteria comprise a large and diverse group of unicellular microorganisms. Found in virtually any environment, even deep-sea thermal vents and salty bodies of water, bacteria are critical for the Earth's ecosystem. Bacteria are often used in industrial and agricultural applications, and certain strains are even used in food applications, most notably for producing fermented foods such as sauerkraut and yogurt.

Of the countless species of bacteria that exist, most are harmless to humans. In fact, many types of beneficial bacteria symbiotically live on or in human hosts as normal flora. However, some bacteria are pathogenic and cause disease when they gain access to the host in numbers too great for the immune system to eliminate. Sometimes, bacteria that constitute a host's normal flora can cause infections when the body's normal defense mechanisms are compromised, or if the bacteria gain access to other parts of the body. For example, *Escherichia coli,* which normally lives in the colon and provides much of the vitamin K needed by humans, can cause urinary tract infections. *Staphylococcus aureus,* part of the normal flora of the skin, can cause infections through cuts or other breaks in the skin. Deep skin infections, called cellulitis, are frequently caused by bacteria from the genus *Staphylococcus* or *Streptococcus* that normally reside on the skin surface.

Bacterial infections may be classified by location (e.g., urinary tract infection) or by the pathogen type (e.g., mycobacterial infection). Any organ or organ system is susceptible to bacterial infection, and each has unique physical, mechanical, humoral, and cellular immune defenses against infection.[1] Such defenses include physical barriers (e.g., skin, mucus), enzymes (e.g., in tears), and chemicals (e.g., stomach acids). The immune system may also initiate specific responses to bacterial infections. If uncontrolled, bacterial infections may disrupt normal cellular functions and cause disease or even death.

The immune system reacts to the presence of the invading pathogen by releasing *cytokines,* hormonelike substances that regulate the intensity and duration of the immune response. White blood cell (WBC) production is increased, and specific WBCs are directed to *phagocytize* (ingest) the bacteria. The process, known as *phagocytosis,* is an important defense mechanism that ultimately destroys the bacteria. Antibodies may also recognize specific components of a bacterium, such as proteins in the bacterial wall. The immune response is in fact responsible for many of the signs and symptoms of infections. Associated symptoms include pain, erythema (redness), edema (swelling), and fever. Some infections produce a purulent discharge containing dead WBCs, which may require medical intervention to assist drainage. Severe infections sometimes result in *sepsis,* a systemic inflammatory response to bacteria, viruses, or toxins. Severe sepsis is associated with hypotension and organ dysfunction. *Septic shock* is sepsis with hypotension that does not respond to intravenous fluid administration. Without immediate treatment, sepsis can be fatal.

Antimicrobials are substances that either kill or inhibit the growth of microbes such as bacteria, parasites (see Chapter 28), or viruses (see Chapter 29). Many plants produce compounds with antimicrobial activity to fight fungal or bacterial pathogens (Figure 27-1).[2] Similarly, microorganisms themselves (including fungi and bacteria) also produce antimicrobial compounds in order to compete with other microorganisms, especially bacteria. Antimicrobials used specifically to treat bacterial infections are known as *antibiotics,* many of which are derived from fungi or other bacteria. The antibiotic properties of microorganisms have been used medicinally by many cultures for thousands of years; the first record of such use occurred over 2,500 years ago in China, where moldy soybean curds were used to treat infections.[3] However, the discovery of penicillin, a compound produced by the *Penicillium* fungi, led to the modern era of mass-produced antibiotic drugs.[4] The mechanism of action, concentration of antibiotic

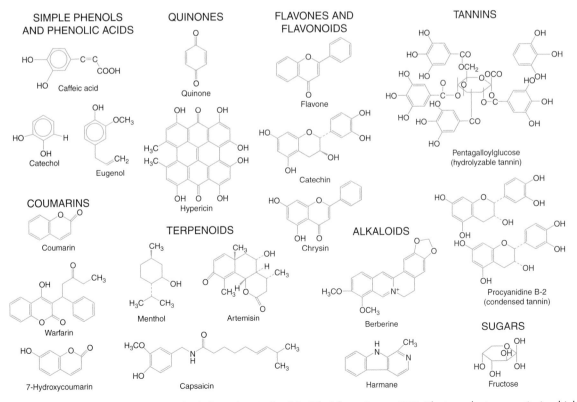

Figure 27-1 Structures of common antimicrobial plant chemicals. (Modified from Cowan MM: Plant products as antimicrobial agents, *Clin Microbiol Rev* 12(4):564-582, 1999.)

Bacterial Diseases*

DISEASE	BACTERIAL CAUSE(S)	DISEASE	BACTERIAL CAUSE(S)
Actinomycosis	*Actinomyces israelii, Actinomyces gerencseriae, Propionibacterium propionicus*	Listeriosis	*Listeria monocytogenes*
		Lyme disease	*Borrelia burgdorferi, Borrelia afzelii, Borrelia garinii*
Acute prostatitis	*Escherichia coli, Klebsiella, Proteus, Pseudomonas, Enterobacter, Enterococcus, Serratia, Staphylococcus aureus*	Melioidosis (Whitmore disease, nightcliff gardener's disease)	*Burkholderia pseudomallei*
		Meningococcal disease	*Neisseria meningitidis*
Anthrax	*Bacillus anthracis*	Necrotizing fasciitis (NF, fasciitis necroticans, flesh-eating disease, flesh-eating bacteria	*Streptococcus* spp., *Staphylococcus aureus, Vibrio vulnificus, Clostridium perfringens, Bacteroides fragilis*
Bacterial pneumonia	*Streptococcus pneumoniae, Staphylococcus aureus, Haemophilus influenzae, Klebsiella pneumoniae, Escherichia coli, Pseudomonas aeruginosa, Moraxella catarrhalis, Coxiella burnetti, Chlamydophila pneumoniae, Mycoplasma pneumoniae, Legionella pneumophila*		
		Paratyphoid fever (enteric fevers)	*Salmonella paratyphi*
		Pertussis (whooping cough)	*Bordetella pertussis*
		Pinta	*Treponema carateum*
		Plague (bubonic plague, pneumonic plague)	*Yersinia pestis*
Bartonellosis (Carrion's disease, trench fever, cat-scratch disease)	*Bartonella* spp.	Pseudomembranous colitis	*Clostridium difficile*
		Pseudotuberculosis	*Yersinia pseudotuberculosis*
		Psittacosis (parrot disease, parrot fever, ornithosis)	*Chlamydophila psittaci*
Bejel (endemic syphilis)	*Treponema pallidum*		
Botryomycosis (bacterial pseudomycosis)	*Staphylococcus aureus, Pseudomonas aeruginosa*	Pyomyositis	*Staphylococcus aureus*
		Q fever	*Coxiella burnetii*
Brazilian purpuric fever (BPF)	*Haemophilus influenzae*	Rat-bite fever (sodoku, Haverhill fever, epidemic arthritic erythema)	*Spirillum minus*
Brucellosis (undulant fever, Malta fever, Bang's disease)	*Brucella abortus*		
Campylobacteriosis	*Campylobacter* spp.	Rocky Mountain spotted fever	*Rickettsia rickettsii*
Caries	*Lactobacillus* spp., *Streptococcus mutans, Actinomyces* spp.	Scarlet fever	*Streptococcus pyogenes*
		Southern tick–associated rash illness (STARI), Masters' disease	*Amblyomma americanum*
Cellulitis	*Staphylococcus aureus, Streptococcus pyogenes*		
Chancroid	*Haemophilus ducreyi*	Streptococcal pharyngitis (streptococcal sore throat, strep throat)	*Streptococcus pyogenes*
Chlamydia	*Chlamydia trachomatis*		
Cholera	*Vibrio cholerae*		
Diphtheria	*Corynebacterium diphtheriae*	Syphilis	*Treponema pallidum*
Donovanosis (granuloma inguinale)	*Klebsiella granulomatis*	Tetanus	*Clostridium tetani*
		Tuberculosis (TB, consumption)	*Mycobacterium tuberculosis*
Epiglottitis	*Haemophilus influenzae, Streptococcus pneumoniae, Streptococcus pyogenes*	Tularemia (rabbit fever, deerfly fever, Ohara fever, Francis disease)	*Francisella tularensis*
Gonorrhea	*Neisseria gonorrhoeae*		
Impetigo	*Staphylococcus aureus, Streptococcus pyogenes*	Typhoid fever (enteric fever, bilious fever, yellow Jack)	*Salmonella enterica*
Legionellosis (Legionnaires' disease, Pontiac fever)	*Legionella pneumophila*	Ulcers	*Helicobacter pylori*
		Waterhouse-Friderichsen syndrome (WFS)	*Neisseria meningitidis, Staphylococcus aureus, Streptococcus pyogenes*
Lemierre's syndrome (Lemierre's disease)	*Fusobacterium necrophorum*		
Leprosy (Hansen's disease)	*Mycobacterium leprae*	Yaws (Pétasse tropica, thymosis, polypapilloma tropicum, pian, parangi)	*Treponema pertenue*
Leptospirosis (Weil's disease, canicola fever, canefield fever, nanukayami fever, 7-day fever)	*Leptospira* spp.		
		Yersiniosis	*Yersinia enterocolitica*

*This information is not an all-inclusive or comprehensive list of bacterial diseases.

at the site of infection, and other factors (including sensitivity of the bacteria to the antibiotic) may determine what effect the antibiotic will have. Antibiotics may be administered orally, topically, or intravenously. The route of administration varies depending on the type and severity of the infection, and the patient's immunity. Because antibiotic therapy often depletes the body of its normal bacterial flora (such as those in the intestines), *secondary infections* by "opportunistic" bacteria sometimes occur after primary infections are treated.[5]

Bacterial pathogens are often classified by the makeup of their cell walls and by their shape, and may be identified through direct microscopic observation. A common technique uses the *Gram staining* method which differentiates between bacteria with thick, complex cell walls (*gram positive*) and bacteria with thinner cell walls (*gram negative*). Gram staining reveals bacterial morphology (shape), and observations are typically reported as "cocci" (round shape) or "bacilli" (rod shaped), with additional descriptions such as "in chains" or "in pairs."

Gram-Positive Bacteria

The cell walls of gram-positive bacteria have a thick layer of *peptidoglycan,* a sugar-protein complex, and appear violet or dark blue by Gram staining. Some classes of antibiotics function by cleaving the peptidoglycan layer of the bacterial cell wall, thus inhibiting bacterial growth. Common gram-positive cocci that infect humans are streptococci and staphylococci. The *Streptococcus* genus comprises various gram-positive bacteria responsible for a variety of diseases, including acute pharyngitis ("strep throat"), pneumonia, otitis media, rheumatic fever, scarlet fever, glomerulonephritis, and invasive fasciitis. *Staphylococcus* is a separate genus of gram-positive cocci that form grapelike clusters. Most staphylococcal infections are caused by *Staphylococcus aureus* or *Staphylococcus epidermidis*. Staphylococci can cause many diseases, including soft tissue infections, endocarditis, osteomyelitis, and toxic shock syndrome. Gram-positive bacilli (rods) can be divided according to their ability or inability to produce spores. Important diseases caused by the sporulating rods include anthrax *(Bacillus anthracis),* tetanus *(Clostridium tetani),* gangrene *(Clostridium perfringens),* and botulism *(Clostridium botulinum). Corynebacterium diphtheriae,* which causes diphtheria, is a group of nonsporulating rods.

Gram-Negative Bacteria

Gram-negative bacteria have thin peptidoglycan layers in their walls. Unlike gram-positive bacteria, gram-negative bacteria do not retain the dark Gram stain, thus appearing pink after the staining procedure. Many gram-negative bacteria are pathogenic. Gram-negative cocci include organisms that cause meningitis *(Neisseria meningitidis)* and gonorrhea *(Neisseria gonorrhoeae).* Gram-negative bacilli (rods) can cause a number of diseases, including urinary tract infections *(Escherichia coli);* gastrointestinal problems *(E. coli, Helicobacter pylori, Salmonella enteritidis, Shigella* spp.*, Vibrio cholerae);* skin infections *(Pseudomonas aeruginosa);* and respiratory infections *(Haemophilus influenzae, Klebsiella pneumoniae, P. aeruginosa).*

Mycobacteria

Mycobacteria are rod-shaped microorganisms with waxy cell walls (Latin *myco,* meaning "fungus" or "wax"). Members of the genus *Mycobacterium* are referred to as *acid-fast bacilli* because they are impermeable to usual stains but can be detected using an acid-fast stain. Further differentiation of mycobacteria can be done with nucleic acid amplification (e.g., polymerase chain reaction), also called *genotyping.* Several serious diseases, most notably tuberculosis and leprosy, are caused by mycobacteria. *Mycobacterium avium* complex (MAC) is another common mycobacterial infection, especially in patients with acquired immunodeficiency syndrome (AIDS).

Mycobacteria are notoriously difficult to culture, which has significantly hindered research. The species *Mycobacterium leprae,* which causes leprosy, is particularly challenging to study; it grows very slowly, taking 2 to 3 weeks to complete one division cycle (vs. 20 minutes for some strains of gram-negative *E. coli*). Further, *M. leprae* cannot be cultured in vitro; propagation in the laboratory is restricted to animal models such as the armadillo, the only other significant host (besides humans) of *M. leprae* in nature.[6] Mycobacterial infections may also be difficult to treat with antibiotics because of the thick, hydrophobic cell walls and slow growth.

Drug resistance may develop during treatment of these infections, so drug regimens typically use more than one drug for an extended time.

Oxygen Dependence

Bacteria may also be classified by their dependence on oxygen for growth. The dependence on oxygen is determined by culturing the bacteria in an *aerobic* (oxygen present) or *anaerobic* (oxygen absent) environment. Blood, sputum, cerebrospinal fluid, urine, and other fluids, as well as tissues, are used for culture. Bacteria that need oxygen are called *aerobes;* those that do not need oxygen, and may even die in the presence of oxygen, are called *anaerobes.* Some bacteria can grow in either environment and are known as *facultative anaerobes.*

Types of Infections
Bacterial Conjunctivitis

Bacterial conjunctivitis is an extremely contagious infection of the *conjunctiva,* a thin protective membrane that covers the inner surface of the eyelids. This condition is marked by bacterial invasion and inflammation of the tissue, and can be easily spread by sharing eye makeup with an infected person or by touching or rubbing the eyes with contaminated hands. Bacteria that cause conjunctivitis include *Staphylococcus aureus, Streptococcus pneumoniae,* and *Haemophilus influenzae.* Common organisms in sexually transmitted diseases (STDs) may also cause conjunctivitis, including *Neisseria gonorrhoeae* and *Chlamydia trachomatis.*

Bacterial conjunctivitis can occur at any age, and may take 3 to 7 days from transmission to become evident. If left untreated, the infection may take weeks to resolve. Conjunctivitis is rarely threatening to eyesight unless the infection spreads to the cornea. Use of ophthalmic antibiotics usually cures the infection within 7 to 10 days. Good ocular hygiene and handwashing aids recovery and helps to minimize the spread of infection.

Signs and Symptoms

The telltale signs of bacterial conjunctivitis are swollen, red, irritated, and itchy eyes. The patient may also have increased lacrimation (tearing) and a thick mucus discharge that causes the eyelashes to mat and that may impair vision. Patients may also complain of ocular pain and photophobia (sensitivity to light), which suggests corneal involvement (keratitis). Bacterial conjunctivitis usually begins as a unilateral infection that affects only one eye; however, it often spreads to the other (contralateral) eye. In some cases, bacterial conjunctivitis is accompanied by upper respiratory tract infections; in these patients, the offending pathogen is likely to be the same for both infections.

Diagnosis

Diagnosis of bacterial conjunctivitis is typically based on conclusions from the ocular examination and medical history. Although uncommon in new conjunctivitis cases, culture of the ocular exudate may be used to identify the causative pathogen.

Bacterial Meningitis

Meningitis is an infection of the *meninges* (lining of brain and spinal cord) that may be caused by bacteria or viruses. In either case, if not properly treated, meningitis may lead to permanent brain damage. In some patients, death occurs within days after onset of symptoms. Medical care should be sought immediately if meningitis is suspected.

Bacterial meningitis is most often caused by either *Streptococcus pneumoniae* or *Neisseria meningitidis* in adults. In newborns, however, the most common organisms are group B streptococci, *Escherichia coli*, *Listeria monocytogenes*, and *Klebsiella pneumoniae*. Children usually develop infections through contact with respiratory secretions from infected people. Bacteria that infect children include *S. pneumoniae* and *N. meningitidis*. *Haemophilus influenzae* type B formerly was the most common cause of bacterial meningitis in children; however, with childhood vaccination against that organism, it is now a rare cause of infection. Pneumococcal conjugate vaccine is effective against *S. pneumoniae*, and meningococcal conjugate vaccine protects individuals from *N. meningitidis*. These vaccines have recently been incorporated into the childhood vaccination schedule. Vaccines should also dramatically reduce the incidence of these organisms as the cause of bacterial meningitis and other infections.

Signs and Symptoms

Common symptoms of bacterial meningitis are headache, nausea, vomiting, stiff neck, lethargy, fever, meningismus (discomfort from irritated meninges), confusion, and irritability. The severity and type of symptoms and the rapidity of onset can vary based on the pathogen and the patient's age and immune status. In very young patients, symptoms include inability to maintain eye contact, seizures, lethargy, photophobia, anorexia (loss of appetite), skin rash, bulging fontanels (soft spaces between skull bones), opisthotonos (muscular spasm in which spine arches), and coma. Older patients may have more subtle symptoms.

Diagnosis

A medical history and physical examination should be conducted to differentiate bacteria from other causes, such as viruses. A lumbar puncture is the primary test for meningitis and helps distinguish a bacterial from a viral cause. A spinal needle is inserted between the third and fourth lumbar vertebrae under sterile conditions, and approximately 3 to 4 mL of cerebrospinal fluid (CSF) is withdrawn into several separate test tubes. During the process, CSF opening pressure is measured. The CSF then undergoes laboratory analysis for bacteria, viruses, and other etiologic agents. In addition, CSF is analyzed for the presence of white blood cells (WBCs), red blood cells (RBCs), protein, and glucose. As with any suspected infection, a laboratory analysis of the patient's blood is conducted, including a WBC count and differential. The blood, urine, sputum, and other suspected sites of infection are cultured and compared with CSF culture results. Polymerase chain reaction (PCR) is a highly sensitive and specific test used to determine viral causes of meningitis; it can be used to exclude a bacterial etiology and support discontinuation of antibiotics. Radiography, ultrasonography, and computed tomography (CT) of the chest, head, or other organs may suggest or rule out pathology suggestive of the origin of infection.

Cholera

Cholera is a bacterial infection of the small intestine caused by *Vibrio cholerae* that results in severe, watery diarrhea. The bacteria are usually spread through contaminated water or food. *V. cholerae* secretes an *enterotoxin* (toxin secreted into intestinal tract) that causes fluid and electrolyte loss from the small intestine. Some humans may act as a reservoir for *V. cholerae*, shedding bacteria in their stool for years. Risk factors for acquisition include drinking contaminated water, introducing hands into containers used for drinking water storage, drinking beverages from street vendors, and drinking beverages with contaminated ice cubes in areas with poor water hygiene and where cholera has been reported. Boiling the water for drinking kills the bacteria. Patients receiving antacids are at increased risk of infection because an acidic environment suppresses growth of the organism.

Cholera is most frequently found in underdeveloped areas that have poor sanitation, such as sub-Saharan Africa. Most patients with cholera require oral or intravenous hydration and should receive supportive care. Antibiotics have a secondary role in the management of cholera and can reduce stool discharge and duration of symptoms. If patients with severe forms of cholera do not receive supportive care, renal failure and death may occur.

Signs and Symptoms

In addition to diarrhea, cholera patients may experience dehydration, abdominal cramps, nausea, and vomiting. Severe dehydration may occur within a few hours. Electrolyte and acid-base abnormalities are usually present.

Diagnosis

Cholera is diagnosed after the bacteria from a stool sample are microscopically identified. In endemic areas, diagnosis is based on the clinical presentation.

Foodborne Illness

Foodborne illnesses are common and sometimes life-threatening conditions that affect millions of people worldwide. Food contaminated with pathogenic bacteria can produce mild to severe gastrointestinal symptoms, potentially leading to permanent organ damage and fatalities. Individuals who are very young, elderly, or immunocompromised are at increased risk of foodborne illness. Common bacterial pathogens in foodborne infections include *Campylobacter, Salmonella, Shigella,* and *Listeria* spp., as well as *Escherichia coli* and *Clostridium botulinum*.[7] In the past the primary vehicles for the foodborne illnesses were improperly prepared or cooked meat, pork, and poultry products, which were contaminated with feces during processing. Recent outbreaks, however, have also been linked to fruits and vegetables.[8] It is suspected that the animal byproducts used as fertilizer are major sources of contamination.

Substandard food storage, handling, and preparation are major health concerns, even in developed countries where proper sanitation is widely available. Outbreaks of foodborne illness are monitored by the U.S. Centers for Disease Control and Prevention (CDC). Prevention of foodborne disease requires proper handling of food products "from farm to table." At home, careful cooking and storage can minimize exposure to these pathogens. Patients at risk for foodborne illness should be counseled to avoid consuming those products likely to contain pathogens.

Signs and Symptoms

Patients may be symptom free or may complain of mild to severe gastric distress (upset stomach), nausea, vomiting, cramping, and diarrhea that present within 48 hours of consuming a contaminated food or drink. Patients often develop fever, dehydration, and diarrhea; those with severe infection may experience mental status changes, paralysis, and sepsis.

Diagnosis

Foodborne pathogens can be differentiated by signs and symptoms, onset of disease, and blood/stool cultures. A history of the outbreak, physical examinations, and interviews with other persons consuming the same food help to confirm the diagnosis. Leftover food may be collected and tested to establish the etiology of infection. However, identification of the causative agent is not always practical or even possible in isolated cases. For outbreaks, it is more critical to identify and trace the pathogen to the source.

Leprosy

Leprosy, or *Hansen's disease,* is characterized by infiltrative skin lesions, hypoesthesia (decreased sensation), and peripheral neuropathy (numbness of hands and feet). Before identification of *Mycobacterium leprae* as the causative agent, many people believed that leprosy was inherited. Genetics may in fact determine susceptibility to *M. leprae* infection; specific gene variations have been identified as risk factors for leprosy.[9] Leprosy can be successfully controlled with aggressive antibiotic therapy; however, despite effective antibiotic treatments, leprosy continues to be a public health concern in underdeveloped countries.

Clinical leprosy is categorized into two groups by the number of lesions present: *paucibacillary* (indeterminate, tuberculoid, and borderline tuberculoid) and *multibacillary* (midborderline, borderline lepromatous, and lepromatous). *Tuberculoid* leprosy is characterized by one or several skin lesions, whereas patients with *lepromatous leprosy* have numerous lesions. Both forms are associated with skin lesions and peripheral sensory neuropathy. Nerve damage is caused by the organism as well as by the immune response to the infection. Lepromatous leprosy is the more severe form. The predominant mode of transmission is through respiratory or nasal discharge.

The three established antibiotics for leprosy are dapsone, rifampin, and clofazamine. A multidrug regimen given for 3 to 5 years is recommended to increase the cure rate and prevent treatment failure. Treatment of leprosy may result in *reversal reactions,* in which new lesions appear where previous lesions have subsided; in rare cases, reversal reactions can be fatal or lead to permanent nerve damage.

Signs and Symptoms

Patients with tuberculoid leprosy may have the sole complaint of white, flat lesions with scales. Lepromatous leprosy typically causes many skin nodules without scales. Peripheral sensory neuropathy is more common in patients with lepromatous leprosy and can lead to the development of blisters and skin wounds on the soles of the feet. Wounds that go unnoticed eventually progress to disfiguring sores and eruptions.

If left untreated, leprosy may lead to serious complications: permanent nerve damage, physical deformities, eye damage that may lead to blindness, erectile dysfunction, infertility (in males), generalized inflammation that may be painful, chronic nasal congestion, and decreased quality of life. Without treatment, the skin, nose, and appendages may become damaged and scarred. Eventually, this may lead to sloughing of skin, complete collapse of the nose, and loss of fingers or toes.

Diagnosis

Leprosy is diagnosed by histological examination of a skin scraping. *Mycobacterium leprae* stains red with an acid-fast stain (Ziehl-Neelsen), and identification of the pathogen is necessary to distinguish leprosy from other skin conditions. Clinical examination should focus on careful assessment of skin and peripheral nerves as well as loss of sensation.

Methicillin-Resistant *Staphylococcus aureus*

Staphylococcus aureus is a species of small, round bacteria that grow in clusters. Methicillin-resistant *Staphylococcus aureus* (MRSA) infections are becoming increasingly common, which is particularly concerning because these strains are resistant to most first-line antibiotics.[8] Patients may fail multiple courses of therapy until infection with MRSA is confirmed, allowing the infection to spread and possibly acquire resistance to more antibiotics. Until recently, MRSA was primarily observed in hospitalized patients or intravenous (IV) drug users; however, MRSA can now be a community-acquired infection, known as CA-MRSA. MRSA can live on most surfaces and objects. Colonization with MRSA occurs in persons with a history of the infection, recent hospital admission, or contact with an infected person. MRSA can be carried in the nasal passages, skin, and bowel; the infection is transmitted by physical contact or with inhalation of aerosolized bacteria. MRSA can infect the skin, lungs, blood, bone, kidneys, and other organs. MRSA infections are treated with antibiotics such as sulfamethoxazole-trimethoprim (Bactrim) and vancomycin (Vancocin).

Signs and Symptoms

Symptoms of an MRSA infection are generally similar to those of other infections and vary based on the site or type of infection. When *Staphylococcus aureus* is the likely pathogen, MRSA should be suspected if improvement in signs and symptoms does not occur with standard antibiotic therapy.

Diagnosis

A MRSA infection is confirmed with bacterial cultures and antibiotic susceptibility testing.

Mycobacterium avium Complex

Mycobacterium avium complex (MAC) infections involve two species of mycobacteria; *Mycobacterium avium* and *M. intracellulare*. These organisms are classified under a subgroup of mycobacteria called *nontuberculous mycobacteria* (NTM). Although NTM are ubiquitous and found in most humans, most carriers do not usually develop infections. However, immunocompromised patients, such as those infected with human immunodeficiency virus (HIV), can develop MAC infections.

MAC infections may be limited to one part of the body or may enter the bloodstream and spread throughout the body. *Disseminated* MAC (DMAC) is a condition in which MAC bacteria are present in several organs. The most common complication of DMAC is iron deficiency anemia, because mycobacteria require iron to survive and proliferate. DMAC infection may become life threatening. MAC pneumonia can cause respiratory failure and death.

Signs and Symptoms

Infection with MAC produces lymphadenopathy (swollen, enlarged lymph nodes), fever, drenching sweats, diarrhea, weight loss, abdominal pain, fatigue, weakness, shortness of breath, enlarged breasts, inflamed muscle tissue, hepatosplenomegaly, and skin lesions. A brain abscess may also form, producing neurological symptoms such as headache, dizziness, neck pain, confusion, drowsiness, irritability, decreased responsiveness, seizures, and loss of coordination. Patients usually experience fatigue and have pale skin, anemia, leukopenia (decreased WBC count), and thrombocytopenia (low platelet count).

Diagnosis

Blood and bone marrow cultures are the most sensitive diagnostic tests for MAC. Extracting bone marrow for culture is an invasive and painful procedure, and thus a blood culture is more often used to make the diagnosis.

Otitis Media

Otitis media (OM) is an inflammation of the middle ear, including the *tympanic membrane* (eardrum). Acute bacterial OM occurs when fluid resulting from a cold, allergy, or upper respiratory infection (URI) develops behind the tympanic membrane. The space behind this membrane is normally sterile; however, if bacteria are present in the accumulating fluid, this can lead to obstruction of the *eustachian tube* (small tube connecting ear to back of nose).

Otitis media is the most frequently diagnosed childhood illness in the United States. More than 3 of 4 children have had at least one ear infection by age 3 years.[10] Adults can also contract the condition, although much less often than children. The eustachian tubes in a child are narrower and shorter than in an adult; thus, eustachian tube dysfunction occurs more frequently, and fluid is more likely to accumulate in the middle ear of a child.

In severe cases of OM, large amounts of fluid accumulate, increasing pressure on the eardrum until it ruptures and the fluid drains out. This is usually very painful. The ruptured eardrum typically heals within a couple of weeks without intervention. Multiple bouts of OM can result in clinically significant hearing loss because of scarring that occurs with repeated healing of the eardrum. OM is not contagious.

Symptoms of OM often start 2 to 7 days after a cold or other URI. Acute ear infections usually resolve in 1 or 2 weeks, depending on the treatment. An infection that does not resolve with multiple courses of antibiotic treatment (or that recurs frequently) is termed *chronic otitis media*.

Signs and Symptoms

Symptoms of OM in very young patients (<3 years) include increased irritability, difficulty sleeping, tugging or pulling at one or both ears, ear pain, fever, fluid draining from the ear, loss of balance, and signs of hearing loss. Older children and adults can have similar symptoms but are able to vocalize the location and severity of pain. In some cases, OM may be asymptomatic. Some patients complain of ear fullness or "popping."

Diagnosis

The diagnosis of otitis media requires a history of the onset of signs and symptoms, the presence of middle ear effusion (e.g., bulging of tympanic membrane), and signs and symptoms of middle ear inflammation (e.g., erythema of tympanic membrane). Although not normally part of the clinical OM workup, blood tests, including WBC counts, can be used to determine if the immune system is functioning appropriately and to confirm the presence of an infection.

Periodontal Disease

Periodontal (gum) diseases include gingivitis and periodontitis. *Gingivitis* is inflammation of the gums that causes them to bleed and swell. It is very common and becomes more common as people age. Most people show signs of the disease by their mid-30s. Gingivitis is caused by infection or plaque around the teeth and is a common cause of tooth loss after age 35. Gingivitis may progress to *periodontitis,* which affects the underlying bone structure that supports the teeth in addition to the soft gum tissues. Periodontitis is the more severe form of gum disease and may lead to tooth loss.

Plaque hardens into calculus (tartar) when left on the teeth. As plaque and tartar build up, the gums begin to recede from the teeth, and pockets form between the teeth and gums. The gums recede, and the infection spreads to the jawbone and periodontal ligament. Teeth may become loose and may require extraction.

Gingivitis and periodontitis can be aggravated by numerous behaviors, including tobacco use, clenching or grinding the teeth, poor nutrition, and poor dental hygiene. Heredity also plays a role and is a factor in an estimated 30% of cases. Hormonal changes may also affect gum health, especially during stress, pregnancy, puberty, menopause, and oral contraceptive use. Other medications, such as phenytoin (Dilantin), cyclosporin (Sandimmune), and calcium channel blockers are also known to affect gum health. Conditions that may aggravate periodontal disease include diabetes, HIV infection or AIDS, and certain cancers. A patient may have periodontal disease with no obvious symptoms or warning signs. Regular dental checkups, periodontal examination, and proper oral hygiene can reduce the incidence of periodontal disease.

Signs and Symptoms

In patients with periodontal disease, the gums may be red, swollen, and painful and are likely to bleed. The gums may also recede and expose parts of the tooth not protected by enamel. Other symptoms include persistent bad breath or bad taste, permanent teeth that are loose, changes in bite, and changes in the fit of partial dentures. Pain appears after damage to the tooth has already begun. The pain from tooth decay (dental caries) can be dull or throbbing. The type and intensity of the pain varies depending on the amount of decay. An acute, brief pain may indicate the onset of dental caries. Generally, the pain is triggered by a specific event, such as eating something hot or cold; the deeper the decay, the more intense the pain. When the caries reach the dental pulp, the pain becomes continuous and piercing. Other symptoms associated with dental caries include food deposits between teeth, sensitivity to hot or cold food and beverages, swelling of the gum, and facial swelling with enlarged glands in the neck.

Diagnosis

A dentist will begin by taking a medical history to identify underlying conditions or risk factors that may contribute to gum disease. A number of procedures may be performed to diagnosis periodontal disease. Dentists visually inspect the teeth to determine if dental caries are present. Dental radiographs may be taken to look for dental caries and bone loss.

Trachoma (*Chlamydia* Eye Infection)

Trachoma is an infection of the conjunctiva, cornea, and eyelids caused by *Chlamydia trachomatis* serotypes A, B, and C. Trachoma is spread through direct contact with infected eye, nose, or throat secretions; it may also result from contact with other bodily secretions or contaminated objects, such as towels or clothing. In addition, certain flies (e.g., muscoid flies) can spread the bacteria. The condition is most often found in children, as well as individuals with a history of multiple eye infections, and is endemic in areas of poor sanitation. If left untreated, trachoma may cause corneal scarring or blindness.

Signs and Symptoms

The eyelids of patients with trachoma are severely irritated, which may result in deformities. The irregular surface of the eyelid rubs against the cornea, causing eye ulcers, scarring, vision loss, perforation, and blindness. Eyelid deformities can also cause the eyelashes to turn inward and lead to further scarring of the cornea. In some cases, surgery may be needed to repair deformed eyelids and to prevent long-term scarring. If not properly treated, continued corneal scarring may lead to blindness.

Diagnosis

Trachoma is generally diagnosed clinically, based on the medical history, especially in economically poor areas with limited medical resources where trachoma is endemic. Laboratory analysis may include microscopic evaluation of a swab or scraping, cell culture, or PCR for presence of *Chlamydia trachomatis.*

Tuberculosis

Tuberculosis (TB), previously known as "consumption," is a mycobacterial infection caused by *Mycobacterium tuberculosis*. TB is transmitted through airborne droplets of infected sputum. Initial infection is relatively mild, but even after the patient recovers from this illness, the organism continues to reside in lung tissue as a latent infection. Individuals with latent TB and healthy immune systems are able to suppress active infection; however, latent infections may reactivate if immune function decreases. Active TB can cause serious respiratory problems that can be life threatening, especially if left untreated. *M. tuberculosis* typically causes pneumonia (inflammation of lung) but can also cause meningitis and systemic infections.

Signs and Symptoms

Symptoms of active TB include cough, hemoptysis (coughing up blood), dyspnea (shortness of breath), pleurisy (tenderness and inflammation of chest lining), fever, significant weight loss, night sweats, chills, and anorexia. Latent TB is usually asymptomatic.

Diagnosis

The recommended diagnostic approach with suspected TB begins with a careful history to determine patient risk, followed by physical examination and chest radiograph. Based on radiographic findings suggestive of TB, acid-fast bacilli (AFB) smear and sputum culture should be obtained. A positive AFB smear is predictive of mycobacterial infection; if the test is negative, however, it does not exclude a TB diagnosis if other clinical factors are highly suggestive. Serum samples can also be analyzed for antibodies to *M. tuberculosis*; however, a positive finding (seroconversion) may result in uninfected patients who have received the bacille Calmette-Guérin (BCG) vaccine for preventing TB. Multidrug-resistant TB is also a public health concern; thus antibiotic susceptibility testing may also be performed.

Upper Respiratory Tract Infection (Bacterial)

The upper respiratory tract consists of the nasal passages, pharynx, larynx, and sinuses. Upper respiratory infections (URIs) caused by bacteria include sinusitis (sinus infection), pharyngitis (pharynx infection), laryngitis (larynx infection), and tracheitis (trachea infection). These are the most common acute illnesses seen in outpatient clinics. URIs caused by bacteria involve direct invasion of the mucosal lining of the upper airway. Most URIs are spread by person-to-person transmission; furthermore, a URI may develop as a superinfection after a viral or bacterial URI. A *superinfection* is defined as an infection that follows a previous infection and that is often caused by organisms that have become resistant to a previously used antibiotic. Bacterial inoculation begins when infected secretions are transferred from the hand to the nose or mouth or by directly inhaling respiratory droplets from an infected person who is coughing or sneezing. The incubation time before symptoms develop varies among pathogens, with most bacterial infections ranging from 3 to 10 days after exposure.

Signs and Symptoms

Signs and symptoms of bacterial URI include rhinorrhea (runny nose), nasal congestion, sinus pain, sore throat, dry cough, muscle ache, headache, sneezing, itchy or watery eyes, fever, and fatigue. Nasal discharge may become thicker and discolored (yellow, green, or brown) as the infection progresses.

Diagnosis

A URI is usually self-diagnosed or diagnosed clinically based on symptoms. A throat swab for culture or blood analysis/culture may be done to determine if a streptococcal infection is present. Radiography or CT of the sinuses may be performed in patients with a history of multiple URIs.

Urinary Tract Infection

The urinary tract consists of the kidneys, ureters, bladder, prostate, and urethra (see Chapter 26), all of which are susceptible to acute and chronic infection. The urinary tract is normally a sterile environment that uses a variety of host defenses to minimize infection, including urine pH and osmolality, urine flow and micturition, urinary inhibitors of bacterial adherence, and immune system responses, such as polymorphonuclear neutrophils (PMNs) and cell-mediated immunity.

Cystitis and *urethritis* are infections of the lower urinary tract (bladder and urethra, respectively), and *pyelonephritis* is an infection of the upper urinary tract (kidneys and ureters). Patients with lower UTIs typically have bacteriuria (bacteria in the urine) and pain while urinating; however, many lower UTIs resolve without treatment, and others resolve fully with antibiotic treatment. However, if the patient does not receive treatment, the infection may spread to the kidneys, where it can cause renal cell death and permanent damage. The spread of bacteria from the urinary tract to the blood can lead to *urosepsis*, a serious and a possibly fatal infection.

Risk factors for UTI include obstruction, neurogenic bladder, catheterization, sexual intercourse, pregnancy, diabetes mellitus, poor hygiene, and previous UTI.[1] UTIs can occur at any age, but are more common in women than men.[11] Women are more susceptible because they have a much shorter urethra than men; thus the distance between the unsterile body exterior (especially the anus) and the sterile bladder is much shorter. Pathogens for *uncomplicated* acute UTIs include Enterobacteriaceae such as *Escherichia coli*, *Staphylococcus saprophyticus*, and *Enterococcus* spp. Uropathogenic *E. coli* adheres to urinary bladder cells with surface hairlike fimbriae or pili. *Complicated* UTIs can be caused by the previous bacteria as well as *nosocomial* pathogens contracted in hospitals such as *Pseudomonas aeruginosa* and *Staphylococcus aureus*.

Signs and Symptoms

A patient with bacteriuria or UTI can be asymptomatic. Cystitis symptoms include dysuria, cloudy or foul-smelling urine, urinary frequency and urgency, hematuria (blood in urine), and suprapubic pain. Patients with pyelonephritis may also complain of flank pain, tenderness, and constitutive symptoms such as fever, fatigue, malaise, nausea, and vomiting.

Diagnosis

Urinalysis and urine culture are the standard diagnostic tests for a UTI, although patients with lower UTIs may be presumptively diagnosed without culture. Urinalysis reveals the specific gravity of urine, amount of protein present, presence of bacteria, WBC and RBC count, and *urinary casts* (cylindrical clumps of particles that form in kidney and pass into bladder). A dipstick urinalysis of a midstream clean-catch sample can be done to determine the presence of leukocyte esterase or nitrites, either of which, if positive, suggests the presence of bacteria.

Urine cultures are used to assess if bacteria are present but may be contaminated with improper collection. Urine bacterial count (bacteriuria) of less than 10^5 bacteria/mL, as well as the presence of multiple bacterial strains, may be considered contamination. Thus, bacteriuria counts greater than 10^5 bacteria/mL are indicative of infection.

SELECTED HERBAL THERAPIES

Note

To help make this educational resource more interactive, all pharmacokinetics, adverse effects, and interactions data have been compiled in Appendix A. Safety data specifically related to pregnancy and lactation are listed in Appendix B. Please refer to these appendices when working through the case studies and answering the review questions.

Acacia (*Acacia* spp.)

Grade C: *Unclear or conflicting scientific evidence (dental plaque)*

Mechanism of Action

The usable part of acacia is the gum, which mainly consists of *arabic acid*. When hydrolyzed, arabic acid becomes arabinose, galactose, and arabinosic acid. Acacia gum is highly water soluble and is a common component of chewing gum. Acacia has an antimicrobial activity against *Streptococcus faecalis*.[12-15]

Acacia gum contains fluoride, which has been shown to enhance enamel remineralization and prevent dental caries.[12,13] Acacia gum also contains cyanogenic glycosides and other enzymes (e.g., peroxidases) that exhibit antimicrobial properties, which may help inhibit plaque formation.[16]

Scientific Evidence of Effectiveness

Acacia has been reported anecdotally to be beneficial in the management of plaque and gingivitis. Few studies have been published, although the limited preliminary evidence is promising.[17] Acacia gum lowered plaque and gingival scores after several days of use compared with sugar-free gum.

Dose

Acacia products are not widely standardized to any one constituent. For plaque, daily use of a chewing stick of *Acacia arabica* for 10 minutes five times daily for 7 days has been reported to be effective.[17]

Adverse Effects, Interactions, Pharmacokinetics. See Appendix A.

Andrographis (*Andrographis paniculata*)

Grade A: *Strong scientific evidence (upper respiratory tract infection: treatment)*

Grade C: *Unclear or conflicting scientific evidence (upper respiratory tract infection: prevention)*

Mechanism of Action

Andrographolide, a diterpene lactone compound, is believed to be the principal active agent of andrographis.[18] The aqueous extract of *Andrographis paniculata* has reported bacteriostatic activity. It displayed antimicrobial activity against *Streptococcus mutans* by glucosyltransferase and glucan-binding lectin inhibition.[19]

Scientific Evidence of Effectiveness

BACTERIAL UPPER RESPIRATORY TRACT INFECTION: TREATMENT. *Andrographis paniculata* has traditionally been used as a treatment for fever and infectious illnesses in a number of Asian medical systems. Based on this historical use, it has more recently become popular in Western countries as a treatment for upper respiratory illness, among other treatments. A systematic review of frequently used complementary and alternative medicine (CAM) therapies for UTI in children included *A. paniculata*, *Echinacea*, propolis, ascorbic acid, and homeopathy.[20] Clinical trials, mostly done on the standardized product Kan Jang (Swedish Herbal Institute), collectively suggest that andrographis is effective in reducing the symptom severity and duration of URI, both in children and in adults, if started within 36 to 48 hours of onset of symptoms.[21-26] Although some studies have methodological flaws and almost all lack a standardized outcome measure for assessing patient symptoms of URI, there is good evidence of efficacy. The most significant problem is that almost every trial of andrographis has been conducted with collaboration and support from the manufacturer; further studies should be conducted without such involvement. It is also unclear whether the combination product tested in some trials, which also contains

Eleutherococcus, is more or less effective than the single-herb preparation tested in other studies. Because the investigators did not assess if the infection was bacterial or viral, there is insufficient evidence to recommend this product specifically for the treatment of a bacterial URI.

BACTERIAL UPPER RESPIRATORY TRACT INFECTION: PREVENTION. Based on its apparent effectiveness in treating URIs and possible immunostimulant activity, andrographis has been examined as a possible strategy to prevent URIs during the winter months. Based on the evidence, andrographis may reduce the incidence of URIs during the winter months if taken daily at 200 mg of the standardized extract (Kan Jang, single-herb preparation).[27] Additional studies with larger sample sizes are required to substantiate the effectiveness of andrographis for prevention of URIs. Because the investigators did not assess if the infection was bacterial or viral, there is insufficient evidence to recommend this product specifically for the prevention of a bacterial URI.

Dose

Some commercial products are standardized to contain 4% andrographolides. The most widely tested products are two Kan Jang preparations. One standardized product is a single-herb preparation of the extract SHA-10, standardized to contain 5.25 mg of andrographolide and deoxyandrographolide per tablet; the other product is a combination product containing SHA-10 and the *Eleutherococcus senticosus* extract SHE-3. Standardized extracts of andrographis containing 48 to 60 mg of the andrographolide constituents, divided into three or four daily doses, have been studied for respiratory infections in most clinical trials to date.[21-24,28] According to limited research in children age 4 to 11 years, two tablets of Kan Jang (~30 mg daily of andrographolide and deoxyandrographolide), taken three times daily for 10 days, may improve URI symptoms and were well tolerated.[23] Lower doses of standardized extracts have been evaluated for URI prevention. A single 200-mg to 300-mg standardized tablet has been taken daily for 3 months.[24] Higher doses of andrographis for extended periods may be unsafe, leading to significant side effects.[29]

Adverse Effects, Interactions, Pharmacokinetics. See Appendix A.

Astragalus *(Astragalus membranaceus)*

Grade C: *Unclear or conflicting scientific evidence (tuberculosis)*

Mechanism of Action

In vitro, *Astragalus* has been shown to increase significantly certain antibody classes (IgA and IgG),[30] interleukins, and tumor necrosis factor alpha (TNF-α) by activated macrophages.[31] In mouse study, *Astragalus* polysaccharide fractions activated B cells and macrophages but not T cells.[32]

Scientific Evidence of Effectiveness

Astragalus is typically used in combination with other herbs; therefore it is difficult to evaluate its effectiveness as a monotherapy. Limited clinical evidence suggests that astragalus benefits TB patients. Astragalus (20 mL) was added to 5% glucose solution (500 mL) for intravenous drip once daily in elderly patients with pulmonary TB, which elevated erythrocyte immunity.[33]

Dose

Astragalus, 20 mL in 500 mL 5% glucose solution for IV drip, once daily for 2 months has been used for TB.[33]

Adverse Effects, Interactions, Pharmacokinetics. See Appendix A.

Betel Nut *(Areca catechu)*

Grade C: *Unclear or conflicting scientific evidence (dental caries)*

Mechanism of Action

Betel nut has been shown to slow *Streptococcus mutans* growth by inhibiting glucosyltransferase.[34] Tannic acid from betel nut has also been shown to inhibit the growth of *Staphylococcus aureus, Fusobacterium nucleatum,* and *Streptococcus salivarius.*[35]

Scientific Evidence of Effectiveness

Toothpaste containing betel nut was believed to protect against tooth decay and strengthen the gums; however, the preparation has been discontinued because of safety concerns.[36] Clinical studies are limited. One study assessed the effects of betel nut chewing on dental health in a retrospective analysis.[37] The prevalence of dental caries in subjects who were non–betel nut chewers was compared to regular betel nut chewers. Dental caries occurred in 23% of betel chewers vs. 49% of nonchewers, with statistical significance. In a retrospective analysis of 982 subjects, an inverse relationship was noted between the incidence of dental caries and frequency of betel nut chewing.[38] In a similar study of 301 subjects of New Guinea, the prevalence of dental caries was also found to be inversely proportional to the frequency of betel nut chewing.[39] Because of the known toxicity associated with acute or chronic betel use, however, and the availability of other therapies with demonstrated efficacy against caries development, the risks of betel nut use likely outweigh the potential benefits.

Notably, chewing betel nut alone or with tobacco has been associated with enhanced periodontitis and increased adverse effects on gums and oral hygiene.[40,41] Occurrence of periodontal pockets, gingival lesions, and gum recession was significantly higher in betel nut chewers.[40] Because of conflicting evidence, betel nut chewing should be avoided until further data become available.

Dose

The dose of betel nut for dental caries has not been determined.

Adverse Effects, Interactions, Pharmacokinetics. See Appendix A.

Bloodroot (Sanguinaria canadensis)

Grade B: *Good scientific evidence (plaque/gingivitis)*

Grade C: *Unclear or conflicting scientific evidence (periodontal disease)*

Mechanism of Action

Bloodroot *(Sanguinaria canadensis)* contains several alkaloids, primarily in the rhizomes, which contain approximately 3% to 7% total alkaloid. The major alkaloids include sanguinarine, chelerythrine, chelirubine, sanguirubine, chelilutine, the opium alkaloid protopine, and sanguilutine.[42-44] The chief benzylisoquinoline alkaloid is *sanguinarine*, which is attributed with most of bloodroot's antibacterial and antiinflammatory properties.[45] The root also contains red resin and a large quantity of starch.

Sanguinarine has demonstrated antibacterial activity against gram-positive and gram-negative bacteria.[46-49] The proposed antibacterial mechanism of sanguinarine is its ability to react with nucleophiles.[50] Sanguinarine may also eradicate animal cells by blocking the action of Na^+,K^+-ATPase transmembrane proteins. There is particular interest in the drug sanguinarium's effects on oral bacterial pathogens.[51,52] In clinical split-mouth study, a 7-day treatment with sanguinarium 5% led to significant microbiota changes, such as decreases in antibiotic-resistant bacteria and yeast in periodontal sites as well as in the saliva.[53] The reduction in bacterial growth may result from the inhibition of bacterial adherence and plaque formation, because saguinarine induces bacteria to aggregate and become morphologically irregular in vitro.[45,52,54]

With in vitro screening, sanguinarine and chelerythrine from the roots of *Sanguinaria canadensis* inhibited *Mycobacterium aurum* and *M. smegmatis*.[44] Compared to sanguinarine, chelerythrine was more active against both M. aurum (IC50=7.30 mcg/mL or 19.02 mcM) and M. smegmatis (IC50=29.0 mcg/mL or 75.56 mcM). For most species of plaque bacteria, sanguinarine's minimum inhibitory concentration (MIC) is 1 to 32 mcg/mL.[45]

Scientific Evidence of Effectiveness

PLAQUE/GINGIVITIS. Sanguinarine, a constituent of bloodroot, has been used in multiple clinical trials as a toothpaste or mouthwash ingredient.[55-87] In a 2003 report the U.S. Food and Drug Administration (FDA) Dental Plaque Subcommittee of the Nonprescription Drugs Advisory Committee concluded that "sanguinaria extract at 0.03-0.075% concentration is safe, but there are insufficient data available to permit final classification of its effectiveness in an oral rinse or dentifrice dosage form as an [over-the-counter] antigingivitis/antiplaque active ingredient." Sanguinaria products have been reported to reduce plaque, gingival inflammation, and bleeding parameters for up to six months with no adverse hard tissue effects.[55] Chlorhexidine has been reported as superior to sanguinaria in the prevention of plaque and gingivitis.[88] The antibacterial effects of bloodroot appear to be enhanced by zinc supplementation. Reports of adverse microbiological shifts in the normal oral flora are lacking.

PERIODONTAL DISEASE. The benzophenanthridine alkaloids of bloodroot, including sanguinarine, have displayed anti-inflammatory and antimicrobial activity in vitro.[45-54,89] When tested clinically, sanguinarium 5% reduced pocket depth in deep pockets between teeth and gums compared with controls.[87] However, subgingivally delivered doxycycline hyclate 10% appears to be more effective than sanguinarium chloride 5% in the treatment of periodontitis.[85]

Dose

For gingivitis prevention, oral rinses containing 300 mcg/mL of *Sanguinaria* extract have been used twice daily for up to 6 months in clinical trials,[63,71] as both a manual rinse and under pressure in an oral irrigator.[78] Veadent, a commercially available toothpaste and rinse that contains 0.03% sanguinarine and 0.2% zinc chloride, has been used twice daily for the prevention of gingivitis.

For the treatment of established periodontal disease, oral rinses containing 0.01% sanguinarine have been used daily for up to 6 weeks to reduce plaque formation in patients with established and developing plaque and periodontal disease.[86]

Adverse Effects, Interactions, Pharmacokinetics. See Appendix A.

Bromelain (Bromeliaceae)

Grade C: *Unclear or conflicting scientific evidence (urinary tract infection)*

Mechanism of Action

Bromelains are protease enzymes derived from the plant family Bromeliaceae, which includes the pineapple (*Ananas comosus*).[90,91] In animals, bromelain inhibited *Escherichia coli* in a dose-dependent manner.[92] The exact mechanism of action is not well understood but is likely to involve bromelain's enzymatic activity.

Scientific Evidence of Effectiveness

Results from a randomized controlled study found improvements in subjective symptoms, including pain and urination patterns, in patients with UTIs who used a product containing bromelain (Kimotab).[93] The objective symptoms, such as hematuria and urine protein, WBCs,

RBCs, epithelia, and bacteria, displayed a trend toward improvement.[93]

Dose

The dose of bromelain for UTI has not been determined; however, one study used Kimotab, containing 50 mg (20,000 units) of bromelain and 1 mg (2500 units) of trypsin, to treat UTIs, with some success.[93]

Adverse Effects, Interactions, Pharmacokinetics. See Appendix A.

Cranberry (Vaccinium macrocarpon)

Grade B: *Good scientific evidence (chronic urinary tract infection prophylaxis)*

Grade C: *Unclear or conflicting scientific evidence (urinary tract infection treatment; dental plaque)*

Mechanism of Action

Cranberry was long thought to prevent UTI by means of urinary acidification. However, it has now been demonstrated that cranberry juice inhibits bacterial adherence to uroepithelial cells by 75% for 60 of 77 *Escherichia coli* clinical isolates in vitro when controlling for pH.[94-98] Uropathogenic *E. coli* bacteria adhere to urinary bladder cells because they have substances that mediate adhesion on the fimbriae or pili (threadlike appendages) on cell surfaces. Cranberry juice contains two compounds found to block *E. coli* adhesion.[99] *Fructose* in guava, pineapple, mango, grapefruit, blueberry, and cranberry juice inhibits the mannose-sensitive type 1 fimbrial adhesion in yeast aggregation assays. The second inhibitor is a high-molecular-weight compound called *proanthocyanidin,* found in cranberry and blueberry juices (genus *Ericaceae*), which acts on the mannose-resistant type P fimbriae or pili expressed by uropathogenic *E. coli*.[95,100,101] In vitro this inhibition is irreversible.

Although *E. coli* is the most studied bacterial pathogen treated by cranberry, in vitro examinations of bacterial adherence to urinary epithelial cells have shown that preincubation of *Proteus* and *Pseudomonas* with "cranberry juice cocktail" also results in decreased adhesion to epithelial cells.[102] This effect has been more pronounced in vitro than in vivo, and cranberry juice has not been found to eradicate the most adherent bacteria. Cranberry supplement (Cranactin tablet, 400 mg three times daily for 2 days) and ascorbic acid (500 mg twice daily for 2 days) have decreased deposition rates and numbers of adherent *E. coli* and *Enterococcus faecalis* in vitro; however, they did not exhibit a similar effect with *Pseudomonas aeruginosa, Staphylococcus epidermidis,* or *Candida albicans.*[103] Recently, investigators used a fivefold concentrated preparation of cranberry juice adjusted to pH 7.0 and incubated bacterial strains in broth with cranberry and plain controls. At 24 hours the cranberry-inoculated broth showed no growth of *E. coli, Staphylococcus aureus, Pseudomonas, Klebsiella,* or *Proteus* spp. and decreased growth of *E. faecalis* and *Salmonella* spp.[104] Cranberry has not been shown to be bactericidal.

With consumption of cranberry juice up to 4 L/day, hippuric acid excretion increases, as does urine volume, leading to no changes in urine pH and minimal increases in hippuric acid concentration (to a level insufficient for bacteriostasis).[105] One study showed only transient decreases in urinary pH in three of four subjects.[106] A study in 40 normal subjects found urinary pH to decrease by 0.5, to a minimum of 5.4, with consumption of 250 mL of 80% cranberry juice three times daily for 12 days.[107] A limitation of this study was that the beverage contained 80% cranberry juice, whereas commercially available cocktails contain 25% to 33% juice. Notably, bacteriostasis has been achieved at pH 5.5.

Scientific Evidence of Effectiveness

CHRONIC URINARY TRACT INFECTION PROPHYLAXIS. Although not definitive, highly suggestive evidence supports the use of cranberry for UTI prophylaxis. No single study convincingly demonstrates the ability of cranberry to prevent UTIs. However, despite the poor methodological quality of almost all available studies, the aggregation of favorable evidence combined with a plausible biological mechanism does tend to support this use. Notably, many of the positive and negative studies have been sponsored by the manufacturer Ocean Spray. The effective dose and duration of treatment have not been determined. A properly randomized, double-blind, placebo-controlled trial with adequate follow-up or intention-to-treat analysis could help resolve this question. Additional studies should also be conducted to determine optimal dose.

URINARY TRACT INFECTION TREATMENT. A literature review revealed no reliable evidence to support the use of cranberry for treating UTI. One reason may be that cranberry fails to eradicate the most adherent bacteria in vitro.[107] Without explicit study in this area, a recommendation cannot be made.

DENTAL PLAQUE. In vitro research suggests that reducing the bacterial flora of dental plaque with cranberry may decrease gingival irritation and periodontal disease.[108] However, supportive clinical data are lacking. Commercially available cranberry juice, with its high fructose and dextrose content, may not be suitable for this purpose because of the known contribution of fructose and dextrose to plaque accumulation.

Dose

In general, cranberry juice contains glucose, fructose, ascorbic acid, benzoic acid, citric acid, quinic acid, malic acid, proanthocyanidins, triterpenoids, catechins, lectins, and 90% water. Some cranberry preparations are standardized to 11% to 12% quinic acid per dose.

Studied doses are for *preventing,* not treating, UTI. Cranberry products are not consistently standardized, although 300 mL (10 oz) daily of "cranberry cocktail" (Ocean Spray) was studied in a widely noted trial.[109,110] Recommended doses range from 90 to 480 mL (3-16 oz) of cranberry cocktail twice daily, or 15 to 30 mL of unsweetened 100% cranberry juice daily.

Many experts also recommend one to six 300-mg to 400-mg capsules of hard-gelatin concentrated cranberry extract twice daily, given with water 1 hour before meals or 2 hours after meals. Soft-gelatin capsules contain vegetable oil and a decreased amount of the cranberry compound.[111]

Adverse Effects, Interactions, Pharmacokinetics. See Appendix A.

Eucalyptus (*Eucalyptus* spp.)

Grade C: *Unclear or conflicting scientific evidence (dental plaque/gingivitis)*

Mechanism of Action

Antimicrobial activity of eucalyptus has been studied in animal and basic science research,[112-118] but the exact mechanism of action is not well understood. Studies of medicinal plant extracts have demonstrated broad antimicrobial activity of eucalyptus against *Alicyclobacillus acidoterrestris, Bacillus cereus, Escherichia coli, Enterococcus faecalis,* MRSA, *Propionibacterium acnes, Staphylococcus aureus,*[112-114] and other gram-positive bacteria. Specific activity has been observed against periodontopathic bacteria, such as *Porphyromonas gingivalis, Actinobacillus actinomycetemcomitans, Fusobacterium nucleatum, Streptococcus mutans,* and *Streptococcus sobrinus.*[115-119] Crown gall, a plant tumor obtained from *Eucalyptus globulus,* has shown antibacterial activity against *E. faecalis, Pseudomonas aeruginosa, Bacillus subtilis,* and *Staphylococcus epidermidis.*[119] An in vitro study in rat liver suggested that protonophoric activity may contribute to the cytotoxic and antimicrobial properties of eucalyptus.[120]

Scientific Evidence of Effectiveness

Studies of medicinal plant extracts have demonstrated broad antimicrobial activity of eucalyptus against *E. coli, S. aureus,* and *Candida albicans* isolates,[116] as well as gram-positive and gram-negative oral cariogenic and periodontopathic bacteria.[117,121] Eucalyptol (1,8-cineole), a principal constituent of eucalyptus oil, has a long history of use in endodontics as a solvent, as well as to soften gutta percha (thermoplastic filling material) and various sealers.[122] Several studies have assessed the effects of *Eucalyptus* extract or eucalyptol for the treatment of mouth flora associated with plaque or gingivitis.[123-135] Despite promising preliminary results, the evidence remains equivocal.

Listerine is a broad-spectrum antibacterial mouthrinse that contains a combination of essential oils (eucalyptol, menthol, thymol, methyl salicylate). Although positive results have been obtained using Listerine for reducing plaque and gingivitis, it is difficult to interpret the contribution of eucalyptus to these effects. The mouthwash has been reported to reduce gingivitis and plaque significantly in several additional human studies,[133-135] but to be less efficacious than Peridex (chlorhexidine) against plaque.[136-138] However, Listerine is less likely than Peridex to cause tongue, dental, or restoration stains or supragingival calculus,[139] an effect shown to be caused by Peridex binding to bacterial surfaces. A 2001 human trial conducted by Pfizer, the manufacturer of Listerine, reported that a combination of Listerine mouthwash and a fluoride toothpaste was superior to Colgate Total toothpaste for the reduction of plaque and gingivitis in 316 individuals with plaque after 6 months.[140] Some evidence indicates that Listerine is able to penetrate dental plaque biofilm and kill gram-positive organisms interproximally, in the area most associated with periodontitis and dental caries; this area was previously thought to be cleansed primarily by flossing.[141,142]

Dose

Some suggest that to be medicinally effective, eucalyptus leaf oil must contain 70% to 85% 1,8-cineole (eucalyptol). The Listerine recommendation to reduce gingivitis and plaque is to rinse with a capful (~30 mL) of Listerine twice daily.

Adverse Effects, Interactions, Pharmacokinetics. See Appendix A.

Eyebright (*Euphrasia officinalis*)

Grade C: *Unclear or conflicting scientific evidence (bacterial conjunctivitis)*

Mechanism of Action

Eyebright contains iridoid glycosides, including aucubin,[143,144] as well as flavonoids, including quercetin, apigenin, and tannins. The most studied constituent of eyebright is *aucubin* and its aglycon, *aucubigenin,* shown in vitro to possess antibacterial effects against *Staphylococcus aureus, Proteus mirabilis,* and *Bacillus subtilis.*[145] However, a mechanism of therapeutic action is unknown at this time.

Scientific Evidence of Effectiveness

Eyebright's medicinal properties date from the fourteenth century, when it was believed to "cure all evils of the eye." In Europe, eyebright has been used for centuries as a rinse, compress, or bath against eye infections and other eye-related irritations (a use reflected in many of its vernacular names). Beyond historical and anecdotal reports, clinical trials investigating eyebright for conjunctivitis in children and adults are limited.[146,147] Safety data for this indication are also insufficient, with concerns about potential contamination of products and risk of infection. The German Commission E suggests that eyebright has not been proven safe and effective, and this expert panel does not recommend the topical application of eyebright for hygienic reasons. Eyebright continues to be used as a topical treatment for inflammatory eye disorders such as blepharitis, conjunctivitis, and stye (hordeolum), although safety and efficacy information is lacking.

Dose

There is no widely accepted standardization for eyebright formulations. For adults, 1 drop of eyebright once to five times daily for 3 to 17 days to treat inflammatory or catarrhal conjunctivitis was used in a prospective cohort trial.[146] Traditionally, eyebright has also been applied using compresses.

Children have tolerated four or five homeopathic pills of eyebright 30C daily for 3 days for prevention of viral conjunctivitis in an RCT.[147] However, safety and efficacy data are insufficient to recommend for or against eyebright use in children for any indication.

Adverse Effects, Interactions, Pharmacokinetics. See Appendix A.

Ginseng (Panax spp.)

Grade C: *Unclear or conflicting scientific evidence (methicillin-resistant Staphylococcus aureus)*

Mechanism of Action

The major active components of ginseng are a diverse group of steroidal saponins, labeled *ginsenosides*,[148-150] the mechanisms of which are not fully understood. Every part of the plant has displayed pharmacological activity; however, the root is used most often and has higher ginsenoside content.[151] Generally, the saponin content is higher in *Panax notoginseng* and *Panax quinquefolius* than in *Panax ginseng*.[152]

In mice treated with ginseng before a bacterial challenge of *Staphylococcus aureus*, sepsis was prevented, possibly from early suppression of acute inflammatory responses and later enhancement of macrophage activity.[153] Ginseng has been shown to enhance immune function by stimulating natural killer (NK) cell activity[154-156] and antibody-dependent cellular cytotoxicity,[157,158] as well as intracellular killing in neutrophils and blastogenesis of circulating lymphocytes.[157] However, it is currently unclear how ginseng modulates the immune system, particularly in the context of infection.

Studies have shown ginseng to have various immunomodulatory effects, with either suppression or enhancement of humoral and cellular immunity;[159] these conflicting effects may result from differences in dose levels, composition, and duration of therapy.

Panaxanes and polysaccharides isolated from the roots and culture of *Panax ginseng* have shown analogous immunotropic effects.[160] Prophylactic use of panaxanes increased resistance to *Escherichia coli* sepsis in mice, increased neutrophil and macrophage phagocytosis, stimulated humoral and cell immune factors, and induced important regulating cytokines, interferon gamma and tumor necrosis factor.

Scientific Evidence of Effectiveness

In patients treated with Hochu-ekki-to, which contains ginseng and several other herbs (astragalus, *Atractylodes macrocephala*, dong quai, bupleurum, *Zizyphus spinosa*, citrus peel, licorice, black cohosh, and ginger), urinary MRSA has been reported to decrease after a 10-week treatment period.[161] Further research using ginseng as a monotherapy is warranted.

Dose

The dose of ginseng for MRSA infection has not been determined.

Adverse Effects, Interactions, Pharmacokinetics. See Appendix A.

Goldenseal (Hydrastis canadensis)

Grade C: *Unclear or conflicting scientific evidence (infectious diarrhea; trachoma [Chlamydia trachomatis eye infection])*

Mechanism of Action

The active ingredients of goldenseal include lisoquinoline alkaloids such as berberine, canadine, and hydrastine. The constituent *berberine* has antibacterial activity against *Chlamydia trachomatis, Clostridium tetani, Streptococcus pyogenes, Escherichia coli, Vibrio cholerae, Bifidobacterium longum, Bifidobacterium bifidum, Clostridium perfringens, Clostridium paraputrificum, Actinomyces naeslundii, Porphyromonas gingivalis, Prevotella intermedia, Prevotella nigrescens,* and *Actinobacillus actinomycetemcomitans.*[162-171] This activity appears to increase with pH.[169] Berberine has been found to interfere with the adhesive properties of bacteria by releasing the adhesion lipoteichoic acid (LTA) and preventing adhesion of fibronectin (a glycoprotein) to bacteria.[167,168]

In vitro, an aqueous extract containing berberine had an MIC of 50 mcg/mL for *C. tetani*.[166] The MIC for *S. pyogenes* was 30 mcg/mL; berberine inhibits the adherence of *S. pyogenes* to epithelial cells, possibly by immobilizing fibronectin and hexadecane at concentrations below the MIC.[167] Decreased adhesion to the bladder lining and reduced synthesis of *E. coli* has also been noted.[168] Berberine is bactericidal against *V. cholerae* at concentrations of 35 mcg/mL and against *Staphylococcus aureus* at 50 mcg/mL.[169] Berberine sulfate has been shown to possess antimicrobial activity against gram-positive and gram-negative bacteria in vitro through inhibition of ribonucleic acid (RNA) and protein synthesis.[169] Berberine chloride produced a clear inhibitory effect against *B. longum, B. bifidum, C. perfringens,* and *C. paraputrificum.*[170]

Berberine has a reported inhibitory effect on periodontopathogenic bacteria (*A. naeslundii, P. gingivalis, P. intermedia, P. nigrescens,* and *A. actinomycetemcomitans*) at MIC of 31 to 250 mcg/mL.[171]

Scientific Evidence of Effectiveness

INFECTIOUS DIARRHEA. Berberine, an alkaloid constituent of goldenseal, has been evaluated as a treatment for infectious diarrhea, including choleric diarrhea, in several animal and small preliminary human studies.[172,173] In animals, berberine appears to exert antisecretory effects in diarrhea induced by *E. coli* enterotoxin or *V. cholerae*.[174-178] Berberine sulfate has been suggested to treat diarrhea caused by a number of etiologies.[179] However, data are conflicting from unclear human studies with poor design. Furthermore, because of the small amount of berberine actually available from goldenseal preparations (0.5%-6%), it is not clear whether the concentrations of berberine in goldenseal are sufficient to elicit clinically significant effects. Therefore, the evidence is currently insufficient regarding the efficacy of berberine or goldenseal in the management of infectious diarrhea.

TRACHOMA (*Chlamydia trachomatis* EYE INFECTION). Berberine has been found in vitro and in animals to possess antibacterial properties. Several clinical studies, although of limited methodological strength, have reported favorable effects of berberine ophthalmic preparations on trachoma.[180-183] The effects of berberine appeared to be more effective than sulfacetamide at destroying the organism, but sulfacetamide appeared better in improving short-term symptoms.[180]

Goldenseal is often found in URI remedies that also contain echinacea and may enhance the effects of echinacea. However, the effects of these agents, alone or in combination, are unclear.

Dose

The dose of goldenseal for infectious diarrhea has not been determined. For trachoma, 0.2% berberine drops three times daily for 3 months has been used.[180]

Adverse Effects, Interactions, Pharmacokinetics. See Appendix A.

Horseradish (Armoracia rusticana, syn. Cochlearia armoracia)

Grade C: Unclear or conflicting scientific evidence (urinary tract infection)

Mechanism of Action

Perhaps the most well-known constituent of horseradish is horseradish peroxidase,[184,185] which is widely used in biochemical and histological assays. Other horseradish constituents include glucosinolates (sinigrin, glucobrassicin, neoglucobrassicin, and gluconasturtiin), myrosinase, plastoquinone-9, 6-*O*-acyl-β-d-glucosyl-β-sitosterol, 1,2-dilinolenoyl-3-galactosylglycerol, 3-acyl-sitosterols, and phosphatidylcholines.[186-189] When horseradish cells are damaged by cutting, grating, or chewing, enzymes convert sinigrin to allyl isothiocyanate (mustard oil).

Several early in vitro studies found that some horseradish constituents may have antibacterial activity against gram-negative and gram-positive bacteria.[190-195] The constituent allyl isothiocyanate has been shown to inhibit the growth of food pathogens.[196] The exact mechanism of action is not well understood.

Scientific Evidence of Effectiveness

Several early in vitro studies have indicated that some horseradish constituents have antimicrobial activity.[190-192] An enzyme-glycoside mixture obtained from horseradish roots has been used to treat nonspecific UTIs.[197] According to limited research, the herbal combination drug Angocin Anti-Infekt (containing nasturtium herb and horseradish root) reduced UTI symptoms.[198]

Dose

Horseradish is not widely standardized, and the dose of horseradish for UTI has not been determined. According to secondary sources, a common dose of horseradish is 6 to 20 g daily of the root or equivalent preparations.

Adverse Effects, Interactions, Pharmacokinetics. See Appendix A.

Lime (Citrus aurantifolia)

Grade C: Unclear or conflicting scientific evidence (cholera prevention)

Mechanism of Action

Lime juice has reported protective activity against cholera (*Vibrio cholerae*).[199] However, the exact mechanism of action is not well understood.

Scientific Evidence of Effectiveness

One controlled case study found that lime juice in sauces might aid in the prevention of cholera.[200] Another preliminary case study suggested a protective effect of using limes in the main meal.[201] However, both studies were investigated by the same research group; independent examination is warranted.

Dose

The dose of lime for the prevention of cholera has not been established.

Adverse Effects, Interactions, Pharmacokinetics. See Appendix A.

Lingonberry (Vaccinium vitis-idaea)

Grade C: Unclear or conflicting scientific evidence (urinary tract infection prevention)

Mechanism of Action

A tannin found in lingonberry, epicatechin-(4βbeta→8)-epicatechin-(4βbeta→8, 2βbeta→O→7)-catechin, was found to have strong antimicrobial activity against *Porphyromonas gingivalis* and *Prevotella intermedia*, but not *Actinobacillus actinomycetemcomitans*. Other tannins (unspecified) from lingonberry did not show antimicrobial activity.[202] The exact mechanism of action is not well understood.

Scientific Evidence of Effectiveness

A clinical trial using a combination of cranberry and lingonberry juice determined that this treatment was significantly more effective than no intervention.[203] Although these results are promising, the specific effect of lingonberry on UTI prevention is difficult to interpret.

Dose

The dose of lingonberry for UTI prevention has not been determined.

Adverse Effects, Interactions, Pharmacokinetics. See Appendix A.

Mastic (Pistacia lentiscus)

Grade C: Unclear or conflicting scientific evidence (dental plaque)

Mechanism of Action

The essential oil of mastic gum has been shown to have activity against gram-positive and gram-negative bacteria, although activity was more potent against gram-positive bacteria.[204] Chewing mastic gum reportedly has a broad range of antimicrobial activity against plaque and other oral bacteria.[205,206] Mastic has also exhibited bactericidal activity against isolates of *Helicobacter pylori*.[207,208] Cell wall changes, including morphological abnormalities and cell fragmentation, have been reported.[207]

Scientific Evidence of Effectiveness

Preliminary evidence indicates that chewing mastic gum may reduce the degree of plaque accumulation and gingival inflammation. Compared with placebo gum, mastic gum led to a greater reduction in bacterial colonies after 4 hours of chewing.[206]

Dose

Chewing one piece of mastic gum for 10 to 20 minutes after each meal may help reduce plaque.[206]

Adverse Effects, Interactions, Pharmacokinetics. See Appendix A.

Neem (Azadirachta indica)

Grade C: Unclear or conflicting scientific evidence (dental plaque)

Mechanism of Action

Neem has displayed antimicrobial activity against oral pathogens, including *Streptococcus mutans* and *Lactobacillus*.[209-211] However, the exact mechanism of action is not well understood.

Scientific Evidence of Effectiveness

Several human trials showed that neem has antiplaque properties and antimicrobial activity against oral pathogens.[209-211] Neem extract gel (5% w/w) applied for up to 6 weeks significantly reduced plaque and gingival scores, as effectively as gel containing chlorhexidine gluconate[210] and more effectively than control gel.[209]

Dose

Official standards of neem have been established in the United States. A gel formulation containing neem extract taken twice daily (before bed and after breakfast) for 6 weeks has reduced plaque and gingival scores.[209,210]

Adverse Effects, Interactions, Pharmacokinetics. See Appendix A.

Pycnogenol (Pinus pinaster subsp. atlantica)

Grade C: Unclear or conflicting scientific evidence (dental bleeding/plaque)

Note: Pycnogenol contains oligomeric proanthocyanidins (OPCs) as well as several other bioflavonoids. There has been some confusion in the U.S. market regarding OPC products containing Pycnogenol or grape seed extract (GSE) because one of the generic terms for chemical constituents ("pycnogenols") is the same as the patented trade name (Pycnogenol). Some GSE products formerly were erroneously labeled and marketed in the United States as containing "pycnogenols." Although GSE and Pycnogenol do contain similar chemical constituents (primarily in the OPC fraction), the chemical, pharmacological, and clinical literature on the two products is distinct. The term *Pycnogenol* should therefore be used only when referring to this specific proprietary pine bark extract. Scientific literature regarding this product should not be referenced as a basis for the safety or effectiveness of GSE.

Mechanism of Action

Pycnogenol has been shown in vitro to inhibit gram-positive and gram-negative bacteria,[212] specifically *Escherichia coli*, *Salmonella typhimurium*, *Listeria monocytogenes*, and *Aeromonas hydrophila*.[213,214]

Antioxidants in Pycnogenol gum might minimize gingival inflammation, although the exact mechanism is not well understood.

Scientific Evidence of Effectiveness

Pycnogenol chewing gum was reported to minimize gingival and plaque accumulation.[215] Plaque scores remained unchanged from baseline to after treatment in the Pycnogenol group, whereas it increased in the placebo group. Pycnogenol may be added to toothpaste for its antioxidant effect and astringent taste. Further research is needed to confirm the efficacy of Pycnogenol in promoting gingival health.

Dose

Chewing 5 mg of Pycnogenol gum (six pieces daily) for 14 days has been used to reduce dental plaque.[215]

Adverse Effects, Interactions, Pharmacokinetics. See Appendix A.

Rhubarb (*Rheum* spp.)

Grade B: *Good scientific evidence (gingivitis)*

Mechanism of Action

Anthraquinone glycosides (aloe-emodin, rhein, emodin, chrysophanol, and physcion) found in rhubarb may reduce inflammation and bacterial growth.[216-218] A rhubarb-containing dental product (Parodium) has been found to reduce matrix metalloproteinase type 9 (MMP-9) on fibroblasts and mononuclear cells, which may contribute to its effects on gingival inflammation.[218] Oxalate-containing phytocomplexes extracted from rhubarb reduced dentinal hypersensitivity and pain by producing a layer of crystals that reduces dentinal permeability.[219]

Scientific Evidence of Effectiveness

Pyralvex (containing rhubarb extract and salicyclic acid) has been used for decades as a salve for gingivitis and the oral mucosa. Parodium (containing rhubarb and chlorhexidine) was introduced more recently as a similar treatment. Clinical studies on Pyralvex and Parodium indicate that these combination treatments may be beneficial in treating gingivitis.[220-222] However, more high-quality studies with rhubarb as a monotherapy are needed to discern its role in gingivitis treatment.

Dose

The manufacturer (Laboratoire Pierre Fabre Sane, France) recommends that Parodium gel (containing 0.02 g chlorhexidine and 0.2 g rhubarb extract) be rubbed on the gingival surface for 1 minute three times daily.

The recommended use for Pyralvex solution (rhubarb extract [equivalent to 0.005 g anthraquinone glycosides] and 0.01 g salicylic acid) is to apply to the sore area of the mouth three or four times daily using the provided brush, and to avoid rinsing the mouth or eating for 15 minutes after use.

Adverse Effects, Interactions, Pharmacokinetics. See Appendix A.

Tea (*Camellia sinensis*)

Grade C: *Unclear or conflicting scientific evidence (dental caries prevention; methicillin-resistant* **Staphylococcus aureus** *infection treatment)*

Mechanism of Action

The polyphenol components of black and green tea are thought to exert antibacterial effects against dental plaque;[200] however, the mechanism of this effect is not fully understood.[223] In vitro, extracts of tea *(Camellia sinensis)* reversed methicillin resistance in MRSA isolates and, to some extent, penicillin resistance in beta-lactamase–producing *S. aureus*. *C. sinensis* was found to prevent PBP2′ synthesis and inhibit the secretion of beta-lactamase.[224]

The microbiological effects of black tea compared with green tea were assessed alone and in combination with selected antibiotics against *Escherichia coli*.[225] Both tea extracts inhibited bacterial growth at 5 and 7 hours. Black teas had either synergistic or antagonistic effects at different concentrations, which varied with the antibiotic used.

Scientific Evidence of Effectiveness

DENTAL CARIES PREVENTION. There is limited preliminary evidence suggesting that green and black tea may be effective in decreasing plaque.[223,226] One study found that rinsing with a black tea mouthwash five times for 30 seconds over a 15-minute period inhibited bacterial growth in dental plaque.[223] In another study, individuals rinsing with black tea for 1 minute, 10 times a day, accumulated significantly less plaque than those rinsing with water.[226]

METHICILLIN-RESISTANT *Staphylococcus Aureus* INFECTION: TREATMENT. Inhaled tea catechin, a tannic acid, was temporarily effective in reducing MRSA growth and decreasing the hospital stay in older patients with MRSA in their sputum.[227] However, this limited clinical evidence warrants further investigation of tea use in MRSA infections.

Dose

For dental cavity prevention, 20 mL of black tea has been gargled for 60 seconds daily (duration unspecified). The dose of green tea for dental carries or MRSA has not been determined.

Adverse Effects, Interactions, Pharmacokinetics. See Appendix A.

Tea Tree (*Melaleuca alternifolia*)

Grade C: *Unclear or conflicting scientific evidence (methicillin-resistant* **Staphylococcus aureus** *colonization; dental plaque/gingivitis)*

Mechanism of Action

The antimicrobial activity of tea tree oil has been attributed to the constituent terpinen-4-ol.[228] In vitro studies showed that at concentrations that inhibit the growth of several bacterial species, tea tree oil also inhibited glucose-stimulated leakage of intracellular potassium.[229,230] Tea tree oil has been found to stimulate autolysis of bacterial cells in both the exponential and the stationary growth phase, with greater activity during the exponential phase.[231] The antibacterial activity of tea tree oil may be decreased by the presence of organic matter or certain detergents.[232]

Scientific Evidence of Effectiveness

According to in vitro studies, tea tree oil has antimicrobial activity against MRSA.[233-235] According to preliminary studies, topical tea tree oil may be beneficial in the eradication of MRSA colonization.[236-238] A 4% tea tree oil nasal ointment and 5% tea tree oil body wash appeared to be more effective than a standard treatment of 2% mupirocin nasal ointment and triclosan body wash, although the results were not statistically significant.[239]

Dose
The dose of tea tree oil for the eradication of MRSA colonization has not been determined.

Adverse Effects, Interactions, Pharmacokinetics. See Appendix A.

Thyme (Thymus vulgaris)

Grade C: *Unclear or conflicting scientific evidence (dental plaque)*

Mechanism of Action
The essential oils of thyme include the phenol *thymol*, a key constituent.[240-242] Antimicrobial activities of thyme and thymol have been reported in vitro.[243] Antibacterial efficacy has been noted against several bacterial species, including *Salmonella typhimurium*, *Staphylococcus aureus*, and *Helicobacter pylori*.[244-249] Activity against cariogenic and periodontopathogenic bacteria such as *Porphyromonas gingivalis*, *Selenomonas artemidis*, *Streptococcus sobrinus*, and *Streptococcus mutans* has been reported, possibly related to membrane perforation and rapid efflux of intracellular components.[250,251]

Scientific Evidence of Effectiveness
Thymol shows in vitro activity against *P. gingivalis*, *S. artemidis*, *S. sobrinus*, and *S. mutans*.[250,251] Thymol is included as one of several ingredients in antiseptic mouthwashes, including Listerine (0.064%). Clinical studies have reported efficacy of Listerine in decreasing plaque formation and gingivitis,[251-254] although there is limited evidence that thymol alone is effective.

Dose
For periodontal prophylaxis in adults, it is recommended to steep 5 g dried thyme leaf in 100 mL boiling water for 10 minutes and strain (5% infusion). Thymol is a constituent in some combination mouthwash products such as Listerine, which is demonstrated to be effective in reducing oral bacteria.

For periodontal prophylaxis in children, a combination product containing 1% chlorhexidine/thymol varnish (Cervitec) was well tolerated by 110 healthy children (age 8-10 years) when taken three times daily for 2 weeks.[251]

Adverse Effects, Interactions, Pharmacokinetics. See Appendix A.

Uva Ursi (Arctostaphylos uva-ursi)

Grade C: *Unclear or conflicting scientific evidence (urinary tract infection)*

Mechanism of Action
Arbutin, the main chemical constituent of uva ursi, is a phenolic glycoside that becomes hydrolyzed to hydroquinone. Both chemicals may contribute to antiseptic effects in the urinary tract. Arbutin has been reported to be active against *Staphylococcus aureus* and *Escherichia coli*; it has also been reported to be an effective urinary antibiotic, but only if taken in large doses and if the urine is alkaline.[255] Arbutin and extract from the leaves of uva ursi have an inhibitory effect on glucosidase activity of bacteria in vitro.[256] The minimal bactericidal concentration of arbutin ranges from 0.4% to 0.8%, depending on the species of microorganism. An in vitro study indicated that aqueous extracts from uva ursi leaves increased hydrophobicity of gram-negative bacteria (*E. coli* and *Acinetobacter baumannii*).[257] Thus the bacterial particles might be more easily aggregated and excreted.

Scientific Evidence of Effectiveness
Uva ursi has long been used as a folk remedy to treat UTI; however, supportive clinical evidence is limited. According to preliminary study, a combination of hydroalcoholic extracts from uva ursi leaves (with standardized content of the phenolglycosides arbutin and metylarbutin) and dandelion (UVA-E) may reduce UTI recurrence in women.[258]

Dose
Traditionally, 250 to 500 mg of uva ursi powdered extract (20% arbutin) has been taken three times daily (for no more than 4 days) to treat UTI.

Adverse Effects, Interactions, Pharmacokinetics. See Appendix A.

HERBAL THERAPIES WITH NEGATIVE EVIDENCE

Cranberry (Vaccinium macrocarpon)

Grade D: *Fair negative scientific evidence (chronic urinary tract infection prophylaxis in children with neurogenic bladders)*

Cranberry is widely used to prevent UTIs. However, it does not appear to be effective UTI prophylaxis in children with neurogenic bladder.[259]

HERBAL THERAPIES WITH LIMITED EVIDENCE

Agrimony (Agrimonia spp.)

The ancient Egyptians used agrimony to treat tuberculosis (TB). The antibacterial activity of agrimony may be attributed to certain components from its seed extract.[260]

Currently, evidence evaluating agrimony's efficacy against *Mycobacterium tuberculosis* strains is lacking.

Angostura (*Galipea officinalis*, syn. *Angostura trifoliata*)

Allocspariene, candicine, tetrahydroquinolines, and several other alkaloids have been isolated from angostura trunk bark.[261-263] These alkaloids have displayed activity against *M. tuberculosis* strains.[261]

Bamboo (*Arundinaria japonica*)

In folk medicine, *tabashir*, which is a hardened material inside bamboo, has been used for TB and leprosy. Clinical evidence is lacking.

Beta-Sitosterol (β-Sitosterol), Sitosterol (22,23-dihydrostigmasterol, 24-ethylcholesterol)

Beta-sitosterol and β-sitosterol glucoside have been studied as adjunct treatment for TB.[264] Preliminary study of a small patient sample found improved weight gain and higher lymphocyte and eosinophil counts in pulmonary TB patients receiving sitosterols in addition to an efficacious antituberculosis regimen.

Blessed Thistle (*Cnicus benedictus*)

Laboratory studies report that blessed thistle (and chemicals in blessed thistle such as cnicin and polyacetylene) has activity against several types of bacteria but no effects on other types. Reliable human study is lacking. Further evidence is necessary to draw conclusions.

Chamomile (*Matricaria recutita*, syn. *Matricaria suaveolens*, *Matricaria chamomilla*, *Anthemis nobilis*, *Chamaemelum nobile*, *Chamomilla chamomilla*, *Chamomilla recutita*)

In vitro study results of chamomile's antimicrobial activity have been encouraging, but human data are lacking. Chamomile oil is actively antibacterial and fungicidal at concentrations of at least 25 mg/mL, as is the chamomile constituent *bisabolol* at concentrations of at least 1 mg/mL. Alpha-bisabolol, luteolin, quercitin, and apeginin have been theorized to possess antibacterial properties.[265] The coumarin constituent *hernearin* may also have antibacterial properties in the presence of ultraviolet light. High-molecular-weight polysaccharides with immunostimulating activity have been isolated from German chamomile.[266] Two studies demonstrated that gram-positive bacteria were more susceptible to chamomile oil than gram-negative bacteria.[276] Chamomile oil was most effective against *Staphylococcus aureus*, *Streptococcus mutans*, and *Streptococcus salivarius*, with bactericidal activity against *Bacillus megatherium*, *Leptospira icterohaemorrhagiae*, and *Trichomonas* as well. The hydroalcoholic extract of chamomile completely inhibited growth of group B streptococci.[268] Additional in vitro studies showed that chamomile blocked aggregation of *Helicobacter pylori*[269] and numerous strains of *Escherichia coli*.[257]

Echinacea (*Echinacea* spp.)

Oral preparations of echinacea are popular in Europe and the United States for the prevention and treatment of upper respiratory tract infections (URIs) or the common cold. Its beneficial effects appear to be primarily caused by its immunostimulatory properties, which target both nonspecific and specific immune function. Laboratory studies also suggest that echinacea may have antibacterial effects.[270,271]

Euphorbia (*Euphorbia* spp.)

Euphorbia is reported as having antibacterial activity against pathogenic strains of gram-positive and gram-negative bacteria in animals.[272] The rootstock extracts may have better antibacterial properties than leaf extracts. Glucocerebrosides found in methanolic extracts from the plant *Euphorbia peplis* L. are theorized to contribute to antifungal and antitubercular activity.[273]

Garlic (*Allium sativum*)

Garlic has a long history of use in the treatment of various infectious agents, including bacteria. Garlic has been effective in vitro against numerous gram-negative and gram-positive bacteria, including resistant strains,[274-279] mycobacteria,[280-282] and *Helicobacter* spp.[278,283,284] Heating may adversely affect this benefit, related to a loss of alliinase activity,[285] and different preparations may have variant pharmacological activities against bacteria and mycobacteria.[280-282] Antimicrobial activity of garlic oil is more potent than garlic powder on a unit-weight basis.[286] There is currently a lack of human evidence.

Kudzu (*Pueraria lobata*)

Kudzu root inhibited microbial growth of both gram-negative and gram-positive foodborne pathogens in various foods, especially liquid foods.[287]

Lavender (*Lavandula angustifolia*)

Preliminary data from in vitro studies suggest that lavender oils possess antibiotic activity. Gabbrielli et al[288] demonstrated in vitro activity of lavender oil (*Lavandula angustifolia* and *L. latifolia*) against various strains of nontubercular mycobacteria. Activity of 2% to 0.12% (v/v) lavender oils has been documented against both methicillin-resistant *Staphylococcus aureus* (MRSA) and vancomycin-resistant enterococci (VRE).[289] However, this has not been tested in animal or human studies, and results cannot be considered clinically relevant.

Peppermint (*Mentha* x *piperita*)

Grade C: *Unclear or conflicting scientific evidence (urinary tract infection)*

In vitro, peppermint oil inhibited growth of *Haemophilus influenzae, Streptococcus pyogenes, Streptococcus pneumoniae*, and *Staphylococcus aureus*, but not *Escherichia coli*.[290] However, the exact mechanism of action is not well understood. Peppermint tea, in combination with other therapies, has been traditionally used in the treatment of UTIs,[12] but research is lacking. Peppermint may warrant further investigation for its potential therapeutic efficacy in UTIs.

Sanicle (*Sanicula europaea*)

Potential favorable results of a sanicle *(Sanicula aqua)* heuristic homeopathic preparation have been reported in a case report for recurrent otitis media.[291] High-quality clinical studies are needed before a recommendation can be made.

Seaweed

A lectinlike mucopolysaccharide found in *Fucus vesiculosus* (bladderwrack) has been found to inhibit the growth of multiple *Neisseria meningitidis* and *Escherichia coli* strains in vitro.[292] The mucopolysaccharide inhibited the growth of many *N. meningitidis* strains at a concentration of 5 mcg/mL and was bactericidal at concentrations greater than 10 mcg/mL. The growth of select *E. coli* strains was also inhibited by this mucopolysaccharide at concentrations greater than 10 mcg/mL. However, clinical evidence is lacking.

Sorrel (*Rumex acetosa, Rumex* spp.)

Well-conducted studies that demonstrate antiviral or antibacterial activity of sorrel are lacking. In an in vitro study, sorrel did not demonstrate activity against *Bacillus subtilis, Escherichia coli, Proteus morganii, Pseudomonas aeruginosa, Proteus vulgaris, Serratia marcescens*, or *Staphylococcus aureus*.[293]

Yarrow (*Achillea millefolium*)

Essential oil from yarrow *(Achillea fragrantissima, A. multifida, A. clavennae, A. holosericea)* has been found to contain terpinen-4-ol. This constituent has reported bacteriostatic activity against *Escherichia coli, Salmonella typhosa, Shigella sonnei, Staphylococcus aureus, Klebsiella pneumoniae, Streptococcus pneumoniae*, and *Pseudomonas aeruginosa*.[294-297] Although yarrow's antibacterial effects have been demonstrated in vitro, preliminary research on a herbal combination of yarrow, juniper, and nettle found no benefit in plaque or gingivitis inhibition.[298]

Yerba Santa (*Eriodictyon californicum*)

Yerba santa was used clinically in the United States and Britain starting in the late 1800s, with formalized use ending in the 1960s when drug regulations became more stringent with proof of efficacy. Use of *Eriodictyon* extracts in pulmonary conditions (e.g., bacterial pneumonia, TB) has an extensive clinical history.[299-302] However, there are no available human trials in this area.

ADJUNCT THERAPIES

1. Various dietary supplements, including probiotics, vitamins, and other CAM modalities, may be useful as adjunct therapies to standard antimicrobials. Furthermore, supplements may help optimize immune function, prevent infection, provide symptomatic relief, and improve overall quality of life in patients.
2. The term *probiotics* was first coined in 1965,[303] and refers to beneficial bacteria ("friendly germs") taken as dietary supplements (capsules, tablets, beverages, powders, yogurts, other foods) to help maintain intestinal tract health and aid in digestion. They also are purported to keep potentially harmful bacteria and yeasts in the gut under control. Common probiotics include *Lactobacillus* and *Bifidobacterium* strains. Most probiotics come from food sources, especially cultured milk products. Probiotics may suppress pathogenic microbial growth through competitive inhibition. Systematic reviews and meta-analyses have shown overall benefits for probiotic supplementation in treating infectious diarrhea,[304,305] antibiotic-associated diarrhea,[306] and other infections. Moreover, probiotics display numerous immunomodulatory actions. Probiotics may directly enhance immunity by providing microbial stimuli to gut-associated lymphoid tissue (GALT, critical site of immune maturation); may enhance gut barrier function to assist local immune responses; and may enhance innate immunity (e.g., phagocytic and NK activity)[307] and acquired immunity (e.g., immunoglobulin and cytokine production).[308] Good evidence supports immunomodulating properties for individual probiotic strains, although differences exist, even for the same species. For example, *Lactobacillus rhamnosus* (formerly *L. casei*) strain GR-1 efficiently colonizes the gut and vagina and may offer benefit in urogenital infections. In contrast, *L. rhamnosus* strain GG (LGG) efficiently colonizes and has demonstrated numerous benefits in the intestinal tract, but does not colonize the vagina. Nonetheless, with abundant research on collective probiotic strains, very strong evidence supports the health benefits of probiotics in general. Also, probiotics may be taken to reestablish gastrointestinal microflora after antibiotic ablation.

Herbs with Potential Antibacterial or Antimycobacterial Properties*

HERB	SPECIFIC THERAPEUTIC USE(S)†	HERB	SPECIFIC THERAPEUTIC USE(S)†
Abuta	Cholera, leprosy	Boswellia	Antibacterial, antiseptic, infections
Acerola	Antibacterial	Bromelain	Antibiotic absorption problems in gut, cellulitis, staphylococcal infections
Aconite	Antibacterial, cholera, gonorrhea, scarlet fever, tetanus, tuberculosis		
African wild potato	Tuberculosis	Buchu	Antimicrobial, antiseptic, cholera
Agave	Antibacterial	Buckshorn plantain	Antibacterial
Alfalfa	Antimicrobial	Bugleweed	Tuberculosis
Alkanna	Antibacterial, antimicrobial	Bulbous buttercup	Antibacterial, antimicrobial, antiseptic
Allspice	Antiseptic (teeth and gums)	Bupleurum	Antibacterial, antipseudomonal, antiseptic, tuberculosis (pulmonary)
Aloe	Bacterial skin infections		
Alpinia	Antibiotic, antimicrobial	Burdock	Bacterial infections, gonorrhea
American pawpaw	Antibacterial, scarlet fever	Cajeput	Antibacterial
Andiroba	Antimicrobial	Calamus	Antibacterial, antimicrobial, tuberculosis
Andrographis	Cholera, gonorrhea		
Anise	Antibacterial	Calendula	Bacterial infections, cholera, tuberculosis
Annatto	Antimicrobial, antiseptic, bacterial skin infections, gonorrhea, leprosy		
		California jimson weed	Antibacterial
Apricot	Antibacterial		
Aristolochia spp.	Antibacterial, infections	Cardamom	Antiseptic (pulmonary), bacterial infections (teeth, gum), tuberculosis
Arnica	Antibacterial, antiseptic		
Arrowroot	Antibacterial, cholera, gangrene	Carqueja	Antimicrobial
Ash	Antimicrobial	Cascara	Antibacterial
Ashwagandha	Tuberculosis	Catnip	Antibacterial, antimicrobial
Asparagus	Antimicrobial	Cat's claw	Antibacterial, antimicrobial, gonorrhea
Astragalus	Leprosy		
Bacopa	Antimicrobial	Chaparral	Antibacterial, tuberculosis
Bael	Cholera	Chickweed	Antibacterial
Banaba	Antibacterial	Chicory	Antibacterial
Barberry	Antimicrobial, antiseptic, cholera, infections (*E. coli*), tuberculosis	Chrysanthemum	Antibacterial
		Cinnamon	Antibacterial, antimicrobial, antiseptic
Barley	Antimicrobial		
Bay laurel	Antibacterial, antimicrobial, antiseptic	Clove	Antibacterial, antimicrobial, antiseptic
Belladonna	Scarlet fever	Comfrey	Antimicrobial, gangrene
Betony	Antimicrobial, antiseptic	Cordyceps	Tuberculosis
Bilberry	Antimicrobial, antiseptic, bacterial skin infections	Cramp bark	Skin disinfectant/sterilization
		Daisy (*Bellis perennis*)	Antimicrobial
Birch	Antimicrobial	Damiana	Antibacterial
Bitter almond	Antibacterial	*Datura wrightii*	Antibacterial
Bitter melon	Antimicrobial	Desert parsley	Antibacterial, trachoma, tuberculosis
Black horehound	Antibacterial	Devil's club	Antibacterial, skin infections, tuberculosis
Black pepper	Antibacterial		
Bloodroot	Antibacterial, antimicrobial, antiseptic, bacterial skin infections, leprosy, tuberculosis	Dong quai	Antibacterial, antiseptic, infections
		Elecampane	Antibiotic, antimicrobial, antiseptic, tuberculosis
		Ephedra	Gonorrhea
Blue flag	Cholera, tuberculosis (scrofula)	Fennel	Antibacterial
Boldo	Antiseptic, gonorrhea	Fenugreek	Cellulitis, infections, tuberculosis

Continued

Herbs with Potential Antibacterial or Antimycobacterial Properties—cont'd

HERB	SPECIFIC THERAPEUTIC USE(S)†	HERB	SPECIFIC THERAPEUTIC USE(S)†
Flax	Gonorrhea, skin infections	Noni	Antibacterial, infections, tuberculosis
Fo-ti	Infections, tuberculosis	Nux vomica	Antibacterial, bubonic plague
Garcinia	Antibacterial, antimicrobial	Oleander	Bacterial infections, leprosy
Ginger	Antibacterial, antiseptic, cholera	Olive leaf	Antibacterial
Ginkgo	Antibacterial	Onion	Antibacterial, antimicrobial
Goji	Antimicrobial	Oregano	Antibacterial, including against MRSA
Goldenrod	Infections, antimicrobial, tuberculosis	Pagoda tree	Antimicrobial
Gotu kola	Infections, cellulitis, cholera, leprosy, tuberculosis	Papain	Tuberculosis
		Passion flower	Bacterial infections
Grape seed	Antimicrobial, cholera	Pennyroyal	Antiseptic, leprosy
Grapefruit	Antibacterial, antiseptic	Perilla	Antimicrobial
Greater celandine	Antimicrobial	Podophyllum	Antibacterial
Ground ivy	Antibacterial, antiseptic	Pokeweed	Anthrax, antimicrobial, gonorrhea
Guggul	Leprosy	Pomegranate	Leprosy
Gymnema	Antimicrobial	Populus	Antibacterial
Hawthorn	Antibacterial	Quassia	Antibacterial
Heartsease	Antimicrobial, gonorrhea	Raspberry	Antibacterial/antifungal, infections (chronic)
Hibiscus	Antibacterial (melioidosis)		
Holy basil	Antibacterial, cholera, gonorrhea, tuberculosis	Red clover	Antibacterial, tuberculosis
		Red yeast rice	Anthrax
Hop	Antibacterial, antimicrobial, leprosy, tuberculosis	Rhodiola	Antimicrobial
		Rooibos	Infections
Horny goat weed	Antibacterial, antimicrobial	Rose hip	Antibacterial, antiinfective, antiseptic
Horseradish	Tuberculosis	Rosemary	Antibacterial, antimicrobial
Horsetail	Gonorrhea, tuberculosis	Sage	Antibacterial, antimicrobial, antiseptic
Jackfruit	Antibacterial		
Jequirity	Antimicrobial, gonorrhea, tetanus	Sarsaparilla	Antibacterial, antimicrobial
Jointed flatsedge	Antimicrobial	Saw palmetto	Antibacterial
Katuka	Infections	Scotch broom	Diphtheria
Kava	Gonorrhea, infections, leprosy, tuberculosis	Sea buckthorn	Antibacterial, infections
		Shepherd's purse	Antimicrobial
Kiwi	Antibacterial	Shiitake mushroom	Antimicrobial, infections, tuberculosis
Labrador tea	Tuberculosis	Skullcap	Antibacterial
Lemongrass	Antibacterial, antimicrobial, antiseptic, cholera, infections, sudden acute respiratory syndrome (SARS)	Slippery elm	Tuberculosis
		Spirulina	Antibacterial
		St. John's wort	Bacterial skin infections (topical)
Licorice	Antibacterial, antimicrobial, methicillin-resistant *Staphylococcus aureus* (MRSA)	Star anise	Antibacterial
		Stevia	Antibacterial, antimicrobial
		Stinging nettle	Cholera, gangrene, tuberculosis
Maca	Tuberculosis	Strawberry	Antibacterial
Maitake mushroom	Antiinfective, bacterial infection	Sweet almond	Antibacterial
Mangosteen	Antibacterial, antiseptic, gonorrhea, skin infections, tuberculosis	Sweet Annie	Antibacterial
		Sweet basil	Antibacterial, antimicrobial
Meadowsweet	Antibacterial, cellulitis	Tamanu	Antibacterial, leprosy
Milk thistle	Antibacterial	Tamarind	Antimicrobial, antiseptic, bacterial skin infections (erysipelas), leprosy, skin disinfectant/sterilization
Morus nigra	Antibacterial, tetanus		
Mugwort	Antimicrobial, antiseptic		
Mullein	Antibacterial, antiseptic, tuberculosis	Tangerine	Antibacterial

Herbs with Potential Antibacterial or Antimycobacterial Properties—cont'd

HERB	SPECIFIC THERAPEUTIC USE(S)†	HERB	SPECIFIC THERAPEUTIC USE(S)†
Tansy	Antibacterial, antiseptic, tuberculosis	Watercress	Antibiotic, antimicrobial, skin infections, tuberculosis
Thyme	Cellulitis, MRSA	White horehound	Tuberculosis
Tribulus	Gonorrhea, leprosy	White oak	Antibacterial, antiseptic, tuberculosis (prevention)
Turmeric	Antibacterial, antimicrobial, gonorrhea, infections (MRSA), leprosy	White water lily	Antiseptic, gonorrhea, tuberculosis
Usnea	Antibacterial, tetanus, tuberculosis	Wild arrach	Antimicrobial
Verbena	Antibacterial, antimicrobial	Willow	Antiseptic
Wasabi	Antibacterial	Yohimbe	Leprosy

*This is not an all-inclusive or comprehensive list of herbs with antibacterial or antimycobacterial properties; other herbs and supplements may possess these qualities. A qualified health care provider should be consulted with specific questions or concerns regarding potential immunomodulating effects or interactions.
†Based on expert opinion, anecdote, case reports, and/or preliminary trial evidence.

3. Probiotics should not be confused with *prebiotics,* which are complex sugars (lactulose, lactitol, fructo-oligosaccharides, inulin) that promote the growth of beneficial bacteria in the intestines. In 1995, Gibson and Roberfroid coined the term "prebiotic" to describe "the non-digestible food that beneficially affects the host by selectively stimulating the growth and/or activity of one or more bacteria in the colon."[309] For example, bifidobacteria are promoted by fructo-oligosaccharides and inulin. The term *synbiotic* refers to a product that contains both a probiotic and a prebiotic.
4. *Berberine,* a constituent of plants such as goldenseal, has been studied as an adjunct to standard tetracycline therapy for cholera, with slight to modest benefits over tetracycline alone.[310-312]
5. *Vitamin C* (ascorbic acid), about 1 g daily, has been suggested for women with recurrent UTIs. It is believed that vitamin C acidifies urine and thereby inhibits bacterial growth. Vitamin C may also have a role in the prevention of foodborne disease, because patients with hypochlorhydria are believed to be at greater risk of infection.
6. High doses of *zinc* supplements (80 mg daily) may increase the risk for UTIs and other urological problems. The recommended daily zinc is 8 mg for women and 11 mg for men. Zinc deficiency is associated with reduced absorption and increased secretion of water and electrolytes in an in vitro model of cholera infection.[313] In one study, zinc supplementation significantly reduced the duration of diarrhea and stool output in children with cholera.[314] The authors recommended supplementation with zinc for children with cholera to reduce disease duration and severity.
7. *Selenium* may stimulate immune function by increasing the activity of interleukin-2 and promoting the development of T-helper cells. Preliminary research reports that selenium can be beneficial in the prevention of several types of infection, including recurrence of erysipelas (bacterial skin infection associated with lymphedema), sepsis, and *Mycoplasma pneumoniae.*
8. Various CAM therapies, including natural health products such as herbs and homeopathic remedies, may be beneficial for pain related to infection. In Germany, *sage* mouthwashes and gargles have long been approved for the treatment of sore throat by the German Commission E. Herbal ear drops may contain calendula *(Calendula officinalis)* and lavender *(Lavendula officinalis),* and homeopathic preparations may include belladonna, calendula, capsicum, mullein, and aconite—all of which target the pain of an ear infection (otitis media).
9. *Chiropractic manipulation,* a discipline that focuses on the relationship between spinal structure and body function mediated by the nervous system, has been used to treat infection, particularly recurrent otitis media. Chiropractic may stimulate drainage of the ear in children who build up fluid and consequently acquire infection. However, evidence is lacking to support pediatric use for chiropractic manipulation as a treatment or an adjunct therapy for any infection.
10. Similar to chiropractic manipulation, *osteopathy* utilizes various techniques that are generally less forceful. This practice emphasizes the structural, mechanical, and functional imbalances to provide pain relief. It may also be used as an adjunct to recurrent otitis media care. There are risks of serious adverse effects of chiropractic care. Parents of children with recurrent ear infections must weigh the benefits and risks of these interventions.

INTEGRATIVE THERAPY PLAN

- Discuss the patient's symptoms of possible bacterial infection, including fever, swelling, chills, sweating, redness, and pain.

- Ensure that laboratory tests were performed and accurately interpreted. This will confirm the presence of infection and identify the pathogen. A variety of tests, including WBC count, Gram stain, and culture and sensitivity, should be evaluated.
- Obtain the patient's medical history, including any allergies.
- Review the patient's prescription and nonprescription regimen before adding an antibiotic or antibacterial herb or supplement.
- Determine if the patient has taken or been prescribed any antibiotics (e.g., penicillin, amoxicillin, ciprofloxacin, cephalexin) for an existing infection.
- In patients who are interested, discuss the uses and efficacy of dietary supplements for bacterial infections and enhancing the immune system.
- Cranberry (juice or capsules) may be beneficial for the prevention of UTIs. Most evidence has focused on effects against *Escherichia coli*, although in vitro research also suggests activity against *Proteus, Pseudomonas,* and other species. No clear dosing guidelines exist, but given its safety, moderate amounts of cranberry juice "cocktail" may be recommended to prevent UTI in non–chronically ill individuals.
- The goldenseal component berberine has effects against bacteria and inflammation. Weak human studies have reported favorable effects of berberine ophthalmic preparations on trachoma. Goldenseal is often combined with echinacea to treat URIs, but their effects when combined are scientifically unproven.
- Bloodroot, rhubarb, and thyme may each be found in various dental products. Bloodroot has traditionally been associated with antimicrobial activity; its constituent sanguinarine has been used as a toothpaste or mouthrinse ingredient for gingivitis. Pyralvex and Parodium contain rhubarb, an herb with antiinflammatory and antibacterial properties that may also be beneficial in treating gingivitis. Thymol is one of several ingredients in antiseptic mouthwashes such as Listerine. Clinical studies have reported efficacy of Listerine in decreasing plaque formation and gingivitis, although human evidence for thymol alone is limited.
- Ensure that all patients receiving antibiotics or antibacterial herbs or supplements are being monitored for efficacy, including lowered body temperature, decreased WBC count, and reduced symptoms of infection.
- Discuss antibiotic resistance with the patient and the potential for resistant bacteria with antibiotic use. Instruct the patient to complete the full course even if the patient "feels better." Tell the patient never to share or save antibiotics. Antibiotics for one type of infection may not treat another type of infection, and some individuals may have severe allergic reactions to certain antibiotic classes.
- Advise the patient to avoid close contact with individuals to reduce the risk of acquiring and spreading infections.
- Encourage the patient to consume foods that have a positive effect on the immune system, including nonfat dairy products such as yogurt (containing probiotics), fresh fruits and vegetables, and whole grains.
- Recommend regular exercise as well as vitamins and minerals, including zinc, vitamin C, and selenium, to prevent infection and boost the immune system.
- Various CAM practices, including natural health products and chiropractic and osteopathic manipulation, are popularly used for the prevention and treatment of ear infections. However, supportive research is scarce. Parents of children with recurrent ear infections must weigh the benefits and risks of all interventions.
- Urge the patient to practice good hygiene. Wash hands in warm soapy water after using the bathroom, changing diapers, playing or working outdoors, or handling pets, and before meals, cleaning wounds (before and after), and caring for an infant (before and after). For best results, apply soap and rub hands together for 20 seconds before rinsing thoroughly.

Case Studies

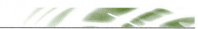

CASE STUDY 27-1

EA is a 32-year-old registered nurse (RN) who works in a local hospital. She scraped her arm on an open cabinet in the utility room, and the wound subsequently became infected. She was "too busy taking care of patients" to attend to what she thought at the time was an inconsequential abrasion. She was given a prescription for cephalexin (Keflex); however, the infection worsened. Culture and sensitivity testing revealed that the infectious organism was methicillin-resistant *Staphylococcus aureus* (MRSA). Her physician advised her to discontinue the cephalexin and admitted her to the hospital for a course of intravenous vancomycin therapy and wound care. EA is willing to explore all options for treating her MRSA infection, including adjuncts to conventional antibiotic therapy. As an attending pharmacist in the hospital, discuss integrative treatment options with EA, and include methods to prevent acquiring or spreading bacterial infections.

Answer: MRSA is a bacterium resistant to certain antibiotics, including many penicillin compounds. Vancomycin is the antibiotic of choice for MRSA. Many herbal agents work against a wide spectrum of bacterial resistance. Herbal agents may act synergistically with antibiotics to kill microbes and reduce drug resistance.

Hospital workers such as EA are at higher risk because these organisms are much more prevalent in hospitals and nursing homes. In general, more antibiotic-resistant bacteria may be found in health care facilities because widespread antibiotic use, combined with patient noncompliance, favors the development of resistant strains. If EA had promptly cleansed the wound with a topical antiseptic such as povidone-iodine (Betadine), MRSA infection may have been prevented. The IV vancomycin, coupled with immediate wound care, is an appropriate treatment for this potentially fatal disease.

Herbal remedies proposed for the treatment of MRSA might augment the effect of vancomycin, increasing survival and shortening EA's hospital stay. Black tea *(Camellia sinensis)* has been shown to function in this regard. The adverse effects are extremely minimal for EA. Ginseng (e.g., *Panax ginseng*) has possible value in the treatment of MRSA, and a serious side effect from ginseng would be unlikely for EA. Lavender *(Lavandula angustifolia)* oil and tea tree oil *(Melaleuca alternifolia)* may possess antibiotic activity when topically applied; however, a potent topical such as povidone-iodine would be more appropriate.

Good hygiene is key in preventing MRSA. The bacteria can live on surfaces for a day or weeks and may be transmitted after a person touches it. Hands should be kept clean by washing thoroughly with soap and warm water or using an alcohol-based sanitizer. Cuts should be covered and kept clean. Clothes and towels should not be shared.

CASE STUDY 27-2

KS is a 22-year-old woman who presents at the pharmacy with a new prescription for nitrofurantoin (Macrodantin), 100 mg QID X 7D, and a refill of her oral contraceptive (OC) Tri-Levlen 28. She says she has yet another bladder infection. KS is frustrated with the recurrent episodes of cystitis and asks about ways to prevent their occurence. On this occasion and in the past, when she first experiences UTI symptoms, she starts drinking cranberry juice; however, she receives no symptomatic relief. On further questioning, KS states that recurrent episodes of cystitis began at age 18 when she went away to college and have persisted until the present. What advice could you give KS regarding integrative options for UTI treatment and prevention?

Answer: KS's cystitis will most likely resolve with her course of nitrofurantoin. Cranberry *(Vaccinium macrocarpon)* has not been proven effective for the treatment of cystitis; however, evidence exists that regular ingestion is good urinary tract prophylaxis. Uva ursi *(Arctostaphylos uva-ursi)* has been used to treat UTIs, but its efficacy is unclear. After completing nitrofurantoin, KS should modify her behavior to reduce the chance of a recurrence. A daily glass of cranberry juice will be beneficial; fructose and proanthocyanidin inhibit attachment of *Escherichia coli* to bladder cells. Cranberry juice also increases fluid intake, which "flushes out" bacteria from the bladder before they can replicate. Bromelain, a sulfur-containing proteolytic enzyme that is extracted from the stem and fruit of the pineapple *(Ananas comosus)*, has been shown to prevent attachment of *E. coli* to intestinal walls in animals.

Her OC use indicates that KS is sexually active. The onset of recurrent cystitis when she went away to college may have coincided with her becoming sexually active. Sexual intercourse can chafe the urethra, facilitating bacterial growth. Urinating shortly after intercourse can reduce the chance of cystitis. All women should be advised to wipe from front to back after a bowel movement. Forward wiping can expose the vagina and urethra to *E. coli* and other bacteria typically found in the gastrointestinal tract. Bathing immediately after sexual intercourse may also reduce the incidence of UTI.

Instruct KS to complete the full course of antibiotics, because incomplete ablation of the bacterial infection may favor the development and growth of antibiotic-resistant strains. Discuss antibiotic resistance with KS and the potential to create resistant bacteria each time an antibiotic is used.

CASE STUDY 27-3

JK is a 53-year-old man who presents at the pharmacy with a prescription for a 10-day course of doxycycline (Vibramycin). He is taking captopril (Capoten, 25 mg/day), hydrochlorothiazide (HydroDiuril, 50 mg/day), and a potassium supplement for control of his hypertension. He has been smoking two packs of cigarettes a day since age 18. He says he has "come down with another damn bug." In recent years, bouts of URIs and bronchitis have recurred with increasing frequency. JK adds that he has tried echinacea but found it was ineffective. He asks whether any other herbal therapies are available that might provide him with long-term relief. JK interrupts his conversation to cough into a tissue and blow his nose.

Answer: One major factor that may contribute to JK's recurring bouts of URIs and bronchitis is his cigarette smoking. He has likely had some pulmonary damage and is at greatly increased risk for emphysema and lung cancer. The doxycycline will probably help resolve his current infection; however, it could progress to pneumonia. His best course of action for long-term improvement is to quit smoking. A number of herbal remedies might help resolve JK's current condition; however, they should not be used in place of the doxycycline.

To date, no herbal remedy has been proven efficacious for the treatment of URIs. Echinacea *(Echinacea* spp.) has been frequently recommended to reduce the duration and severity of URIs. Earlier studies were promising, but recent studies found no benefit. Blessed thistle *(Cnicus benedictus)* and constituent chemicals (cnicin, polyacetylene) reportedly possess broad-spectrum antimicrobial activity, but clinical evidence is lacking. Garlic *(Allium sativum)* reportedly has immunologic activity, including enhanced phagocytosis, lymphocyte proliferation, enhanced NK cell activity and cytokine production, and prevention of immune suppression. Garlic has a long history of use in the treatment of various infectious agents, including bacteria, viruses, and fungi, and studies have reported its efficacy. Small reductions in blood pressure have been documented with garlic use. Garlic's possible efficacy plus its mild hypotensive effect and lack of side effects make it a good choice for JK. Goldenseal *(Hydrastis canadensis)* is a popular treatment for URIs and is often combined with echinacea in commercial herbal cold remedies. Berberine, a constituent of goldenseal, has been found to possess antimicrobial properties in animal studies. However, berberine may decrease the efficacy of tetracycline and is contraindicated while JK is taking doxycycline.

Recommend that JK monitor his blood pressure regularly, because any type of illness (including infection) may cause changes in blood pressure.

References for Chapter 27 can be found on the Evolve website at http://evolve.elsevier.com/Ulbricht/herbalpharmacotherapy/

Review Questions

1. Which of the following statements about bacteria is *false*?
   a. Some bacteria can grow in environments with or without the presence of oxygen.
   b. All bacteria are pathogenic to humans.
   c. Certain bacteria may be identified by Gram staining.
   d. Bacteria may be classified by their shapes (cocci, bacilli).

2. True or false: Arbutin, a constituent of uva ursi, has been shown to inhibit select gram-positive and gram-negative bacteria.

3. Which of the following is *false* regarding cranberry?
   a. Cranberry does not appear to be effective in preventing UTI in children with neurogenic bladder.
   b. Cranberry prevents bacteria adhering to uroepithelial cells that line the bladder.
   c. Cranberry hinders bacterial proliferation in the urinary tract by acidifying urine.
   d. Highly suggestive evidence supports cranberry for UTI prophylaxis.

4. Which of the following therapies has been used as adjunctive therapy for children with recurrent or chronic otitis media?
   a. Calendula
   b. Chiropractic manipulation
   c. Belladonna
   d. All the above

5. Which of the following effects has been reported with bloodroot?
   a. Bloodroot can inhibit the action of Na^+,K^+ATPase.
   b. Sanguinarine is the major constituent of bloodroot with antimicrobial effects.
   c. Bloodroot can inhibit bacterial adherence to teeth and plaque formation.
   d. All the above.

6. True or false: The standardized extract Kan Jang, containing ginseng, may stimulate the immune system and prevent URIs, especially during winter months.

7. Which of the following agents has displayed activity against mycobacteria?
   a. Angostura
   b. Garlic
   c. Lavender
   d. All the above

8. The compound berberine, found in goldenseal, has been studied extensively in humans for which bacterial infection(s)?
   a. Trachoma
   b. Cholera
   c. Vaginitis
   d. Both a and b

9. Which of the following statements regarding Pyralvex (a rhubarb-containing product) is *false*?
   a. The active ingredients are chlorhexidine and rhubarb extract.
   b. It should be applied three to four times daily to the sore area with the provided brush.
   c. It contains rhubarb extract equivalent to 0.005 g anthraquinone glycosides and 0.01 g salicylic acid.
   d. Based on its active ingredients, it may reduce inflammation and bacterial growth.

10. Listerine, a broad-spectrum antimicrobial mouthrinse, contains which essential oils?
    a. Eucalyptol
    b. Sweet orange
    c. Thymol
    d. a and c

Answers are found in the Answers to Review Questions section in the back of the text.

28 Parasitic and Fungal Infections

Outline

OVERVIEW
  Protozoal Infections
    Leishmaniasis
    Malaria
    Giardiasis (Beaver Fever)
  Helminthic Infections
    Hookworm Infection
    Tapeworm Infection
    Ascariasis
    Dracunculiasis (Guinea Worm Disease)
    Loiasis
    Lymphatic Filariasis
    Onchocerciasis (River Blindness)
    Threadworm Infection
    Trichinosis
    Whipworm Infection
    Diagnosis
  Fungal Infections
    Tinea Capitis and Tinea Corporis (Ringworm)
    Tinea Cruris (Jock Itch)
    Tinea Pedis (Athlete's Foot)
    Tinea Unguium (Onychomycosis)
    Fungal Paronychia
    Tinea Versicolor
    Candidiasis
    Histoplasmosis
    Diagnosis
SELECTED HERBAL THERAPIES
  Bishop's Weed *(Ammi majus)*
  Bitter Orange *(Citrus aurantium)*
  Cinnamon *(Cinnamomum* spp.*)*
  Garlic *(Allium sativum)*
  Goldenseal *(Hydrastis canadensis)*
  Pomegranate *(Punica granatum)*
  Tea Tree *(Melaleuca alternifolia)*
  Thyme *(Thymus vulgaris)*
HERBAL THERAPIES WITH LIMITED EVIDENCE
ADJUNCT THERAPIES
INTEGRATIVE THERAPY PLAN
CASE STUDIES
REVIEW QUESTIONS

Learning Objectives

- Identify common fungal, protozoal, and helminthic pathogens
- Know the mechanisms of action, adverse effects, and drug interactions for common herbs used to treat fungal, protozoal, and helminthic infections
- Devise an integrative care plan for patients with fungal, protozoal, or helminthic infections.

OVERVIEW[1-4]

A parasite is an organism that lives on or in another organism, called a *host*, during all or part of its life cycle. In a parasitic relationship, the parasite depends on the host for survival and obtains nourishment and/or protection from its host. A parasite may or may not harm the host, but the host seldom derives any benefits from the parasite. Many organisms, including animals, plants, fungi, insects, worms, protists, bacteria, and viruses, may be considered parasites; however, only a small fraction of these can cause infectious diseases in humans and other animals. Nonetheless, parasites are responsible for the majority of infectious deaths in tropical and subtropical regions of the world.

Parasites that live inside their hosts are called *endoparasites*; they may enter the body through openings in the skin, mucous membranes, or mouth. Parasitic organisms that live on the surface of hosts are called *ectoparasites*; many arthropods (which include insects, lice, ticks, and fleas) may be considered ectoparasites. Some disease-causing parasitic microorganisms are transmitted via ectoparasites; for example, Lyme disease (caused by the bacterium *Borrelia burgdorferi*) may be acquired through tick bites. Although mosquitoes feed on the blood of humans and other animals, they are technically not ectoparasites, as they do not live on a host. However, mosquitoes are major carriers of malaria, which is caused by protozoan parasites of the genus *Plasmodium* and may be acquired through mosquito bites. This chapter will focus on parasites that directly cause disease, primarily endoparasites and parasitic microorganisms other than bacteria (discussed in Chapter 27) or viruses (discussed in Chapter 29).

Each type of parasite affects the human body differently. Some feed on human cells, such as red blood cells (RBCs) in malaria, whereas others live in the intestines and absorb nutrients from food consumed by the host.

Although parasitic infections can cause permanent tissue and organ damage, most patients experience a complete recovery if they are diagnosed and treated quickly. Parasitic infections are treated with prescription antiparasitics, which may be administered orally, intravenously, or topically.

Protozoal Infections

Protozoa (or protozoans) comprise a diverse group of single-celled organisms that are found almost everywhere in the natural environment. Examples of protozoa include amoebas, trypanosomes, sporozoans, and paramecia. Only a small proportion of protozoa are capable of causing human disease. Historically, taxonomists classified protozoa in the kingdom of life called Protista. This diverse group of *protists* includes the slime molds and algae, and is distinct from bacteria (kingdoms Bacteria and Archaea), plants (kingdom Plantae), (kingdom Animalia), and fungi (kingdom Fungi). It has been recently proposed to classify protozoans in a separate kingdom (Protozoa), though this remains a point of controversy among taxonomists.[4]

Leishmaniasis

Leishmaniasis is a parasitic disease that is caused by the protozoal genus *Leishmania*. These protozoa fall under the taxonomical order known as *trypanosomes,* which have a single flagellum (whiplike tail) and are exclusively parasitic. *Leishmania* larvae may be transmitted by sandflies, blood-sucking insects found on beaches and marshes and especially common in Florida. Humans (or animals) become infected with the parasite after they are bitten by sandflies that harbor *Leishmania* larvae. Of the many different types of leishmaniasis, the most common form is a skin disease called *cutaneous leishmaniasis.* This infection causes skin sores, which may or may not be painful. The sores have raised edges and a flat center.

Signs and Symptoms

Patients with leishmaniasis typically develop skin sores weeks to months after the parasite enters the body. The skin may become red or ulcerated or may have lesions, blisters, or pimples. Smaller lesions may be present around one larger ulcer on the skin. Some patients may develop nasal congestion, postnasal drip, nosebleeds, or difficulty breathing or swallowing. Ulcers and sores may also develop in the mouth, tongue, gums, lips, nose, or nasal septum. The parasite may also enter the bloodstream and spread to internal organs; symptoms then may include persistent fever, night sweats, fatigue, weakness, loss of appetite, weight loss, vomiting (most common in children), abdominal pain, scaly skin, gray or dark skin, and thinning hair.

Malaria

Malaria is an infectious disease of the RBCs caused by the protozoan parasites *Plasmodium falciparum, P. vivax, P. malariae,* and *P. ovale.*[1-3] These protozoa spend the first portion of their life cycle inside mosquitoes. When an infected mosquito bites a human, malaria can be transmitted. This life-threatening disease is most common in tropical and subtropical areas, such as Africa, Asia, the Middle East, South America, and Central America. According to the U.S. Centers for Disease Control and Prevention (CDC), about 350 to 500 million patients become infected with malaria each year.[2] More than 1 million of these patients die, most of them young children from sub-Saharan Africa. Malaria can be successfully treated with antimalarial medications. However, drug resistance is a growing problem in many countries.

Signs and Symptoms

Symptoms of malaria include cycles of chills, fever, and sweating. These symptoms occur in cycles every 1, 2, or 3 days if the infection is not treated. Some individuals may also experience diarrhea, jaundice, coughing, nausea, and vomiting.

Giardiasis (Beaver Fever)

Giardiasis is an infection of the small intestine caused by the protozoan parasite *Giardia lamblia* (syn. *Lamblia intestinalis, Giardia duodenalis*). Infection occurs when humans or animals ingest *Giardia* cysts, which are common in natural water sources (lakes and rivers), where they can survive in a dormant state for months.[5] The parasite lives exclusively in the small intestine, and the cysts are expelled in feces. Thus, infection is spread by the fecal-oral route. Giardiasis is commonly known as "beaver fever" because it has been associated with drinking water near beaver dams.

Signs and Symptoms

Giardiasis is asymptomatic in about half of all cases. Any apparent symptoms are usually related to the intestinal inflammation that results when the parasites colonize the intestinal lining,[5] including nonspecific gastrointestinal problems such as nausea, diarrhea, gas, abdominal pain, and steatorrhea (greasy stools). In healthy patients, giardiasis usually resolves on its own. However, some individuals, especially those who are immunocompromised, may experience long-term or recurring infections. This can lead to malnutrition because the intestinal inflammation may interfere with nutrient absorption. Depending on the nutrient deficiencies, chronic malnutrition can cause various ailments, including fatigue, weight loss, and anemia.

Helminthic Infections

Helminthic infections are caused by parasitic worms, which may enter the human body through contact with other humans, plants, insects, or animals. Helminthic infections can also be acquired directly through penetration of the skin. Symptoms vary depending on the type and severity of the infection. Parasitic worms may be successfully treated with antihelminthic (anthelmintic) medications, which expel them from the body. An example of an anthelmintic is albendazole, which may be used to expel hookworms, tapeworms, threadworms, roundworms, and whipworms.

Hookworm Infection

A hookworm infection is caused by one of two roundworms, *Ancylostoma duodenale* or *Necator americanus*. Researchers estimate that about 25% of the world's population is infected with hookworm. Humans become infected with hookworm through contact with contaminated soil or stool. The larvae can enter the skin and travel through the blood to the lungs, eventually reaching the throat, where they are coughed up and swallowed. As the larvae enter the digestive tract, they attach themselves to the wall of the small intestine. Here they mature into adult worms and reproduce. Adult hookworms may live up to 10 years, feeding on the blood of the host. If not treated, hookworm infections can lead to abdominal pain and iron deficiency.

Signs and Symptoms

Most patients with hookworm infections do not experience symptoms. Some patients develop an itchy skin rash where the worms entered the body. When the worms enter the lungs, some patients develop symptoms similar to asthma or pneumonia, such as fever, persistent cough, wheezing, or difficulty breathing. When the worms enter the intestines, patients may experience abdominal pain, decreased appetite, diarrhea, weight loss, and excessive gas.

Tapeworm Infection

A tapeworm infection is a parasitic infection that affects the digestive tract. Humans become infected with tapeworms after they consume food or water that is contaminated with tapeworm larvae. Many different types of tapeworm exist; however, those that infect humans are typically the pork tapeworm (*Taenia solium*), dwarf tapeworm (*Hymenolepis nana*), beef tapeworm (*Taenia saginata*), and fish tapeworm (*Diphyllobothrium latum*). Tapeworm infections typically occur when a person consumes food, water, or soil contaminated with human or animal feces.

Signs and Symptoms

Most tapeworm infections do not cause symptoms. Symptomatic patients typically experience abdominal pain, bloating, nausea, and diarrhea. Some patients might notice small, white tapeworm eggs in their stool.

Ascariasis

Ascariasis is a type of parasitic infection caused by the roundworm *Ascaris lumbricoides*. Humans become infected after they ingest the parasite's microscopic eggs. The parasite can be transmitted when humans eat produce grown in soil contaminated with human feces that contains roundworm eggs. This is more common in developing countries, where sanitation is poor and human feces may be used as fertilizer for crops. When the eggs are ingested, they mature into larvae. The mature adults may reside in the intestines, where they feed on food that enters the body. Adult worms can grow to 15 inches (38 cm) in length and can live up to 2 years. Adult female worms can produce more than 200,000 eggs a day, which are excreted in the patient's feces. Ascariasis is considered the most common type of roundworm infection in humans. Researchers estimate that about 25% of the world's population is infected with this parasite. In the United States, most infections occur in rural areas that have warm climates, such as the southern United States.

Signs and Symptoms

Symptoms of ascariasis can range from mild to severe, depending on the number of parasites in the body and where they colonize. If only a few parasites are consumed, patients generally experience few, if any, symptoms. If the larvae enter the lungs, patients may experience symptoms similar to pneumonia, such as persistent cough, shortness of breath, and wheezing. When the larvae reach the intestines and develop into adults, mild or moderate symptoms include abdominal pain, nausea, diarrhea, and sometimes bloody stools. Severe infections may cause stomach pain, fatigue, vomiting, or weight loss. In some patients the worms may be seen in vomit or stool or may even emerge from the mouth or nose.

Dracunculiasis (Guinea Worm Disease)

Guinea worm disease, also called dracunculiasis, is a painful parasitic infection caused by a roundworm called the guinea worm (*Dracunculus medinensis*), which is found only in Africa. Patients become infected with this worm after drinking water contaminated with water fleas that harbor guinea worm larvae. Once the larvae enter the human, they mature into adults in the gastrointestinal tract. Inside the human host, these adult worms can reach up to 3 feet (90 cm) in length. The adult guinea worms then migrate to another area of the body (typically the legs), from which they will eventually emerge. After about 1 year the adult worm is ready to release its eggs; a small part of the worm emerges through a painful, round blister in the skin. The tip of the adult worm breaks through the skin to release its eggs into water. The adult worm continues to emerge and lay eggs whenever the affected limb is submerged in water. This often causes long-term suffering and sometimes crippling effects in the human host.

Signs and Symptoms

Symptoms of guinea worm disease develop after about 1 year, when the adult guinea worm is ready to release its eggs. Symptoms become apparent a few days to hours before the adult worm emerges through the skin to release its eggs. The patient may develop a fever and have pain and swelling in the area where the worm emerged. A blister, which eventually forms an open wound, may also develop near the area. When the wound is immersed in water, the tip of the worm begins to emerge from the skin to lay its eggs. Although these worms may be present in any area of the body, they are usually found on the legs or feet. After the worm releases its eggs, it goes back inside the body, and the wound typically becomes painful, swollen, and infected.

Loiasis

Loiasis (or loaiasis) is a parasitic infection caused by a roundworm, the African eye worm *(Loa loa)*, and is most prevalent in tropical areas of Africa.[3] Humans become infected with the parasite after being bitten by deerflies (genus *Chrysops*) that harbor immature African eye worms. These deerflies are typically found near the Congo River region, Sudan, and Ethiopia.[3] Once the parasite enters the human host, it migrates toward the eyes, where it causes eye congestion and irritation. Sometimes the worm moves to the brain, where it causes potentially fatal cerebral edema (brain swelling).

Signs and Symptoms

The eyes of patients with loiasis may be irritated, itchy, and watery. Vision may be blurred, and the eyes may become congested. Patients may be able to see the threadlike worms move across their eyeballs.

Lymphatic Filariasis

Filariasis is a type of infection caused by any of the round, threadlike parasitic worms called filariae. Lymphatic filariasis, also called elephantiasis, is caused by worms (*Wuchereria bancrofti* or *Brugia malayi*) that infect the human lymph system. Lymphatic filariasis is transmitted to humans by mosquitoes that harbor parasite larvae. Once this parasite enters the human, it migrates to the lymph nodes, where it develops into an adult. Females release larvae, which circulate in the patient's bloodstream. If not treated with antiparasitic medications, adult filarial worms typically live for about 7 years. Although lymphatic filariasis is rarely fatal, it can cause fevers, frequent infections, and serious inflammation of the lymph system if not treated.

Signs and Symptoms

Humans with lymphatic filariasis generally develop symptoms 5 to 18 months after being bitten by infected mosquitoes. Lymphatic filariasis causes tissue damage that limits the normal flow of lymph fluid through the body. As a result, patients typically experience swelling, scarring, and infections, especially in the legs and groin.

Onchocerciasis (River Blindness)

River blindness, also called onchocerciasis, is a parasitic infection of the eyes that is caused by a worm called *Onchocerca volvulus*. The disease is transmitted to humans by black flies called buffalo gnats. When these flies bite a human, they allow the parasitic larvae to enter the human's body. Once inside the human, the larvae begin to mature into adults. Adult worms then produce millions of tiny worms, called microfilariae, which migrate throughout the human body. River blindness often causes severe itching of the skin and eyes. If left untreated, the worms may cause blindness. Onchocerciasis is considered to be at epidemic levels in more than 25 countries in central Africa.[3]

Signs and Symptoms

Symptoms of onchocerciasis usually develop 1 to 3 years after the larvae enter the body. Besides vision, many symptoms involve the skin, which may develop rashes, lesions, or loss of pigmentation. Patients may also develop enlarged lymph nodes. Researchers estimate that about 18 million people are infected with river blindness each year worldwide. Of those infected, an estimated 6.5 million have severe itching or dermatitis, 770,000 have serious visual impairment, and 270,000 become blind.

Threadworm Infection

Threadworm infection, also called strongyloidiasis, is a parasitic infection of the intestines and skin caused by the roundworm *Strongyloides stercoralis*. The infection is transmitted to humans when a person comes into contact with soil contaminated by threadworm. The larvae may enter the human through the skin, usually when walking barefoot on soil. Once inside the body, the larvae migrate to the lymph nodes, where they are carried into the lungs. From the lungs the larvae may migrate to the patient's throat. When the patient coughs, the larvae are swallowed and then enter the digestive tract, where they mature into egg-producing adults. The eggs are then released in the patient's feces. Adult threadworms may reach 1 to 2 inches (2-2.5 cm) in length. Threadworm infections are rarely fatal, but if left untreated, infections can last for up to 45 years. Although this infection can occur in most areas of the world, it is most prevalent in tropical and subtropical climates.

Signs and Symptoms

The signs and symptoms of threadworm infection vary depending on the stage of the disease. After the larvae enter the body through the skin, the area may be swollen and pruritic (itchy). Patients with long-term threadworm infections may develop a pruritic rash near the buttocks, abdomen, and thighs. Some patients may have only mild diarrhea and cramping, whereas others may have nausea, vomiting, fever, fatigue, and stools containing blood or mucus. When the larvae move to the lungs and airways, the patient may develop a dry cough, fever, or difficulty breathing and may cough up blood or pus.

Trichinosis

Trichinosis is a parasitic infection caused by the roundworm *Trichinella spiralis*. Humans become infected when they eat undercooked meat (usually pork, but sometimes beef) that is contaminated with *Trichinella* larvae. Over several weeks the larvae mature into adult worms inside the intestines. The adults then produce larvae that migrate to various body tissues, including the muscles. Patients generally experience mild (if any) symptoms; however, infection with a large number of worms may cause permanent tissue damage.

Trichinosis can be prevented by cooking meat thoroughly before ingestion. The meat must reach at least 150° F (65.5° C) to ensure that tapeworm eggs and larvae are killed.

Signs and Symptoms

Symptoms of trichinosis range from mild to severe, depending on the number of parasites in the body. Patients with a very mild form may experience no symptoms. When the parasite is in the intestine, common symptoms include diarrhea, abdominal pain, and general discomfort. About 1 week after the parasite enters the body, the females produce larvae that may migrate into other body tissues, including the muscles. Symptoms at this stage may include high fever, muscle pain and tenderness, weakness, swelling of the eyelids or face, sensitivity to light, headache, and conjunctivitis.

Whipworm Infection

Whipworm infection, also called trichuriasis, occurs when *Trichuris trichiura* infects the large intestine. This infection primarily affects children. Humans become infected after they consume foods contaminated with soil containing whipworm eggs. Once inside the body, the eggs hatch and attach themselves to the wall of the large intestine. Whipworms are found around the world, especially in tropical countries with warm, humid weather.

Signs and Symptoms

Common symptoms of whipworm infections include abdominal pain and diarrhea. A severe infection may cause bloody diarrhea or iron deficiency anemia. In some severe cases, rectal prolapse (protrusion of rectum through anus) may occur.

Diagnosis

A parasitic infection (protozoal and helminthic) is suspected if a patient has signs and symptoms of an infection and has inhabited or visited an area known to have certain parasites. A diagnosis is confirmed after the parasite is identified in the body. Samples of blood, stool, urine, or phlegm may be analyzed for the presence of parasites. A tissue biopsy may also be performed. The sample is then analyzed microscopically for the presence of parasites.

Fungal Infections

Fungi are multicellular organisms that form spores and include molds, mildews, mushrooms, and yeasts. They can be found in virtually every type of habitat, including land, fresh water, and salt water. However, they are most common in dark, moist, and warm environments. Fungi are often found in the soil, on food, and on the skin. Many types of fungi are harmless to humans. However, some yeasts and molds may be infectious, and some fungi, including certain mushrooms, are toxic or may cause severe allergic reactions if ingested.

When a fungus enters the human body, it can cause a localized or systemic infection. Disease-causing fungi may enter the body through the skin, nose, vagina, nails, or mouth, and these areas of the body are the most likely to be exposed to fungi. Fungal infections are often classified by the site of infection, rather than the type of organism causing the infection. Certain types of fungi can infect different parts of the body and thus can cause different types of infections. Fungi that infect the skin are collectively known as *dermatophytes* and include more than 40 species in the genera *Microsporum*, *Epidermophyton*, and *Trichophyton*. Fungal infections of the skin are collectively known as *tinea*. Many dermatophytes that can cause infection normally live on the skin in a noninfectious state. Where body areas are frequently moist, however, the fungi may grow uncontrollably. Although anyone can acquire a fungal skin infection, those who perspire heavily (e.g., athletes, overweight people) are most often infected; warm and sweaty environments promote fungal growth.

With fungal infections, symptoms vary depending on the type and severity of the infection, as well as the parts of the body infected. Patients should seek professional medical advice if any of these symptoms develop. Most fungal infections do not cause serious medical problems. If left untreated, however, some fungal infections may damage the skin or nails. The fungi may spread to other parts of the body and even lead to death in severe cases.

Fungal infections are treated with antifungal medications that may be administered topically, orally, or intravenously. If diagnosed and treated quickly, most patients with fungal infections recover completely.

Tinea Capitis and Tinea Corporis (Ringworm)

The term *ringworm* is somewhat misleading because the infectious agent is not a "worm" but rather a fungus that grows in the shape of a circle. *Tinea capitis* refers to ringworm of the scalp, and *tinea corporis* is the same type of infection occurring elsewhere on the body. Both are extremely contagious and can spread through skin-to-skin contact. Patients may be exposed to the fungi after touching an infected animal. Dogs, cats, ferrets, rabbits, goats, and pigs are among the animals that can harbor ringworm. Patients may also become infected after touching objects (towels, clothing, bed linens) that an infected person or animal previously touched.

Signs and Symptoms

Patients with localized fungal infections of the skin (e.g., tinea capitis or corporis) typically develop a swollen, circle-shaped rash on the skin. The skin may be scaly and itchy. Small black dots may appear on the scalp, and patients may lose small patches of hair, which grow back once treatment is started.

Tinea Cruris (Jock Itch)

Tinea cruris, commonly called "jock itch," is a fungal infection that affects the skin of the inner thighs, buttocks, and genitals. Tinea cruris is mildly contagious and may spread through physical contact or after sharing personal items (e.g., towels) that had come into contact with infected skin. Jock itch usually causes mild discomfort and is not a serious medical condition. It may be treated with antifungal agents applied to the skin.

Signs and Symptoms

Patients with tinea cruris have redness and itching of the groin and inner thigh area. They may have swelling, redness, and pustule formation. The associated rash is typically well demarcated from the surrounding normal skin.

Tinea Pedis (Athlete's Foot)

Tinea pedis, commonly called "athlete's foot," is caused by dermatophytes; like all fungi, dermatophytes prefer warm, moist environments. Individuals whose feet are exposed to this environment have an increased risk of developing athlete's foot. Exposure typically occurs when showering barefoot at common facilities, such as locker rooms or college dormitories. If the fungus infects the skin, it begins to reproduce and cause skin inflammation. As a result, the skin on the feet may become thick, scaly, and itchy.

Signs and Symptoms

Tinea pedis may cause burning or itching anywhere on the feet. Symptoms are usually most noticeable between the toes. Patients may also develop itchy blisters or dry skin; the skin may start to crack or peel. If the infection occurs in or near the toenails, they may become thick, crumbly, or discolored.

Tinea Unguium (Onychomycosis)

Onychomycosis, or tinea unguium, is a fungal infection of the nail bed. Patients are most likely to develop onychomycosis if their nails are frequently exposed to warm, damp environments, such as sweaty socks or shower floors. Toenails are more likely to be affected than fingernails. Onychomycosis can be successfully treated with oral antifungal agents.

Signs and Symptoms

Patients who have fungal nail infections may develop thick, brittle, or crumbly fingernails or toenails, which may be painful. The nails may become distorted in shape, flat, or dull. The nails may be yellow, green, brown, or black and may emit a foul odor. In some cases, infected nails may separate from the nail bed, causing *onycholysis*.

Fungal Paronychia

Fungal paronychia is a fungal skin infection that occurs near the nail beds. It causes the skin around the fingernails or toenails to become red and swollen and may also cause pus-filled blisters to form. Fungal paronychia is usually caused by dermatophytes and is common among patients with onychomycosis or diabetes and those who frequently have wet hands for long periods (e.g., swimmers). Biting the nails, hangnails, or pushing back the cuticles also increases the risk of an infection. Patients respond well to oral antifungal agents, although complete resolution of the infection may take several months.

Signs and Symptoms

The main symptom of fungal paronychia is a painful, red, swollen area around the nail, often at the cuticle or at the site of a hangnail or other injury. The nail may look detached, may be abnormally shaped, or may have an unusual color (darkened or opaque).

Tinea Versicolor

Tinea versicolor, also called *pityriasis versicolor,* is the most common type of fungal skin infection and causes small, discolored patches to appear on the skin. The infection generally worsens during hot and humid weather. Tinea versicolor is typically caused by the yeast *Malassezia furfur,* which may be part of the normal flora of the skin. Many factors, including hot and humid weather, immunosuppression, hormonal changes, excessive sweating, and oily skin, may trigger the fungi to multiply uncontrollably and cause an infection. It may take several weeks for antifungal creams and lotions to eliminate the fungus completely from the body.

Signs and Symptoms

Symptoms of tinea versicolor typically include small patches of discolored skin that grow slowly and prevent the skin from tanning. As a result, symptoms are usually most apparent after the skin is exposed to the sun. The patches of scaly skin may be various colors, such as white, pink, tan, or dark brown. The affected skin may also be itchy. The back, chest, neck, and upper arms are most likely to be affected. Symptoms may appear or worsen during hot, humid weather.

Candidiasis

The *Candida albicans* fungus is found almost everywhere in the environment and frequently colonizes the oral cavities of healthy individuals. It may also be found in the normal flora of the vagina. *Candida* infections are often "opportunistic," occurring in individuals with weakened immune systems. Candidiasis can infect the mouth (oral candidiasis, or *oral thrush*), esophagus (esophageal candidiasis), or vagina (vulvovaginal candidiasis, commonly known as a "yeast infection").

The acidity of the stomach (pH 1 to 2) is normally sufficient to suppress the growth of most fungi. However, drugs that suppress stomach acid production, such as H_2 blockers (e.g., ranitidine) and proton pump inhibitors (e.g., pantoprazole), may predispose some patients to fungal infections of the upper gastrointestinal tract, such as infectious *Candida* esophagitis.

Vaginal candidiasis (yeast infection) is common in both healthy and immunocompromised patients. Researchers estimate that about 75% of all women have at least one vaginal *Candida* infection during their lifetime, and up to 45% experience two or more. Several factors are associated with increased risk of developing vaginal yeast infections, including pregnancy, antibiotic use, high-estrogen birth control, diabetes mellitus, tight-fitting clothes, or having a sexually transmitted disease (STD).

Candidal infections are commonly treated with antifungals applied topically to the area of infection. Treatment generally lasts 10 to 14 days. Single-dose treatments are also available. Some patients receive a systemic medication for candidiasis.

Signs and Symptoms

The symptoms of candidiasis vary, depending on the body part affected. Symptoms of oral thrush may develop suddenly and typically involve creamy-white lesions on the tongue, inner cheek, gums, and roof of the mouth. The tonsils may also be affected. These lesions are often painful and may bleed when rubbed. Severe cases of oral thrush may spread into the esophagus (esophageal candidiasis), stomach, and lung. This is more likely to occur if oral thrush is left untreated or if the patient is extremely immunocompromised. Common symptoms of esophageal candidiasis include throat pain or difficulty swallowing. A fever may indicate that the infection has spread beyond the esophagus.

Common symptoms of vulvovaginal candidiasis include itching, watery or curdlike whitish vaginal discharge, vaginal erythema (redness), dyspareunia (pain during sexual intercourse), painful urination, swollen labia and vulva, and vaginal lesions. Symptoms generally worsen during menstruation because the hormonal changes provide a better environment for fungal growth.

If left untreated, severe candidiasis may spread to the bloodstream and affect other organs, including the intestines, kidneys, or heart; this condition is called *candidemia*. Fever and hypotension (low blood pressure) often occur in patients with candidemia. Additional symptoms depend on which body parts are affected. For example, infection of the heart may cause a heart murmur.

Histoplasmosis

Histoplasmosis is caused by the fungus *Histoplasma capsulatum*, typically found in damp soil that is rich in organic material. Histoplasmosis typically begins in the lungs and may spread to other organs and tissues of the body. Healthy patients who develop histoplasmosis often experience no symptoms and require no treatment. However, patients with weakened immune systems, especially infants and patients with human immunodeficiency virus (HIV), are vulnerable to developing infections in the lungs and systemically. Histoplasmosis may spread to virtually any part of the body, including the liver, bone marrow, eyes, skin, adrenal glands, and/or intestinal tract; this condition is called *disseminated histoplasmosis*, which may be fatal if untreated.

Patients with underlying pulmonary diseases, such as emphysema, are also vulnerable to developing a long-term histoplasmosis infection that primarily affects the lungs. Patients with this type of infection, called *chronic pulmonary histoplasmosis*, may require lifelong treatment with antifungal drugs. If exposed to large amounts of the fungus, otherwise healthy individuals may develop *Histoplasma* infections that require treatment. For example, farmers who are frequently exposed to soil or guano (bird or bat droppings) have an increased risk of developing infection.

Signs and Symptoms

Symptoms of histoplasmosis typically develop about 17 days after the fungal spores are inhaled. Common symptoms include fever, headache, dry cough, chills, chest pain, weight loss, and sweats. Symptoms of disseminated histoplasmosis vary depending on which organs are infected. When a fungal infection enters the bloodstream and affects multiple body tissues and organs, the condition may lead to severe and potentially fatal complications, including pneumonia, pericarditis, meningitis, and adrenal insufficiency.

Diagnosis

Most fungal infections are diagnosed after the fungi are identified in the patient's blood or tissue. Localized infections of the skin and nails and candidal infection of the mouth or vagina can often be diagnosed based on physical examination. If further workup is needed, a scraping or biopsy of the affected tissue may be examined for the presence of fungi. Blood tests can also be performed to detect serum antibodies against a specific fungus.

SELECTED HERBAL THERAPIES

Note

To help make this educational resource more interactive, all pharmacokinetics, adverse effects, and interactions data have been compiled in Appendix A. Safety data specifically related to pregnancy and lactation are listed in Appendix B. Please refer to these appendices when working through the case studies and answering the review questions.

Bishop's Weed (Ammi majus)

Grade C: *Unclear or conflicting scientific evidence (tinea versicolor)*

Mechanism of Action

Photoreactive furocoumarins *(psoralens)*, including 8-methoxypsoralen, have been identified in *Ammi majus*.[6-9] Psoralens have well-established photosensitizing properties and have been widely used to stimulate melanin production and accelerate suntanning.[10] Thus, psoralens may be useful for treating skin hypopigmentation caused by numerous skin conditions, such as tinea versicolor. However, their mutagenic potential has been linked to increased melanoma incidence among psoralen-based suntan accelerators, so psoralens have since been banned from tanning lotions.[10]

Scientific Evidence of Effectiveness

The compound 8-methoxypsoralen (8-MOP) is used in photochemotherapy for several skin disorders, including vitiligo and psoriasis. Preliminary evidence suggests that oral 8-MOP may be useful for repigmenting skin discoloration in the treatment of tinea versicolor.[11] Additional research is needed before a firm recommendation can be made. The potential for increased melanoma risk warrants caution when using any psoralens to accelerate skin pigmentation.[10]

Dose

There is no well-known standardization for bishop's weed. For tinea versicolor, the therapeutic effective dose was 0.25 mg/kg body weight by mouth, followed 30 minutes later by exposure to ultraviolet A (UVA) light for 35 to 55 minutes. Repigmentation was achieved after 12 sittings.[11]

Adverse Effects, Interactions, Pharmacokinetics. See Appendix A.

Bitter Orange (Citrus aurantium)

Grade C: *Unclear or conflicting scientific evidence (fungal infections)*

Mechanism of Action

Bitter orange extract comes from the *Citrus aurantium* plant, which contains synephrine alkaloids and *p*-octopamine.[12-14] These molecules are usually cited as "active ingredients" on product labels. Flavonoids, including limonene, hesperidin, neohesperidin, naringin, and tangaretin, are also present in bitter orange peel, flowers, and leaves.[15] The flavonoid content of bitter orange is noted as being higher in the flowers than the leaves.[16] Bitter orange also contains the furocoumarins bergapten and oxypeucedanin,[17-19] which have well-established photosensitizing and photoreactive properties. Bitter orange preparations are reported to have a variety of antimicrobial properties. In vitro study has found oil of bitter orange to exert fungistatic and fungicidal activity against a variety of pathogenic dermatophyte species.[20]

Scientific Evidence of Effectiveness

There is some clinical evidence that supports using bitter orange oil as a topical antifungal agent.[20] Patients with various dermatophyte infections were cured within 3 weeks of treatment using bitter orange oil as an emulsion or alcohol mixture or in its pure form.

Dose

Bitter orange extract has been standardized to 4% to 6% synephrine for thermogenic action.[21] Dosages of bitter orange used to treat dermatological fungal infections such as tinea corporis, tinea cruris, and tinea pedis have included 25% emulsion of bitter orange oil three times daily, 20% bitter orange oil in alcohol three times daily, and 100% bitter orange oil once daily for 2 to 3 weeks.[22]

Adverse Effects, Interactions, Pharmacokinetics. See Appendix A.

Cinnamon (Cinnamomum spp.)

Grade C: *Unclear or conflicting scientific evidence (oral candidiasis)*

Mechanism of Action

Cinnamon oil had a significant inhibitory effect against several fungi in vitro.[23-25] *Trans*-cinnamaldehyde, a component in the oil of *Cinnamomum zeylanicum*, was the most active against 17 micromycetes.[26] The essential oils of several *Cinnamomum* species showed anticandidal and antidermatophytic activity in vitro.[27,28] *C. zeylanicum* has potent in vitro activity against both fluconazole-resistant and fluconazole-susceptible *Candida* isolates.[29]

Scientific Evidence of Effectiveness

In vitro evidence of the activity of cinnamon against fluconazole-resistant and fluconazole-susceptible *Candida* isolates led to a pilot study using cinnamon to treat oral candidiasis in HIV-positive patients.[29] Symptomatic and clinical improvements were noted in three of the five patients taking cinnamon lozenges for 1 week.

Dose

In a pilot study, eight lozenges of a commercially available cinnamon candy (not further specified) were taken daily for 1 week by patients with HIV and oral candidiasis.[29]

Adverse Effects, Interactions, Pharmacokinetics. See Appendix A.

Garlic (Allium sativum)

Grade C: *Unclear or conflicting scientific evidence (topical antifungal)*

Mechanism of Action

The antimicrobial activity of garlic has been attributed to the sulfur-containing compounds in garlic oil. The strong-smelling oil was termed "allicin" in the mid-1900s.[23,30] The sulfur compound *alliin* (*S*-allyl-l-cysteine sulfoxide) produces *allicin* (diallyl thiosulfinate) through the enzyme *allinase* when the bulb is crushed or ground. Other potentially active ingredients derived from garlic include peptides, steroids, terpenoids, flavonoids, phenols, and other sulfur-containing compounds[31-33] that form when allicin is metabolized. The exact mechanism of action underlying garlic's effects remains unclear and may vary according to the preparation[34] and the therapeutic effect.

Garlic has been demonstrated in vitro to exert activity against multiple pathogens,[33,35-41] including fungi.[42,43] Alliin and allinase are found in separate but adjacent compartments of the garlic clove; when the garlic is crushed, the antimicrobial compound allicin is produced. Allicin may inhibit thiol-containing compounds and various enzyme systems, DNA, RNA, and protein synthesis.[32,38,44,45] Garlic oil's antimicrobial activity may be more potent than garlic powder on a unit-weight basis.[46]

The minimum inhibitory concentration (MIC) of aqueous garlic extract (AGE) against six clinical yeast isolates ranged from 0.8 to 1.6 mg/mL in one study.[45] Garlic appeared to alter the structure and integrity of the outer surface of yeast cells and to decrease their total lipid content. Garlic was also shown to increase phosphatidylserine content of the cell wall (while decreasing phosphatidylcholine). Oxygen consumption of yeast cells was also reduced by garlic. The anticandidal activity of AGE was antagonized by thiols, including L-cysteine, glutathione, and 2-mercaptoethanol. The effect of AGE on the macromolecular synthesis of *Candida albicans* revealed that protein and nucleic acid synthesis was inhibited and lipid synthesis arrested.[47] Antagonism of lipid synthesis may be a component of the anticandidal activity of garlic.

Scientific Evidence of Effectiveness

A trial of topical *ajoene* (a garlic constituent) in patients with tinea pedis reported "complete cure" in 27 of 34 patients after 1 week of treatment.[48] A follow-up study reported ajoene to be equivalent to terbinafine (Lamisil) treatment in 60 patients with tinea cruris and/or tinea corporis.[49] A separate trial reported similar results for tinea pedis.[50] Case studies have reported successful treatment of *Microsporum canis*[51] and sporotrichosis[52] with fresh-cut garlic and garlic oil, respectively.

Garlic has been used topically to treat fungal infections,[32,53] and antifungal effects have been demonstrated in vitro against *Candida*,[54,40] *Aspergillus*,[55] *Cryptococcus neoformans*,[56] and other dermatophytes.[57] Diminished adherence of *Candida* to buccal epithelial cells has been demonstrated.[58]

Dose

For tinea cruris, tinea corporis, or tinea pedis, subjects treated for 1 week with topical ajoene (0.6%-1.0%) had equivalent healing rate to standard treatment (1% terbinafine).[48-50] In case reports, culture-confirmed lesions of *Microsporum canis* or sporotrichosis were successfully healed with freshly cut garlic applied topically for 10 days.[51,52] Acute antifungal activity (against *Candida*, *Cryptococcus*, *Aspergillus*, and other genera) was observed in subjects 30 to 60 minutes after ingesting 10 to 25 mL of garlic extract.[43]

For ascaridiasis, infected children were given a daily infusion of 8 g garlic for 5 days; results failed to show efficacy.[59] Children infected with *Hymenolepis nana* (dwarf tapeworm) or *Giardia lamblia* were given 5 mL crude garlic extract in 100 mL water twice daily, or a commercial preparation of 1.2 mg garlic twice daily for 3 days; garlic treatment was reported to shorten the duration of conventional treatment.[60]

Adverse Effects, Interactions, Pharmacokinetics. See Appendix A.

Goldenseal (Hydrastis canadensis)

Grade C: *Unclear or conflicting scientific evidence (chloroquine-resistant malaria; parasitic infection [Leishmania])*

Mechanism of Action

Berberine has displayed activity against various types of parasites and fungi, including *Alternaria* spp., *Candida albicans*, *Curvularia* spp., *Drechslera* spp., *Fusarium* spp., *Mucor* spp., *Rhizopus oryzae*, *Aspergillus flavus*, *Aspergillus fumigatus*, *Entamoeba histolytica*, *Giardia lamblia*, *Trichomonas vaginalis*, and *Leishmania donovani*.[61-64] However, in vitro research has reported no activity of berberine against *Plasmodium* in malaria.[65] The mechanism of action of berberine has not been clearly established.

Scientific Evidence of Effectiveness

CHLOROQUINE-RESISTANT MALARIA. Preliminary research suggests that berberine has antiprotozoal activity, although no laboratory or animal study has shown activity against pathogens that cause malaria. A low-quality randomized trial assessed the use of berberine in combination with pyrimethamine in the treatment of chloroquine-resistant malaria.[66] Clearance of asexual parasitemia was seen after 4 days of treatment, which was greater than that seen with pyrimethamine plus tetracycline or pyrimethamine plus cotrimoxazole. It was suggested that combining berberine-containing herbs such as goldenseal with conventional antimalarial agents may result in synergistic effects. However, no statistical analysis was performed in the available study to determine if the results are significant. Because of the small amount of berberine actually available from goldenseal preparations (0.5%-6%), it is unclear if goldenseal contains enough berberine to be an effective treatment for chloroquine-resistant malaria.

PARASITIC INFECTION (*Leishmania*). The benefits of berberine in the treatment of leishmaniasis are widely accepted. One study found berberine to be as effective in cutaneous leishmaniasis as the standard drug treatment antimonate.[67] The lack of standardized use probably results from the limited methodological design of available studies.

Dose

The dose of goldenseal for chloroquine-resistant malaria has not been determined.

For leishmaniasis, intralesional injections of 1% berberine at weekly intervals for 2 months have been used.[68]

Adverse Effects, Interactions, Pharmacokinetics. See Appendix A.

Pomegranate *(Punica granatum)*

Grade C: *Unclear or conflicting scientific evidence (antifungal)*

Mechanism of Action

Clinical studies have shown *Candida albicans* to be sensitive to pomegranate.[69-71] However, the exact mechanism of action of pomegranate for fungal infections is not well understood.

Scientific Evidence of Effectiveness

The extract of pomegranate was shown to be as effective as miconazole (Daktarin) oral gel when used topically to treat candidiasis associated with denture stomatitis in a randomized controlled trial (RCT).[69] The gel was applied three times daily for 15 days. Also, pomegranate extract in combination with *Centella asiatica* extract was found to have a statistically significant benefit in plaque reduction compared with placebo.[70]

Dose

Pomegranate gel has been used three times daily for 15 days to treat denture stomatitis.[69]

Adverse Effects, Interactions, Pharmacokinetics. See Appendix A.

Tea Tree *(Melaleuca alternifolia)*

Grade C: *Unclear or conflicting scientific evidence (pityriasis capitis [dandruff]; Candida albicans [oral thrush]; onychomycosis; tinea pedis [athlete's foot]; vaginal yeast infections)*

Mechanism of Action

The tea tree is related to *Melaleuca quinquenervia* and *Melaleuca cajuputi*, which are trees that produce oils often used in aromatherapy and that are similar to camphor and peppermint. However, tea tree oil comes exclusively from *Melaleuca alternifolia* and should not be confused with cajeput oil, niauouli oil, kanuka oil, or manuka oil obtained from other *Melaleuca* species. Their composition is quite different, and these other species contain higher concentrations of cineole, a skin irritant that may decrease the antiseptic activity of the purported active ingredient of tea tree oil (terpinen-4-ol).[1,23]

Tea tree oil inhibits the in vitro conversion of *Candida albicans* from yeast to mycelial form.[105] In vitro studies have shown that terpinen-4-ol is the component most likely responsible for its antimicrobial properties of tea tree oil.[106]

Tea tree oil is toxic when ingested orally and therefore should not be swallowed.

 Sweet Annie *(Artemisia annua)*

Artemisinin is the major active constituent of *Artemisia annua*, and related species. Derivatives of this compound include arteether, artemether, artemotil, artenimol, artesunate, and dihydroartemisinin, which, along with artemisin, are currently being used to treat drug-resistant and non–drug-resistant malaria.[72-79] The aerial parts of *A. annua* contain 0.01% to 0.8% artemisinin per dry weight.[80,81] Other constituents of *A. annua* include deoxyartemisinin, artemisinic acid, arteannuin-B, stigmasterol, friedelin, friedelan-3β beta-ol, artemetin, and quercetagetin 6,7, 3'',4''-tetramethyl ether.[82,83]

According to laboratory tests using nuclear magnetic resonance (NMR) spectroscopy, *Artemisia annua* extracts have antimalarial properties.[84,85] In one study in mice infected with *Plasmodium berghei*, a gelatin capsule of *A. annua* had an ED_{50} of 11.9 ±2.4 g (crude drug) for clearance of parasitemia and a therapeutic index of 13.6, which was 3.5 times greater than that of artemisinin.[86] A combination of *A. annua* and chloroquine was more effective in fever subsidence and resolution of malarial symptoms, but the recrudescence (recurrence of symptoms) rate was still high. This rate was reduced by increasing the therapeutic dose or combining with primaquine.

The antimalarial effect of artemisinins has been attributed to its ability to enter the parasite food vacuole and increased oxidative stress.[87] Artemisinins have also been reported to alter intracellular calcium in parasites.[88]

Artemisinin has shown rapid antimalarial activity in humans, especially when used as an adjuvant with standard antimalarial drugs.[89-97] Derivatives of artemisinin, including arteether, artemether, artemotil, artenimol, artesunate, and dihydroartemisinin, are also currently being used to treat drug-resistant and non–drug-resistant malaria.[72-79,98-101] *Artemisinin-based combination therapies* (ACTs) are recommended by the World Health Organization (WHO) to treat malaria, especially multidrug-resistant strains.[102]

Although there has been some interest in using the *Artemisia annua* herb as an antimalarial, little clinical evidence is currently available. Of the limited studies conducted,[103-104] one showed resolution of parasitemia, and another showed a lower rate of parasitemia with a high recrudescence rate.

The dose of sweet Annie for malaria has not been determined.

Scientific Evidence of Effectiveness

PITYRIASIS CAPITIS (DANDRUFF). A placebo-controlled trial reported that a 5% tea tree oil shampoo (used daily for 4 weeks) was more effective than placebo for the treatment of dandruff.[107] Further research is needed before a firm conclusion can be made.

CANDIDA ALBICANS (ORAL THRUSH). It has been hypothesized that tea tree oil may be efficacious as a gargle for the treatment of thrush. One open-label study reported promising early results with oral thrush in patients with acquired immunodeficiency syndrome (AIDS).[108] After 4 weeks, eight of 12 evaluable patients had responded to the treatment with tea tree oil oral solution four times daily, and two patients were cured of oral candidiasis. The overall clinical response rate was 67%. A case series of 14 AIDS patients with oral thrush reported five cures and five improvements after 4 weeks of treatment with Melaleuca Oral Solution M (Breathaway).[108] Although these results are promising, additional studies are needed before concrete conclusions can be made.

ONYCHOMYCOSIS. Tea tree oil has been proposed as a potential topical therapy for onychomycosis. Although methodologically flawed, initial human trials have reported positive results.[109,110] A double-blind, randomized trial reported 100% tea tree oil to be equivalent in effectiveness to 1% clotrimazole cream for the treatment of lower-extremity onychomycosis.[109] Another double-blind, randomized trial reported that a cream containing a combination of 2% butenafine and 5% tea tree oil was superior to a cream with an unspecified amount of tea tree oil.[110] Lack of placebo and insufficient methodological design in these studies mean that further clinical research is required before a recommendation can be made.

TINEA PEDIS (ATHLETE'S FOOT). Tea tree oil has also been proposed as a potential topical therapy for tinea pedis. Literature review reveals a single human study with equivocal results.[33] According to one study, tea tree oil cream (10% w/w) reduced the symptomatology of tinea pedis as effectively as tolnaftate 1% but was no more effective than placebo in achieving a mycological cure.[111] Therefore, at this time, reliable human evidence is insufficient to draw a firm conclusion in this area.

VAGINAL YEAST INFECTIONS. In vitro studies have demonstrated tea tree oil to possess antimicrobial activity against pathogens that typically cause vaginal infections.[105,112-118] When tested clinically, 20% tea tree oil applied with a saturated tampon for 24 hours was as effective as standard therapy for trichomonal vaginitis.[119]

Dose

In 1996, the International Organization for Standardization specified the component limits for 14 of the almost 100 elements that make up tea tree oil (ISO 4730 Oil of *Melaleuca*, terpinen-4-ol).[120] Tea tree oil must contain terpinolene (1.5%-5%); 1,8-cineole (≤15%); α-terpinene (5%-13%); γ-terpinene (10%-28%); *p*-cymene (0.5%-12%); terpinen-4-ol (≥30%); α-terpineol (1.5%-8%); limonene (0.5%-4%); sabinene trace (3.5%); aromadendrene trace (7%); δ-cadinene trace (8%); globulol trace (3%); viridiflorol trace (1.5%); and α-pinene (1%-6%). Before the development of the international standard (ISO 4730), an Australian standard existed (AS2782-1985) that required tea tree oil preparations to contain more than 30% terpinene-4-ol and less than 15% 1,8-cineole.[121] Although 100% tea tree oil is sometimes used, it is often diluted with inert diluents.

For the treatment of dandruff, 5% tea tree oil shampoo has been used daily for 4 weeks.[107]

For thrush, clinical trials have used tea tree oral mouthwash four times daily for 2 to 4 weeks, or *Melaleuca* Oral Solution M (Breathaway) four times daily for 4 weeks.[108]

For tinea pedis, doses have included a 10% tea tree oil cream (Pharmaco Pty, Sydney, Australia) applied twice daily after thoroughly washing and drying feet, or 25% to 50% tea tree oil solution applied twice daily to the affected area for up to 4 weeks.[122]

For onychomycosis, doses have included daily applications of 100% tea tree oil,[109] or a combination cream containing 2% butenafine and 5% tea tree oil.[110]

For vaginal yeast infection, a 20% solution of tea tree oil has been applied with a saturated tampon for 24 hours.[119] After that time, a daily douche with 0.4% tea tree oil in 1 quart of water was used.

Adverse Effects, Interactions, Pharmacokinetics. See Appendix A.

Thyme (*Thymus vulgaris*)

Grade C: Unclear or conflicting scientific evidence (paronychia/onycholysis/fungal infections)

Mechanism of Action

The key constituents of thyme include essential oils, such as the phenols thymol and carvacrol, glycosides, flavonoids, *p*-cymene, borneol, linalool, alcohols, rosmarinic acid, saponins, tannins, and terpenoids.[123-125] Four acetophenone glycosides have been isolated from the butanol-soluble fraction of thyme extracts, with weak cytotoxic and antioxidant effects in vitro.[126]

Antimicrobial activities of thyme and thymol have been demonstrated in vitro.[127] Thymol has exhibited activity against some fungi and yeast, including *Aspergillus parasiticus*, *Aspergillus flavus*, and *Candida albicans*, and suppressed fungal growth and aflatoxin synthesis in vitro at doses of 250 ppm.[127-131]

Scientific Evidence of Effectiveness

Topical thymol has been used traditionally in the treatment of paronychia and onycholysis. In vitro studies suggest that thyme essential oil and thymol exert activity against a number of fungi, including *Aspergillus parasiticus* and *A. flavus*, and may completely suppress growth and aflatoxin synthesis.[127-131] In the 1930s, five patients with actinomycosis were successfully treated to resolution with thymol in oral doses, ranging from 1 g twice weekly to 2 g once daily.[132] Three of the five patients received additional thymol as a 10% to 25% injection into the sinus tract. A sixth patient received local thymol injection only and subsequently died of fungemia. Adverse effects were not clearly reported, and in light of the known toxicity of thymol and the current availability of other antifungal agents with demonstrated efficacy and more favorable therapeutic indices, thymol may not be advisable for such patients.

A 1965 review article suggested that 1 drop of 1% or 2% thymol in chloroform can be used for acute paronychia, and that chronic cases can be treated with 4% thymol applied three times daily.[133] The author noted more than 20 years of personal experience treating patients with these formulations with good results and excellent tolerance. However, controlled clinical trials are lacking.

Dose

Standardized amounts of thyme oil may be found in commercial products, such as topical cosmetic formulations or mouthwash.[127] Standardized extracts may contain 0.6% to 1.2% volatile oil and 0.5% phenol content. Common thyme contains a greater quantity of volatile oil (0.4%-3.4%) than Spanish thyme (0.7%-1.38%).

For paronychia, 1 drop of 1% to 2% thymol in chloroform to the affected area (or 1 drop of 4% thymol in chloroform to a chronically affected area) three times daily has been used.[133] For *Actinomyces*, oral doses ranging from 1 g twice weekly to 2 g daily have been used in a small 1930s study of five patients.[132] Three of the five patients received additional thymol as a 10% to 25% injection into the sinus tract.

Adverse Effects, Interactions, Pharmacokinetics. See Appendix A.

HERBAL THERAPIES WITH LIMITED EVIDENCE

Alfalfa (Medicago sativa)

Alfalfa may possess antimicrobial properties.[134] Compound G2 has been isolated from alfalfa roots and has displayed a high degree of activity against *Cryptococcus neoformans*, with MIC of 2 mcg/mL in vitro.[135] G2 exhibits activity against a wide range of yeast strains and appears to induce lethal ion leakage from yeast cells.[136] Medicagenic acid, hederagenin glycosides, and soyasapogenols may contribute to the antifungal actions of alfalfa, including against *Aspergillus niger*, *Candida albicans*, and *Candida tropicalis*.[137]

Barberry (Berberis spp.)

The barberry constituent berberine has been demonstrated to completely inhibit the in vitro growth of promastigotes at a concentration of 5 mg/mL while inhibiting endogenous respiration of the organism as well as nucleic acid and protein synthesis.[61] Subsequent research showed that berberine chloride interacts with *Leishmania donovani* nuclear DNA, inhibiting the multiplication of amastigotes in macrophage culture in vitro and decreasing the parasite load in animals.[62]

Bitter Melon (Momordica charantia)

Bitter melon's constituents include *Momordica charantia* peroxidase,[138] MAP30,[139-142] and 9*cis*,11*trans*,13*trans*-conjugated linolenic acid.[143] In an assay using free-living nematodes, a crude extract of *M. charantia* produced 96% mortality.[144]

Corydalis (Corydalis spp.)

Corydalis may offer a potential benefit in patients with the tapeworm infection *Echinococcus granulosus*.[145-149]

Cranberry (Vaccinium macrocarpon)

Cranberry juice at 40% concentration inhibits the growth in vitro of *Microsporum* spp. and some species of *Trichophyton* and *Epidermophyton*.[150] *Candida albicans* growth has not been inhibited. The clinical significance of these findings is unclear. There is a lack of clinical evidence supporting the use of cranberry as an antifungal agent.

Elecampane (Inula helenium)

In vitro a 5% aqueous extract of elecampane killed eggs and larvae of *Ascaris lumbricoides*.[151] In animal study a boiled-water extract of elecampane suppressed egg-laying capacity of *Clonorchis sinensis*.[152] The same author found that a boiled-water extract of elecampane induced degeneration, atrophy, necrosis, and dilation of the viscera of these worms.[153] Secondary reports indicate the use of alantolactone for worm infections in humans.

Greater Celandine (Chelidonium majus)

Researchers studied *Chelidonium majus* and two other Papaveraceae organisms for their fungitoxic alkaloids. Ten alkaloids (two of which were found to be new compounds) were isolated, identified, and tested.[154] Aqueous extracts of *C. majus* demonstrated considerable inhibitory action against 10 strains from the *Fusarium* genus of filamentous fungi. However, methanolic extracts of *C. majus* showed the best results. Root extracts inhibited *Fusarium* growth more efficiently than shoot extracts. Because most *Fusarium* strains have high resistance to conventional fungicides, *C. majus* was proposed as a potential treatment of *Fusarium* fungal infections.[155]

Holy Basil (Ocimum sanctum)

The essential oil of *Ocimum sanctum* and eugenol, tested in vitro, showed potent anthelmintic activity.[156] The clinical efficacy is unclear.

Kiwi (Actinidia deliciosa, Actinidia chinensis)

A potential allergen of kiwi[157] with a partial N-terminal sequence is a thaumatin-like protein (TLP) with concanavalin A–binding ability. TLP (isoelectric points of 9.4 and 9.5 and molecular weight of 24 kD) showed antifungal activity toward *Saccharomyces carlsbergensis* and *Candida albicans*.

Lingonberry (Vaccinium vitis-idaea)

Extracts from dry red bilberry fruit (*Vaccinium vitis-idaea*) have shown vermifugal (anthelminthic) activity.[158]

Noni (Morinda citrifolia)

In vitro study showed that a noni leaf ethanol extract induced paralysis and death of the nematode *Ascaris lumbricoides* within 24 hours.[159]

Oregano (Origanum vulgare)

Oregano has exhibited antifungal properties against *Aspergillus niger*, *Aspergillus terreus*, *Candida albicans*, *Fusarium* spp., *Blastocystis hominis*, *Entamoeba hartmanni*, and *Endolimax nana*.[160-164] Studies suggest that both carvacrol and eugenol consistently affect the envelope of *Candida* cells.[161]

Rhubarb (Rheum spp.)

In animals, emodin, an active component in the root and rhizome of *Rheum palmatum*, delayed the development of subcutaneous abscesses caused by *Trichomonas vaginalis* in mice.[165] Emodin also was effective against intravaginal infection of trichomonads when taken orally. In cell cultures, *Rheum* reduced the cytotoxic effect of *T. vaginalis* toward mammalian cells. This inhibition was reversed by the coexistence of free-radical scavengers, indicating the possible mediation of free radicals.

Rosemary (Rosmarinus officinalis)

In turkey poults an oral herbal product with extracts from cinnamon, garlic, lemon, and rosemary reduced the mortality of birds infected with the protozoan parasite *Histomonas meleagridis*.[166]

Seaweed

Preclinical studies have reported antifungal effects of seaweed.[167] Currently, however, high-quality clinical studies investigating the antifungal activity of seaweed are lacking. A lectinlike mucopolysaccharide isolated from *Fucus vesiculosus* has been found to be specific for complex carbohydrates. This mucopolysaccharide causes agglutination of the yeast *Candida guilliermondii* and inhibits its growth by 99.2%.[167] Clinical evidence is currently lacking.

Shiitake Mushroom (Lentinus edodes)

Lentin, isolated from *Lentinula edodes*, inhibits mycelial growth in a variety of fungal species, including *Physalospora piricola*, *Botrytis cinerea*, and *Mycosphaerella arachidicola*.[168]

Tamanu (Calophyllum inophyllum)

Extracts of de-oiled, powdered *Calophyllum inophyllum* have anthelmintic properties against root-knot larvae in suspension.[169]

Yerba Santa (Eriodictyon californicum)

Preclinical studies showed that flavanones such as eriodictyol are active against malaria and trypanosomes.[170-172]

ADJUNCT THERAPIES

1. *Zinc* is a mineral that has been used since ancient Egyptian times to enhance wound healing. Zinc pyrithione shampoo is a standard treatment option for pityriasis versicolor (tinea versicolor),[173] and efficacy is supported by clinical trials.[174,175] Results are contradictory regarding the effect of zinc on malaria symptoms. Some randomized, double-blind clinical trials suggest no effect of zinc supplementation on the severity of malaria. Other studies suggest that zinc supplementation may reduce hospitalization time and mortality caused by *Plasmodium falciparum* infection. Further well-designed RCTs are required to address these discrepancies.
2. In a few studies of varying quality, patients with cutaneous leishmaniasis were given six weekly injections of 2% zinc sulfate ($ZnSO_4$) intralesionally. One study found that zinc sulfate was better than standard treatment (meglumine antimoniate) for the first 4 weeks, but no statistical differences were observed after 6 weeks.[176] Another study found that zinc sulfate was less effective than meglumine antimoniate.[177] Zinc may decrease the severity of infection and reinfection of *Schistosoma mansoni*, but 30-mg to 50-mg doses of zinc orally for 12 months do not seem to prevent initial infection.[178] More research is needed to examine how zinc affects the *S. mansoni* life cycle and whether these data can be extrapolated to other *Schistosoma* spp. Conflicting results indicate the need for further study before zinc can be recommended for the treatment of parasites.
3. *Propolis* is a natural resin created by bees to make their hives. Propolis is made from the buds of conifer and poplar trees combined with beeswax, resins, and other plant-derived constituents, which vary depending on available plants and geographical region. The Brazilian commercial ethanol propolis extract, also formulated to ensure physical and chemical stability, was found to inhibit oral candidiasis in 12 denture-wearing patients with prosthesis stomatitis candidiasis.[179] Severe allergic reactions have

Herbs with Potential Antifungal, Antiprotozoal, and/or Anthelmintic Properties*

HERB	SPECIFIC THERAPEUTIC USE(S)†	HERB	SPECIFIC THERAPEUTIC USE(S)†
Abuta	Malaria	Bulbous buttercup	Helminthic infections, candidal infections
Acacia	Visceral leishmaniasis	Bupleurum	Fungal infections, malaria
Acerola	Fungal infections	Burdock	Fungal infections, ringworm
Aconite	Fungal infections	Calamus	Fungal infections
Agave	Parasitic infections	Calendula	Tinea pedis (athlete's foot), fungal infections
Aloe	Candidal skin infections, helminthic infections	Capers	Helminthic infections
Alpinia	Fungal infections, helminthic infections, protozoal infections	Carob	Helminthic infections
American pawpaw	Fungal infections	Carrot	Parasitic infections (intestinal)
Andiroba	Parasitic infections (fungal infections, malaria)	Cascara	Parasitic infections
Andrographis	*Ascaris lumbricoides* (in vitro), malaria	Cat's claw	Fungal infections, parasitic infections, candidal infections
Angostura	Malaria	Chamomile	Fungal infections, malaria, parasitic infections, helminthic infections
Anise	Parasitic infections, fungal infections		
Annatto	Parasitic infections, ascaridiasis (pediatric)	Chaparral	Parasitic infections
Aristolochia spp.	Helminthic infections, fungal infections, antifungal, trypanosomes	Chasteberry	Fungal infections
		Chicory	Malaria
		Chrysanthemum	Fungal infections
Arnica	Fungal infections	Clove	Antifungal, tinea pedis (athlete's foot), oral candidiasis (thrush), parasitic infections
Asarum	Fungal infections		
Ashwagandha	Fungal infections		
Astragalus	Fungal infections	Comfrey	Fungal infections
Bael fruit	Fungal infections, malaria	Daisy	Fungal infections
Bamboo	Ringworm	Dandelion	Fungal infections
Bay leaf	Fungal infections	Desert parsley	Fungal infections
Berberine	Fungal infections, yeast infections (vaginal)	Devil's claw	Malaria
		Devil's club	Fungal infections
Betel nut	Helminthic infections (veterinary), parasitic infections	Dong quai	Fungal infections, malaria
		Echinacea	Candidiasis, malaria
Betony	Helminthic infections	Elecampane	Fungal infections, roundworm, threadworm, hookworm, whipworm
Bilberry	Fungal infections		
Black cohosh	Malaria		
Black horehound	Helminthic infections (intestinal)	English ivy	Parasitic infections
Blessed thistle	Malaria	Eucalyptus	Hookworm, parasitic infection, ringworm, tinea
Bloodroot	Fungal infections (tinea pedis, athlete's foot), parasitic infections, ringworm		
		Euphorbia	Fungal infections, parasitic infections, helminthic infections
Blue flag	Helminthic infections (intestinal), tinea pedis (athlete's foot)	Eyebright	Helminthic infections
		Fennel	Fungal infections
Boldo	Helminthic infections	Fo-ti	Tinea pedis (athlete's foot)
Boneset	Malaria, parasitic infections, helminthic infections	Garcinia	Helminthic infections, fungal infections
Boswellia	Fungal infections, typanosomiasis	Germanium	Malaria
Bromelain	Helminthic infections	Ginger	Fungal infections, tinea pedis (athlete's foot), parasitic infections (intestinal), malaria
Buckshorn plantain	Malaria		

Continued

Herbs with Potential Antifungal, Antiprotozoal, and/or Anthelmintic Properties—cont'd

HERB	SPECIFIC THERAPEUTIC USE(S)†	HERB	SPECIFIC THERAPEUTIC USE(S)†
Ginkgo	Fungal infections, parasitic infections, filariasis	Noni	Helminthic infections, fungal infections, malaria
Ginseng	Fungal infections	Nux vomica	Helminthic infections
Globe artichoke	Fungal infections	Oleander	Parasitic infections (veterinary), malaria, ringworm
Goji	Fungal infections		
Goldenrod	Fungal infections, yeast infections	Olive leaf	Fungal infections, parasitic infections
Gotu kola	Fungal infections, malaria	Onion	Fungal infections
Grapefruit	Fungal infections, parasitic infections	Oregano	Fungal infections (including activity against candidiasis and foodborne pathogens), parasitic infections, tinea pedis (athlete's foot, [topically]), ringworm
Ground ivy	Helminthic infections		
Guarana	Malaria		
Gymnema	Malaria		
Heartsease	Ringworm	Papain	Malaria, parasitic infections
Hibiscus	Fungal infections	Passion flower	Fungal infections
Hop	Fungal infections, parasitic infections	Podophyllum	Helminthic infections
		Pokeweed	Helminthic infections, ringworm, schistosomiasis (tropical parasitic infection)
Horseradish	Helminthic infections (in children)		
Horsetail	Malaria		
Hydrangea	Fungal infections, malaria	Psyllium	Parasitic infections
Hyssop	Helminthic infections, fungal infections	Pycnogenol	Parasitic infections
		Pygeum	Malaria
Jackfruit	Fungal infections	Quassia	Fungal infections, parasitic infections
Jequirity	Helminthic infections, malaria, schistosomiasis (urinary)	Raspberry	Malaria
		Rehmannia	Fungal infections
Jointed flatsedge	Fungal infections	Sage	Fungal infections
Juniper	Helminthic infections	Sandalwood	Fungal infections
Katuka	Helminthic infections	Sanicle	Fungal infections
Kava	Fungal infections, filariasis, parasitic infection	Sarsaparilla	Fungal infections
		Sassafras	Fungal infections
Lavender	Fungal infections, parasitic infection	Sea buckthorn	Helminthic infections
		Skullcap	Fungal infections
Lemongrass	Fungal infections, tinea pedis (athlete's foot), parasitic infections (intestinal, skin), malaria, ringworm	Skunk cabbage	Parasitic infections, helminthic infections, ringworm
		Slippery elm	Helminthic infections
		Sorrel	Ringworm
Maitake mushroom	Fungal infections	Soy	Fungal infections
Mangosteen	Helminthic infections, fungal infections, malaria	Spirulina	Fungal infections
		St. John's wort	Malaria
Mastic	Fungal infections, ringworm	Star anise	Fungal infections
Milk thistle	Malaria	Stinging nettle	Helminthic infections, fungal infections
Morus nigra	Helminthic infections, antifungal		
Mugwort	Helminthic infections, fungal infections, malaria	Tamarind	Helminthic infections
		Tansy	Helminthic infections, fungal infections
Muira puama	Hookworm		
Mullein	Fungal infections	Tea	Fungal infections
Neem	Fungal infections, malaria, parasitic infections, tinea pedis (athlete's foot)	Tribulus	Helminthic infections
		Turmeric	Fungal infections, parasitic infections, ringworm

Herbs with Potential Antifungal, Antiprotozoal, and/or Anthelmintic Properties—cont'd

HERB	SPECIFIC THERAPEUTIC USE(S)†	HERB	SPECIFIC THERAPEUTIC USE(S)†
Usnea	Fungal infections, parasitic infections	Wild yam	Fungal infections
		Willow	Malaria
Watercress	Helminthic infections, fungal infections	Yellow dock	Fungal infections, candidal infection
		Yucca	Fungal infections
White horehound	Helminthic infections		
White water lily	Thrush		

*This is not an all-inclusive or comprehensive list of herbs with possible antifungal, antiprotozoal, and/or anthelmintic properties; other herbs and supplements may possess these qualities. A qualified health care provider should be consulted with specific questions or concerns regarding potential antiparasitic effects or interactions.
†Based on expert opinion, anecdote, case reports, and/or preliminary trial evidence.

been reported.[1] There has been one report of kidney failure with the ingestion of propolis that improved on discontinuing therapy and deteriorated with reexposure.[180] Use of propolis during pregnancy or breastfeeding is not recommended because of the high alcohol content in some propolis products.

4. *Selenium* is a mineral found in soil, water, and some foods. Commercially available 1% selenium sulfide shampoo has been reported as equivalent to sporicidal therapy in the adjunctive treatment of tinea capitis infection.[181] Selenium sulfide shampoo has also been studied as a possible treatment for tinea versicolor.[175,182]

5. *Probiotics* are beneficial bacteria that help to maintain the health of the intestinal tract and aid in digestion. They also help keep potentially harmful organisms in the body under control. Most probiotics come from food sources, especially cultured milk products. Probiotics can be consumed as capsules, tablets, beverages, powders, yogurts, and other foods. Some clinical studies have supported the use of probiotics for vaginal *Candida* infections,[183] though efficacy remains unclear.

6. *Vitamin A* is a fat-soluble vitamin derived from two sources: pre-formed retinoids and provitamin carotenoids. Retinoids such as retinal and retinoic acid are found in animal sources, including liver, kidney, eggs, and dairy produce. Carotenoids such as beta-carotene (which has the highest vitamin A activity) are found in plants, including dark or yellow vegetables and carrots. Numerous reports suggest that vitamin A may reduce fever, morbidity, and parasite blood levels in patients with malaria (*Plasmodium falciparum* infection).[184-190]

7. *Riboflavin* (vitamin B$_2$) is a water-soluble vitamin involved in vital metabolic processes in the body. It is necessary for normal cell function, growth, and energy production. Small amounts of riboflavin are present in most animal and plant tissues. Riboflavin deficiency has been associated with lower parasite counts in malaria patients; however, the recovery time was longer in riboflavin-deficient patients despite lower levels of *Plasmodium*.[191] Although the relationship among the host, riboflavin levels, and the virus itself is still unclear, riboflavin may play an important role in immune function and disease susceptibility.

INTEGRATIVE THERAPY PLAN

- Patients with parasitic infections may present with a variety of complaints. Symptoms vary depending on the type and severity of the infection, as well as the parts of the body that are infected. Patients should first undergo a thorough medical examination by a physician.
- A thorough travel and exposure history should be collected to diagnose a parasitic infection accurately, because many causative agents have distinct distribution around the world and in specific environments.
- To diagnose the parasitic infection, various laboratory tests may be performed, including ova and parasite test (O&P) or fecal examination, blood tests (serologic assays, antigen detection tests, blood smear), pelvic examination (vaginal infections), endoscopy, colonoscopy, bronchoscopy, blood tests, radiography, magnetic resonance imaging (MRI), and computed tomography (CT).
- Record the patient's medication regimen and use of nonprescription agents, including dietary supplements.
- Prescription drugs and over-the-counter agents that are available for parasitic infections include praziquantel (Biltricide), albendazole (Albenza), mebendazole (Vermox), terbinafine (Lamisil), ketoconazole (Nizoral), clotrimazole (Lotrimin), and miconazole (Monistat).
- Currently, herbal or integrative therapies are not strongly recommended for treating fungal, protozoal, or helminthic infections. Evidence suggests that some herbal therapies may be effective for some indications. For example, tea tree oil has been used successfully to treat certain fungal infections, and derivatives of artemisinin (a constituent of sweet Annie) are

currently used along with standard antimalarial treatments. Further research is required before herbs can be strongly recommended for fungal, protozoal, or helminthic infections.
- Because many parasitic infections are transmitted through physical contact, patients should be advised to maintain good hygiene.
- Travelers to areas where malaria is highly prevalent should protect themselves by wearing long-sleeved shirts and pants and using N,N-diethylmetatoluamide (DEET)–containing insect repellents. Patients who are visiting tropical areas of the world where malaria is common should sleep with a bednet to prevent mosquitoes and other bugs from transmitting diseases during the night.
- If an individual is traveling to an area where malaria is common, taking antimalarial drugs exactly as prescribed by a physician is important. For preventive therapy, individuals generally take the prescribed drug 1 to 2 weeks before leaving, throughout the trip, and for 4 weeks after return.
- Urge patients to limit their exposure to warm, moist environments. Individuals should wear shower shoes (e.g., flip-flops, sandals) when they are exposed to wet or moist surfaces at public settings, including public showers and swimming pools at gyms and workout clubs. Patients should change their socks if they become sweaty.
- Individuals who are in areas of the world with poor sanitation should only drink bottled water. If this is not possible, individuals should boil their water before drinking it. This kills any parasites that may be living in the water.
- Recommend that patients wash all produce before eating to prevent exposure to disease-causing organisms. Raw or undercooked meat should not be eaten. Individuals should be especially careful when preparing pork, venison, or lamb because these contain the most dangerous parasites.
- Probiotics have been extensively studied for treating fungal infections, especially vaginal candidiasis. Probiotics are bacterial strains that normally colonize humans (in the skin, mouth, colon, and vagina) and are thought to confer beneficial effects by inhibiting the growth of harmful microbes. Probiotic strains are found in cultured products such as yogurt and buttermilk and may be taken by mouth, gargled, or applied topically. Vaginal suppositories containing probiotics have also been used to treat or prevent vaginal infections such as candidiasis.

Case Studies

CASE STUDY 28-1

GK is a 22-year-old woman who was sent home from missionary work in Zanzibar, Africa, after contracting *Plasmodium falciparum* malaria. She was initially given a course of chloroquine (Aralen), but she recently suffered a relapse. GK is prescribed mefloquine (Lariam), five 250-mg tablets in a single 1250-mg dose. She is extremely disappointed that she has contracted the disease and even more disappointed the chloroquine therapy was unsuccessful; furthermore, she is concerned that she has contracted a drug-resistant form of malaria. GK is willing to try adjunctive treatments for malaria, including alternative treatment options. Her current herbal medications include St. John's wort for depression and ginseng for energy. Discuss an integrative treatment plan for GK, taking into consideration her medical history and her current medications (conventional and herbal).

Answer: Drug-resistant strains of malaria are increasing, and failure of chloroquine therapy is not unusual. A number of herbal remedies have been proposed for the treatment of malaria, but there is limited convincing evidence of efficacy. GK should therefore be counseled to complete her course of mefloquine.

Two herbal products might be beneficial: goldenseal *(Hydrastis canadensis)* and sweet Annie *(Artemisia annua)*. Of the two, sweet Annie holds the most promise. The main active constituent of sweet Annie is artemisinin, a sesquiterpene lactone thought to damage the malaria parasite within the RBCs. Artemisinin and its derivatives have demonstrated antimalarial activity in humans. Artemisinin-based combination therapies (ACTs) are recommended by WHO to treat malaria, especially multidrug-resistant strains.[102]

Sweet Annie alone is not recommended as a primary treatment for malaria; rather, artemisinin should be taken in conjunction with mefloquine and might actually enhance the drug's effects. Cures and reduced mortality have been reported with sweet Annie, which is considered to be relatively safe with few drug or herbal interactions.

Limited research supports the use of goldenseal as treatment for drug-resistant malaria. The antimalarial effect of goldenseal is thought to be caused by berberine. Only a trace amount of berberine is found in most goldenseal preparations, however, and it is unclear whether the herb can be beneficial. Goldenseal has anticoagulant activity, which may act synergistically with ginseng to increase the risk of bleeding. Goldenseal, St. John's wort, and ginseng all inhibit the cytochrome P450 enzymes and may have synergistic effects.

Serious side effects have been reported for mefloquine, but the risk is low for GK because she is young and in good health aside from her malaria. The side effects of mefloquine often involve the central nervous system and may include nightmares, dizziness, headache, and insomnia. Mefloquine has also been reported to cause seizures, peripheral neuropathy, vestibular damage, and severe depression. Because GK has a history of depression, her physician should monitor her closely for an exacerbation.

CASE STUDY 28-2

AM is a 32-year-old woman who visits the pharmacy accompanied by her 2-year-old daughter. After a recent course of ampicillin, the daughter complained of a sore mouth. Her mother noted white lesions on the daughter's tongue and inner cheeks and immediately called her pediatrician. The pediatrician diagnosed oral thrush and prescribed miconazole oral gel (Monistat). However, on the advice of a friend who is a proponent of herbal medicine, AM inquires about the efficacy of tea tree oil for oral thrush. What guidance can you offer to AM regarding the various treatment options for her daughter's oral thrush?

Answer: Tea tree oil inhibits the in vitro conversion of *Candida albicans* from yeast to mycelial form and may therefore resolve oral thrush. However, large-scale clinical trials have not been performed. Adults have gargled with tea tree oil and cured oral thrush; however, they were strongly cautioned not to swallow it. Tea tree oil is not recommended for AM's daughter because it can be toxic if swallowed. Oral thrush in children can often be resolved with the ingestion of yogurt or buttermilk. Both contain lactobacilli, which are probiotics that may limit the growth of harmful organisms. If yogurt or buttermilk is not effective, miconazole can be used; it is very effective, has minimal side effects, and can resolve the condition. If AM's mother insists on an herbal remedy, an extract of pomegranate *(Punica granatum)* has been shown to be as effective as miconazole. However, pomegranate can potentiate the effects of many drugs. Advise AM that she should not rely on these natural remedies if her daughter's oral thrush does not seem to improve.

CASE STUDY 28-3

JW is a 24-year-old male athlete who comes to you after his family physician diagnosed him with onychomycosis of the left great toenail. He was prescribed oral terbinafine (Lamisil). JW has heard that terbinafine can cause serious side effects and asks if an herbal product or a topical product is available. He also inquires about preventing future infections. His current medications include valerian and kava for anxiety and metoprolol (Lopressor) for hypertension.

Answer: Onychomycosis is a strong infection that requires long-term treatment. Oral agents such as terbinafine have the highest cure rate but can be hepatotoxic and can affect blood cell counts. A complete blood count (CBC) and liver function tests should be done before and at intervals during the therapy, which can last for months. Systemic lupus erythematosus has appeared or flared up in patients taking terbinafine. Onychomycosis lodges deep in the nail bed, and topical preparations do not penetrate well. Research is ongoing for effective topical preparations. Terbinafine is available as a topical product and is effective for more superficial fungal infections, such as tinea corporis, cruris, and pedis.

No topical herbal remedies have been demonstrated to be consistently effective in clinical trials; however, anecdotal evidence warrants further investigation. Tea tree oil *(Melaleuca alternifolia)* and thyme *(Thymus vulgaris)* have been used topically, but no definitive studies proving efficacy have yet emerged. Povidone-iodine (Betadine) is an effective fungicide. Daily soaking on a long-term basis with povidone-iodine might be effective. Other topical nonprescription products include Listerine and vinegar.

The potential hepatotoxic effects of terbinafine and kava are important to discuss with JW. If he begins terbinafine treatment, he should discontinue kava. JW's liver function should be monitored throughout treatment, and he should seek professional medical advice should he choose to reinitiate kava after terbinafine treatment. JW should also be counseled of the potential for interaction between metoprolol and valerian; concomitant use has been associated with reduced mental performance (see Appendix A). Alternative stress-relieving practices may be suggested, such as meditation and massage.

References for Chapter 28 can be found on the Evolve website at http://evolve.elsevier.com/Ulbricht/herbalpharmacotherapy/

Review Questions

1. Preclinical studies have shown thyme to interact with which of the following hormones?
   a. Estrogen
   b. Prolactin
   c. Testosterone
   d. Cortisol

2. Which of the following is true regarding the use of tea tree oil?
   a. Tea tree oil is derived from the *Camellia sinensis* plant.
   b. Thymol is the component most likely responsible for its antimicrobial properties.
   c. Tea tree oil is toxic when ingested.
   d. Tea tree oil may be safely ingested with meals.

3. Which of the following statements about sweet Annie is *false*?
   a. The *Artemisia* derivative artemisinin has antiparasitic effects in vitro and in vivo.
   b. Sweet Annie may inhibit angiogenesis and should be avoided in patients recovering from surgery and in those with other wounds.
   c. Based on results from preclinical studies, sweet Annie may have immunosuppressive effects.
   d. Sweet Annie should be avoided in patients taking antiplatelet or anticoagulant medications because of potential thrombotic effects.

4. What constituent(s) of bladderwrack may exert antifungal effects?
   a. Beta-glucan
   b. Thymol
   c. A lectinlike mucopolysaccharide
   d. b and c

5. True or false: Pomegranate extract has been shown to be effective in the treatment of vaginal candidiasis.

6. Berberine is a constituent in which of the following herbs:
   a. Goldenseal
   b. Barberry
   c. a and b
   d. None of the above

7. Berberine may interact with all of the following drugs *except*:
   a. Warfarin
   b. Metoprolol
   c. Cyclosporine
   d. Levothyroxine

8. Which of the following statements is *incorrect* regarding the antiparasitic activity of garlic?
   a. Garlic is primarily used topically when treating parasitic infections.
   b. It has been suggested that the antimicrobial activity of garlic powder is more potent than garlic oil on a unit weight basis.
   c. Alliin and allinase are found in separate but adjacent compartments of the garlic clove.
   d. All the above are incorrect.

9. What is the primary active constituent of bitter orange oil?
   a. Synephrine alkaloids
   b. Para-octopamine.
   c. Furocoumarins
   d. All the above

10. True or false: Bishop's weed psoralens are considered safe for treating skin discolorations, such as those caused by tinea versicolor.

Answers are found in the Answers to Review Questions section in the back of the text.

29 Viral Infections

Outline

OVERVIEW
  Types of Viral Infections
    Common Cold
    Human Immunodeficiency Virus
    Herpesviruses
    Measles, Mumps, and Rubella

SELECTED HERBAL THERAPIES
  Astragalus (*Astragalus membranaceus*)
  Beta-Sitosterol (β-Sitosterol), Sitosterol
    (22,23-Dihydrostigmasterol, 24-Ethylcholesterol)
  Bitter Melon (*Momordica charantia*)
  Blessed Thistle (*Cnicus benedictus*)
  Boneset (*Eupatorium* spp.)
  Boxwood (*Buxus sempervirens*)
  Chamomile (*Anthemis nobilis*, *Chamaemelum nobile*, *Chamomilla chamomilla*, *Chamomilla recutita*)
  Echinacea (*Echinacea* spp.)
  Elder (*Sambucus nigra*)
  Garlic (*Allium sativum*)
  Licorice (*Glycyrrhiza glabra*)
  Mistletoe (*Viscum album*)
  Sage (*Salvia officinalis*)
  Shiitake Mushroom (*Lentinus edodes*)

HERBAL THERAPIES WITH NEGATIVE EVIDENCE
HERBAL THERAPIES WITH LIMITED EVIDENCE
ADJUNCT THERAPIES
INTEGRATIVE THERAPY PLAN
CASE STUDIES
REVIEW QUESTIONS

Learning Objectives

- Understand the role of herbal agents for viral infections.
- Develop an integrative patient care plan to manage or prevent viral infections.

OVERVIEW

Viruses are small infectious particles (even smaller than bacteria) that multiply within host organisms. Although they contain genetic material (DNA or RNA) and can reproduce, they do not meet the criteria for classification as "living" organisms. Nonetheless, viruses are known to infect virtually any type of organism, including bacteria, fungi, plants, insects, and animals.[1]

More than 400 different viruses are known to cause infections in humans. Viral infections can affect most parts of the body, including the liver, immune system, and skin. However, most viruses infect specific types of cells in the body. For example, the human immunodeficiency virus (HIV-1 and HIV-2) primarily attacks cells with the CD4 receptor on their cell surfaces, or CD4-positive (CD4+) cells. Because the CD4+ cells fight against disease and infection, HIV weakens the immune system and may progress to acquired immunodeficiency syndrome (AIDS), less frequently in adults. If left untreated, flu symptoms can worsen and lead to complications such as pneumonia, as such as the common cold, may cause mild symptoms that disappear in a few days. Other viral infections, such as hepatitis, may be life threatening (see Chapter 25). Some viruses, such as Kaposi's sarcoma–associated herpesvirus, primarily infect immunocompromised individuals such as AIDS patients.

Depending on the specific virus, the infection may be transmitted in various ways. Many infections, such as the common

Of the estimated 25 to 50 million annual cases of flu in the United States, 30,000 to 40,000 are fatal.[2] Worldwide, influenza afflicts more than 1 billion people and causes 300,000 to 500,000 fatalities. Fatal infections are more common in children, elderly people, and immunocompromised individuals.

Human Immunodeficiency Virus

As the virus that causes AIDS, HIV primarily attacks the immune system, making the patient extremely vulnerable to opportunistic infections. These opportunistic infections are caused by pathogens (infectious organisms) that generally do not affect those with healthy immune systems. HIV primarily infects and destroys CD4+ T cells. Healthy individuals have a CD4+ cell count between 600 and 1200 cells per microliter (mcL) of blood. HIV patients have less than 600 CD4+ cells/mcL blood; the lower the CD4+ count, the weaker the immune system.

Infection with HIV progresses to AIDS if CD4+ cell counts drop below 200 cells/mcL. This may occur if an infected patient receives inadequate treatment or develops a major infection. Patients with a CD4+ cell count lower than 200 have the greatest risk of developing opportunistic infections, such as *Mycobacterium avium* complex (MAC) infections (see Chapter 27) or Kaposi's sarcoma.

According to the U.S. Centers for Disease Control and Prevention (CDC), approximately 56,300 patients in the United States were newly infected with HIV in 2006, a 40% increase from the 40,000 annual estimate used for past years.[3] The increased number may reflect more accurate testing and new statistical methods, not an actual worsening of the epidemic. In fact, AIDS fatalities continue to decline. Advanced treatments contribute to increased survival, resulting in more people living with AIDS in the United States. Worldwide AIDS-related deaths are also on the decline; in sub-Saharan Africa (an area with the highest AIDS prevalence), efforts to combat AIDS have lowered death rates by as much as 10.5% in focus countries.[4]

Signs and Symptoms

Many patients are asymptomatic when first infected with HIV. From 1 to 2 months after infection, almost all HIV patients develop flulike symptoms that last about 1 week. For the next several months or years, patients usually have no symptoms of the disease. Once this asymptomatic period ends, symptoms may include enlarged lymph nodes, fatigue, weight loss, frequent fevers and sweats, persistent or frequent yeast infections of the mouth or vagina, persistent skin rashes, flaky skin, pelvic inflammatory disease (PID) in women, and short-term memory loss. As the immune system continues to weaken, patients may eventually progress to AIDS. During this stage, patients have the greatest risk of developing life-threatening opportunistic infections.

Herpesviruses

Herpesviruses (family Herpesviridae) comprise more than 100 viruses that infect humans and other animals, causing various conditions with many unique signs and symptoms. The viruses fall into the following three subfamilies:

- Alpha-herpesvirinae: includes herpes simplex viruses 1 and 2 (HSV-1, HSV-2) and human herpesvirus 3 (HHV-3), also known as varicella-zoster virus (VSV).
- Beta-herpesvirinae: includes HHV-5 (cytomegalovirus), HHV-6 (human B-cell lymphotrophic virus and roseolovirus), and HHV-7.
- Gamma-herpesvirinae: HSV-4 (Epstein-Barr virus), lymphocryptovirus, and HSV-8 (Kaposi's sarcoma–associated herpesvirus).

All herpesviruses share some common properties, including a pattern of active symptoms followed by latent (inactive) periods with no symptoms. This latent period may last for months, years, or even a lifetime. The severity of herpes symptoms depends on the type of virus that causes the infection.

Herpes infections spread when the carrier is producing (or "shedding") active viruses, which are transmitted various ways. With HSV-1, which causes the majority of "cold sores" (also known as *oral* herpes), contact and infection can occur through direct contact such as mouth-to-mouth contact, hand-to-mouth contact, or through the use of everyday objects that have come in contact with the virus, including razors, towels, dishes, and glasses. HSV-1 may also cause sores in the genital area; however, genital herpes is primarily caused by HSV-2, and is contracted through direct sexual contact (genital-to-genital, mouth-to-genital, or hand-to-genital contact, not kissing) with an infected partner. Occasionally, oral-genital contact can spread oral herpes to the genitals (and vice versa). Individuals with active herpes lesions on or around their mouths or on their genitals should avoid oral sex. The varicella-zoster (chickenpox) virus spreads through the humidity in the air when inhaled and mainly spreads during the incubation period, which is just before an outbreak of symptoms.

During the latent period, the virus hides in nerves that connect to the area of the original viral outbreak. During illness or times of stress, the virus may reactivate; viral particles are produced in the nerve cells, then transported outwardly via the nerve to the skin. Thus, the virus begins to multiply and becomes transmissible again. This process of viral shedding may or may not be accompanied by symptoms.

The ability of the herpesvirus to become latent and reactive explains the chronic (long-term), recurring nature of a herpes infection. Recurrence of the viral symptoms is usually milder than the original infection. Recurrence may be triggered by menstruation, sun exposure, febrile illness, stress, or immune system imbalances.

Signs and Symptoms

HERPES SIMPLEX VIRUS TYPE 1 (HSV-1 OR HHV-1). HSV-1 is the primary cause of *oral herpes* infections (also called *herpes labialis*). It is easily transmitted and is the most common form of the herpes simplex virus. Oral herpes (cold sores or fever blisters) affects 15% to 30% of the population, and most people become infected between 6 months and 3 years of age. The primary symptoms of oral herpes are cold sores or blisters located on or around the lips and edge of the mouth. Often, tingling, burning, or itching occurs before the cold sore appears. HSV-1 may also cause a subset of genital herpes infections.

HERPES SIMPLEX VIRUS TYPE 2 (HSV-2 OR HHV-2). HSV-2 is the primary cause of *genital herpes* infections. Signs of genital herpes tend to develop within 3 to 7 days of skin-to-skin contact with an infected person. Genital herpes infections appear as small blisters or ulcers (circular areas of broken skin) on the genitals. HSV-2 also causes a subset of oral herpes infections.

VARICELLA-ZOSTER VIRUS (VSV). VSV causes a condition known as *varicella* or "chickenpox," which is perhaps the most well known of all childhood diseases. Individuals with chickenpox may notice several symptoms before the typical chickenpox rash appears. The *prodromal* (early) symptoms include fever, a vague feeling of sickness, and decreased appetite. Within a few days, a rash that includes small, red pimples or blisters appears. The rash appears in batches over the next 2 to 4 days. It usually starts on the trunk and then spreads to the head, face, arms, and legs. Blisters may also be found in the mouth or the genital areas because the virus can affect mucous membranes. Before the introduction of the vaccine in 1995, about 4 million cases of chickenpox were reported in the United States each year. According to the CDC, some regions currently report fewer than 50% of the pre-1995 disease rates.

Infection with VSV generally confers lifelong resistance to further VSV infections; however, anyone who has had chickenpox (90% of U.S. adults) is at risk for shingles later in life. This condition is caused by the same virus that causes chickenpox; however, instead of contracting the virus from someone else, people develop shingles when the latent virus reactivates. About 500,000 cases of shingles occur in the United States each year, in about 10% to 20% of adults who have had chickenpox, generally during times of stress or weakened immunity. Thus, shingles risk increases with age and declining immunity. It usually begins with prodromal (nonspecific) symptoms, such as itching, burning, tingling, aching, or a painful sensation in a bandlike area. As the rash progresses, it may begin to blister; during this phase, direct contact with the sores may transmit VSV to those who do not have immunity to the virus (either through previous VSV infection or immunization). The rash may also lead to a painful condition called *postherpetic neuralgia*, which may cause lingering nerve pain long after the rash subsides. Shingles is painful and often debilitating, but symptoms may be lessened with early treatment, usually with antiviral drugs such as valacyclovir (Valtrex) and oral corticosteroids such as prednisone. A shingles vaccine (Zostavax), which is similar to the chickenpox vaccine (Varivax), may be given to individuals age 60 or older to help prevent shingles.

EPSTEIN-BARR VIRUS (EBV). Epstein-Barr virus (EBV) is implicated in *mononucleosis*. EBV can cause fever, sore throat, swollen lymph glands (especially in the neck), and extreme fatigue. Although typically caused by EBV, mononucleosis (commonly called "mono") can also be caused by other herpesviruses, including cytomegalovirus (CMV). Infection with EBV during adolescence or young adulthood results in mononucleosis in 35% to 50% of cases.

CYTOMEGALOVIRUS (CMV). In people with weakened immune systems, such as HIV or AIDS patients, CMV can cause a number of infections, including retinitis (inflammation of retina), pneumonia, colitis (inflammation of colon), encephalitis (inflammation of brain), mononucleosis, pneumonia, hepatitis, and uveitis.

Measles, Mumps, and Rubella

Measles, mumps, and rubella are highly contagious viral infections that are rare in countries such as the United States, where a combination vaccine for all three viruses (MMR vaccine) is given routinely to children. *Measles* is a viral infection of the respiratory tract; prior to successful vaccination efforts in the United States, measles was a serious concern for childhood illness and death. *Mumps* is a viral infection of the salivary glands that causes swelling. *Rubella,* also called "German measles," is a mild infection of the respiratory tract that often goes unnoticed. However, if a pregnant woman develops rubella, it may lead to birth defects in the infant. These infections are transmitted through airborne droplets. People become infected with the viruses when they inhale particles of infected sputum from the air. The viruses become airborne when infected people expel saliva when coughing, sneezing, talking, or spitting.

Although measles was declared to be eliminated from the United States in 2001,[5] recent outbreaks have occurred in unvaccinated children.[6] A decline in MMR vaccination has been attributed to a controversial study that linked the MMR vaccine to autism.[7] This report was later partially retracted by the study's coauthors,[8] and the lead author was accused of data falsification.[9]

Signs and Symptoms

Measles is a virus that causes a rash, cough, runny nose, eye irritation, and fever in most patients. In severe cases, patients may develop pneumonia, seizures, brain damage, and death. The mumps virus typically causes fever, headache, and swollen glands. In severe cases, mumps may lead to deafness, meningitis (infection of the membranes that surround the brain and spinal cord), swollen testicles or ovaries, and death. Rubella is generally a mild disease but may cause serious birth defects if a pregnant mother becomes infected.

Diagnosis

Many common viral infections, such as the common cold or influenza, are usually *self-limiting* (the symptoms resolve on their own) and often self-diagnosed based on symptoms. Medical advice may be sought if symptoms are severe or prolonged. If a serious infection is suspected, an *antibody titer* may be performed to determine if the patient has developed antibodies to a particular virus. A blood sample, urine sample, or swab from the gums is taken. The sample is sent to a laboratory for analysis. If antibodies are present, a positive diagnosis is made. Antibody testing is time sensitive because the immunological response and time to mount significant levels of antibodies are delayed.

Unlike the antibody titer, *antigen detection* can be used to diagnose an infection before the patient has had time to develop antibodies. However, this test is much more expensive and less often used than an antibody test. The antigen test can determine if a virus is present in the body and requires a blood sample, nasal swab, or throat swab. The sample is sent to a laboratory for analysis. Results are usually available within 30 minutes.

A herpes viral culture may be taken from the blister fluid or sometimes cerebrospinal fluid (CSF). The samples are sent to a laboratory for analysis; it takes 1 to 14 days to detect the virus in the preparation made from the specimen.

A throat culture, sputum culture, or blood culture may be performed to rule out a secondary infection from a bacterium, such as *Streptococcus* (which causes "strep throat"), or pneumonia.

SELECTED HERBAL THERAPIES

 Note

To help make this educational resource more interactive, all pharmacokinetics, adverse effects, and interactions data have been compiled in Appendix A. Safety data specifically related to pregnancy and lactation are listed in Appendix B. Please refer to these appendices when working through the case studies and answering the review questions.

Aloe (Aloe vera)

Grade B: *Good scientific evidence (genital herpes)*

Grade C: *Unclear or conflicting scientific evidence (HIV infection)*

Mechanism of Action

Aloe vera has both antiviral and immune-enhancing properties, attributed to its water-soluble polysaccharide constituent *acetylmannan* (acemannan).[10,11] Aloe has been shown to stimulate the immune system by activating macrophages. The macrophage-stimulating principle of acetylmannan appears to reside in the high-molecular-weight polysaccharide aloeride.[11]

The antiviral effects of aloe may result from the interference with DNA synthesis.[12] According to in vitro research, acemannan acts synergistically with azidothymidine (AZT) (antiretroviral drug) and acyclovir (antiviral) to inhibit the replication of HIV-1 and HSV-1. Antiviral effects appear to be associated with modification of the glycosylation of viral glycoproteins.[13] Acetylmannans also demonstrate a direct virucidal effect on HSV and inhibition of replication.[13,14]

Acetylmannans have been shown to increase lymphatic response to alloantigens by enhancing the release of interleukin-1 from monocytes.[15]

Scientific Evidence of Effectiveness

HERPES SIMPLEX VIRUS (HSV). According to available randomized controlled trials (RCTs), topical application of *Aloe vera* may be beneficial for the first genital herpes episode in men.[16,17] A shorter-than-average healing time was noted with aloe cream versus gel (4.8 vs. 7 days).[16] A relapse occurred in six of the 49 healed patients.[17]

HUMAN IMMUNODEFICIENCY VIRUS (HIV). Preliminary studies indicate potential benefits of aloe in combination with other antivirals (e.g., AZT) for treatment of HIV. Acemannan raised CD8+ levels but had no effect on CD4+ counts in HIV-infected patients.[18-20] Increases were also noted in circulating monocytes and macrophages, phagocytic activity, and absolute T4, T8, and p24 core antigen levels. Other clinical research found no beneficial effects when acemannan was used as an adjunct to antiretroviral therapy.[21]

Dose

For genital herpes, patients have been treated with topical application of *Aloe vera* 0.5% hydrophilic cream or gel three times daily for up to 2 weeks.[16,17] Extracts of standardized acetylmannan (acemannan) have been administered orally in dosages ranging from 800 to 1600 mg daily in conjunction with standard antiretroviral therapy.[18-22]

Adverse Effects, Interactions, Pharmacokinetics. See Appendix A.

Andrographis (Andrographis paniculata)

Grade C: *Unclear or conflicting scientific evidence (influenza; HIV)*

Mechanism of Action

Andrographolide, a diterpene lactone compound, is believed to be the principal active agent of andrographis.[23] In general, *Andrographis paniculata* exerts its beneficial antiviral effects through immunomodulation. Andrographis may stimulate immune function by increasing antibodies and antibody-activated phagocytosis by macrophages,[24] offering a potential benefit in the broad-spectrum management of viral infections.

Data derived from HIV studies reveal that 14-dehydroandrographolide succinic acid monoester (DASM, active constituent of andrographis) may inhibit proteolytic cleavage of the HIV envelope glycoprotein, thus acting as a protease inhibitor for HIV (in vitro).[25]

Scientific Evidence of Effectiveness

INFLUENZA. Andrographis has become popular in Scandinavia as a remedy for influenza. Clinical research using a standardized andrographis preparation (Kan Jang) has reported a significant reduction in duration and severity of symptoms, as well as a decrease in time off from work, in patients treated for influenza.[26]

HUMAN IMMUNODEFICIENCY VIRUS (HIV). In a Phase I dosing trial in HIV positive patients, andrographolide raised CD4+ cells from baseline values.[27] However, the dose (5 mg/kg daily for 3 weeks, followed by 10 mg/kg for 3 weeks) did not appear to be well tolerated in most patients. Adverse reactions included multiple cases of allergic reactions, fatigue, headache, painful lymphadenopathy, nausea, diarrhea, and elevated liver transaminases.[27]

Dose

Most clinical studies have tested products standardized to the andrographolide fraction. Some commercial products contain 4% andrographolides. The most widely tested products are the two Kan Jang preparations (Swedish Herbal Institute): a single-herb preparation containing the extract SHA-10, standardized to contain 5.25 mg andrographolide and deoxyandrographolide per tablet, and a combination product containing SHA-10 with the *Eleutherococcus senticosus* extract SHE-3.

Two tablets of SHA-10 andrographis extract (Kan Jang) three times daily for 3 to 5 days has been used for influenza.[26]

In HIV-positive adults, 5 mg/kg oral andrographolide daily for 3 weeks, followed by 10 mg/kg for 3 weeks, has been tested, but this dose was not well tolerated.[27]

Adverse Effects, Interactions, Pharmacokinetics. See Appendix A.

Astragalus (Astragalus membranaceus)

Grade C: *Unclear or conflicting scientific evidence (antiviral activity)*

Mechanism of Action

Active constituents of astragalus root have been identified and characterized and include: polysaccharide cycloartane glycoside fractions (astragalosides I-IV and trigonosides I-III), four major isoflavonoids (formononetin, ononin, calycosin, and its glycoside) and several minor isoflavonoids, gamma-aminobutyric acid (GABA) and other biogenic amines.[28-33]

Astragalus was shown to increase T- and B-lymphocyte proliferation in vivo, increase the number of macrophages, and enhance T-cell transformation from suppressor to helper cells. It may also promote the immune system's ability to produce interferon (IFN).[34-36] Astragalus can inhibit the replication of Coxsackie B virus, an infection that can lead to viral myocarditis; however, the mechanism did not appear to involve IFN-β.[37]

Scientific Evidence of Effectiveness

Astragalus is thought to boost the body's immune system, and has been used to treat a host of medical conditions. Experimental evidence indicates that astragalus induces endogenous IFN production in vitro and in vivo and is effective for the treatment of several types of viral illness (e.g., Coxsackie B viral myocarditis, HSV-1).[38,39] Available clinical data support this hypothesis, particularly in HSV patients and immunocompromised patients with hepatitis C.[40] In contrast, the clinical data do not support the efficacy of astragalus in treating hepatitis B or viral myocarditis.[41-43]

Dose

The dose of astragalus for viral infections is not clear. For herpes simplex cervicitis, 0.5 mL of astragalus (1:1 extract) has been applied topically twice weekly for 3 weeks.[35]

Adverse Effects, Interactions, Pharmacokinetics. See Appendix A.

Beta-Sitosterol (β-Sitosterol), Sitosterol (22,23-Dihydrostigmasterol, 24-Ethylcholesterol)

Grade C: *Unclear or conflicting scientific evidence (HIV)*

Mechanism of Action

Beta-sitosterol is one of the most common dietary phytosterols (plant sterols) found and synthesized exclusively by plants.[44-56] Beta-sitosterol glucoside is attached to β-sitosterol.[48,57,58] Other phytosterols include campesterol and stigmasterol.[44,47-53,59,60] Stanols are saturated derivatives of sterols.[61] A possible mechanism for effects in maintaining CD4+ counts is an increase in T-helper cell type 1 (Th1) cellular response, which may inhibit viral replication.[48]

Scientific Evidence of Effectiveness

Data suggest that beta-sitosterol and beta-sitosterol glucoside have immunomodulating effects. Therefore, these sterols have been studied in combination in HIV treatment.[62] According to preliminary research, Moducare (proprietary mixture containing 20 mg β-sitosterol and 0.2 mg β-sitosterol glucoside) maintained CD4+ cell count in HIV-positive patients who were not taking retroviral medications.[48]

Dose

HIV patients have taken one capsule of a proprietary mixture of sterol/sterolin supplement (Moducare; 20 mg β-sitosterol, 0.2 mg glucoside) three times daily by mouth, 30 minutes before meals.[48]

Adverse Effects, Interactions, Pharmacokinetics. See Appendix A.

Bitter Melon (Momordica charantia)

Grade C: *Unclear or conflicting scientific evidence (HIV)*

Mechanism of Action

Antiviral activity observed in vitro has been attributed to a 30-kD protein called MAP30, which has been isolated from bitter melon seeds.[63-66] This protein has been reported to inhibit HIV viral integrase and cause irreversible relaxation of supercoiled viral nucleic acids.[67] These changes are thought to inhibit viral integration into host cell genomes. Rates of

T-lymphocyte infection with HIV-1 and reduced rates of viral replication in infected cells have also been reported in vitro.[65,66]

Scientific Evidence of Effectiveness

In a case report, CD4+ count and CD4+/CD8+ ratio improved in an HIV-infected man after he drank bitter melon juices (or a combination of juices and decoction) for 1 year.[68] Because of the bad taste, the patient then used an enema, holding an inserted bag or rectal syringe until the juice/decoction was absorbed. After 7 days of the rectal therapy, his energy rapidly increased, and his physical stamina and appetite improved. After 1 year of therapy, his CD4+ count greatly increased, and his CD4+/CD8+ ratio later returned to normal. He no longer has acute sinusitis or recurrent respiratory infections and had no serious side effects from the bitter melon therapy.

Dose

The dose of bitter melon for HIV has not been determined. However, in one case report, 10 oz of bitter melon juices (or a combination of juices and decoction) was taken 5 days a week for 1 year; alternatively, a rectal retention enema (16 oz daily) was used.[68]

Adverse Effects, Interactions, Pharmacokinetics. See Appendix A.

Blessed Thistle (Cnicus benedictus)

Grade C: *Unclear or conflicting scientific evidence (viral infections)*

Mechanism of Action

The lignan constituents of blessed thistle are under investigation as antiviral agents, particularly in HIV.[69-72] However, the exact mechanism of action is not well understood.

Scientific Evidence of Effectiveness

In vitro studies suggest a broad spectrum of antimicrobial activity for blessed thistle. *Cnicus benedictus* lignans have been investigated as anti-HIV agents.[73] However, blessed thistle has exhibited no antiviral activity against herpes, influenza, or polioviruses.[74] Reliable human trials assessing blessed thistle as treatment for viral infections are currently lacking. In one case report an HIV-infected woman used an herbal mixture that included blessed thistle.[75] Although she reportedly felt symptomatic improvement after using this preparation, she subsequently died of pneumonia. Additional details, such as viral load or CD4+ counts, are not available. The potential effects of other herbs in the preparation are not known.

Dose

The dose of blessed thistle for viral infections has not been determined.

Adverse Effects, Interactions, Pharmacokinetics. See Appendix A.

Boneset (Eupatorium spp.)

Grade C: *Unclear or conflicting scientific evidence (colds/flu)*

Mechanism of Action

Boneset contains sesquiterpene lactones, which have been shown to have immunostimulating activities.[76,77] However, the antiviral mechanism of action of boneset is not well understood.

Scientific Evidence of Effectiveness

Traditionally, boneset has been used to treat influenza and other infectious diseases. According to clinical research, homeopathic boneset was as effective as aspirin, as measured by subjective complaints and laboratory findings for patients with common cold.[78]

Dose

Traditionally, 1 to 3 tsp of boneset (steeped in 1 cup boiling water for 10-15 minutes) has been used every ½ hour to every 2 hours; up to 6 cups has been taken daily for 2 days for fever or influenza.[10]

Adverse Effects, Interactions, Pharmacokinetics. See Appendix A.

Boxwood (Buxus sempervirens)

Grade C: *Unclear or conflicting scientific evidence (HIV/AIDS)*

Mechanism of Action

The mechanism of action for SPV-30, an extract of boxwood being studied for HIV, is not well understood.[79-81]

Scientific Evidence of Effectiveness

An extract of boxwood, SPV-30 (Arkopharma, France), has been studied for its potential effects in HIV and AIDS; however, available clinical evidence is inconclusive.[79-88] A review mentions a study in which SPV-30 showed no statistical difference in new AIDS-defining events, CD4+ cell counts, or viral load compared with placebo.[88] However, the authors noted that an earlier pilot trial found a positive effect of SPV-30 on the CD4+ cell count; this remains unsubstantiated. Other unsubstantiated reports have noted that SPV-30 may increase CD4+ and CD8+ cell counts and reduce HIV viral load; however, data are limited, and the mechanism of action for SPV-30 is currently unknown.[79-81]

The U.S. Food and Drug Administration (FDA) has disciplined the manufacturer of SPV-30 regarding unsubstantiated claims about changes in CD4+ and viral load values in product labeling.[79,80,84,85]

Dose

There is no well-known standardization for boxwood. The dose of boxwood for HIV/AIDS has not been clearly established.

Adverse Effects, Interactions, Pharmacokinetics. See Appendix A.

Chamomile (*Matricaria recutita*, syn. *Matricaria suaveolens, Matricaria chamomilla, Anthemis nobilis, Chamaemelum nobile, Chamomilla chamomilla, Chamomilla recutita*)

Grade C: *Unclear or conflicting scientific evidence (common cold)*

Mechanism of Action

High-molecular-weight polysaccharides with immunostimulating activity have been isolated from German chamomile.[89] An ethanolic extract of the entire plant has been reported to inhibit the growth of poliovirus and herpesvirus.[90] The exact mechanism of chamomile in viral infections is not well understood.

Scientific Evidence of Effectiveness

According to preliminary research, inhaling steam with chamomile extract (Kneipp Kamillen-Konzentrat) may relieve common cold symptoms.[91]

Dose

The dose of chamomile for common cold has not been determined.

Adverse Effects, Interactions, Pharmacokinetics. See Appendix A.

Echinacea (*Echinacea* spp.)

Grade B: *Good scientific evidence (treatment of upper respiratory tract infections in adults)*

Grade C: *Unclear or conflicting scientific evidence (prevention of upper respiratory tract infections in adults and children)*

Mechanism of Action

Immunostimulatory properties of echinacea appear to target both nonspecific and specific immune function. Nonspecific effects include increases in macrophage proliferation and phagocytosis, as well as secretion of interferon (IFN), tumor necrosis factor (TNF), and interleukin-1 (IL-1), in vitro and in vivo.[92-101] Specific immune responses include the activation of alternate complement pathway components and elevated levels/activity of T lymphocytes and natural killer (NK) cells.[102-106] *Echinacea purpurea* is believed to exert its strongest potency on the immune system.[107]

Immunostimulation may depend on the dosage and frequency of administration. Cell-mediated immunity may be stimulated by one therapeutic administration followed by a "free" interval of 1 week, but immunity can be depressed by the daily administration of higher doses.[108] Other studies have failed to elicit these responses.[109]

Constituents of echinacea (e.g., dicaffeoylquinic acids) have been reported to have antiviral activity, but reports of antiviral effects on viral respiratory pathogens are currently lacking.[110-112]

Scientific Evidence of Effectiveness

PREVENTION OF UPPER RESPIRATORY TRACT INFECTIONS IN ADULTS AND CHILDREN. The evidence for echinacea's efficacy in the prevention of upper respiratory infections (URIs) remains equivocal and controversial. Some studies report that echinacea may help prevent URIs.[113-117] Recent meta-analysis has shown that echinacea decreased the risk of developing the common cold.[118] However, data from more rigorous trials have been negative.[119,120] Additional studies sponsored by the U.S. National Center for Complementary and Alternative Medicine (NCCAM) are in progress. Pending additional results, however, the evidence for echinacea in URI prevention appears less promising. If the results of ongoing trials of echinacea are similarly negative, this will suggest a lack of efficacy. For now, the evidence remains indeterminate.

TREATMENT OF UPPER RESPIRATORY TRACT INFECTIONS IN ADULTS. Oral echinacea is frequently recommended to reduce the duration and severity of URIs or the "common cold." Numerous trials have been conducted in this area. Recent meta-analysis has shown that echinacea decreases the duration of a cold by 1.4 days compared with placebo.[118] However, most other positive trials were published before 2001 and were largely of limited methodological quality or used combination products. High-quality studies have reported negative results in adults and children[119-121] and have raised controversy in this area.[122] Although NCCAM-sponsored studies are in progress, current evidence for this use of echinacea appears less promising than that of previous studies. If results of ongoing trials of echinacea are similarly negative, a lack of efficacy will be more firmly established. At present, the evidence remains indeterminate. Future research should consider the possible differential efficacy of various *Echinacea* species and their different plant parts (root vs. above-ground herb).

Dose

For URI prevention in adults, a 1.5-mL tincture containing the equivalent of 300 mg *Echinacea angustifolia* root has been taken three times daily for a 7-day course before experimental infection, or starting on the day of experimental infection and continuing for 5 days.[119] Echinacea at 2.5 mL three times daily has also been used for 7 days before and 7 days after intranasal inoculation.[123]

For the treatment of URIs in adults, the dose recommended most often is 500 to 1000 mg three times daily for 5 to 7 days.[124] A total daily dose of 900 mg has been shown to be superior to 450 mg daily for the improvement of cold or flu symptoms.[102] The recommended dose of expressed juice is 6 to 9 mL daily in divided doses, for 5 to 7 days. Experts recommend a tincture dosage of 0.75 to 1.5 mL (equivalent of 900 mg dried *Echinacea* root), gargled then swallowed, two to five times daily for 5 to 7 days.

Adverse Effects, Interactions, Pharmacokinetics. See Appendix A.

Elder (Sambucus nigra)

Grade C: *Unclear or conflicting scientific evidence (influenza)*

Mechanism of Action

There are multiple chemical and biochemical studies of chemical constituents in *Sambucus nigra*, including α-amyrenone, α-amyrin, betulin, oleanolic acid, β-sitosterol,[125] rutin, mucilage, tannins, and organic acids. *S. nigra* reduced hemagglutination of red blood cells (RBCs) and inhibited replication of several strains of influenza A and B in vitro.[126]

Scientific Evidence of Effectiveness

Oral elderberry may also be beneficial in the treatment of influenza A and B viruses. Fever, fatigue, headache, sore throat, cough, and aches improved in less than half the time than for normal recovery from the flu (4 days earlier), and patients who received elderberry used less rescue medication.[126] Other evidence suggests that elder may reduce mucus production and may possess antiinflammatory and antiviral effects.[127]

Dose

For treating influenza A and B infections, patients received 15 mL of elderberry four times daily for 5 days. The standardized elderberry product Sambucol (containing 38% black elderberry extract and three flavonoids) has also been used to improve flulike symptoms. Children received 2 tbsp daily and adults received 4 tbsp daily for 3 days.[126]

Adverse Effects, Interactions, Pharmacokinetics. See Appendix A.

Garlic (Allium sativum)

Grade C: *Unclear or conflicting scientific evidence (upper respiratory tract infection)*

Mechanism of Action

In vitro studies have demonstrated effects of garlic against several viruses, including influenza B virus, HSV-1,[128] HSV-2, parainfluenza virus type 3, vaccinia virus, vesicular stomatitis virus, human rhinovirus type 2,[129,130] and cytomegalovirus.[131] The compound ajoene, found in oil macerates of garlic, reportedly possesses a high level of antiviral activity, followed by allicin, allyl methyl thiosulfinate, and methylallyl thiosulfinate.[132] However, the exact mechanism of action is not well understood.

Scientific Evidence of Effectiveness

According to clinical studies, daily garlic supplementation may reduce the severity and duration of symptoms associated with viral URIs.[133,134] However, evidence remains equivocal.

Dose

For URI, the European Scientific Cooperative on Phytotherapy (ESCOP) 1997 monograph recommends 2 to 4 g of dried garlic bulb or 2 to 4 mL of garlic tincture (1:5, 45% ethanol) three times daily.

Adverse Effects, Interactions, Pharmacokinetics. See Appendix A.

Lemon Balm (Melissa officinalis)

Grade B: *Good scientific evidence (herpes simplex virus infections)*

Mechanism of Action

The tannins found in lemon balm are reported to possess antiviral properties,[135-139] as are the polyphenolic compounds rosmarinic, caffeic, and ferulic acids.[135,140] Studies report that aqueous extracts of lemon balm exhibit antiviral effects against Newcastle disease virus, Semliki Forest virus, influenza virus, myxoviruses, vaccinia, and HSV.[135-140] Lemon balm extract and its constituent rosmarinic acid have demonstrated antiviral properties against HIV-1.[141] Studies conducted to assess the antiviral effects of lemon balm on HSV-1 have suggested that different extracts of the herb (M1, M2, M3, and M4) have different effects on the virus.[140] Studies assessing the antiviral effects of lemon balm on HSV-2 suggest that the volatile oil components of lemon balm inhibit its replication.[142]

Scientific Evidence of Effectiveness

In Europe, lemon balm has been widely used as a topical antiviral treatment for genital and oral herpes, applied at the first sign of a herpes flare-up, or regularly for prevention. According to clinical studies, cream containing 1% of a standardized 70:1 lemon balm extract (Lomahephan) lowers symptoms scores, shortens healing time, prevents the spread of infection, and reduces HSV recurrence.[143-146]

Dose

Cream containing 1% of a standardized 70:1 extract (Lomahephan), topically up to four times daily for 5 to 10 days, has shown effectiveness in the treatment of active viral herpes (HSV).[144-146]

Adverse Effects, Interactions, Pharmacokinetics. See Appendix A.

Licorice (Glycyrrhiza glabra)

Grade C: *Unclear or conflicting scientific evidence (herpes simplex virus; herpes zoster; HIV/AIDs)*

Mechanism of Action

Glycyrrhizin is a glycoside and the major constituent of licorice. According to animal research, glycyrrhizin may offer a protective effect against influenza by inducing the production of interferon by T cells.[147,148] Glycyrrhizin has been reported to inhibit HIV replication. It also has shown antiviral activity against varicella-zoster virus.[149] Glycyrrhizin has been reported to induce interferon, inactivate viruses, and enhance NK cell effects.[149-151]

Scientific Evidence of Effectiveness

HERPES SIMPLEX VIRUS (HSV). Carbenoxolone, a succinate derivative of glycyrrhetinic acid popular for peptic ulcers, has been studied in HSV-infected patients. Studies have been small but suggest that topical application of carbenoxolone cream may improve healing and prevent HSV recurrence.[152,153]

HERPES ZOSTER (VSV). Preliminary research has shown glycyrrhizin to be beneficial as an alternative or adjunct antiviral agent for herpes zoster.[154] When patients received glycyrrhizin with acyclovir, patients experienced pain relief earlier than with acyclovir alone.

HUMAN IMMUNODEFICIENCY VIRUS (HIV). Clinical research found that glycyrrhizin helps prevent the progression of HIV to AIDS by increasing the number of CD4+ T lymphocytes.[150]

Dose

The dose of glycyrrhizin for herpes zoster has not been determined.

A 2% carbenoxolone cream or gel has been applied five times daily for 7 to 14 days for HSV skin lesions.

For HIV/AIDS, 5 mg/kg of the glycyrrhizin formulation Stronger Neo-Minophagen C (SNMC), which contains 40 mg glycyrrhizin, was administered by drip infusion.

Adverse Effects, Interactions, Pharmacokinetics. See Appendix A.

Mistletoe (Viscum album)

Grade C: Unclear or conflicting scientific evidence (HIV)

Mechanism of Action

Animal studies have shown that mistletoe increases the production of IFN-α, TNF, and IL-1 and increases both the activity and the number of NK cells.[155-158]

Scientific Evidence of Effectiveness

Patients with HIV infection have been treated with mistletoe in Europe since the beginning of the AIDS epidemic in the early 1980s. Mistletoe has been shown to inhibit disease progression, prevent patient deterioration, and improve quality of life.[159-162] However, not all mistletoe preparations appear to have equal effects. Further research is needed to clarify the effects of mistletoe in HIV infection.

Dose

For HIV, doses of 0.01 to 10 mg *Viscum album* extract (*V. album* Quercus Frischsaft [Qu FrF]), standardized for its lectin and viscotoxin content, were administered subcutaneously twice weekly in gradually increasing doses for 2 to 17 weeks.[159]

Adverse Effects, Interactions, Pharmacokinetics. See Appendix A.

Rhubarb (Rheum spp.)

Grade C: Unclear or conflicting scientific evidence (herpes)

Mechanism of Action

The exact mechanism of rhubarb in herpes is not well understood. In vitro research showed that the ethanol extract from the root and rhizome of rhubarb had low cytotoxicity, tended to promote cell growth, and had a minimum inhibitory dose for HSV of 100 micromol/mL.[163] The extract also seemed to prevent cells from being infected and had some direct effect on viral particles. In another in vitro study, *emodin*, an anthraquinone compound derived from rhubarb, significantly blocked the S protein and angiotensin-converting enzyme 2 (ACE-2) interaction of the sudden acute respiratory syndrome (SARS) virus in a dose-dependent manner.[164] Emodin also inhibited the infectivity of S protein–pseudotyped retrovirus to green monkey kidney cells.

Scientific Evidence of Effectiveness

According to clinical research, a cream made from rhubarb root and sage appears to be useful in the treatment of recurrent herpes labialis.[165] The rhubarb-sage cream decreased skin swelling and reduced pain and appeared to be as effective as acyclovir (Zovirax) cream.

Dose

The dose of rhubarb for herpes has not been determined.

Adverse Effects, Interactions, Pharmacokinetics. See Appendix A.

Sage (Salvia officinalis)

Grade B: Good scientific evidence (acute pharyngitis; herpes)

Mechanism of Action

Based on in vitro research, sage extracts affect HSV before adsorption, but have no effect on intracellular virus replication.[166] However, the exact effects of sage on the herpesvirus are not well understood.

Scientific Evidence of Effectiveness

ACUTE PHARYNGITIS. Sage mouthwashes and gargles have been approved for use against sore throat in Germany by the German Commission E for many years. According to preliminary research, sage may be beneficial for patients with acute viral pharyngitis.[167] The change in throat pain intensity was documented every 15 minutes for the first 2 hours after the first application compared to baseline, using a visual analog scale. The 15% spray was significantly superior to placebo in reducing the throat pain intensity score.

HERPES. According to clinical research, a cream made from sage leaf and rhubarb root appears to be useful in the treatment of recurrent herpes labialis.[165] The combination preparation appeared to be more efficacious than sage alone. The rhubarb-sage cream decreased skin swelling and reduced pain and appeared to be as effective as acyclovir (Zovirax) cream.

Dose

For acute pharyngitis, a 15% sage spray (Valverde Salvia Rachenspray; containing 140 mcL *Salvia officinalis* fluid extract) for 3 days, has been used, with 6 to 9 sprays daily as needed.[167]

The dose of sage for herpes has not been determined.

Adverse Effects, Interactions, Pharmacokinetics. See Appendix A.

Shiitake Mushroom (Lentinus edodes)

Grade C: Unclear or conflicting scientific evidence (genital warts; HIV [adjunct to conventional therapy])

Mechanism of Action

In vitro, an extract of a culture medium of *Lentinus edodes* mycelia inhibited the replication and infectivity of HIV and had cytopathic effects on the virus-infected cells.[168,169] Lentin, isolated from *L. edodes*, inhibits HIV-1 reverse transcriptase.[170,171] Lentin has also been shown to modulate the immune system in human studies.[172-182]

Scientific Evidence of Effectiveness

GENITAL WARTS. Based on information from in vitro, animal, and human studies, lentinan and *L. edodes* have immunomodulatory effects.[173,176,182-195] In preliminary clinical research, lentinan modulated the cellular immune function of patients with genital warts. Significant increases in CD4+/CD8+ and serum IL-2 were noted.[196]

HUMAN IMMUNODEFICIENCY VIRUS (HIV) ADJUNCT THERAPY. In vitro, animal, and human studies have shown that lentinan and *Lentinus edodes* have immunomodulatory effects.[173,176,182-195] Shiitake has been shown to have antiviral activity against HIV.[197,198] Administration of lentinan with didanosine significantly increased CD4+ levels for up to 38 weeks.[198]

Dose

A weekly 2-mg intravenous dose of lentinan for 24 to 80 weeks (following 400 mg/day oral didanosine for 6 weeks) has been used in patients with HIV.[198]

Adverse Effects, Interactions, Pharmacokinetics. See Appendix A.

Tea Tree (Melaleuca alternifolia)

Grade C: Unclear or conflicting scientific evidence (recurrent oral herpes infection)

Mechanism of Action

Tea tree oil has been found to alter the herpesvirus before and during adsorption, but not after penetration into the host cell.[199] However, the exact antiviral effects of tea tree oil are not well understood.

Scientific Evidence of Effectiveness

Tea tree oil has been proposed as a potential topical therapy for genital HSV infections based on in vitro findings of antiviral activity.[199] According to preliminary research, tea tree oil administered to patients with recurrent herpes labialis resulted in a trend toward reduced duration of positive cultures; however, there was no difference compared with placebo.[200]

Dose

The dose of tea tree oil for recurrent herpes labialis has not been determined.

Adverse Effects, Interactions, Pharmacokinetics. See Appendix A.

Turmeric (Curcuma longa)

Grade C: Unclear or conflicting scientific evidence (HIV/AIDS)

Mechanism of Action

Curcumin, a polyphenol compound responsible for the bright-yellow color of turmeric, is believed to be the principal pharmacological agent. In vitro studies suggest that curcumin may inhibit HIV-1 and HIV-2 proteases[201-205] and HIV-1 integrase.[205,206]

Scientific Evidence of Effectiveness

Human evidence regarding the use of turmeric or curcumin is mixed.[207,208] According to a conference abstract reporting a Phase I/II trial, no improvement in viral load or CD4+ count was noted after 8 weeks of high-dose curcumin (4800 or 2700 mg).[207] However, it was previously reported that HIV patients receiving curcumin had increased CD4+ counts compared with placebo.[208]

Dose

Patients with HIV receiving 2000 mg of curcumin daily reportedly had increased CD4+ counts compared with those taking placebo.[208]

Adverse Effects, Interactions, Pharmacokinetics. See Appendix A.

Wild Indigo (Baptisia australis, Baptisia tinctoria)

Grade C: Unclear or conflicting scientific evidence (respiratory tract infections)

Mechanism of Action

Several preliminary in vitro studies have shown immunostimulatory properties in *Baptisia tinctoria* extracts.[209-213] Researchers have described wild indigo's activity as either "immunobalancing"[214] or immunostimulating, which may result from increased macrophage activity.[209,215] Antiviral effects of wild indigo are not well understood.

Scientific Evidence of Effectiveness

Available clinical studies have been conducted using the combination called Esberitox N (*Echinacea purpurea, Echinacea pallida, Baptisia tinctoria,* and *Thuja occidentalis*).[214,216] Although showing improvement in symptoms, studies had significant weaknesses that may have introduced bias to the results. More studies using wild indigo as a monotherapy are needed to define wild indigo's role in the treatment of respiratory tract infections.

Dose

No well-known standardization is available for wild indigo. The dose of wild indigo for respiratory tract infections has not been determined.

Adverse Effects, Interactions, Pharmacokinetics. See Appendix A.

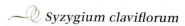

Syzygium claviflorum

> Panacos Pharmaceuticals is developing a new oral treatment for HIV infection derived from the Chinese herb *Syzygium claviflorum*, a member of a diverse genus of over 1000 plant species that includes the clove (*Syzygium aromaticum,* syn. *Eugenia aromaticum*). The herb contains betulinic acid, which has been found to inhibit HIV replication.[217,218] The experimental drug bevirimat (PA-457) is a novel inhibitor of HIV-1 maturation and currently undergoing Phase IIb trials. Researchers suggest that because the agent works differently than currently available treatment options, bevirimat may be effective in patients resistant to standard therapy.

HERBAL THERAPIES WITH NEGATIVE EVIDENCE

St. John's Wort (Hypericum perforatum)

Grade D: *Fair negative scientific evidence (HIV)*

A variety of in vitro studies has documented St. John's wort's antiviral properties.[219-228] However, these studies have not been substantiated by clinical research.[229] Furthermore, multiple reports of significant adverse effects and interactions with protease inhibitors (PIs) and nonnucleoside reverse-transcriptase inhibitors (NNRTIs) may preclude any use in patients with HIV/AIDS. Therefore the evidence recommends against using St. John's wort in the treatment of HIV/AIDS patients.

Echinacea (Echinacea spp.)

Grade D: *Fair negative scientific evidence (treatment of upper respiratory tract infections in children; genital herpes)*

TREATMENT OF UPPER RESPIRATORY TRACT INFECTIONS IN CHILDREN. Initial research suggests that echinacea may not be helpful in children for the alleviation of cold symptoms.[120,122] This finding may result from the parents' inability to recognize early symptoms of the common cold and initiate early treatment, or from the lack of a well-established pediatric dose for echinacea.[230,231] Also, echinacea may be more effective in adults than children because of distinguishing features of childhood URIs. For example, respiratory infections are more frequently caused by bacteria than by viruses in children. Certain viruses, such as respiratory syncytial virus (RSV), are also much more common in children than in adults. Until additional research is available, echinacea is generally not considered to be an effective URI treatment in children. Furthermore, many incidents of a rash outbreak have been reported with echinacea; therefore the risks may outweigh the potential benefits in the pediatric population.

GENITAL HERPES. A small clinical trial assessing the potential benefit of oral echinacea for recurrent herpes genitalis found no effect.[232] Echinacea failed to reduce the number of recurrences and other indicators of disease status (visual analog scale of pain, CD4+ counts, neutrophil counts).

Licorice (Glycyrrhiza glabra)

Grade D: *Fair negative scientific evidence (genital herpes)*

Carbenoxolone, a semisynthetic derivative of glycyrrhetinic acid (active compound of licorice), has not been found beneficial when applied topically to the skin to treat genital herpes infections.[233]

HERBAL THERAPIES WITH LIMITED EVIDENCE

Cranberry (Vaccinium macrocarpon)

In a series of in vitro studies, a commercially available cranberry fruit juice drink had a nonspecific antiviral effect toward unrelated viral species, including bacteriophages T2 and T4 and the simian rotavirus SA-11.[234] In addition, high-molecular-weight materials from cranberry dose-dependently inhibited influenza virus A and B from hemagglutinating RBCs and reduced the infectivity of the viruses in vitro.[235]

Sorrel (Rumex acetosa, Rumex spp.)

Although sorrel has been suggested as a treatment for viral infections, definitive studies that demonstrate these properties are lacking. Sorrel demonstrated no activity against HSV-1, HSV-2, or HIV in vitro.[236]

Herbs with Potential Antiviral Properties*

HERB	SPECIFIC THERAPEUTIC USE(S)†	HERB	SPECIFIC THERAPEUTIC USE(S)†
Abuta	Rabies	Eyebright	Antiviral, measles
Ackee	Yellow fever	Garcinia	Antiviral, Ebola virus
Aconite	Dengue fever, measles, mumps	Germanium	Epstein-Barr virus
African wild potato	Antiviral	Ginger	Antiviral
Agrimony	Antiviral	Goldenseal	Diphtheria, antiviral
Alkanna	Antiviral, measles, smallpox	Grape seed	Antiviral, smallpox
American pawpaw	Antiviral	Greater celandine	Antiviral
Annatto	Measles	Ground ivy	Antiviral
Ash	Antiviral	Hibiscus	Antiviral
Bamboo	Measles	Hop	Hepatitis C virus, rhinovirus, herpesvirus, Epstein-Barr virus
Barberry	Antiviral		
Belladonna	Measles, mumps	Horny goat weed	Antiviral, polio
Betel nut	Diphtheria	Hyssop	Antiviral
Bilberry	Antiviral	Jackfruit	Antiviral
Bitter orange	Rotavirus, peste des petits ruminants (goat plague)	Jequirity	Rabies (prevention)
		Jewelweed	Measles
Black bryony	Antiviral	Kudzu	Measles
Black cohosh	Yellow fever	Lingonberry	Antiviral
Black pepper	Measles	Maitake mushroom	Antiviral
Boneset	Antiviral, dengue fever, yellow fever	Mangosteen	Antiviral
		Mugwort	Antiviral
Bromelain	Antiviral	Mullein	Antiviral
Bulbous buttercup	Antiviral	Noni	Antiviral (polio)
Bupleurum	Poliovirus	Nopal	Antiviral
Burdock	Measles	Nux vomica	Rabies
Calendula	Antiviral	Olive leaf	Antiviral
Capers	Antiviral	Papain	Antiviral
Carob	Antiviral	Passion flower	Epstein-Barr virus
Carqueja	Antiviral	Peppermint	Antiviral
Cascara sagrada	Herpes simplex virus 2, vaccinia	Perilla	Antiviral
		Pokeweed	Antiviral, rabies
Catnip	Poliovirus	Pomegranate	Mumps
Cat's claw	Antiviral	Quassia	Antiviral
Chaparral	Antiviral	Raspberry	Antiviral (febrile stages), measles
Chia	Antiviral	Reishi mushroom	Antiviral, Epstein-Barr virus
Chrysanthemum	Epstein-Barr virus	Sanicle	Antiviral
Cinnamon	Antiviral	Saw palmetto	Epstein-Barr virus
Clove	Antiviral	Seaweed	Antiviral
Dandelion	Antiviral	Skullcap	Antiviral
Danshen	Antiviral	Spirulina	Antiviral, cytomegalovirus, measles, mumps
Desert parsley	Antiviral, Epstein-Barr virus (mononucleosis)		
		Stinging nettle	Antiviral
Devil's club	Antiviral, diphtheria, measles	Sweet Annie	Antiviral
Dong quai	Antiviral	Sweet basil	Antiviral
Elecampane	Antiviral	Tamanu	Antiviral
Ephedra	Antiviral	Tamarind	Antiviral
Eucalyptus	Antiviral	Usnea	Antiviral
Euphorbia	Antiviral		

Continued

Herbs with Potential Antiviral Properties—cont'd

HERB	SPECIFIC THERAPEUTIC USE(S)†	HERB	SPECIFIC THERAPEUTIC USE(S)†
Valerian	Antiviral, measles	Yarrow	Measles, smallpox
White horehound	Rabies	Yerba santa	Antiviral
White oak	Antiviral	Yew	Rabies
Wild yam	Antiviral	Yucca	Antiviral
Willow bark	Antiviral		

*This is not an all-inclusive or comprehensive list of herbs with possible antiviral properties; other herbs and supplements may possess these qualities. A qualified health care provider should be consulted with specific questions or concerns regarding potential adverse effects or interactions with other therapies.
†Based on expert opinion, anecdote, case reports, and/or preliminary trial evidence.

ADJUNCT THERAPIES

1. Some viral infections, such as the common cold and influenza, are self-limiting, resolving on their own. Treatment usually involves relieving the symptoms. Fevers may be reduced with fluid intake, warm baths, and cool compresses. Over-the-counter (OTC) medications such as acetaminophen (Tylenol) may be helpful for pain as well as body aches and fever associated with viral infections. Adequate fluid intake, rest, and good nutrition are important for patients with viral infections such as influenza. Vaporizers at night may relieve much of the congestion and sinus-related symptoms of flu patients. To avoid spreading influenza, patients should practice good hygiene, including proper handwashing.

2. Many other common viral infections also have OTC remedies. For example, docosanol (Abreva) is an OTC antiviral agent specifically for herpes simplex virus. Povidone-iodine (Betadine) will dry out the blisters and help prevent secondary infection. Epsom salt baths may help ease discomfort in patients with genital herpes.

3. Individuals presenting with chronic viral infections, particularly HIV infections, require longer-term adjunctive therapy designed to increase immune defenses, promote adherence to and compliance with treatment regimens, and promote general psychological well-being. Adjunctive therapies in the management of patients with viral infections include dietary supplementation, adequate nutritional intake, and mind-body techniques.

4. Vitamins and minerals may become depleted in patients with viral infections, especially in HIV infections. Deficiencies, notably in carotenoids (pigments related to vitamin A), selenium, zinc, and B vitamins, may worsen as the disease progresses because of inadequate dietary intake, altered metabolism, and diarrhea. Supplementation may be beneficial in nutrition deficiencies and may slow the rate of HIV progression to AIDS.

5. Nutritional interventions from the American Dietary Association include assessing HIV patients for level of nutritional risk and including registered dietitians in management of patients' daily intake plan. Ingestion of foods known to enhance overall health (and possibly immune function), such as fruits and vegetables high in phytoestrogens and antioxidants, are recommended.

6. Progressive involuntary weight loss in HIV patients is a serious problem caused by inadequate oral intake of food, altered metabolic state, and malabsorption. Nutritional supplements (Ensure, Sustacal, Resource) may help prevent wasting, especially in patients who find eating large meals difficult. Ingestion of alpha-linolenic acid (derived from flax) in combination with arginine and yeast RNA has also been associated with weight gain in HIV patients.[237] According to a small preliminary study, antineoplastons, a group of naturally occurring peptide fractions, may also increase weight as well as energy in HIV patients.[238] A decrease in opportunistic infections and increase in CD4+ cell counts have also been noted with antineoplaston use.

7. Various mind-body techniques (relaxation techniques, hypnotherapy, meditation) may be beneficial complementary therapies for patients with viral infections, particularly HIV. These therapies may help reduce the related stress as well as enhance the patient's coping ability and overall quality of life. Prayer and other therapies with a spiritual component (tai chi, Qi gong, Reiki, yoga) can promote total body relaxation and improve mental health. However, there is limited documentation on the effectiveness of these CAM therapies.

INTEGRATIVE THERAPY PLAN

- The clinical presentation of viral infections may vary, but the most common symptoms include fatigue, fever, sore throat, myalgias, and rash.
- Determine the patient's current medication history, including herbal preparations and OTC medications, with dosage and frequency.

- Collect laboratory data according to recommendations for the given viral infection. Baseline serum chemistry panels, including serum electrolytes, liver function tests, renal function tests, and serum glucose, should be obtained, particularly for HIV patients. A throat culture, sputum culture, or blood test may be performed to rule out a secondary bacterial infection such as *Streptococcus* ("strep throat") or pneumonia. Additional baseline tests include a complete blood cell count (CBC) with differential, a CD4+ count, and CD4+/CD8+ ratio.
- For patients with HIV, make a nutritional risk assessment and a care plan to include nutritional consultation and a physical exercise routine. Recommendations for adjunctive treatments, such as meditation, yoga, acupuncture, support groups, and cognitive-behavioral therapy, should be developed.
- Natural products such as beta-sitosterol, mistletoe, echinacea, and licorice may have antiviral and immunostimulating effects, which may be beneficial in various viral infections.
- Echinacea is popular for the prevention and treatment of upper respiratory infections (URIs) or the common cold. However, the evidence concerning its efficacy is conflicting. Echinacea may reduce the odds of developing the common cold and the duration of cold.
- Lentinan from shiitake mushroom, beta-sitosterol, and licorice have been reported to increase CD4+ counts in HIV patients and possibly prevent progression of disease.
- Integrative therapies should not replace antiretroviral therapy in HIV patients. Patients should consult their health care provider before taking any herbs or supplements because these may interact with treatment. In particular, HIV patients should not take St. John's wort because of possible interactions with antiretroviral medications (see Appendix A).
- Recommend bed rest, adequate fluids, and good nutrition for patients with viral infections such as influenza.
- Advise the patient to try OTC therapies for viral infections. Docosanol (Abreva) is an OTC antiviral agent specifically for herpes simplex virus. Povidone-iodine (Betadine) will dry out the blisters and help prevent secondary infection. Epsom salt baths may help ease discomfort in patients with genital herpes.
- Fevers may be lowered significantly with oral rehydration therapy (preferably water), warm baths, and cool compresses. These measures for reducing fever may prevent the need for other antiinflammatory and antipyretic therapy. Acetaminophen (Tylenol) may be helpful for pain as well as body aches and fever associated with viral infections.
- Vaporizers at night may relieve much of the congestion and sinus-related symptoms of flu patients.
- Urge the patient to practice good hygiene, including proper handwashing, to lower the risk of spreading infection.
- Monitor for improvements in signs and symptoms of the viral infection (sinus congestion, fever, sweating, chills, myalgia, fatigue).
- Assess the patient's response to prescription and nonprescription therapy. If no response is apparent, the particular agent should be discontinued and an alternate therapy considered. Most HIV patients are taking multiple therapies, so any additional therapy should be carefully assessed for drug interactions, efficacy, and toxicity.
- Stress the importance of adherence to integrative treatment regimens, particularly in HIV patients who require chronic therapy with multiple medications.
- Patients with viral infections may find symptomatic relief by targeting specific complaints, such as congestion or fatigue. Recommend dietary evaluation and management, preferably with involvement of a registered dietitian; exercises and conditioning designed to increase physical strength; and health and wellness initiatives, such as group support, cognitive-behavioral therapy, and meditation, to strengthen resolve and well-being.
- Recommend that patients receive the influenza vaccine. This vaccination, which lasts only 1 year, may be injected or sprayed intranasally. Research has shown that both forms of the vaccination are equally effective. The flu vaccine is approved for all age groups 6 months and older, including healthy people and patients with chronic medical conditions such as diabetes, asthma, and heart disease. The flu vaccine is recommended in children age 6 months to 5 years, adults in close contact with these children (teachers, daycare workers), people age 50 years and older, health care workers, all caregivers of high-risk patients (HIV/AIDS, cancer), patients with chronic health conditions (e.g., asthma), and pregnant women. The best period to receive any influenza vaccine is soon after the vaccine becomes available each fall.

Case Studies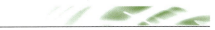

CASE STUDY 29-1

Your hospital is sponsoring a community influenza vaccine program. As hospital pharmacist, you are stationed at a help desk to address the questions and concerns of the patients. KW, a 67-year-old woman, has been taking sorrel for its anticancer and antiviral properties. She asks if you are aware of any other herbs that will reduce her chances of contracting influenza. She takes chlorpropamide (Diabinase, 250 mg/day) for type 2 diabetes and warfarin (Coumadin, 5 mg/day) for the past month after being diagnosed with a deep venous thrombosis (DVT) of her left leg. In addition to her recent hospitalization for DVT and for childbirth, she was hospitalized 2 years ago for a kidney stone. Drawing on the evidence regarding herbal antivirals, and considering KW's medical history, what advice can you offer?

Answer: Sorrel (*Rumex acetosa*, *Rumex* spp.) has no proven efficacy in the treatment or prevention of cancer, viral infections, or bacterial infections. Furthermore, the oxalates in sorrel increase the risk of nephrolithiasis and kidney damage.

KW should discontinue sorrel and consider other herbal remedies.

Astragalus (*Astragalus membranaceus*) has been used to treat a wide variety of health conditions, and may help boost the body's immune system. However, the herb may potentiate the effects of oral hypoglycemic drugs, including chlorpropamide; thus, it could lower KW's blood glucose levels. Chlorpropamide is a long-acting sulfonylurea with a high risk of hypoglycemia. Advise KW to consult her physician about lowering her chlorpropamide dose. Of more concern is the possibility that astragalus could potentiate anticoagulant therapy with warfarin. Unless KW can obtain a standardized dose of astragalus, it should not be used with warfarin. In any event, her prothrombin time should be closely monitored when initiating astragalus therapy.

Andrographis (*Andrographis paniculata*) has been reported to be effective for influenza treatment, reducing the duration and severity of symptoms. Though andrographis was reportedly well tolerated in most clinical studies, andrographolide (an active constituent) was not well tolerated in daily doses of 5 to 10 mg/kg. Furthermore, because of potential antithrombotic, hypotensive, and hypoglycemic effects of andrographis (see Appendix A), KW should be aware of potential interactions with the medications she is currently taking.

CASE STUDY 29-2

BD, a 37-year-old man, presents at the pharmacy with new prescriptions for indinavir (Crixivan), zidovudine (Retrovir), and lamivudine (Epivir). He also requests a refill of glyburide (Micronase) for his type 2 diabetes. He has been newly diagnosed as HIV positive. He is extremely depressed about his condition and has increased his intake of St. John's wort. He began taking the herb 2 years ago for mild depression and feels that current circumstances warrant a dosage increase. He is also interested in adjunct therapies (including herbal remedies) that may help his immune status and improve his outlook. Given BD's current drug regimen and medical status, what advice could you offer?

Answer: Of concern is BD's use of St. John's wort. Despite evidence that the herb possesses antiviral properties, St. John's wort is a cytochrome P450 3A4 inducer and thus decreases the effectiveness of indinavir. BD should therefore discontinue St. John's wort.

A number of herbal remedies have been proposed for HIV/AIDS. None has proved to be efficacious, although studies suggest benefit. Aloe (*Aloe vera*) has been reported to improve immune function and accelerate wound healing. Human studies also show that aloe is effective when used with other antiviral agents, such as zidovudine; thus, BD needs to continue taking his current antiretroviral therapy. Aloe's effect may be caused by acemannan, the major carbohydrate fraction in aloe gel. Antiretroviral activity also has been reported with acemannan (HIV is a retrovirus). Aloe might potentiate the hypoglycemic effect of glyburide; therefore, if BD takes aloe, his blood glucose should be more closely monitored.

Mistletoe (*Viscum album*) has been shown to inhibit the progression of HIV/AIDS; it also possesses hypoglycemic properties. Bitter melon (*Momordica charantia*) contains MAP30, which may have antiviral activity; however, human studies are lacking. Boxwood (*Buxus sempervirens*) contains SPV-30, which may decrease the viral load in HIV/AIDS patients. Turmeric (*Curcuma longa*) contains curcumin, which may inhibit HIV-1 and HIV-2 proteases, as well as HIV-1 integrase. Turmeric may decrease blood glucose levels. Flax (*Linum usitatissimum*) contains a number of constituents, including gamma-linolenic and eicosapentaenoic acids, which may slow the progression to AIDS.

CASE STUDY 29-3

ML is a 27-year-old woman who presents at the pharmacy with a prescription for acyclovir (Zovirax). She also requests a refill of her oral contraceptive, Ortho Tri-Cyclen. Her first outbreak of genital herpes occurred 3 years ago, and since then she has had recurring episodes two or three times a year. Several days before an outbreak, she experiences genital itching. She has smoked a pack of cigarettes a day for the past 10 years. For the past year, on the advice of a friend, she has been taking blessed thistle for her herpes but has noted no improvement. She asks if other available herbal remedies might be more effective. How do you counsel?

Answer: Acyclovir has proven efficacy for genital herpes. It is generally well tolerated but may cause diarrhea, nausea, and a general ill feeling. Positive evidence that blessed thistle (*Cnicus benedictus*) can reduce the recurrence, decrease the duration, or reduce the severity of a herpes outbreak is lacking. Two topical herbal remedies might be beneficial, and application can begin when ML experiences the early symptom of genital itching. Aloe (*Aloe vera*) is readily available, but its antiviral effect has been studied only in men during the first genital herpes episode. Astragalus (*Astragalus membranaceus*) has been reported to reduce the severity and duration of a herpes outbreak.

Beyond herbal remedies, the topical antiseptic povidone-iodine (Betadine) can be beneficial. It can dry out the blisters and help in managing symptomatic recurrences of herpes simplex infection.

Cigarette smoking suppresses the immune system. Advise ML to quit smoking to improve her health and reduce the recurrence and duration of her outbreaks. All the severe side effects of oral contraceptives, such as stroke and heart attack, are much more frequent in smokers than nonsmokers.

References for Chapter 29 can be found on the Evolve website at http://evolve.elsevier.com/Ulbricht/herbalpharmacotherapy/

Review Questions

1. The HIV virus targets which of the following types of cells?
   a. B cells
   b. CD4+ T cells
   c. Red blood cells
   d. None of the above

2. Which of the following triggers is associated with recurrent herpes outbreaks?
   a. Stress
   b. Menstruation
   c. Sun exposure
   d. All the above

3. True or false: Sage alone appears to be as effective as acyclovir for the treatment of recurrent herpes labialis.

4. According to experimental studies, aloe may have which of the following effects?
   a. Inhibition of viral replication
   b. Interference with DNA synthesis
   c. Modification of the glycosylation of viral glycoproteins
   d. All the above

5. True or false: Administration of lentinan with didanosine has been reported to significantly increase CD4+ levels.

6. True or false: Immunostimulatory properties of echinacea may target both nonspecific and specific immune function.

7. Which of the following is *true* regarding St. John's wort?
   a. St. John's wort may be applied topically to treat genital herpes.
   b. There is currently strong supportive evidence for the use of St. John's wort for influenza.
   c. Significant adverse effects and interactions with protease inhibitors (PIs) and nonnucleoside reverse transcriptase inhibitors (NNRTIs) have been reported with concurrent use of St. John's wort.
   d. There is strong evidence supporting its use for influenza.

8. Elderberry has been reported to cause which of the following?
   a. Reduced mucus production
   b. Some relief in flulike symptoms
   c. Requirement of less rescue medication
   d. All the above

9. Which of the following statements regarding licorice is supported by some evidence?
   a. Glycyrrhizin, a glycoside of licorice, has been reported to inhibit HIV replication
   b. Glycyrrhizin may be beneficial as an alternative or adjunct to antiviral therapy in patients with herpes zoster
   c. a and b
   d. None of the above

10. True or false: According to experimental studies, mistletoe has been found to increase production of IFN-α, TNF, and IL-1, and the activity and number of NK cells.

Answers are found in the Answers to Review Questions section in the back of the text.

30 Cancer

Outline

OVERVIEW
  Signs and Symptoms
    Nonspecific Symptoms
    Specific Symptoms
  Diagnosis
    Screening
    Diagnostic Tests
    Staging
  Safety Concerns
    Antioxidant Interference
    Drug Interactions
    Perioperative Considerations
  Cancer Remission
SELECTED HERBAL THERAPIES
  Aloe (*Aloe vera*)
  American Pawpaw (*Asimina triloba*)
  Astragalus (*Astragalus membranaceus*)
  Black Cohosh (*Actaea racemosa*, formerly *Cimicifuga racemosa*)
  Boswellia (*Boswellia serrata*)
  Bromelain (Bromeliaceae)
  Bupleurum (*Bupleurum* spp.)
  Cat's Claw (*Uncaria* spp.)
  Chaparral (*Larrea tridentata, Larrea divaricata*)
  Chrysanthemum (*Chrysanthemum* spp.)
  Echinacea (*Echinacea* spp.)
  Evening Primrose (*Oenothera biennis*)
  Flax (*Linum usitatissimum*)
  Garlic (*Allium sativum*)
  Ginkgo (*Ginkgo biloba*)
  Ginseng (*Panax* spp.)
  Goji (*Lycium* spp.)
  Greater Celandine (*Chelidonium majus*)
  Jiaogulan (*Gynostemma pentaphyllum*)
  Lavender (*Lavandula angustifolia*)
  Maitake Mushroom (*Grifola frondosa*)
  Milk Thistle (*Silybum marianum*)
  Mistletoe (*Viscum album*)
  Modified Citrus Pectin
  Oleander (*Nerium oleander, Thevetia peruviana*)
  Peony (*Paeonia* spp.)
  Podophyllum (*Podophyllum* spp.)
  PSK (*Coriolus versicolor*)
  Psyllium (*Plantago* spp.)
  Red Clover (*Trifolium pratense*)
  Reishi Mushroom (*Ganoderma lucidum*)
  Rhodiola (*Rhodiola rosea*)
  Rhubarb (*Rheum* spp.)
  Sage (*Salvia officinalis*)
  Saw Palmetto (*Serenoa repens*)
  Shiitake Mushroom (*Lentinus edodes*)
  Skullcap (*Scutellaria* spp.)
  Slippery Elm (*Ulmus rubra*, syn. *Ulmus fulva*)
  Sorrel (*Rumex acetosa, Rumex* spp.)
  Soy (*Glycine max*)
  Spirulina (*Arthrospira* spp.)
  Strawberry (*Fragaria* spp.)
  Sweet Annie (*Artemisia annua*)
  Tea (*Camellia sinensis*)
  Turmeric (*Curcuma longa*)
HERBAL THERAPIES WITH NEGATIVE EVIDENCE
HERBAL THERAPIES WITH LIMITED EVIDENCE
MANAGEMENT OF TOXICITY AND SIDE EFFECTS
  Chemotherapy
    Nausea and Vomiting
    Constipation
  Radiotherapy
    Xerostomia
    Mucositis and Stomatitis
    Leukopenia and Anemia
    Dermatitis
ADJUNCT THERAPIES
INTEGRATIVE THERAPY PLAN
CASE STUDIES
REVIEW QUESTIONS

Learning Objectives

- Understand the role of herbal agents in cancer chemotherapy.
- Identify herbs used for cancer treatment and secondary prevention.
- Understand the mechanism of action, adverse effects, and drug interactions for common herbs used for cancer.
- Identify, assess, and recommend appropriate herbal pharmacotherapy for common complications of cancer including nausea and vomiting, infection, and anemia.
- Develop an integrative patient care plan to manage and prevent cancer.

OVERVIEW

Cancer is the second leading cause of death among Americans, surpassed only by heart disease.[1] In 2005, of the estimated 58 million all-cause mortalities worldwide, 7.6 million were caused by some form of cancer. Based on projections by the World Health Organization (WHO), cancer deaths will continue to increase, with an estimated 9 million people dying from cancer in 2015 and 11.4 million in 2030.[2] Table 30-1 lists American Cancer Society (ACS) estimates of cancer cases and deaths for 2008.

Normal human cells divide a finite number of times before entering a state called *senescence* in which they cease to divide. After cells become senescent, they undergo *apoptosis* (programmed cell death). Cells may also stop dividing when they come in close contact with other cells, a phenomenon known as *contact inhibition*. All these processes are normal parts of the tightly regulated cell cycle, which is influenced by many different genes and external factors (e.g., hormones, immune system, environment). Some cells escape the normal control of the cell cycle and fail to respond to internal or external cues to cease cellular division. When cells divide uncontrollably, they may form a tumor, which may then progress to cancer. By its simplest definition, cancer is an uncontrolled growth of cells that has become *malignant*, meaning these cells have gained the capacity to infiltrate other tissues and interfere with normal function. When cancerous cells detach from the primary tumor and spread to other parts of the body, this is known as *metastasis*.[3-6]

It is important to note that not all tumors are cancerous. *Benign* tumors do not metastasize (or spread) to other parts of the body and, with rare exceptions, are not life threatening. Malignancy may develop from a previously benign tumor but may also develop *de novo*, that is, directly from normal cells with no clinically evident intervening period of precancerous growth.

Cancer occurs in all racial and ethnic groups, although the rate of occurrence may vary among populations. Cancer

TABLE 30-1 New Cancer Cases and Deaths—2008 Estimates

ESTIMATED NEW CASES					
MALE			FEMALE		
Prostate	186,320	25%	Breast	182,460	26%
Lung/bronchus	114,690	15%	Lung/bronchus	100,330	15%
Colon/rectum	77,250	10%	Colon/rectum	71,560	10%
Urinary/bladder	51,230	7%	Uterine corpus	40,100	6%
Non-Hodgkin's lymphoma	35,450	5%	Non-Hodgkin's lymphoma	30,670	4%
Melanoma of skin	34,950	5%	Thyroid	28,410	4%
Kidney/renal pelvis	33,130	4%	Melanoma of skin	27,530	4%
Oral cavity/pharynx	25,310	3%	Ovary	21,650	3%
Leukemia	25,180	3%	Kidney/renal pelvis	21,260	3%
Pancreas	18,770	3%	Leukemia	19,090	3%
All sites	745,180	100%	All sites	692,000	100%
ESTIMATED NEW DEATHS					
MALE			FEMALE		
Lung/bronchus	90,810	31%	Lung/bronchus	71,030	26%
Prostate	28,660	10%	Breast	40,480	15%
Colon/rectum	24,260	8%	Colon/rectum	25,700	9%
Pancreas	17,500	6%	Pancreas	16,790	6%
Liver/intrahepatic bile duct	12,570	4%	Ovary	15,520	6%
Leukemia	12,460	4%	Non-Hodgkin's lymphoma	9370	3%
Esophagus	11,250	4%	Leukemia	9250	3%
Urinary bladder	9950	3%	Uterine corpus	7470	3%
Non-Hodgkin's lymphoma	9790	3%	Liver/intrahepatic bile duct	5840	2%
Kidney/renal pelvis	8100	3%	Brain/nervous system	5650	2%
All sites	294,120	100%	All sites	271,530	100%

Modified from *Cancer facts & figures 2008*, American Cancer Society.

affects more men (~50%) than women (~33%) and is more prevalent in the elderly population. Two thirds of individuals diagnosed with cancer are over age 65. Certain lifestyle choices (e.g., smoking, alcohol consumption) may also impact the risk of cancer.

Many factors may incite the development of cancer, but almost all cancerous cells have some form of abnormality in their genetic material (DNA). These abnormalities, which may include gene mutations, translocations, deletions, or amplifications, can allow cancer cells to divide indefinitely. These genetic changes may be spontaneous, inherited, or environmentally induced (e.g., excessive sunlight) or caused by exposure to certain mutagenic agents (e.g., cigarette smoke, certain chemicals). Infection with certain viruses, such as human papillomavirus, may also lead to cancer.

In healthy cells, DNA abnormalities are usually corrected by DNA repair enzymes. Damaged DNA may not be repaired in cancer cells, possibly because of genetic mutations affecting proteins required for DNA repair. Many other types of mutations may also lead to the development of cancer; for example, damage to genes involved in regulation of the cell cycle may lead to uncontrolled growth. In many cases, cancer does not develop from a single genetic mutation; rather, multiple factors are required before cells become cancerous.

In addition to defending against invasion by pathogens, the immune system usually recognizes and attacks abnormal cells in the body. In some cases, this means the immune system will resolve an abnormal growth of cells before it becomes cancerous. However, both benign and cancerous growths are often composed of cells that are only slightly different from normal cells, and these cells may evade the immune system. Immunosuppressed individuals are at an increased risk of cancer, presumably because of the faulty immune response to abnormal cells and external pathogens (including cancer-causing viruses).

Symptoms and treatment depend on the specific type and stage of the cancer. Cancers that are early in development and localized may often be asymptomatic, because the cancer growth may not be extensive enough to impinge on adjacent structures or organ function. Conversely, advanced metastatic cancer may produce a wide range of symptoms related to mass effect both at the primary and at distant sites of tumor involvement.

Treatment plans may include surgery, radiation, and chemotherapy. In some types of cancer, these therapies can be curative, whereas in many cancers (especially those at advanced stages) the only benefit (if any) may be prolonged survival. All of these methods carry a high risk of serious adverse effects, especially because anticancer treatments may also damage a significant amount of healthy tissue. Regardless of the therapy used, the goal is to control the cancer while limiting the damaging effects on normal, healthy tissue.

Signs and Symptoms

Different types of cancer have unique symptoms and characteristics depending on the organs and tissues involved. Although cancers differ greatly, some nonspecific symptoms are usually experienced by most cancer patients; these include pain, fatigue, fever, and unexplained weight loss. Some cancers may have more specific symptoms, such as unusual bleeding from the vagina (vaginal cancer) and difficulty swallowing (esophageal cancer).[3-6]

Nonspecific Symptoms

Depression. Cancer patients often experience depression, which may be psychological and related to a fear of dying, loss of independence, or the symptoms of the illness. Also, some cancers may physiologically cause depression by affecting normal brain function.

Fatigue. Extreme tiredness is one of the most common symptoms of cancer. Fatigue may occur early in cancers that cause a chronic loss of blood, including leukemia and colon or stomach cancer. Fatigue may become more common and severe as cancer progresses.

Fever. Most cancer patients experience fever at some point, particularly if the cancer or its treatment (e.g., chemotherapy, radiation) impairs the immune system. Less often, fever may be an early sign of cancer, as with leukemia or lymphoma.

Neuromuscular symptoms. Cancer may compress or grow directly on nerves, causing various neurological and muscular symptoms, such as changes in sensation or muscle weakness. When a cancer grows in the brain, symptoms may include confusion, dizziness, headaches, nausea, changes in vision, and seizures.

Pain. Pain is normally present when cancer progresses, caused by mass effect on normal tissues and nerve impingement. However, pain can be present early in some cancers (e.g., bone, testicular).

Respiratory symptoms. Cancer can compress or block physical structures, such as the airways in the lungs or trachea, causing shortness of breath, cough, or pneumonia. Cancer cells that contain fluid may accumulate in the space between the lung and the chest wall (known as *pleural effusion*), which can cause shortness of breath.

Skin changes. Skin changes such as jaundice, hyperpigmentation (skin darkening), abnormal hair growth, erythema, boils, and pruritus can indicate certain types of cancers, most often those involving the liver, gallbladder, or hematopoietic system.

Weight loss. Most individuals with cancer will lose weight at some time during the course of the disease. Unintentional weight loss can be one of the first symptoms experienced with cancer, particularly cancers of the pancreas, stomach, esophagus, or lung.

Specific Symptoms

Bladder cancer. Blood in the urine, pain or burning on urination, frequent urination, and cloudy urine.

Bone cancer. Pain in the bone or swelling around the affected site. Bone cancer may also weaken the bones, resulting in fractures.

Brain cancer. Dizziness, drowsiness, abnormal eye movements or changes in vision, weakness, loss of feeling in arms or legs or difficulties in walking, fits or convulsions, headaches that tend to be worse in the morning and ease during the day, headaches that may be accompanied by nausea or vomiting, and changes in personality, memory, or speech.

Breast cancer. Although most lumps are not cancerous, the most common sign of breast cancer for both men and women is a lump or thickening in the breast. Often, the lump is painless. Other symptoms may include spontaneous clear or bloody discharge from the nipple often associated with a breast lump, retraction or indentation of the nipple, change in the size or contours of the breast, flattening or indentation of the skin over the breast, and redness or pitting of the skin over the breast (similar to skin of orange).

Colorectal cancer. Rectal bleeding (red blood in stools or black stools), abdominal cramps, constipation alternating with diarrhea, other changes in bowel habits, and weight loss.

Kidney cancer. Blood in urine, dull ache or pain in the back or side, or a lump in the kidney area, sometimes accompanied by high blood pressure or abnormality in red blood cell (RBC) count.

Leukemia. Although leukemia is a very specific form of cancer that affects white blood cells (WBCs), the symptoms tend to be nonspecific. Leukemia patients often experience aches; weakness; flulike symptoms; bruising and prolonged bleeding; enlarged lymph nodes, spleen, and liver; and night sweats. Because WBCs carry out important immune functions, patients may experience frequent infections.

Lung cancer. Wheezing cough for months, blood-streaked sputum, persistent ache in chest, congestion in lungs, and enlarged lymph nodes in neck.

Melanoma. A form of skin cancer, melanoma often presents as a mole or other bump on the skin that bleeds or changes in size, shape, color, or texture.

Non-Hodgkin's lymphoma. Group of cancers affecting the immune system; painless swelling in the lymph nodes in the neck, underarm, or groin. The spleen, an important site of immune maturation, may also become enlarged.

Oral cancer. Lump in the mouth; ulceration of the lip, tongue, or inside of the mouth that does not heal in 2 weeks. Other symptoms include dentures that no longer fit well, oral pain, oral bleeding, foul breath, loose teeth, and changes in speech.

Ovarian cancer. Abdominal swelling, abnormal vaginal bleeding (in rare cases), and digestive discomfort.

Pancreatic cancer. Upper abdominal pain and unexplained weight loss; pain near the center of the back; inability to eat fatty foods without experiencing gas, bloating, nausea, or vomiting; yellowing of the skin; and abdominal masses or enlargement of liver and spleen.

Prostate cancer. Urination difficulties caused by blockage of the urethra, urinary retention creating frequent feelings of urgency to urinate (especially at night), incomplete bladder emptying, burning or painful urination, bloody urine, tenderness over the bladder, and dull ache in the pelvis or back.

Stomach cancer. Indigestion or heartburn, discomfort or pain in the abdomen, nausea and vomiting, diarrhea or constipation, bloating after meals, loss of appetite, and bleeding, such as vomiting blood or blood in the stool.

Uterine cancer. Abnormal vaginal bleeding, a watery bloody discharge in postmenopausal women, painful urination, pain during intercourse, and pain in the pelvic area.

Diagnosis

Cancer diagnoses are generally based on a combination of the patient's symptoms, physical examination results, and histological, laboratory, and radiographic testing results. Screening tests are often the initial method of evaluation for cancer. Screening tests are not diagnostic and are used either to evaluate the patient with a suspected malignancy, as based on physical examination and history, or to screen the general public for cancers that may be asymptomatic, allowing earlier diagnosis.[3-6]

Screening

Screening tests help to detect a cancer before symptoms occur and are important prophylactic measures for early cancer detection. If a screening test is positive, diagnostic tests are performed to confirm a diagnosis of cancer.

Although screening tests can potentially save lives, they can be costly and can produce false-positive results; these may create undue psychological stress and can lead to other tests that are expensive and risky. Screening tests can also produce false-negative results, which fail to detect the cancer. However, cancer screening is important for individuals with risk factors for cancer involving age, race, heredity, and lifestyle (e.g., smoking, lack of exercise, overweight). The ACS has cancer screening guidelines that are widely used by health care providers.[5]

Specific recommendations for cancer screening depend on many factors, including age, gender, race, previous medical/family history, and lifestyle. These screening recommendations are for individuals with no symptoms and with an average risk of cancer. For individuals at higher risk, such as those with a strong family history of certain cancers or those with previous cancer diagnoses, screening may be recommended more frequently or at a younger age. Screening tests other than those listed here may also be recommended, depending on the individual's family history, environmental exposures, and other risk factors.[3-6]

Breast Cancer

Breast self-examination (BSE) is recommended monthly after age 20. A physical examination by a health care provider is recommended every 3 years between ages 20 and 39, then yearly. A yearly mammogram is recommended for women starting at age 40; mammograms should be started earlier in women with family histories of breast cancer.

Cervical Cancer

A Papanicolaou (Pap) test/smear is recommended for all women, beginning 3 years after onset of sexual intercourse or at age 21, whichever comes first. Women between ages 21 and 29 should have an annual Pap test. For women over age 30, testing can be performed every 2 to 3 years if they have a history of normal Pap tests. Some women age 65 to 70 or older who have had three or more consecutive normal Pap tests may choose to stop having cervical cancer screening. Tests can also detect the DNA of certain human papillomavirus (HPV) strains that cause most cervical cancer cases.

Lung Cancer

Although there are no standard recommendations for regular lung cancer screening, researchers are investigating the clinical utility of measuring exhaled organic compounds for detecting lung cancer.[7] One proposed method uses dogs to detect subtle changes in breath scent imparted by the volatile organic compounds.[8] Although breath screenings may prove to be highly accurate, findings should be confirmed with histological tests. If a patient presents with symptoms of lung cancer, such as persistent hoarseness or cough, chest radiography, sputum cytology, or computed tomography (CT) may be performed.

Prostate Cancer

A rectal examination is recommended yearly for men after age 50. Prostate-specific antigen blood test is also recommended yearly after age 50, or for men with benign prostatic hyperplasia (BPH, enlarged prostate).

Rectal and Colon Cancer

A stool examination for occult (hidden) blood should be performed yearly after age 50. Beginning at age 50, a sigmoidoscopic examination should be performed every 5 years, or a colonoscopic examination should be performed every 10 years. Genetic testing may also be performed to identify mutations in the adenomatosis polyposis coli (APC) gene, which causes familial adenomatous polyposis (FAP) and greatly increases the risk of early-onset colorectal cancer. For patients with FAP or other genetic predispositions for colorectal cancer, earlier physical examinations are recommended.

Skin Cancer

A dermatological assessment should be part of a routine checkup to screen for potentially cancerous growths (e.g., moles) on the skin. More frequent examinations may be needed for individuals at high risk for developing skin cancer, such as those with fair skin or frequent sunburns. Whole-body photography is not routinely needed, although it may be helpful in patients with multiple moles, or if examination of the skin is difficult.

Diagnostic Tests

The tests used to diagnose cancer depend on the type of cancer suspected. Imaging studies, such as radiography, ultrasonography, CT, and magnetic resonance imaging (MRI), may be performed for most types of cancer. Although these tests can show the presence, location, and size of an abnormal mass, they usually cannot confirm that cancer is the cause. Usually, a biopsy or fine-needle aspiration is performed to evaluate the histological appearance of the cells. Tumors that are difficult to locate visually are often biopsied under ultrasound or CT guidance.

For patients with findings on examination or imaging that suggest cancer, measuring blood levels of tumor markers may provide additional evidence for or against the diagnosis of cancer. *Tumor markers* are substances produced by tumor cells or by other cells of the body in response to cancer or certain benign conditions.[3-6] Tumor markers can be found in the blood, the urine, the tumor tissue, or in other tissues. Different tumor markers are found in different types of cancer, and levels of the same tumor marker can be altered in more than one type of cancer. In addition, tumor marker levels are not altered in all people with cancer, especially in early-stage cancer. Some tumor marker levels can also be altered in patients with noncancerous conditions. Common cancer tumor markers include the following:

- Adenomatosis polyposis coli mutations cause FAP and greatly increase the risk of colorectal cancer.
- Prostate-specific antigen (PSA) is used to screen for prostate cancer.
- Alpha-fetoprotein (AFP) level may be elevated in patients with testicular or liver cancer.
- Loss of β_2-microglobulin may occur in patients with multiple myeloma or chronic lymphocytic leukemia.
- Carcinoembryonic antigen (CEA) may be elevated in individuals with colon cancer.
- CA 125 (carbohydrate antigen 125) may be elevated in patients with some types of ovarian cancer, as well as in patients with cancer of the uterus, cervix, pancreas, liver, colon, breast, lung, and digestive tract.
- CA 19-9 may be elevated in patients with cancer of the pancreas, colon, stomach, and bile duct.
- CA 27-29 may be elevated in patients with breast cancer, as well as in patients with cancer of the colon, stomach, kidney, lung, ovary, pancreas, uterus, and liver.
- CA 15-3 may be elevated in patients with breast cancer, as well as those with advanced breast cancer, and in patients with cancer of the ovary, lung, and prostate.

Tumor markers are rarely used alone for cancer diagnosis and are generally used in conjunction with other laboratory tests, radiographic findings, and tissue biopsy. More often, tumor markers are used to follow a patient's response to treatment and to monitor for recurrence.[3-6]

Staging

Staging is the process of determining how far the cancer has spread. Staging the cancer is a vital step in determining cancer treatment choices and also assists in prognosis. Each type of cancer has its own staging system; common factors that affect staging include the size of the tumor, the depth of invasion into the native tissue, invasion into adjacent structures, and metastasis to distant sights.

The TNM system is the most widely used staging method. The "T" describes the size of the tumor and whether the cancer has invaded nearby tissues and organs. The "N" describes the degree of spread to the lymph nodes. The "M" describes whether the cancer has metastasized (spread) to other organs of the body. Once established, the TNM descriptions can be grouped together into a simpler set of stages, stages 0 through stage IV (0-4). In general, the lower the number, the less the cancer has spread. A higher number, such as stage IV (4), means a more serious, widespread cancer. A T1N2M0 cancer would be a cancer with a T1 tumor, N2 involvement of the lymph nodes, and no metastases.[3-6]

Safety Concerns

Several studies suggest that over 80% of U.S. cancer patients have used complementary therapies, including herbal and vitamin therapies.[9-12]

Many forms of complementary and alternative medicine (CAM) for cancer are associated with minimal or no risk.[3,4] However, some CAM therapies have the potential for drug interactions or adverse outcomes. Potential morbidity and cost may be indirectly associated with direct toxicity and herb/supplement-drug interactions, including increased emergency department (ED) visits, outpatient clinic visits, and perioperative complications.[9-12] However, these costs have not been ascertained; furthermore, it remains unclear how these CAM-related interactions and adverse effects contribute to the overall morbidity and mortality of cancer.

Antioxidant Interference

Because oxidative damage to cells may increase the risk of cancer, botanical antioxidants such as those found in green tea and soy have been suggested for cancer treatment or prevention. Concern has been raised that antioxidants may interfere with radiation therapy or some chemotherapy agents (e.g., alkylating agents, anthracyclines, platinums), which themselves may depend on oxidative damage to be cytotoxic to tumor cells. Studies of antioxidant effects on cancer therapies report mixed results ranging from antagonistic effects to synergism, and most suggest no significant interaction. In contrast, others have noted that the possible harm from antioxidants is only hypothetical, and that protecting normal cells from the effects of chemotherapy and radiation may have an overall benefit. Whether antioxidants are beneficial or harmful is currently unclear and remains controversial.[13,14]

Drug Interactions

Though many botanical agents are pharmacologically active, there is still little definitive evidence supporting efficacy in treating cancer; furthermore, there are numerous potential interactions between specific herbs/vitamins and drugs.[15-23] Therefore, the potential for negative interactions should be considered before integrating herbs, vitamins, or nutritional supplements during chemotherapy.

Common chemotherapy agents metabolized through enzymes in the cytochrome P450 (CYP450) system, and the specific isoenzymes responsible for drug metabolism may indicate possible interactions. St. John's wort *(Hypericum perforatum)* is of particular concern and has multiple well-documented drug interactions. This herb appears to inhibit the hepatic enzyme CYP450 3A4 acutely, then induce it with repeated administration. A study of individuals given irinotecan (CPT-11) chemotherapy reports a greater than 50% reduction in serum levels of the active metabolite SN-38 after concomitant administration of St. John's wort.[24] St. John's wort should be used cautiously in combination with other drugs with similar modes of metabolism.

Based on preclinical evidence, other herbs that may induce CYP450 3A4 include hop *(Humulus lupulus)*, chasteberry *(Vitex agnus-castus)*, bloodroot *(Sanguinaria canadensis)*, oregano *(Origanum* spp.*)*, damiana *(Turnera* spp.*)*, and yucca *(Yucca* spp.*)*. Agents that may inhibit CYP450 3A4 include cannabinoids, grapefruit juice, milk thistle *(Silybum marianum)*, the chaparral component nordihydroguaiaretic acid (NDGA), goldenseal *(Hydrastis canadensis)*, cat's claw *(Uncaria* spp.*)*, *Echinacea angustifolia* root, wild cherry *(Prunus serotina)*, chamomile *(Matricaria chamomilla)*, and licorice *(Glycyrrhiza glabra)*.[3,25]

Perioperative Considerations

An increased risk of bleeding is an adverse effect of many herbs and supplements. Multiple case studies have reported clinically significant bleeding with the use of *Ginkgo biloba* either alone or with aspirin or warfarin, and there have been isolated case reports of bleeding with the use of saw palmetto *(Serenoa repens)* and garlic *(Allium sativum)*. With the prevalent use of herbal supplements by cancer patients, surgical personnel should carefully screen patients preoperatively for use of agents that may affect blood coagulation.

Cancer Remission

Remission is a period when the cancer is responding to treatment or is under control. In a *complete* remission, all the signs and symptoms of the disease disappear. Patients may also have a *partial* remission, in which the cancer does not completely disappear. Remissions can last several weeks to many years. Complete remissions may continue for years and the cancer considered cured. If the disease returns, another remission often can occur with further treatment. A cancer that has recurred may respond to a different type of therapy, including a different drug combination. Recurrent cancer may not respond to the same medications and treatments as the cancer before remission. *Spontaneous* remission of cancer refers to exceptional and unexplained partial or complete disappearance of cancer without medical intervention.

SELECTED HERBAL THERAPIES

Note
To help make this educational resource more interactive, all pharmacokinetics, adverse effects, and interactions data have been compiled in Appendix A. Safety data specifically related to pregnancy and lactation are listed in Appendix B. Please refer to these appendices when working through the case studies and answering the review questions.

Aloe (Aloe vera)

Grade C: *Unclear or conflicting scientific evidence (cancer prevention)*

Mechanism of Action

Antioxidant properties have been attributed to aloesin, a component of *Aloe vera*.[26-28] APS-1, a polysaccharide from *Aloe vera*, also showed free-radical scavenging and other antioxidant properties in vitro.[29] Antileukemic and antimutagenic effects of aloe in vitro have been attributed to di(2-ethylhexyl)phthalate (DEHP).[30] Promotion of apoptosis has been reported in vitro as a possible antineoplastic mechanism.[31] Aloe appears to affect detoxification of reactive metabolites by the liver and other organs.[27] Studies suggest that aloe polysaccharides might have a radioprotective effect on nonmalignant cells through its ability to modulate the cell cycle.[32,33]

Scientific Evidence of Effectiveness

Preliminary epidemiological evidence suggests that dietary aloe consumption *(Aloe arborescens)* may prevent human carcinogenesis at various sites, such as the lung.[34] Although compelling, the methodological difficulties of case-control studies apply to this report. The possible effect of confounders not detected by the study questionnaire is prominent. Also, it is unclear whether this effect is generalizable to other *Aloe* species.

Dose

The dose of aloe for cancer prevention is not established.

Adverse Effects, Interactions, Pharmacokinetics. See Appendix A.

American Pawpaw (Asimina triloba)

Grade C: *Unclear or conflicting scientific evidence (cancer treatment)*

Mechanism of Action

Various compounds derived from American pawpaw show selective tumor cytotoxicity against tumor cell lines[35,36] in breast,[37-39] colon,[38-40] prostate,[40,41] pancreatic,[41] and lung[37-39] cells, with some studies showing equivalent or increased potency compared with doxorubicin (Adriamycin).[35,36,40,42] Active antineoplastic properties have been reported for the constituent asimicin,[43-45] as well as for its structural isomers asimin, asiminacin, and asiminecin.[46] Trilobacin and asimicin showed potent and selective cytotoxicities in the U.S. National Cancer Institute human tumor cell line screen.[47]

The *acetogenins* in pawpaw may inhibit adenosine triphosphate (ATP) synthesis in cells in two ways. First, the disruption of a mitochondrial proton pump theoretically results in the generation of reactive oxygen species that trigger cellular pathways to apoptosis. This rationale for the selectivity of acetogenins is based on the rapid respiration rates of cancer cells compared with surrounding tissue. It is thought that acetogenins at low levels can trigger apoptosis in cancer cells while not affecting normal cells. A second possible mechanism against refractory cancer cells is that efflux pumps, such as the P-glycoprotein pump, may also be inhibited by the acetogenins. If this is one of their mechanisms of action, acetogenins may enhance the effectiveness of other chemotherapeutic drugs.

Scientific Evidence of Effectiveness

Evidence supporting the use of American pawpaw for treating cancer is largely anecdotal and subjective. One clinical trial evaluated the use of American pawpaw in patients with solid tumors.[48] Details of this unpublished study were not clear, and many of the patients were also receiving concomitant chemotherapy and/or radiation.

Dose

In an unpublished study, patients with various forms of cancer took 12.5 to 50 mg of American pawpaw standardized extract daily for 18 months.[48]

Adverse Effects, Interactions, Pharmacokinetics. See Appendix A.

Astragalus (Astragalus membranaceus)

Grade C: *Unclear or conflicting scientific evidence (cancer treatment)*

Mechanism of Action

In vitro evidence indicates that astragalus may potentiate efficacy and reduce adverse effects of chemotherapy through stimulation of immune function.[49-51] Astragalus extract has been shown to significantly increase in vitro cytokine secretion and gene expression in blood mononuclear cells of lung cancer patients.[52] Astragalus extracts have also been shown to induce lymphokine-activated killer (LAK) cell activity in the lymphocytes of cancer patients and patients with human immunodeficiency virus (HIV) and to stimulate the blastogenic response of lymphocytes to mutagens in patients with various cancers.[53-58] An astragalus-containing herbal preparation inhibited tumor growth in vivo while augmenting macrophage and LAK cell activity.[59] Herbal remedies containing astragalus also inhibited tumor growth and prolonged survival in rats compared to those treated with conventional chemotherapy alone. Other studies report potentiation of interleukin-2–generated cytotoxicity in animal models[53,60] and reduction of mutagenesis.[61]

Scientific Evidence of Effectiveness

Astragalus has been used in Chinese medicine for centuries for its purported immune-enhancing properties. Clinical trials have shown improved survival, immune function, and quality of life in cancer patients. According to preclinical research, astragalus improved survival and enhanced immune response in patients with cancer.[58] In advanced non–small cell lung cancer patients, intravenous (IV) infusion of astragalus improved quality of life and survival compared with chemotherapy alone.[62] Huangqi Zengmian Powder (HQZMP), an astragalus-containing product, was reported to induce histological evidence of increased immune response in esophageal cancer patients.[63] More rigorous clinical trials are needed to determine whether astragalus is effective as a cancer treatment.

Dose

The percentage and relative proportions of astragalosides, trigonosides, and flavonoid constituents of dried astragalus root vary with the age, size, and growing conditions of the root.[64] Commercially available astragalus products are standardized to 70% polysaccharides, 0.3% astragaloside content, or 0.5% triterpenoids glycoside content.

For advanced non–small cell lung cancer, an IV drip of 60 mL daily was used for two or three treatment cycles of 21 to 28 days per cycle, along with unspecified forms of chemotherapy.[62]

Adverse Effects, Interactions, Pharmacokinetics. See Appendix A.

Black Cohosh (*Actaea racemosa*, formerly *Cimicifuga racemosa*)

Grade C: *Unclear or conflicting scientific evidence (breast cancer prevention)*

Mechanism of Action

In vitro studies have shown that black cohosh possesses inhibitory effects on estrogen-responsive cancer cell lines and breast cancer cells.[65-69] Furthermore, in vitro research showed that relatively low concentrations of either actein or the methanol/water fraction of black cohosh caused synergistic inhibition of human breast cancer cell proliferation when combined with different classes of chemotherapy agents (paclitaxel, 5-fluorouracil, or doxorubicin).[70] The constituents actaealactone and cimicifugic acid may also have a stimulating effect on the growth of breast cancer cell proliferation.[71] In vitro the extract killed hormone-responsive or hormone-unresponsive prostate cancer cells by inducing apoptosis and activating caspases.[72] Research conducted in mice demonstrated inhibition of PC3 prostate cancer tumor growth with black cohosh and other herbal extracts.[73] The mechanism behind tumor inhibition appeared to be antiangiogenic and caused a decrease in intratumoral microvessel density. Antiangiogenic action may be beneficial for preventing cancer and other diseases of blood vessel growth, such as retinopathy and macular degeneration.

Scientific Evidence of Effectiveness

Black cohosh may have antiestrogenic effects that inhibit breast carcinogenesis.[74] According to a retrospective analysis, black cohosh may lower breast cancer risk. However, supportive clinical evidence is lacking.

Dose

The dosage of black cohosh is often based on its triterpenes content, calculated as 27-deoxyactein. The German product Remifemin, used in the majority of clinical studies, contains an alcoholic extract of black cohosh rhizome standardized to contain 1 mg of 27-deoxyactein per 20-mg tablet.[75] The manufacturing process and dosing recommendations for Remifemin have changed over time, and doses used in different studies may not be comparable. A standardized liquid formulation of Remifemin was used in some studies. The dose of black cohosh for breast cancer prevention has not been determined.

Adverse Effects, Interactions, Pharmacokinetics. See Appendix A.

Boswellia (*Boswellia serrata*)

Grade B: *Good scientific evidence (brain cancer treatment)*

Mechanism of Action

Several triterpenoid acids have been isolated from *Boswellia serrata* and *Boswellia carterii* and evaluated for their antiproliferative, cytotoxic, and cytostatic effects.[76] Both in vivo and in vitro studies have demonstrated apoptotic, cytostatic, and antiproliferative activity against a number of cancer cell lines through different mechanisms.[77,78] Acetyl-11-keto-beta-boswellic acid (AKBA), a pentacyclic triterpenoid isolated from the resin of *B. serrata*, was shown to potentiate apoptosis induced by tumor necrosis factor (TNF) and chemotherapeutic agents, suppress TNF-induced invasion, and inhibit receptor activation of nuclear factor kappa B (NF-κB) ligand–induced osteoclastogenesis.[79] Therefore, AKBA may enhance apoptosis induced by cytokines and chemotherapeutic agents, inhibit invasion, and suppress osteoclastogenesis through inhibition of NF-κB–regulated gene expression. Some studies suggest that the cytotoxic action of AKBA on meningioma cells may be mediated, at least in part, by the inhibition of the ERK signal transduction pathway.[77,80] However, other studies found that *Boswellia* extract with a defined boswellic acid content was more effective at inhibiting cancer cell growth than pure 3-O-AKBA.[81]

Investigations using *B. carterii* suggest that the mechanism of cytotoxic effects of a 1:1 mixture of alpha-boswellic acid acetate and beta-boswellic acetate resulted from capsase-8–induced expression of death receptors 4 and 5.[82] Moreover, activated capsase-8 directly activated capsase-3, resulting in decreased mitochondrial membrane potential. Of the several triterpenoid acids isolated from *B. carterii* resin, seven potently inhibited the induction of Epstein-Barr virus early antigens.[83] Moreover, 15 acid compounds exhibited potent cytotoxic activities with IC_{50} values of 4.1 to 82.4 mcM against human neuroblastoma cells.

In vitro evaluation of the anticancer effects of BC-4, an isometric compound isolated from *B. carterii* extract, demonstrated cytostatic activity, as evidenced by inhibition of cell population in the G1 phase and topoisomerase II activity, cell differentiation, and antimigratory activity.[84]

In human colon cancer cells, the acetyl-keto-beta form of boswellic acid exerted potent apoptotic activity, primarily through caspase-8 activation–dependent increases in cytoplasmic DNA-histone complex and pre-G1 peak.[85] Boswellic acid also inhibited [^{3}H]-thymidine incorporation and cell viability. Earlier research by the same group demonstrated that boswellic acid induced time-dependent and dose-dependant apoptosis in human leukemia cells.[86]

Scientific Evidence of Effectiveness

In vitro and in vivo studies have shown that extracts of *Boswellia* species exert anticarcinogenic, antiproliferative, antitumor, cytostatic, and apoptotic activity.[81,84-93] In rats, boswellia reduced the rate of skin tumors and aberrant crypt foci.[87]

Boswellia has been popularly used as a brain cancer treatment, specifically to reduce intracranial tumors or edema caused by these tumors. It has been reported to reduce intracranial edema and to induce clinical improvements in general health in a case series.[91,94] In one case report, metastatic brain lesions regressed in a patient taking *Boswellia serrata*.[95] Additional research is ongoing.

Dose

Studies have reported using H15, a proprietary combination of boswellic acids, in patients with brain tumors.[94,96] In a case series, patients received a maximum dose of 126 mg/kg of H15 daily for a median of 9 months.[94]

Adverse Effects, Interactions, Pharmacokinetics. See Appendix A.

Bromelain (Bromeliaceae)

Grade C: *Unclear or conflicting scientific evidence (cancer treatment, cancer prevention)*

Mechanism of Action

Bromelain is a sulfur-containing proteolytic enzyme found in the stem and the fruit of the pineapple plant *(Ananas comosus)* and other plants of the family Bromeliaceae. Bromelains are glycoproteins with one carbohydrate chain per protein molecule and an active site represented by the reactive sulfhydryl group of cysteine.[97] Bromelain also contains peroxidase, acid phosphatase, several protease inhibitors, and organically bound calcium.[98]

In vitro, bromelain was able to induce leukemic cells to differentiate and to reduce tumor growth; this was attributed to the proteolytic activity of bromelain.[97] Bromelain has been studied as a skin cancer prevention agent in mice.[99]

Scientific Evidence of Effectiveness

CANCER TREATMENT. Female patients who had received surgical therapy for breast cancer were given 400 mg of bromelain twice daily for 10 days and were evaluated for bromelain cytotoxicity.[100] After analysis the interleukin-activated killer cells and the natural killer (NK) cells did not show significant changes. However, basal macrophage killer cells and macrophage interferon-activated killer cells showed significant effects in both cell lines.

Another study examined the immunological effects of an oral bromelain preparation on 16 breast cancer patients compared with healthy donors.[101] Oral bromelain increased activity of cytotoxic lymphocytes in breast cancer patients. Possible explanations of the anticancer effects of bromelain include disruption of adhesion molecules on tumor and endothelial cells through its proteolytic activity and inhibition of signaling by ERK-2 and p21*ras*. It has also been speculated that bromelain may play a role in the differentiation of malignant cells.

Preliminary research involving patients with advanced cancer treated with bromelain reported regression of tumor mass in two breast cancer patients.[102]

Dose

Bromelain is standardized to milk clotting unit (mcu) or gelatin-digesting unit (gdu) activity. The mcu measurement is officially recognized by the Food Chemistry Codex. Anecdotal reports have recommended using a bromelain product that has been standardized to contain at least 2000 mcu/g per dose.

Clinical studies have used Extranase (bromelain) at 600 mg daily for up to several years (unspecified).[102] The dosage of bromelain for cancer prevention and treatment has not been established.

Adverse Effects, Interactions, Pharmacokinetics. See Appendix A.

Bupleurum (*Bupleurum* spp.)

Grade C: *Unclear or conflicting scientific evidence (hepatocellular carcinoma prevention)*

Mechanism of Action

Bupleurum scorzonerifolium has shown anticancer properties in vitro and in vivo.[103-105] This effect has been attributed to isochaihulactone, a constituent of *B. scorzonerifolium*, which has been shown to inhibit tubulin polymerization, arrest the cell cycle at the G2/M phase, and to induce apoptosis in a concentration-dependent manner.[103] Rotundiosides extracted from *Bupleurum rotundifolium* have also shown antiproliferative activity against human gastric adenocarcinoma (MK-1) cell growth.[106] A *Bupleurum*-containing combination supplement, sho-saiko-to, has been shown to inhibit cell differentiation,[107] an effect that has been attributed baicalein and glycyrrhetinic acid from *Scutellaria baicalensis* and *Glycyrrhiza glabra*, respectively.[108]

Scientific Evidence of Effectiveness

Sho-saiko-to, a Japanese combination herbal formula that contains bupleurum, may slow the growth of tumor cells and stimulate a person's immune system to help kill tumor cells. A clinical trial reported a possible role of this product in preventing the development of hepatocellular carcinoma in patients with cirrhosis. From this trial, sho-saiko-to did not prevent the development of hepatocellular carcinoma, but it did appear to improve survival in patients with cirrhosis.[109] After 5 years, 75% of patients receiving sho-saiko-to were alive versus 61% receiving only the conventional medicines. Currently, a Phase II trial is underway to study the effectiveness of sho-saiko-to in treating liver cancer patients after hepatic artery embolization.[110]

Dose

A safe and effective dose of bupleurum has not been determined. Bupleurum is typically taken in combination formulas with other herbs and has not been well studied as a monotherapy.

The combination therapy sho-saiko-to has been administered at a dose of 7.5 g daily, in combination with conventional treatment, to patients with hepatocellular carcinoma cirrhosis.[109]

Adverse Effects, Interactions, Pharmacokinetics. See Appendix A.

Cat's Claw (*Uncaria* spp.)

Grade C: *Unclear or conflicting scientific evidence (cancer prevention)*

Mechanism of Action

The pentacyclic oxindole alkaloid constituents of cat's claw have been reported to enhance the cellular immune system and to regulate specific immune system cytokines, which may help improve the body's defense system against cancer.[111,112] Research conducted in vitro has shown cat's claw to inhibit tumor cell proliferation and inflammatory responses.[113] However, the extract does not interfere with interleukin-2 (IL-2) production or IL-2 receptor signaling. Cat's claw may also modulate immune responses that target abnormally proliferating cells. In mice, cat's claw extract prolonged lymphocyte half-life and increased spleen cell number.[114] The extract also induced cell proliferation arrest and inhibited activation of the transcriptional regulator NF-κB in vitro. Cat's claw extracts and fractions have exerted direct antiproliferative activity on several cell lines, including MCF7 breast cancer, glioma, neuroblastoma, premyelocytic leukemia, and acute lymphoblastic leukemia.[115-119]

Scientific Evidence of Effectiveness

Cat's claw has been shown to prevent mutagenic activity in nonsmokers and to decrease mutagenic activity in smokers.[120,121] Healthy volunteers showed enhanced immune response when treated with C-Med-100 (aqueous extract of cat's claw) concurrently with the influenza vaccine.[122] C-Med-100 increased WBC counts in healthy subjects[123] and decreased chemotherapy-induced DNA damage in healthy volunteers.[124]

Dose

For cancer, 6.5 g of the dried bark of cat's claw (boiled in water for 3 hours) was taken for 15 days.[121]

Adverse Effects, Interactions, Pharmacokinetics. See Appendix A.

Chaparral (*Larrea tridentata, Larrea divaricata*)

Grade C: *Unclear or conflicting scientific evidence (cancer)*

Mechanism of Action

Lignans isolated from the flowering tops of *Larrea tridentata* have demonstrated growth-inhibitory effects against human breast cancer, human colon cancer, and human melanoma cell lines.[125]

The chaparral constituent nordihydroguaiaretic acid (NDGA) has been theorized to block cellular respiration and exert antioxidant effects.[3] NDGA also has been shown to inhibit cell metabolism; furthermore, it may modulate apoptosis, cellular immune system responses, and biological responses to a variety of chemicals (including hormones). NDGA has been demonstrated to have antitumor effects as well as mutagenic potential.[126] Stimulation of tumor growth was reported in a preliminary study using NDGA to treat cancer.[127] According to anecdotal and in vitro evidence, NDGA possesses dose-dependent cytotoxic activity.[126]

In PC3 human prostate cancer cells, NDGA released stored calcium from the endoplasmic reticulum and caused a calcium influx, thereby inducing a calcium increase in the cells.[128] NDGA caused cytotoxicity in these prostate cancer cells at higher concentrations. In the same cell line, NDGA reduced vascular endothelial growth factor expression, suggesting that it has antiangiogenic effects.[129]

A combination of nonsteroidal antiinflammatory drugs (NSAIDs), butyrate, indomethacin, and NDGA was effective in inhibiting cell proliferation in the colon cancer cell line HT29.[130]

Tetra-O-methyl-NGDA is a global transcription inhibitor.[131] In nude mice with xenografts of five human tumor types (hepatocellular carcinoma, prostate carcinoma, colorectal carcinoma, breast carcinoma, and erythroleukemia cells), oral and intravenous tetra-O-methyl-NGDA suppressed tumor growth, particularly in four of the five tumor lines.[132] In another nude mouse study, tetra-O-methyl-NGDA and maltose-tri-O-methyl-NGDA both reversed the multidrug resistance of xenografted tumor cells, and a combination of tetra-O-methyl-NGDA or maltose-tri-O-methyl-NGDA with paclitaxel synergistically inhibited tumor growth.[133]

Scientific Evidence of Effectiveness

A case series reported 25% tumor regression in 4 of 59 cancer patients.[134] A case report documented regression of metastatic melanoma in a patient self-treating with chaparral tea.[135] Rigorous clinical evidence is lacking. Because of the known toxicity of chaparral, the risks of this therapy may outweigh the potential benefits. Chaparral has been associated with multiple serious and potentially fatal adverse effects.[136] The U.S. Food and Drug Administration (FDA) removed chaparral from the "generally recognized as safe" (GRAS) list in 1970 and now considers chaparral to be unsafe.

Dose

The chaparral constituent nordihydroguaiaretic acid (NDGA) is potentially toxic or fatal when taken orally,[126,136-139] and is not recommended for general use.

Adverse Effects, Interactions, Pharmacokinetics. See Appendix A.

Chrysanthemum (*Chrysanthemum* spp.)

Grade C: *Unclear or conflicting scientific evidence (cancer prevention; treatment of precancerous lesions)*

Mechanism of Action

Chrysanthemum may exhibit anticancer effects by modulating cell proliferation and/or apoptosis. According to *in vitro* research using human prostate cancer LNCaP and DU145 cells, linarin (isolated and purified from *Chrysanthemum awadskii*), linarin acetate (chemically synthesized from linarin), and acacetin (obtained commercially) induced apoptosis and arrested cell development in various stages.[140]

Scientific Evidence of Effectiveness

Note: Chrysanthemum was an ingredient in PC-SPES, a combination product used for prostate cancer, which was recalled from the U.S. market after tests showed that it contained the prescription blood thinner warfarin.[5]

CANCER PREVENTION. Research conducted in vitro showed that chrysanthemum extracts inhibit cancer cell proliferation and tumor promoter activity.[141] The effect of chrysanthemum in human cancer prevention is unknown.

CANCER TREATMENT (PRECANCEROUS LESIONS). There is limited preliminary evidence that hua-sheng-ping (which includes *Chrysanthemum morifolium, Glycyrrhiza uralensis*, and *Panax notoginseng*) may be beneficial for patients with precancerous lesions.[142] However, rigorous clinical studies are lacking.

Dose

Combination products containing chrysanthemum have been used clinically; studies using chrysanthemum monotherapy are lacking.

Adverse Effects, Interactions, Pharmacokinetics. See Appendix A.

Echinacea (*Echinacea* spp.)

Grade C: *Unclear or conflicting scientific evidence (cancer)*

Mechanism of Action

Constituents of the root oil of *Echinacea angustiflora* and *Echinacea pallida* have been shown to possess antitumor activity in vivo.[143] Echinacea extracts produce cytotoxic effects in colon and pancreatic cancer cell lines.[144] Intravenous echinacea was reported to increase chemotherapy-induced WBC counts in gastric cancer patients.[145]

In contrast to these findings, another study reported that echinacea extract had no effect on metastatic tumors in a mice lung cancer model and increased tumor growth.[146] This study also reported that a hydrophilic polysaccharide complex isolated from echinacea had antitumor effects in a rat lung cancer model. Echinacea extracts have also been reported to interfere with the cytotoxicity of doxorubicin (Adriamycin), a standard chemotherapeutic agent.[147]

Scientific Evidence of Effectiveness

Clinical evidence is lacking regarding the efficacy of echinacea in cancer therapy. No change in WBC count or cytokine production was seen in brain tumor patients treated with 3 mL of a 40% *Echinacea angustifolia* herbal therapy daily for 4 weeks.[148] A study of 15 patients with metastatic colon cancer treated with low-dose cyclophosphamide, thymostimulin, and Echinacin[149] reported a mean survival of 4 months. In a case series, five patients with advanced hepatocellular carcinoma were treated with a combination regimen including Echinacin, and mean survival was 10 weeks.[150]

Dose

Some manufacturers standardize echinacea extracts to 4% to 5% echinacoside, whereas others standardize to cichoric acid. Because the active constituent(s) has not been identified, standardization may not be clinically relevant in predicting effectiveness. Furthermore, the dosing of echinacea for cancer has not been determined.

Adverse Effects, Interactions, Pharmacokinetics. See Appendix A.

Evening Primrose (Oenothera biennis)

Grade C: *Unclear or conflicting scientific evidence (breast cancer treatment, cancer prevention)*

Mechanism of Action

In mice with breast carcinoma xenografts, evening primrose oil (EPO) reduced tumor size more than olive oil and placebo but less than fish oil.[151] EPO showed cytotoxic effects in vitro and in vivo associated with increases in superoxide generation.[152] One study showed EPO to induce apoptosis in rat ascites tumor cells, associated with a rapid increase in intracellular peroxide levels, loss of mitochondrial membrane potential, and mitochondrial release of cytochrome c; no effect was seen on normal cells.[153] EPO was reported to have cytotoxic effects on melanoma cells in vitro but promoted tumor growth in a melanoma mouse model.[154] The compound oenothein A, isolated from the leaves of *Oenothera biennis*, is also reported to have antitumor activity.[155]

Scientific Evidence of Effectiveness

BREAST CANCER TREATMENT. Breast cancer patients taking tamoxifen (a primary treatment for estrogen-dependent breast cancer) and gamma-linolenic acid (GLA, a component of EPO) experienced a faster clinical response than those taking tamoxifen alone.[156] These preliminary data warrant further study.

CANCER PREVENTION. Preliminary animal research suggested that EPO reduces mammary tumorigenesis over corn oil.[157] These apparent cancer-preventive effects warrant further analysis.

Dose

Breast cancer patients have taken 3.8 g GLA (active ingredient in EPO) by mouth daily as an adjunct to tamoxifen therapy.[156]

Adverse Effects, Interactions, Pharmacokinetics. See Appendix A.

Flax (Linum usitatissimum)

Grade C: *Unclear or conflicting scientific evidence (breast cancer prevention and treatment)*

Mechanism of Action

Flaxseed (not flaxseed oil) is a rich source of plant lignans[158-160] and is a particularly concentrated food source of the lignan secoisolariciresinol diglycoside (SDG).[161] Lignans are often referred to as *phytoestrogens* and may possess ER agonist or antagonist properties that have unclear effects on hormone-sensitive cancers such as breast, uterine, and prostate cancer.[160]

Flaxseed has been shown to inhibit tumor growth in several studies using mouse models of breast cancer.[162-167] In mice, the flaxseed constituents enterodiol and enterolactone reduced estradiol-induced growth and angiogenesis in solid tumors, presumably by decreasing serum levels of vascular endothelial growth factor (VEGF).[167] Flaxseed may also enhance the effects of tamoxifen, an ER antagonist commonly used in breast cancer treatment.[162] Lignans isolated from flaxseed inhibited breast cancer cell adhesion, invasion, and migration in vitro alone and in combination with tamoxifen.[168] In a mouse model of prostate cancer, flaxseed supplementation showed no significant difference in tumor grade after 20 weeks; at 30 weeks, however, the flaxseed-treated mice had significantly less aggressive tumors than controls.[169]

Enterolactone and enterodiol (metabolized from flaxseed in the bowel) may decrease cell proliferation and inhibit aromatase, 5α-reductase, and 17β-hydroxysteroid dehydrogenase activity, which may reduce the risk of breast, prostate, and other hormone-sensitive cancers.[161] In humans, flaxseed consumption has been reported to reduce significantly serum levels of 17β-estradiol and estrone sulfate, increase prolactin levels, increase sex hormone–binding globulin (SHBG) synthesis,[161] increase the urinary ratio of the two estrogen metabolites 2-hydroxyestrogen and 16α-hydroxyestrone,[170,171] increase urinary excretion levels of enterodiol and enterolactone,[171] and increase fecal excretion of enterodiol, enterolactone, and matairesinol.[172] Flaxseed may have more potent effects on estrogen metabolism than soy.[173] The effects of these hormonal changes on cancer or cancer therapy are uncertain.

Scientific Evidence of Effectiveness

BREAST CANCER PREVENTION. Few clinical studies have evaluated the effect of flaxseed on breast cancer. To date, most clinical trials have examined the effect of flaxseed ingestion on hormone levels in healthy premenopausal and postmenopausal women. Clinical research has shown that flaxseed ingestion reduced 17β-estradiol and estrone sulfate levels and increased prolactin levels in healthy postmenopausal women.[161] Also, flaxseed increased the urinary ratio of the two estrogen metabolites 2-hydroxyestrogen and 16α-hydroxyestrone in postmenopausal women,[170,174] a finding proposed as linked to reduced breast cancer risk. A dose of 10 g of flaxseed daily (vs. a low-fiber diet) for three menstrual cycles produced prolongation of the luteal phase and a decrease in anovulatory cycles.[175] Flaxseed consumption significantly increased the fecal excretion of enterodiol, enterolactone, and matairesinol (compared to baseline values).[172] How these effects on hormone levels translate to breast cancer prevention is unclear.

There is preliminary evidence that flaxseed may improve the symptoms of cyclical mastalgia.[176] Although cyclical mastalgia may be a risk factor for breast cancer,[177] it is not clear that flaxseed reduces this risk.

BREAST CANCER TREATMENT. One study reported that large tumor size and low level of alpha-linoleic acid (ALA, found in flaxseed oil) were associated with the a risk of metastasis in breast cancer.[178] However, it is unclear from this study whether low ALA levels have any clinical relevance and whether supplementation with ALA would confer any benefit.

Dose

The dose of flaxseed for breast cancer prevention or treatment has not been determined. However, a clinical study showed possible hormone-regulating effects in women taking 10 g of flaxseed daily for three menstrual cycles.[175]

Adverse Effects, Interactions, Pharmacokinetics. See Appendix A.

Garlic (Allium sativum)

Grade C: *Unclear or conflicting scientific evidence (cancer prevention)*

Mechanism of Action

Animal studies have demonstrated protective effects of garlic against hepatotoxins,[179-182] cyclophosphamide,[183] doxorubicin (Adriamycin),[184] methylcholanthrene,[185] gentamicin,[186] 4-nitroquinoline 1-oxide,[187] and bromobenzene.[188,189] Garlic strongly inhibits cancer development in the presence of known tumor promoters, including 12-O-tetradecanoylphorbol-13-acetate,[190,191] 7,12-dimethylbenzanthracene,[192] and phorbol-myristate-acetate,[193] as well as tumor inducers such as 7,12-dimethylbenzanthracene[191] and 1,2-dimethylhydrazine.[194,195] Some evidence indicates that molecules containing allyl groups may be responsible for chemoprotective properties.[196] Research has provided evidence of antiproliferative effects of garlic on human cancer cell lines,[197] including induction of apoptosis,[198-202] regulation of cell cycle progression,[203] and signal transduction modification. Both cellular proliferation[204,205] and immune function[206,207] appear to be affected.

Scientific Evidence of Effectiveness

A review of epidemiological literature found conflicting results, with most of the 22 studies reporting reduced cancer risk with garlic consumption, but with many of these risks failing to reach statistical significance.[208] However, raw garlic appeared to have a greater benefit than commercial garlic supplements. Four of five reports found that garlic decreased the risk of gastric cancer,[209-213] and six of seven studies reported reduced risk of colon cancer with garlic.[214-216] Two studies reported reduced risk of breast cancer.[217,218] A subsequent meta-analysis by the same author reported reduced risk of gastric and colon cancer, but significant methodological flaws were found in most studies.[219]

Numerous case-control and population-based studies have examined the relationship between diet and cancer incidence. The effects of garlic on cancer incidence remain unclear, and prospective intervention trials are warranted.

Dose

The dose of garlic for cancer prevention is unknown. The European Scientific Cooperative on Phytotherapy (ESCOP) 1997 monograph recommends 3 to 5 mg of allicin daily (1 garlic clove or 0.5-1.0 g dried garlic powder) for prophylaxis of atherosclerosis. The WHO 1999 monograph recommends 2 to 5 g of fresh garlic, 0.4 to 1.2 g of dried garlic powder, 2 to 5 mg of garlic oil, 300 to 1000 mg of garlic extract, or other formulations corresponding to 2 to 5 mg of allicin.

Adverse Effects, Interactions, Pharmacokinetics. See Appendix A.

Ginkgo (Ginkgo biloba)

Grade C: *Unclear or conflicting scientific evidence (colorectal cancer; gastric cancer; pancreatic cancer; ovarian cancer)*

Mechanism of Action

The *Ginkgo biloba* extract kaempferol inhibited pancreatic cancer cell proliferation and induced cancer cell apoptosis in vitro.[220] Ginkgo extract and its components, quercetin and ginkgolides A and B, had antiproliferative effects in serous ovarian cancer cells but minimal effect in mucinous ovarian cancer cells;[221] the ginkgolides also appeared to inhibit the cell cycle at the G0/G1 to S phase. The ginkgo extract EGb 761 decreased the expression of the peripheral-type benzodiazepine receptor (PBR), which is upregulated in some cancers, and inhibited the proliferation of breast, glioma, and hepatocellular carcinoma cell lines.[222] Ginkgo extract also decreased growth of xenografted breast and glioma cells in mice.[222] EGb 761 inhibited cellular proliferation and induced caspase-dependent apoptosis in oral cavity cancer cells.[223] Ginkgo extracts inhibited tumor cell growth without affecting normal cells in vitro.[224]

In hepatocellular carcinoma cell lines, ginkgo extracts inhibited cell proliferation, decreased proliferating cell nuclear antigen (PCNA), and increased p53 expression.[225] Another study reported that *Ginkgo biloba* polysaccharides actually increased apoptosis in hepatocellular carcinoma cell lines.[226] In mouse fibrosarcoma, ginkgo extract increased radiosensitivity without damaging normal tissue.[227]

Scientific Evidence of Effectiveness

COLORECTAL CANCER. In a Phase II clinical trial, 44 colorectal cancer patients were pretreated with 5-fluorouracil (5-FU) conventional therapy, then treated with 5-FU and *Ginkgo biloba* extract (GBE 761 ONC) every 3 weeks; after the fourth course of treatment with 5-FU and GBE 761 ONC, data from 32 available patients showed partial response to therapy in two patients, with survival times similar to known second-line treatments.[228] Although the effects of ginkgo were unclear, the results suggested a good benefit-risk ratio of 5-FU and GBE 761 ONC combination therapy.

GASTRIC CANCER. Thirty patients with gastric cancer were treated with *Ginkgo biloba* exocarp polysaccharide (GBEP).[229] Compared with baseline measures, tumor areas decreased with an effective rate of 73.4%. Ultrastructural changes of the cells suggested that GBEP induced apoptosis and differentiation in gastric cancer patients. Cell culture studies suggested that GBEP inhibited the growth of human gastric cancer by altering the expression of *c-myc*, *bcl-2*, and *c-fos* genes, which may in turn inhibit proliferation and induce apoptosis and differentiation of tumor cells.

PANCREATIC CANCER. A Phase II trial of parenteral GBE 761 ONC combined with 5-FU showed results equivalent to those seen with conventional therapy.[230]

OVARIAN CANCER. Epidemiological findings suggested a protective effect of ginkgo on the development of ovarian cancer, particularly nonmucinous tumors.[221] Clinical evidence is lacking.

Dose

Ginkgo products referred to as "EGb 761" contain 24% ginkgo flavone glycosides and 6% terpenoids. Products referred to as "LI 1370" contain 25% ginkgo flavone glycosides and 6% terpenoids.

The dose of ginkgo for cancer treatment or prevention has not been established. Patients with gastric carcinoma treated with oral *Ginkgo biloba* exocarp polysaccharides (0.25 g per capsule) received two capsules twice daily for 30 days.[229]

Adverse Effects, Interactions, Pharmacokinetics. See Appendix A.

Ginseng (*Panax* spp.)

Grade C: Unclear or conflicting scientific evidence (cancer prevention; gastric cancer)

Mechanism of Action

Numerous anticancer mechanisms of action have been proposed for ginseng.[231-248] *Panax ginseng* apparently mitigates cancer through antiinflammatory, antioxidant, and apoptotic mechanisms; additional mechanisms of action include modulating neurotransmission and immune parameters.

In vitro, American ginseng root has been shown to dose-dependently inhibit MCF-7 cell proliferation.[249] Ginsenosides Rc and Re stimulated *c-fos* expression in human breast carcinoma cell lines, but not through estrogen receptors (ERs).[250]

The oral ginsenoside Rh2 has been shown to inhibit the growth of human ovarian cancer cells in animal cancer models.[251] The anticancer effect of ginseng may be attributed to ginsenosides, which are thought to interfere with tumor cell processes.[252]

In vitro, ginsenosides extracted from *P. ginseng* have inductive differentiation effects on all types of acute nonlymphocytic leukemia cells in primary culture.[253] This effect may result from increased intracellular cyclic adenosine monophosphate (cAMP) and interferon.

Antineoplastic effects of ginseng have been found with in vitro, in vivo,[254-264] and epidemiological studies.[265] The nature of this mechanism is poorly understood, but ginsenosides Rg3, Rg5, and Rh2 are active components that may prevent cancer either singularly or synergistically.[266] One study reported a reduction of oxidative DNA damage and protein oxidation in smokers taking ginseng supplements,[267] suggesting antioxidative properties. The compounds that mediate such effects remain unclear. Saponins, polysaccharides, and polyacetylenes are likely to contribute and may act in synergy on neoplastic processes[268] and as immunomodulators.[269] The saponin extract of *P. ginseng* inhibited the production of tumor necrosis factor in mouse skin.[234]

Panax quinquefolius was found to inhibit cancer cell growth synergistically when used with breast cancer agents (e.g., cytoxan, doxorubicin, fluorouracil, methotrexate).[270] Triol saponins in combination with polysaccharides from Korean red ginseng exhibit a protective effect on the formation and growth of tumors in mice. One study found that the intestinal bacterial metabolite M1 of protopanaxadiol saponins of ginseng exhibited antimetastatic activity.[271] *Panax ginseng* had an inductive differentiation effect on all types of acute nonlymphocytic leukemia cells, possibly by increasing intracellular cAMP and inducing interferon.[253] Korean red ginseng administered to mice prevented cancer-causing and proliferative effects of DMBA, urethane, and aflatoxin compared with controls.[272] Lipid-soluble components of *P. ginseng* were found to block cell cycle progression and thus inhibit the proliferation of human renal cancer cell lines.[273]

In mice transplanted with sarcoma and melanoma, treatment with red ginseng and paclitaxel increased life span by inducing the secretion of interleukin-6, restoring the proliferation of splenocytes and NK cell activity, and increasing tumoricidal activity of macrophages.[238] In vitro, renal carcinoma cell proliferation was inhibited by lipid-soluble components of *P. ginseng* roots, which blocked cell cycle progression at the G1 to S phase transition.[273] Ginsenoside-Rh2 inhibited the growth of MCF-7 human breast carcinoma cells by inducing protein expression of p21 and reducing the protein levels of cyclin D, which downregulated cyclin/Cdk complex kinase activity, decreased phosphorylation of pRb, and inhibited E2f release.[239] Panaxytriol from *P. ginseng* accelerates mitomycin C cellular accumulation in vitro.[274]

A study of 101 patients with various cancers was described in a secondary review. It reported that in patients treated with ginseng plus chemotherapy, 70% showed symptomatic improvement in their general condition (fewer symptoms, improved appetite, weight gain) as well as improvements in various clinical parameters (hemoglobin, immunoglobulin, lymphocytes).[275] The positive effects of supplemental treatment with ginseng were observed especially in patients with colon and stomach cancer. However, this has not been confirmed with the primary source.

Based on animal and laboratory studies, differentiation of HL-60 (promyelocytic cells) is induced in Rh2- and Rh3-treated cells. Rh2 appears to cause arrest of B16-BL6 melanoma cells at the G1 phase along with suppression of cyclin-dependent kinase-2. Studies with Rh2 show inhibited growth of human ovarian cancer xenografts and prolonged survival in nude mice.[276] Use of *Panax ginseng* for chemoprevention may reduce the incidence of chemically induced lung, liver, skin, and ovarian cancers in mice.

Scientific Evidence of Effectiveness

CANCER PREVENTION. The preventive effect of ginseng intake has been suggested for various human cancers based on the data from a case-control study.[277] The findings supported the view that ginseng consumers had a decreased risk for most cancers compared with nonconsumers. Several studies that used medium-term and long-term anticarcinogenesis models in animals showed that ginseng extracts have a tumor-inhibitory effect in mice exposed to chemical carcinogens.[272,278,279] Epidemiological and prospective studies have been conducted with some showing that ginseng *(Panax ginseng)* consumers had a lower risk for gastric and lung cancer, suggesting that ginseng may have a non–organ-specific anticarcinogenic effect.[240,280,281]

GASTRIC CANCER. As an adjunct to surgical resection and chemotherapy, ginseng has been reported to improve patient survival and immune parameters in gastric cancer patients.[282]

Dose

The dose of ginseng for cancer prevention and treatment has not been determined. Ginseng extracts may be standardized to 4% to 7% total ginsenosides content,[283] and a typical dose is 100 to 200 mg daily.[284] As a result of controlled studies, the official German pharmacopeia prescribes daily dosages of 1 to 2 g dried ginseng root or 20 to 30 mg ginsenosides.[285] Based on historical and common use of gingseng, the typical daily dose may be 1 to 2 g of raw herb (root) or 100 to 200 mg of a standardized extract containing 4% to 7% ginsenosides.

Adverse Effects, Interactions, Pharmacokinetics. See Appendix A.

Goji (*Lycium* spp.)

Grade C: *Unclear or conflicting scientific evidence (cancer)*

Mechanism of Action

In vitro research has demonstrated that *Lycium barbarum* extract (LBE) inhibits proliferation and stimulates apoptosis in cultured hepatocarcinoma cells.[286,287] It was surmised that the antiproliferative activity of LBP may occur by inducing cell cycle arrest and increasing intracellular calcium.

Scientific Evidence of Effectiveness

Polysaccharide constituents, such as the alpha-glucans and beta-glucans from a variety of plants, are reported to have immune system–enhancing properties. Some clinical evidence suggests that *Lycium barbarum* polysaccharide (LBP) has synergistic effects in the treatment of various cancers when administered with LAK/IL-2.[288] Patients treated with combination therapy showed greater increases in NK and LAK cell activity and longer mean remission.

Dose

The dose of goji in cancer prevention and treatment has not been established. A typical dose is 6 to 15 g daily of *Lycium* berries.[289] According to anecdotal reports, 3 to 4 oz of goji juice has been taken for a variety of conditions. Traditionally, the goji leaf has been taken as a tea. A typical daily dose is one or more cups of tea of varying strength.

Adverse Effects, Interactions, Pharmacokinetics. See Appendix A.

Greater Celandine (*Chelidonium majus*)

Grade B: *Good scientific evidence (cancer)*

Grade C: *Unclear or conflicting scientific evidence (esophageal cancer, lung cancer, pancreatic cancer)*

Mechanism of Action

The pharmacological actions of the Chinese herb *Chelidonium majus* have been studied extensively in animals.[290] Human clinical trials have focused primarily on the use of the semisynthetic drug Ukrain (thiophosphoric acid derivative of a sum of the alkaloids isolated from *C. majus*) in the treatment of cancer. These studies have uniformly administered Ukrain via IV injection and demonstrate its anticancer and immunomodulating properties. Investigations into Ukrain's mechanism of action suggest cytotoxic and apoptotic effects against malignant cells but not against normal cells, although limited research has found similar effects against both cancer cells and normal cells in vitro.[291,292] These cytotoxic effects have been attributed to Ukrain's potential to inhibit tubulin polymerization, leading to impaired microtubule dynamics and a metaphase block.[293] The immunomodulating effects of Ukrain include improvements in total T, T-helper (Th), and NK cell counts; decrease in T-suppressor (Ts) cells; and normalization of the H/S ratio.[294,295]

Ukrain induced apoptosis in a panel of cancer cell lines (including HeLa cervical cancer cells) through activation of the intrinsic cell death pathway, as demonstrated by the cleavage of caspase-9 and caspase-3 and the upregulation of caspase-3. Although it did activate NF-κB, Ukrain's effects were not mediated by NF-κB, in contrast to other antineoplastic drugs.[296]

A secondary source reported potential antineoplastic and immunomodulatory properties of Ukrain, which has purportedly demonstrated inhibition of cancer cell growth in vitro, reductions in tumor size in vivo, and partial and complete remissions in cancer patients. Suggested mechanisms of action include disruption of cancer cell metabolism and induction of apoptosis in malignant cells. In addition, Ukrain appears to improve host immunological response through an increase in total T-cell count as well as normalization of the Th/Ts ratio.[297] IV Ukrain was found to be effective in delaying tumor growth in Balb/C mice with genetically identical mammary carcinoma.[298] Ukrain induced cell cycle arrest at the G2/M phase and apoptosis in carcinoma cells, but not in normal human keratinocytes.[299,300] Overexpression of Bcl-2 protein appeared to protect keratinocytes against apoptosis, whereas Bcl-2 expression did not change substantially in ME180 and A431 carcinoma cells.[299]

Scientific Evidence of Effectiveness

CANCER (GENERAL). Clinical trials have resulted in consistently positive outcomes, with Ukrain demonstrating immune system–modulating and immunostimulating properties, cytotoxic effects on malignant cells, and improvements in the clinical course of disease.[292,294,301] A systematic review of randomized clinical trials (RCTs) on Ukrain found that this medicine has promise as an anticancer agent for many types of cancer.[302]

ESOPHAGEAL CANCER. *Chelidonium majus*, with or without the standard chemotherapeutic agent cyclophosphamide, was studied in patients with advanced esophageal cancer.[303] Compared to patients treated with surgery alone or with herbs plus cyclophosphamide, the herbal treatments increased lymphocyte infiltration and apparent cancer cell apoptosis.

LUNG CANCER. The effects of Ukrain in lung cancer patients are comparable to its effects in other types of cancer. It appears to improve immune system function in cancer patients who concurrently demonstrate clinical improvement.[295]

PANCREATIC CANCER. Ukrain combined with the chemotherapeutic drug gemcitabine doubled the median survival time in patients with unresectable pancreatic cancer compared to gemcitabine alone.[304]

Dose

Ukrain is a semisynthetic *Chelidonium majus* alkaloid derivative, consisting of three chelidonine alkaloids combined to form triaziridide.[305] Results of several chemical analyses were inconsistent with the proposed trimeric structure and suggested that at least some commercial preparations of Ukrain are, in fact, a mixture of *C. majus* alkaloids, including chelidonine.

CANCER (GENERAL). Ukrain has been given intravenously to cancer patients in doses of 10 mg every other day or every 3 days, or 20 mg weekly. Ukrain has been used for up to 2 months in clinical trials.[292] The dose of greater celandine for advanced esophageal cancer is not well understood. For lung cancer, IV Ukrain at 10 mg every 3 days was found to improve immunological parameters in men with lung cancer.[295] One course of treatment consisted of 10 injections of 10 mg each. For pancreatic cancer, Ukrain at 20 mg weekly almost doubled the median survival time in pancreatic cancer patients compared with patients given gemcitabine alone.[304]

For stage III cancer patients, intravenous Ukrain at 10 mg every second day had a cytostatic effect on malignant cells and a normalizing effect on the immune system.[292] Each patient received 300 mg of IV Ukrain (30 injections).

Adverse Effects, Interactions, Pharmacokinetics. See Appendix A.

Jiaogulan (*Gynostemma pentaphyllum*)

Grade C: *Unclear or conflicting scientific evidence (cancer)*

Mechanism of Action

In vitro studies have reported that gypenosides extracted from *Gynostemma pentaphyllum* decreased cancer cell viability, arrested the cell cycle, and induced apoptosis in human colon cancer cells and induced apoptosis in human hepatoma cells.[306-308] *G. pentaphyllum* also showed antiproliferative activity against human lung adenocarcinoma cells.[309]

Scientific Evidence of Effectiveness

A clinical study assessed the effects of *G. pentaphyllum* Makino on the immunological function of cancer patients,[310] but study details are unclear.

Dose. Insufficient available evidence.

Adverse Effects, Interactions, Pharmacokinetics. See Appendix A.

Lavender (*Lavandula angustifolia*)

Grade C: *Unclear or conflicting scientific evidence (advanced cancer treatment)*

Mechanism of Action

Components of lavender appear to have cytotoxic properties. It has been demonstrated that perillyl alcohol (POH) modulates cell proliferation in smooth muscle cell cultures.[311] Both limonene and POH have been shown to inhibit tumor growth in rats by blocking initiation and by promoting apoptosis.[312-314] In an in vitro model of lung carcinogenesis, POH had an inhibitory effect on farnesylation, a step toward activation of the oncogene K-ras.

Scientific Evidence of Effectiveness

In clinical studies evaluating POH in patients with various advanced malignancies, no objective tumor responses were seen, despite basic evidence showing potential anticancer effects; however, disease stabilization was reported in some patients. In a Phase II clinical trial of POH in refractory prostate cancer, no objective responses occurred.[315] Similarly, no change in disease progression was seen in metastatic colorectal carcinoma patients treated with POH in another Phase II trial.[316] Thus far, the evidence does not support the use of POH for the treatment of advanced prostate or colorectal cancer. Its effects in other types of cancer (particularly in earlier stages) remain unclear.

Dose

In phase I and II clinical trials, doses of POH 800 to 1600 mg/m^2 four times daily in a 50:50 POH/soybean oil preparation were tolerated with minimal adverse effects; however, clinical effects were not observed.[315-318]

Adverse Effects, Interactions, Pharmacokinetics. See Appendix A.

Maitake Mushroom (Grifola frondosa)

Grade C: *Unclear or conflicting scientific evidence (cancer)*

Mechanism of Action

The polysaccharide fractions of maitake have demonstrated antitumor effects in vitro.[319,320] Furthermore, based on in vitro evidence, the relatively low-molecular-mass polysaccharides isolated from mycelia of *Grifola frondosa* may enhance innate immunity by promoting phagocytosis and increasing NK cell cytotoxicity, thereby serving as biological response modifiers.[321] In preclinical studies, the D-fraction of maitake (β-glucan extract) has been associated with activation of cellular immunity (specifically Th cells); decreased activation of B cells; increased production of interferon-gamma (IFN-γ), interleukin-12 (IL-12), p70, and IL-18; and suppression of IL-4.[319,322] Proposed antitumor mechanisms based on in vitro and animal research include induction of nitric oxide synthase by maitake D fraction,[319,320] enhanced TNF production by macrophages (induced by β-glucan "grifolan" or gel-forming (1→3)-β-D-glucan),[323-325] antiangiogenesis with increased VEGF levels induced by D fraction,[326] oxidative damage and induced apoptosis by β-glucan,[327] increased Kupffer cell activity against neoplastic cells stimulated by a branched-type gel-forming (1→3)-β-D-glucan,[325] enhanced lymphocyte activity,[328] and alternate complement pathway activation.[329]

Scientific Evidence of Effectiveness

In a small case series, therapy with maitake powder and β-glucan MD fraction was associated with tumor regression in greater than 50% of patients with stage II to IV breast, lung, and liver cancer; no improvements were observed in leukemia, gastric cancer, or brain tumors.[330] This series was not well described, with limited information regarding patient baseline characteristics.

Dose

The dosage of maitake for cancer has not been determined.

Milk Thistle (Silybum marianum)

Grade C: *Unclear or conflicting scientific evidence (cancer prevention)*

Mechanism of Action

A flavonoid complex called *silymarin* can be extracted from the seeds of milk thistle and is believed to be the biologically active component. The terms *milk thistle* and *silymarin* are often used interchangeably. A standard milk thistle extract contains 70% silymarin, which is composed of flavonolignans (silydianin, silychristine) and silibinin. According to in vitro assays, the *silibinin* fraction of silymarin has the most biological activity. It has been proposed that silymarin mediates suppression of a nuclear transcription factor through regulation of genes involved in inflammation and carcinogenesis.[331]

Ongoing research on the anticarcinogenic effects of silymarin and silibinin in human breast, cervical, and prostate cancer cells reports significant inhibition of cell and DNA growth; growth of human breast and prostate carcinoma cells was almost completely inhibited by silymarin, and cyclin-dependent kinase inhibitor Cip1/p21 expression drastically increased, resulting in G1 arrest.[332-335] In human leukocytes, silymarin has been found to protect against DNA damage caused by hydrogen peroxide. In a mouse skin model, topical silymarin dramatically reduced UVB and chemically induced carcinogenesis, an effect that may be attributable to the strong antioxidant properties of silymarin.[336,337] Almost complete ablation of chemically induced tumor promotion in rats by silymarin was accompanied by inhibition of the hypothetical endogenous tumor promoter TNF-α.[338] Hydrolysis of glucuronides may expose the intestinal mucosa to carcinogens, and inhibition of β-glucuronidase by silymarin, as demonstrated in rats,[339] may play a preventive role against intestinal carcinogenesis. Silymarin was shown to protect against chemically induced bladder carcinogenesis in mice[340] and to inhibit mitogenic signaling pathways involved in proliferation of androgen-independent and androgen-dependent prostate cancer cells.[341,342]

Scientific Evidence of Effectiveness

Ongoing research on the anticarcinogenic effects of silymarin and silibinin in human breast, cervical, and prostate cancer cells reports that silibinin may inhibit cell growth and DNA replication.[336,337] Investigators at M.D. Anderson Cancer Center have proposed that silymarin suppresses a nuclear transcription factor that activates genes involved in inflammation and carcinogenesis.[331] With human clinical trials lacking, insufficient evidence exists to recommend milk thistle in cancer treatment.

Dose

Milk thistle capsules, tincture, and powder are often standardized to contain 70% to 80% silymarin. In general, up to 450 mg is taken daily in three divided doses.[343] The dose of milk thistle for cancer prevention has not been determined; however, there is a case report of "spontaneous" regression of biopsy-proven unresectable hepatocellular carcinoma in a 52-year-old man after self-medication with 450 mg of silymarin daily.[344]

Adverse Effects, Interactions, Pharmacokinetics. See Appendix A.

Mistletoe (Viscum album)

Grade C: *Unclear or conflicting scientific evidence (cancer)*

Mechanism of Action

Mistletoe is widely used as a medicinal herb and has shown some promise in cancer therapy. Extensive clinical research has evaluated its mechanisms of action and efficacy in treating various cancers. The main active constituent is *mistletoe lectin-1* (ML-1, viscumin), which is a ribosome-inactivating protein that demonstrates potent cytotoxic and antitumor activity in vitro and in vivo.[345-353] The lectins may also target the carbohydrates on the cell's surface, causing agglutination.[354-360] One such lectin, *aviscumine* (recombinant mistletoe lectin), has been the subject of numerous clinical studies.

Mistletoe has been demonstrated to modulate several immune parameters. In tumor patients, twice weekly subcutaneous (SC) injections of 1 mg/kg of ML-1 yielded statistically significant increases in certain acute-phase reactants (C-reactive protein, haptoglobin, ceruloplasmin, C3, albumin, IgM) after 4 weeks of therapy.[361] In tumor patients, mistletoe extracts elicited a humoral response. Immunoglobulin G (IgG, but not IgM) antibodies were detected against lectins and other components. Injection of mistletoe extract in eight cancer patients also caused changes in the levels of TNF-α, IL-1, and IL-6. Enhanced NK cytotoxicity has been observed using *Viscum album* extracts (Iscador) in cytotoxicity assays with human peripheral mononuclear cells and human K562 erythroleukemia cells, as well as in animal studies.[362-364] Rhamnogalacturan from mistletoe also enhanced cytotoxicity of NK cells to erythroleukemia cells in vitro.[365] Induction of increased beta-endorphin plasma levels, which correlated with enhanced activities of blood NK and T cells (correlation between immune and neuroendocrine systems), has been noted with ML-1. Breast cancer patients treated with Iscador displayed increased activity in NK cells and granulocyte phagocytosis.[366-370]

Mistletoe may also exert antitumor effects by inducing apoptosis. A lectin-induced increase in apoptotic nuclei was observed in human peripheral blood lymphocytes and monocytes, murine thymocytes, and human monocytic THP-1 cells when incubated in the presence of *Viscum album* agglutinin-1 (VAA-1).[371,372] Viscotoxins resulted in the generation of reactive oxygen intermediates in human lymphocytes and caused cell death.[373]

Scientific Evidence of Effectiveness

Mistletoe is one of the most widely used alternative cancer treatments in Europe. Results of a 1995 national survey in Germany by the Society for Biologic Cancer Defense found that mistletoe preparations represented 80% of biological drug prescriptions. Studies have examined mistletoe for treating bladder, breast, cervical, central nervous system (CNS), colorectal, head and neck, liver, lung, lymphatic, ovarian, and renal cancers, as well as melanoma and leukemia. However, efficacy has not been conclusively proved for any one condition. In fact, some studies have shown lack of efficacy of certain preparations for a variety of cancers. Larger, well-conducted, randomized trials are needed to provide evidence of efficacy for mistletoe as a cancer treatment or adjuvant therapy.

The National Cancer Institute (NCI) monograph *Mistletoe Extracts* provides a CAM information summary and overview of the use of mistletoe as a treatment for cancer.[6] NCI noted the following: (1) in animal studies, mixed results have been obtained using mistletoe extracts for slowing tumor growth; (2) well-designed clinical trials using mistletoe or its components have not been sufficient to prove efficacy in the treatment of human cancers; and (3) mistletoe plants and berries are toxic to humans, and their extracts are not sold in the United States.

A 2008 systematic review of 21 RCTs concluded that overall methodological quality was poor and results indeterminate.[374] However, some evidence suggests that mistletoe may improve quality of life during breast cancer chemotherapy. Mistletoe products used in clinical trials include Abnoba viscum, Eurixor, Helixor, Iscador (with added copper, mercury, and silver), Isorel, and Vysorel.

Dose

Iscador is marketed as IscadorM (from apple trees), IscadorP (from pine trees), IscadorQ (from oak trees), and IscadorU (from elm trees). Helixor, which is standardized by its biological effect on human leukemia cells in vitro, is marketed as HelixorA (from spruce trees), HelixorM (from apple trees), and HelixorP (from pine trees).

INDUCTION PHASE. According to the manufacturer's directions, each 1-mL ampule is injected subcutaneously two or three times a week or every 2 to 3 days during the induction phase. The series pack is labeled in the order 1 to 7 and the ampules must be administered in numerical order of increasing strength. After 14 injections, there is a 7-day pause before resuming treatment. If the induction phase is well tolerated, the maintenance phase should be started. In the rare event of an overreaction to the induction phase (skin reaction ~5 cm), treatment should be stopped at least 2 to 3 days before resuming administration using the lowest strength.

MAINTENANCE PHASE. The maintenance phase of Iscador offers a choice of two types of treatments: basic therapy with Iscador special or standard therapy with Iscador series.

Basic therapy. Basic therapy is a newer preparation with standardized lectin content. The recommended dosage for Iscador special is IscadorM 5 mg special (for women) and IscadorQu 5 mg special (for men). Iscador special is prescribed in packs of 7 × 5-mg ampules. Each 1-ml ampule is injected subcutaneously two or three times a week or every 2 to 3 days continuously, without treatment pause.

Standard therapy. Standard therapy with Iscador series contains increasing concentrations of active ingredients. Treatment is continued after the induction phase with 2 packs (7 ampules per pack) of series 0, I, or II, selected according to the individual patient's reaction. Each pack contains three strengths: series 0 consists of 2 ampules of 0.01 mg, 2 ampules 0.1 mg, and 3 ampules 1 mg; series I consists of 2 ampules of 0.1 mg, 2 ampules 1 mg, and 3 ampules 10 mg; series II consists of 2 ampules of 1 mg, 2 ampules 10 mg, and 3 ampules 20 mg. Each 1-mL ampule is injected subcutaneously two or three times a week or every 2 to 3 days. The series pack is labeled in the order 1 to 7, and the ampules must be administered in numerical order of increasing strength. After 14 injections, there is a 7-day pause before resuming treatment. The type of Iscador is selected according to the primary tumor site.

PREOPERATIVE AND POSTOPERATIVE TREATMENT. According to the manufacturers, Iscador can be used to reduce the risk of developing cancer recurrences or metastases and to promote the activation of the immune system to improve recovery.

Basic therapy (Iscador special). Preoperative therapy begins 14 days before surgery with an induction phase of series 0 (1 × 7 ampules). Postoperative therapy begins 14 days after surgery with an induction phase of series 0 (2 × 7 ampules, then 7-day pause). Maintenance phase begins using basic therapy of Iscador special (if induction phase is well tolerated).

Standard therapy (Iscador series): Preoperative therapy begins 14 days before surgery with an induction phase of series 0 (1 × 7 ampules). Postoperative therapy begins 14 days after surgery with induction phase of series 0 (2 × 7 ampules, then 7-day pause). The maintenance phase begins using standard therapy of Iscador series (when tolerated as long-term therapy). Iscador (mistletoe) has been used in various clinical trials for cancer at doses of 1 ng/kg body weight.[375]

Adverse Effects, Interactions, Pharmacokinetics. See Appendix A.

Modified Citrus Pectin

Grade C: *Unclear or conflicting scientific evidence (prostate cancer)*

Mechanism of Action

Pectins are gel-forming polysaccharides from plant cell walls, especially found in apple and citrus fruits. Although pectins are not digestible by humans, modified citrus pectin (MCP) is altered to increase its absorbability. In animal models of breast, colon, and lung cancers, oral MCP significantly inhibited carbohydrate-mediated tumor growth, angiogenesis, and metastasis, presumably through its effects on the galactose-specific lectin 3 (galectin-3) molecules on the surface of cancer cells. Galectin-3 binds to galactose, allowing cells to aggregate and adhere to other cells.[376-379] Galectin-3 may be pivotal in mitosis and proliferation, especially because metastatic cells of specific cancers (e.g., prostate, lung, breast) have more galectin-3 on their surface than healthy cells. Galactose-rich MCP is thought to saturate the galactose-binding sites on the cancer cell surface by tightly binding with galectins.[380-383] With MCP bound to the cell surface, the cancer cell is thought to be unable to aggregate with other cancer cells or adhere to normal cells, thereby reducing the ability to metastasize. This provides preclinical evidence for a possible mechanism of action in prostate cancer. In vitro, the addition of MCP to the media of cultured androgen-independent human prostatic JCA-1 cells reduced cell growth and correspondingly [^{3}H]-thymidine incorporation into DNA.[377] This also provides preclinical evidence for a possible mechanism of action in prostate cancer.

Scientific Evidence of Effectiveness

According to preliminary research, MCP significantly slowed the progression of prostate cancer in 9 of 12 patients, as measured by changes in PSA levels. Notably, although PSA doubling time is believed to be a surrogate marker for progression of disease, it has not been proven that PSA doubling time correlates with true clinical outcomes, such as survival or pain.

Dose

The recommended oral dose of PectaSol brand MCP is 15 g daily in three divided doses.[384] However, an effective dose has not yet been determined for cancer treatment.

Adverse Effects, Interactions, Pharmacokinetics. See Appendix A.

Oleander (Nerium oleander, Thevetia peruviana)

Grade C: *Unclear or conflicting scientific evidence (cancer)*
Note: All parts of the oleander plant (including flowers, leaves, and nectar) are considered toxic and are not recommended for consumption.

Mechanism of Action

The main active constituents of oleander, oleandrin and oleandrigenin, possess cytotoxic properties. The inhibition of the sodium-potassium adenosine triphosphatase (Na^+,K^+-ATPase) exchange pump, with resulting increased intracellular calcium (Ca^{2+}) is thought to cause a release of mitochondrial cytochrome *c*, activation of the caspase cascade, and PARP cleavage. Fibroblast growth factor 2 (FGF-2), a cellular protein involved in cell differentiation and tumor growth, is exported from the cell through alpha-subunit binding to the Na^+,K^+-ATPase pump; thus, pump inhibition may decrease FGF-2 release from the cell.[385,386] Oleandrin also blocks activation of the transcription factor NF-κB, which may also contribute to its antitumor effects.

Scientific Evidence of Effectiveness

The term *oleander* refers to two common plant species, *Nerium oleander* (common oleander) and *Thevetia peruviana* (yellow oleander), which grow in temperate climates throughout the world. However, purported medicinal effects are largely attributed to *N. oleander*. The anticancer effects of oleander extracts are being investigated largely using in vitro cell line models. Anvirzel (Ozelle Pharmaceuticals), an aqueous *N. oleander* extract, is currently being studied in Phase I trials for its antitumor effects. In November 2006 the manufacturer's website discussed the status of this investigational drug, including the lack of safety and efficacy data. Before this, in March 2000, the FDA issued a warning to Ozelle after claims on the Ozelle website that Anvirzel was safe and effective based on preliminary and inconclusive data.

A Phase I trial of parenteral Anvirzel reported no antitumor response in patients with advanced, refractory solid tumors.[387] Despite the lack of efficacy data, oleander is promoted on a number of websites as an anticancer or antiviral agent.

Dose

In a Phase I clinical trial, Anvirzel was administered to patients with refractory solid tumors by intramuscular injection in doses of 0.1, 0.2, and 0.4 mL/m²/day (with subsequent patients receiving 0.8 or 1.2 mL/m²/day sequentially).[387] No antitumor activity was observed; the recommended Phase II dose was 0.8 mL/m²/day.

Peony (*Paeonia* spp.)

Grade C: Unclear or conflicting scientific evidence (lung cancer)

Mechanism of Action

In vitro research has demonstrated several anticancer mechanisms of action for various peony preparations. These include antiangiogenic effects for 1,2,3,4,6-penta-*O*-galloyl-β-D-glucose (PGG), found in peony root, apoptotic effects for *Paeonia* radix root-derived resveratrol and its derivatives, and cytotoxic and antimutagenic effects for stilbenes found in seeds.[388-391]

Scientific Evidence of Effectiveness

In one case report a lung carcinoma patient was treated with a traditional Chinese formula *Ninjin Yoei To* (dried extract obtained from peony, ginseng, cinnamon bark, Japanese angelica root, astragalus root, peony root, citrus unshiu peel, rehmannia root, polygala root, atractyloides rhizome, schisandra fruit, *Poria sclerotium*, and glycyrrhiza) for 7 weeks.[392] After 7 weeks there was a decrease in the patient's CEA and CA 19-9 (tumor marker) levels. In addition, appetite improved and cough disappeared. Despite these favorable results, the effects of peony are difficult to distinguish from the other constituents of this combination therapy.

Dose

The dose of peony as a monotherapy for lung cancer has not been determined.

Adverse Effects, Interactions, Pharmacokinetics. See Appendix A.

Podophyllum (*Podophyllum* spp.)

Grade C: Unclear or conflicting scientific evidence (uterine cancer)

Mechanism of Action

According to case reports and clinical evidence, podophyllum seems to be cytotoxic by interrupting cellular mitosis at metaphase.[393-395] It also appears to exert antiproliferative effects by inhibiting mitochondrial function,[396] DNA synthesis,[397-399] premitotic microtubule assembly,[397,398] and protein synthesis.[397]

In mice, the aqueous extract of podophyllum, RP-1, which provided significant protection to whole-body–irradiated animals, exerted tumoricidal effects.[396] RP-1 at 0.5 to 10 mcg/L reduced colonogenic survival, increased the free-radical generation, induced cell cycle arrest, and increased apoptosis. Mitochondrial antiapoptotic proteins Bcl-2 and Hsp-70 levels were also reduced by RP-1 treatment in a dose- and time-dependent manner.

Although promising in the treatment of cancer, podophyllum (podophyllin) may be toxic to healthy cells. Podophyllin has demonstrated neurotoxic,[400-402] hepatoxic,[397] and necrotic[403] effects.

Scientific Evidence of Effectiveness

Podophyllum has been used in traditional Ayurvedic medicine for the treatment of genital warts, Hodgkin's disease, Non-Hodgkin's lymphoma, and other types of cancers. However, there is a lack of supportive clinical evidence for these indications. The available evidence, although preliminary, suggests that podophyllum increased survival when used as an adjunct to radiation therapy for uterine cancer.[404]

Dose

Standardized doses of podophyllum have not been rigorously tested in human trials. One clinical study used 1 g of parenteral podophyllum daily after radiation therapy, for a total dose of 30 to 50 g over the course of treatment.[404]

Adverse Effects, Interactions, Pharmacokinetics. See Appendix A.

PSK (*Coriolus versicolor*)

Grade C: *Unclear or conflicting scientific evidence (cancer adjuvant [colorectal; esophageal; gastric; leukemia; liver; lung; nasopharyngeal])*

Mechanism of Action

The *Coriolus versicolor* mushroom has been used in traditional Chinese medicine (TCM) since the Ming Dynasty of China. The *polysaccharide K* (PSK) *fraction*, obtained from cultured mycelia of the mushroom, is thought to have antitumor properties. PSK (biological response modifier) extracts are available for clinical use in Japan, where they are currently the best-selling cancer treatment, used in conjunction with surgery, chemotherapy, and radiation therapy. Its active ingredient can be administered as a tea or a capsule. A similar product labeled simply *"Coriolus versicolor extract"* is available in limited supply in the United States.

Potential antitumor modes of PSK action include induction of cell cycle arrest, apoptosis, caspase-3 expression,[405,406] cytochrome *c* release, and decreased expression of Bcl-2 and cyclin B1.[407] PSK showed antitumor effects in a lung carcinoma mouse model and enhanced the antitumor effect of tegafur/uracil (UFT) with leucovorin in a sarcoma mouse model.[408]

Injection of PSK increased tumor rejection and survival in neonatal mice, but no effect was seen in athymic mice, suggesting an immunomodulatory role for PSK.[409] PSK decreased production of IL-4 and IL-10 and slightly increased production of TNF-α and INF-γ, as well as activity of NK and cytotoxic T cells.[410] Several other studies (in vitro, in vivo, human) have demonstrated the apoptotic and cytotoxic potential of PSK.[411-417]

Scientific Evidence of Effectiveness

In humans, PSK inhibited NF-ϰB in tumor cells and independently improved prognosis in colon cancer patients.[418] Colorectal cancer patients treated with PSK showed increased serum levels of collagen type IV, which were attributed to increased vascular basement membrane degradation by PSK.[419] PSK treatment may also exert immunomodulatory effects, as evidenced by increased DNA synthesis in peripheral lymphocytes isolated from gastric and colorectal cancer patients.[420]

There is some evidence that *Coriolus versicolor* may be effective in inducing regression of low-grade squamous intraepithelial lesions (LSILs), which often precede cervical cancer. In a study conducted by Mycology Research Laboratories,[421] *C. versicolor* (or placebo) was administered to patients infected with human papillomavirus (HPV) subtypes associated with cervical cancer. Treatment was associated with greater reversion to normal cytology (72.5%, vs. 47.5% placebo). Furthermore, most recipients reverted to a negative HPV status after treatment, versus only 8.5% in the control group. These encouraging results warrant further research to ascertain the efficacy of *C. versicolor* in cancer treatment or prevention.

An uncontrolled trial reported improved survival in cancer patients compared with historical controls.[422] PSK has been reported to improve survival in colorectal,[423-427] gastric,[428-434] breast,[435,436] esophageal,[437,438] lung,[439-441] hepatocellular,[442] and nasopharyngeal[443] carcinoma and in acute leukemia.[444] Other trials have reported no benefit.[422,445-449] PSK improved survival in a subset of colorectal cancer patients with histological evidence of diffuse beta-catenin activation within tumor cells.[418] Preoperative CEA and PPD values were reported to be predictive of colorectal cancer response to PSK therapy.[450]

In gastric cancer, PSK improved survival in patients with a preoperative granulocyte/lymphocyte ratio of 2.0 or higher, but had no effect in patients with lower ratios.[451] HLA-A$_2$ antigen in gastric cancer patients correlated with a better postoperative response to PSK than to chemotherapy.[452]

Two breast cancer trials reported improved survival with PSK.[435,436] However, other studies have reported no survival benefit with PSK as an adjuvant therapy.[436,453] In breast cancer patients, presence of the HLA-B40 allele corresponded to increased disease-free survival in PSK-treated patients.[454]

Dose

For tumors, PSK has been used at 3 g daily (or every other day), either alone or with conventional therapy. PSK has also been administered at 2 g/m^2 daily in three divided doses for 1 month. HPV-infected women with LSILs were supplemented with *Coriolus versicolor* (3 g daily) for 1 year.

Adverse Effects, Interactions, Pharmacokinetics. See Appendix A.

Psyllium (*Plantago* spp.)

Grade C: *Unclear or conflicting scientific evidence (colon cancer)*

Mechanism of Action

As with other forms of dietary fiber, psyllium is thought to help maintain intestinal health, and may help maintain normal cell proliferation in the colon.[455,456] Psyllium alone does not appear to affect the absorption of carcinogens in the gastrointestinal tract, and the soluble fiber formed by psyllium does not bind to carcinogens; rather, it is widely believed that psyllium's benefits are due to its metabolic products. Soluble fibers such as psyllium fiber are metabolized to butyrate[457] and propionic acid[458] in the colon, which appear to have anticarcinogenic effects. Some evidence suggests that psyllium might improve the chemoprotective effect of wheat bran.[459]

Dietary supplementation with a 4%:4% mixture of an insoluble (wheat bran) fiber and a soluble (psyllium) fiber to a high-fat diet inhibited tumorigenesis in a mouse mammary tumor model.[460]

Scientific Evidence of Effectiveness

Preliminary clinical research has demonstrated that psyllium increases the concentration of butyrate by 42% in postsurgical patients.[457] The effects of psyllium on survival and prognosis in cancer patients remain to be established.

Dose

For colon cancer, an oral dose of 20 g of *Plantago ovata* seeds was used daily for 3 months.[457]

Adverse Effects, Interactions, Pharmacokinetics. See Appendix A.

Red Clover (Trifolium pratense)

Grade C: *Unclear or conflicting scientific evidence (prostate cancer)*

Mechanism of Action

The red clover isoflavones biochanin A and genistein have been shown to inhibit cell proliferation in vitro; apoptosis is believed to be the primary mechanism of action, based on demonstrated DNA fragmentation.[461-463] Genistein inhibits cell proliferation through inhibition of tyrosine kinases and DNA synthesis.[464] It has been speculated that genistein's cytotoxicity may also be the result of disrupted RNA synthesis.[465] Coumestrol, another isoflavone found in high quantities in red clover, has been shown in vitro to exhibit both mutagenic and clastogenic (chromosome-breaking) properties in cultured human lymphoblastoid cells.[466] Isoflavones such as genistein are believed to have estrogen-like effects in the body and thus are sometimes called "phytoestrogens," which may exert antiandrogenic properties. These effects have also been proposed as possibly beneficial in prostatic hyperplasia or prostate cancer.[467]

Scientific Evidence of Effectiveness

A small clinical study reported increased apoptosis in prostate specimens of men acutely exposed to red clover preoperatively.[468] A case report of a patient who took red clover supplements (Promensil) for 7 days before prostate cancer surgery reported histological changes in the postsurgical prostate suggestive of androgen deprivation.[469] These reports indicate a possible cytotoxic effect of red clover in prostate cancer, but further clinical evidence is required before a recommendation can be made.

Dose

The dose of red clover for cancer treatment or prevention has not been determined. In one case report, however, postsurgical histological changes were observed in a patient who took four 40-mg red clover isoflavone tablets (Promensil) daily for 7 days before surgery.[469]

Adverse Effects, Interactions, Pharmacokinetics. See Appendix A.

Reishi Mushroom (Ganoderma lucidum)

Grade C: *Unclear or conflicting scientific evidence (cancer)*

Mechanism of Action

Numerous in vitro studies have shown *Ganoderma lucidum* to inhibit growth in various tumor cell lines.[470-480] In vivo studies also demonstrated a potential anticancer effect of *G. lucidum*. Multiple mechanisms have been proposed, including apoptosis induction[481] through caspase-3 activation[482] or upregulation of Bax.[483,484] Potential cytotoxic mechanisms include lipid peroxidation and free-radical inactivation,[485-488] TNF-α induction and interleukin production,[481,489,490] enhanced neutrophil phagocytosis and chemotaxis,[491] and enhanced NK cell activity.[492,493] *G. lucidum* has also been shown to have antiangiogenic effects[470] and to inhibit tumor cell migration and invasion.*

Scientific Evidence of Effectiveness

A case of complete regression of advanced-stage lymphoma after *Ganoderma lucidum* treatment has been reported.[497] Treatment with reishi mushroom extract (Ganopoly) for 12 weeks resulted in a significant increase in plasma levels of IL-2, IL-6, and IFN-γ, decreased IL-1 and TNF-α levels, and increased NK cells in advanced-stage cancer patients.[492] Well-designed long-term studies are needed to confirm these results and to examine potential side effects.

Dose

For cancer, 600 to 1800 mg of reishi has been taken three times daily for 12 weeks.[492,493,498]

Adverse Effects, Interactions, Pharmacokinetics. See Appendix A.

Rhodiola (Rhodiola rosea)

Grade C: *Unclear or conflicting scientific evidence (bladder cancer)*

Mechanism of Action

Antimutagenic activity has been shown for *Rhodiola rosea* in vitro.[499,500] *Rhodiola* extract inhibited proliferation and induced cell cycle arrest in erythroleukemic cells[501] and promyelocytic leukemia cells without harming normal human lymphocytes.[502] In animals with transplantable

---

*References 477, 478, 480, 483, 484, 494-496.

tumors, *R. rosea* increased survival and decreased metastasis.[503-505]

Scientific Evidence of Effectiveness

Limited clinical evidence suggests that *Rhodiola rosea* may offer some benefits for patients with superficial bladder cancer, with improvement seen in the characteristics of the urothelial tissue integration, parameters of leukocyte integrins, and T-cell immunity; however, no effects on frequency of relapse were observed.[506]

Dose

Rhodiola extracts may be standardized to contain a minimum of 3% rosavins and 1% salidroside. Doses of 200 to 600 mg *Rhodiola rosea* are generally recommended by natural medicine experts; high doses are considered to be daily intakes of 1000 mg and higher. Although not supported by available clinical evidence, it is recommended to take *Rhodiola* on an empty stomach and to take a break from treatment every 1 to 2 weeks. *Rhodiola* extract was examined for its effect on superficial bladder cancer recurrence;[507] however, the effective dose is unclear.

Adverse Effects, Interactions, Pharmacokinetics. See Appendix A.

Rhubarb (*Rheum* spp.)

Grade C: Unclear or conflicting scientific evidence (nasopharyngeal carcinoma)

Mechanism of Action

Rhapontin, derived from rhubarb, inhibited growth and induced apoptosis in cultured human stomach cancer cells.[508] *Emodin*, a constituent of rhubarb, inhibited *c-myc* messenger RNA expression in vitro.[509] In another in vitro study, emodin (50 micromol) induced CH27 cell apoptosis.[510] This apoptosis does not involve modulation of endogenous Bcl-X(L) protein expression, but appears to be associated with the increased expression of cellular Bak and Bax proteins. Emodin has been reported to act through the tyrosine kinases, phosphoinositol-3-kinase (PI3K), protein kinase C (PKC), NF-κB, and mitogen-activated protein kinase (MAPK) signaling cascades.[511,512] Emodin also inhibits matrix metalloproteases (MMPs) in cancer cell lines.[512] *Aloe-emodin,* another anthroquinone isolated from rhubarb, exerts antitumor effects through modulation of the p53 and p21 pathway, cAMP-dependent protein kinase, PKC, Bcl-2, caspase-3, caspase-8, caspase-9, p38 protein expression, and cytochrome *c* release.[511,513,514] Another constituent, *rhein,* affects cellular glucose uptake and membrane function, resulting in cell death.[511] Rhein induces apoptosis in hepatoblastoma cells through increased expression of p53 and p21/WAF1 proteins and enhanced CD95 and CD95 ligand activity.[515] There is limited evidence that the hydroxyanthraquinone compound emodin from rhubarb blocks ERK phosphorylation of prostate cancer cells, suggesting anticancer potential.[516]

Scientific Evidence of Effectiveness

Nasopharyngeal carcinoma patients treated with radiotherapy with or without *shenlong* oral liquid, which contains rhubarb and other herbs, showed no effects on remission or survival rate, but did have decreased adverse effects and a decreased dose of radiation at remission.[517] Because shenlong contains multiple herbs, the direct effects of rhubarb are difficult to determine.

Dose

The dose of rhubarb as a monotherapy for cancer has not been determined.

Adverse Effects, Interactions, Pharmacokinetics. See Appendix A.

Sage (*Salvia officinalis*)

Grade C: Unclear or conflicting scientific evidence (lung cancer prevention)

Mechanism of Action

An aqueous and 50% ethanolic extract of *Salvia officinalis* exhibited strong cytotoxic activity in vitro, greater than that of the antibiotic tetracycline.[518] Quinones from *S. officinalis* roots, called *royleanones,* displayed marked protonophoric activity on artificial bilayer lipid membranes in vitro and exerted an uncoupling action on oxidative phosphorylation in isolated rat liver mitochondria.[519] The results suggest that biological membranes are the primary targets of royleanones, and that the protonophoric activity may contribute to the cytotoxic and antimicrobial properties of sage.

In vitro, three diterpenoid quinones, royleanone (SAR 3), horminone (SAR 26), and acetyl horminone (SAR 43), isolated from the roots of *S. officinalis* were tested for their cytotoxic and DNA-damaging activity in human colon carcinoma (Caco-2) cells and human hepatoma (HepG2) cells cultured in vitro.[520] Although all the quinones tested decreased the viability of the cells in a dose-dependent manner, the rate of apoptosis (equal to a topoisomerase I inhibitor) was demonstrated only in HepG2 cells treated with 1×10^{-4} mol/L SAR 26 or SAR 43. There was minimal or no increase in the levels of apoptotic nuclei in SAR 3–treated HepG2 cells and in the Caco-2 cells treated with SAR 3, SAR 26, or SAR 43. All compounds tested induced DNA strand breaks in both cell types at concentrations greater than 1×10^{-7} to 1×10^{-6} mol/L. The authors noted that the kinetics of DNA break repair revealed that SAR-induced DNA breaks were repaired very slowly.

Scientific Evidence of Effectiveness

Epidemiological evidence suggests sage may have chemoprotective effects and may decrease lung cancer risk. According to a case-control study, patients who use sage as a spice in cooking have a 54% lower risk of lung cancer than those who do not use sage as a spice.[521] Additional clinical evidence is warranted.

Dose

Sage used daily as a spice in foods has been associated with a lower risk of lung cancer in the Mediterranean diet.[521] The exact quantity or frequency of consumption has not been determined in relation to this effect.

Adverse Effects, Interactions, Pharmacokinetics. See Appendix A.

Saw Palmetto *(Serenoa repens)*

Grade C: *Unclear or conflicting scientific evidence (cancer prevention, prostate cancer treatment/prevention)*

Mechanism of Action

Note: Saw palmetto is an ingredient in PC-SPES, a combination product used for prostate cancer, which was recalled from the U.S. market after it was found to contain small amounts of an undeclared prescription drug (warfarin).[5]

An in vitro study of cultured fibroblasts and epithelial cells derived from prostate, epididymis, testes, skin, and breast tissue suggested that saw palmetto (Permixon) may selectively act to disrupt intracellular nuclear membranes of prostate cells, thereby increasing apoptosis.[522] Antiproliferative and proapoptotic properties have been attributed to saw palmetto based on the results of other in vitro studies that demonstrated inhibition of growth factor–induced hyperplasia.[523-527] In human urological cancer cell lines, saw palmetto extract inhibited urokinase-type plasminogen activator, an enzyme implicated in tumor cell invasion.[528] In vitro data demonstrated that the antiproliferative effect exerted by the ethanolic extract of *Serenoa repens* is at least triggered by the induction of apoptosis.[529] The effect of an ethanolic extract of *S. repens* (10-1000 mcg/mL) was tested in hormone-sensitive LNCaP, MCF-7, and hormone-insensitive DU-145, renal Caki-1, urinary bladder J82, colon HCT-116, and lung A549 cancer cells, as well as MDA-MB231 prostate and breast carcinoma cell lines. The *S. repens* extract induced a dose-dependent antiproliferative effect on all human malignant cells tested, with GI_{50} values between 107 and 327 mcg/mL. In hormone-sensitive prostate LNCaP and breast MCF-7 cell lines, the effect of the ethanolic extract of *S. repens* expressed in GI_{50} was 2.2- and 2.5-fold more potent than in hormone-insensitive DU-145 and MDA-MB231 cells. The proportion of apoptotic cells, except in A549 cells, was 22.5% to 36.3%. *S. repens* extract did not induce apoptosis in lung cancer A549 cells.

In vitro and in vivo research demonstrated a biological response to homeopathic preparations of *Sabal serrulata* (another name for saw palmetto), *Thuja occidentalis*, and *Conium maculatum*, as manifested by cell proliferation and tumor growth. This biological effect was significantly stronger for *S. serrulata* than for control, and the response was specific to human prostate cancer.[530] Treatment with *S. serrulata* in vitro resulted in a 33% decrease of PC-3 cell proliferation at 72 hours and a 23% reduction of DU-145 cell proliferation at 24 hours. The difference in reduction is likely caused by the specific doubling time of each cell line. No effect was observed on MDA-MB231 human breast cancer cells. In vivo, prostate tumor xenograft size was significantly reduced in *S. serrulata*–treated mice compared with untreated controls. No effect was observed on breast tumor growth. In other in vitro study, researchers investigated the effect of the homeopathic preparations *C. maculatum*, *S. serrulata*, *T. occidentalis*, Asterias, Phytolacca, and Carcinosin on prostate and breast cancer cell (DU-145, LNCaP, MAT-LyLu, MDA-MB231) growth and on gene expression that regulates apoptosis, using MTT and multiprobe ribonuclease protection assay.[531] None of the tested homeopathic remedies in different potencies produced significant inhibitory or growth-promoting activity in either prostate or breast cancer cells. Also, gene expression studies by ribonuclease protection assay produced no significant changes in mRNA levels of bax, bcl-2, bcl-x, caspase-1, caspase-2, caspase-3, Fas, or FasL after treatment with homeopathic medicines. Based on these results, the authors concluded that the highly diluted anticancer remedies used by homeopathic practitioners show no measurable effects on cell growth or gene expression in vitro using currently available methodologies.

Scientific Evidence of Effectiveness

CANCER PREVENTION. In homeopathy, *Sabal serrulata* is often prescribed for many types of prostate conditions, including prostate cancer.[530] A prospective cohort study found no association between saw palmetto use and the development of prostate cancer.[532] However, limited human data are available on the efficacy of saw palmetto to prevent prostate cancer. Additional, well-designed studies are needed before a firm conclusion can be made.

PROSTATE CANCER TREATMENT/PREVENTION. More studies are required before saw palmetto can be recommended for prostate cancer patients. The scientific evidence is insufficient to recommend the discontinued combination product PC-SPES, which contains saw palmetto, for prostate cancer. The FDA issued a warning not to use PC-SPES, and it is no longer commercially available because it was found to contain the anticoagulant warfarin.[5]

Dose

Insufficient data exist for an effective dosage of saw palmetto for prostate cancer prevention or treatment.

Adverse Effects Interactions, Pharmacokinetics. See Appendix A.

Shiitake Mushroom *(Lentinus edodes)*

Grade C: *Unclear or conflicting scientific evidence (chemotherapy adjuvant)*

Mechanism of Action

Chemopreventive effects of plant polysaccharides from *Lentinus edodes* have been shown with in vitro screening assays.[533] Lentin, isolated from *L. edodes*, is a beta-glucan shown to inhibit leukemia cell proliferation in vitro.[534] In animal models, *lentinan* displayed antitumor activity against allogeneic, syngeneic, and autochthonous tumors.[535,536] In an animal model, oral administration of *L. edodes* mycelia increased IL-1 levels in liver and spleen;[537] this was suggested as one possible antimetastatic mechanism of shiitake. Beta-(1→6)-branched beta-(1→3)-glucohexaose (the basic unit of lentinan), as well as several of its analogs, inhibited U(14) noumenal tumors in mice.[538]

In animals the lipid and polysaccharide fractions of shiitake were thought to have antitumor and immune-potentiating (increased macrophages and NK activity) effects.[539] Mice treated orally with lentinan had smaller tumors compared with tumors from non–lentinan-fed mice.[540] Also, when lymphocytes from these mice were given to athymic nude mice, smaller tumors were also formed in the nude mice. According to animal research, the polysaccharide L-II, isolated from the fruiting body of *Lentinus edodes*, may have antitumor activity in mice mediated by T-cell and macrophage-dependent immune system responses.[541]

In vitro, lentinan bound to monocytes from healthy subjects.[542] This binding was completely inhibited by a combination of anti-CR1 and anti-CR3 monoclonal antibodies. Also, lentinan-bound monocytes in the peripheral blood of the healthy subjects increased within 3 to 4 hours after intravenous (IV) administration of 2 mg lentinan (in 3 mcg/mL solution) and returned to low levels by 5 hours after injection. There was no increase in lentinan-bound neutrophils or lymphocytes.

In vitro, ethanol extracts of *Lentinus edodes* induced a transient G1 arrest in murine skin carcinoma cells (CH72) with no changes in nontumorigenic epidermal cells (C50).[543] In vitro a xylose-rich heteroglycan-protein fraction prepared from the culture medium of *L. edodes* also stimulated the production of IFN-γ and nitrite in mouse splenic cells.[544]

In vitro experiments using human and murine tumor cell lines showed that sulfated *Lentinus edodes*–derived alpha-(1→3)-D-glucan had antiproliferation activity at a concentration of 20 mcg/mL toward four tumor cell lines.[545] In vitro, *L. edodes* mycelia inhibited growth of human breast carcinoma–derived cells (MCF-7 cells).[546]

The potential antitumor activity of shiitake mushroom appears to be protein dependent. In an animal model, lentinan accelerated tumor growth in protein-deficient animals.[547-549] There was no beneficial effect of lentinan in patients with low serum protein levels (<5.9 g/dL).

Intraperitoneal administration of lentinan enhanced an interstitial response and resulted in the development of reticular fibers.[550] In gastric cancer patients, lentinan administration resulted in fragmentation of cancer cell nests with infiltrated T lymphocytes. In animals and breast cancer patients, lentinan injection (dosage unclear) after surgical therapy induced atrophy of tumors.[551] This was accompanied by infiltration of T cells, B cells, and macrophages into the stroma around the tumor.

Scientific Evidence of Effectiveness

Shiitake is used traditionally in Asia as a food and medicine. Combination therapy of lentinan with chemotherapeutic agents has resulted in reduced tumor size, improved symptoms, and improved survival time in various clinical trials and case studies.[552-569] One RCT suggests that intramuscular (IM) injection of lentinan (2 mg weekly for inpatients, or 4 mg every 2 weeks for outpatients) in combination with oral tegafur chemotherapy (400-800 mg daily) may offer survival benefit in prostate cancer.[570] In an open study, there was no effect of lentinan on PSA levels.[571] Further well-designed clinical trials are required to confirm these results.

Dose

Shiitake is not widely standardized, though lentinan is thought to be its main pharmacologically active constituent. As a chemotherapy adjunct, 1 mg of lentinan has been administered twice weekly (or 2 mg once weekly).[570] A dose of 1 to 4 mg of IM or IV lentinan has been used weekly.[572-575] In limited clinical research, duration of this dosage was 4 weeks.

For prostate cancer, shiitake-containing capsules have been administered based on weight, with a dose of 8 g/day for a 70-kg man.[571]

Adverse Effects, Interactions, Pharmacokinetics. See Appendix A.

Skullcap (*Scutellaria* spp.)

Grade C: *Unclear or conflicting scientific evidence (cancer prevention; cancer treatment)*

Mechanism of Action

Barbat skullcap (*Scutellaria barbata*) and Baikal skullcap (*Scutellaria baicalensis*) have been used in numerous in vitro and animal studies examining hepatocellular carcinoma, hepatoma, uterine cancer, skin cancer, leukemia, renal cell carcinoma, hepatoblastoma, breast cancer, lung cancer, cervical cancer, nasopharyngeal cancer, oral epidermoid cancer, colorectal cancer, pancreatic cancer, and prostate cancer.[576-595] Most studies indicate that barbat skullcap inhibits cellular proliferation and induces apoptosis, possibly in a time-dependent and dose-dependent manner. Barbat skullcap may also induce differentiation in uterine carcinoma cells.[583] Another study found that combined treatment with cyclophosphamide modulated cytotoxic activity of NK cells and peritoneal macrophages during tumor growth.[587] A third study found that barbat skullcap dose-dependently augmented a macrophage oxidative burst to inhibit tumor growth.[590] In addition, Baikal skullcap showed antimetastatic activity in rats with lymphosarcoma, with a possible relationship between functional activity of thrombocytes and the degree of tumor advancement and its metastatic activity.[596]

Scientific Evidence of Effectiveness

Note: Baikal skullcap is an ingredient in PC-SPES, a combination product used for prostate cancer, which was recalled from the U.S. market after it was found to contain small amounts of an undeclared prescription drug (warfarin).[5]

CANCER TREATMENT. In TCM, barbat skullcap *(Scutellaria barbata)* has been used with *Oldenlandia diffusa* for liver, lung, and rectal tumors.[590] In vitro and animal studies have found anticancer properties for both barbat and Baikal skullcap, but limited human clinical evidence is currently available.[576-601] According to a Phase I trial, barbat skullcap aqueous extract (BZL 101) stabilized disease progression and reduced tumor size in patients with advanced breast cancer.[602]

CANCER PREVENTION. In preclinical studies, Baikal skullcap inhibited the development of precancerous breast lesions and inhibited the growth of gynecological cancer cell lines.[576] Evidence of cancer prevention in humans is lacking.

Dose

An oral dose of 350 mL of BZL101 (aqueous extract of barbat skullcap) daily has been used as a sole therapy in patients with advanced breast cancer.[602]

Adverse Effects, Interactions, Pharmacokinetics. See Appendix A.

Slippery Elm (*Ulmus rubra*, syn. *Ulmus fulva*)

Grade C: *Unclear or conflicting scientific evidence (cancer)*

Mechanism of Action

Fatty acids and fatty acid esters similar to those in slippery elm have been reported in animal and in vitro studies to possess immunomodulatory potential and cytostatic and proapoptotic activity in tumor models.[603,604]

Scientific Evidence of Effectiveness

Slippery elm is found as a common ingredient in a purported herbal anticancer product called Essiac and a number of Essiac-like products (see box on p. 474). Essiac (Resperin Canada Limited, Waterloo, Ontario, Canada) contains slippery elm and at least three other herbs (burdock, Indian rhubarb, and sheep sorrel); it is one of the most popular herbal remedies for breast cancer treatment, particularly as an adjunct to the side effects of conventional treatment.[605] However, the mechanisms underlying the purported anticancer effects of Essiac and its constituents remain unclear. Human evidence is limited regarding the efficacy or safety of Essiac or Essiac-like products.[606]

Quality clinical data are lacking on the effects of Essiac or slippery elm for the treatment of cancer.

Dose

Traditional doses of slippery elm are based on historical practice, with no established or universally accepted dosing regimen. Further, no widely accepted standardization exists for slippery elm preparations. Amounts of slippery elm used in Essiac and Essiac-like products are proprietary and therefore not disclosed by the manufacturers.

Because of the lack of human data in cancer patients, dosing for Essiac in cancer is unknown. The most common current use of Essiac is as a tea, although it has also been used historically in tablet/capsule form or as an injection. Anecdotally, 30 mL of Essiac tea has been taken one to three times daily on an empty stomach.

Adverse Effects, Interactions, Pharmacokinetics. See Appendix A.

Sorrel (*Rumex acetosa*, *Rumex* spp.)

Grade C: *Unclear or conflicting scientific evidence (cancer)*

Mechanism of Action

Emodin, a constituent of sorrel, inhibited tumor cell proliferation and showed antimutagenic properties in vitro.[607] *Rumex acetosa*–derived polysaccharides depressed aniline hydroxylase and aminopyrine demethylase activities, prolonged the duration of pentobarbital-induced narcosis, and significantly enhanced the phagocytic and C3 activity in sarcoma-bearing mice.[608]

Scientific Evidence of Effectiveness

Reliable human evidence evaluating sorrel monotherapy as a cancer treatment is currently lacking.[608,609] Sorrel is included as an ingredient in the combination herbal formula Essiac and in several Essiac-like products used in the management of cancer (see box on p. 474). However, reliable research on these formulas is limited,[603,606,610-613] and whether cancer patients receive any benefit remains unclear.

Dose

The most common current use of Essiac is as a tea, although it has also been used historically in tablet/capsule form or as an injection. Anecdotally, 30 mL of Essiac tea has been taken one to three times daily on an empty stomach. Reliable published clinical data of Essiac or Essiac-like products are currently unavailable, and safety or effectiveness has not been established scientifically for any dose. Instructions for tea preparation and dosing vary from product to product.

Adverse Effects, Interactions, Pharmacokinetics. See Appendix A.

Soy (*Glycine max*)

Grade C: *Unclear or conflicting scientific evidence (breast cancer prevention, prostate cancer prevention, colon cancer prevention, endometrial cancer prevention, cancer treatment, gastric cancer treatment)*

Mechanism of Action

Soy and soy components called *isoflavones* have been studied for numerous health conditions. Soy *isoflavones* such as genistein are structurally similar to estradiol, and are believed to have estrogenic effects. Although soy isoflavones are classified as "plant estrogens" or *phytoestrogens,* it remains uncertain whether they exert estrogenic or antiestrogenic effects.[3]

Components of soy thought to have anticancer effects include saponins, phytates, protease inhibitors, phenolic acids, and lecithin[614,615] in addition to the isoflavones (phytoestrogens).[616] Administration of soy isoflavones to rats during early life promotes maturation and differentiation of mammary glands[617,618] and decreases the rate of mammary tumors.[615,619] Diets high in soy decreased oxidative DNA damage[620,621] and decreased lipid peroxidation[622] in healthy human subjects. Soy isoflavones reportedly induced phase II enzymes,[619] thought to be associated with cancer prevention. Diets high in concentrated soy proteins prevented the development of liver and colon cancer in rats.[623,624]

Scientific Evidence of Effectiveness

BREAST CANCER PREVENTION. There is considerable public and scientific interest in the role of soy foods in the prevention of breast cancer, although clinical evidence in support for such a role is limited. The interest stems from epidemiological observations that soy foods are consumed in most Asian countries, where the rates of breast cancer are lower than in the United States and other Western countries. Epidemiological studies in Asian-American populations also suggest that soy food intake may decrease the risk of breast cancer. Soy contains high levels of plant isoflavones, which exert a variety of anticancer activities in laboratory studies. These effects in hormone-sensitive cancers remain unclear, and use in patients with estrogen receptor–positive breast cancer is particularly controversial. It is generally recommended to use these agents cautiously in this population, although some authors assert that antagonistic effects of certain herbs may actually be beneficial.

Perhaps because soy has the potential to produce both estrogenic and antiestrogenic effects, studies on soy and breast carcinogenesis have produced conflicting results. Although current epidemiological and laboratory evidence suggests that it is safe to consume an amount of soy found in typical Asian diets, it is unclear whether increasing soy intake may result in beneficial effects. This amount would be provided by as many as three servings per day of soy foods, such as tofu and soy milk. However, because higher doses of soy may have estrogenic effects, and because higher levels of estrogens clearly increase the risk for breast cancer progression, it is prudent for breast cancer survivors to avoid high doses of soy and soy isoflavones that are provided by more concentrated sources, such as soy powders and isoflavone supplements.[625] Nonetheless, preliminary evidence suggests that soy is safe to use in breast cancer patients, although the pending results of ongoing research may provide more definitive safety data.[626] Short-term use of soy isoflavones is likely safe.

PROSTATE CANCER PREVENTION. Increased soy consumption is a common self-care strategy among prostate cancer survivors, because of the purported antiandrogenic activity of phytoestrogens. Although soy has been suggested to decrease the risk for prostate cancer, it remains unclear whether the effects of soy or other phytoestrogens are beneficial in prostate cancer; studies are currently under way. A few studies suggest that diets rich in phytoestrogens have effects on PSA in men diagnosed with prostate cancer.[627,628] However, it is not known whether these findings result in better prognoses.

COLON CANCER PREVENTION. A review of epidemiological studies identified 13 reports evaluating the effect of soy consumption on colon cancer prevention.[629] The results were conflicting, with some studies reporting a decreased rate of colorectal cancer and others finding no benefit.

ENDOMETRIAL CANCER PREVENTION. Low rates of endometrial cancers in countries with high-soy diets have suggested a protective effect. However, there is a lack of high-quality clinical or epidemiological evidence supporting this effect.

PROSTATE CANCER TREATMENT. In men with primary and recurrent prostate cancer, soy slowed the rise of PSA in several small trials.[627,630-632] It is unclear whether this effect on PSA level translates into a survival benefit.

GASTRIC CANCER TREATMENT. There is a lack of strong clinical evidence regarding the safety and efficacy of soy in gastric cancer.

Dose

The dose of soy for cancer treatment or prevention has not been determined.

Adverse Effects, Interactions, Pharmacokinetics. See Appendix A.

Spirulina (*Arthrospira* spp.)

Grade C: *Unclear or conflicting scientific evidence (oral cancer)*

Mechanism of Action

Spirulina is the common name for several species of algae in the genus *Arthrospira* (formerly classified under the genus *Spirulina*). Spirulina induces apoptosis and inhibits proliferation in hepatocellular carcinoma[633] and chronic myeloid leukemia cell lines.[634] Spirulina increased doxorubicin sensitivity in hepatocellular cells.[633] These effects were associated with cytochrome *c* release, decreased membrane potential, caspase-3 activation, downregulation of the antiapoptotic protein Bcl-2, and upregulation of the proapoptotic Bax (Bcl-2–associated X protein).

One study found that the application of a *Spirulina-Dunaliella* combination algae extract to buccal pouch carcinoma in hamsters induced TNF-α production and promoted tumor regression.[635] In a similar study, animals given oral *Spirulina-Dunaliella* algae extract three times weekly did not develop experimentally induced buccal pouch tumors while control animals developed gross tumors; however, microscopic examination revealed localized dysplasia.[636] Through a series of in vitro experiments, calcium spirulan, a sulfated polysaccharide from *Spirulina platensis*, has been shown to inhibit the invasion, migration, and adhesion of tumor cells.[637] Spirulina may also exert anticancer effects through enhanced NK cell activity and IFN-γ, as demonstrated in vitro.[638]

Scientific Evidence of Effectiveness

There is some clinical evidence that *Spirulina fusiformis* treatment may cause regression of precancerous oral leukoplakia in tobacco and alcohol users.[639] However, additional clinical evidence is warranted.

Dose

For oral leukoplakia, 1 g of *Spirulina fusiformis* has been used daily for up to 1 year.[639]

Adverse Effects, Interactions, Pharmacokinetics. See Appendix A.

Strawberry (Fragaria spp.)

Grade C: *Unclear or conflicting scientific evidence (colorectal cancer prevention)*

Mechanism of Action

Individual compounds in strawberries have demonstrated anticancer activity in several different studies Proposed mechanisms include blocking initiation of carcinogenesis, dose-dependently inducing apoptosis, and suppressing progression and proliferation of tumors.[640-644] This activity may result from the antioxidant properties of strawberry extracts and their ability to reduce oxidative stress.[643,645-652] The antioxidant effects from strawberries may be caused by ellagic acid and certain flavonoids, such as anthocyanin, catechin, quercetin, and kaempferol.[641,648]

Scientific Evidence of Effectiveness

Many in vitro studies report antioxidant properties of strawberries.[643,645-652] Evidence from a survey indicates that strawberries and other fruits (mandarin, persimmon) may reduce the risk of adenoma with mild dysplasia in women;[650] however, this evidence is insufficient to support a cancer-preventive effect.

Dose

The dose of strawberry for cancer has not been determined.

Adverse Effects, Interactions, Pharmacokinetics. See Appendix A.

Sweet Annie (Artemisia annua)

Grade C: *Unclear or conflicting scientific evidence (cancer)*

Mechanism of Action

Artemisinin and quercetagetin 6,7,3′,4′-tetramethyl ether, constituents of *Artemisia annua*, have shown cytotoxic activity against cancer cells.[651,652] Two analogs of *A. annua* constituents also have anticancer properties in vitro. The artemisinin analog *dihydroartemisinin* (DHA) has significantly reduced the number of Molt-4 cells (human lymphoblastoid leukemia cell line)[653,654] but did not significantly affect the number of normal human lymphocytes also in the culture.[653] When sodium butyrate was added, the combination killed the Molt-4 cells but did not affect the lymphocytes. When analyzed for its anticancer activity against 55 cancer cell lines, artesunate (a derivative of artemisinin, the active constituent *A. annua*) was most active against leukemia and colon cancer cell lines.[655] Artesunate's cytotoxicity was comparable to that of standard cytostatic drugs. In addition, artesunate induced apoptosis in human umbilical vein endothelial cells in vitro.[656]

Scientific Evidence of Effectiveness

In vitro, artesunate has shown cytotoxic effects in several cancer cell lines.[651-659] In case reports, artesunate in combination with standard chemotherapy seemed to inhibit tumor growth at least temporarily and increase survival time in patients with uveal melanoma.[657] Although these cases offer hope for patients with terminal cancer, more clinical evidence is needed to assess the safety and potential of this herbal therapy.

Dose

The dose of sweet Annie for cancer has not been determined.

Adverse Effects, Interactions, Pharmacokinetics. See Appendix A.

Tea (Camellia sinensis)

Grade C: *Unclear or conflicting scientific evidence (cancer prevention; cancer treatment)*

Mechanism of Action

The polyphenols found in tea have been studied for various health-promoting effects, including antioxidant and antitumor activities. *Catechins* are major polyphenolic compounds derived from green (unoxidized) tea leaves; these are oxidized to *theaflavins* during the manufacture of black and oolong teas.[660] Both the catechins of green tea and the theaflavins of black tea have demonstrated antioxidant effects in numerous studies. Tea polyphenols have been shown to inhibit cytochrome P450 (CYP450) activation of carcinogens; increase tissue antioxidant capacity; enhance the activity of antioxidant enzymes (glutathione reductase and glutathione-S-transferase); induce apoptosis in cancer cells; inhibit cancer cell growth; inhibit *N*-nitrosomethylbenzylamine–induced tumorigenesis; inhibit ultraviolet

A (UVA) light–induced photochemical damage; inhibit testosterone-mediated induction of ornithine decarboxylase; and inhibit toposiomerase I activity, telomerase activity, and oncogene expression.[661-695]

GREEN TEA. In addition to inhibiting cell growth, green tea polyphenols also suppressed the invasive behavior of MDA-MB-231 cells in vitro.[696] Anecdotally, green tea inhibits tumor-associated quinol oxidase but does not inhibit quinol oxidase activity of healthy cells. Quinol oxidase is found on cell surfaces and is required for cell growth.

The green tea component *epigallocatechin gallate* (EGCG) is a potent free-radical scavenger. EGCG inhibits the proteolytic enzyme urokinase, which is involved in tumor invasion and metastasis.[697] EGCG has been shown to inhibit the growth of human lung cancer cell lines (PC-9 cells) by cell cycle G2/M arrest[698] and to regulate tissue necrotic factor gene expression by modulating NK-κB activation.[699] Green tea extracts (GTEs) have been shown to modulate the expression of human CYP450-1A, a gene thought to play a role in aryl hydrocarbon–induced cancers; this effect was not attributed to a single tea catechin, but suggested to result from the effects of a complex mixture.[700]

Aqueous GTEs induced a concentration-dependent inhibition of the Aroclor 1254–hepatic S9–mediated mutagenicity of heteroclinical amines (IQ and Glu-p-1), benzo[a]pyrene and 7,12-dimethylbenz[a]anthracene, and the isoniazid-induced S9-mediated mutagenicity of nitrosopiperidine and nitrosopyrrolidine. Green tea induced a concentration-dependent decrease in the O-dealkylation of methoxyresorufin, ethoxyresorufin, and pentoxyresorufin. In addition, GTE inhibited NADPH-dependent reduction of cytochrome *c*.[701]

One cup of green tea contains approximately 50 mg of caffeine, and excessive tea consumption may lead to adverse effects or toxicity. Green tea supplement capsules usually contain less caffeine (~5 mg of caffeine in 500 mg).

BLACK TEA. Black tea has shown numerous anticancer effects, mostly attributed to the polyphenolic theaflavins and thearubigins. Numerous in vitro[702,703] and in vivo[704-708] studies have demonstrated the anticarcinogenic effects of black tea polyphenols (BTPs). Inhibition of carcinogenesis was reported to act synergistically with concomitant milk ingestion.[709,710] The anticarcinogenic effects of BTPs include inhibition of cell proliferation in vitro[707,711-714] and in vivo. BTPs have also been shown to induce apoptosis in vitro[703,715,716] and in vivo,[710,714] as well as enhance cytotoxicity against cancer cells in vitro[716,717] and in vivo.[718] Other reported anticancer effects include inhibition of cyclooxygenase-2 (COX-2),[710,713] angiogenesis,[707] and DNA damage.[719-721]

Scientific Evidence of Effectiveness

CANCER PREVENTION. Several large case-control and cohort studies have largely focused on prevention of gastrointestinal and breast cancers with green tea.[722-727] Results are variable, with some suggesting chronic tea consumption may decrease cancer risk and others reporting no benefits. Epidemiological studies have shown reduced risks of stomach cancer associated with green tea consumption.[723,728] A large cohort study reported a decreased risk of cancer and later age at cancer onset associated with green tea consumption, particularly with intake greater than 10 cups daily.[729] A separate study found no decrease in gastric cancer risk with green tea ingestion.[722] In a prospective study of green tea consumption and cancer incidence in Japan, researchers found no statistically significant decrease in cancer occurrence related to green tea consumption.[730] A protective effect against esophageal cancer was reported in women, but not men, who drank green tea regularly.[726] In another population-based control study, increasing green tea consumption was associated with decreased risk of colon, rectal, and pancreatic cancer.[731] Overall, the epidemiological evidence suggests that green tea consumption may protect against cancer; however, these studies have been mostly observational, and other lifestyle choices of tea drinkers may confound these results.

In smokers, consumption of decaffeinated green tea (4 cups daily for 4 months) resulted in decreased urinary 8-hydroxydeoxyguanosine (8-OHdG),[732,733] suggesting decreased oxidative DNA damage. Consumption of green tea by smokers was associated with decreased sister-chromatid exchange compared with smokers who did not drink green tea.[734]

A recent randomized, placebo-controlled study in 60 volunteers with high-grade prostate intraepithelial neoplasia revealed that green tea catechins are safe and effective for treating premalignant lesions before prostate cancer develops. After 1 year, only one tumor was diagnosed among the 30 men treated with catechins, whereas nine cancers were found among the 30 placebo-treated men. The total PSA levels were not significantly different between the two arms. The International Prostate Symptom Score was significantly improved (9.12 vs. 11.12 at baseline) in the catechin-treated men. No significant side effects or adverse effects were documented.[727]

Several studies have also explored a possible association between regular consumption of black tea and rates of cancer in populations. This research has yielded conflicting results, with some studies suggesting benefits[735,736] and others reporting no effects.[737] Laboratory and animal studies report that components of tea (e.g., polyphenols) have antioxidant properties and effects against tumors. Effects in humans remain unclear, and these components may be more common in green tea than black tea. Some animal and laboratory research suggests that components of black tea may actually be carcinogenic, although effects in humans are not clear. Overall, the relationship between black tea consumption and human cancer remains undetermined.

CANCER TREATMENT. Several large population-based studies examined the possible association between green tea consumption and cancer incidence. Cancers of the digestive system (stomach, colon, rectum, pancreas, esophagus) have been primarily tracked, although risk of breast cancer in women has also been studied. Across these prospective and retrospective studies, relative risks of 0.5 to 1.5 and odds ratios of 0.5 to 0.8 have been reported. Preliminary clinical trials suggest that green tea does *not* appear to be effective in the treatment of cancer. Additional human research is needed before a recommendation can be made for or against the use of green tea in cancer prevention or treatment.

In a breast cancer study, green tea ingestion was associated with improved prognosis in stage I and II cancers, but no effect was seen on grade III cancers.[738]

A small clinical trial similarly reported no effect of GTE on prostate cancer progression.[739] No change in serum PSA was found among men with preexisting PSA elevations treated with green tea versus placebo.[740] In contrast, a decreased occurrence of prostate cancer was reported among healthy men treated with GTE versus placebo.[727]

No difference in lesion size or abnormal cell proliferation was found among patients with precancerous esophageal lesions treated with green tea versus placebo.[741] No response was seen in 17 advanced lung cancer patients treated with GTE.[742]

Supplementation with green tea (1.42 L daily for 5 days) in men scheduled for surgical prostatectomy resulted in a reduction in ex vivo prostate cancer cell proliferation when cells were grown in media containing patient serum collected after green tea consumption.[743]

Dose

GREEN TEA. GTEs from some of the major supplement manufacturers have considerable variation in the amount of GTE milligrams per capsule, ranging from 100 to 750 mg per capsule.[744] GTEs may be standardized to 60% to 97% polyphenols.[745]

For cancer prevention, studies have used daily doses of 1 to 10 cups.[726,728,746-748] Epidemiological studies in Japan state that cancer patients who consumed more than 10 cups of green tea daily extended their survival by approximately 4 to 6 years compared with those who drank fewer than 3 cups daily.[749] For cancer treatment, patients with prostate neoplasia have received 200 mg of green tea catechins.[727]

BLACK TEA. The dose of black tea for cancer prevention has not been established.

Adverse Effects, Interactions, Pharmacokinetics. See Appendix A.

Turmeric (Curcuma longa)

Grade C: *Unclear or conflicting scientific evidence (cancer prevention; cancer treatment)*

Mechanism of Action

Multiple preclinical studies have explored potential anticancer mechanisms of curcumin.[750-781] In vitro, curcumin derivatives demonstrated antiproliferative and proapoptotic effects in numerous cell lines,[756] including multidrug-resistant cell lines,[772] rat aortic smooth muscle cells,[773] leukemic cells,[767,774] human breast cancer cells,[771,772] and human epidermoid carcinoma cells.[775] These effects may occur through modulating aryl hydrocarbon receptors[776] or ornithine decarboxylase activity.[772] The protective role of curcumin against carcinogenesis has also been attributed to antioxidant effects.[777] Extracts of turmeric and curcumin are nonmutagenic using the Ames test and serve protective roles against experimental mutagenesis induced by capsaicin, chili extract, and tobacco-derived mutagens.[778]

In rodents, diets containing 0.2% to 5% curcumin were preventive, therapeutic, and proapoptotic in numerous models of cancer, including chemically induced colon cancer,[766,779,780] prostate cancer,[761] gastric cancer,[767,781] radiation-induced lung cancer,[782] and skin cancer.[767,781] Topical application of curcumin has also been shown to inhibit chemically induced tumors in mouse skin,[783] which may be attributable to suppression of protein kinase C activity.[784]

Scientific Evidence of Effectiveness

CANCER PREVENTION. A combination of turmeric and quercetin decreased the number and size of polyps in five patients with familial adenomatous polyposis, a genetic condition that increases the risk of early-onset colorectal cancer.[785] Evidence from controlled clinical research is lacking.

CANCER TREATMENT. A case series reported topical turmeric to decrease pain and exudate from topical cancer in 50% and 70% of patients, respectively; furthermore, turmeric decreased lesion size in 10% of patients.[752] Another case series reported a decrease in urinary mutagens in healthy smokers treated with oral turmeric.[786] Additional clinical evidence is required to establish the effect of tumeric on cancer prevention or treatment.

Dose

Turmeric may be standardized to contain 95% curcuminoids per dose. The dried root of turmeric is reported to contain 3% to 5% curcumin.[787]

In clinical trials, patients with colorectal cancer have ingested 450 to 3600 mg of curcumin for 7 days[750] and a 750-mg tablet of turmeric twice daily[786] and have applied topical turmeric ethanol extract or 0.5% curcumin ointment three times daily for up to 4 weeks.[752]

Adverse Effects, Interactions, Pharmacokinetics. See Appendix A.

Essiac Herbal Combination Tea

Essiac is a combination herbal tea originally developed in the 1920s by the Canadian nurse Rene Caisse ("Essiac" spelled backward). The original proprietary formula contained burdock root (*Arctium lappa*), sheep sorrel (*Rumex acetosella*), slippery elm inner bark (*Ulmus fulva*), and Turkish rhubarb (*Rheum palmatum*). The recipe is said to be based on a traditional Ojibwa (Native-American) remedy. Later formulations added other herbs, including blessed thistle (*Cnicus benedictus*), red clover (*Trifolium pratense*), kelp (*Laminaria digitata*), and watercress (*Nasturtium officinale*).[3,4,25]

In general, pharmacological data for Essiac formulations are primarily based on theoretical or empirical knowledge of the individual constituents. According to anecdotal reports, activity of Essiac is through enlargement and hardening of tumors, followed by softening and final expulsion of the contents as pus and fleshy material. Caisse believed that Essiac induced the cancerous cells to retreat to the original site of the tumor, shrink, and discharge to the exterior. In addition, intramuscular injection of the herbs is reported to result in localization of the tumor, with additional symptom relief, including an increase in appetite, alleviation of pain, and enhanced well-being.[3,4]

Caisse administered the formula orally and parenterally to numerous cancer patients during the 1920s and 1930s. Reliable, published research of Essiac is currently lacking. Rodent studies at Memorial Sloan-Kettering Cancer Center in the 1970s were not formally published, and 86 human case reports collected retrospectively in 1988 by the Canadian Department of National Health and Welfare yielded unclear results.[4] Recently, some concern was raised with Flor-Essence and Essiac Herbal Tonics about a potential to stimulate the growth of human breast cancer cells through the estrogen receptor (ER) and ER-independent mechanisms.[52] This is in contrast to previous reports that both Essiac and Flor-Essence herbal teas demonstrated antiproliferative properties in vitro at high concentrations. A systematic review found no published clinical trials evaluating this herbal complex in patients with cancer. However, Essiac did not seem to cause serious adverse effects. Despite this lack of evidence, Essiac and Essiac-like products (which may add additional herbs) remain popular among cancer patients.[4]

Six ounces of Essiac tea three times daily has been used to treat advanced cancer. There is no well-known standardization for Essiac. Because the exact formula for Essiac is proprietary, it is not clear what standards for manufacturing are followed. Some brands of Essiac disclose the amounts of herbal constituents, although the basis for standardization is not always clear. One suggested Essiac recipe consists of 6.5 (measuring cup) oz cut burdock root, 16 (scale weight) oz powdered sheep sorrel herb, 4 (scale weight) oz powdered slippery elm inner bark, and 1 (scale weight) oz powdered Turkish rhubarb root.

HERBAL THERAPIES WITH NEGATIVE EVIDENCE

Apricot (*Prunus armeniaca*)

Grade D: *Fair negative evidence (cancer)*

Apricot pit contains *amygdalin*, a plant compound that contains sugar and produces cyanide. Laetrile, an alternative cancer drug marketed in Mexico and other countries outside the United States, is derived from amygdalin. Based on a 1982 Phase II trial, the U.S. National Cancer Institute concluded that laetrile ("*l*aevorotatory mandeloni*trile*") is not an effective chemotherapeutic agent. Nonetheless, many people still travel to international clinics offering this therapy. Multiple cases of cyanide poisoning, including deaths, have been associated with laetrile therapy.[788,789]

Laetrile remains unapproved by the FDA, which is also seeking a permanent injunction against three corporations for unlawfully promoting and marketing on their websites injectable and oral formulations of laetrile and apricot kernels for treating cancer.

Bitter Almond (*Prunus amygdalus*)

Grade D: *Fair negative scientific evidence (cancer)*

The almond is closely related to the apricot (classified as *drupes*). Unlike apricot, however, the outer layer of the almond is not edible. The compound, amygdalin, differentiates the bitter almond from the sweet almond. Laetrile, derived from amygdalin found in the pits of fruits and nuts such as apricots and bitter almonds, has not been shown to be an effective chemotherapeutic agent (see Apricot).

Flax (*Linum usitatissimum*)

Grade D: *Fair negative evidence (prostate cancer treatment)*

Several case-control studies[790,791] and a prospective cohort study[792] found an association between the intake of alpha-linolenic acid (ALA, present in flaxseed) and an increased risk of developing prostate cancer. One brief, small case series in patients with prostate cancer found that flaxseed supplementation decreased serum total testosterone, free androgens, and total cholesterol with no effect on serum PSA levels.[791] This same study reported a reduction in prostate cell proliferation and increased rates of apoptosis. Until better human evidence is available, based on the available research, flaxseed and ALA supplements should be avoided in patients with or at risk for prostate cancer.

PSK (Coriolus versicolor)

Grade D: *Fair negative evidence (breast cancer [adjuvant])*
The available evidence does not support the use of PSK, in conjunction with hormone therapy, chemotherapy, or surgery, to increase survival in breast cancer patients.

HERBAL THERAPIES WITH LIMITED EVIDENCE

Bitter Melon (Momordica charantia)

Preclinical evidence suggested that bitter melon prevented stomach tumor development in mice.[793] MAP30, a protein isolated from bitter melon extract, has been reported to possess antineoplastic effects in vitro.[794-797] These effects have been attributed to the reduced expression of growth factor receptors such as the transmembrane tyrosine kinase receptor HER2 (also known as *neu* or *c-erb*-2), which has been implicated in breast cancer.[795] MAP30 was originally identified as a single-chain ribosome-inactivating protein (SCRIP), but its in vitro activities appear to be unrelated to its effect on ribosomes. Bitter melon has been suggested to potentiate the function of NK cells in cancer patients.[798,799] In addition, *cis*-9, *trans*-11, *trans*-13-conjugated linolenic acid extracted from bitter melon seed has shown antineoplastic effects in human colon cancer cell lines.[800] An in vivo study reported cytostatic activity in IM9 human leukemic lymphocytes resulting from inhibition of RNA synthesis by an unidentified bitter melon constituent.[801] Another study associated the cytotoxicity of bitter melon extract on leukemic lymphocytes with the inhibition of guanylate cyclase, an enzyme normally present in normal and leukemic lymphocytes. This blockade in leukemic lymphocytes correlates with cell death.[802] In rats, the constituent *cis*(c)9, *trans*(t)11, t13-conjugated linolenic acid inhibited the development of azoxymethane-induced colonic aberrant crypt foci.[803]

Chlorella (Chlorella spp.)

Algae in the genus *Chlorella* have been shown to have anticancer effects in various in vitro studies. In a toll-like receptor (TLR) knockout mouse study, the glycoprotein ARS-2, purified from the culture medium of *Chlorella vulgaris*, has shown antitumor activity that may be caused by effects on TLR-2 signaling.[804] In another study, monogalactosyl diacylglycerols isolated from *C. vulgaris* inhibited tumor promotion.[805]

Chlorella has been reported to inhibit lymphocyte proliferation and matrix metalloproteinase activity in vitro.[806] Clinical evidence is required before chlorella can be recommended for the prevention of cancer.

Cranberry (Vaccinium macrocarpon)

Several in vitro and animal studies using various cancer cell lines (oral cancer, prostate cancer, colon carcinoma, human liver cancer, human breast cancer, and glioblastoma) have shown that cranberry extracts arrest tumor cell proliferation and induce apoptosis.[807-812] One animal study showed that the extract of cranberry presscake (product remaining after removing juice from berry) was effective in inducing apoptosis and blocking cell cycle progression in mice bearing human breast cancer tissue cells.[813] Cranberry may induce antiproliferation through cell cycle arrest.[810,814] The *Vaccinium* subspecies, including lowbush blueberry, bilberry, cranberry, and lingonberry, have been shown to possess anticarcinogenic activity.

Clinical evidence is lacking. Cranberry should be used cautiously to treat cancer, because cranberry supplementation has been strongly associated with bladder cancer;[815] however, a causal relationship has not been established.

Dandelion (Taraxacum officinale)

Several laboratory studies report antineoplastic properties of dandelion and other *Taraxacum* species.[816-821] Dandelion extract has been reported to have antioxidant and cytotoxic effects in vitro.[822,823] Eleven triterpenoids (1-11) from the roots of *Taraxacum japonicum* were found to have inhibitory effects on Epstein-Barr virus early antigen (EBV-EA) induced by the tumor promoter 12-*O*-tetrade-canoylphorbol-13-acetate (TPA).[821] Limited animal research has not clearly established the effects of dandelion on tumor growth.[816,817] High-quality clinical evidence is lacking in this area.

Grape Seed (Vitis spp.)

In vitro and in vivo studies suggest that oligomeric proanthocyanidins (OPCs) from grape seed may promote apoptosis of cancer cells while providing chemoprotective effects for nonmalignant cells.[824-828] Scientific reviews have discussed the use of polyphenolic antioxidants, such as (−)-epigallocatechin gallate, found in grape seed extract, for certain types of skin cancer.[829]

PC-SPES

Note: PC-SPES and SPES were voluntarily withdrawn from the U.S. market in 2002 and should not be used.[5]

PC-SPES is an herbal combination product that contains Da Qing Ye (*Isatis indigotica*), licorice (*Glycyrrhiza glabra, G. uralensis*), San Qi (*Panax pseudoginseng*), reishi mushroom (*Ganoderma lucidum*), baikal skullcap (*Scutellaria baicalensis*),

Hoxsey Formula

> "Hoxsey formula" is a misleading name because it is not a single formula but rather a therapeutic regimen consisting of an oral tonic, topical preparations, and supportive therapy. The tonic is individualized for cancer patients based on general condition, location of cancer, and previous history of treatment. The ingredient usually received by every patient is *potassium iodide*. Other ingredients are then added and may include licorice, red clover, burdock, stillingia root, berberis root, pokeroot, cascara, aromatic USP 14, prickly ash bark, and buckthorn bark. A red paste may be used, which tends to be caustic (irritating), and contains antimony trisulfide, zinc chloride, and bloodroot. A topical yellow powder may be used and contains arsenic sulfide, talc, sulfur, and a "yellow precipitate." A clear solution may also be administered and contains trichloroacetic acid.
>
> There is a lack of quality human evidence regarding the safety or effectiveness of Hoxsey formula.

chrysanthemum *(Dendranthema morifolium)*, *Rabdosia rubescens*, and saw palmetto *(Serenoa repens)*. It was produced and marketed by BotanicLab for use in prostate cancer (PC, and Latin *spes*, "hope").

Because the prescription drug warfarin (Coumadin) was detected in PC-SPES, the product was removed from the U.S. market.[830]

Seaweed

Bladderwrack *(Fucus vesiculosus)* appears to suppress the growth of various cancer cells in animal and laboratory studies. Fucoidans from bladderwrack strongly blocked breast carcinoma cell adhesion to platelets, which may have inhibitory effects on tumor cell metastasis.[831] Fucoidan increased the viability of dendritic cells, production of IL-12 and TNF-α, and expression of major histocompatibility complex classes I and II, CD54, and CD86 molecules.[832] In rats, kelp *(Laminaria* spp.) showed endocrine-modulating effects that may suggest a role in prevention of hormone-dependent tumors.[833]

Currently, there is a lack of reliable data to support use of seaweed in cancer.

MANAGEMENT OF TOXICITY AND SIDE EFFECTS

Chemotherapy

Several herbal therapies have been used or evaluated to prevent or alleviate chemotoxicity, although clear benefits have not been consistently demonstrated. In China, danshen *(Salvia miltiorrhiza)* and dong quai *(Angelica sinensis)* have been used to treat bleomycin-induced pulmonary toxicity, but scientific evidence is currently unavailable to support their use for chemotherapy toxicity.

A meta-analysis of 30 randomized studies reported astragalus-based Chinese herbal medicine may increase effectiveness of platinum-based chemotherapy such as cisplatin (Platinol).[834] Astragalus is also used to reduce side effects of cancer treatments, such as fatigue and weight loss. However, the effectiveness of astragalus as an adjunct to cancer therapy has been debated,[835] and remains controversial.

Based on animal research, *Scutellaria baicalensis* extract may ameliorate 5-fluorouracil–induced myelotoxicity.[836] A related species, *Scutellaria barbata* extract, may potentiate the antimetastatic effect of cyclophosphamide.[587,837]

Other approaches used (but not well studied) for chemotoxicity, include *Ginkgo biloba*, Essiac tea, and *Panax ginseng*.

Nausea and Vomiting

Chinese herbs may help reduce chemotherapy-induced nausea and include decoctions of Huang qi (astragalus) compounds. When given in addition to chemotherapy, these Chinese herbs reportedly caused a significant reduction in the proportion of patients who experienced nausea and vomiting.[838]

Other herbal approaches used (but not well studied) include calendula *(Calendula officinalis)*, clove *(Eugenia aromatica)*, elder *(Sambucus nigra)*, lavender *(Lavandula angustifolia)*, marshmallow *(Althaea officinalis)*, oleander *(Nerium oleander, Thevetia peruviana)*, peppermint *(Mentha x piperita)*, tea *(Camellia sinensis)*, valerian *(Valeriana officinalis)*, white horehound *(Marrubium vulgare)*, and wild yam *(Dioscorea villosa)*.

Constipation

Numerous natural derivatives are used for constipation and are often recommended by physicians. Strong evidence supports the laxative effects of oral senna or *Aloe vera*, and there is good evidence for other fiber-rich sources such as psyllium *(Plantago* spp.) and flax *(Linum usitatissimum)*. Patients also use many other natural sources of fiber for constipation.

Radiotherapy

Prunus amygdalus dulcis, Medicago sativa, bladderwrack *(Fucus vesiculosus)*, *Panax ginseng*, milk thistle *(Silybum marianum)*, and spirulina *(Arthrospira* spp.) have been used for nonspecific symptoms related to radiation therapy. *Salvia miltiorrhiza* has been used in patients with radiation pneumonitis.

Xerostomia

Xerostomia ("dry mouth"; salivary secretions abnormally low) is a permanent and troublesome side effect of head and neck irradiation. Studies have shown that acute administration of yohimbine, an α_2-adrenoceptor antagonist, is able to increase salivary secretion in animals and in humans.[839-842] Although not systematically evaluated for treating xerostomia, betel

Herbs with Potential Antineoplastic Properties*

HERB	SPECIFIC THERAPEUTIC USE(S)†	HERB	SPECIFIC THERAPEUTIC USE(S)†
Acacia	Cancer	Burdock	Cancer
Acai	Cancer	Calamus	Cancer, tumors
Acerola	Cancer	Calendula	Cancer, colon cancer, leukemia
Aconite	Cancer, Hodgkin's disease, scirrhus (hard tumor)	Cardamom	Antimutagenic, colon cancer
African wild potato	Cancer, lung cancer, prostate cancer	Carrot	Cancer
Agrimony	Tumors	Cascara sagrada	Leukemia
Alfalfa	Cervical cancer	Celery	Cancer
Alizarin	Leukemia	Chamomile	Cancer
Alkanna	Cancer	Cherry	Bladder cancer, cancer, colon cancer
Allspice	Anticarcinogenic	Chia	Cancer, tumors
Alpinia	Cancer, leukemia	Chickweed	Anticarcinogenic
Amaranth	Cancer, lung cancer prevention	Chicory	Breast cancer, cancer, colon cancer
Andiroba	Tumors	Cinnamon	Antimutagenic, tumors, cancer
Andrographis	Cancer	Cleavers	Cancer (bone marrow)
Angostura	Cancer	Clove	Antimutagenic, cancer
Anise	Cancer	Club moss	Cancer
Annatto	Cancer	Codonopsis	Cancer, gastric cancer
Aristolochia spp.	Cancer	Coleus	Cancer
Arnica	Cancer, tumors	Comfrey	Cancer
Asafoetida	Cancer	Cordyceps	Cancer
Asarum	Cancer	Corydalis	Cancer
Ashwagandha	Tumors	Cramp bark	Cancer
Asparagus	Tumors	Cranberry	Cancer treatment
Avocado	Cancer	Dandelion	Breast cancer, leukemia
Babassu	Leukemia, tumors	Danshen	Tumors, cancer, leukemia, liver cancer
Bael fruit	Tumors	Date palm	Cancer
Bamboo	Cancer prevention	Devil's claw	Skin cancer
Banaba	Tumors	Devil's club	Cancer prevention
Barberry	Antimutagenic, cancer	Dogwood	Cancer
Barley	Cancer, colon cancer	Dong quai	Tumors, cancer, stomach cancer
Bay leaf	Cancer, leukemia	Elder	Cancer
Bellis perennis	Breast cancer, cancer	Elecampane	Cancer
Bilberry	Antiangiogenic, cancer, leukemia	English ivy	Cancer
Birch	Cancer	Eucalyptus	Cancer, leukemia
Bitter melon	Tumors	Euphorbia	Cancer, leukemia, tumors
Bitter orange	Cancer, leukemia	Eyebright	Cancer
Black currant	Tumors (hemorrhoidal)	False pennyroyal	Cancer
Blackberry	Cancer	Fennel	Cancer prevention, prostate cancer
Blessed thistle	Cervical dysplasia	Fenugreek	Cancer, colon cancer, leukemia
Bloodroot	Cancer	Feverfew	Antiangiogenic, breast cancer, cancer, colorectal cancer, leukemia, pancreatic cancer, skin cancer
Blue cohosh	Cervical dysplasia, liver cancer		
Blue flag	Cancer, tumors		
Borage	Cancer	Fig	Cancer
Buckshorn plantain	Leukemia	Fo-ti	Cancer
Bulbous buttercup	Antimutagenic, tumors, cancer, leukemia, skin cancer	Garcinia	Cancer, tumors

Continued

Herbs with Potential Antineoplastic Properties—cont'd

HERB	SPECIFIC THERAPEUTIC USE(S)†	HERB	SPECIFIC THERAPEUTIC USE(S)†
Ginger	Cancer, leukemia, neuroblastoma	Neem	Antimutagenic, cancer, gastric cancer, glioblastoma, melanoma
Goldenrod	Tumors		
Goldenseal	Astrocytoma, cancer, leukemia, glioblastoma	Noni	Cancer
Gotu kola	Bladder lesions, cancer	Nux vomica	Cancer, liver cancer
Grape seed	Breast cancer, colorectal cancer, prostate cancer, skin cancer	Onion	Cancer, lung cancer, stomach cancer, antimutagenic, anticarcinogenic
Grapefruit	Cancer	Papain	Cancer
Ground ivy	Cancer	Parsnip	Cancer
Guggul	Tumors	Passion flower	Cancer
Gymnema	Cancer	PC-SPES	Breast cancer, cancer prevention, colon cancer, leukemia, lymphoma, melanoma, pancreatic cancer
Hawthorn	Cancer		
Hibiscus	Cancer, leukemia		
Holy basil	Adaptogen, anticarcinogenic, tumors, cancer		
Hop	Breast cancer, cancer, leukemia (HL-60)	Peppermint	Cancer
		Perilla	Cancer, leukemia
Horny goat weed	Cancer, prostate cancer	Peyote	Tumor
Horse chestnut	Antiangiogenic	Pokeweed	Cancer, leukemia
Horseradish	Antimutagenic, cancer	Polypodium	Cancer
Horsetail	Cancer	Pycnogenol	Cancer prevention, cancer treatment, leukemia, lung cancer
Hoxsey formula	Lymphoma, melanoma, sarcomas		
Hyssop	Cancer, Kaposi's sarcoma, leukemia, melanoma	Pygeum	Prostate cancer
		Quassia	Leukemia
Jequirity	Tumors, cancer, leukemia	Raspberry	Antimutagenic, cancer
Juniper	Cancer	Red yeast rice	Cancer, ovarian cancer
Katuka	Cancer	Rehmannia	Cancer pain, lung cancer, sarcomas, bone cancer
Kava	Cancer		
Kiwi	Cancer prevention	Rooibos	Cancer
Kudzu	Cancer, leukemia	Rose hip	Cancer, prostate cancer
Lemon balm	Cancer	Rosemary	Cancer prevention
Lemongrass	Antineoplastic, cancer	Safflower	Prostate cancer, tumors
Licorice	Tumors, aplastic anemia, breast cancer, cancer, colorectal cancer, liver cancer, lung cancer, melanoma, prostate cancer	St. John's wort	Cancer
		Sarsaparilla	Cancer, leukemia
		Scotch broom	Cancer
		Sea buckthorn	Cancer, leukemia
Lime	Cancer	Shepherd's purse	Cancer
Lingonberry	Cancer	Skunk cabbage	Cancer
Lousewort	Cancer	Squill	Cancer
Maca	Adaptogen, cancer, leukemia	Stevia	Antimutagenic, tumors
Mangosteen	Cancer	Stinging nettle	Cancer
Marshmallow	Cancer	Sweet almond	Bladder cancer, breast cancer, colon cancer, mouth and throat cancers
Meadowsweet	Antineoplastic, cervical cancer, cervical dysplasia		
		Tamanu	Cancer
Morus nigra	Cancer	Tangerine	Cancer, cancer prevention
Mugwort	Cancer	Tansy	Tumors
Muira puama	Cancer	Tea tree	Melanoma

*This is not an all-inclusive or comprehensive list of herbs with potential antineoplastic properties; other herbs and supplements may possess these qualities. A qualified health care provider should be consulted with specific questions or concerns regarding potential antineoplastic effects or interactions.
†Based on expert opinion, anecdote, case reports, and/or preliminary trial evidence.

nut chewing has been noted to produce copious salivation in users, possibly from the muscarinic agonist activity of betel components. However, based on the known toxicities associated with betel use, the risks likely outweigh any potential benefits.

Mucositis and Stomatitis

Oral mucositis (inflammation of mucosa) has been reported in approximately 60% of patients receiving radiation therapy. Radiotherapy may damage the lining of the mouth and cause redness or severe ulceration. Patients may have significant discomfort when eating and swallowing. Clinical trials have suggested using licorice for radiation-induced oral mucositis, and the use of curcumin showed positive results in a rat model of radiation therapy. However, specific guidelines are not available. Analysis of the available research revealed several methodological flaws, which precluded the recommendation of these therapies for preventing or treating of mucositis.[3]

A small, randomized, placebo-controlled double-blind clinical trial conducted in 32 patients showed that a homeopathic combination remedy, TRAUMEEL S, significantly reduced the severity and duration of chemotherapy-induced stomatitis in patients undergoing bone marrow transplantation. A larger, multisite pediatric trial commenced after this trial.[843]

Leukopenia and Anemia

Radiation therapy may cause low white blood cell (WBC) count, especially in patients also receiving chemotherapy. Patients with low WBC counts may be more susceptible to infections. Symptoms of infection include fever of 100° to 105° F (37.7°-40.5° C) or higher, chills, and sweating. Cancer therapy may also affect red blood cell (RBC) count. *Aplastic anemia* refers to low levels of all blood cell types, including WBCs, RBCs, and platelets. An herbal mixture that includes astragalus improved blood cell counts in patients with aplastic anemia.[844] However, evidence is currently insufficient to recommend astragalus for the treatment of aplastic anemia.

There is conflicting evidence from a small number of randomized trials using *Echinacea* for treating radiation-induced leukopenia. Studies have used the combination product Esberitox, which includes extracts of *Echinacea* (*E. purpurea* and *E. pallida*) root, white cedar *(Thuja occidentalis)* leaf, and wild indigo *(Baptisia tinctoria)* root.[845]

Dermatitis

Radiation dermatitis (radiodermatitis) is a common side effect of radiation therapy. Radiation skin irritation may begin a few weeks after beginning treatment. Common skin changes include redness, pruritus, and swelling.

Homeopathic application of belladonna (based on the "like cures like" rationale of homeopathy) can be traced to the observed similarities between radiodermatitis symptoms and belladonna side effects. A randomized trial reported modest benefits of a homeopathic oral belladonna preparation for radiodermatitis.[846] However, due to the minute (even negligible) amounts of the purported active constituents in homeopathic preparations, there is no clear biochemical basis for any observed effects.

Topical preparations used to minimize radiation skin reactions include chamomile, for which there is inconclusive evidence.[847] However, good evidence from an open Phase III trial indicates that topical *Calendula officinalis* extract may help prevent dermatitis, pain, and erythema during radiation therapy.[848]

Reports published in the 1930s described topical aloe's beneficial effect on radiodermatitis and triggered widespread use in dermatological and cosmetic products.[849] Some practitioners recommend aloe gel for radiation dermatitis; however, recent Phase III clinical trials have shown that aloe is not beneficial for this indication.[850-853]

ADJUNCT THERAPIES

1. Patients diagnosed with cancer often experience additional health consequences. The stress of a cancer diagnosis can lead to anxiety, depression, and difficulty sleeping. Most cancers are associated with some degree of fatigue and weakness. Depending on the tumor's location, patients may also have pain, increased susceptibility to infection, or difficulty eating and breathing. Cancer treatments, such as chemotherapy or radiotherapy, may also carry adverse effects; they may increase the risk of infection, induce nausea and vomiting, and decrease appetite. Because of the multitude of secondary symptoms associated with cancer, complementary and alternative therapies are often employed in adjunct to standard care.[9-12]

2. After primary cancer treatment (chemotherapy, surgery, radiation), *adjuvant therapy* is often used in an effort to prevent cancer recurrence. *Shiitake mushroom* has been used as adjuvant therapy for a number of cancers with some success. *Lentinan* (shiitake beta-glucan) combined with chemotherapeutic agents has reduced tumor size, improved symptoms, and improved survival time in liver, gastric, and ovarian cancer.[552-569] Results from both animal and in vitro studies support these findings.* Intramuscular injection of lentinan with chemotherapy may offer survival benefits in prostate cancer, and lentinan has had no effect on prostate specific antigen (PSA) levels. Further well-designed clinical trials are required to confirm these results.

3. *Coriolus versicolor* (PSK) has shown some success as an adjuvant therapy for colorectal cancer, esophageal cancer, gastric cancer, leukemia, liver cancer, lung cancer, nasopharyngeal carcinoma, non–small cell lung cancer, and breast cancer.†

---

*References 533, 535, 536, 538-541, 543, 545, 546.
†References 416, 423, 440, 446, 449, 453, 454, 854-861.

4. *Podophyllum* has been traditionally used in Ayurvedic medicine for Hodgkin's disease, non-Hodgkin's lymphoma, and other cancers. Although clinical trials are limited, preliminary research suggests that podophyllum increases survival when used as an adjunct to radiotherapy for uterine cancer.[404]
5. *Rehmannia,* an herb traditionally believed to nourish the blood, has been found to mitigate duration and severity of aplastic anemia, a condition associated with various cancers (such as leukemia).[862,863]
6. *Psychotherapy* is a counseling process between a person and a qualified mental health professional (psychiatrist, psychologist, clinical social worker, licensed counselor). Approaches include supportive-expressive therapy, cognitive-behavioral therapy, and group therapy. There is strong scientific evidence that psychotherapy can improve the quality of life and reduce stress in cancer patients. Some studies also report that psychotherapy improves self-esteem, anxiety, and self-satisfaction, but these reports have not been substantiated.[864] Psychotherapy has not been shown to improve prognosis or survival in cancer patients.
7. *Focusing* (experiential therapy) is a method of psychotherapy that involves being aware of one's feelings about a particular issue and understanding the meaning of associated words or images. Preliminary evidence suggests that focusing may improve the mood and body attitude of cancer patients.[864]
8. *Energy therapies* are based on the theory that manipulating "energy fields" around a patient has therapeutic value. Energy therapies include a variety of modalities, such as Reiki, therapeutic touch, HT, and external Qi gong. There is a lack of convincing evidence that energy therapy is beneficial, or that these energy fields even exist.[865]
9. Preliminary data suggest that *healing touch* (HT) may benefit cancer patients by inducing relaxation and improving quality of life. Because of methodological weaknesses in a small number of studies, however, data are insufficient to make definitive recommendations.[865]
10. Research is limited with mixed results on *acupuncture* for cancer pain. Small studies have reported reduced nausea and vomiting in chemotherapy patients with acupuncture at the P6 point on the wrist.[865]
11. *Aromatherapy* is often used in people with chronic illnesses, frequently in combination with massage, to improve quality of life or well-being. Scientific evidence in this area is insufficient to form a firm conclusion about the effectiveness of aromatherapy.[866]
12. *Art therapy* involves the application of a variety of art modalities, including drawing, painting, clay, and sculpture. Art therapy enables the expression of inner thoughts or feelings when verbalization is difficult or not possible. Limited evidence suggests that family caregivers of cancer patients may benefit from art therapy to help them cope with the stress of caregiving. Art therapy may reduce stress and anxiety while improving emotions and communication with cancer patients and health care professionals. Art therapy may also reduce pain and other symptoms in cancer patients.[867]
13. *Yoga* is an ancient system of relaxation, exercise, and healing with origins in Indian philosophy. Several studies in cancer patients report enhanced quality of life, less sleep disturbance, decreased stress symptoms, and changes in cancer-related immune cells after patients received relaxation, meditation, and gentle yoga therapy.[868] Yoga is not recommended as a sole treatment for cancer but may be helpful as an adjunct therapy.
14. *Massage therapy* applies pressure to muscle and connective tissue to reduce musculoskeletal tension and pain and to improve circulation and relaxation; types include Swedish massage, Thai massage, and shiatsu. Massage therapy is generally safe when practiced by licensed practitioners. Serious adverse events are rare but may occur with inexperienced massage therapists or exotic types of massage.[869] Massage therapy may help relieve anxiety and pain in cancer patients when used appropriately.[4,870,871]
15. *Mind-body modalities* attempt to use the connection among the intellect, emotions, and body to provide physical and mental healing. Types of mind-body techniques include meditation, hypnosis, relaxation techniques, cognitive-behavioral therapy, biofeedback, and guided imagery. A meta-analysis found mind-body therapies to be beneficial in cancer patients, particularly in the reduction of anxiety, depression, and mood disturbances, and in the improvement of coping skills.[872] Mind-body techniques also may provide relief from physical symptoms (chronic low back pain, joint pain, headache, procedural pain, nausea, vomiting) and improve quality of life, sleep, and overall physical symptoms.[868]
16. *Moxibustion* is a healing technique employed across the diverse traditions of acupuncture and Oriental medicine for more than 2000 years. Moxibustion uses the principle of heat to stimulate circulation and break up congestion or stagnation of blood and *chi*. Moxibustion is applied to specific acupuncture points. Moxibustion has been suggested as a treatment for cancer pain, though the efficacy is still unclear.[873]
17. *Prayer* is often used by cancer patients for psychological well-being and in the hope of improving survival.[874] Studies of ill patients report variable effects on disease progression or death rates when intercessory prayer is used.[875] Because of methodological limitations when designing clinical trials of alternative modalities such as prayer, it may be difficult to ascertain clinical efficacy.
18. Studies have suggested that *melatonin* may offer therapeutic benefits in different cancers, particularly as an adjunct to chemotherapy.[876]
19. *Vitamin A* is a fat-soluble vitamin that is a metabolite of preformed retinoids and provitamin carotenoids in the

diet. All-*trans*-retinoic acid (ATRA, Vesanoid) is a prescription vitamin A derivative and treatment for acute promyelocytic leukemia.[877] Vitamin A supplements should not be used simultaneously with ATRA due to a risk of vitamin A toxicity.[3]

20. *Antineoplastons* are naturally occurring peptide fractions found in human blood and urine, reported to be absent in the urine of cancer patients. Scientific evidence is inconclusive regarding the effectiveness of antineoplastons in cancer treatment. Preliminary clinical studies (case series, Phase I/II trials) have examined antineoplaston types A2, A5, A10, AS2-1, and AS2-5 for a variety of cancer types.[878-880] It remains unclear if antineoplastons are effective or what doses may be safe.

21. *Arabinoxylan* is made by altering the outer shell of rice bran using enzymes from *Hyphomycetes* mycelia mushroom extract. Arabinoxylan has been shown to exert anticancer effects in animals and in vitro.[881-885] Arabinoxylan products may contain high calcium and phosphorus levels, which may be harmful for patients with compromised renal (kidney) function.[3]

22. There is some evidence that *bee pollen* may exert some anticancer effects,[886,887] but the evidence is equivocal. Caution is advised when taking bee pollen supplements because allergic reactions may occur in sensitive individuals. Bee pollen should not be used if the patient is pregnant or breastfeeding, unless otherwise directed by a physician.[3]

23. *Gerson therapy* involves a lactovegetarian diet that is low in sodium and high in potassium, fruit juices, and vitamins; in addition, coffee enemas are used. Gerson therapy attempts to alter electrolyte "imbalances" that are hypothesized to promote tumor growth.[4] This treatment is administered at a clinic in Tijuana, Mexico, and is coordinated by the Gerson Institute U.S. office in California. Limited research has been conducted on Gerson therapy. A briefly described retrospective analysis of melanoma patients reported favorable results compared to historic controls.[888] Additional prospective trials are necessary before a conclusion can be drawn. Risks associated with coffee enemas include caffeine toxicity from systemic absorption, infection from mucosal damage, and bowel perforation.[4]

24. *Copper* is a mineral present naturally in many foods, including vegetables, legumes, nuts, grains, fruits, shellfish, avocado, and beef (organs such as liver). Preliminary research reports that lowering copper levels theoretically may arrest the progression of cancer by inhibiting blood vessel growth (angiogenesis).[889-892] Copper intake has not been identified as a risk factor for the development or progression of cancer. Copper is potentially unsafe when used orally in higher doses than the recommended dietary allowance (RDA) of 0.9 mg (for adults).

25. *Hydrazine* is an industrial chemical marketed to repress weight loss and cachexia associated with cancer and to improve appetite. Preclinical studies have shown that hydrazine induces tumor regression.[4] Clinical trials have not supported the claims that hydrazine improves quality of life or survival in cancer patients.[893,894] Adverse effects reported with hydrazine include hepatotoxicity, nausea, vomiting, fatigue, neuropathy, and reduced quality of life in cancer patients.

26. High levels of *lycopene* are found in tomatoes and in tomato-based products. Several laboratory and human studies examining tomato-based products and blood lycopene levels suggest that lycopene may stimulate the immune system and may be associated with reduced cancer risk.[895]

27. *Omega-3 fatty acids* are essential fatty acids found in some plants and fish. Because of their antioxidant activity, omega-3 fatty acids have been suggested to benefit cancer treatment or prevention.[896] Caution is advised when taking omega-3 supplements because of the potential for numerous adverse effects (e.g., increased bleeding) and drug interactions. Omega-3 supplements should not be used if the patient is pregnant or breastfeeding, unless otherwise directed by a physician.[3]

28. *Selenium,* a trace mineral found in soil, water, and some foods, is an essential element in several metabolic pathways. Studies suggest that low levels of selenium may place individuals at risk for developing cancer, particularly prostate cancer. Population studies suggest that people with cancer are more likely to have low selenium levels than healthy matched individuals, but whether the low selenium levels are a cause or a consequence of disease is usually not clear.[897] It also remains unclear whether selenium supplementation is beneficial in the treatment of any type of cancer.

29. For several decades, *shark cartilage* has been proposed as a cancer treatment. Studies have shown that shark cartilage and the shark cartilage product AE-941 (Neovastat) have antiangiogenic properties.[898] There have also been several reports of successfully treating end-stage cancer patients with shark cartilage. However, these studies were not well designed and did not make reliable comparisons to accepted treatments. Preclinical studies of shark cartilage demonstrated antiangiogenic properties.[899,900] Human case reports and early-phase trials also have been reported,[901] but a Phase III trial in advanced breast and colorectal carcinoma patients found no benefit.[902] In the United States, shark cartilage products cannot claim to "cure cancer," and the FDA has sent warning letters to companies that promote products in this way. Without further evidence from well-designed human trials, it remains unclear whether shark cartilage is of any benefit in cancer, and patients are advised to check with their physicians and pharmacists before taking shark cartilage.

30. *Transcutaneous electrical nerve stimulation* (TENS) is a noninvasive technique in which a low-voltage electrical

current is delivered through wires from a small power unit to electrodes on the skin. Although TENS has been used with some success for pain associated with cancer,[903] the available evidence is equivocal.

31. *Thiamine* deficiency has been observed in some cancer patients, possibly from increased metabolic needs. However, lowered levels of thiamine may actually be beneficial in patients with cancer.[904] Currently, it remains unclear whether thiamine supplementation plays a role in the management of any particular type(s) of cancer.

32. *Traditional Chinese Medicine* (TCM) is based on the ancient Chinese philosophy of Taoism. TCM uses more than 120 different herbs in cancer treatment, depending on the type and cause of the cancer. Reported benefits include reduced tumors, reduced treatment side effects, and improved response to treatment.[905] More rigorous studies are needed before TCM can be recommended with confidence as an adjunct to cancer treatment, although centuries of traditional use in cancer cannot be discounted.

33. Dietary intake of fruits and vegetables high in *vitamin C* has been associated with a reduced risk of various types of cancer in population studies, particularly cancers of the mouth, esophagus, stomach, colon, and lung. Vitamin C also has a long history of adjunctive use in cancer therapy, and although no definitive studies have used intravenous (or oral) vitamin C, evidence suggests it has benefit in some patients. However, it is not clear whether the vitamin C is the beneficial component of various foods, and vitamin C supplements have not been associated with this protective effect.[906] Experts have recommended increasing dietary consumption of fruits and vegetables high in vitamin C, such as apples, asparagus, berries, broccoli, cabbage, melon (cantaloupe, honeydew, watermelon), cauliflower, citrus fruits (lemons, oranges), fortified breads/grains/cereal, kale, kiwi, potatoes, spinach, and tomatoes. Large doses (>2 g) may cause diarrhea and gastrointestinal upset.

34. *Antioxidant* use is often discouraged in patients undergoing treatment with chemicals or radiation, which depend on oxidative damage and cytotoxicity to exert anticancer effects. For this reason, it has been proposed that high-dose antioxidants may actually reduce the effectiveness of chemotherapy and radiotherapy. This remains an area of controversy, with variable research results.[907] Patients interested in using high-dose antioxidants such as *vitamin E* during chemotherapy or radiation should discuss this decision with their medical oncologist or radiation oncologist. Besides potentially interfering with chemotherapy or radiation therapy, numerous adverse effects and drug interactions are possible.

35. *Probiotics* have been shown to be effective in treating a number of gastrointestinal symptoms, including colitis and diarrhea,[908] and may offer some benefits for relieving radiation-induced colitis and diarrhea.

INTEGRATIVE THERAPY PLAN

- Cancer symptoms are highly variable and depend on the location of the primary and metastatic lesions. General symptoms that should prompt a medical evaluation include unexplained weight loss, fatigue, loss of appetite, and fever.
- Signs of specific types of cancer include blood in the stool or vomit (gastrointestinal cancer), vaginal bleeding (uterine and cervical cancer), difficulty breathing (lung cancer or anemia from other type of tumor), lymph node swelling (lymphoma), or headaches with vomiting and mental status changes (brain cancer).
- Diagnostic workup varies depending on the type of cancer suspected. Physical examination and basic laboratory values are initially ordered. Additional studies may include radiographic examination and biopsy. Genetic testing may be performed for cancers with known underlying genetic causes, such as BRCA1/BRCA2 mutations in breast cancer and adenomatosis polyposis coli gene in familial adenomatous polyposis.
- Once a diagnosis of cancer has been made, patients should be treated with the standard of care for the particular cancer and its stage. Treatments have traditionally included chemotherapy, radiation, and surgery.
- Patients should be counseled that herbal therapies have not been proven to treat or prevent cancer. Additionally, herbs with antioxidant properties may interfere with the effects of chemotherapy and radiation on neoplastic cells. Before beginning any herbal therapy, patients should discuss their plans with their oncologist in detail.
- Mistletoe is one of the most widely used unconventional cancer treatments in Europe. Extracts have been studied for a variety of human cancers including bladder, breast, cervical, CNS, colorectal, head and neck, liver, lung, lymphatic, ovarian, and renal (kidney) cancers, as well as melanoma and leukemia. Efficacy has not been conclusively proved for any one condition, and some studies even showed a lack of efficacy in certain preparations for a variety of cancers.
- Several human studies suggest that Asian ginseng (*Panax ginseng*) may reduce the risk and progression of various organ cancers, especially if ginseng powder or extract is used. Results may have been affected by other lifestyle choices in people who use ginseng, such as exercise or dietary habits. Asian ginseng is also reported to help protect against radiation damage, increase immunity and well-being, and decrease fatigue. Additional trials are necessary before making a conclusion.
- Patients may benefit from psychotherapy or mind-body techniques to aid in the treatment of depression, stress, and decreased quality of life.
- Counsel patients regarding controlling weight and exercising regularly, which can reduce the risk of developing cancer. The American Cancer Society recommends at least 30 minutes of physical activity 5 or more days a week if the individual can tolerate it.

- Recommend to the patient to eat 5 or more servings of fresh fruits and vegetables every day. Fruits, vegetables, and whole grains contain vitamins, minerals, fiber, and antioxidants and may help protect the patient from developing various types of cancer. A variety of types of produce, such as kale, chard, spinach, dark-green lettuce, peppers, and squashes, should be included in the diet.
- Advise patients to limit high-fat diets, which may be linked to a higher rate of cancer (e.g., colon). It is important to limit saturated fats from animal sources such as red meat. Other foods that contain saturated fat include milk, cheese, ice cream, and coconut and palm oils. It is best to restrict the total fat intake to about 30% of the daily calories, with no more than 10% coming from saturated fats.
- Advise patients to limit tobacco use, as well as alcohol intake (especially in women). According to a well-publicized study, women who drank at least two drinks daily had more than twice the breast cancer rate as women who drank less.[909] Excess alcohol and tobacco use is also linked to increased risk of cancer in the digestive tract, respiratory system, and liver.[910]

Case Studies

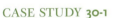

CASE STUDY 30-1

PK is a 75-year-old man recently diagnosed with stage 1 prostate cancer. He comes to your clinic and seeks your advice. His physician has recommended "watchful waiting" initially. PK takes glipizide for type 2 diabetes and aspirin for heart disease prevention. His blood sugar is well controlled. His last HbA$_{1c}$ value was less than 6%. He also uses St. John's wort for mild depression and licorice for upset stomach. He expresses interest in flaxseed because his neighbor, who had breast cancer 15 years ago, takes flaxseed and has not had a recurrence of her disease. PK is also interested in any other herbal therapies that might prevent a progression of his disease. Considering PK's condition and his current medications (including herbal supplements), discuss complementary treatment options for prostate cancer.

Answer: Flaxseed is *not* recommended for the treatment of prostate cancer. Several studies have associated the intake of alpha-linolenic acid, present in flaxseed, with an increased risk of developing prostate cancer. Although other herbal remedies have been proposed for the treatment of prostate cancer, to date their benefits remain controversial.

American pawpaw *(Asimina triloba)* contains asitrocin and asitrocinones, which have exhibited potent bioactivity against prostate (PC-3) cell lines at 10 to 100 times the potency of the anticancer drug doxorubicin (Adriamycin). Because it contains cytotoxic substances, American pawpaw should be taken under a physician's supervision. Because of this, coupled with the early stage of PK's disease, American pawpaw is not recommended at present.

Chrysanthemum *(Chrysanthemum awadskii)* has been suggested to have anticancer properties. However, allergic reactions are very common with this herb. Chrysanthemum may improve fasting blood glucose and postprandial glucose in type 2 diabetic patients; thus it may improve PK's diabetes but may also act synergistically with glipizide and cause hypoglycemia. If PK does use this herb, his glipizide dosage might require adjustment.

Cranberry *(Vaccinium macrocarpon)* might be beneficial and is considered nontoxic. One or two glasses of unsweetened cranberry juice can be added to his regimen. Modified citrus pectin might be beneficial because it reportedly decreases the doubling time of PSA. Red clover contains isoflavones (phytoestrogens). The effects of red clover have been evaluated in human prostate cancer cell lines in vitro, but clinical evidence is limited.

Saw palmetto *(Sarenoa repens)* is often taken for prostate problems, including benign prostatic hyperplasia (BPH) and prostate cancer. In vitro studies have demonstrated saw palmetto to inhibit the growth of prostatic cancer cells and may actually destroy cancer cells. Saw palmetto may artificially lower PSA levels; thus, it may interfere with monitoring PK's PSA levels. Furthermore, the combined use of saw palmetto and aspirin may increase the risk of bleeding.

PK should be counseled on the potential adverse interactions of these therapies, and that none of these herbal remedies are supported by significant clinical evidence of efficacy for prostate cancer.

PK should be especially counseled about the effects of St. John's wort on glucose control. Although he has good glucose control, this herb may alter glucose metabolism, and PK should therefore continue to monitor his blood sugar carefully. Because it is metabolized by the CYP450 system, St. John's wort may have effects on a variety of medications and herbal therapies. The patient should also be advised to take his licorice several hours before or after his other medications, because licorice may inhibit absorption of other drugs if taken together.

CASE STUDY 30-2

AP explains that her 54-year-old father has undergone surgery for lung cancer and a course of chemotherapy with cisplatin (Platinol) and vinblastine (Velbe). He also takes ginseng for energy, bacopa for memory enhancement, and valerian for anxiety. He has smoked two packs of cigarettes a day since high school and is still smoking because "it doesn't matter now." He complains of fatigue, hair loss, nausea, vomiting, decreased appetite, and weight loss, which are common side effects of chemotherapy. AP read on the Internet that astragalus may be beneficial for his cancer. How would you counsel this patient's daughter?

Answer: Astragalus-based Chinese herbal medicine may increase the effectiveness of platinum-based chemotherapy with agents such as cisplatin. Astragalus has been occasionally used with the goal of reducing side effects, such as fatigue and weight loss; however, neither astragalus nor any other herbal therapy has definitely proved to be beneficial.

The ginseng AP's father takes for energy may have cytotoxic effects, as demonstrated in numerous laboratory and clinical studies. Therefore, ginseng may benefit his cancer treatment. However, if decides to take astragalus, he should be counseled about possible interactions with ginseng. Both herbs may decrease blood sugar and cholesterol, and their additive effects are unknown. Additionally, both have anticoagulant activity and may place him at an increased risk of bleeding. AP's father should be aware of signs of unusual bleeding, including severe bruising, nosebleeds, or blood in the urine. Ginseng has been shown to induce hypertension, whereas astragalus may produce hypotension. These two drugs' effect on blood pressure is unknown, so it should be monitored closely.

Ginger may also be recommended to AP's father based on some evidence that it may reduce nausea and vomiting associated with chemotherapy.

CASE STUDY 30-3

CS is a 70-year-old woman who recently underwent a partial mastectomy for breast cancer. She comes with her daughter to have her prescriptions refilled. Besides tamoxifen for breast cancer chemotherapy, CS is taking atorvastatin for hyperlipidemia, atenolol for hypertension, a low-dose aspirin for heart disease protection, and a multivitamin. In addition to her drug regimen, CS is taking herbal supplements containing cat's claw and feverfew for osteoarthritis. According to her last lipid profile, her total cholesterol was 180 mg/dL. Her monitored blood pressure in the morning was 125/70 mm Hg. CS is interested in dietary phytoestrogens to prevent a remission of her breast cancer. A friend told her that black cohosh would be beneficial. How do you counsel this patient?

Answer: In vitro, black cohosh has been shown to inhibit the growth of estrogen receptor–positive breast cancer cells. However, this finding has yet to be reproduced in human studies, and black cohosh cannot be recommended as beneficial at this time. More importantly, CS should be counseled on the potential interactions between her current medications and herbs or supplements.

Cat's claw and feverfew both have antiplatelet effects, which may have additive effects with aspirin and may increase her risk of bleeding. Black cohosh contains salicylic acid, which is a chemical precursor to acetylsalicylate (aspirin). If CS decides to take black cohosh, she may theoretically further increase her bleeding risk. Cat's claw also has blood pressure–lowering effects and, when used with atenolol, may have additive effects. If CS decides to use cat's claw, her blood pressure may be further reduced, placing her at risk for dangerously low blood pressure. CS should monitor her blood pressure closely and be aware of any sudden drop or symptoms such as dizziness or fainting. She should also consult her physician regarding her medication treatment plan.

Notably, antioxidants typically found in multivitamins are thought to reduce the cytotoxic effects of chemotherapy such as tamoxifen. CS should be advised to limit the number of antioxidant-containing supplements and herbs taken, such as vitamin E, lycopene, and quercetin.

References for Chapter 30 can be found on the Evolve website at http://evolve.elsevier.com/Ulbricht/herbalpharmacotherapy/

Review Questions

1. All the following are true of aloe *except*:
   a. Antimutagenic effects are attributed to di(2-ethylhexyl)phthalate (DEHP).
   b. The half life of aloe-emodin is 4 to 6 hours.
   c. Preliminary studies suggest antiviral effects of aloe.
   d. Promotion of apoptosis in vitro has been reported as a possible antineoplastic mechanism.

2. True or false: The percentage and relative proportions of astragalosides, trigonosides, and flavonoid constituents of dried astragalus root vary with the age, size, and growing conditions of the root.

3. Which of the following statements is true regarding chaparral?
   a. The chaparral constituent nordihydroguaiaretic acid (NDGA) has been theorized to block cellular respiration.
   b. NDGA induces endoplasmic reticulum calcium release.
   c. Chaparral may have mutagenic properties; stimulation of tumor growth was reported in an early study using NDGA to treat cancer.
   d. All the above.

4. True or false: Cranberry has shown some benefit in the treatment of bladder cancer.

5. Ginseng may interact with which of the following chemotherapeutic agents?
   a. Cytoxan
   b. Doxorubicin
   c. Fluorouracil
   d. All the above

6. PSK is derived from which of the following?
   a. Shiitake mushroom
   b. Reishi mushroom
   c. Coriolus versicolor mushroom
   d. Maitake mushroom

7. All the following are true of shiitake *except*:
   a. Lentinan, derived from shiitake, has been administered by injection in clinical studies.
   b. Shiitake lentinan has not been shown to benefit mean survival time in cancer patients.
   c. Shiitake does not appear to affect prostate-specific antigen (PSA) levels.
   d. For prostate cancer, shiitake-containing capsules have been administered based on weight, with a dose of 8 g per day for a 70-kg man.

8. Which of the following statements concerning mistletoe is *true*?
   a. Mistletoe is a widely used cancer treatment in Europe.
   b. Clinical studies have consistently shown mistletoe to be an effective treatment of human cancer.
   c. Mistletoe extracts and berries are available as dietary supplements in the United States.
   d. All the above.

9. Turmeric has shown which of the following activities in laboratory tests?
   a. Antiproliferative and/or proapoptotic effects in numerous cell lines
   b. Mutagenic effects, shown by the Ames test
   c. Induction of protein kinase C activity
   d. Oxidative cytotoxicity against tumor cells

10. What is considered to be the active constituent of milk thistle?
    a. Silica
    b. Salicylic acid
    c. Silymarin
    d. Aviscumine

Answers are found in the Answers to Review Questions section in the back of the text.

A Safety: Adverse Effects, Interactions, Pharmacokinetics

This appendix contains information on the pharmacokinetics and adverse effects of select herbal products, as well as known or potential interactions between herbs and drugs, other herbs/supplements, and foods. This is not an all-inclusive or comprehensive list of known or potential interactions. Concurrent use of substances with similar effects (e.g., antiinflammatory, estrogenic, hepatotoxic) should be approached with caution. A qualified health care practitioner should be consulted with specific questions or concerns regarding potential interactions.

Acacia (Acacia senegal)

Pharmacokinetics: Insufficient available evidence.

Adverse effects

There are minimal adverse effects associated with acacia gum (gum arabic). The most common reported side effects are allergic asthma and rhinitis[1-15] and gastrointestinal complaints.[16] The bark of certain *Acacia* species, such as *Acacia catechu*, contains a high percentage of tannins.[17] The oral toxicity of plant tannins is low, as tannins are readily hydrolyzed in the gut to gallic acid and other metabolites. However, liver and kidney toxicity has occurred with high tannin doses used topically or intravenously.[18] Tannin consumption has been associated with certain cancers, such as esophageal cancer; however, it is unclear whether this is due to the tannins themselves or other compounds associated with tannins.[19]

Interactions

ALCOHOL: According to secondary sources, acacia is insoluble in solutions greater than 50% ethyl alcohol.

AMOXICILLIN: Acacia has been shown to affect the absorption of amoxicillin when taken concurrently;[20] this is likely attributable to the fiber in acacia, which may impair the absorption of oral agents. Doses should be separated by at least 4 hours.

ANTINEOPLASTIC AGENTS: Based on in vitro evidence,[1] use of acacia as a surfactant may increase the intestinal absorption of some antineoplastic agents through P-glycoprotein (P-gp) inhibition and thus improve bioavailability for P-gp substrate.

IRON: According to secondary sources, acacia can be gelatinized by solutions of ferric iron salts.

KIDNEY AND LIVER FUNCTION TESTS: *Acacia catechu* contains high levels of tannins;[17] overuse may result in tannin toxicity, which may be reflected in kidney and/or liver function tests.

ORAL AGENTS: According to secondary sources, the fiber content of acacia gum may impair the absorption of oral agents.

P-GLYCOPROTEIN SUBSTRATES: P-gp is a cell membrane–associated protein that transports a variety of drug substrates. Interaction with P-gp, including activation, inhibition, and induction, can lead to altered plasma or brain levels of P-gp substrates. Use of acacia as a surfactant may increase the intestinal absorption of some antineoplastic agents through P-gp inhibition, thus improving bioavailability for P-gp substrate, as suggested by uptake of epirubicin by Caco-2 cells in vitro.[21] However, clinical reports of such drug interactions are lacking.

Aconite (Aconitum napellus)

Pharmacokinetics

According to animal research, the esophagus absorbs the alkaloid aconitine with greater ability than the stomach.[1] Aconite appears to be metabolized in the liver; however, the route of metabolism has not been fully elucidated. Cytochrome P450 (CYP450) may be involved in aconite's metabolism. *Aconitum* alkaloids (aconitine, mesaconitine, hypaconitine, and their metabolites) were detected in urine 6 days after ingestion. These alkaloids are thought to be excreted in a time-dependent manner.[2] Because of aconite's lipid solubility and molecular weight of 645.7 kD, its elimination is unlikely to be enhanced by hemodialysis, peritoneal dialysis, hemoperfusion, or hemofiltration.[3]

Adverse effects

Aconite is unsafe when used orally or topically. Aconite alkaloids may cause serious cardiovascular and central nervous system (CNS) adverse effects. Based on clinical and animal data, aconite may cause hypotension, irregular pulse, various arrhythmias, or first-degree heart block.[3-17] Aconite poisoning causes prolonged repolarization of the myocardium, which may lead to abnormal depolarizations and ventricular tachyarrhythmias, including ventricular ectopy, ventricular tachycardia, and ventricular fibrillation.[18,19]

Aconite has also been reported to cause nausea, vomiting, epigastric pain, and diarrhea in clinical and animal studies.[1,5,17,20-24] It should be avoided in patients with gastrointestinal disorders, stomach ulcers, duodenal ulcers, reflux esophagitis, ulcerative colitis, spastic colitis, and diverticulosis. Aconite may lower blood sugar levels, based on limited human research.[5,20] It should be avoided in patients with diabetes.

Interactions

BLOOD PRESSURE: Aconitine has purported hypotensive effects.[3,5-7,12] Concomitant use with blood pressure–lowering agents may result in additive effects.

DIGITALIS: Cardiac glycosides may alter aconitine's effects on cardiac tissue, producing an unclear pharmacological effect. The manifestations of digitalis and aconite poisoning are similar,[25] and thus, simultaneous use of these agents could be extremely dangerous and could result in additive effects for both agents.

ELECTROLYTES: Aconitine purportedly has diuretic effects, likely from the high water content of homeopathic preparations. Overuse may lead to electrolyte imbalance.

Agrimony (Agrimonia spp.)

Pharmacokinetics: Insufficient available evidence.

Adverse effects

Reports of significant adverse effects of agrimony are currently lacking. The high amount of tannins (up to 21%) in agrimony may lead to gastrointestinal upset and nausea; it should be taken with food to avoid such effects. Agrimony should be used only for mild and acute diarrhea. Patients who are prone to constipation should avoid agrimony.[1] Agrimony contains up to 21% tannins.[2] The oral toxicity of plant tannins is low, as tannins are readily hydrolyzed in the gut to gallic acid and other metabolites. However, liver and kidney toxicity has occurred with high tannin doses used topically or intravenously.[3] Tannin consumption has been associated with certain cancers, such as esophageal cancer; however, it is unclear whether this is due to the tannins themselves or other compounds associated with tannins.[4]

Interactions

ANTICOAGULANTS/ANTIPLATELETS: Isocoumarins can be found in the roots of agrimony.[2] Concomitant use of coumarins and anticoagulants/antiplatelets may increase the risk of bleeding. However, clinical reports of such drug interactions are lacking.

BLOOD GLUCOSE: Agrimony has demonstrated insulin-like effects in mice,[3,4] so it may alter blood glucose readings. Concurrent use with other agents that lower blood sugar might increase the risk for hypoglycemia.

BLOOD PRESSURE: Hypotensive effects in anesthetized cats have been documented for agrimony extract given by intravenous injection; blood pressure was lowered by more than 40%.[5] Agrimony thus may lower blood pressure; concurrent use with other blood pressure–lowering agents may cause additive effects.

ESTROGENIC AGENTS: Agrimony may contain estrogen-like constituents,[6] which could interact with concurrent estrogen/phytoestrogen use. However, clinical reports of such drug interactions are lacking.

KIDNEY AND LIVER FUNCTION TESTS: Because agrimony contains up to 21% tannins, chronic ingestion may result in nephrotoxicity (kidney damage) or hepatotoxicity (liver damage). Kidney and/or liver function tests may be altered. Caution is warranted in patients taking other agents that may also cause kidney or liver damage.

Alfalfa (Medicago sativa)

Pharmacokinetics: Insufficient available evidence.

Adverse effects

Alfalfa has long been used with few adverse effects. In the few human case reports available, alfalfa appears to be generally well tolerated. Lupus-like effects have been associated with alfalfa use.[1-4] Symptoms included arthralgias (joint pain), myalgias (muscle pain), and rash; positive antinuclear antibodies (ANAs) were seen 3 weeks to 7 months after initiating alfalfa therapy. Symptoms resolved upon discontinuation of alfalfa tablets in all patients. It is unclear what other environmental or genetic factors may have affected these individuals, and the association with alfalfa is unclear. Nonetheless, caution is warranted in patients with systemic lupus erythematosus (SLE) or other autoimmune diseases due to insufficient safety data.

Alfalfa has been associated with reduced serum glucose levels in rat studies.[5,6] Also, alfalfa contains constituents, including coumestrol, with reported estrogenic activity.[7-9] Effects in humans are unclear.

A case report documented hypokalemia (low potassium level) in a woman who had been drinking a "cleansing tea" containing alfalfa, licorice, and nettles.[10] Her potassium level returned to normal after she stopped drinking the tea and took potassium supplements. The specific cause of the hypokalemia was not clear. Notably, both the other constituents have been associated with hypokalemia (nettles may exert a diuretic effect, and licorice may decrease potassium through an aldosterone-like effect).

Interactions

ANTICOAGULANTS/ANTIPLATELETS: Alfalfa contains significant amounts of vitamin K[11,12] and therefore may reduce the effects of anticoagulants/antiplatelets that rely on depletion of vitamin K. However, clinical reports of such drug interactions are lacking.

BLOOD ALCOHOL: Many alfalfa tinctures and liquid extracts contain high levels of alcohol and may affect blood alcohol levels. Typical drug-alcohol reactions are possible.

BLOOD GLUCOSE: Alfalfa may lower blood glucose levels[5,6,13] and interact with other hypoglycemic agents.

BLOOD LIPIDS: Based on clinical and animal data, alfalfa may lower total cholesterol, low-density lipoprotein (LDL), and triglyceride concentrations.[14-17]

CALCIUM: Mean serum calcium levels decreased significantly in patients taking 40 g of heat-prepared alfalfa seed three times daily for 8 weeks.[14] However, the alfalfa constituent L-canavanine was shown to elevate intracellular calcium levels in vitro.[18] Alfalfa may interact with calcium supplementation.

CHLORPROMAZINE (THORAZINE): Chlorpromazine diminished the adenylate cyclase activity of alfalfa in vitro.[19] The clinical relevance of this effect is not clear.

ESTROGENIC AGENTS: Alfalfa has been reported to contain coumestrol, a phytoestrogen that may possess estrogenic properties.[7,8] Excessive amounts of alfalfa may interact with estrogen/phytoestrogen therapy. However, clinical reports of such drug interactions are lacking.

IRON: Alfalfa and other fibers have been shown in vitro to bind iron[20] and may thereby decrease its absorption.

PHOTOSENSITIZING AGENTS: High amounts of alfalfa may potentiate photosensitization. Concomitant use with other photosensitizing agents might increase the likelihood of photosensitivity reactions.

POTASSIUM: Anecdotally, alfalfa has been reported to lower serum potassium concentrations.[10]

THYROID HORMONES: Immunoreactive thyrotropin-releasing hormone–like material has been found in alfalfa, although its biological action is unclear.[21]

URIC ACID: Alfalfa may increase serum urate levels.[14]

VITAMIN E: Alfalfa contains saponins, which may interfere with the absorption or activity of vitamin E. In addition, vitamin E may potentiate the effects of L-canavanine, a component of alfalfa associated with the development of lupus-like syndrome or exacerbation of lupus.[3] Data are limited in this area.

VITAMIN K: Alfalfa contains vitamin K[11,12] and may alter levels in the blood, which in turn may affect clotting time and anticoagulant therapy.

WHITE BLOOD CELL COUNTS: Lupus-like effects have been associated with alfalfa use.[1-4] It has also been shown to stimulate the immune system.[1,22,23]

Aloe (Aloe vera)

Pharmacokinetics

Aloe latex contains anthraquinone glycosides (aloin, aloe-emodin, barbaloin), which are absorbed well only after digestion by intestinal bacteria and are eliminated in the urine, bile, feces, and breast milk. The half-life of aloe-emodin is about 48 to 50 hours.[1]

Adverse effects

Aloe leaf is used topically for burns and wound healing. Aloe latex is used systemically (internally); it is commonly used as a laxative and may cause abdominal cramping and diarrhea.[2,3] Excessive use may cause potassium loss.[4] Combined use of oral aloe latex and other laxatives or diuretics may exacerbate hypokalemia, dehydration, metabolic alkalosis, and other electrolyte abnormalities. Chronic use has been associated with an increased risk of colorectal cancer.[5] Aloe has been implicated in thyroid dysfunction.[6]

Interactions

ANTIDIABETIC AGENTS: Oral aloe gel has been associated with reduced blood glucose when used with glibenclamide (also known as glyburide in the United States).[7] Concurrent use of aloe with other agents that lower blood sugar, such as insulin,[7] may increase the risk of hypoglycemia.

ELECTROLYTES: Laxatives such as aloe may cause fluid and potassium loss[2,3] and may lead to hypokalemia. Concurrent use of aloe, diuretics, and/or laxatives may increase the risk of dehydration, hypokalemia, and electrolyte imbalance.

ESTROGENIC AGENTS: Methanolic extracts from *Aloe* spp. contain hydroxyanthraquinones such as emodin. These phytoestrogens have an affinity for human estrogen receptors[16] and may alter the effects of other estrogenic agents; however, clinical reports of such drug interactions are lacking.

HISTOLOGICAL TESTS: Numerous laboratory studies suggest that aloe-emodin and aloe extracts may have cytotoxic or anticancer effects.[8-11] Aloe has been suggested as an adjunct to standard chemotherapies and may affect histological tests.

ORAL AGENTS: When taken orally, the high mucilage content in aloe may interfere with the absorption of foods and oral agents. Malabsorption may occur after prolonged oral use of aloe. However, clinical reports of such drug interactions are lacking.

SEVOFLURANE (ULTANE): Excess bleeding was reported when a patient took aloe before surgery; a possible interaction was suggested with the anesthetic agent sevoflurane, which also has antiplatelet effects.[17] Aloe should be discontinued 1 week before surgery.

THYROID HORMONES: Aloe has been linked to thyroid dysfunction.[6] Theoretically, aloe may interact with thyroid hormones and test results.

VIRAL LEVELS: Acemannan, the major carbohydrate fraction in aloe gel, has been shown in vitro to possess antiretroviral activities.[12-14] Preliminary clinical reports suggest that azidothymidine (AZT) may be boosted by aloe ingestion.[15]

VITAMINS C AND E: Aloe has been shown to affect the absorption of vitamins C and E in humans.[18]

American Ginseng. See Ginseng (*Panax* spp.)

American Hellebore (*Veratrum viride*). See False Hellebore (*Veratrum* spp.)

American Pawpaw (*Asimina triloba*)

Pharmacokinetics: Insufficient available evidence

Adverse effects

Rigorous studies on the long-term effects of pawpaw use are lacking. The safety and efficacy of America pawpaw has not been established.

Interactions

HISTOLOGICAL TESTS: Many compounds in American pawpaw were found to have cytotoxic effects on cancer cell lines,[1-13] which may alter the outcome of histological tests.

American Pennyroyal (*Hedeoma pulegioides*). See False Pennyroyal (*Hedeoma* spp.)

Anapsos. See Polypodium (*Polypodium leucotomos*)
Andrographis (*Andrographis paniculata*)

Pharmacokinetics

In humans, maximum plasma levels of andrographolide (active constituent of andrographis) are reached within 1½ to 2 hours of a typical therapeutic dose (20 mg, or four tablets of Kan Jang preparation).[1] After oral administration, andrographolide undergoes extensive first-pass metabolism.[2] Andrographolides are excreted primarily in urine. The half-life of andrographolide is approximately 6.6 hours.[1]

Adverse effects

At usual recommended doses, andrographis appears to be safe and well tolerated. Adverse effects reported in trials have been mild, infrequent, and self-limiting. However, most trials have been brief (≤2 weeks), and the safety of long-term use remains unclear. Doses of 5 mg/kg andrographolide daily for 3 weeks, followed by 10 mg/kg for 3 weeks, were not well tolerated. Side effects included multiple cases of allergic reactions, fatigue, headache, painful lymphadenopathy, nausea, diarrhea, and elevated liver transaminases.[3] Animal studies suggest that andrographis may have antifertility or contraceptive effects at high doses.[4]

Interactions

ANTIBODY LEVELS: Several systematic reviews and randomized controlled trials (RCTs) indicate that andrographis may effectively treat upper respiratory infections (URIs), purportedly by enhancing immune function.[5-14] Antibody tests thus may be altered. Interactions with immunomodulators may occur.

ANTICOAGULANTS/ANTIPLATELETS: Andrographis been shown to inhibit platelet aggregation in vitro,[15] which may account for its purported antithrombotic activity. Theoretically, concomitant use of andrographis with anticoagulants/antiplatelets may increase the risk of bleeding. However, clinical reports of such drug interactions are lacking.

BLOOD GLUCOSE: Andrographis has been shown to lower blood glucose in animals.[16]

BLOOD PRESSURE: Based on animal studies, andrographis may lower blood pressure[17] and may therefore interact with antihypertensive agents.

CYTOKINES AND INFLAMMATORY MARKERS: Based on several in vitro and in vivo studies,[18-24] andrographis its constituents may have antiinflammatory effects.

HISTOLOGICAL TESTS: Based on several in vitro studies, andographolide may have antineoplastic effects[25-27] and may alter the outcome of histological tests.

VIRAL LEVELS: Andrographis may act as a protease inhibitor[3,28] and may decrease viral load in patients infected with human immunodeficiency virus (HIV). Andrographis thus has been suggested to improve clinical outcome in HIV patients when combined with antiretroviral agents.

WHITE BLOOD CELL COUNTS: Several systematic reviews and RCTs indicate that andrographis may effectively treat URIs,[5-14] reportedly by enhancing immune function. WBC counts and activity may be altered. Andrographis may act as a protease inhibitor and may increase CD4+ cells in HIV-infected patients.[3,28] Andrographis thus has been suggested to improve clinical outcome in HIV patients when combined with antiretroviral agents.

Apricot (Prunus armeniaca)

Pharmacokinetics

After intravenous (IV) administration of laetrile (amygdalin-derived alternative cancer agent), amygdalin has been shown to be excreted primarily unchanged, with urinary recovery as high as 100%. Peak plasma levels after a 6-g intramuscular (IM) dose of laetrile were 180 mcg/L.[1] Prunasin, a metabolite of amygdalin, has a bioavailability of approximately 50%. Prunasin's volume of distribution and clearance are greater than those of amygdalin.[2]

Adverse effects

Apricot is generally well tolerated when consumed in normal amounts as food. Apricot pits are toxic at low to moderate dosing levels due to the cyanogenic compound amygdalin. Apricot kernels may cause chronic poisoning, with symptoms of increased blood thiocyanate level, goiter, thyroid cancer, optic nerve lesions, blindness, ataxia, hypertonia, cretinism (stunted physical and mental growth in infants and children caused by a lack of thyroid hormone), and mental retardation. Demyelinating lesions and neuromyopathies reportedly occur after chronic exposure, according to unsubstantiated sources. Laetrile is considered unsafe in any form because of its potential for causing cyanide toxicity. Reactions appear to be more severe with oral than with IV or IM administration.

Interactions

BLOOD GLUCOSE: Apricot contains a variety of sugars, which may increase blood glucose levels and interact with agents used to lower blood sugar.

BLOOD PRESSURE: Apricot kernels may cause hypotension.

ELECTROLYTES: Apricot is rich in potassium. High levels of potassium, or hyperkalemia, can lead to harmful effects, including cardiac arrhythmia. However, potassium overdose is generally not a concern with using apricot as food.

IRON: Apricot is rich in iron, which may be reflected in blood tests.

VITAMINS: Apricot is rich in various water-soluble vitamins, including thiamine, niacin, and vitamin C. These may be reflected in blood tests; excessive amounts may be detected in the urine.

Arnica (Arnica spp.)

Pharmacokinetics

The pharmacokinetics of arnica is not well understood. It appears that 30% to 50% of sesquiterpene lactones, the active constituents of arnica, are bound to plasma.[1]

Adverse effects

Based on historical use and available research, arnica is generally well tolerated when used in recommended highly dilute homeopathic doses for up to 2 weeks. Allergic skin reactions and numerous cases of contact dermatitis have been reported.[2-9] To avoid contact dermatitis, arnica should not be used on open wounds or near the eyes or mouth. It should be avoided in patients with known allergies to arnica or any plant in the Asteraceae (Compositae) family.

Ingestion of oral nondiluted *Arnica montana*–containing extracts has induced severe gastroenteritis, nervousness, accelerated heart rate, muscular weakness, and death.[10]

Interactions

ANALGESIC AND ANTIINFLAMMATORY AGENTS: Arnica may have antiinflammatory and analgesic activity[11-14] and theoretically may interact with similar agents. In clinical research involving healthy human subjects, topical arnica increased hydroxyethyl salicylate's analgesic effects.[15]

ANESTHETICS: According to one survey of 601 children presenting for day surgery, herbal products may have serious interactions with anesthetic drugs. Arnica was one of the most common herbals used by children, which may have implications for the perioperative management of children presenting for surgery.[16]

ANTICOAGULANTS/ANTIPLATELETS: Because of its theoretical inhibition of platelet activation, arnica may enhance bleeding if taken with other anticoagulants. *Arnica montana* has been shown to increase bleeding time by inhibition of platelet aggregation in vitro,[17] although no change in bleeding time was observed in a clinical trial using a homeopathic dose of arnica.[18]

BELLIS PERENNIS: Arnica used with *B. perennis* has been suggested to reduce postpartum blood loss.[19]

BLOOD LIPIDS: Sesquiterpene lactones block lipogenesis, resulting in reduced serum lipid levels in mice.[20]

BLOOD PRESSURE: Based on anecdotal evidence, arnica may reduce effectiveness of antihypertensive agents.

Arrowroot (Maranta arundinacea)

Pharmacokinetics: Insufficient available evidence.

Adverse effects

There is limited available evidence on the adverse effects of arrowroot. Based on limited available scientific literature, the most common adverse effect of arrowroot was constipation and exacerbation of dyspepsia.[1] Based on its historical use as food, arrowroot appears to be well tolerated.

Interactions
Insufficient available evidence.

Ash (Fraxinus spp.)

Pharmacokinetics: Insufficient available evidence.

Adverse effects

Documentation of severe adverse effects other than allergic responses is lacking.

Interactions

ANALGESIC AND ANTIINFLAMMATORY AGENTS: According to a review, the hydroxycoumarin components present in ash may inhibit the arachidonic acid cascade.[1] Because arachidonic acid serves as precursor in the synthesis of prostaglandins, ash may interact with antiinflammatory or analgesic agents.

ANTICOAGULANTS/ANTIPLATELETS: Ash contains hydroxycoumarins;[1,2] concurrent use of coumarins and anticoagulants/antiplatelets may increase the risk of bleeding. However, clinical reports of such drug interactions are lacking.

URIC ACID: Based on animal and clinical studies, treatment with a combination product containing ash (Rebixiao granule, RBXG) may reduce blood uric acid concentrations.[3]

WHITE BLOOD CELL COUNTS: According to a review, the hydroxycoumarin components present in ash may inhibit activation of T-cells.[2]

Ashwagandha (Withania somnifera)

Pharmacokinetics: Insufficient available evidence.

Adverse effects

There are few reports of adverse effects associated with ashwagandha. Occasionally, clinical trials have reported dermatitis, diuresis, diarrhea, hypoglycemia, nausea, and abdominal discomfort.[1-4]

Interactions

ANDROGENIC AGENTS: Based on rat evidence of increased testicular weight and spermatogenesis, ashwagandha may possess androgenic (testosterone-like) properties.[5] Concurrent use with antiandrogens, androgens, or testosterone may result in interactions.

ANTICOAGULANTS/ANTIPLATELETS: Ashwagandha has been reported to increase coagulation time greatly in rats,[6] although the significance in humans is not clear. Theoretically, concurrent use of ashwagandha and anticoagulants/antiplatelets may increase the risk of bleeding. However, clinical reports of such drug interactions are lacking.

BLOOD GLUCOSE: Ashwagandha was shown to decrease blood sugar in patients with type 2 diabetes, although the mechanism is unclear.[3,4]

BLOOD LIPIDS: Ashwagandha may have cholesterol-lowering effects.[3]

BLOOD PRESSURE: Ashwagandha may lower systolic and diastolic blood pressures based on dog studies.[7]

CHOLINERGIC AGENTS: Ashwagandha has been associated with cholinesterase inhibition in biochemical studies.[8] Because common Parkinson's disease drugs are present in some combination ashwagandha products,[9] it should be used cautiously in patients with Parkinson's disease.

PACLITAXEL: Although clinical data are lacking, evidence from animal studies suggests that ashwagandha may enhance the effects of paclitaxel.[10-13] Ashwagandha may also prevent paclitaxel-induced neutropenia in mice.[14]

SEDATIVES AND CENTRAL NERVOUS SYSTEM DEPRESSANTS: Based on animal research, ashwagandha may cause sedation and possibly life-threatening respiratory depression[15-17] as well as additive effects when used with sedatives, hypnotics, or other CNS depressants.[18]

THYROID HORMONES: Based on mouse research, ashwagandha may cause thyroid stimulation and increased T_4 serum levels;[19,20] thus, it may alter test results.

Asian Ginseng. See Ginseng (Panax spp.)

Asparagus (Asparagus officinalis)

Pharmacokinetics

The pharmacokinetics of asparagus is not well understood, but it appears to be excreted in urine.[1]

Adverse effects

Allergic reactions have been documented with asparagus, sometimes with cross-reactivity to other members of the Liliaceae family, which includes onions, garlic, leeks, and chives. Reactions include itchy conjunctivitis, runny nose, tightness of the throat and coughing during preparation of fresh asparagus,[2] acute urticaria after ingestion of asparagus,[3] contact dermatitis,[4,5] and occupational asthma caused by asparagus inhalation.[6-10]

Interactions

ELECTROLYTES: According to secondary sources, asparagus is a diuretic and may cause fluid loss and electrolyte imbalance.

Astragalus (Astragalus membranaceus)

Pharmacokinetics

The pharmacokinetics of astragalus is not well understood. Clinical research indicates that *Astragalus* flavonoids may be absorbed in the gastrointestinal tract and that the major metabolites of the flavonoid constituents are glucuronides.[1]

Adverse effects

Astragalus in recommended doses is considered to be safe and well tolerated. The most common adverse events are diarrhea and other mild gastrointestinal effects.[2,3]

Interactions

ANTICOAGULANTS/ANTIPLATELETS: Clinical studies have shown astragalus to inhibit platelet aggregation,[4] which may increase the risk of bleeding when used with anticoagulants/antiplatelets. However, clinical reports of such drug interactions are lacking.

BLOOD GLUCOSE: Astragalus may reduce blood sugar, as suggested by its historical use as an antidiabetic agent.[5] Concurrent use with antidiabetic agents may increase the risk of hypoglycemia.

BLOOD LIPIDS: Astragalus may have cholesterol-lowering effects.[5] Blood lipid levels may be altered.

BLOOD PRESSURE: According to canine experiments, astragalus may reduce blood pressure[6] and thus may cause additive effects when used with hypotensive agents.

ELECTROLYTES: According to animal research, astragalus may possess diuretic properties.[7] Excessive use may lead to fluid loss and electrolyte imbalance.

IMMUNOSUPPRESSANTS: Astragalus inhibited the actions of cyclophosphamide in animal studies.[8-11] Similar interactions are possible in humans, although clinical evidence is lacking.

RECOMBINANT INTERFERON-1: Activity of recombinant interferon-1 may be potentiated by astragalus, as suggested by animal studies.[12-14]

STANOZOLOL: Clinical research has demonstrated that astragalus enhances the effect of stanozolol in treating chronic aplastic anemia.[15]

Avocado (Persea americana)

Pharmacokinetics: Insufficient available evidence.

Adverse effects

Based on historical use and available research, avocado appears to be well tolerated. Headache, migraine with fever, and drowsiness have been reported. One patient with severe cardiovascular disease developed hemiplegia during a trial evaluating the effects avocado/soybean unsaponifiables (ASU) in the treatment of osteoarthritis.[1]

Cross-allergy between avocado and latex proteins has been reported in several studies and case reports.[2-10] Allergy symptoms include urticaria, bronchospasm, and intestinal spasms. Research also suggests potential cross-sensitivity among avocado, chestnut, and banana allergies.[5,10,11]

Interactions

ANTICOAGULANTS/ANTIPLATELETS: Anecdotally, avocado has been reported to reduce the anticoagulant effect of warfarin.[12] However, clinical reports of such drug interactions are lacking.

BLOOD LIPIDS: Several clinical studies have shown that avocado has the potential to lower plasma lipid levels,[13-17] presumably because of its beta-sitosterol content.

CYTOKINES AND INFLAMMATORY MARKERS: In vitro studies have demonstrated that ASU can decrease proinflammatory mediators.[18-20]

MONOAMINERGIC AGENTS: Large amounts of avocado may potentiate effects of MAO inhibitors and may lead to hypertensive crisis, as demonstrated by a clinical case report.[21]

Bacopa (Bacopa monnieri)

Pharmacokinetics

The pharmacokinetics of bacopa is not well understood. In clinical studies the effects of *Bacopa monnieri* were significant only after 12 weeks of treatment.[1,2]

Adverse effects

Adverse effects of bacopa may include palpitations, nausea, dry mouth, thirst, and fatigue. Bacopa should be used cautiously in patients with thyroid disorders because it may increase thyroid hormone levels.[3]

Interactions

CYTOCHROME P450 SUBSTRATES: In animals, bacopa has been shown to increase CYP450 enzyme activity and should be used cautiously with all agents metabolized by CYP450.[4]

SEDATIVES AND CENTRAL NERVOUS SYSTEM DEPRESSANTS: As suggested by animal research, bacopa has anxiolytic[5] and CNS depressant[6,7] effects. Interactions between similarly acting agents may occur.

THYROID HORMONES: Animal research suggests that bacopa may increase thyroid hormone levels.[8]

Baikal Skullcap (Scutellaria baicalensis). See Skullcap (Scutellaria spp.)

Banaba (Lagerstroemia speciosa)

Pharmacokinetics

Soft-gel formulations of banaba may have better bioavailability than dry-powder formulations.[1]

Adverse effects

Reports of adverse effects with banaba are currently lacking in the available literature.

Interactions

ANTICOAGULANTS/ANTIPLATELETS: Banaba has been shown to produce antithrombin activity in vitro.[2] Concurrent use of banaba with anticoagulants/antiplatelets may increase risk of bleeding. However, clinical reports of such drug interactions are lacking.

BLOOD GLUCOSE: According to clinical and animal data, banaba may lower blood glucose.[1,3]

URIC ACID: Compounds in banaba have been found to inhibit xanthine oxidase stronger than allopurinol in vitro.[4] Banaba thus may alter uric acid levels.

Barbat Skullcap (Scutellaria barbata). See Skullcap (Scutellaria spp.)

Barberry. See Berberine

Barley (Hordeum vulgare)

Pharmacokinetics

Barley contains greater amounts of soluble and nonsoluble starches than do other cereals, and approximately 17% of the carbohydrates in barley are not absorbed. This leads to fermentation in the colon by microflora, measurable by the H_2 breath test.

Adverse effects

Barley appears to be generally well tolerated in healthy adults in recommended doses for short periods, or as a cereal or in beer. Frequent cases of allergy have been reported, and cross-reactivity may occur with allergy to grass or wheat. The most common complaint is abdominal fullness.[1]

Interactions

BLOOD GLUCOSE: Barley contains more fermentable carbohydrates than other cereals such as rice. Fermentation of undigested carbohydrates produces short-chain fatty acids, some of which may reduce hepatic glucose production and affect postprandial glycemia.[2,3] Barley may result in lowered blood glucose concentrations, and when taken with hypoglycemic agents, theoretically it may result in lower-than-expected blood glucose values. Based on clinical research, a high dose of barley/beta-glucan supplement may improve glucose control when taken with high-carbohydrate foods, but not when added to high-carbohydrate beverages.[4]

BLOOD PRESSURE: Barley may decrease blood pressure, especially when consumed with other whole grains (rice, wheat).[5]

CATECHOLAMINERGIC AGENTS: Hordenine, an aminophenol in the root of germinating barley, is a sympathomimetic[6,7] and in theory may interact with catecholamines such as epinephrine (adrenaline), norepinephrine (noradrenaline), and dopamine. Blood pressure may be affected. Clinical data are lacking in this area.

ORAL AGENTS: Because of its fiber content, barley may reduce the absorption of some agents by reducing gastrointestinal transit time.

TRICLABENDAZOLE: Barley has been suggested to alter the metabolism of triclabendazole, a benzimidazole anthelmintic drug, in sheep.[8,9]

Beet (Beta vulgaris)

Pharmacokinetics

The pharmacokinetics of beet is not well understood. However, research has shown that intact betalins (the water-soluble chromoalkaloids responsible for beet color) are excreted rapidly and in relatively high volume.[1] This suggests that the bioavailability of betalins is low or that renal excretion is the primary route of elimination for these compounds. Sugar beet fiber increases cholesterol and decreases bile acid excretion by the small bowel.[2]

Adverse effects

Allergic skin reactions and skin diseases following exposure to beets have been reported in the general population and among people who work with beets in agricultural or factory settings.[3-6] Ingestion of beetroot is known to produce red or pink urine (beeturia) in approximately 10% to 14% of the population.[7,8]

Several cases of occupational illness, including asthma, anaphylaxis, toxic poisoning, respiratory infections, and tularemia, have been described among beet farmers and workers in beet sugar–processing facilities.[3-6,9-15] Most of these illnesses were not directly caused by beet exposure, but rather by exposure to the environmental bacteria, fungi, pollutants, or chemical insecticides present in such settings.

According to the American Academy of Pediatrics, beets should be avoided in infants younger than 3 months because of the high nitrate content and the risk of nitrate poisoning. However, breastfed infants of mothers who ingest beets and other foods high in nitrates are *not* at risk of nitrate poisoning because nitrate concentration does not increase significantly in breast milk.[16]

Interactions

BLOOD GLUCOSE: Although studies evaluating the effects of beet fiber on glucose metabolism have yielded inconsistent results, several clinical studies have shown that beet fiber supplementation may reduce postprandial glucose and insulin levels and impact other parameters of glucose metabolism in some patients.[17-20]

MINERALS: Studies evaluating the effects of vegetables or their fiber supplements on zinc, iron, and copper status in human subjects indicate that ingestion of beet in its pure vegetable form or as a fiber supplement does not affect the absorption or bioavailability of dietary minerals.[21,22]

ORAL AGENTS: Clinical research has shown that the addition of sugar beet fiber to the diet significantly decreases gastrointestinal transit time.[23] Contrarily, increased secretion of motilin, a gastrointestinal hormone, was observed after meals in a subset of obese patients with non-insulin-dependent diabetes who were taking a beet fiber supplement, suggesting that increased beet fiber in the diet may increase transit time.[17] Increased or decreased transit time could impact the absorption and bioavailability of some orally ingested agents.

PROBIOTICS: Arabino-oligosaccharides are derivatives of beet pectin that have demonstrated the ability to stimulate growth of colonic bacteria in vitro, including *Bifidobacterium*, *Bacteroides*, and *Lactobacillus*, and to decrease growth of *Clostridium*, suggesting their potential value as prebiotics in the human gut.[24]

STARCHES: In clinical research evaluating the effects of sugar beet and pea fibers on the absorption of wheat bread, both supplements increased the fraction of unabsorbed starch, affected the amount of starch absorbed by the small intestine, and increased meal transit time.[25] Beet and pea fiber reportedly altered wheat starch absorption and increased the amount of starch available for colonic fermentation.

Belladonna (Atropa spp.)

Pharmacokinetics

Pharmacokinetics data have been obtained from several cases of accidental belladonna ingestion.[1] The belladonna constituent atropine had a reported half-life of several hours and was rarely detectable in the plasma after 24 hours. Elimination half-life of atropine from raw or cooked belladonna berries was approximately 120 to 140 minutes. Atropine was primarily excreted by the kidneys.

Adverse effects

There is extensive literature on the adverse effects and toxicity of belladonna, principally related to its known anticholinergic actions. Common adverse effects include dry mouth, constipation, urinary retention, flushing, tachycardia, mydriasis, photophobia, blurred vision, dilation of pupils, dizziness, lightheadedness, drowsiness, unsteadiness, confusion, hallucinations, slurred speech, sedation, hyperreflexia, convulsions, and vertigo.[1-12] Many effects may occur at therapeutic doses.

Tachycardia has been reported in cases of toxicity.[1,4-6,9,11] Belladonna contains atropine, which is typically used in hospitals to increase heart rate. In one case report, infants who received hyoscyamine sulfate developed heart rates of 155 to 220 beats/min when given 2 to 4 mL of hyoscyamine.[13] Death in children may occur at 0.2 mg/kg of atropine.[14]

Interactions

ALCOHOL: Concomitant use of alcohol with belladonna has been suggested to result in additive central nervous system (CNS) depression.[15,16]

ANTICHOLINERGIC AGENTS: Belladonna displays anticholinergic effects and may cause additive effects when used with other anticholinergic agents (especially tricyclic antidepressants).[15,16] Dry mouth, constipation, urinary retention, mydriasis, and tachycardia may be exacerbated.

CISAPRIDE (PROPULSID): Cisapride enhances distal esophageal motor activity, presumably by means of a muscarinic receptor mechanism. In humans, these effects were completely blocked by atropine when it was administered before cisapride; the effect did not occur when atropine was administered after cisapride.[17]

TACRINE (COGNEX): In mice, cognitive deficits associated with belladonna alkaloid administration were attenuated by tacrine,[18] a cholinesterase inhibitor.

Berberine

Pharmacokinetics

After receiving 500 mg/kg of berberine (the main constituent of goldenseal and *Berberis* spp. such as barberry) whole-blood concentrations were 0.8 mcg/mL at 8 hours in rabbits.[1] Berberine appears to be metabolized in the liver, undergoing phase I hepatic metabolism and phase II glucuronidation.[2] It also seems to be a substrate of P-glycoprotein and organic cation transporter, which may limit oral bioavailability.[2,3] Berberine is excreted through the urine and feces.[1] Peak urinary excretion of berberine is seen between 12 and 24 hours, and peak fecal excretion is seen after 48 hours.

Adverse effects

Berberine may cause transient gastrointesinal effects, including constipation.[4,5] Headache, bradycardia, nausea, vomiting, and leukopenia have been noted in both animals and humans.[6-11] Berberine has also been associated with ventricular arrhythmias in patients with congestive heart failure (CHF).[7] Rarely, it may cause drying of mucous membranes, respiratory failure, and paresthesias.[12] Functional liver or kidney damage has not been observed in patients.[4] Berberine-containing herbs, such as goldenseal, have been suggested historically as abortifacients, although published research is lacking.

Interactions

ACETAMINOPHEN: In rats, berberine has demonstrated hepatoprotective effects when administered before toxic doses of acetaminophen.[13,14]

ANTICOAGULANTS/ANTIPLATELETS: Based on clinical research, berberine bisulfate may stimulate platelet formation and reduce bleeding.[15,16] Theoretically, berberine may decrease the effects of anticoagulants/antiplatelets, although clinical evidence of drug interaction is lacking.

BLOOD GLUCOSE: Based on both human and animal studies, berberine may decrease blood sugar levels.[4,5,17,18]

BLOOD LIPIDS: Based on both human and animal studies, berberine may decrease total and LDL cholesterol, as well as triglycerides.[4,5,19,20]

BLOOD PRESSURE: Based on animal studies, berberine lowers blood pressure.[6,21] Theoretically, concurrent use of berberine with antihypertensive agents may cause additive blood pressure lowering.

CARMUSTINE (BICNU): Based on in vitro research, berberine and carmustine may have additive effects.[22]

CYCLOSPORINE: In transplant patients, berberine has been shown to elevate the blood concentration of cyclosporin A, attributed to inhibition of CYP3A4 by berberine.[23] This inhibition is supported by in vitro studies, which demonstrate 3A4 inhibition by berberine.[24,25]

CYTOKINES AND INFLAMMATORY MARKERS: Berberine has been shown to inhibit interleukin-1 (IL-1) and decrease IL-8.[26,27] In vitro and in animals, berberine has been shown to have antiinflammatory effects; some studies have demonstrated COX-2 inhibitory activity.[26,28-33] Thus, berberine may interact with other antiinflammatory agents; however, clinical reports of such drug interactions are lacking.

FLUCONAZOLE: Berberine was shown in vitro to enhance the antifungal properties of fluconazole against clinical isolates of *Candida albicans*.[34] However, reports of synergistic clinical effects are lacking.

HEART RATE: Berberine has been shown to mitigate aconitine-induced arrhythmia.[35] This antiarrhythmic activity is supported by in vitro studies.[36-39] However, in clinical research, berberine was associated with the development of ventricular arrhythmias in CHF patients.[7] Caution is advised in patients using antiarrhythmic agents.

L-PHENYLEPHRINE: In animals, berberine and L-phenylephrine were shown to have additive effects when administered concurrently; each reduced the net enterotoxin-induced secretion of water.[40]

LIVER FUNCTION TESTS: Based on clinical research, berberine may decrease ALT, AST, and GGT.[19] Berberine has also been shown to displace bilirubin from albumin, increasing serum total and direct bilirubin concentrations.[41]

NEOSTIGMINE (PROSTIGMIN): In animals, berberine has been shown to reverse the secretory properties of neostigmine;[40] this antisecretory effect of berberine may be mechanistically similar to alpha-2-adrenergic agonists, opiates, and anticholinergic agents. Although clinical evidence is lacking, similar interactions may occur in humans.

P-GLYCOPROTEIN INHIBITORS: Based on in vitro and in vivo research, P-gp may contribute to the poor intestinal absorption of berberine.[3] Theoretically, P-gp inhibitors may be of therapeutic value by improving its bioavailability.

SEDATIVES AND CENTRAL NERVOUS SYSTEM DEPRESSANTS: Based on animal studies, berberine may have sedative effects.[16,41-43] Theoretically, concomitant use of berberine and other agents that have sedative properties may cause additive effects.

TETRACYCLINE: Based on clinical evidence, berberine may enhance the efficacy of tetracycline against *Vibrio cholerae*.[44]

TYRAMINE-CONTAINING FOODS: Based on clinical evidence, tyramine-containing foods (e.g., wine, cheese, chocolate) may interact with berberine.[45]

VITAMIN B: Berberine may decrease the metabolism of vitamin B, and concomitant use should be avoided.

WHITE BLOOD CELL COUNTS: Based on clinical research, berberine may increase leukocyte counts.[46]

YOHIMBINE: Based on in vitro research, berberine may competitively inhibit the binding of yohimbine to platelets.[47]

Beta-Glucan (β-Glucan)

Pharmacokinetics

Beta-glucan is a nondigestible soluble fiber, which is fermented in the colon and excreted in feces.[1]

Adverse effects

Orally, yeast-derived beta-glucans seem to be well tolerated, with minimal adverse effects. Rarely, they may cause constipation, nausea, and vomiting. Beta-glucan is listed by the U.S. Food and Drug Administration (FDA) as "generally recognized as safe" (GRAS).[2]

In a case series, 6 of 20 patients with acquired immunodeficiency syndrome (AIDS) or AIDS-related complex developed keratoderma of the palms and soles after IV infusion of soluble glucan (beta-1-3 polyglucose). Because none of the untreated 735 patients developed similar hyperkeratosis, the correlation to beta-glucan was significant; however, it was suggested that this reaction may be limited to patients with AIDS.[3]

Interactions

ANTIINFLAMMATORY AGENTS: Although clinical evidence is lacking, severe GI damage resulting in enteric-induced bacterial peritonitis has been associated with intake of beta-glucan and NSAIDs/aspirin in mice.[4,5]

BACTERIAL LEVELS: Yeast-derived beta-glucan has been suggested to have antibactercial properties, and alpha lipoic acid (ALA) has been suggested to enhance the antibacterial qualities of beta-glucan;

however, the daily use of beta-glucan for infections has been controversial.[6]

BLOOD GLUCOSE: Beta-glucan supplementation may reduce blood glucose levels because of the known postprandial effects of nondigestible carbohydrates.

BLOOD LIPIDS: Beta-glucan–containing sources have been used to treat hyperlipidemia.[7-18]

CATECHOLAMINERGIC AGENTS: Hordenine, an aminophenol in the root of germinating barley, is a sympathomimetic[19,20] and in theory may interact with catecholamines such as epinephrine (adrenaline), norepinephrine (noradrenaline), and dopamine. Blood pressure may be affected. Clinical evidence for this theoretical interaction is lacking.

CYTOCHROME P450 SUBSTRATES: Studies demonstrate that lentinan, a constituent of beta-glucan, suppresses hepatic CYP450-1A.[21] The effects of 1A substrates may be altered.

ORAL AGENTS: Fiber may affect the absorption of other oral agents by reducing gastrointestinal transit time. Oral agents should be taken 2 hours before or 2 hours after taking beta-glucan.

QUERCETIN: Quercetin has been suggested to enhance the antibacterial qualities of beta-glucan.[6]

SELENIUM: Selenium has been suggested to enhance the antibacterial qualities of beta-glucan.[6]

VITAMINS A, C, AND E: Vitamins A, C, and E have been suggested to enhance the antibacterial qualities of beta-glucan.[6]

WHITE BLOOD CELL COUNTS: Beta-glucans have been shown in numerous in vitro and animal studies to possess macrophage-specific immunomodulatory effects.[22-26] Clinical studies have also demonstrated immunomodulating effects.[27-29] Beta-glucan has been suggested as an adjunct to vaccines and other immunotherapies.

Beta-Sitosterol (β-Sitosterol), Sitosterol (22,23-Dihydrostigmasterol, 24-Ethylcholesterol)

Pharmacokinetics

Plant sterols are poorly absorbed because they are bound to the fibers of the plant.[1-3] Plasma plant sterol contents change in parallel with cholesterol and fat absorption; the lower the cholesterol absorption, the lower the plasma beta-sitosterol level.[4-13] Beta-sitosterol is structurally similar to cholesterol.[14,15] In vitro research suggests that beta-sitosterol is converted into cholic acid in the intestinal tract.[16] Beta-sitosterol passes through the intestine in the same physicochemical state as cholesterol and is lost to the same extent as cholesterol in the feces.[1] Beta-sitosterol is also excreted in bile, with minimal urinary excretion.[17-22] Data from some clinical trials suggest that beta-sitosterol may reduce progesterone levels in healthy males and females, although the extent and significance of the reduction are unclear.[23,24]

Adverse effects

Based on available evidence, beta-sitosterol is well tolerated in recommended doses for up to 6 months.[24-31] Both diarrhea and constipation have been reported.[25,32]

Interactions

ACARBOSE (GLUCOBAY, PRANDASE, PRECOSE): The impact of starch malabsorption on colon carcinogenesis has been examined clinically, and it was found that the antidiabetic drug acarbose decreased fecal concentration of beta-sitosterol by approximately 40%, indicating that absorption may be increased.[33]

ACTIVATED CHARCOAL: Data from clinical trials indicate that activated charcoal (8 g three times daily) may slightly decrease serum levels of beta-sitosterol.[34]

ALPHA-ADRENERGIC AGENTS: Clinical studies suggest that beta-sitosterol may relieve symptoms of benign prostatic hyperplasia (BPH) through mechanisms similar to those of finasteride and alpha blockers.[35-37] The combination of the sterols and these agents may result in synergistic effects, though clinical evidence for this interaction is lacking.

ANTIBIOTICS: Beta-sitosterol has been demonstrated in vivo to protect and improve the oral absorption of acid-labile antibiotics, particularly the potassium salts of penicillin G, penicillin V, and erythromycin lactobionate.[38]

ANTIBODY LEVELS: In vivo studies show that beta-sitosterol and beta-sitosterol glucoside may decrease immunoglobulin E (IgE) plasma levels.[39]

ANTICOAGULANTS/ANTIPLATELETS: Certain plant species that contain beta-sitosterol exhibit antiplatelet aggregation activities in vitro. The exact contribution of beta-sitosterol to this activity is unclear. However, caution should be used when combining beta-sitosterol with these agents because of the theoretical risk of increased bleeding.[40] Clinical reports of such drug interactions are lacking.

BLOOD GLUCOSE: In animals, fractions obtained from the leaves of *Morus insignis* demonstrated pronounced hypoglycemic effects. Beta-sitosterol was a constituent of this plant, so it may exhibit hypoglycemic effects.[41] Furthermore, clinical research has suggested that plant sterol use may result in hypoglycemic effects.[42]

BLOOD LIPIDS: Beta-sitosterol has been shown to lower total cholesterol and LDL cholesterol in several RCTs.[6,23,26,28-30,43-54] Beta-sitosterol may lower cholesterol levels by interfering with the intestinal absorption of cholesterol and increasing bile acid secretion. Another possible mechanism for this effect, demonstrated in vitro, is the inhibition of sterol (24)-reductase and HMG-CoA reductase, essential enzymes in the process of cholesterol biosynthesis.[6,19,56-59] Beta-sitosterol may interfere with the uptake of micellar cholesterol, leading to decreased plasma membrane cholesterol influx and cholesteryl ester secretion.[60,61] In cultured adrenal cells, addition of stigmasterol, but not sitosterol, inhibited SREBP-2 processing and reduced cholesterol synthesis. Stigmasterol also activated the liver X receptor in a cell-based reporter assay. These data indicate that certain dietary plant sterols disrupt cholesterol homeostasis by affecting two critical regulatory pathways of lipid metabolism.[62] Biliary cholesterol saturation may also decrease with increased consumption of beta-sitosterol.[63,64]

CAROTENOID LEVELS: Clinical research demonstrated that beta-sitosterol in doses of up to 1.5 g daily may reduce blood levels of lutein and lycopene.[65] Clinical trials demonstrated that beta-sitosterol doses up to 9 g daily may reduce beta-carotene blood levels,[6,26,27,31,54,65-68] presumably from reductions in LDL by beta-sitosterol.[58] Data from RCTs indicate that the lowering of beta-carotene may be counterbalanced by consuming an additional daily serving of a high-carotenoid vegetable or fruit when consuming spreads containing sterol or stanol esters.[69]

CHOLESTYRAMINE (QUESTRAN): Cholestyramine (up to 32 g daily) has been shown to reduce beta-sitosterol concentrations in patients with sitosterolemia.[70-72]

CORTISOL: Beta-sitosterol and beta-sitosterol glucoside may decrease serum levels of cortisol and cause a slight decrease in cortisol/DHEA-S ratio, as suggested by a clinical trial testing beta-sitosterol as an adjuvant for pulmonary tuberculosis.[73]

CYCLOOXYGENASE INHIBITORS: In vitro analysis of some plant species containing beta-sitosterol suggests that components of the plants may exhibit anticyclooxygenase effects.[74] Thus, beta-sitosterol may interact with COX inhibitors.

CYTOKINES AND INFLAMMATORY MARKERS: Beta-sitosterol and beta-sitosterol glucoside may decrease levels of proinflammatory cytokines interleukin-2 (IL-2) and IL-6 in the blood.[73,75]

DIOSGENIN: Although clinical evidence is lacking, animal research suggests that coadministration of beta-sitosterol and diosgenin, a steroid sapogenin, may affect the uptake of diosgenin by the liver.[76]

ESTROGENIC AGENTS: Beta-sitosterol has demonstrated estrogenic/antiestrogenic activity in vitro and in animal studies.[77,78] Thus, beta-sitosterol may alter the effects of estrogen therapies. However, clinical reports of such drug interactions are lacking.

EZETIMIBE (ZETIA): Ezetimibe has been shown clinically to decrease plasma plant sterol concentrations in individuals with sitosterolemia.[79]

FINASTERIDE (PROSCAR): Clinical studies suggest that beta-sitosterol may relieve BPH symptoms through mechanisms similar to those of finasteride and alpha blockers.[35-37] The combination of the sterols and these agents may result in synergistic effects.

HIGH-LIPASE PANCREATIN: High-lipase pancreatin treatment may alter fecal excretion of beta-sitosterol.[80] However, clinical reports of interactions are lacking.

HMG-CoA REDUCTASE INHIBITORS: In clinical research, simvastatin has been shown to elevate the ratio of plant sterol to cholesterol in patients with the highest baseline campestanol levels.[81] Simvastatin and niacin in combination have been shown in an RCT to elevate beta-sitosterol levels in patients with low levels of high-density lipoprotein (HDL) cholesterol.[9] Atorvastatin and simvastatin have been shown independently to elevate the plant sterol/cholesterol ratio in patients with coronary heart disease,[82] and atorvastatin has been suggested to increase levels of plasma plant sterols in diabetic patients.[83] In vitro studies suggest that beta-sitosterol may decrease the activities of HMG-CoA reductase and thereby have synergistic effects if taken in combination with these agents.[84]

LACTATE DEHYDROGENASE: In vitro bioassays demonstrate that sterol beta-D-glucosides may activate the release of LDH.[85]

LIFIBROL: Lifibrol, a lipid-lowering drug used to treat hypercholesterolemia, has been shown in clinical trials to reduce sterols, including lanosterol, lathosterol, beta-sitosterol, and campesterol.[86]

NMDA RECEPTOR ANTAGONISTS: NMDA receptor antagonists may block the neurotoxic actions of sterol glucosides according to in vitro bioassays, although they do not compete for binding at the NMDA receptor.[85]

OLESTRA: Olestra, a nonabsorbable fat substitute that comprises long-chain fatty acid esters of sucrose, has been shown in clinical trials to decrease the amount of beta-sitosterol in stools.[87]

PROGESTOGENIC AGENTS: Data from some clincial trials suggest that beta-sitosterol may reduce progesterone levels in healthy men and women, although the extent and significance of the reduction are unclear.[23,24] Thus, beta-sitosterol may alter the effects of progestins and phytoprogestins. However, clinical reports of such drug interactions are lacking.

UBIQUINOL-10 LEVELS: RCTs demonstrate that absolute plasma ubiquinol-10 concentrations can be lowered by up to 15.4% versus control with beta-sitosterol supplementation of 2.6 to 3.7 g daily.[58]

VITAMINS: Clinical trials demonstrated that bioavailability of alpha-tocopherol (vitamin E) may be decreased with concurrent administration of beta-sitosterol.[88] Clinical trials demonstrate no effect of beta-sitosterol in doses of up to 9 g daily on blood levels of fat-soluble vitamins A (retinol) and D.[6,26,50,89]

WHITE BLOOD CELL COUNTS: Beta-sitosterol and beta-sitosterol glucoside may increase WBC (lymphocyte, eosinophil, neutrophil) levels from baseline when used in combination with various antituberculosis agents. Beta-sitosterol and beta-sitosterol glucoside may cause an increase in CD3+ and CD4+ cells.[73]

Betel Nut (Areca catechu)

Pharmacokinetics

The pharmacokinetics of betel nut is not well understood. Minutes after mastication (chewing) of betel, the onset of effects occurs, lasting a mean of 17 minutes.[1]

Adverse effects

Betel nut is not considered safe for human use, particularly when used chronically or in high doses. Constituents of betel nut are potentially carcinogenic.[2-9] Long-term use has been associated with oral submucous fibrosis (OSF), precancerous oral lesions, and squamous cell carcinoma.[10-19] Wheezing, bronchoconstriction, dyspnea, and pulmonary edema have been noted anecdotally in users of betel nuts. Acute toxicity of betel nut has resulted in tachypnea and dyspnea.[20] Aggravation of asthma with a decrease in forced expiratory volume has been reported in patients who chew betel nuts.[21-23] Patients chewing betel nuts have reported acute chest pain, ventricular arrhythmias, tachycardia, palpitations, and hemodynamic instability (hypotension/hypertension).[20,24-28] Extrapyramidal symptoms (EPS), such as tremor and stiffness, have been reported in patients who chewed betel while receiving antipsychotic agents.[29,30]

Interactions

ANTIPSYCHOTIC AGENTS: Tremor and stiffness have been reported in patients who chewed betel while receiving anti-psychotic agents.[29,30] The cholinergic effect of betel nut may increase the incidence of EPS of antipsychotic agents.

BLOOD GLUCOSE: The arecoline fraction from betel nuts has been found to reduce blood sugar in diabetic rabbits.[31] Although clincial evidence is lacking, concomitant use of betel nut with blood sugar–lowering agents may theoretically increase the risk of hypoglycemia.

CHOLINERGIC AGENTS: Anticholinergic effects may be reduced when used in combination with betel nut because of the cholinergic properties of the betel constituent arecoline.[29] However, clinical reports of such drug interactions are lacking.

COPPER: Patients who chewed betel nuts have been shown to have increased copper levels in oral mucosal tissue.[32,33]

FECAL TESTS: Anecdotal reports have noted that chewing areca nuts can stain feces red and may interfere with fecal laboratory tests.

KIDNEY FUNCTION TESTS: In type 2 diabetic patients, betel nut chewing was associated with urinary albumin excretion rate and albuminuria, indicating nephrotoxicity.[34]

LIVER FUNCTION TESTS: In animals, arecoline may up regulate hepatotoxic marker enzymes (AST/SGOT and ALT/SGPT) in scrum.[35]

THYROID HORMONES: Betel nut has exhibited both stimulatory and inhibitory effects on thyroid function in male mice.[36] Thyroid function may also be altered in humans.

Bilberry (Vaccinium myrtillus)

Pharmacokinetics

The gastrointestinal absorption of bilberry was reported to be 5% of the administered dose, and bioavailability appears to be low. After oral doses in rats, plasma levels of bilberry reached a peak at 15 minutes and declined rapidly within 2 hours, and the absolute bioavailability was 1.2% of the administered dose.[1] Anthocyanosides found in bilberry appear to have a high affinity for tissues high in collagen concentration, including the skin, liver, and kidneys.[2] Bilberry appears to be eliminated in bile (15%-20%) and urine (25%-30%).[3]

Adverse effects

The long-term safety and side effects of bilberry have not been extensively studied. Safety is often presumed based on bilberry's history as a food source. According to postmarketing surveillance data from 2295 individuals who used bilberry extract, adverse effects were experienced by 4% overall, with 1% complaining of gastrointestinal discomfort and less than 1% experiencing nausea or heartburn.[4]

Interactions

ANTICOAGULANTS/ANTIPLATELETS: Thoeretically, bilberry may potentiate the effects of anticoagulants/antiplatelets because of antiplatelet effects.[3,5-8] However, clinical reports of such drug interactions are lacking.

ANTIDIABETIC AGENTS: In a recent cross-sectional, point-of-care survey of 1818 patients, three cases were identified as potentially clinically significant interactions between bilberry and antidiabetic agents.[9]

BACTERIAL LEVELS: Based on in vitro research, bilberry leaves may have antibacterial properties.[10] Bilberry anthocyanidins may have antiulcer activity, as evidenced by animal and clinical studies.[11-13] However, the mechanism of action is not understood.

BLOOD GLUCOSE: Based on animal studies, bilberry may lower blood sugar levels.[14-17]

BLOOD PRESSURE: Bilberry has been theorized potentially to lower blood pressure.[18-21]

ESTROGENIC AGENTS: Based on in vitro comparative research, bilberry extract may inhibit absorption of estrogens.[22] However, clinical reports of such drug interactions are lacking.

HISTOLOGICAL TESTS: Based on in vitro research, bilberry may inhibit cancer cell growth.[23] Histological assays may be affected.

Bishop's Weed (Ammi majus)

Pharmacokinetics: Insufficient available evidence.

Adverse effects

Photoreactive furocoumarins (psoralens) have been identified in bishop's weed.[1-4] Psoralens may be phototoxic, potentially causing photosensitivity,[5] phototoxic skin damage,[1] contact urticaria,[6] phototoxic dermatitis,[3,6] pigmentary retinopathy,[7] and increased melanoma risk.[8]

Interactions

ANTICOAGULANTS/ANTIPLATELETS: Because of the photoreactive furocoumarins in bishop's weed, concurrent use with anticoagulants/antiplatelets (aspirin) may increase risk of bleeding. However, clinical reports of such drug interactions are lacking.

CYTOCHROME P450 SUBSTRATES: Theoretically, bishop's weed may increase the effects of agents metabolized by CYP450. The bergaptens found in bishop's weed are similar to those in grapefruit, bitter orange, and oil of bergamot, which inhibit CYP450. Concurrent use of bishop's weed and CYP450 substrates may lead to increased serum levels of the substrates.

PHOTOSENSITIZING AGENTS: According to a review and several case reports, bishop's weed may be photoreactive and phototoxic, potentially causing photosensitivity,[5] phototoxic skin damage,[1] contact urticaria,[6] phototoxic dermatitis,[3,6] pigmentary retinopathy,[7] and increased melanoma risk.[8] Reports of such drug interactions are lacking, but additive effects may occur when using bishop's weed with other photosensitizers. Exposure to sunlight should be limited.

Bitter Almond (Prunus amygdalus)

Pharmacokinetics

The kernels of bitter almond are about 3% to 4% amygdalin, which is hydrolyzed to poisonous hydrocyanic acid. After IV administration of laetrile (amygdalin-derived alternative cancer agent), amygdalin has been shown to be excreted primarily unchanged, with urinary recovery as high as 100%. Peak plasma levels following a 6-g IM dose of laetrile were 180 mcg/L.[1] Prunasin, a metabolite of amygdalin, has a bioavailability of approximately 50%. Prunasin's volume of distribution and clearance are greater than those of amygdalin.[2]

Adverse effects

Laetrile, derived from the amygdalin found in bitter almonds, is considered unsafe in any form because of its potential for causing cyanide toxicity.[3-8] Reactions appear to be more severe with oral than with IV or IM dosing.

Interactions

ALCOHOL: Almond oil was shown in mice to be an inducer of hepatic alcohol dehydrogenase,[9] which may result in a buildup of the toxic metabolic intermediate (acetaldehyde). This finding suggests a possible adverse interaction between almond oil and alcohol, because of a possible disulfiram-like flushing reaction with concomitant use.

ANALGESICS: According to animal research, amygdalin, a compound found in bitter almonds, has antiinflammatory and analgesic effects.[10,11]

RAW ALMONDS: When using bitter almond products or laetrile, concomitant ingestion of raw almonds has been suggested in several cases to increase the incidence of cyanide poisoning.[7,12]

SEDATIVES AND CENTRAL NERVOUS SYSTEM DEPRESSANTS: Theoretically, depressant effects caused by bitter almond may be potentiated when administered with CNS depressants.

Bitter Melon (Momordica charantia)

Pharmacokinetics

The pharmacokinetics of bitter melon is not well understood. It appears to be excreted in urine.[1]

Adverse effects

A few adverse effects, including headache, have been associated with bitter melon in humans. Individuals with glucose-6-phosphate dehydrogenase (G6PD) deficiency are at risk of developing "favism" after ingestion of bitter melon seeds. Favism is defined by the onset of hemolytic anemia with symptoms that include headache, fever, stomach pain, and coma.[2] In animals, bitter melon has been shown to exert abortifacient effects,[3-5] reduce fertility rates,[6] or inhibit spermatogenesis.[7] Thus, bitter melon may alter fertility.

Interactions

ANTIVIRAL AGENTS: In HIV patients, MAP30 (isolated from bitter melon extract) was reported to enhance the effects of dexamethasone and indomethacin.[8]

BLOOD GLUCOSE: Based on animal experiments, several methodologically weak clinical studies, and case reports, bitter melon may lower blood glucose levels.[2,28-46] Theoretically, concomitant use of bitter melon with other hypoglycemic agents may cause additive effects.

BLOOD LIPID LEVELS: Based on animal data and clinical evidence, bitter melon may reduce apolipoprotein B and lower triglyceride levels.[9-12]

HISTOLOGICAL TESTS: As suggested by in vitro, animal, and clinical studies, bitter melon may have antineoplastic effects and may reverse chemotherapy drug resistance.[13-23] Thus, bitter melon has been suggested for use as a chemotherapy adjunct.

LIVER FUNCTION TESTS: Based on research conducted in animals, bitter melon may significantly increase gamma-glutamyl transferase (GGT) and alkaline phosphatase levels, although these increases were not associated with significant histopathological changes in the liver.[27] Theoretically, concurrent use of bitter melon with hepatotoxic agents may increase the risk of liver damage.

P-GLYCOPROTEIN SUBSTRATES: P-glycoprotein is a cell membrane–associated protein that transports a variety of drug substrates. Interaction with P-gp, including activation, inhibition, and induction, can lead to altered plasma or brain levels of P-gp substrates. Based on in vivo research, 1-monopalmitin found in bitter melon may inhibit P-gp–mediated efflux[47,48] and thus may alter the levels of P-gp substrates.

SEMEN TESTS: In animals, bitter melon has been shown to inhibit spermatogenesis. Sperm counts may be altered.[7]

VIRAL LEVELS: As suggested by in vitro, animal, and clinical studies, bitter melon and MAP30 (isolated from bitter melon extract) may have antiviral activity, specifically against human immunodeficiency virus (HIV).[14,16,24-26] Thus, bitter melon has been suggested for use as adjunct to antiviral and antiretroviral therapy.

WHITE BLOOD CELL COUNTS: Anecdotally, bitter melon has been reported to increase CD4+ count and CD4+/CD8+ T-lymphocyte ratios in patients with HIV.[26]

Bitter Orange (Citrus aurantium)

Pharmacokinetics

Meta-synephrine, an alkaloid constituent of bitter orange, is readily absorbed after oral administration. Approximately 80% of oral doses is excreted in the urine within 24 hours. After single oral doses, peak plasma concentration typically occurs in 1 to 2 hours. Plasma half-life is 2 to 3 hours.

Adverse effects

Research evaluating the effects of a dietary supplement containing bitter orange (Advantra ZR, Nutratech) on exercise tolerance found no significant adverse events.[1] However, synephrine, a constituent of bitter orange, is similar to phenylephrine and ephedra. Theoretically, synephrine may cause cardiovascular adverse effects similar to phenylephrine and ephedra. In clinical research and case reports, tachycardia, tachyarrhythmia, QT prolongation, and myocardial infarction have been noted with bitter orange use.[2-5] In healthy young adults, systolic blood pressure, diastolic blood pressure, and heart rate were higher for up to 5 hours after a single dose of bitter orange (900 mg dietary supplement extract standardized to 6% synephrine) compared with placebo.[6] Dizziness, concentration problems, memory loss, syncope, seizure, and stroke have been noted in case reports.[3-7] Photosensitivity may occur, particularly in fair-skinned people.[8] Because of its synephrine content, bitter orange may theoretically worsen glaucoma and alter thyroid function.

Interactions

Note: Interactions may be similar to those of ephedra.

ALPHA-ADRENERGIC AGENTS: Bitter orange may be antagonized by alpha-blocking agents.

ANTIDEPRESSANTS: Based on preliminary animal and clinical research, synephrine may have antidepressant effects, possibly by promoting norepinephrine release.[9,10] Additionally, bitter orange contains monoamine oxidase (MAO) substrates: tyramine, octopamine, and synephrine.[11-14] Concomitant use of MAO inhibitors with bitter orange may increase the hypertensive effects of synephrine and potentially cause hypertensive crisis.

BETA-ADRENERGIC AGENTS: Bitter orange appears to have beta-adrenergic properties and theoretically may interact with beta-blocking agents.

BLOOD PRESSURE: Based on animal and clinical research, bitter orange may increase systolic and diastolic blood pressure.[6,15,16]

CENTRAL NERVOUS SYSTEM STIMULANTS: Because of its synephrine content,[11,17] other CNS stimulants may adversely interact with bitter orange.

CYTOCHROME P450 SUBSTRATES: Bitter orange juice may inhibit CYP450-3A4,[18] causing increased drug levels and potentially increasing the risk of adverse effects.

CYTOKINES AND INFLAMMATORY MARKERS: Based on animal research, bitter orange peel may have antiinflammatory activity.[19] Theoretically, bitter orange may affect the inflammatory marker levels and may interact with other antiinflammatory agents.

HEART RHYTHM: Bitter orange might prolong the QT interval, especially when used in combination with other stimulants.[3]

HISTOLOGICAL TESTS: Based on preliminary research, bitter orange constituents auraptene, marmin, tangeretin, and nobiretin, as well as a psoralen compound, may have antitumor effects.[19] Histologic tests may be affected.

HONEY: Honey has been suggested to reduce the absorption of naringin, a flavone glycoside of bitter orange.[20]

PHOTOSENSITIZING AGENTS: Based on secondary reports, oil of bergamot from Citrus aurantium may cause hyperpigmentation or dermatitis and make a patient more sensitive to laser treatment. Bitter orange oil also contains the furocoumarins bergapten and oxypeucedanin,[21] which may also increase sensitivity to light.

THYROID HORMONES: Theoretically, bitter orange may interact with thyroid agents or may worsen hyperthyroidism as a result of its synephrine content.[23]

VIRAL LEVELS: Based on laboratory research, bitter orange fruit may have antiviral activity against rotavirus.[24] Theoretically, bitter orange may interact with antiviral agents.

Black Cohosh (Actaea racemosa, formerly Cimicifuga racemosa)

Pharmacokinetics

The pharmacokinetics of black cohosh is not well understood. However, it does not appear to modulate P-glycoprotein (P-gp).[1]

Adverse effects

Safety and efficacy data beyond 6 months are not available, although recent reports suggest safety of short-term use, including in menopausal women not on estrogen replacement therapy.[2,3] Nonetheless, because long-term follow-up is lacking, caution is advised until improved safety data are available.

In studies, black cohosh is generally well tolerated in recommended doses for up to 6 months.[2,4-14] The most common side effects seem to be gastrointestinal upset and rash.[4] The potential effects of black cohosh on estrogen-sensitive conditions such as breast cancer, uterine cancer, or endometriosis are unclear.

Various cases of liver damage have been reported with the use of black cohosh.[15-19] Based on these data, the Dietary Supplement Information Expert Committee determined that black cohosh products must be labeled with a warning statement.[19]

Interactions:

ALCOHOL: Tonic-clonic seizures were reported in a 45-year-old woman taking black cohosh, chaste tree (berries and seeds), and primrose oil for 4 months, who also consumed alcohol.[20] The relative contribution of each agent and risk of the combination are not clear. Tinctures of black cohosh may contain high alcohol content, which may be reflected in blood tests.

AMERICAN (FALSE) PENNYROYAL: Pennyroyal *(Hedeoma pulegioides)* and black cohosh are sometimes taken together to induce abortion, although the concomitant may have potential for increased toxicity and death. In one case report a 24-year-old woman took 48% to 56% pennyroyal herb in an alcohol base and an unclear amount of black cohosh root for 2 weeks to induce abortion.[21] The patient died within 48 hours of taking a single subsequent dose of this combination.

ANTICOAGULANTS/ANTIPLATELETS: Native black cohosh contains small amounts of salicylic acid and may potentiate the antiplatelet effects of other agents. This is a theoretical concern, and it is not clear if therapeutic amounts of salicylates are present in commercial or processed black cohosh products. Clinical reports of such drug interactions are lacking.

BLOOD PRESSURE: There have been reports of hypotension in animals, although clinical data are limited in this area. Increased peripheral blood flow was associated with black cohosh administration in a 1962 study.[22] Because of theoretical hypotensive effects,[22,23] black cohosh should be used cautiously with other hypotensive agents. Clinical reports of interactions are lacking.

BLUE COHOSH: Both black cohosh and blue cohosh *(Caulophyllum thalictroides)* are often used by nurse-midwives in the United States to assist birth. There is a report of severe multi-organ hypoxic injury in a child delivered "naturally" with the aid of both blue and black cohosh. The child, who was not breathing at birth,[24] survived with permanent central nervous system damage. Notably, blue cohosh possesses a vasoconstrictive glycoside, which may have been responsible for the adverse effects.

BONE MARKERS: Isopropanolic extract of black cohosh significantly diminished the urinary content of pyridinoline and deoxypyridinoline (specific markers for bone loss) and the morphometric correlates of bone loss associated with ovariectomy in rats.[25] Based on in vitro and animal studies, black cohosh may increase osteogenesis,[25-27] which may be reflected in bone marker assays.

CHASTEBERRY: Tonic-clonic seizures were reported in a woman taking black cohosh, chaste tree (berries and seeds), and primrose oil for 4 months; she also consumed alcohol.[20] The relative contribution of each agent and risk of the combination are not clear.

CYTOCHROME P450 SUBSTRATES: The effects of black cohosh on CYP450 enzymes are unclear. Evidence suggests black cohosh may inhibit CYP450-2D6.[28] However, contradictory evidence suggests that black cohosh has no clinically significant effects on substrates of 2D6 and 3A4.[29]

DOPAMINERGIC AGENTS: Recent studies suggest that the mechanism of action of black cohosh may be centrally mediated and may occur at dopamine receptors.[30,31] Thus, black cohosh may interact with dopamine agonists or antagonists.

ESTROGENIC AGENTS: The estrogenic activity of black cohosh remains controversial. Specific estrogenic constituents have not been identified, and it is not clear how (or if) black cohosh interacts with estrogens/estrogen receptors or progestins. Recent publications suggest that there may be no direct effects on estrogen receptors, although this is an area of active controversy.[4,26,30-35] Therefore, caution is warranted in individuals taking both black cohosh and estrogens, because of unclear effects and the lack of interactions data.

EVENING PRIMROSE OIL: Tonic-clonic seizures occurred in a 45-year-old woman taking black cohosh, chaste tree (berries and seeds), and primrose oil for 4 months and who also consumed alcohol.[20] The relative contribution of each agent and risk of the combination are unclear.

HISTAMINE: In vitro, black cohosh has been shown to inhibit histamine release.[36]

HISTOLOGICAL TESTS: In vitro, black cohosh has demonstrated antiproliferative effects.[37,38] Based on in vitro research, relatively low concentrations of actein or the methanol/water fraction of black cohosh may cause synergistic inhibition of human breast cancer cell proliferation when combined with different classes of chemotherapy agents.[39] Histological tests may be affected.

LIVER FUNCTION TESTS: Black cohosh has been associated with various cases of liver damage.[15-19] Theoretically, black cohosh may increase the risk of hepatotoxicity when used with other agents that adversely affect the liver. Liver function tests may be altered.

ORAL AGENTS: Extracts of black cohosh moderately (but significantly) inhibited estrone-3-sulfate uptake, which suggests that coadministration may decrease the absorption of orally administered substrates of organic anion-transporting polypeptide B. Polypeptide B is thought to be involved in the intestinal absorption of various agents.[40]

SEROTONERGIC AGENTS: Animal and in vitro studies suggest that the mechanism of action of black cohosh may be centrally mediated, with possible action at the level of serotonin receptors.[30,31] Theoretically, black cohosh may interact with agents that affect serotonin, such as the selective serotonin reuptake inhibitors (SSRIs) citalopram and fluoxetine, although the exact effects are unclear. However, clinical reports of such drug interactions are lacking.

TAMOXIFEN: Controversy surrounds the ability of black cohosh to reduce tamoxifen-induced hot flashes; clinical trials have produced conflicting results.[3,41]

Black Currant *(Ribes nigrum)*

Pharmacokinetics

The pharmacokinetics of black currant is not well understood. The gamma-linolenic acid (GLA) constituent of black currant is turned into dihomo-GLA.[1] Metabolites are primarily excreted in urine.[2]

Adverse effects

Based on historical information and data from several studies, black currant appears to be well tolerated in doses up to 1000 mg three times daily.[3,4] Diarrhea and mild gastrointestinal upset occur rarely.[5]

Interactions

ANTICOAGULANTS/ANTIPLATELETS: Theoretically, concomitant use of black currant and anticoagulants/antiplatelets may increase the risk of bleeding, although clinical reports of such drug interactions are lacking. Black currant contains GLA and alpha-linolenic acid, which inhibit thromboxane B_2 production and increase prostacyclin production.[6]

BLOOD PRESSURE: Black currant may have hypotensive effects[7] and may cause additive blood pressure lowering when used with hypotensive agents.

CYTOKINES AND INFLAMMATORY MARKERS: Black currant has been shown to reduce prostaglandin E_2 production and to cause modest immune-enhancing effects.[8]

MONOAMINERGIC AGENTS: Based on secondary sources, black currant may have MAO inhibitor effects and theoretically may interact with other monoaminergic agents. However, clinical reports of such drug interactions are lacking.

VIRAL LEVELS: Black currant has been shown to inhibit influenza and herpes simplex type 1 viruses.[9,10]

Black Pepper (Piper nigrum)

Pharmacokinetics: Insufficient available evidence.

Adverse effect

Black pepper has a long safety history when used as a spice. According to clinical research, however, ingestion of black pepper may cause dyspepsia and other gastrointestinal adverse effects.[1,2] Based on case reports, inhalation of black pepper has caused respiratory irritation and edema, and even respiratory arrest, severe anoxia, and death.[3-5] Reviews and case-control studies also suggest a link between ingestion of black pepper and nasopharyngeal or esophageal cancer.[6-8] Caution is advised with excessive use. Black pepper may cause adverse respiratory effects.[3-5] Caution is warranted in patients with asthma.

Interactions

ANALGESICS: In vitro research using whole-cell patch-clamp electrophysiology showed that piperine (pungent alkaloid found in black pepper) had similar agonist effects on the human vanilloid receptor TRPV-1 as capsaicin.[10]

CHOLINERGIC AGENTS: In vitro, black pepper extracts have been shown to inhibit acetylcholinesterase.[12] Caution is warranted with concomitant use of cholinergic agonists and antagonists.

CYCLOSPORINE: Based on in vitro research, piperine may inhibit cyclosporine transport in intestinal cells.[13]

CYTOCHROME P450 SUBSTRATES: Based on in vitro research, constituents isolated from black pepper, including piperine and dipiperamides D and E, may potently inhibit some CYP450 metabolic pathways, including 2D6[13] and 3A4.[13,14] Caution is advised in patients using CYP450 substrates.

CYTOKINES AND INFLAMMATORY MARKERS: Black pepper may have antiinflammatory activity[11] and may reduce inflammatory marker assays; theoretically, it may interact with antiinflammatory agents.

DIGITALIS: Based on in vitro research, piperine may inhibit digoxin transport in intestinal cells.[13] Interactions with digitalis are possible.

FOOD: In a literature review, consumption of black pepper was suggested to lead to greater satiety.[9]

GREEN TEA: Based on animal research, piperine from black pepper may enhance the bioavailability of EGCG, a polyphenol constituent from green tea *(Camellia sinensis)*.[15]

ORAL AGENTS: Based on clinical research of intestinal peristalsis in healthy volunteers, consumption of black pepper may increase orocecal transit time,[16] thus potentially improving the absorption and bioavailability of oral agents. Several clinical studies have shown altered drug bioavailability with concomitant black pepper use.

PHENYTOIN: Based on animal and clinical trials, piperine from black pepper may significantly enhance the bioavailability of the antiepileptic medication phenytoin, possibly by increasing its absorption.[17-19]

PROPRANOLOL: Based on clinical research in healthy volunteers, piperine may increase the bioavailability of the beta-adrenergic agent propranolol.[18]

RIFAMIPICIN (RIFAMPIN): Based on clinical research in patients with pulmonary tuberculosis, piperine may increase plasma concentrations of the antibiotic rifamipicin (rifampin).[18]

THEOPHYLLINE (BRONKODYL, ELIXOPHYLLIN, SLO-BID): Based on clinical research in healthy volunteers, piperine may increase the bioavailability of the bronchodilator theophylline.[18]

Black Tea. See Tea (Camellia sinensis)

Bladderwrack (Fucus vesiculosus). See Seaweed

Blessed Thistle (Cnicus benedictus)

Pharmacokinetics

The pharmacokinetics of blessed thistle is not well understood. After oral ingestion of blessed thistle, the lignans arctiin and tracheloside are metabolized to genins, arctigenin and trachelogenin. Peak serum levels have been reached at 4 hours for arctigenin and at 8 hours for trachelogenin.[1]

Adverse effects

Blessed thistle is generally considered to be safe when used in recommended doses for short periods, with few reported adverse effects. Cross-reactivity may occur with the Asteraceae (Compositae) family, including bitter weed, blanket flower, chrysanthemum, coltsfoot, daisy, dandelion, dwarf sunflower, goldenrod, marigold, prairie sage, and ragweed.[2]

Anecdotally, blessed thistle taken in high doses (>5 g per cup of tea) may cause stomach irritation and vomiting. Blessed thistle contains approximately 8% tannins; notably, chronic ingestion of plants that contain 10% tannins or greater may cause gastrointestinal upset. The oral toxicity of plant tannins is low, as tannins are readily hydrolyzed in the gut to gallic acid and other metabolites. However, liver and kidney toxicity has occurred with high tannin doses used topically or intravenously.[3] Tannin consumption has been associated with certain cancers, such as esophageal cancer; however, it is unclear whether this is due to the tannins themselves or other compounds associated with tannins.[4]

Interactions

ACIDITY: Traditionally, blessed thistle is believed to stimulate gastric acid secretion and may antagonize the effects of certain medications, such as antacids, H_2-receptor antagonists, proton pump inhibitors, and sucralfate.

ANTICOAGULANTS/ANTIPLATELETS: Blessed thistle has been shown to possess platelet-activating factor (PAF) antagonist properties, which in theory may reduce PAF-stimulated platelet aggregation, increasing the risk of bleeding.[1] However, clinical reports of such drug interactions are lacking.

BACTERIAL LEVELS: Blessed thistle may have antibacterial effects[5-7] and theoretically may interact with antibacterial agents.

CYTOKINES AND INFLAMMATORY MARKERS: Constituents of blessed thistle (e.g., cnicin, arctigenin) have displayed antiinflammatory effects. Markers of inflammation may be reduced; furthermore, blessed thistle may interact with antiinflammatory agents.

HISTOLOGICAL TESTS: Cnicin and arctigenin, constituents of blessed thistle, have exhibited cytotoxic activity against some tumor cell lines, including leukemia (HL-60), hepatomas, and sarcomas, through inhibition of cellular DNA, RNA, or protein synthesis.[7-13] Blessed thistle is included in some brands of the unproven anticancer herbal remedy Essiac. Blessed thistle is thus suggested as an adjunct to standard antineoplastic agents.

VIRAL LEVELS: Lignans in blessed thistle may have antiviral activity, particularly anti-HIV integrase, and have been suggested for use in combination antiviral therapies.[14]

Bloodroot (Sanguinaria canadensis)

Pharmacokinetics

The pharmacokinetics of bloodroot in humans is unclear. Evidence from in vitro research suggests that cytochrome P450-80B1 may be involved in the metabolism of sanguinarine (main constituent of bloodroot).[1]

Adverse effects

Chronic use of sanguinarine oral products may cause leukoplakia in sites other than the buccal vestibule, or keratoses similar to non-sanguinaria dysplastic lesions of the lip and mucosa.[2,3] According to anecdotal evidence, ingestion of more than 300 mg of bloodroot results in vomiting, intense thirst, diarrhea, and abdominal cramping. Prolonged use of sanguinaria extract as an oral rinse may result in impaired sensation of taste, as well as staining of the tongue, teeth, and fillings.[4] These side effects reverse after treatment stops.

An expert panel on the safety of sanguinaria extract used in Viadent oral rinse and toothpaste products found that published literature suggesting an association between human exposure to sanguinaria extract and potential reproductive, cardiovascular, or ocular toxicity, or carcinogenicity, was anecdotal, unfounded, and not corroborated by or consistent with the substantial database subjected to peer review.[5] Bloodroot may cause tissue damage when applied topically, which may cause other topical agents used at the same time to be absorbed systemically, possibly resulting in unwanted adverse effects.

Interactions

BACTERIAL LEVELS: Based on in vitro studies, sanguinarine may have antibacterial activity against both gram-positive and gram-negative bacteria.[6-9] Methanol extracts of *Sanguinaria canadensis* rhizomes may inhibit the growth of *Helicobacter pylori*.[6] Based on in vitro screening, sanguinarine and chelerythrine from the roots of *S. canadensis* may inhibit *Mycobacterium aurum* and *M. smegmatis*.[10]

BLOOD PRESSURE: Based on anecdotal reports, large doses of sanguinaria may cause low blood pressure.

CYTOCHROME P450 SUBSTRATES: CYP80B1 may be involved in the metabolism of sanguinarine. CYP1A has also been implicated in sanguinarine metabolism based on in vitro research.[11] Sanguinarine also inhibits activity of NADPH/CYP reductase, an enzyme required for CYP activity.

HORMONAL AGENTS: Based on anecdotal evidence, bloodroot may interact with hormonal agents.

PARASITIC INFECTIONS: Based on in vitro studies, sanguinarine may have antifungal activity against *Candida* and dermatophytes, as well as antiprotozoal activity against *Trichomonas*.[12]

SEDATIVES AND CENTRAL NERVOUS SYSTEM DEPRESSANTS: Bloodroot contains sanguinarine, a morphine-like alkaloid that may cause sedation, faintness, and vertigo and may impair decision making and increase response time. These effects may be more pronounced when bloodroot is used with agents that act similarly. Clinical reports of such drug interactions are lacking.

Boneset (Eupatorium spp.)

Pharmacokinetics: Insufficient available evidence.

Adverse effects

The adverse effects of boneset are not well understood because clinical data are lacking. Traditionally, boneset in large doses has been reported to cause nausea, vomiting, and diarrhea and even coma or death. This herb may also contain hepatotoxic unsaturated pyrrolizidine alkaloids.

Interactions

BACTERIAL LEVELS: Based on in vitro research, boneset may have weak antibacterial activity against gram-positive bacteria.[1] Theoretically, boneset may interact with certain antibacterial agents.

CYTOKINES AND INFLAMMATORY MARKERS: Based on secondary sources, boneset may have antiinflammatory effects and may interact with antiinflammatory agents.

ELECTROLYTES: Based on secondary sources, boneset may cause excessive fluid loss from the body, possibly disrupting electrolyte balance.

LIVER FUNCTION TESTS: According to secondary sources, hepatotoxic unsaturated pyrrolizidine alkaloids are common in this genus and might be in boneset as well. Theoretically, boneset may have additive adverse effects to the liver when used with other hepatotoxic agents.

VIRAL LEVELS: Based on limited clinical evidence, homeopathic boneset may have antiviral effects[2] and may thus interact with antiviral agents.

WHITE BLOOD CELL COUNTS: Based on animal research, boneset may increase phagocytosis.[3]

Borage (Borago officinalis)

Pharmacokinetics

The pharmacokinetics of borage is not well understood. The gamma-linolenic acid (GLA) constituent of borage is metabolized into dihomo-GLA.[1] Metabolites are primarily excreted in urine.[2]

Adverse effects

Borage may cause diarrhea and bloating.[3] Numerous studies have suggested that borage may lower the seizure threshold.[4]

Interactions

AGENTS THAT LOWER SEIZURE THRESHOLD: Borage may lower the seizure threshold, and concomitant use with similar-acting agents may increase the risk of seizure. Epileptic individuals should avoid borage because it may increase the risk of seizure or alter the effects of antiseizure medications.

ANTICOAGULANTS/ANTIPLATELETS: Borage seed oil has been suggested to increase the risk of bleeding or potentiate the effects of warfarin therapy.[5,6] However, in clinical research involving healthy volunteers, the therapeutic dosage of 3 g daily of borage oil supplementation did not affect platelet aggregation.[7] Nonetheless, caution is still warranted when using borage with anticoagulant/antiplatelet agents.

BLOOD PRESSURE: Borage may lower blood pressure, cause reflex vasodilation, and augment arterial baroreflex control of vascular resistance.[8] Caution is warranted with cardiovascular agents.

CYTOKINES AND INFLAMMATORY MARKERS: Based on a review, borage oil may have antiinflammatory properties[2] and theoretically may interact with antiinflammatory agents.

WHITE BLOOD CELL COUNTS: Based on in vitro, animal, and clinical studies, GLA from borage oil may dose-dependently reduce WBC proliferation.[9-12] Thus, borage oil may affect WBC counts.

Boswellia (Boswellia serrata)

Pharmacokinetics

The pharmacokinetics of boswellia is not well understood. After a single 333-mg dose of *Boswellia serrata* extract, the mean elimination half-life was reported as 5.97 ± 0.95 hours.[1] Pharmacokinetics data revealed poor bioavailability of boswellic acids, the active ingredients of boswellia. Food appears to alter the pharmacokinetic profile of boswellia.[2] 11-Keto-β-boswellic acid, but not 3-acetyl-11-keto-β-boswellic acid, undergoes extensive phase I metabolism. Oxidation to hydroxylated metabolites is the principal metabolic route.[3] Metabolites of boswellia appear to be excreted in urine.[4]

Adverse effects

Boswellia is generally believed to be safe when used as directed, although there is a lack of safety studies in humans. Mild gastrointestinal effects, including abdominal fullness, epigastric pain, gastroesophageal reflux symptoms, diarrhea, and nausea, have been reported in 6 of 34 patients with ulcerative colitis.[5] Dermatitis has also been reported in 3 of 42 patients using a combination product containing boswellia and other potentially active herbal agents; the independent role of boswellia in these reactions could not be determined.[6,7]

Interactions

ANALGESICS: Based on animal research, *Boswellia serrata* gum resin exhibits an analgesic effect similar to that of morphine (4.5 mg/kg).[8] Boswellia may interact with other analgesic agents.

BACTERIAL LEVELS: Based on laboratory tests, boswellia may have antibacterial activity.[9]

BLOOD LIPIDS: The gum resin of boswellia has been reported to lower cholesterol and triglyceride levels.[10]

CYTOCHROME P450 SUBSTRATES: *Boswellia carterii, B. frereana, B. sacra,* and *B. serrata* have been shown to be moderate to potent, nonselective inhibitors of CYP450 enzymes 1A2, 2C8, 2C9, 2C19, 2D6, and 3A4.[11] Theoretically, boswellia may increase concentrations of agents metabolized by these enzymes.

CYTOKINES AND INFLAMMATORY MARKERS: Based on in vitro and animal studies, boswellia may have antiinflammatory activity.[12-22] Boswellia has been found to inhibit the release of proinflammatory leukotriene B_4 in vitro,[23-26] thus potentially decreasing inflammatory markers. Interactions with LTB_4 inhibitors are possible.

FUNGAL LEVELS: The essential oil from *B. serrata* has been reported to possess antifungal activity and weak activity against human fungal pathogens in vitro, but greater effect against plant fungal pathogens.[27]

GLYCOSAMINOGLYCANS: Boswellia has been reported to reduce the degradation of GAGs in rats[28] and may interact with agents that effectively treat osteoarthritis, such as glucosamine and chondroitin.

HIGH-FAT FOODS: Studies demonstrate that food intake has a profound effect on the pharmacokinetic parameters of boswellic acids.[2] Meals that are high in fat seem to increase the concentration of boswellia in the body, whereas certain boswellic acids are undetectable after boswellia is taken in a fasting state.

HISTOLOGICAL TESTS: Numerous in vitro preclinical studies have shown that boswellic acids have potent cytotoxic and antiproliferative activity against numerous cancer cell lines.[29-38] Concomitant use with other antiproliferative agents may increase the effects or toxicity of boswellia.

LIVER FUNCTION TESTS: In mice, high doses of boswellia caused pronounced hepatomegaly and steatosis.[39] Although clinical reports of boswellia-associated toxicity are lacking, similar liver toxicity and subsequent changes in laboratory values may theoretically occur in humans taking boswellia formulations. Toxin-induced transaminitis in mice was reduced by administration of boswellia, although effects on normal liver or on humans are not clear.[25]

SEDATIVES AND CENTRAL NERVOUS SYSTEM DEPRESSANTS: Boswellia has exhibited sedative effects comparable to chlorpromazine (7.5 mg/kg) in animals.[8] Concomitant use of boswellia with sedative agents may have additive effects.

WHITE BLOOD CELL COUNTS: Research has shown that boswellic acids have immunostimulant activity in that they modify lymphocyte response and release of inflammatory mediators.[40,41]

Boxwood (Buxus sempervirens)

Pharmacokinetics: Insufficient available evidence.

Adverse effects

The literature contains a few reports of adverse effects associated with boxwood. Based on anecdote, boxwood has been associated with allergic contact dermatitis.[1]

Interactions

BLOOD PRESSURE: Based on animal and in vivo research, boxwood may slightly increase and then dramatically decrease blood pressure.[2]

CHOLINERGIC AGENTS: Based on in vitro research, boxwood may inhibit acetylcholinesterase.[2,3] Theoretically, boxwood may have additive effects when used with cholinergic or anticholinergic agents.

STEROIDS: According to laboratory assays, boxwood contains steroidal alkaloids,[4,5] which may be reflected in blood or urine tests.

VIRAL LEVELS: Boxwood may modify effects of antiretroviral agents and has been suggested as an adjunct to standard therapy. SPV-30 (extract of boxwood) may lower viral load in HIV-infected patients; however, available clinical evidence is inconclusive.[6-15]

WHITE BLOOD CELL COUNTS: Boxwood may have immunomodulatory properties. SPV-30 may increase CD4+ and CD8+ cell count in HIV-infected patients, but clinical evidence is inconclusive.[6-15]

Bromelain (Bromeliaceae)

Pharmacokinetics
Oral bromelain tablets have a bioavailability of 2% to 4% in humans.[1] Bromelain is best taken 1 hour before or after food.[2] Bromelain is distributed in plasma,[3] but its metabolism and excretion are not well understood. The elimination half-life of bromelain was found to be 6 to 9 hours.[3]

Adverse effects
Bromelain appears to be well tolerated, although it has been reported to cause diarrhea and gastrointestinal upset.[4] Cases of bromelain allergy have also been reported.[5-7] Bromelain should be used cautiously in patients allergic to pineapple or related plants in the Bromeliaceae family.

Interactions
ANTIBIOTICS: Clinical studies suggest that bromelain may increase the absorption of some antibiotics (notably amoxicillin and tetracycline) and increase levels of these drugs in the body.[9-12] However, one study showed no effect on absorption of tetracycline when patients were coadministered bromelain (80 mg) with tetracycline (500 mg).[13]

ANTICOAGULANTS/ANTIPLATELETS: Bromelain has exhibited platelet aggregation inhibition in vitro[14] and may increase the risk of bleeding if taken concurrently with anticoagulant/antiplatelet agents. However, clinical reports of such drug interactions are lacking.

BLOOD PRESSURE: Animal studies have demonstrated hypotensive effects of bromelain.[8] Interactions with other hypotensive agents are possible.

HEART RATE: Bromelain increases heart rate and therefore may theoretically interact with agents that affect heart rate.[15]

HISTOLOGICAL TESTS: Because of its fibrinolytic and antitumor effects,[16] bromelain may enhance the efficacy of certain chemotherapeutic agents such as 5-fluorouracil and vincristine.

MAGNESIUM: Magnesium acts as a reducing agent, which may theoretically lead to activation of bromelain.

PROTEIN: Foods or supplements that are high in protein, such as soy, may inhibit the effects of bromelain by saturating its enzymatic activity.

SEDATIVES AND CENTRAL NERVOUS SYSTEM DEPRESSANTS: Bromelain may cause additive effects when used with sedative agents.

TRYPSIN-CONTAINING FOODS, HERBS, AND SUPPLEMENTS: Bromelain and trypsin are thought to have synergistic effects.[17] Bromelain may react with other proteases (e.g., papain), some grass pollens, and wheat and rye flour.[18,19]

ZINC: Zinc acts as an oxidizing agent and may theoretically inhibit bromelain activity when used together.

Bupleurum (*Bupleurum* spp.)

Pharmacokinetics
Saikosaponins in bupleurum are minimally absorbed after oral absorption.[1] Saikosaponins absorption may vary with food intake.[2,3] Saikosaponins are hydrolyzed to saikogenins (active metabolites) and prosaikogenins by intestinal bacteria in humans.[4] Saikosaponins undergo enterohepatic circulation and largely undergo fecal excretion.[1] Bupleurum was undetectable 1½ hours after oral administration.[2]

Adverse effects
In recommended doses (1.5-6 g of dried-root decoction daily), many practitioners agree that bupleurum is well tolerated. However, systematic collection and analysis of safety data are lacking. Some reports of bupleurum adverse effects are from combination therapy, making it difficult to attribute the effect to bupleurum alone. Unverified reports have noted sedation, drowsiness, and lethargy as frequent side effects. Rare instances of fatigue and paresthesia were noted in one study that investigated combination therapy sho-saiko-to.[5]

Interactions
ADRENOCORTICOTROPIC HORMONE: Saikosaponins from bupleurum were shown to raise plasma ACTH (corticotropin) concentrations in rats.[6]

ANTICOAGULANTS/ANTIPLATELETS: Bupleurum has been shown to inhibit human platelet activation in vitro.[7] Theoretically, bupleurum may increase the risk of bleeding when used with anticoagulant/antiplatelet agents. However, clinical reports of such drug interactions are lacking.

BACTERIAL LEVELS: *Bupleurum* has displayed antibacterial activity against *Helicobacter pylori*.[8]

BLOOD GLUCOSE: Saikosaponins, constituents of bupleurum, have been shown to increase plasma glucose concentrations in rat studies.[6,9] Theoretically, bupleurum may antagonize the effects of blood sugar–lowering agents.

BLOOD LIPIDS: Bupleurum and saikosaponins have been shown to reduce cholesterol and triglyceride levels in animals.[10,11]

BLOOD PRESSURE: Because of the possibility of adrenal stimulation,[12] bupleurum may increase blood pressure.

CORTICOSTEROIDS: Because of possible adrenal stimulation,[12] combination of corticosteroids with bupleurum may result in interactions.

HISTOLOGICAL TESTS: *Bupleurum* has displayed anticancer and antiproliferative activity in animal, in vitro, and in vivo studies.[13-16] Theoretically, bupleurum may interact with antineoplastic agents.

IMMUNOMODULATORS: Bupleurum has displayed both immune-inhibitory and immune-stimulating effects[17-19] and theoretically may interact with immunomodulating agents.

LIVER FUNCTION TESTS: Bupleurum has been shown to decrease serum aspartate transaminase (AST, SGOT) and alanine transaminase (ALA, SGPT).[20] Saikosaponins were shown to increase the activity of liver tyrosine aminotransferase.[21]

SEDATIVES AND CENTRAL NERVOUS SYSTEM DEPRESSANTS: Bupleurum may cause increased drowsiness and have additive effects when used with sedative agents.[22]

TOLBUTAMIDE: In animal and in vitro experiments, a combination product containing bupleurum was shown slightly to increase the gastrointestinal absorption of the potassium channel blocker tolbutamide.[23] Caution is warranted when using bupleurum with tolbutamide.

VIRAL LEVELS: Sho-saiko-to, a combination that contains bupleurum, was found to enhance the anti-HIV-1 activity of lamivudine in vitro.[24]

Burdock (*Arctium lappa*)

Pharmacokinetics
The pharmacokinetics of burdock is not well understood. The burdock constituent arctiin remains stable in gastric juice and is rapidly transformed into arctigenin metabolite 1, followed by conversion to its metabolite 2 through C3 methylation. After an oral dose of 200 mg/kg in rats, the arctiin metabolite 1 reaches its peak serum level after 4 hours.[1]

Adverse effects

Based on traditional use, oral burdock is generally believed to be safe. It should be used cautiously in patients taking diuretics or in those with electrolyte imbalances or dehydration, because diuretic effects of burdock have been observed in limited research.[2] Handling the plant or using topical preparations has occasionally been associated with contact dermatitis.[3] Atropine-like (anticholinergic) reactions such as bradycardia have been reported after consumption of burdock products.[4-7] These cases are believed to result from contamination with belladonna alkaloids, which resemble burdock during harvesting. Burdock itself has not been found to contain atropine or other constituents that would be responsible for these reactions.

Interactions

ANTICOAGULANTS/ANTIPLATELETS: Lignans in burdock have been found to inhibit the binding of platelet-activating factor (PAF) in rabbits[8] and theoretically may increase the risk of bleeding with other anticoagulants/antiplatelets. However, clinical reports of such drug interactions are lacking.

CYTOKINES AND INFLAMMATORY MARKERS: Constituents of burdock may have antiinflammatory effects.[8,9] Reports of clinical drug interactions are lacking.

BACTERIAL LEVELS: Burdock has been reported to exhibit in vitro activity against gram-negative bacteria.[10]

BLOOD ALCOHOL: Tinctures of burdock may contain high concentrations of alcohol (ethanol), which may affect blood alcohol levels. Concomitant use with disulfiram (Antabuse) or metronidazole (Flagyl) may cause adverse effects.

BLOOD GLUCOSE: Burdock fruit extracts have demonstrated hypoglycemic activity in rats[11] and may lower blood glucose levels in humans.[12-14] Theoretically, concomitant use of burdock with other agents that lower blood sugar may cause additive effects and increase the risk of hypoglycemia.

ELECTROLYTES: Oral burdock use has been associated with diuretic effects, as shown in animal and clinical studies.[1,2] Excessive use may lead to electrolyte imbalance.

ESTROGENIC AGENTS: Oral burdock use has been associated with estrogenic effects in HIV patients[1] and, in theory, may interact with estrogens or estrogen-like compounds. However, there is insufficient clinical evidence of this potential interaction.

HISTOLOGICAL TESTS: In vitro, burdock has been shown to exhibit anticancer and antitumor effects.[15-18] Histological findings may be affected.

URIC ACID LEVELS: Burdock has been historically used to eliminate uric acid. Altered uric acid levels may be present in blood and urine.

VIRAL LEVELS: Inhibition of HIV-1 infection has been demonstrated in vitro.[19] Theoretically, burdock may interact with antiretroviral agents.

Butterbur (Petasites hybridus)

Pharmacokinetics

The pharmacokinetics of butterbur is not well understood. Petasins have been reported to be bioavailable and have a half-life of 4 to 6 hours.

Adverse effects

Raw, unprocessed butterbur plant should not be ingested because of the potential for hepatotoxicity of pyrrolizidine alkaloids with long-term use (specifically, concern of venoocclusive disease) and possible carcinogenicity, based on animal studies.[1] This includes any teas, capsules of raw herb, or unprocessed tinctures or extracts. Use should be limited to commercially available products that are free of pyrrolizidine alkaloids. These products are generally believed to be well tolerated, although long-term safety (>12-16 weeks of use) is not well studied. Butterbur should *not* be used to relieve acute asthma exacerbations.[2]

Interactions

CYTOKINES AND INFLAMMATORY MARKERS: Butterbur has been shown in vitro to inhibit cyclooxygenase-2 (COX-2) by directly binding the enzyme.[3] Interactions with other COX-2 inhibitors are possible, although clinical reports of such drug interactions are lacking.

LIVER FUNCTION TESTS: In a clinical trial, subjects supplemented with butterbur showed increased liver enzyme levels.[4]

Caffeine (Black Tea, Cola Nut, Green Tea, Guarana, Yerba Mate)

Pharmacokinetics

Caffeine is well absorbed and distributed quickly. After absorption, caffeine passes into the brain. Caffeine is extensively metabolized in the liver, where primary metabolism is carried out by cytochrome P450-1A2. Caffeine is metabolized to more than 25 metabolites in humans. It is eliminated in urine. Less than 5% of caffeine is found in the urine as unchanged drug. The half-life of caffeine ranges from 1 to 10 hours, and studies have shown that smoking cigarettes decreases the half-life of caffeine.[1-3]

Adverse effects

Caffeine is a central nervous system (CNS) stimulant and may cause insomnia in adults, children, and infants, including nursing infants of mothers taking caffeine. Caffeine acts on the kidneys as a diuretic, increasing urine and urine sodium/potassium levels and potentially decreasing blood sodium/potassium levels, and may worsen incontinence. Caffeine-containing beverages may increase the production of stomach acid and may worsen ulcer symptoms. Tannin in tea can cause constipation. Caffeine in certain doses can increase heart rate and blood pressure, although people who consume caffeine regularly do not seem to experience these effects long term.

An increase in blood sugar levels may occur after ingesting high levels of caffeine. Caffeine-containing beverages such as black tea should be used cautiously in patients with diabetes. People with severe liver disease should use caffeine cautiously because levels of caffeine in the blood may build up and last longer. Skin rashes have been associated with caffeine ingestion. In laboratory and animal studies, caffeine has been found to affect blood clotting, although effects in humans are unclear.

The effects of caffeine are likely more pronounced at extreme ages, such as in the elderly and in children.[4] The chronic use of caffeine, especially in large amounts, may produce tolerance, habituation, and psychological dependence. Abrupt discontinuation of caffeine can result in physical withdrawal symptoms that include headache, irritation, nervousness, anxiety, and dizziness.

Interactions

ADENOSINE: Caffeine has been shown to inhibit the hemodynamic and antiarrhythmic effects of adenosine in humans.[5]

ALCOHOL: Alcohol consumption may increase serum concentrations of caffeine.[6]

ANTICOAGULANTS/ANTIPLATELETS: Caffeine may have antiplatelet activity[7,8] and may theoretically increase the risk of bleeding when used with anticoagulant/antiplatelet agents.

BENZODIAZEPINES: In humans, doses of 125 to 500 mg of caffeine counteracted the reduced anxiety and reduced mental performance associated with 2.5 mg of lorazepam (Ativan).[9]

BITTER ORANGE: Theoretically, concomitant use of bitter orange and caffeine may increase blood pressure and heart rate and increase the risk of serious cardiovascular effects.

BLOOD GLUCOSE LEVELS: Caffeine might increase or decrease blood sugar levels.[10]

CATECHOLAMINERGIC AGENTS: Caffeine overdose has been associated with elevated levels of plasma catecholamines.[11] An increase in catecholamine levels was found when caffeine was administered as an adjunct to aerobic exercise.[12] A catecholamine test may be performed to help diagnose a tumor in the adrenal glands (pheochromocytoma).

CYTOCHROME P450 SUBSTRATES: Caffeine has been reported to induce CYP450 enzymes 1A1, 1A2, and 2B1.[13] In theory, clinically significant alterations of the metabolism of concomitant agents may occur.

DIPYRIDAMOLE (PERSANTINE): Caffeine has been shown to inhibit dipyridamole-induced vasodilation in humans.[14]

ECHINACEA: Echinacea may reduce the oral clearance of caffeine, likely caused by the inhibition of CYP450-1A2 by echinacea.[15]

EPHEDRINE: Caffeine has been shown to enhance the thermogenic activity of ephedrine in clinical and animal studies.[16-18] Other adverse effects caused by the combination of caffeine and ephedrine include abnormal heart rhythms, insomnia, anxiety, headache, irritability, poor concentration, blurred vision, and dizziness. Fatalities have been associated with simultaneous caffeine and ephedrine use.[19,20]

ESTROGENIC AGENTS: Estrogen has been found to inhibit caffeine metabolism in female patients.[21]

GINSENG: There is controversy over whether caffeine and other stimulants are safe to take with ginseng. Some experts believe that Asian ginseng is considered safe when taken in the recommended dosages;[22] others disagree.[23] Ginseng may cause insomnia and headaches and enhance the effects of caffeine. Commercial ginseng preparations are said to contain methylxanthines (e.g., caffeine, theophylline, theobromine) in widely varying amounts, which may influence experimental results.[24] Although the herb itself does not contain caffeine, some commercial ginseng supplements test positive for caffeine.

GRAPEFRUIT: Theoretically, concomitant administration of caffeine with grapefruit juice may increase caffeine levels and the risk of adverse effects. However, clinical studies show that the ingestion of grapefruit juice should not alter pharmacokinetics or pharmacodynamics when coadministered with caffeine.[25-27] There was no significant difference in ambulatory systolic and diastolic blood pressure or heart rate when grapefruit juice was coadministered with caffeine.[25]

HOMOCYSTEINE: A dose-dependent relationship between coffee consumption and plasma homocysteine levels has been reported.[28,29]

LITHIUM: Caffeine withdrawal has been shown to increase serum lithium levels in humans[30] and may increase the risk of lithium toxicity.

LIVER FUNCTION TESTS: Regular daily coffee consumption may dose-dependently lower levels of liver enzymes, such as gamma-glutamyl transferase (GGT), alanine transferase (ALT), and alkaline phosphatase (ALP).[31]

MEXILETINE (MEXITIL): In humans, mexiletine has been shown to decrease caffeine elimination by 50%.[32]

QUINOLONES: Caffeine clearance was decreased in patients treated with norfloxacin.[33] Quinolones may inhibit the N-demethylation pathway of caffeine. Ciprofloxacin slightly increases the half-life of caffeine from 5.2 to 8.2 hours.[34,35] Ofloxacin had no effect on the clearance of caffeine.[36,37]

TERBINAFINE (LAMISIL): Terbinafine has been shown in healthy volunteers to decrease the clearance of caffeine[38] and may increase the risk of adverse effects associated with caffeine.

THEOPHYLLINE (BRONKODYL, ELIXOPHYLLIN, SLO-BID): In healthy volunteers, caffeine has been shown to decrease clearance of the bronchodilator theophylline, increase its elimination half-life, and increase serum levels.[39]

URIC ACIDS: Caffeine may falsely elevate uric acid concentrations.[40]

URINE TESTS: Caffeine may increase 5-hydroxyindoleacetic acid concentrations and urine test results for serotonin analysis.[41]

VERAPAMIL (ISOPTIN): Clinically significant interactions between caffeine and the calcium channel blocker verapamil have been noted.[42] Verapamil may increase plasma caffeine concentrations and increase the risk of adverse effects associated with caffeine.

YOHIMBE (PAUSINYSTALIA YOHIMBE): Caffeine-containing agents such as coffee, tea, cola, guarana, and mate may theoretically increase the risk of hypertensive crisis when taken with yohimbine.

Caper (Capparis spinosa)

Pharmacokinetics: Insufficient available evidence.

Adverse effects

In a 6-month study evaluating the effects of Liv-52, an herbal preparation containing *Capparis spinosa*, no adverse effects were reported.[1] Theoretically, *C. spinosa* may induce allergic reactions in people allergic to mustard oil (methyl isothiocyanate) because it contains significant amounts of this substance.[2] Cross-sensitivity is possible in people allergic to members of the Capparaceae family, such as sweet vernal grass (*Apophyllum anomalum*) or *Steriphoma paradoxum*.

Interactions

BACTERIAL LEVELS: In vitro, extracts of the aerial parts of *C. spinosa* exhibited antibacterial activity against gram-positive and gram-negative bacteria and theoretically may interact with antibacterial agents.[3]

BLOOD GLUCOSE: Based on ethnobotanical data, *C. spinosa* may have hypoglycemic effects[4] and theoretically may cause additive effects when used with blood sugar–lowering agents.

BLOOD PRESSURE: Based on tradition, *C. spinosa* may have antihypertensive effects[5] and theoretically may have additive effects when used with other blood pressure–lowering agents.

CYTOKINES AND INFLAMMATORY MARKERS: Extracts of *C. spinosa* were shown to counter the effects of inflammatory stress in vitro[4] and theoretically may interact with antiinflammatory agents.

ELECTROLYTES: Based on clinical data, Liv-52 (herbal preparation containing extracts of *C. spinosa, Cichorium intybus, Solanum nigrum, Terminalia arjuna,* and *Achillea millefolium*) displayed diuretic effects.[1] Although its contribution to the diuretic effects remains unclear, excessive use of caper may lead to electrolyte imbalance.

FUNGAL LEVELS: In vitro, extracts of the aerial parts of *C. spinosa* have exhibited antifungal activity.[3]

IRON: In addition to capers, Liv-52 also contains iron, which may affect blood levels.

LIVER FUNCTION TESTS: *C. spinosa* is one of several ingredients in a combination drug, Liv-52 (Himalayan Co., India), associated with improved clinical outcomes in liver cirrhosis.[1] Thus, caper may affect hepatic assays.

VIRAL LEVELS: *C. spinosa* bud extract was shown to interfere with herpes simplex virus type 2 (HSV-2) replication in human peripheral blood mononuclear cells in vitro.[6] Theoretically, caper may interact with other antiviral agents.

Carob (Ceratonia siliqua)

Pharmacokinetics
Carob contains a large proportion of insoluble fiber, which is not digested and passes through the gut unchanged. The pharmacokinetics of the other constituents of carob is not well understood.

Adverse effects
Carob appears to be well tolerated. Hypersensitivity reactions, including urticaria, asthma, and rhinitis, have been reported in workers exposed to carob.[1,2]

Interactions
BLOOD GLUCOSE: According to clinical and animal studies, carob bean gum decreased the glucose response and glycemic index.[3,4] Theoretically, carob may interact with agents that lower blood sugar.

BLOOD LIPIDS: Carob may reduce total and LDL cholesterol.[5-7]

CHROMIUM: Based on animal research, carob bean gum may reduce the absorption of chromium.[8]

COBALT: Animal research suggests that carob bean gum may reduce the absorption of cobalt.[8]

COPPER: In animals, carob bean gum has been shown to reduce copper absorption.[8]

CREATININE: In patients with renal failure, carob bean gum has been shown to reduce creatinine levels.[9]

ELECTROLYTES: Carob bean gum may act as a laxative as a result of its fiber content.[10-12] Excessive use may lead to water loss and electrolyte imbalance.

IRON: In vitro, carob bean gum has been shown to reduce the bioavailability of iron.[13-15]

ORAL AGENTS: Carob contains a large proportion of insoluble fiber, which is not digested and passes through the gut unchanged. In animals carob bean gum has been shown to decrease bowel transit time[4,16] and interfere with the absorption of oral agents. It may be ideal to separate doses of carob bean gum and oral agents by several hours.

URIC ACID: In animals, carob bean gum has been shown to decrease serum uric acid concentration.[17]

VIRAL LEVELS: Based on in vitro research, carob bean gum polysaccharides may block a step in rubella virus replication subsequent to virus attachment.[18] Theoretically, carob may interact with some antiviral agents.

ZINC: In vitro and in vivo, carob bean gum has been shown to reduce the absorption of zinc.[8,13-15]

Cascara (Rhamnus purshiana)

Pharmacokinetics
Based on unsubstantiated reports, orally administered cascara laxatives usually produce a bowel movement within 6 to 8 hours, although the effect may not occur for 24 hours. After oral administration, the anthraquinone glycosides are purported to be poorly absorbed until they are hydrolyzed by colonic bacteria; then moderate absorption of cascara occurs at the intestinal wall, to an unclear extent.[1] Anthranoids are readily transformed to corresponding glucuronide and sulfate derivatives. The colon and jejunum also exert an anthraquinone-conjugating activity. At least a part of these compounds undergoes extrahepatic metabolism.[1] After oral administration and hydrolysis by colonic bacteria, the anthraquinones are partially eliminated renally.

Adverse effects
Orally, cascara may cause mild abdominal discomfort, colic, and cramps.[2] Long-term use may lead to potassium depletion, albuminuria, hematuria, disturbed heart function, muscle weakness, finger clubbing, and cachexia. Purportedly, cascara bark must be aged for 1 year or heat-treated to remove harsh constituents (anthrones), which produce severe vomiting, intestinal cramping, and possibly spasms.[3]

Interactions
ANTICOAGULANTS/ANTIPLATELETS: Theoretically, cascara may potentiate anticoagulant therapy by reducing the absorption of vitamin K from the gut.[3] However, clinical reports of such drug interactions are lacking.

CORTICOSTEROIDS: Concomitant use of corticosteroids with cascara may increase the risk of potassium depletion.[3]

ELECTROLYTES: As a laxative, cascara may prevent nutrient absorption from the gut. Chronic or excessive use may lead to fluid loss and electrolyte balance. Concomitant use with other laxatives, diuretics, or electrolyte-depleting agents (e.g., licorice) may exacerbate electrolyte imbalance.

ORAL AGENTS: As a laxative, cascara may prevent absorption from the gut. The cathartic action of cascara may hasten the passage of all oral agents through the gut, thereby inhibiting their action. Because of its anthranoid content, cascara has been suggested to inhibit the absorption of oral agents.[4] However, clinical reports such of drug interactions are lacking.

SQUILL (URGINEA MARITIMA, SYN. SCILLA MARITIMA): Cascara may inhibit the absorption of digitalis glycosides and decrease their cardiac action. However, cathartic-induced hypokalemia increases the toxicity and potency of absorbed digitalis.[3]

URINE TESTS: Cascara can discolor urine (pink, red, purple, orange, rust), interfering with diagnostic tests that depend on a color change, as a result of its anthraquinone content.[3]

VITAMIN K: Cascara induces increased speed of intestinal emptying, which theoretically may result in decreased absorption of vitamin K and altered coagulation.[3]

Cat's Claw (Uncaria spp.)

Pharmacokinetics: Insufficient available evidence.

Adverse effects
In various clinical studies (including manufacturer's website study), cat's claw appears to be well tolerated.[1-3] Although clinical safety data are limited, long-standing historical use shows limited reports of adverse events. Rarely, cat's claw may cause diarrhea, changes in bowel movements, abdominal pain, gastrointestinal problems, nausea, dizziness, and increased risk of bleeding.[4,5] In a case report, cat's claw was linked to acute renal failure in a patient with systemic lupus erythematosus (SLE).[6] Cat's claw is reported to contain tannins. The

oral toxicity of plant tannins is low, as they are readily hydrolyzed in the gut to gallic acid and other metabolites. However, liver and kidney toxicity has occurred with high tannin doses used topically or intravenously.[7] Tannin consumption has been associated with certain cancers, such as esophageal cancer; however, it is unclear whether this is due to the tannins themselves or other compounds associated with tannins.[8]

Interactions

ANALGESICS AND ANESTHETICS: Various studies have demonstrated antiinflammatory and pain-reducing effects of cat's claw.[9,10] In animal studies, *Uncaria tomentosa* produced dose-related antinociception in several models of chemical and thermal pain through mechanisms that involve an interaction with serotonin receptors.[10] Theoretically, cat's claw may interact with analgesic agents.

ANTICOAGULANTS/ANTIPLATELETS: Cat's claw contains rhynchophylline, which may inhibit platelet aggregation.[11,12] Based on animal studies, the antiplatelet effect of cat's claw may increase the risk of bleeding.[5] Although clinical reports of such drug interactions are lacking, caution is warranted when using cat's claw with anticoagulants/antiplatelets because of an increased risk of bleeding.

BLOOD ALCOHOL: Many tinctures of cat's claw contain high levels of alcohol and may affect blood alcohol levels. Adverse interactions may occur when taken with disulfiram (Antabuse) or metronidazole (Flagyl).

BLOOD LIPIDS: Cat's claw contains rhynchophylline, which may lower blood cholesterol.

BLOOD PRESSURE: Cat's claw contains rhynchophylline, which may cause hypotension and decrease heart rate.[11,12] Geissoschizine methyl ether, an indole alkaloid extracted from *Uncarie ramulus*, is a potent vasorelaxant.[13] Theoretically, cat's claw may affect blood pressure and vascular resistance.

CHONDROCYTE MARKERS: Based on in vitro research using human cartilage, coadministration of extracts from *Uncaria guianensis* and maca (*Lepidium meyenii*) may promote chondrocyte growth.[14]

CYTOCHROME P450 SUBSTRATES: Preliminary in vitro evidence suggests that cat's claw may inhibit CYP450-3A4 enzymes.[15] Theoretically, cat's claw may increase levels of agents metabolized by 3A4 enzymes.

CYTOKINES AND INFLAMMATORY MARKERS: According to in vitro and clinical studies, the antiinflammatory effects of cat's claw may inhibit production of tumor necrosis factor alpha (TNF-α) and, to a lesser extent, prostaglandin E_2 (PGE_2).[9-18] Theoretically, cat's claw may interact with other antiinflammatory agents.

DIAGNOSTIC RADIOPHARMACEUTICALS: Based on animal studies, the oral ingestion of *Uncaria tomentosa* extract may alter the biodistribution of the radiobiocomplex sodium pertechnetate ($Na^{99m}TcO_4$), particularly in the heart, pancreas, and muscles.[19] Theoretically, cat's claw may interact with certain diagnostic radiopharmaceuticals.

ELECTROLYTES: Based on unsubstantiated reports, the mytraphylline constituent of cat's claw may have diuretic properties that may lead to electrolyte imbalances when used with other diuretics.

ESTROGENIC AGENTS: Serum estrogen concentrations may be reduced after cat's claw ingestion.[20] Theoretically, cat's claw may interfere or reduce the effects of estrogen therapy.

HEART RATE: Hirsutine, an indole alkaloid component of *U. tomentosa*, has been shown in vitro to have antiarrhythmic activity.[21,22]

HISTOLOGICAL TESTS: According to in vitro and animal studies, C-Med-100 inhibits tumor cell proliferation and inflammatory responses,[22] induces prolonged lymphocyte half-life, increases spleen cells,[24] and has direct antiproliferative activity on several cell lines.[25-29] Theoretically, cat's claw may interact with antineoplastic agents.

IRON: Cat's claw is purported to contain tannins. Tannins bind to and decrease absorption of iron,[30] which may affect levels in the blood.

KIDNEY FUNCTION TESTS: Cat's claw has been linked to acute renal failure in a patient with SLE.[6] Caution is warranted when using cat's claw with nephrotoxic agents.

MACA: Based on in vitro research using human cartilage, coadministration of extracts from *Uncaria guianensis* and maca (*Lepidium meyenii*) may promote chondrocyte growth.[11]

MUSHROOM: According to in vitro and in vivo studies, cat's claw water extract and medicinal mushroom extract are synergistic and do not exhibit metabolic competition.[31]

PROGESTOGENIC AGENTS: Serum progestin concentrations may be reduced after cat's claw ingestion.[20] Theoretically, cat's claw may alter or reduce the effects of progestin therapy.

VIRAL LEVELS: In vitro, quinovic acid glycosides from *U. tomentosa* exhibited antiviral properties when tested against two RNA viruses, vesicular stomatitis virus, and rhinovirus 1B.[32] Theoretically, cat's claw may interact with antiviral agents.

WHITE BLOOD CELL COUNTS: Cat's claw has exhibited lymphocyte-stimulatory activity in vitro.[33-35]

Chamomile (Matricaria recutita, syn. Matricaria suaveolens, Matricaria chamomilla, Anthemis nobilis, Chamaemelum nobile, Chamomilla chamomilla, Chamomilla recutita)

Pharmacokinetics: Insufficient available evidence.

Adverse effects

Except in patients sensitive to plants in the Asteraceae family, chamomile is generally well tolerated. Patients with allergies or hypersensitivities to plants in the Asteraceae (Compositae) family, including ragweed, mugwort, asters, and chrysanthemums, as well as to celery (Umbelliferae) and onion (Amaryllidaceae) should not use chamomile; cross-sensitivity may provoke allergic reactions.

Interactions

ADRENOCORTICOTROPIC HORMONE: ACTH levels were decreased by chamomile in animals.[1]

ANTICOAGULANTS/ANTIPLATELETS: Because of its coumarin content,[2,3] chamomile may increase risk of bleeding when ingested concomitantly with anticoagulants/antiplatelets. It remains unclear whether this potential interaction is clinically significant, but caution is advised when using chamomile concomitantly with anticoagulant/antiplatelet agents.

BLOOD ALCOHOL: Many chamomile tinctures contain high levels of alcohol and thus may affect blood alcohol levels. Adverse interactions may occur when taken with disulfiram (Antabuse) or metronidazole (Flagyl).

BLOOD GLUCOSE: Based on laboratory research, the flavonoid glucoside chamaemeloside found in *Chamaemelum nobile* has in vivo hypoglycemic activity.[4] Caution is advised when using chamomile with other agents that may lower blood sugar.

BLOOD PRESSURE: Based on animal research, the chamomile constituent apigenin may have hypotensive properties,[5] likely by suppressing the calcium influx through both voltage-operated and receptor-operated calcium channels.[6] This may affect blood pressure. Caution is advised when using chamomile with other agents that may lower blood pressure.

CYTOCHROME P450 SUBSTRATES: In vitro, chamomile has demonstrated inhibition of CYP450 enzymes (1A2, 2C9, 2D6, 3A4).[7,8]

ESTROGENIC AGENTS: In vitro, an extract containing *Matricaria chamomile, Sideritis euboea, Sideritis clandestine,* and *Pimpinella anisum* was associated with selective estrogen receptor modulator (SERM) properties against osteoporosis.[9] Interactions with estrogenic agents are thus possible, and bone marker tests may be altered. However, clinical reports of such drug interactions are lacking.

HEART RATE: Apigenin, a constituent of chamomile, relaxed thoracic aorta in rats by suppressing calcium influx through both voltage-operated and receptor-operated calcium channels.[6] This may affect heart rate.

SEDATIVES AND CENTRAL NERVOUS SYSTEM DEPRESSANTS: Benzodiazepines and other sedatives that may cause drowsiness should be used cautiously with chamomile because of an increased risk of additive effects.[3,10] Apigenin, an extract of chamomile, has been shown to have central benzodiazepine receptor affinity and anxiolytic and sedative effects in mice.[11]

Chaparral *(Larrea tridentata, Larrea divaricata)*

Pharmacokinetics

Nordihydroguaiaretic acid (NDGA) is the active metabolite of chaparral. Other metabolites include secoisolariciresinol, enterodiol, enterolactone, matairesinol, and guaiaretic acid diquinone.[1] Reportedly, NDGA is metabolized to an *o*-quinone derivative[2,3] and could be further metabolized by conjugation to glutathione.[2] NDGA is absorbed in the bloodstream, filtered by the glomeruli, and retained by the proximal tubules, where it accumulates.[1,3] Free NDGA is not found in the rat kidney but is found in the feces.[1]

In female mice, intravenous NDGA at 50 mg/kg yielded a primary half-life ($T_{1/2}\alpha$) of 30 minutes and a secondary half-life ($T_{1/2}\beta$) of 135 minutes, with the peak plasma concentration (C_{max}) of 15 mcg/mL.[2,4]

Adverse effects

Chaparral was removed from the FDA's "generally recognized as safe" (GRAS) list in 1970. Chaparral and NDGA are generally considered unsafe and are not recommended for use. Exposure to lignans, which may yield toxicity, appears to be greater from capsule or tablets than from decoctions of chaparral tea.[5]

Multiple reports have detailed serious adverse reactions associated with chaparral, including liver cirrhosis/failure, kidney cysts/failure, and kidney cancer.[1,6-15] The most serious outcomes of liver toxicity include several case reports of cirrhosis. In most cases, symptoms arose 3 to 52 weeks after initiating chaparral and resolved within 1 to 17 weeks after discontinuation.[6] Symptoms reported include fatigue, right upper quadrant abdominal pain, dark urine, light stools, nausea, diarrhea, anorexia, weight loss, icterus, fatigue, pedal edema, and increased abdominal girth. Elevations in ALP, ALT, AST, total bilirubin, and GGT have also been reported.

Interactions

ANTICOAGULANTS/ANTIPLATELETS: In theory, there may be an increased risk of bleeding with concurrent use of chaparral and other agents. The chaparral component NDGA diminishes platelet aggregation in aspirin-treated patients and delayed its onset.[16]

BLOOD GLUCOSE: In theory, chaparral may have additive effects when taken concurrently with hypoglycemic agents. In mouse models of type 2 diabetes, NDGA was shown to decrease plasma glucose concentrations, without a change in insulin concentration.[17] NDGA improved glucose tolerance and the ability of insulin to decrease glucose concentration.

CYTOCHROME P450 SUBSTRATES: NDGA inhibits CYP450-mediated monoxygenase activity in rat hepatic microsomes.[18] In theory, chaparral, which contains NDGA, may interact with other agents metabolized by the CYP450 pathway and may raise the levels of P450 substrates.

HISTOLOGICAL TESTS: Based on in vitro and animal studies, lignans from *Larrea tridentata*, including NDGA, may have antineoplastic effects.[19-25] Histological findings may be affected.

KIDNEY FUNCTION TESTS: The use of chaparral with other agents known to induce renal toxicity should be avoided. In case reports, chaparral has been implicated in kidney failure,[6] renal cell carcinoma, and renal cystic disease.[7]

LIVER FUNCTION TESTS: Chaparral has been implicated in numerous case reports of acute liver injury.[6,11,13-15] The use of chaparral with other hepatotoxic agents should be avoided.

MONOAMINERGIC AGENTS: Chaparral has been reported anecdotally to pose a risk of reacting with MAO inhibitors. However, there is limited evidence supporting this interaction.

SEDATIVES AND CENTRAL NERVOUS SYSTEM DEPRESSANTS: It has been hypothesized that NDGA may inhibit barbiturate metabolism and interact with phenobarbital.[2]

VIRAL LEVELS: Based on in vitro research, NDGA may have antiviral activity, especially against the influenza virus.[26]

WHITE BLOOD CELL COUNTS: It has been suggested that chaparral contains immune-stimulating polysaccharides.[2] Certain immune parameters, such as WBC counts, may be affected.

Chasteberry *(Vitex agnus-castus)*

Pharmacokinetics: Insufficient available evidence.

Adverse effects

Chasteberry appears to be generally well tolerated, with few adverse events reported.[1-3] Side effects reported in clinical trials have been mostly nonspecific (headache, acne, eczema, itching, rash, skin eruptions, urticaria, diarrhea, nausea, gas/flatulence, heartburn, vomiting).[1,4-6] Rare cases of menstrual bleeding, altered hormone levels, vertigo, and nosebleed have also occurred.[1-3,6-8]

Interactions

DOPAMINERGIC AGENTS: Chasteberry competitively binds to D_2 receptors in vitro[9,10] and may alter dopaminergic effects. Clinical drug interactions are unclear.

ESTROGENIC AGENTS: In vitro, constituents in chasteberry bind selectively to estrogen receptor beta[11,12] and may interact with other estrogenic agents. However, clinical reports of drug interactions are unclear.

PROLACTIN: In humans, low doses of chasteberry have been observed to increase serum prolactin levels, and higher doses of chasteberry have resulted in the inhibition of prolactin secretion and lower serum levels of prolactin.[5,13] In vitro, chasteberry was found to inhibit prolactin secretion.[9,10]

Cherry (Prunus avium, Prunus cerasus and various Prunus spp.)

Pharmacokinetics: Insufficient available evidence.

Adverse effects

Cherries are known to contain cyanide,[1] and two species of cherry (*Prunus padus* and *Prunus serotina*) have been discussed in reports of toxic plants.[2] There have been case reports of cyanide poisoning after ingesting choke cherries.[1]

Allergy to cherry is a common component of multifood allergies.[3] All members of the Prunoideae subfamily, which includes plum, peach, cherry, and apricot, are known to cross-react both in vitro and in vivo because of a shared allergen.[4] The major allergen reported in cherry is Pru av 1, which is similar in structure to the major birch (*Betula verrucosa*) allergen, Bet v 1.[5,6] Novel isoforms of Pru av 1 with different combinations of epitopes are also known to exist.[7] Because of the structural similarity of their allergenic proteins, individuals sensitive to birch pollens may also exhibit allergic reactions to cherry, and vice versa.[8-18]

The variable allergenicity to cherry reported worldwide[19,20] is believed to result from the proteins eliciting the allergic response. Although the oral allergic response is elicited by a reaction with a protein similar to an allergen present in birch pollen, systemic allergic response is elicited by a different class, lipid transfer proteins (LTPs).[9] The LTPs have been demonstrated to be more stable relative to the birch pollen homologs in vitro, and some evidence suggests that this stability is related to the more severe reactions associated with LTP allergic response.[21]

Interactions

CYTOKINES AND INFLAMMATORY MARKERS: Studies have demonstrated cherry consumption to reduce plasma C-reactive protein (CRP) and nitric oxide (NO) concentrations in healthy subjects.[22,23] In vitro, cherry has also been shown to inhibit cyclooxygenase enzymes and lipid peroxidation.[24,25]

HISTOLOGICAL TESTS: Cherry has been shown to inhibit tumor cell proliferation in vitro and in vivo.[24,26,27]

URIC ACID: A study investigating the effects of cherry consumption on plasma urate concentrations reported that the consumption of cherries led to a decrease in plasma urate 5 hours after consumption, with a noted increase in urinary urate.[23]

Chia (Salvia hispanica)

Pharmacokinetics: Insufficient available evidence.

Adverse effects

Based on a report of 100 healthy subjects who were divided into four groups and given either 4 g of sunflower seeds (control) or 2.5, 5, or 10 g of chia seeds daily for 4 weeks, toxicological safety of chia was deemed satisfactory for use in human and animals by the U.K. Committee for Novel Foods and Processes. No significant adverse effects were reported. The same report also noted potential chia protein allergenicity, as demonstrated by specific IgE binding and immunoblot analysis. It was proposed that chia-containing products should carry statements cautioning consumers with food sensitivities, particularly those with allergies to sesame or mustard seeds.

Other safety data are limited, although the seeds *of Salvia hispanica* (chia) and *Salvia columbariae* (golden chia) have been used for centuries as a food staple. Gastrointestinal side effects were reported in clinical research that used Salba as a dietary supplement.[1] The roots of *S. columbariae* have been historically used by Native Americans to treat stroke,[2] and the roots of *Salvia miltiorrhiza* (danshen) are widely accepted as a safe and effective stroke treatment in China and other countries.[3] However, safety data on the roots of the genus *Salvia* are limited.

Interactions

ANTICOAGULANTS/ANTIPLATELETS: In theory, the roots of chia may interact with warfarin; pharmacokinetic and pharmacodynamic interactions have been reported between warfarin and roots of the related species *Salvia miltiorrhiza* (danshen).[4,5] However, clinical reports regarding the specific drug interactions of *Salvia hispanica* are lacking.

BLOOD LIPIDS: The clinical evidence that shows lipid-lowering effects of the *S. hispanica* variety Salba[1] are supported by animal studies.[6]

BLOOD PRESSURE: Salba may lower blood pressure.[1] Theoretically, concurrent use of chia and antihypertensive agents may cause additive blood pressure–lowering effects.

CYTOCHROME P450 SUBSTRATES: Drug-metabolizing enzymes have been shown to be affected by extracts of *S. miltiorrhiza* in vivo and in vitro.[7]

HISTOLOGICAL TESTS: Chia has been reported to inhibit tumor growth in a murine model of adenocarcinoma.[8] Theoretically, chia may affect histological findings.

Chicory (Cichorium intybus)

Pharmacokinetics: Insufficient available evidence.

Adverse effects

Chicory appears to be generally well tolerated, but skin rash and contact dermatitis have been reported with its use.[1-3] Weight loss, loss of appetite, and myalgic encephalomyelitis (chronic, multisystemic inflammatory disease that primarily affects nervous system) have also been associated with chicory use.[4]

Interactions

CALCIUM: Chicory extract (inulin) may marginally increase the absorption of dietary calcium.[5]

CYTOCHROME P450 SUBSTRATES: Biochemical studies have suggested that chicory may interact with CYP450-metabolized agents.[6]

Chrysanthemum (Chrysanthemum spp.)

Pharmacokinetics

Pyrethrins found in the seed casings of *Chrysanthemum* appear to be readily absorbed through the gut and lung and poorly absorbed through skin contact.[1,2] Normally, the liver rapidly and extensively metabolizes pyrethrins; thus, they have a relatively low risk of chronic accumulation.

Adverse effects

Chrysanthemum flowers may cause allergic reactions in individuals sensitive to members of the Asteraceae (Compositae) family.[3-6] Patients allergic to feverfew, tansy, chamomile, *Artemisia vulgaris*, Liliaceae plants, tulip, Easter lily (*Lilium longiflorum*), *Gerbera*, lettuce, *Senecio cruentus*, *Aster*, *Matricaria*, *Solidago*, daisy, dandelion, *Parthenium hysterophorus*, *Xanthium strumarium*, *Helianthus annuus*, *Frullania dilatata*, *Frullania tamarisci*, *Arnica longifolia*, *Arnica montana*, primrose, sunflower, ragweed, pollen of the Amaryllidaceae family (*Alstroemeria* and *Narcissus*), or mugwort should avoid *Chrysanthemum*.[5,7-27] Allergic symptoms include pollinosis, rhinoconjunctivitis, asthma, urticaria, contact dermatitis, eczema (ranging from localized and seasonal to generalized and persistent), actinic reticuloid, and photosensitivity.*

Pyrethrins found in the seed casings of *Chrysanthemum cinerariifolium* and *C. coccineum* are used as insecticides and insect repellents. Adverse effects associated with pyrethrin poisoning are related to toxicity in the nervous system, specifically related to the sodium channels of nerve cell axons, which may lead to convulsions. Ocular exposure to pyrethrins has resulted in corneal erosions.[2]

Interactions

ANESTHETICS: Based on laboratory research, *Chrysanthemum* may have anesthetizing activity[46] and may interact with anesthetic agents.

BLOOD GLUCOSE: The *Chrysanthemum* product jiangtangkang has been shown to improve glucose levels and insulin sensitivity in patients with non-insulin-dependent diabetes.[47]

CYTOKINES AND INFLAMMATORY MARKERS: Based on in vitro studies, *Chrysanthemum* flowers may inhibit lipopolysaccharide-induced prostaglandin E_2 production[48] and may interact with antiinflammatory agents. However, clinical reports of such drug interactions are lacking.

HISTOLOGICAL TESTS: Based on in vitro studies, *Chrysanthemum* may have antineoplastic activity[49,50] and may affect histological findings.

PHOTOSENSITIZING AGENTS: In case reports, *Chrysanthemum* has been suggested to cause photosensitization[7,8,29,30] and may have additive effects when used with similarly acting agents.

URIC ACID: *Chrysanthemum* has been shown to inhibit the enzyme xanthine oxidase in vitro,[51] which may in turn affect uric acid levels.

VIRAL LEVELS: *Chrysanthemum* has demonstrated anti-HIV activity in vitro[52-55] and theoretically may affect viral counts.

WHITE BLOOD CELL COUNTS: Based on in vitro studies, *Chrysanthemum* may inhibit the behavior of human polymorphonuclear leukocytes[56] and may stimulate the proliferation of splenocytes.[52] WBC counts thus may be affected by chrysanthemum.

Cinnamon (*Cinnamomum* spp.)

Pharmacokinetics

A pharmacokinetic study measured the absorption of orally administered procyanidin B_2 and procyanidin B_3 isolated from cinnamon bark in rat plasma.[1] In animals, cinnamaldehyde (a component of cinnamon) administered intraduodenally is absorbed quickly, and its effects are long-lasting.[2] The metabolism of *o*-methoxycinnamaldehyde from cinnamon was studied in rats. The major metabolic pathway (approximately two thirds of the dose) was oxidation to the corresponding cinnamic and phenylpropionic acids (C6-C3 acids), which were largely excreted as glycine conjugates. Intermediate amounts (~10% of dose) of the *o*-demethylated C6-C3 acids were excreted. Urinary excretion of metabolites was rapid (91% in 24 hours and 98% in 48 hours).[3]

Adverse effects

Reports of adverse effects are lacking in clinical trials evaluating cinnamon for diabetes.[4,5] Asthma and other chronic respiratory symptoms were observed from inhalation of cinnamon dust in spice-factory workers.[6-8]

Allergic reactions are common with the use of cinnamon, its constituents, members of the Lauraceae family, or Balsam of Peru.[9-13] Dermatitis, stomatitis, glossitis, gingivitis, perioral dermatitis, oral lesions, and cheilitis have been noted in case reports after external application of cinnamon (e.g., cinnamon oils), as well as after use of flavored chewing gums, mints, or toothpastes.[14-34]

Interactions

ANTIBIOTICS: In theory, the antimicrobial properties of cinnamon seen in vitro[35-41] may enhance the effects of common antibacterial agents. On the contrary, cinnamon bark powder has been suggested to *slow* tetracycline absorption and consequently reduce blood levels.[42]

ANTIBODIES: In animal and in vitro studies, aqueous cinnamon extracts inhibited allergic and complement-related antibody responses.[43,44]

ANTICOAGULANTS/ANTIPLATELETS: Based on animal research, cinnamon bark may cause a significant decrease in platelet counts after long-term use.[45,46] Theoretically, concomitant use of cinnamon with anticoagulants/antiplatelets may increase risk of bleeding; however, clinical reports of such drug interactions are lacking.

ANTISPASMODIC AGENTS: Based on secondary sources, cinnamon may have antispasmodic effects and may interact with other antispasmodics.[47]

BLOOD GLUCOSE: Based on in vitro and animal studies, cinnamon may lower blood glucose levels and act as an insulin mimetic.[48-56] Theoretically, concurrent use of hypoglycemic agents with cinnamon may cause additive effects.

CYTOCHROME P450 SUBSTRATES: Cinnamon or its constituents may interact with hepatic microsomal CYP450[57-59] and may interact with agents metabolized by this system.

HEART RATE: Cinnamon may have antiarrhythmic properties;[60,61] heart rate may be affected.

KIDNEY FUNCTION TESTS: In rodents, cinnamon extracts reduced blood urea nitrogen (BUN) levels induced by experimental glomerulonephritis.[44]

VIRAL LEVELS: Clinical research has shown that cinnamon bark extract interferes with HIV-1 and HIV-2 replication,[62] suggesting possible use as an adjunct to antiretroviral agents.

WHITE BLOOD CELL COUNTS: Based on in vitro and animal studies, cinnamon may have stimulatory or inhibitory effects on lymphocyte proliferation.[63,64] WBC counts may be affected.

Clove (*Syzygium aromaticum*, syn. *Eugenia aromaticum*)

Pharmacokinetics

The pharmacokinetics of clove is not well understood. It appears that eugenol (a constituent of clove) is metabolized in the liver.

Adverse effects

Clove has "generally recognized as safe" (GRAS) FDA status for use as a food. However, when clove is ingested in large doses, as undiluted oil (eugenol), or in the form of clove cigarettes, it may cause numerous adverse effects, such as seizures, CNS depression, bronchospasm, pulmonary edema, disseminated intravascular coagulation (DIC), and hepatotoxicity. Ingesting as little as 10 mL of clove oil has been implicated in hepatotoxicity.[1]

The American Dental Association has accepted clove for professional use but not for nonprescription use because it may damage soft tissues. Contact dermatitis has been reported after exposure to clove.[2-4] Painful sensations are possible, believed to be mediated through TRPA-1 (cold ion channel) activation.[5] Allergic stomatitis secondary to eugenol exposure has also been reported.[6] Some people may experience skin irritation or painful sensations from clove, which

---
*References 3, 4, 7, 8, 10, 17, 20-22, 24, 26-45.

may lead to rash, hives, burning, irritation, dry peeling lips, blanching, chemical burns, lack of feeling, and sweating on exposed skin.

Interactions

ANALGESICS: The clove component eugenol may inhibit prostaglandin biosynthesis and thereby depress pain sensory receptors.[7] Based on clinical research, clove gel may be as effective as the oral anesthetic benzocaine 20% gel.[8] Theoretically, additive effects may occur when clove is used with other analgesics or anesthetics.

ANTICOAGULANTS/ANTIPLATELETS: Clove has been shown to inhibit platelet aggregation in vitro[9-11] and was clinically implicated in increased international normalized ratio (INR).[12] Therefore, use with other anticoagulant/antiplatelet agents may result in additive effects and increased bleeding risk.

BLOOD GLUCOSE: Hypoglycemia was noted after the administration of 1 tsp of clove oil to a 7-month-old infant.[13] Caution is warranted in infants and in patients using clove with blood sugar–lowering agents.

BLOOD PRESSURE: Based on animal research, eugenol from clove may have vasorelaxant properties[14] and may affect blood pressure.

CYTOCHROME P450 SUBSTRATES: Based on rat research, clove may reduce levels of CYP450 enzymes.[15] Caution is warranted when using clove with other agents metabolized by CYP450.

CYTOKINES AND INFLAMMATORY MARKERS: Eugenol may act as an antiinflammatory agent and may interact with other antiinflammatory agents.[17]

HISTAMINE: Based on animal research, clove (specifically the eugenol component) may have antihistamine activity.[16]

HISTOLOGICAL TESTS: In vitro, eugenol has been shown to cause apoptosis (cell death)[18] and may theoretically interact with antineoplastic agents.

KIDNEY FUNCTION TESTS: Based on case study, ingested clove oil may be nephrotoxic[13] and should be used cautiously with other nephrotoxic agents.

LIVER FUNCTION TESTS: Based on case reports, ingested clove oil may be hepatotoxic.[1,19] Liver function tests may be affected, and comcomitant use with hepatotoxic agents should be discouraged.

Coleus (Coleus forskohlii)

Pharmacokinetics

The pharmacokinetics of coleus is not well understood. Bioavailability appears to be poor after oral administration.[1]

Adverse Effects

Few adverse effects have been reported with the use of coleus. Coleus has been traditionally used to treat cardiovascular disorders and may cause increased heart rate, flushing, and hypotension.[2,3]

Interactions

ACIDITY: Theoretically, coleus may interact with acidic foods and beverages. Coleus barbatus has been reported to increase intestinal movement and decrease gastric pH in rats.[4] Coleus should be used cautiously when taken concurrently with agents that are dependent on pH and gastric action for breakdown and activation, such as newer cephalosporin antibiotics, itraconazole, ketoconazole, and warfarin.

ANTICOAGULANTS/ANTIPLATELETS: Coleus is a potent inhibitor of platelet aggregation in vivo and in vitro.[5,6] Concomitant use of coleus with anticoagulant/antiplatelet agents, including nonsteroidal antiinflammatory drugs (NSAIDs), may increase the risk of bleeding. However, clinical reports of such drug interactions are lacking.

BLOOD GLUCOSE: Colenol, a compound isolated from coleus, has been shown to stimulate insulin release in rats.[7] Its use with hypoglycemic agents or exogenous insulin may result in additive effects.

BLOOD PRESSURE: Forskolin has been shown to lower blood pressure through vasodilatory effects.[8] The positive inotropic activity of forskolin has been shown on the isolated guinea pig heart, on the isolated left atrium of the guinea pig heart, and on the dog and cat heart.[9]

BRONCHODILATORS: Forskolin has been studied for its effects in asthma. Theoretically, its use with bronchodilators or other asthma agents may result in additive effects. One in vitro study, however, showed that forskolin causes an apparent reversal of tachyphylaxis to the bronchodilator effects of albuterol.[10]

CHOLINERGIC AGENTS: In rodents, forskolin was shown to possess tricyclic antidepressant (TCA)–like activities 150 times more potent than amitriptyline.[11] Interactions with other antidepressants are possible.

ESTROGENIC AGENTS: Forskolin has been reported to stimulate luteinizing hormone (LH) release in animals, an effect that was reversed by administering estrogen.[12] It is likely that estrogenic agents may reverse forskolin-induced LH secretion.

HEART RATE: In animals, forskolin was shown to increase heart rate, an action that was not inhibited by beta blockers.[9]

HISTAMINE: Forskolin caused a dose-dependent inhibition of antigen-induced histamine release from human basophil leukocytes, as well as of histamine release from human lung mast cells.[13] Forskolin's use with other antihistamines may result in additive effects. Forskolin caused a concentration-related inhibition of IgE-mediated release of histamine and peptide leukotriene C_4 (LTC_4) from human basophils and lung mast cells.[14]

INTRAOCULAR PRESSURE: Topical forskolin has been shown to reduce IOP significantly in rabbits, monkeys, and humans through a mechanism distinct from other glaucoma drugs.[15] This action was shown to be a reduction in aqueous inflow, which was not inhibited by the beta-blocking glaucoma drug timolol (Timoptic).[16] Additive effects are thus possible, although clinical reports are lacking.

LUTEINIZING HORMONE: Forskolin has been reported to stimulate LH release in animals.[12]

THYROID HORMONES: Forskolin stimulates thyroid function in animals[17] and in vitro.[18] Levels of thyroid hormones may be affected by forskolin.

Comfrey (Symphytum spp.)

Pharmacokinetics

In animal research, topical application of a crude alcoholic extract of comfrey resulted in very low absorption of pyrrolizidine alkaloids.[1] From 0.1% to 0.4% of the dose was recovered in the urine over the next 24 hours.

Adverse effects

The potential toxicity of comfrey is well documented.[2] Pyrrolizidine alkaloids found in comfrey[3-5] may be hepatotoxic and carcinogenic in both animals and humans.[6] Specifically, they may cause acute liver failure, cirrhosis, pneumonitis, or pulmonary hypertension and have been shown to induce tumors in experimental animals.[7] Pyrrolizidine alkaloids have also been linked to the development of hepatocellular and skin squamous cell carcinomas, as well as liver angiosarcoma. Human exposure to pyrrolizidine alkaloids may occur through consumption of herbal dietary supplements (e.g., comfrey) and contaminated livestock products (e.g., milk). Topical exposure to comfrey may also result in absorption of pyrrolizidine alkaloids.[8]

On the basis of currently available data, the small but significant long-term risk associated with the consumption of comfrey justifies the need to limit its intake. In Australia and the United States, creams containing comfrey are required to include labels warning customers not to use on broken skin.[9] In the United States, oral comfrey products have been removed from the market.[10]

Oral use of comfrey has caused hepatotoxic effects in humans.[6,11-14] Budd-Chiari syndrome (clotting of hepatic vein) has been suggested to be caused by comfrey use.[15] Clinical manifestations of hepatonecrosis include abdominal pain, ascites, hepatomegaly, portal hypertension, and elevated serum transaminase levels.[8,13] Abdominal pain, diarrhea, or abdominal swelling may be seen in subacute toxicity.

Death by liver failure from comfrey ingestion has been reported in humans.[16] Death rates from comfrey toxicity have been estimated at 20% to 50%.[8,13]

Interactions

CYTOCHROME P450 SUBSTRATES: Agents that induce CYP450-3A4 may increase the conversion of compounds in comfrey to toxic metabolites (dehydroalkaloids and pyrroles).[8] It should, therefore, be used cautiously with agents such as phenytoin, phenobarbital, and non-nucleoside reverse-transcriptase inhibitors (NNRTIs).

CYTOKINES AND INFLAMMATORY MARKERS: In clinical trials, topical comfrey has demonstrated antiinflammatory effects.[17-21] Theoretically, it may interact with antiinflammatory agents (e.g., NSAIDs); however, clinical reports of such drug interactions are lacking.

LIVER FUNCTION TESTS: Because of comfrey's documented hepatotoxicity, primarily from toxic pyrrolizidine alkaloids,[2-5,7] liver function tests may be affected. Combined use with other hepatotoxic agents may increase the risk of adverse effects.

ROSEMARY (ROSMARINUS OFFICINALIS): Based on in vitro assay, rosemary and comfrey extracts may induce glutathione.[22] The clinical significance is unclear.

SASSAFRAS (SASSAFRAS ALBIDUM): Based on in vitro assay, sassafras and comfrey extracts may induce glutathione.[22] The clinical significance is unclear.

Cordyceps (Cordyceps sinensis)

Pharmacokinetics

The kinetics of two galactomannans (CI-P and CI-A) isolated from *Cordyceps cicadae* were studied in laboratory animals.[1] CI-P was found to have low affinity for concanavalin A (Con-A) and exhibited potent carbon-clearance activity in mice.

Adverse effects

Minimal side effects, such as dry mouth, nausea, loss of appetite, diarrhea, and drowsiness, have been reported with the use of cordyceps in humans.[2,3]

Interactions

ANTIBIOTICS: Based on clinical research, concomitant administration of cordyceps and aminoglycoside antibiotics may reduce amikacin-induced nephrotoxicity in older people.[4]

ANTICOAGULANTS/ANTIPLATELETS: Cordyceps has been reported to increase bleeding time by inhibiting platelet aggregation in vitro and in laboratory animals[5-7] and may cause similar interactions in humans. However, clinical reports of such drug interactions are lacking.

BLOOD GLUCOSE LEVELS: Based on animal and in vitro studies, cordyceps may have blood sugar–lowering effects.[8-11] Clinical evidence is lacking.

BLOOD LIPIDS: Based on traditional use of cordyceps to treat hyperlipidemia,[2] cordyceps may lower blood lipid levels.

BLOOD PRESSURE: Based on in vitro data,[12] cordyceps may have hypotensive and vasodilatory effects and may have additive effects when used with antihypertensive agents.

CREATININE: Based on clinical reports and laboratory data, the use of cordyceps may alter creatinine levels.[13-15]

HEART RATE: Based on animal research, cordyceps may have significant counteraction against aconitine-induced arrhythmia, by reducing heart rate and contractility of the papillary muscles or atria, and theoretically may interact with antiarrhythmic agents.[16]

KIDNEY FUNCTION TESTS: Based on clinical reports and laboratory data, the use of cordyceps may alter BUN levels.[13-15]

LIVER FUNCTION TESTS: Cordyceps may alter hepatic enzymes, based on in vitro studies and clinical data.[9,17,18] In clinical research, cordyceps decreased ALT enzyme levels.[18]

MONOAMINERGIC AGENTS: Based on in vitro data, cultured cordyceps mycelium extracts may exhibit a significant inhibition of MAO type B.[19,20]

STEROIDS: Animal studies suggest that cordyceps may induce sex steroid–like effects, act on the hypothalamic-pituitary-adrenocortical axis, and interfere with hormone therapies.[21-23]

WHITE BLOOD CELL COUNTS: Based on animal and in vitro data, cordyceps may stimulate the proliferation and activity of phagocytic lymphocytes and decrease autoimmunity.[24-28] Tests for immune parameters may be altered.

Cornflower (Centaurea cyanus)

Pharmacokinetics: Insufficient available evidence.

Adverse effects

Safety data for cornflower are limited. It should be avoided in patients with known allergy or hypersensitivity to cornflower *(Centaurea cyanus)*, its constituents, or members of the Asteraceae (Compositae) family, such as dandelion, goldenrod, ragweed, sunflower, and daisies.[1]

Interactions

CYTOKINES AND INFLAMMATORY MARKERS: Based on animal studies, cornflower flowers may have antiinflammatory properties and may interact with similarly acting agents.[2]

Cowhage (Mucuna pruriens)

Pharmacokinetics

The pharmacokinetics of cowhage is not well understood. However, two does of *Mucuna* (15 g and 30 g) were compared with the standard Parkinson's disease treatment levodopa/carbidopa.[1] The 30-g *Mucuna* preparation led to a considerably faster onset of effect than levodopa/carbidopa (34.6 vs. 68.5 minutes).

Adverse effects

Few adverse effects have been reported. In humans, cowhage has caused mild, mainly gastrointestinal adverse effects.[2] In one clinical case report, cowhage also caused acute toxic psychosis, possibly from its levodopa content.[3] Presumably, in therapeutic doses, adverse effects are similar to those of commercially available agents that contain levodopa.

Interactions

BLOOD GLUCOSE: Cowhage has the potential to lower blood sugar levels[4] and should be used cautiously in patients with diabetes or those taking hypoglycemic agents.

DOPAMINERGIC AGENTS: Because it contains levodopa, cowhage may interact with dopamine agonists/antagonists. Based on clinical research in Parkinson's patients,[1] cowhage may increase serum levodopa concentrations. Cowhage may also cause hypotensive effects,[5] which may interact with methyldopa (Aldomet). Patients being treated for Parkinson's disease should speak with their treating clinician before taking prescribed Parkinson's agents and cowhage simultaneously.

Cranberry (Vaccinium macrocarpon)

Pharmacokinetics: Insufficient available evidence.

Adverse effects

Consuming more than 3 L daily of cranberry juice may cause gastrointestinal distress and diarrhea. Consuming more than 1 L daily may increase the risk of kidney stones.[1] Because cranberry juice blends may contain high amounts of sugar (in the form of high-fructose corn syrup), diabetic patients should drink sugar-free or artificially sweetened juice.

Interactions

ACIDITY: Because of its acidity, cranberry may lower the pH of urine[2] and other body fluids. Cranberry juice has been suggested to counteract the the acid-lowering effects of proton pump inhibitors (PPIs).[3]

ANTICOAGULANTS/ANTIPLATELETS: Consumption of cranberry with warfarin (Coumadin) has been associated with increased INR, suggesting a possible interaction.[4,5] In healthy subjects, cranberry was found to alter the pharmacodynamics of warfarin, potentially increasing its effects significantly.[6] Concurrent use is cautioned.

BACTERIAL LEVELS: Because of its common use, cranberry juice may decrease bacterial levels in urinary tract infections.

SALICYLATE: Consuming more than 250 mL of cranberry juice daily may increase serum and urine salicylate levels.[7]

VITAMIN B_{12}: Cranberry juice has been noted to increase the absorption of vitamin B_{12} in patients using PPIs,[3] which are used to reduce gastric acid production.

Curcumin. See Turmeric (Curcuma longa)

Daisy (Bellis perennis)

Pharmacokinetics: Insufficient available evidence.

Adverse effects

Bellis perennis appears to be well tolerated when used at extremely minute homeopathic doses.[1]

Interactions

ANTICOAGULANTS/ANTIPLATELETS: Based on historical and homeopathic use, *Bellis perennis* may reduce blood loss.[1] Theoretically, daisy may antagonize the effects of anticoagulants/antiplatelets; however, clinical evidence is lacking.

IRON: Based on in vitro research, daisy may be hemolytic[2,3] and may interact with iron supplementation.

Damiana (Turnera diffusa)

Pharmacokinetics: Insufficient available evidence.

Adverse effects

Adverse effects reported with damiana include diarrhea, headaches, insomnia, and hallucinations.[1]

Interactions

BLOOD GLUCOSE: According to conflicting animal studies, damiana may affect (increase or decrease) blood sugar levels.[2,3]

PROGESTOGENIC AGENTS: Among commonly consumed herbs, damiana showed high relative capacity to compete with estradiol and progesterone binding to intracellular receptors in cultured human breast cancer cells, but it showed minimal estrogenic activity.[4] The clinical significance of this effect is unclear, although it suggests potential interactions with sex hormones.

Dandelion (Taraxacum officinale)

Pharmacokinetics: Insufficient available evidence.

Adverse effects

Historically, dandelion has been generally well tolerated. Dandelion should be avoided in individuals with known allergies to dandelion,[1,2] honey,[3] chamomile, chrysanthemums, yarrow, feverfew, or any members of the Asteraceae (Compositae) plant family (ragweed, sunflower, daisies).[4] The most common type of allergy to dandelion is dermatitis, with itching, rash, and red, swollen or eczematous areas with direct skin contact.[5-8] Sesquiterpene lactones are believed to be responsible for these allergic reactions. A patch test has been developed to assess a person's likelihood for dandelion allergy.[9-11]

Interactions

ACIDITY: Lactones in dandelion may increase gastric acid secretion.[12] Dandelion may reduce the effectiveness of antacids or agents typically used to treat peptic ulcer disease, such as famotidine (Pepcid) or esomeprazole (Nexium).

ANTIBIOTICS: Dandelion has high mineral content, which may interfere with the absorption of quinolone antibiotics. Dandelion has been shown to reduce the effectiveness of ciprofloxacin in animals.[13] Although clinical reports of antibiotic interactions are lacking, concomitant use of dandelion with quinolone antibiotics should be avoided.

ANTICOAGULANTS/ANTIPLATELETS: Dandelion leaf extracts contain coumarins and have been shown to inhibit platelet aggregation in vitro.[14] Theoretically, concomitant use of dandelion with anticoagulant or antiplatelet agents may increase risk of bleeding; however, clinical reports of such drug interactions are lacking.

BLOOD ALCOHOL: Many dandelion tinctures contain high amounts of alcohol and may affect blood alcohol levels. Adverse interactions may occur when taken with disulfiram (Antabuse) or metronidazole (Flagyl).

BLOOD GLUCOSE: Animal studies have produced conflicting data on whether dandelion may lower blood sugar levels, with some studies showing hypoglycemic effects[15,16] and other data showing no changes.[17]

CAROTENOIDS: Dandelion leaves contain various carotenoids (e.g., lutein). Consumption of dandelion may alter serum carotenoid levels; excess amounts may increase the risk of vitamin A toxicity.

CORTICOSTEROIDS: Corticosteroids may deplete the potassium contained in dandelion.

CYTOCHROME P450 SUBSTRATES: Dandelion may inhibit CYP450 1A2 and 2E.[18] Theoretically, concurrent use of dandelion with agents metabolized by 1A2 or 2E may increase levels of these agents.

CYTOKINES AND INFLAMMATORY MARKERS: Based on laboratory research, dandelion flower extract may suppress COX-2 protein expression.[22] Theoretically, dandelion may interact with antiinflammatory agents; however, clinical reports of drug interactions are lacking.

ELECTROLYTES: Dandelion leaves contain high amounts of potassium.[19] Excessive amounts may lead to hyperkalemia.

HISTOLOGICAL TESTS: Based on laboratory research, eugenol may display features of apoptosis[20] and theoretically may interact with antineoplastic agents.

HORMONAL AGENTS: Based on clinical and animal studies, dandelion may upregulate estrogen receptors (alpha and beta), progesterone receptors, and follicle-stimulating hormone (FSH) receptor expression, but decrease dehydroepiandrosterone (DHEA), DHEA sulfate, androstenedione, and estrone sulfate levels.[20,21] Test results may be altered, and interactions with hormonal agents are possible.

LITHIUM: In theory, dandelion may increase the effects and toxicity of lithium because of sodium depletion.

ORAL AGENTS: Theoretically, the nondigestible oligosaccharides (fiber) in dandelion may impair the absorption of oral agents. However, clinical reports of drug interactions are lacking.

URINE TESTS: According to traditional use, dandelion has an alkalinizing effect on urine. Substance abusers have historically used dandelion to mask illicit substances in urine drug screens. However, reliable research in this area is currently lacking.

Danshen (Salvia miltiorrhiza)

Pharmacokinetics

The pharmacokinetics of danshen is not well understood. After oral administration the extent of lithospermic acid recovered from the entire gastrointestinal tract at 24 hours ranged from 23.3% to 41.2%. Danshen appears to be partially renally excreted.[1]

Adverse effects

Danshen generally seems to be well tolerated. Reports of adverse effects of danshen are rare, with the most common being increased bleeding when used with anticoagulants or agents that inhibit platelet aggregation and adhesion.[2-4] Danshen may also cause stomach discomfort and reduced appetite.[5]

Interactions

ALCOHOL: In animal studies, danshen and miltirone (constituent of danshen) reduced alcohol intake and reduced alcohol blood levels.[6-8]

ANTICOAGULANTS/ANTIPLATELETS: In animals, prothrombin time (PT) and steady-state plasma concentration of warfarin increased when used concomitantly with danshen.[9] In case reports, overanticoagulation from danshen use[3] and prolonged PT/INR[4] were reported. Caution is warranted when using danshen with blood thinners.

ASTRAGALUS: In humans a combination of danshen and Astragalus membranaceus improved liver fibrosis indices and portal hypertension.[10] Based on clinical research, a combination of danshen and astragalus root may improve vision and visual fields in glaucoma patients.[11]

BENZODIAZEPINES: Danshen has been shown to bind benzodiazepine receptors in vitro.[12] Theoretically, danshen may interact with benzodiazepines.

BLOOD LIPIDS: In humans, danshen in combination with a lipid-lowering medication (unspecified) decreased total, very-low-density lipoprotein (VLDL) and LDL cholesterol and triglycerides and increased HDL cholesterol.[13,14] The effects of danshen alone are not clear.

BLOOD PRESSURE: In animals, danshen has been shown to produce dose-dependent hypotension.[15]

CAPTOPRIL: In animals the dose-dependent hypotension of danshen was potentiated by administration of captopril, an angiotensin-coverting enzyme (ACE) inhibitor.[15]

CREATINE KINASE: In humans, danshen use during anesthesia decreased plasma creatine kinase (CK) in children undergoing cardiopulmonary bypass for congenital heart defects.[16] Tests for CK levels may be altered.

CYTOCHROME P450 SUBSTRATES: In animal studies, the ethyl acetate extract of danshen induced CYP activity.[17] Caution is warranted when using danshen with CYP450-metabolized agents.

CYTOKINES AND INFLAMMATORY MARKERS: In animals, danshen has been shown to inhibit interleukin-12 (IL-12) and interferon-γ gene expression and production.[18] In children with primary nephritic syndrome, combined use of steroidal agents and danshen decreased levels of serum endothelin and soluble interleukin-2 receptor (sIL-2R) to a greater extent than steroidal agents alone.[19] Cytokine assays may be affected.

HEART RATE: Danshen may have positive inotropic effects.[20] Theoretically, danshen may thus affect heart rate.

INTRAOCULAR PRESSURE: In humans, danshen reduced IOP in glaucoma patients; this effect was potentiated by astragalus.[11] Diagnostic test results may be affected.

LIGUSTICUM CHUANXIONG: Based on clinical research, a combination of danshen and Ligusticum chuanxiong rhizome may improve vision and visual fields in glaucoma patients.[11]

LIGUSTRUM LUCIDUM: Based on clinical research, a combination of danshen and Ligustrum lucidum fruit may improve vision and visual fields in glaucoma patients.[11]

LIVER FUNCTION TESTS: In clinical research, danshen reduced levels of ALT and AST.[21] In humans, danshen is associated with normalization of transaminases.[22,23]

POLYPORUS UMBELLATUS: Based on clinical research, danshen and Polyporus umbellatus may normalize ALT levels in patients with hepatitis B.[22]

SERISSA: In a case study, use of danshen with serissa caused complex neurological manifestations, primarily convulsions, mental changes, and dystonia syndromes.[24]

SOPHORA SUBPROSTRATA: In a case report, use of danshen with Sophora subprostrata root caused complex neurological manifestations, primarily convulsions, mental changes, and dystonia syndromes.[24]

STEROIDS: In children with primary nephritic syndrome, combined use of steroidal agents and danshen decreased levels of serum endothelin and sIL-2R to a greater extent than steroidal agents alone.[19]

WHITE BLOOD CELL COUNTS: In clinical research, danshen was associated with enhanced cell-mediated immunity.[25] WBC counts may be altered.

YUN ZHI: In humans, a combination of yun zhi and danshen offered immunological benefit in terms of enhanced cell-mediated immunity.[25]

Deglycyrrhizinated Licorice (DGL). See Licorice *(Glycyrrhiza glabra)*

Devil's Claw *(Harpagophytum procumbens)*

Pharmacokinetics

Harpagoside is stable in artificial gastric juices for about 3 hours and in intestinal juices for 6 hours.[1-4] Nonetheless, gastric digestion may decrease the potency of devil's claw, and enteric-coated preparations may maintain efficacy despite exposure to gastric acids. Harpagoside elimination half-life has been reported as 5.6 hours.[5]

Adverse effects

Devil's claw is generally well tolerated for up to 12 weeks. Studies evaluating the long-term effects are currently lacking. Adverse effects reported in clinical trials include mild gastrointestinal upset, hypotension, diarrhea, loss of taste, anorexia, headache, and tinnitus.[6,7]

Interactions

ACIDITY: Anecdotal reports note that devil's claw may increase stomach pH and therefore may interact with antacids, sucralfate, H_2 antagonists, or proton pump inhibitors.

ANTICOAGULANTS/ANTIPLATELETS: The combination of devil's claw and warfarin (Coumadin) has been associated with purpura in a case report.[8] Devil's claw should be avoided with anticoagulant agents because of increased risk of bleeding.

BLOOD GLUCOSE: In anecdotal reports, devil's claw has been associated with hypoglycemia.[9] Therefore, use with other oral hypoglycemic agents may result in additive effects. Caution is advised.

CYTOKINES AND INFLAMMATORY MARKERS: Devil's claw appears to have antiinflammatory effects and theoretically may interact with similar agents.[9]

HEART RATE: Devil's claw has been shown to decrease heart rate in rats;[10] thus, use with other agents that have similar properties may theoretically result in additive effects. In rabbits, devil's claw (harpagoside constituent) caused mild positive inotropic effects in lower doses and marked negative inotropic effects in higher doses. The harpagoside component resulted only in negative inotropy[10] and therefore may diminish or potentiate the effects of other inotropic agents.

URIC ACID LEVELS: Anecdotal reports have indicated that devil's claw may reduce high uric acid concentrations. Diagnostic tests may be affected.

Devil's Club *(Oplopanax horridus)*

Pharmacokinetics: Insufficient available evidence.

Adverse effects

Chronic ingestion of a devil's club infusion may cause too much weight gain. Diarrhea has been reported in humans taking an aqueous extract of devil's club inner root bark. The spines on the stems and leaves are known to cause a topical allergic reaction.[1]

Interactions

BACTERIAL LEVELS: Purified polyenes, especially falcarinol, falcarindiol, and oplopandiol, from finely ground inner root bark displayed antibiotic activity against gram-negative bacteria, gram-positive bacteria, *Mycobacterium tuberculosis*, and isoniazid-resistant *Mycobacterium avium* in vitro.[2]

BLOOD GLUCOSE: Devil's club had hypoglycemic effects in rabbits fed a diet of greens; this disappeared when the diet was changed to oats and bran.[3] Two cases were reported of altered blood glucose in individuals who took devil's club.[4]

HISTOLOGICAL TESTS: In rats, devil's club extracts inhibited large-bowel neoplasia induced by the carcinogen azoxymethane.[5] In vitro an ethanolic extract of *Oplopanax horridus* has displayed antiproliferative effects and antioxidant activity on several cancer cell lines.[6] Histological results may be altered by devil's club.

Dong Quai *(Angelica sinensis)*

Pharmacokinetics: Insufficient available evidence.

Adverse effects

Although dong quai is accepted as being a safe food additive in the United States and Europe, its safety in medicinal doses is unclear.[1] Reliable long-term studies evaluating its safety are currently lacking.

Interactions

ANTICOAGULANTS/ANTIPLATELETS: Because of anticoagulant and antiplatelet effects,[2] components of dong quai may increase the risk of bleeding when taken with agents believed to increase risk of bleeding. However, clinical reports of such drug interactions are lacking. In a recent cross-sectional, point-of-care survey of 1818 patients, one case was identified as a potentially clinically significant interaction between dong quai and anticoagulant/antiplatelet agents.[3]

ESTROGENIC AGENTS: Dong quai contains phytoestrogens; however, it remains unclear whether it has estrogen-like activity, blocks the activity of estrogens, or has no significant hormonal effects.[4] It is unclear if taking dong quai increases or decreases the effects of oral contraceptives (OCs), hormone replacement therapy (HRT; e.g., Premarin), or selective estrogen receptor modulators (SERMs; e.g., tamoxifen).

HEART RATE: Based on in vitro data, dong quai may increase the effects of agents that affect heart rhythm (e.g., digoxin, beta blockers, calcium channel blockers) or antiarrhythmic agents.[4]

PHOTOSENSITIZING AGENTS: Chemicals in dong quai may cause increased sun sensitivity with a risk of severe skin reactions (photosensitivity).[4] Thus, dong quai should be avoided with other agents that cause photosensitivity, such as tretinoin (Retin-A, Renova) and some types of antidepressants, cancer agents, antibiotics, and antipsychotic agents.

Echinacea *(Echinacea spp.)*

Pharmacokinetics

The pharmacokinetics of echinacea is not well understood. Echinacea may inhibit intestinal cytochrome P450-3A4, but induces hepatic 3A4.[1-3]

Adverse effects

Echinacea has been well tolerated in clinical practice and in trials, with few adverse events reported.[4-6] Gastrointestinal upset and rashes occur most frequently. In rare cases, echinacea has been associated with possibly severe allergic reactions.[4] In children, three studies of 257 subjects (infants to 14-year-olds with whooping cough) found no adverse effects with 1 to 2 mL of squeezed aqueous extract (0.1 g/2 mL) given intramuscularly twice daily for 3 to 21 days.[7-12]

Interactions

ALCOHOL: Echinacea tinctures often contain high alcohol content (15%-90%) and may affect blood alcohol levels. Adverse interactions may occur when taken with disulfiram (Antabuse) or metronidazole (Flagyl).

AMOXICILLIN: In an obscure case study, a 19-year-old patient ingesting amoxicillin and an unclear echinacea preparation developed rhabdomyolysis, shock, and death. Further details were not provided.[13]

ANESTHETICS: Potential interactions may occur between echinacea and anesthetics.[14] However, clear evidence is lacking.

ANTIBODY LEVELS: *Echinacea purpurea* significantly reduced secretory immunoglobulin A (sIgA) and the secretion rate of sIgA at the beginning of a mucosal immunity test in humans. Echinacea did not significantly decrease sIgA or secretion rate of sIgA after intervention.[15]

CAFFEINE: Echinacea may reduce the oral clearance of caffeine, likely caused by the inhibition of CYP450-1A2 by echinacea.[16]

CYCLOPHOSPHAMIDE: Animal and laboratory studies have identified hydrophilic compounds in *Echinacea purpurea*, *E. simulata*, and *E. paradoxa*.[17,18] Based on animal research, a hydrophilic polysaccharide complex isolated from echinacea increased the antitumor and antimetastatic activity of cyclophosphamide.[18]

CYTOCHROME P450 SUBSTRATES: The effects of echinacea on CYP activity appear to be minor. However, further research into the interaction potential is merited.[19] In laboratory research and systematic reviews, echinacea has both mildly inhibited[2] and induced CYP3A4 activity.[1] Echinacea reduced the oral clearance of substrates of CYP1A2 but not the oral clearance of substrates of 2C9 and 2D6. Echinacea selectively modulated the catalytic activity of CYP3A at hepatic and intestinal sites.[16]

ECONAZOLE NITRATE (SPECTAZOLE): Preliminary evidence suggests that the use of echinacea with topical econazole may decrease the recurrence rate of vaginal *Candida* infections.[20]

HISTOLOGICAL TESTS: Echinacea may have additive effects when taken in combination with antineoplastics because constituents of the root oil of *Echinacea angustifolia* and *E. pallida* have been shown to possess antitumor activity in vivo.[21]

KAVA: Multiple reports detail hepatotoxicity associated with kava, most often with heavy or chronic use. Caution should be exercised with concomitant use of echinacea, which some natural medicine practitioners have warned may cause liver toxicity as well. However, no clear evidence from basic science or human reports indicates that echinacea causes significant liver toxicity. This potential interaction remains theoretical.

LIVER FUNCTION TESTS: Natural medicine practitioners often caution that echinacea may cause hepatotoxicity and recommend avoiding concomitant use with other potentially hepatotoxic agents (e.g., anabolic steroids, amiodarone, methotrexate, ketoconazole). However, there is no clear evidence from basic science or clinical reports that echinacea causes significant liver toxicity. Some have noted that echinacea lacks the 1,2 unsaturated necrine ring system that causes hepatotoxicity of pyrrolizidine alkaloids.[22]

VITAMIN B: Echinacea itself has not been found to interact with vitamin B, but many echinacea preparations are combined with goldenseal (*Hydrastis canadensis*), a purported antibacterial agent that may decrease intestinal microflora and vitamin B absorption. These preparations may have low levels of echinacea and may not be efficacious against viral-induced upper respiratory tract infections.

WHITE BLOOD CELL COUNTS: Echinacea may affect lymphocyte subpopulations, specifically, the number of CD8+ T lymphocytes and natural killer cells.[23]

Elder *(Sambucus nigra)*

Pharmacokinetics

Anthocyanins, which are potent flavonoid antioxidants found in elder, are not absorbed in their unchanged glycosylated forms in humans.[1] The maximum concentration of anthocyanins found in blood after injection of a highly concentrated solution was 35 mg/mL at 1 hour, followed by a quick decay.[2] The elimination of plasma anthocyanins appears to follow first-order kinetics, and most anthocyanin compounds are excreted in urine within 4 hours of ingestion.[1] After ingestion of about 30 mL of elderberry extract (147.3 mg total anthocyanins), half-life was 1.74 hours.[3] The urinary excretion rate of intact anthocyanins was rapid and appeared to be monoexponential with high variability. Flowers are believed to be safe for use in food, provided HCN levels are below 25 ppm.

Adverse effects

There are reports of gastrointestinal distress, diarrhea, vomiting, abdominal cramps, and weakness after drinking elderberry juice made from crushed leaves, stems, and uncooked elderberries.[4-6] Elder may also possess laxative effects. Cyanide toxicity is possible with elder.[4,5] The berries must be cooked to prevent nausea or cyanide toxicity.

Interactions

BLOOD GLUCOSE: Based on in vitro data, elder may lower blood sugar levels.[7] Caution is advised when using other agents that may lower blood sugar levels.

BLOOD LIPIDS: Elder has been shown to lower postprandial serum lipids in healthy human subjects.[8]

CAFFEINE: The flavonoid quercetin, which is found in elder, has been reported to inhibit xanthine oxidase[9] and may affect the levels of caffeine and other methylxanthines, such as theophylline.

HISTOLOGICAL TESTS: In vitro data suggest that elder may increase the antineoplastic effects[10,11] of some cancer chemotherapies.

English Ivy *(Hedera helix)*

Pharmacokinetics: Insufficient available evidence.

Adverse effects

The most frequently reported adverse effects related to English ivy are allergy symptoms, including contact dermatitis, asthmatic bronchitis, and allergic rhinoconjunctivitis. Gardeners and those with frequent exposure to English ivy may have a high risk of sensitization and should wear appropriate protective clothing.[1]

Interactions

HISTOLOGICAL TESTS: Based on laboratory studies, *Hedera helix* may have antimutagenic properties.[2,3] Theoretically, English ivy may interact with antineoplastic agents.

Ephedra (Ephedra sinica)

Pharmacokinetics

Ephedrine is well absorbed after oral administration, with a reported half-life of 3 to 6 hours. After oral administration, 88% is excreted in the urine within 24 hours and 97% within 48 hours. Ephedrine and pseudoephedrine are excreted more rapidly with urinary acidifiers (e.g., ammonium chloride) and more slowly with urinary alkalinizers (e.g., disodium bicarbonate).[1,2]

According to anecdotal reports, the onset of bronchodilatory effects with oral ephedrine occurs within 15 to 60 minutes and lasts 2 to 4 hours. Oral ephedrine causes pressor and cardiac effects for 4 hours. Intramuscular or subcutaneous administration of ephedrine results in cardiac effects that last 1 hour.[1,2]

The natural and synthetic forms of ephedrine have similar absorption and pharmacokinetics in adults, but the available natural products contain considerably different concentrations of active alkaloids.[3] Pharmacokinetics has not been extensively studied in children.

Adverse effects

The FDA has collected more than 800 reports of serious ephedra toxicity, including more than 22 deaths. Ephedra is not considered safe despite its possible effectiveness for treating certain conditions. Before the official ban of ephedra sales, the FDA issued a policy that ephedrine products be labeled with possible adverse effects, contain no more than 8 mg of ephedrine per serving, and be used for no longer than 7 days.[1,2] When ephedra is used for prolonged periods, even at recommended doses, chronic toxicity may lead to weight loss, difficulty sleeping, high blood pressure, dry mouth, irregular heart rhythm, rapid heartbeat, anxiety, obsessive-compulsive disorder, flare, nervousness, and heart damage.

A review of 140 reports of adverse events between 1997 and 1999 related to ephedra use was submitted to the FDA.[4] A standardized rating system for assessing causation was applied to each adverse event; 31% of cases were considered to be "definitely" or "probably" related to the use of supplements containing ephedra alkaloids, and an additional 31% were deemed to be "possibly" related. Among these adverse events, 47% involved cardiovascular symptoms and 18% involved the central nervous system (CNS). Hypertension was the single most frequent adverse effect (17 reports); others included palpitations, tachycardia, a combination of palpitations and tachycardia,[5] stroke,[6] and seizures.[7] Ten events resulted in death and 13 events produced permanent disability. Both the ephedrine and the pseudoephedrine constituent of ephedra may induce hypertension, chronotropic, and inotropic effects in humans.[8-11]

A 2003 report by the RAND Southern California Evidence-based Practice Center for the Agency for Healthcare Research and Quality, U.S. Department of Health and Human Services[12,13] reviewed available clinical trials, adverse event reports to the FDA, and reports to the manufacturer Metabolife. Although most prospective trials were not sufficiently large and most adverse event reports were not sufficiently detailed, the authors identified three deaths, two myocardial infarctions, two cerebrovascular accidents, one seizure, and three psychiatric cases that were considered to be "sentinel events" (i.e., strongly tied to ephedra use within 24 hours without other plausible explanations). In addition, 50 other possible sentinel events were identified.

A 2003 analysis in *Annals of Internal Medicine* showed that products containing ephedra account for 64% of all adverse reactions to herbs in the United States, but only represent 0.82% of herbal product sales.[7,14-18] The relative risk for an adverse reaction was extremely high in a person using ephedra compared with other herbs, ranging from 100 (95% CI, 83-140) for kava to 720 (95% CI, 520-1100) for *Ginkgo biloba*. It was concluded that ephedra use greatly increases risk of adverse reactions compared with other herbs. A 2003 analysis in *Neurology* also demonstrated an increased risk of stroke associated with ephedra-containing products.[6,19]

Interactions

ALCOHOL: A 32-year-old man experienced a brief episode of acute psychosis after consumption of alcohol, caffeine, and Vigueur Fit tablets containing ephedra alkaloids.[20]

ALPHA-ADRENERGIC AGENTS: Ergot alkaloids exert alpha-adrenergic vasoconstrictive effects that may increase hypertensive effects when used in combination with ephedra.[1,2]

ANESTHETICS: In clinical studies, propofol anesthesia enhanced the pressor response to IV ephedrine,[21] and ephedrine accelerated the regression of epidural block.[22]

ANTIADRENERGIC AGENTS (ALPHA BLOCKERS): Sympathomimetic effects of ephedrine (e.g., mydriasis, hypertension) may be antagonized by antiadrenergic agents (e.g., clonidine, reserpine, terazosin).[1,2]

BLOOD GLUCOSE: Ephedra may raise blood glucose levels and reduce the effectiveness of hypoglycemic agents.[23]

BLOOD PRESSURE: Both the ephedrine and the pseudoephedrine constituent of ephedra can induce hypertension.[8-11,24,25]

BRONCHODILATORS: Both ephedrine and pseudoephedrine cause bronchodilation,[8] and use with other bronchodilators or asthma agents may lead to additive effects.

CAFFEINE: Use of ephedra with caffeine, theophylline, or other methylxanthines may result in additive neurological, cardiovascular, and psychiatric adverse effects or toxicity. Fatalities have been associated with simultaneous caffeine and ephedrine use.[26,27] Brief acute psychosis occurred in a man after consumption of alcohol, caffeine, and Vigueur Fit tablets containing ephedra alkaloids.[20] Notably, many commercial products contain both ephedra and caffeine. Theophylline combined with ephedrine may induce insomnia, anxiety, and adverse gastrointestinal effects, including vomiting.[28]

CENTRAL NERVOUS SYSTEM STIMULANTS: Cola, guarana, and mate all have CNS-stimulating effects, and combination with ephedra may increase the risk of cardiovascular, neurological, or psychiatric adverse effects. Fatalities have been associated with simultaneous caffeine and ephedrine use.[26,27] Concomitant use of ephedra and guarana has been associated with a case of cerebral infarction.[29] Both ephedrine and pseudoephedrine cause CNS stimulation,[8,30] and use with other CNS stimulants may lead to additive effects.

CHOLINERGIC AGENTS: Concomitant use of the tricyclic antidepressant (TCA) amitriptyline and ephedrine was reportedly associated with hypotension in a 61-year-old woman undergoing ovarian cancer surgery.[31]

ELECTROLYTES: The ephedra constituents ephedrine and pseudoephedrine possess diuretic properties[1,2] and may add to the effects of other diuretics.

HEART RATE: Both the ephedrine and the pseudoephedrine constituent of ephedra may induce hypertension as well as chronotropic and inotropic effects in humans.[8,9] Heart rate may be affected; concomitant use with cardiac agents should be avoided.

LIVER FUNCTION TESTS: Increases in transaminase levels have been noted anecdotally, although in one study, ALT and AST were found to decrease significantly from baseline in patients using ephedrine and caffeine.[32]

MONOAMINERGIC AGENTS: When ephedra is administered in combination with MAO inhibitors, increased sympathomimetic activity may increase the risk of hypertension. One case report noted a 28-year-old woman who developed encephalopathy, neuromuscular irritability, hypotension, tachycardia, rhabdomyolysis, and hyperthermia after taking a combination tablet containing ephedrine, caffeine, and theophylline (a "Do-Do") 24 hours after discontinuing phenelzine treatment.[33]

PHENOTHIAZINES: Phenothiazines may block the alpha-adrenergic effects of ephedra.[34,35]

PULMONARY FUNCTION TESTS: Because of the bronchodilator effects of ephedra, PFT results may be affected.[1,2]

STEROIDS: Ephedrine has been reported in clinical trials to increase clearance and reduce effectiveness of dexamethasone.[36,37] Caution is warranted when using ephedra with steroid agents.

THYROID HORMONES: Ephedra may increase serum T_3 levels, and combination use with thyroid hormones may result in additive effects. In one study, the serum T_3/T_4 ratio was significantly increased after 4 weeks of treatment with ephedra, although this ratio decreased after 12 weeks.[38]

Essiac Herbal Combination Tea

Pharmacokinetics

In general, pharmacodynamic/kinetic data for Essiac are primarily based on theoretical or empirical knowledge of the individual constituents. The original proprietary formula contained burdock root (*Arctium lappa*), sheep sorrel (*Rumex acetosella*), slippery elm inner bark (*Ulmus fulva*), and Turkish rhubarb (*Rheum palmatum*). The recipe is said to be based on a traditional Ojibwa (Native-American) remedy. Later formulations added other herbs, including blessed thistle (*Cnicus benedictus*), red clover (*Trifolium pratense*), kelp (*Laminaria digitata*), and watercress (*Nasturtium officinale*).[3,4,25]

Adverse effects

In general, safety and efficacy data for Essiac are lacking. Adverse effects and toxicities may be anticipated based on theoretical or empirical knowledge of the tolerability of the individual herbal constituents.

Interactions

Note: Drug interactions with Essiac are primarily based on theoretical or empirical knowledge of the individual herbal constituents. In theory, precipitation of some agents may occur when taken concomitantly with sorrel. Therefore, separate administration is recommended.

CANCER THERAPY: Anecdotally, concomitant use of Essiac with chemotherapy and radiotherapy may render the compound ineffective. However, clinical evidence of this potential interaction is insufficient.

CYTOCHROME P450 SUBSTRATES: Based on a case report, a patient taking the experimental drug DX-8951f (metabolized by CYP3A4 and CYP1A2) experienced toxic side effects and drug clearance that was four to five times slower than in other patients.[17] This patient was also reportedly taking "essiac tea," although further details are not available, and it is not clear if the patient was taking Essiac or generic "essiac" formulations.

Eucalyptus (*Eucalyptus* spp.)

Pharmacokinetics

Eucalyptus appears to be readily absorbed orally. Absorption of eucalyptus is likely enhanced by lipids and milk. Metabolism may require induction of the cytochrome P450 enzyme system. Eucalyptus has been reported to be excreted in urine.[1]

Adverse effects

Significant and potentially lethal toxicity has been consistently reported with internal (oral) use of eucalyptus oil in children and adults. In adults, topical or inhaled use is likely safer than oral use but may also pose a risk of toxicity.[2,3] In children, topical use or inhalation has caused severe toxicity and death and should be avoided. It may be safe for adults to consume small amounts of diluted eucalyptus oil or to use topical or inhaled eucalyptus for brief periods, although caution is warranted. The signs and symptoms of eucalyptus toxicity include epigastric burning, nausea, vomiting, dizziness, muscular weakness, constricted pupils, a feeling of suffocation, cyanosis, delirium, and convulsions. Strains of bacteria found on eucalyptus may cause infection.[4] Eucalyptus may also cause allergic reactions in sensitive people.[5-12]

Interactions

5-FLUOROURACIL: Eucalyptus has been found to enhance permeation of topical 5-FU through rat skin.[13] Using topical 5-FU and eucalyptus concomitantly may potentiate the effects of 5-FU.

AMPHETAMINES: In vivo and in vitro studies have demonstrated reductions in amphetamine levels when used with eucalyptol.[14] Clinical data are lacking.

BLOOD GLUCOSE: Eucalyptus has been shown to lower blood glucose concentrations in diabetic animals.[15] Use with hypoglycemic agents may result in additive effects.

CYTOCHROME P450 SUBSTRATES: Cineole has been found to possess CYP450-inducing activity in animals[16] and in vivo and in vitro. Preliminary evidence suggests that cineole is a substrate of CYP450-3A.[15] Other research has isolated the metabolite of eucalyptol, 2-exo-hydroxy-1,8-cineole, as a substrate of CYP450.[17,18]

MILK: The absorption of eucalyptus may be increased in the presence of milk or dietary fats.[19,20]

PYRROLIZIDINE ALKALOID–CONTAINING HERBS: Based on anecdote, eucalyptus may potentiate the toxicity of plants containing pyrrolizidine alkaloids.[19,20]

SEDATIVES AND CENTRAL NERVOUS SYSTEM DEPRESSANTS: In vivo and in vitro studies have demonstrated reductions in pentobarbital levels when used with eucalyptol, a component of eucalyptus.[14] Clinical evidence is lacking; however, interactions are possible.

Eugenol. See Clove (*Syzygium aromaticum*, syn. *Eugenia aromaticum*)

Euphorbia (*Euphorbia* spp.)

Pharmacokinetics: Insufficient available evidence.

Adverse effects

The sap or latex from *Euphorbia* can cause contact dermatitis and injury to the eye, therefore, *Euphorbia* should be handled cautiously with gloves and eye protection.[1-11] Orally, *Euphorbia* may cause nausea and vomiting.

Reports describe *Euphorbia* as a contributor to enhancing African Burkitt's lymphoma and Epstein-Barr virus (EBV). One study suggested that both diseases can be enhanced by *Euphorbia tirucalli*.[12] Another study reported reduction in EBV-specific cellular immunity.[13] A third study reported that *Euphorbia lathyris* or *E. tirucalli* might affect induction of EBV,[14] whereas a fourth study reported that *E. tirucalli* may activate the EBV lytic cycle.[15]

Interactions

ANTICONVULSANT AGENTS: Theoretically, *Euphorbia* may interact with other anticonvulsant agents, although there is no mention of any interactions or mechanism in the available literature.

BLOOD GLUCOSE: Based on in vitro research, *Euphorbia balsamifera* may lower blood sugar levels.[16] Caution is warranted in patients using blood sugar–lowering agents because of an increased risk of hypoglycemia.

CASTOR OIL: Based on research conducted in animals, the aqueous leaf extract of *Euphorbia hirta* may decrease the effect of castor oil–induced diarrhea.[17]

HORMONAL AGENTS: Theoretically, *Euphorbia tirucalli* may decrease prostaglandin E_2 levels in patients with elevated levels caused by tumors, and it may interact with hormone-regulating agents.[18]

VIRAL LEVELS: *Euphorbia* may enhance African Burkitt's lymphoma and EBV.[12-15] Caution is warranted in patients using immunomodulating agents.

Evening Primrose Oil *(Oenothera biennis)*

Pharmacokinetics

After administration of evening primrose oil (EPO), t_{max} of linoleic acid is approximately 3 to 5 hours.[1] Metabolic effects may occur within hours of ingestion and may persist for months. Gamma-linolenic acid (GLA), the active constituent of evening primrose oil, is metabolized to di-homo-GLA, which may be broken down further to arachidonic acid by delta-5 desaturase in small amounts.[2,3] DGLA is cyclooxygenated into prostaglandin E_1 and thromboxane A_1. It is also metabolized into 15-hydroxy-DGLA by 15-lipoxygenase.[2,4,5]

Adverse effects

Evening primrose oil has been well tolerated when taken in doses up to 3 g daily for as long as 1 year.[6] Review of animal research and clinical studies, involving approximately 500,000 users of EPO in the United Kingdom, did not reveal significant toxicity.[7] Several case reports described seizures associated with EPO use in patients with or without known seizure disorders.[8,9]

Interactions

AGENTS THAT LOWER SEIZURE THRESHOLD: Because of several case reports of seizures associated with EPO use in patients with/without known seizure disorders,[8,9] patients taking antiepileptic drugs or agents that may lower the seizure threshold should avoid EPO use.

ANTICOAGULANTS/ANTIPLATELETS: In a recent cross-sectional, point-of-care survey of 1818 patients, two cases were identified as potentially clinically significant interactions between EPO and anticoagulant/antiplatelet agents.[10]

BLOOD PRESSURE: In several rat studies, GLA has been found to decrease central venous blood pressure,[11-16] although preliminary clinical evidence is equivocal.[17,18]

Eyebright *(Euphrasia officinalis)*

Pharmacokinetics

The pharmacokinetics of eyebright is not well understood. Aucubin, a constituent of eyebright, has shown linear pharmacokinetic behavior when administered intravenously to rats. The half-life of aucubin has been reported to be 42.5 minutes.[1]

Adverse effects

Reported side effects with topical and oral use of eyebright include mental confusion, headache, conjunctivitis, increased eye pressure with lacrimation, itching, pruritus, redness and swelling of the eye, vision changes, dim vision, photophobia, weakness, toothache, sneezing, yawning, insomnia, and diaphoresis.[2,3]

Interactions

BLOOD GLUCOSE: Theoretically, eyebright may interact with agents that alter blood glucose levels. In animals, eyebright was found to reduce glucose levels in chemically induced diabetic rats.[4]

CYTOCHROME P450 SUBSTRATES: Theoretically, eyebright may interact with agents that are metabolized by CYP450. In research on rat livers, eyebright demonstrated inhibition of CYP450 by the aglycon of aucubin.[5] However, this effect has not been evaluated in humans.

False Hellebore *(Veratrum spp.)*

Pharmacokinetics: Insufficient available evidence.

Adverse effects

Toxicologists consider the false (American) hellebore plant to be poisonous because of its cardiotoxic effects.[1,2] False hellebore or its alkaloidal constituents may cause adverse effects to the heart.[3,4]

Based on clinical data, false hellebore and its isolated constituents may cause arrhythmias, bradycardia, and hypotension.[1,5-12] Severe poisoning has been reported after ingestion of all parts of the false hellebore plant.[1,9-13]

Interactions

BLOOD PRESSURE: The isolated constituent of false hellebore, O-acetyljervine, has been reported to have beta-agonist activity in vitro.[14] Hypotensive effects have been observed in case reports.[3,4]

CREATININE: False hellebore or its alkaloidal constituents may alter creatinine levels.[3]

KIDNEY FUNCTION TESTS: False hellebore or its alkaloidal constituents may decrease GFR and alter renal function and BUN levels.[3]

Fennel *(Foeniculum vulgare)*

Pharmacokinetics: Insufficient available evidence.

Adverse effects

Fennel is generally well tolerated. Side effect information in infants is currently lacking.

Interactions

CIPROFLOXACIN (CIPRO): Concurrent use of fennel and ciprofloxacin may lead to decreased bioavailability of ciprofloxacin. Fennel contains high amounts of minerals, and formation of a ciprofloxacin-cation complex results. This formation reduces ciprofloxacin absorption, as shown in rodents;[1] however, clinical evidence of this interaction is lacking.

Fenugreek (Trigonella foenum-graecum)

Pharmacokinetics: Insufficient available evidence.

Adverse effects

Fenugreek has traditionally been considered safe and well tolerated. The most frequently reported adverse effects in clinical trials include diarrhea and flatulence.[1-4]

Interactions

ANALGESIC AGENTS: Based on animal data, fenugreek extract may have analgesic effect comparable to NSAIDs.[5,6] Interactions with other analgesic agents are possible, although clinical evidence is lacking.

ANTICOAGULANTS/ANTIPLATELETS: Fenugreek preparations may contain coumarin derivatives that can increase prothrombin time (PT) or international normalized ratio (INR) and risk of bleeding.[6-10] In animals, a fenugreek extract inhibited platelet aggregation.[7] Although clinical evidence of this interaction is insufficient, concomitant use of fenugreek and anticoagulant/antiplatelet agents is not advised.

BLOOD GLUCOSE: Fenugreek has demonstrated hypoglycemic effects in numerous in vitro, in vivo, and clinical studies.[3,11-24] Glucose levels should be monitored closely when using fenugreek.

BLOOD LIPIDS: Based on human, animal, and in vitro studies, fenugreek may lower triglycerides, total cholesterol, and LDL levels.[25-33]

CARBOHYDRATES: Review of the literature reveals no reported serious reactions in humans, although fenugreek may affect key enzymes of carbohydrate metabolism.[34] The effects of domestic processing and cooking methods on total HCL extractable iron from fenugreek leaves have been studied in vitro.[35]

CORTICOSTEROIDS: Fenugreek may reduce corticosteroid effectiveness.[36]

ESTROGENIC AGENTS: Fenugreek contains diosgenin, a phytoestrogen compound.[37] Theoretically, fenugreek may interact with estrogen or estrogen-like compounds; however, clinical evidence is lacking.

ETHANOL: Based on in vitro research, fenugreek seeds may protect the liver from alcohol-induced damage.[38]

HISTOLOGICAL TESTS: Based on rat and in vitro studies, fenugreek seeds may inhibit carcinogenesis by inducing apoptosis and inhibiting cell growth.[39-42] Fenugreek may be useful as an adjunct to standard antineoplastic agents.

MONOAMINERGIC AGENTS: Theoretically, fenugreek may potentiate the activity of MAO inhibitors.

ORAL AGENTS: Products rich in fenugreek fiber may alter the absorption of oral agents as a result of its mucilaginous fiber content and high viscosity in the gut. Agents should be taken 2 hours before or 2 hours after taking fenugreek.

POTASSIUM: A fenugreek aqueous extract was found to reduce potassium levels[19] and may antagonize potassium-containing agents.

THYROID HORMONES: Decreased serum T_3 and T_3/T_4 ratio and increased T_4 levels have been observed in mice and rats given fenugreek.[43] Theoretically, fenugreek may interact with thyroid agents.

URINE TESTS: Because Fenugreek causes the excretion of sotolone, the compound responsible for the aroma in maple syrup urine disease (MSUD), false diagnoses of MSUD have been published in case reports.[44,45] Fenugreek has also been implicated in the production of a body odor similar to that of MSUD in an infant.[46]

Feverfew (Tanacetum parthenium)

Pharmacokinetics

In a human colonic cell line parthenolide, the active constituent in feverfew, was shown to be absorbed via a passive diffusion mechanism.[1]

Adverse effects

Feverfew appears to be generally well tolerated. Mild and transient side effects, including indigestion, nausea, flatulence, constipation, diarrhea, abdominal bloating, and heartburn, have been reported.[2,3] Feverfew may elicit allergic responses in patients who are sensitive to chrysanthemums, daisies, or marigolds. There is potential cross-reactivity with other members of the Compositae family, including ragweed.[4]

Interactions

ANTICOAGULANTS/ANTIPLATELETS: Feverfew has been shown to inhibit platelet secretory and aggregatory activity[5-11] and may theoretically increase the risk of bleeding if used concomitantly with anticoagulant/antiplatelet agents. It is unclear if this potential interaction is clinically significant. In a recent cross-sectional, point-of-care survey of 1818 patients, two cases were identified as potentially clinically significant interactions between feverfew and anticoagulant/antiplatelet agents.[12]

CYTOKINES AND INFLAMMATORY MARKERS: Feverfew has been demonstrated to inhibit prostaglandins,[13-14] but not cyclooxygenase. Theoretically, feverfew may interact with antiinflammatory agents, although this potential interaction has not been well documented.

PHOTOSENSITIZING AGENTS: Feverfew may increase the risk of photosensitivity. Caution is advised with concomitant use of other photosensitizing agents.

Fig (Ficus carica)

Pharmacokinetics: Insufficient available evidence.

Adverse effects

There are few reports of adverse effects associated with fig.[1] Fig leaf tanning lotions have been associated with sunburn, hemolytic anemia, and retinal hemorrhage.[2]

Interactions

ANTICOAGULANTS/ANTIPLATELETS: Fig leaf contains furocoumarins and may increase the risk of bleeding when taken with anticoagulants/antiplatelets. In one case report, hemolytic anemia and retinal hemorrhage presented as systemic complications from the furocoumarins present in the fig leaf decoction.[2] However, clinical reports of such drug interactions are lacking.

BLOOD GLUCOSE: Fig leaf may lower blood glucose, according to anecdotal reports.

PHOTOSENSITIZING AGENTS: Fig leaf tanning lotions have been associated with multiple cases of sunburn, likely caused by the furocoumarin content.[2] Interactions with other photosensitizing agents (e.g., statins) are possible.

Flax (Linum usitatissimum)

Pharmacokinetics

The pharmacokinetics of flaxseed is not well understood. Flaxseed lignan metabolites appear to be excreted in the urine.[1-4]

Adverse effects

Flaxseed and flaxseed oil appear to be well tolerated. Although limited clinical safety data exist, there is long-standing historical use with few reports of adverse events in the available literature. Rarely, flaxseed (not flaxseed oil) may cause diarrhea, nausea, vomiting, abdominal pain, and gastrointestinal distress.[5-9] Based on available research, consumption of flaxseed (not flaxseed oil) may increase episodes of mania and hypomania in bipolar patients.[5]

Interactions

ALKALINE PHOSPHATASE: The use of flaxseed (not flaxseed oil) may decrease ALP levels.[10]

ANTICOAGULANTS/ANTIPLATELETS: Based on trial evidence of decreased platelet aggregation[11,12] and increased bleeding time,[13] flaxseed (not flaxseed oil) may increase risk of bleeding when taken with anticoagulants or antiplatelets. However, clinical cases have not been reported in the available literature.

BLOOD GLUCOSE: The omega-3 fatty acids in flaxseed and flaxseed oil may cause hyperglycemia. In one clinical study, six men with type 2 diabetes experienced increases in fasting glucose levels after 1 month of treatment with omega-3 fatty acids.[14]

BLOOD LIPIDS: Flaxseed and flaxseed oil have been demonstrated to possess lipid-lowering properties in vitro and in animals.[15-17] Multiple preliminary clinical studies have administered flaxseed products and measured effects on lipids, with mixed results.[18-33] Reportedly, defatted flaxseed (equivalent to the fiber component of flaxseed) can significantly reduce levels of total and LDL cholesterol.[20]

BLOOD PRESSURE: Because flaxseed contains alpha-linolenic acid (ALA), it has been proposed that flaxseed may lower blood pressure. In theory, flaxseed may potentiate the effects of antihypertensive agents. Preliminary evidence suggests that higher levels of linolenic acid in human adipose tissue may correlate with lower blood pressure.[34] Flaxseed-supplemented diets have had mixed effects on blood pressure in rats.[34,35] Limited clinical evidence suggests that 2 weeks of flaxseed supplementation may lower blood pressure.[18]

ESTROGENIC AGENTS: Flaxseed (not flaxseed oil) is a rich source of plant lignans.[36,37] Lignans are often referred to as phytoestrogens and may possess estrogen receptor agonist or antagonist properties,[38] with unclear interactions with OCs or HRT.

FLAXSEED-CONTAINING FOODS: Processing and cooking may alter the lipid content and stability of ALA in pasta containing ground flaxseed.[39]

HEMATOCRIT: Based on animal research, flaxseed (not flaxseed oil) may increase total red blood cell (RBC) counts and hemoglobin levels.[10] Hematocrit may be affected.

LUTEINIZING HORMONE: In theory, the use of flaxseed (not flaxseed oil) may increase serum LH levels.[40]

ORAL AGENTS: Consumption of flaxseed (not flaxseed oil) may decrease the absorption of coadministered oral agents, vitamins, or minerals. Oral agents should be taken 1 hour before or 2 hours after flaxseed to prevent decreased absorption.

TESTOSTERONE: In theory, the use of flaxseed (not flaxseed oil) may alter serum levels of testosterone.[40]

VITAMIN E: Consumption of flaxseed (not flaxseed oil) may result in increased vitamin E levels in the liver.[10]

Garcinia (Garcinia cambogia)

Pharmacokinetics: Insufficient available evidence.

Adverse effects

Garcinia has been well tolerated for up to 12 weeks in available human trials. Daily doses up to 4.7 g of hydroxycitric acid (HCA) have been reported as safe with no treatment-related adverse effects.[1] In one case report, a patient experienced rhabdomyolysis in response to a weight loss medicine containing ma huang (ephedrine), guarana (active alkaloid caffeine), chitosan, *Gymnena sylvestre*, *Garcinia cambogia* (50% HCA), and chromium.[2] The contribution of garcinia to this adverse effect is unclear.

Interactions

CREATINE KINASE: Rhabdomyolysis was reported after ingestion of a garcinia-containing weight loss herbal medicine in an otherwise healthy 54-year-old woman.[2] The patient had chest pain, and laboratory investigation showed rhabdomyolysis with peak serum CK of 1028 IU/L, which gradually decreased and normalized after the herbal medicine was discontinued. CK elevation indicated that the muscle breakdown may be one of the mechanisms by which this preparation induces weight loss. The authors suggested monitoring serum CK in patients using herbal weight loss formulas.

HMG-CoA REDUCTASE INHIBITORS: A case report cited the incidence of rhabdomyolysis in a patient taking a weight loss herbal medicine that contained 50% HCA.[2] Thus, taking garcinia may increase the risk of statin-related rhabdomyolysis; however, clinical evidence for this interaction is lacking.

LIPOGENIC DIET: HCA was shown to be a potent inhibitor of adenosine triphosphate (ATP) citrate lyase, which catalyzes the extramitochondrial cleavage of citrate to oxaloacetate and acetyl coenzyme A (CoA). The inhibition of this reaction limits the availability of acetyl-CoA units required for fatty acid synthesis and lipogenesis during a lipogenic diet.[1,3-6] Extensive animal studies have indicated that HCA suppresses fatty acid synthesis, lipogenesis, and food intake.[3] HCA has been suggested to increase fat metabolism, which may be associated with a decrease in glycogen utilization during exercise.[5]

PEAK EXPIRATORY FLOW RATE: PEFR was increased in male patients who consumed garcinia.[7]

Garlic (Allium sativum)

Pharmacokinetics

The pharmacokinetics of garlic and all its constituents is not well understood. The pharmacokinetics of the vinyldithiins, transformation products of allicin, has been described as having maximal concentrations 15 to 30 minutes after oral absorption.[1] S-allyl-cysteine sulfoxide (SAC) constituents of garlic have demonstrated a first-pass effect after rapid gastrointestinal absorption with liver and kidney metabolism.[2] The elimination half-life of N-acetyl-S-allyl-L-cysteine (allylmercapturic acid, ALMA), a urinary metabolite of garlic, was about 6 hours.[3]

Adverse effects

A review of 45 randomized trials and 73 other clinical trials of garlic use found limited detailed information relating to adverse effects.[4] Malodorous breath, body odor, and allergic reactions appear to be the most common effects.[5] Excessive use has been associated with spontaneous epidural hematoma.[6] Potential reactions associated with oral garlic use include bleeding (multiple case reports and a scientific basis) and hypoglycemia (likely not clinically significant); topical exposure may elicit dermatitis or burns (multiple reports).

Interactions

ANTICOAGULANTS/ANTIPLATELETS: Bleeding has been associated with oral garlic use in several studies and case reports, including intraoperatively, possibly related to impaired platelet aggregation or increased fibrinolysis.[7-20] Reduced platelet aggregation was observed in 308 cases of garlic use.[21] There have been anectodal reports of elevated INRs and PTs in warfarin-stabilized patients after taking garlic.[22] In a recent cross-sectional, point-of-care survey of 1818 patients, 25 cases were identified as potentially clinically significant interactions between garlic and anticoagulants/antiplatelets.[23]

BLOOD GLUCOSE: Possible interactions with hypoglycemic agents have not been systematically evaluated; however, garlic has the potential to decrease glucose concentration.[24,25]

BLOOD LIPIDS: Multiple trials have demonstrated modest lipid-lowering properties of oral garlic supplementation, including decreases in total and LDL cholesterol.[26]

BLOOD PRESSURE: Numerous studies have reported small mean reductions in systolic and diastolic blood pressure associated with the use of oral garlic versus placebo.[4,17,20,26-58]

CYTOCHROME P450 SUBSTRATES: Although animal studies suggest possible induction or inhibition of various CYP450 enzymes, including 3A4 and 2E1,[59,60] other evidence shows no effect.[61] Caution should be used with garlic and agents that affect this enzyme system.

FISH OIL AND EICOSAPENTAENOIC ACID: EPA is found in deep-sea fish oils. Garlic may potentiate antithrombotic effects of EPA, and theoretically, concomitant use of these agents may increase the risk of bleeding. Garlic and fish oil may have additive lipid-lowering effects.

HORMONE LEVELS: Garlic and Pycnogenol have been shown to increase human growth hormone secretion in laboratory experiments.[62] Hypothyroidism and reduced iodine uptake by the thyroid have been reported anecdotally with garlic use; thyroid hormone levels may be affected.

IODINE: Hypothyroidism and reduced iodine uptake by the thyroid have been reported anecdotally with garlic use; thyroid hormone levels may be affected.

PROTEASE INHIBITORS: Garlic supplementation was shown to cause a significant decrease in plasma concentrations of the protease inhibitor saquinavir taken at 1200 mg three times daily by 10 healthy volunteers.[62-64] Combination use may result in diminished effects of saquinavir (Invirase or Fortovase).

PYCNOGENOL: Garlic and Pycnogenol have been shown to increase human growth hormone secretion in laboratory experiments.[62]

THYROID HORMONES: Hypothyroidism and reduced iodine uptake by the thyroid have been reported anecdotally with garlic use; thyroid hormone levels may be affected.

Ginger (Zingiber officinale)

Pharmacokinetics: Insufficient available evidence.

Adverse effects

Ginger has a long history of oral and topical use with minimal reports of toxicity or serious reactions. Adverse effects have usually been reported for dosage amounts exceeding (usually far exceeding) recommended doses.[1] According to a systematic review, 3.3% of 777 patients (from 15 studies) experienced slightly mild side effects that mainly included mild gastrointestinal symptoms.[2] Oral and esophageal irritation described as "pepper-like," heartburn,[3] belching,[4] bloating, flatulence, nausea, "bad taste," abdominal discomfort, and transient burning sensation of the tongue have been reported occasionally, primarily with powdered forms of ginger.[5-10] The mild gastrointestinal symptoms may be reduced by ingesting encapsulated (rather than powdered) ginger.[11] According to a systematic review, up to 6 g of ginger daily does not appear to cause many side effects.[2] The U.S. Food and Drug Administration (FDA) lists ginger on its "generally recognized as safe" (GRAS) list, although this does not support ginger's safety as a medicinal agent.

Interactions

ACIDITY: In vitro evidence suggests that ginger rhizome (underground stem) decreases stomach acid production.[12] Gastroprotective effects have been demonstrated in animal models of gastric ulcers.[13,14]

ANTICOAGULANTS/ANTIPLATELETS: In theory, because ginger has been observed to inhibit thromboxane synthetase, and because decreased platelet aggregation has been reported in clinical trials, concurrent use of ginger with agents that predispose to bleeding could enhance their effect and increase the risk of bleeding.[15-18] In addition, there is also a European case report of a 75 year-old woman taking chronic warfarin whose INR rose after initiating therapy with ginger, complicated by epistaxis.[19] Her INR normalized after discontinuation of ginger and treatment with vitamin K. It is not clear to what extent ginger was responsible for this rise in INR. Another case report described a 76-year-old woman who experienced erratic anticoagulation after taking ginger.[20] In other clinical studies, normal and hypertensive patients experienced synergistic antiplatelet effects when nifedipine (Adalat, Procardia) and ginger were used. Nifedipine and ginger had a synergistic effect on the inhibition of platelet aggregation.[21] In one clinical trial, ginger did not affect the pharmacokinetics or pharmacodynamics of warfarin in healthy subjects.[22] However, in a recent cross-sectional, point-of-care survey of 1818 patients, seven cases were identified as potentially clinically significant interactions between ginger and anticoagulants/antiplatelets.[23]

BACTERIAL LEVELS: In vitro evidence indicates that ginger has immunomodulatory effects and is an effective antimicrobial and antiviral agent.[24,25]

BLOOD LIPIDS: Oral ingestion of ginger extract has been shown to have hypocholesterolemic, hypolipidemic, and antiatherosclerotic effects in cholesterol-fed rabbits[26] and in rats.[27] Inhibition of LDL oxidation and attenuated development of atherosclerosis has also been observed in apolipoprotein E–deficient mice.[28]

BLOOD GLUCOSE: Ginger has been shown to decrease blood glucose.[29] Theoretically, because of its purported hypoglycemic effects, ginger may interact with diabetes therapy, potentially requiring dosing adjustments.

BLOOD PRESSURE: Anecdotally, some experts report hemodynamic effects of large ginger doses, including hypertension or hypotension, although scientific data are lacking in this area.

BODY WEIGHT: Ginger has been suggested as a possible weight loss aid.[30,31]

CALCIUM LEVELS: Ginger or ginger extracts may stimulate calcium uptake in both skeletal and cardiac muscle. In vitro studies of gingerol involving canine cardiac tissue and rabbit skeletal muscle demonstrated gingerol to activate the Ca^{2+}-ATPase pump in a dose-dependent manner.[32] Ginger may also have dose-dependent positive inotropic effects.[33] In theory, ginger combined with high serum levels of calcium could cause hyperexcitability of cardiac muscle.

CYTOCHROME P450 SUBSTRATES: The Chinese herbal medicine sho-saiko-to, which contains ginger and six other herbs (bupleurum, *Pinellia* tuber, *Scutellaria* root, jujube fruit, ginseng, licorice root), has been associated in healthy subjects with reduced activity of CYP1A2, CYP3A, and xanthine oxidase (in 26 healthy subjects).[34] The contribution of ginger to this effect is not clear.

CYTOKINES AND INFLAMMATORY MARKERS: Ginger has been shown to suppress prostaglandin synthesis through inhibition of cyclooxygenase (COX-1 and COX-2), as well as suppress leukotriene biosynthesis by inhibiting 5-lipoxygenase.[35,36] Inhibition of prostaglandin and thromboxane formation by human platelets and the subsequent production of lipid peroxides have been proposed as possible mechanisms by which ginger might provide relief of rheumatoid arthritis symptoms.[36] Interactions between other COX or lipoxygenase inhibitors may occur.

HEART RATE: Arrhythmias are theoretically possible at high ginger doses, based on in vitro and in vivo studies showing components of ginger to activate Ca^{2+}-ATPase and to have dose-dependent positive inotropic effects.[37] Anecdotally, some experts report hemodynamic effects of large doses, including hypertension or hypotension, although scientific data are lacking.

HISTOLOGICAL TESTS: The constituents isolated from ginger species, including curcumin, 6-gingerol, and labdane-type diterpene compounds, were found to have positive effects on cell proliferation and the induction of apoptosis in the cultured human T-lymphoma Jurkat cells.[38] Ginger in food may interfere with cell-signaling pathways.[39]

P-GLYCOPROTEIN SUBSTRATES: P-glycoprotein is a cell membrane–associated protein that transports a variety of drug substrates. Interaction with P-gp, including activation, inhibition, and induction, can lead to altered plasma or brain levels of various drugs that are P-gp substrates. 6-Gingerol has been reported to have inhibitory effects of P-gp,[40] a carrier mechanism that transports agents across cell membranes and plays a major role in the distribution and elimination of many therapeutic substances. Theoretically, ginger may interfere with the absorption and action of certain agents to sites of action.

SEDATIVES AND CENTRAL NERVOUS SYSTEM DEPRESSANTS: In theory, because large doses of ginger have been reported to depress the central nervous sytem, it may enhance the CNS depressant effects of other agents, including barbiturates or benzodiazepines.[41,42]

VIRAL LEVELS: In vitro evidence indicates that ginger has immunomodulatory effects and is an effective antimicrobial and antiviral agent.[24,25]

Ginkgo (Ginkgo biloba)

Pharmacokinetics

The pharmacokinetics of *Ginkgo* has been studied in animals as well as humans.[1,2] Oral bioavailability of the terpene lactones ginkgolide A, ginkgolide B, and bilobalide (constituents of *Ginkgo*) is 98% to 100%, 79% to 93%, and 70%, respectively. Absorption has been found to occur principally through the small intestine. Half-life of ginkgolide A, ginkgolide B, and bilobalide is 4.5, 10.6, and 3.2 hours, respectively, with peak plasma levels at 2 to 3 hours. Approximately 70% of ginkgolide A, 50% of ginkgolide B, and 30% of bilobalide are excreted unchanged in urine, with seven other metabolites: 4-hydroxybenzoic acid conjugate, 4-hydroxyhippuric acid, 3-methoxy-4-hydroxyhippuric acid, 3,4-dihydroxybenzoic acid, 4-hydroxybenzoic acid, hippuric acid, and 3-methoxy-4-hydroxybenzoic acid (vanillic acid); these are detectable in the urine but not in serum. Toxicity is low, with an oral LD_{50} in rodents of 7725 mg. Duration of action has been reported as 7 hours.

Adverse effects

Ginkgo appears to be well tolerated in most healthy adults at recommended doses for 6 months to 1 year. In several reviews, *Ginkgo* use was associated with similar rates of adverse effects as placebo.[3-7] Postmarket surveillance of more than 10,000 subjects found a 1.69% incidence of minor symptoms, including headache, nausea, and gastrointestinal complaints.[8] The potential complication of most concern is bleeding, which has been life threatening in a small number of case reports. Infrequent mild GI discomfort has been reported in clinical studies, particularly when *Ginkgo* is taken with SSRIs.[9] *Ginkgo* may also alter blood sugar levels. Rarely, *Ginkgo* may cause allergic hypersensitivity, including Stevens-Johnson syndrome.[10-12] Eating *Ginkgo* seeds may be deadly because of the risk of tonic-clonic seizures and loss of consciousness.[13-15]

Interactions

5-FLUOROURACIL: 5-FU–induced adverse effects may be alleviated by *Ginkgo*, as suggested by a Phase II clinical trial.[16]

AGENTS THAT LOWER THE SEIZURE THRESHOLD: Ingestion of *Ginkgo* seeds has been associated with lower seizure threshold and may antagonize the effect of antiseizure therapies.[17] The protective effects of sodium valproate and carbamazepine on seizures in mice was diminished with the administration of G*inkgo*.[18]

ANTICOAGULANTS/ANTIPLATELETS: Based on several case reports of spontaneous bleeding in patients using *Ginkgo* as a monotherapy or concomitantly with warfarin or aspirin,[19-22] concurrent use of *Ginkgo* with agents that increase clotting time or inhibit platelet function may increase risk of bleeding.

ANTIPSYCHOTIC AGENTS: Based on secondary sources, *Ginkgo* may reduce some side effects of antipsychotic agents, although scientific data are not available.[23]

BLOOD GLUCOSE: *Ginkgo* has been found to increase plasma insulin concentrations in healthy volunteers[24] and to decrease these concentrations in subjects with type 2 diabetes.[25] Effects on serum glucose concentrations have not been evaluated, and possible interactions with hypoglycemic agents are not clear.

C-PEPTIDE: *Ginkgo* has been found to increase C-peptide concentrations in preliminary clinical research with healthy volunteers.[24]

CHOLINERGIC AGENTS: Theoretically, agents such as donepezil (Aricept) and tacrine (Cognex) may have additive effects when used concurrently with *Ginkgo*, potentially precipitating cholinergic effects. However, *Ginkgo* supplementation did not have a major impact on the pharmacokinetics and pharmacodynamics of donepezil in one study.[26]

COLCHICINE: Colchicine has been isolated in commercial preparations of *Ginkgo* and may increase serum concentrations in patients using colchicine.[27]

CYCLOSPORINE (NEORAL, SANDIMMUNE, GENGRAF): Cyclosporine nephrotoxicity may be alleviated by *Ginkgo*, although evidence is preliminary in this area.[28]

FLUOXETINE (PROZAC): G*inkgo* has been used to treat erectile dysfunction[29] and may interact with other agents used in the management of vascular ED. *Ginkgo* has also been reported to relieve sexual dysfunction associated with the selective serotonin reuptake inhibitor (SSRI) fluoxetine (Prozac).[30]

MONOAMINERGIC AGENTS: MAO inhibition by *Ginkgo* was reported in preliminary research conducted in animals[31] but was not confirmed by subsequent animal research[32] or in humans.[33] Based on preclinical research, *Ginkgo* may act additively with MAO inhibitors and may cause serotonin syndrome, a condition characterized by rigidity, tachycardia, hyperthermia, restlessness, and diaphoresis.[34]

NIFEDIPINE (ADALAT, PROCARDIA): The effects of *Ginkgo* leaf extract on the pharmacokinetics and pharmacodynamics of nifedipine, a calcium channel blocker, were studied in healthy volunteers.[35,36] Maximal plasma nifedipine concentration was approximately doubled by *Ginkgo* in two subjects, who had more severe and longer-lasting headaches with *Ginkgo* than without *Ginkgo*. Oral administration of nifedipine with *Ginkgo* also increased heart rate over *Ginkgo* alone.

THIAZIDES: Although paradoxical hypertension was documented in a male patient taking a thiazide diuretic and *Ginkgo*, it has been found to decrease systolic and diastolic blood pressure in healthy volunteers.[24,37] Caution is warranted with concomitant use.

TYRAMINE-CONTAINING FOODS: Based on the possible MAO inhibitor properties of *Ginkgo* (suggested in animal research but refuted in other animal and clinical studies), high doses of *Ginkgo* may lead to hypertensive crisis when ingested with tyramine-containing foods (e.g., cheese) or drinks (e.g., wine). Clinical evidence of this potential interaction is lacking.

Ginseng (*Panax* spp.)

Pharmacokinetics

The ginsenosides found in ginseng appear to be poorly absorbed after oral absorption.[1-3] Compound K is the main metabolite of ginseng. The metabolism and excretion of the constituents of ginseng have not been extensively studied. It appears that ginsenosides are excreted in the urine only in trace amounts.

Adverse effects

Clinical trials have indicated that *Panax ginseng* and American ginseng, when used in recommended doses for a short period, do not seem to be associated with serious long-term side effects.[4] Based on limited evidence, long-term ginseng use may be associated with skin rash or spots, itching, diarrhea, sore throat, loss of appetite, excitability, anxiety, depression, or insomnia. Less common side effects include headache, fever, dizziness/vertigo, blood pressure abnormalities (increases or decreases), chest pain, difficult menstruation, heart palpitations, rapid heart rate, leg swelling, nausea/vomiting, and manic episodes in patients with bipolar disorder. Stevens-Johnson syndrome has occurred in one patient and may have been caused by contaminants in a ginseng product. High intake of American ginseng may result in hypoglycemia in both diabetic and nondiabetic persons.[5]

Interactions

ADRENOCORTICOTROPIC HORMONE: Ginseng may stimulate ACTH and thereby increase plasma cortisol levels.[6]

ANALGESICS: *Panax ginseng* potentiates the antinociceptive effects of pentazocine and aspirin in mice[7] and also appears to have independent effects, based on pharmacological data.[8]

ANTIBIOTICS: Preliminary clinical evidence suggests that ginseng synergistically accelerates bacterial clearance of sputum in bacterial bronchitis treated with antibiotics (amoxicillin, clavulanic acid).[9]

ANTIBODY LEVELS: Ginseng is purported to have numerous immunomodulatory effects. It has been shown to increase antibody titers after influenza immunization while reducing the incidence of cold symptoms and influenza.[10] Ginseng potentiates the effect of vaccines for porcine parvovirus and *Erysipelothrix rhusiopathiae* infections.[11] Ginseng has also been shown to decrease plasma level of IgA.[12]

ANTICOAGULANTS/ANTIPLATELETS: Ginseng may inhibit platelet activity[13-15] and potentiate the action of NSAIDs (e.g., aspirin). Based on in vitro research, nonsaponin lipophilic fraction from the roots of *Panax ginseng* inhibited the aggregation of human platelets induced by thrombin (0.1 unit/mL) in a dose-dependent manner.[15] Ginseng reduced platelet adhesiveness in rat studies;[14] however, the mechanism is not clear because warfarin pharmacokinetics has been shown to be unaltered by a single 2-mg/kg dose of ginseng in rats.[16] In humans a ginseng-gingko combination has been shown to reduce platelet aggregation.[13] One case report of a 47-year-old man stabilized on warfarin for a mechanical heart valve experienced a drop from 3.1 to 1.5 in his INR 4 weeks after starting ginseng capsules three times daily.[17] Two weeks after discontinuation of ginseng, the patient's INR returned to 3.3.[18] Because of conflicting data, it is unclear how ginseng may act when used in combination with anticoagulant/antiplatelet agents; it may increase bleeding or clotting risk. Nonetheless, caution is warranted.

ANTIDIABETIC AGENTS: In a recent cross-sectional, point-of-care survey of 1818 patients, six cases were identified as potentially clinically significant interactions between ginseng and antidiabetic agents.[19]

BLOOD ALCOHOL: *Panax ginseng* may reduce blood concentration of alcohol (ethanol) and enhance blood alcohol clearance.[4,20-22]

BLOOD GLUCOSE: High intake of American ginseng has been shown to lower blood glucose.[5,23-26]

BLOOD LIPIDS: Ginseng has been shown to have cholesterol-lowering effects in animals and humans.[14]

BLOOD PRESSURE: Based on in vitro evidence, extracts of *P. ginseng* (G115) may inhibit angiotensin-converting enzyme (ACE) activity, but may not affect nitric oxide (NO) production.[27] Preliminary evidence suggests that ginseng may increase the QT_c interval (thus increasing risk of abnormal heart rhythms) and decrease diastolic blood pressure 2 hours after ingestion in healthy adults.[28] Hypotensive effects have been observed;[29,30] however, based on clinical trials, American ginseng does not affect blood pressure in hypertensive individuals.[31,32]

CENTRAL NERVOUS SYSTEM STIMULANTS: Controversy surrounds whether caffeine and other stimulants are safe to take with ginseng. Some experts believe that Asian ginseng is safe when taken in the recommended dosage;[23] others disagree.[34] Ginseng may cause insomnia and headaches and enhance the effects of caffeine. Commercial ginseng preparations are said to contain methylxanthines (e.g., caffeine, theophylline, theobromine) in widely varying amounts, which may influence experimental results.[34] Although the herb itself does not contain caffeine, some commercial ginseng supplements test positive for caffeine. Based on animal studies, ginseng has been shown to inhibit the formation of tolerance to psychostimulants.[35,36] It has also inhibited cocaine-induced hyperactivity in mice.[37] Because it is a nonspecific CNS stimulant, *P. ginseng* may increase the effects and side effects of prescription agents that also stimulate the CNS. If *P. ginseng* or *Panax quinquefolius* is taken concomitantly with other known stimulants, additive adverse effects may occur. Clinical evidence of drug interactions is unclear.

CISPLATIN (PLATINOL): In ferrets, Korean red ginseng total extract significantly attenuated the cisplatin-induced nausea and vomiting when administered 1 to 2 hours before cisplatin.[33]

CORTISOL LEVELS: Ginseng may stimulate ACTH and thereby increase plasma cortisol levels, according to animal research data.[6] Anecdotal evidence has suggested that ginseng lowers cortisol levels in diabetic patients but increases cortisol levels in nondiabetic persons.

CYTOCHROME P450 SUBSTRATES: *Panax ginseng* has been shown to inhibit CYP450 2D6 and 3A4.[38,39]

DEHYDROEPIANDROSTERONE: Ginseng may enhance the effectiveness of DHEA supplementation.[40]

DIGOXIN (LANOXIN): Some clinical evidence indicates that ginseng may enhance the effects of digoxin (Lanoxin) in congestive heart failure.[41]

DIHYDROTESTOSTERONE LEVELS: Men treated with ginseng have experienced increases in DHT concentrations.[42]

ESTROGENIC AGENTS: Ginseng has been reported to have estrogen-like effects.[43-45] Mycotoxins in root extracts of American and Asian ginseng bind estrogen receptors alpha and beta in vitro.[46] However, one study found that no estrogenic activity was evident in the sample of *P. ginseng* extract tested, or in a sample of the combination product ArginMax.[47] Clinical relevance of this potential interaction remains unclear.

FOLLICLE-STIMULATING HORMONE: Men treated with ginseng have experienced increased FSH concentrations.[42]

FUROSEMIDE (LASIX): In one case report of a patient taking furosemide, ginseng was suspected of inducing diuresis resistance.[48]

GINKGO BILOBA: Ginseng is often combined with *Ginkgo biloba* in formulas. When used in combination, ginseng may cause decreases in systolic pressure at low or high doses and decreases in diastolic pressure at high doses.[13] Theoretically, the combination of *Ginkgo* and ginseng may lead to additive effects.

LIVER FUNCTION TESTS: Ginseng has been suggested to increase the toxicity of hepatotoxic agents.[49] Concurrent use of ginseng with hepatotoxic agents may lead to adverse effects on the liver, which may be reflected in LFTs.

LUTEINIZING HORMONE: Men treated with ginseng had increased LH concentration.[42]

MITOMYCIN (MUTAMYCIN): Based on in vitro research, panaxytriol from *Panax ginseng* may interact synergistically with mitomycin C.[50]

MONOAMINERGIC AGENTS: *P. ginseng* or *P. quinquefolius* has been suggested to interact with MAO inhibitors.[49] *P. ginseng* has documented and theoretical interactions with phenelzine that cause mania, headache, tremors, and insomnia.[4,20,24,49,51,52]

NIFEDIPINE (PROCARDIA): Based on case reports, ginseng may interact with blood pressure or heart agents, including calcium channel blockers such as nifedipine (Procardia). Ginseng increased serum levels of nifedipine in healthy volunteers.[39]

NONSTEROIDAL ANTIINFLAMMATORY DRUGS: Ginseng may inhibit platelet activity[13-15] and potentiate the action of NSAIDs such as aspirin. However, clinical evidence of this potential interaction is lacking.

OPIATES: In mice, ginseng has been shown to inhibit tolerance to opioids.[35,36] Total saponins of *P. notoginseng* may possess some agonist activities at opioid-like peptide receptors.[53]

PACLITAXEL (TAXOL): Based on animal data, red ginseng may interact synergistically with paclitaxel.[54]

PHENYTOIN: *Panax ginseng* may affect the concentration of the anticonvulsant drug phenytoin via human liver CYP450 enzyme interaction.[49,55]

PHOTOSENSITIZING AGENTS: Evidence from in vitro studies indicates that *P. ginseng* acts as a photoprotector in low concentrations and as a photosensitizer in high concentrations.[56]

POSTERIOR PITUITARY HORMONE LEVELS: Intravenous administration of *P. ginseng* in rats showed that the physiological effect of ginseng is not affected by translation, conversion rate, or the chemical structure of hormones from the posterior pituitary.[57]

PROLACTIN: Men treated with ginseng had decreased prolactin concentration.[42]

P-GLYCOPROTEIN SUBSTRATES: P-glycoprotein is a cell membrane–associated protein that transports a variety of drug substrates. Interaction with P-gp, including activation, inhibition, and induction, can lead to altered plasma or brain levels of P-gp substrates. Certain HIV protease inhibitors have been demonstrated in vitro to be substrates for P-gp and CYP3A4;[49,58] thus, concomitant use with ginseng should be avoided.

RHUBARB: In a clinical trial, rhubarb and sanchi powder (*Panax notoginseng*) were used together for hemorrhgic fever from nephritic syndrome.[59]

RITONAVIR: In vitro, ginseng was shown to enhance the antiviral activity of ritonavir. P-gp and CYP450 enzyme inhibition was proposed to potentiate these interactions.[58]

SEDATIVES AND CENTRAL NERVOUS SYSTEM DEPRESSANTS: Ginseng may interact with sedatives, although clinical evidence is lacking. Based on research conducted in animals, ginseng may inhibit tolerance formation to opioids and psychostimulants.[35,36] It has also inhibited cocaine-induced hyperactivity in mice.[37] Because it is a nonspecific CNS stimulant, *P. ginseng* may increase the effects and side effects of prescription CNS stimulants.

TESTOSTERONE: Men treated with ginseng had increased testosterone concentration.[42] Rats fed with ginseng for 60 days showed significant increases in blood testosterone level and significantly reduced prostate weight.[59]

URINE TESTS: An International Olympic Committee (IOC) urine drug test of athletes ingesting Cold-fX was not positive for any IOC-banned or restricted substances.[60]

VIRAL LEVELS: Ginseng has traditionally been used as an antiviral agent, although clinical evidence is equivocal.

WHITE BLOOD CELL COUNTS: In humans, ginseng significantly ($p < 0.05$) increased CD4+ T-lymphocyte counts.[12]

Globe Artichoke (Cynara scolymus)

Pharmacokinetics

Several metabolites detected in human plasma have been identified as being derived from mono- and di-caffeoylquinic acids and flavonoids that are known active phenolic constituents of artichoke leaf extract.[1] The metabolites caffeic acid, ferulic acid, and isoferulic acid achieved peak plasma concentrations within 1 hour and declined over 24 hours, demonstrating a near-biphasic profile. The hydrogenated metabolites dihydrocaffeic acid and dihydroferulic acid were detected after 6 to 7 hours, suggesting the involvement of more than one pathway in processing caffeoylquinic acids. Peak plasma concentrations of luteolin were reached within 30 minutes, with elimination showing a biphasic profile. The active constituents of artichoke extract have not been identified in human plasma or urine.[1]

Adverse effects

Patients should avoid globe artichoke if they have known allergies or hypersensitivities to *Cynara scolymus*, its constituents, or members of the Asteraceae or Compositae family, including chrysanthemums, daisies, marigolds, ragweed, and arnica, because of possible cross-reactivity.

The adverse effects associated with artichoke are generally mild gastrointestinal symptoms, including flatulence, diarrhea, hunger, and nausea.[2-4] Severe asthma[5,6] and nephrotoxicity[7,8] have also been reported.

Interactions

ANTICOAGULANTS/ANTIPLATELETS: Artichoke may increase the risk of bleeding, based on a case report of significantly reduced platelet aggregation (both spontaneous and ADP-induced) in 62 men taking an artichoke extract (Cynarex) for 2 years (dose not reported), who were also chronically exposed to carbon disulfide.[9] It is not clear whether artichoke or other agents were the cause of this reaction.

BLOOD LIPIDS: There are multiple published reports of cholesterol-lowering effects of artichoke.[10-23]

HMG-CoA REDUCTASE INHIBITORS: In vitro, the artichoke constituent luteolin has been shown to have similar effects to statin agents and inhibit cholesterol synthesis by HMG-CoA reductase.[15] Therefore, artichoke may interact with statins, possibly magnifying their adverse effects. However, clinical evidence of this potential interaction is lacking.

LIVER FUNCTION TESTS: Based on a case series, use of artichoke extracts and products containing artichokes may alter bilirubin and transaminase levels.[2]

Goji (Lycium spp.)

Pharmacokinetics

Plasma zeaxanthin concentrations increased significantly ($p = 0.05$) after volunteers consumed a 5-mg dose of goji.[1] Peak absorption occurred between 9 and 24 hours. Native 3R,3'R-zeaxanthin from wolfberry was determined to be more bioavailable than the nonesterified form.

Adverse effects

Information is lacking on the adverse effects of goji. According to anecdotal reports, high doses of goji berry extract may induce alertness at bedtime, may interact with sleep, and may cause nausea and vomiting.[2]

Interactions

ANTIBODY LEVELS: Lycium may increase in serum IgA and IgG levels, based on evidence from animal research.[3]

ANTICOAGULANTS/ANTIPLATELETS: Goji fruit was shown to elevate international normalized ratio (INR) in a patient stabilized on warfarin.[4]

BLOOD GLUCOSE: In animals, Lycium barbarum has been shown to decrease plasma glucose[5-8] and also increase insulin sensitivity.[6]

BLOOD LIPIDS: In animals, L. barbarum has been shown to decrease plasma cholesterol and plasma triglycerides.[6,7]

BLOOD PRESSURE: Lycium may have antihypertensive effects, according to animal models of hypertension.[9] Theoretically, combined use of Lycium with other agents that decrease blood pressure may increase the risk of hypotension.

CYTOCHROME P450 SUBSTRATES: Based on in vitro assessment, a tea of L. barbarum may weakly inhibit CYP2C9.[4]

HEMATOCRIT: Based on research involving chemotherapy-induced myelosuppressive and irradiated mice, L. barbarum polysaccharide may enhance peripheral RBC counts.[10,11]

HISTOLOGICAL TESTS: Based on several in vitro and animal studies, L. barbarum may have antineoplastic activity.[12-18] Goji has thus been suggested as an adjunct to standard antineoplastic agents.

IRON: In animals, L. barbarum polysaccharide (LBP-4) has been shown to increase the level of iron in muscle and bone.[19]

LIVER FUNCTION TESTS: Based on animal research, Lycium chinense Miller (Solanaceae) fruit may have hepatoprotective effects and may decrease levels of serum aspartate and alanine transaminase (AST and ALT) and alkaline phosphatase (ALP).[20]

MONOAMINERGIC AGENTS: Based on in vitro evidence, L. chinense may inhibit MAO-B.[10] Theoretically, concurrent use of goji and MOA inhibitors may increase the risk of hypertensive crisis.

RADIATION THERAPY: In animals a combination of L. barbarum polysaccharide and radiation has been shown to have significant radiosensitizing effects.[21]

VITAMIN C: The fruits of L. barbarum contain 0.5% of a novel stable precursor of ascorbic acid, which could theoretically increase serum ascorbic acid levels and cause additive effects.[22,23]

WHITE BLOOD CELL COUNTS: In irradiated mice, intraperitoneal L. chinense root has been shown to increase leukocyte counts.[21] In animals, L. barbarum polysaccharide has been shown to increase significantly the numbers of CD4+ and CD8+ T-cells.[24]

ZEAXANTHIN: In healthy volunteers, consumption of goji has been shown to increase plasma zeaxanthin levels.[25]

ZINC: In animals, L. barbarum polysaccharide has increased the zinc level in muscle and bone.[10]

Goldenseal (Hydrastis canadensis). See Berberine

Gotu Kola (Centella asiatica)

Pharmacokinetics

The triterpenoid saponins of gotu kola contain three main components: asiatic acid, madecassic acid, and asiaticoside.[1,2] Peak plasma levels have been reached 2 to 4 hours after oral ingestion, intramuscular (IM) injection, or topical application of gotu kola.[3] After chronic treatment for 7 days with either 30 mg or 60 mg total triterpenic fraction of Centella asiatica (TTFCA) twice daily, peak plasma concentrations, AUC_{0-24}, and half-life were significantly higher than after single-dose administration.[1] Gotu kola is predominantly eliminated in the feces within 24 to 76 hours, with a small, unspecified amount metabolized by the kidneys.

Adverse effects

Gotu kola is not related to the cola nut and does not contain caffeine. Gotu kola is generally reported as safe for short-term use in humans.[4-13] Infertility has occurred after ingestion of gotu kola in animals.[14] Hepatotoxicity has also been reported in animal research with gotu kola use. In rats, liver function tests were elevated after taking gotu kola for 20, 30, and 60 days.[15] Nausea and gastric irritation have also been reported after oral administration of gotu kola.[5]

Interactions

BLOOD GLUCOSE: Gotu kola in large doses has been found to elevate blood glucose levels in animals[16] and may counteract the effects of agents that reduce serum glucose levels. Similar effects may occur in humans, so careful monitoring and dose adjustments may be necessary.

NONSTEROIDAL ANTIINFLAMMATORY DRUGS: In animals the beneficial effects of IM administration of asiaticoside (triterpine glycoside from gotu kola) on wound healing were antagonized by subcutaneous administration of phenylbutazone (an NSAID), implicating a possible interaction with this class of agents.[13] The application to humans is not clear, and IM administration of asiaticoside has not been demonstrated as safe or efficacious for wound healing.

SEDATIVES AND CENTRAL NERVOUS SYSTEM DEPRESSANTS: In animals,[16] gotu kola has been shown to possess sedative qualities; thus it may cause additive effects with other sedatives.

Grape Seed (*Vitis* spp.)

Pharmacokinetics

Oligomeric proanthocyanidins (OPCs) are rapidly absorbed from the gastrointestinal (GI) tract, with maximum blood levels achieved in 45 minutes. The half-life is estimated at 5 hours. Primary routes of excretion are through stool (ethylcatechol) and urine (hippuric acid, ethylcatechol, hydroxyphenylpropionic acid).[1]

Adverse effects

Grape seed extracts (GSEs) are generally well tolerated.[2-4] Reported side effects from clinical trials include dry itching scalp, nausea, indigestion, and other GI disturbances.[5-8] Other clinical adverse effects associated with GSE include dizziness and hypertension.[6]

Interactions

ANTICOAGULANTS/ANTIPLATELETS: Based on clinical research and in vitro evidence, OPC preparations may significantly and dose-dependently reduce platelet aggregation.[9-11] Theoretically, grape seed may increase the risk of bleeding when used with anticoagulants/antiplatelets; however, clinical evidence of this potential interaction is lacking.

BLOOD LIPIDS: Based on animal studies, OPCs may decrease total cholesterol.[12,13] However, other animal studies have provided conflicting evidence on whether grape seed increases, decreases, or maintains HDL concentration. In clinical studies, grape seed did not significantly affect HDL.[12,14,15]

BLOOD PRESSURE: Based on animal and in vitro research, OPCs may inhibit ACE activity by noncompetitive inhibition.[16-18] In clinical studies, however, adverse effects associated with grape seed included dizziness and hypertension.[6]

CHROMIUM: The combination of chromium and GSE may significantly decrease LDL.[14]

CYTOCHROME P450 SUBSTRATES: Based on in vitro research, GSE may reduce CYP2E1 activity.[19] In vitro research also showed that grape seed can inhibit CYP2C9 and CYP3A4 at 10 mcM.[20] Caution is warranted when using grape seed with CYP450-metabolized agents.

FOLATE: Based on in vitro research, OPCs may inhibit xanthine oxidase, which may affect folate metabolism.[21]

HISTOLOGICAL TESTS: GSE has been studied extensively in animal and laboratory research to determine possible mechanisms of action for its potential chemotherapeutic effects, focusing mainly on proanthrocyanidin and gallic acid constituents of grape seed.[22-30] Grape seed has been suggested as an adjuvant for standard antineoplastic agents.

LACTOBACILLUS ACIDOPHILUS: Based on secondary sources, concomitant administration of grape seed and *Lactobacillus acidophilus* may prevent *L. acidophilus* colonization of the GI tract.

METHOTREXATE (RHEUMATREX): Based on in vitro research, the ability of OPCs to inhibit xanthine oxidase may lead to methotrexate toxicity.[21]

URIC ACID: Based on in vitro research, OPCs may be strong and noncompetitive inhibitors of xanthine oxidase.[21] Levels of certain metabolites, such as uric acid, may be altered.

VITAMINS: Although limited research showed Leucoselect-phytosome (OPC preparation) to have no effect on vitamin C or vitamin E levels,[31] anecdotal reports indicate that flavonoids from grape seed may enhance their absorption and effectiveness.

Grapefruit (*Citrus* x *paradisi*)

Pharmacokinetics

The pharmacokinetics of grapefruit are not well understood. However, it is well known that grapefruit juice is a potent inhibitor of the intestinal cytochrome P450 system (specifically CYP3A4-mediated drug metabolism), which is responsible for the first-pass metabolism of many agents. It may also inhibit CYP1A2, 2C9, and 2C19, as well as the drug transporters P-glycoprotein (P-gp) and organic anion transporting peptide (OATP). For these reasons, grapefruit has a high potential for interaction with drugs and other agents.

Adverse effects

Grapefruit appears to be well tolerated. Consumption of large amounts of grapefruit may increase the risk of breast cancer.[1] Grapefruit may increase or decrease the development of kidney stones; research results are conflicting.

Interactions

GENERAL: Grapefruit juice appears irreversibly to inhibit the intestinal CYP450-3A4 system, responsible for the first-pass metabolism of many agents. The inhibition of this enzyme system leads to an elevation in blood serum concentration of certain drugs when administered concurrently with grapefruit juice.

ANESTHETICS: Theoretically, the ability of grapefruit to inhibit CYP3A4 may lead to delayed recovery from anesthesia when these agents are used for this purpose.

ANGIOTENSIN-CONVERTING ENZYME (ACE) INHIBITORS: Concomitant use of grapefruit juice and the ACE inhibitor losartan (Cozaar) has been shown clinically to reduce the effectiveness of losartan.[2]

ANTIBIOTICS: The bioavailability of erythromycin was shown in clinical studies to be increased by grapefruit, likely caused by the inhibitory effect of grapefruit on CYP3A4-mediated metabolism in the small intestine.[3,4] Grapefruit may increase the absorption and plasma concentrations of erythromycin.

ANTICOAGULANTS/ANTIPLATELETS: Grapefruit has been reported to potentiate the antiplatelet effects of cilostazol.[5] After ingestion of grapefruit juice, urinary excretion of 7-hydroxycoumarin after oral administration of 10 mg coumarin was decreased for up to 8 hours.[6] It appears that grapefruit flavonoids inhibit CYP2A-dependent metabolic pathways, but the mechanism of this inhibition is not understood.

ANTICONVULSANTS: Based on clinical evidence, grapefruit may increase the absorption and plasma concentrations of some (but not all) anticonvulsants.[7,8] In patients with epilepsy, grapefruit juice has been shown to increase the bioavailability of carbamazepine (Tegretol) by inhibiting CYP3A4 enzymes in the gut wall and the liver.[7]

ANTIDEPRESSANTS: Based on in vitro, in vivo, and preliminary human evidence, grapefruit may inhibit the metabolism of antidepressants, thereby increasing drug levels and the risk of adverse effects.[9,10]

ANTIFUNGAL AGENTS: There is clinical evidence that grapefruit decreases the systemic availability of itraconazole, possibly by presystemic intestinal metabolism via CYP3A4.[11,12]

ANTIHISTAMINES: Based on in vitro and clinical evidence, grapefruit may increase the bioavailability and side effects associated with antihistamines.[13-19] In clinical studies the administration of grapefruit juice concomitantly with terfenadine (Seldane) was shown to increase terfenadine bioavailability, thus increasing the risk of cardiotoxicity.[14,15,18]

ANTIMALARIAL AGENTS: Grapefruit juice has been shown to increase the bioavailability of antimalarial agents such as artemether and halofantrine.[20-22] However, grapefruit juice has been found to have no effect on quinine pharmacokinetics.[23]

ANTINEOPLASTIC AGENTS: Based on clinical and in vivo studies, grapefruit may reduce the effectiveness of some antineoplastic agents.[19,24,25] Evidence from a clinical crossover study indicates that grapefruit juice coadministered with oral etoposide can reduce the AUC of etoposide (Etopophos, Vepesid) on average by 26.2%.[24] Grapefruit juice may decrease the absorption and plasma concentrations of etoposide. According to the manufacturer, grapefruit juice may inhibit CYP3A4 metabolism of sunitinib (Sutent) in the intestinal wall, possibly resulting in increased drug levels and risk of adverse events.

ANTIPSYCHOTIC AGENTS: Antipsychotic drugs, such as clozapine[26-28] and haloperidol,[29] have not been shown to be altered by grapefruit ingestion in clinical studies. However, according to the manufacturer of aripiprazole (Abilify), because of the ability of grapefruit to inhibit CYP3A4, the levels/effects of aripiprazole may be increased. It is recommended that the dose of aripiprazole be decreased by 50%.

BENZODIAZEPINES: Grapefruit has been shown clinically to increase the plasma concentrations of the benzodiazepines midazolam[30-35] and triazolam.[36,37] However, the effects of these drugs did not appear to be enhancd by grapefruit juice.[38]

BETA-ADRENERGIC AGENTS: Grapefruit juice has been shown clinically to decrease concentrations of beta-blocking agents.[39-41] Clinical research has shown that grapefruit juice decreases plasma concentrations of acebutolol (Sectral) and diacetolol by interfering with GI absorption.[39]

CALCIUM CHANNEL BLOCKERS: Numerous biochemical, in vitro, in vivo, and clinical studies have shown that grapefruit increases the adverse effects associated with some calcium channel blockers.[42-70] The basis for this interaction appears to relate to both flavonoid and nonflavonoid components of grapefruit juice interfering with enterocyte CYP3A4 activity.

CARDIAC GLYCOSIDES: Modest changes in digoxin pharmacokinetics have been observed after concurrent administration of grapefruit juice in humans.[71,72] Inhibition of intestinal P-glycoprotein does not appear to play an important role in drug interactions involving grapefruit juice and digoxin.

CHOLINERGIC AGENTS: Theoretically, grapefruit juice may inhibit the hepatic metabolism of oxybutynin (Ditropan), leading to increased drug levels and associated adverse events. A clinical study showed that the AUC was increased to 30% when scopolamine was administered with grapefruit juice; t_{max}, half-life were also increased.[73] This interaction is likely caused by CYP3A4 inhibition in the intestine.

CORTICOSTEROIDS: In vivo evidence suggests that the dietary flavonoids in grapefruit juice may inhibit the enzyme 11β-hydroxysteroid dehydrogenase, which oxidizes cortisol to inactive cortisone in a concentration-dependent manner.[74] Grapefruit juice has been shown to increase plasma concentration of orally administered methylprednisolone in healthy subjects. Grapefruit juice (200 mL three times daily) increased the half-life of methylprednisolone by 35%, C_{max} by 27%, and total AUC by 75%.[75]

CYTOCHROME P450 SUBSTRATES: Preliminary evidence suggests that grapefruit juice may inhibit CYP1A2,[76] CYP2C9,[76,77] or CYP2C19.[76] However, clinical evidence of these interactions is lacking. Grapefruit juice has been shown in vitro, in vivo, and clinically to inhibit CYP3A4 metabolism of drugs, causing increased drug levels and potentially increasing the risk of adverse effects.[2,44,66,77-91]

DRUG TESTS: Grapefruit juice decreases metabolism and increases plasma concentrations and test results of various agents, including praziquantel,[92] clomipramine,[10,93] artemether and halofantrine,[20-22] amiodarone,[94] amlodipine,[95] diltiazem,[51] felodipine,* nifedipine,† nimodipine,[60] verapamil,[43,57,62] buspirone,[96] midazolam and triazolam,[30-38] diazepam,[97] carbamazepine,[7] dextromethorphan,[98] cyclosporine,[99-101] methylprednisolone,[75] tacrolimus,[102] digoxin,[71,72] erythromycin,[2] clarithromycin,[3] sildenafil,[79,103] atorvastatin,[78,104] lovastatin,[105] simvastatin,[80,106-109] 17β-estradiol,[110] ethinylestradiol,[110] methadone,[111,112] cisapride,[113-115] amprenavir,[116] saquinavir,[117,118] terfenadine,[14,15] quinidine,[119] scopolamine,[73] and theophylline.[120]

ELECTROLYTES: In vivo study has found that the dietary flavonoids in grapefruit juice may inhibit the enzyme 11β-hydroxysteroid dehydrogenase, which oxidizes cortisol to inactive cortisone.[121] High doses were observed to cause an apparent mineralocorticoid effect, and theoretically, some individuals may increase their potassium clearance if they drink large amounts of grapefruit juice.

ESTROGENIC AGENTS: Grapefruit may increase the bioavailability and side effects associated with estrogen therapy.[110,122,123] The most likely mechanism of action of the flavonoids of grapefruit juice on 17β-estradiol metabolism is inhibition of the CYP3A4 enzyme, which catalyzes the reversible hydroxylation of 17β-estradiol into estrone and further into estriol.[110]

HEART RATE: Grapefruit may interact with antiarrhythmic agents through the intestinal CYP3A4 system.[44,94,124]

HEMATOCRIT: Research suggests that grapefruit may lower RBC count in people with an elevated hematocrit.[125] Conversely, in people with a low hematocrit, grapefruit may increase hematocrit. The effect appears to be the same with one-half or one whole grapefruit daily. The grapefruit constituent naringin may be responsible for this effect.

HMG-CoA REDUCTASE INHIBITORS: Grapefruit is known to inhibit P-gp–mediated transport of HMG-CoA reductase inhibitors in vitro.[126] Numerous in vitro, in vivo, and clinical studies have shown that grapefruit increases the absorption and plasma concentrations of these agents.§ Clinical studies show that grapefruit increases plasma levels of simvastatin.[80,106-109] The mean increase in simvastatin AUC was 3.6-fold, and the increase in mean C_{max} was 3.9-fold.[107]

IMMUNOSUPPRESSANTS: Based on animal and clinical studies, grapefruit may increase the absorption and plasma concentrations of immunosuppressants.ǁ Animal and clinical studies have reported increased blood levels of cyclosporine when taken with grapefruit.[75,99,100,102,129-135] A furanocoumarin found in grapefruit,

*References 46-48, 50, 53, 53, 55, 63-65.
†References 42, 46, 54, 56, 58, 65, 68.
§References 44, 78, 80, 82, 104-109, 127, 128.
ǁReferences 44, 75, 99, 100, 102, 129-136.

6′,7′-dihydroxybergamottin, does not appear to be responsible for the effects of grapefruit juice on cyclosporine; rather, inhibition of P-gp activity by other compounds in grapefruit juice may be responsible.[132] The bioavailability of tacrolimus (Prograf) has been shown clinically to double when coadministered with the CYP3A4 inhibitor ketoconazole.[102] In one case report, a liver transplant recipient experienced a considerable increase in the trough blood concentration of tacrolimus after concomitant ingestion of grapefruit juice.[136]

LEVOTHYROXINE: In humans, grapefruit juice may slightly delay the absorption of levothyroxine (Levoxyl, Synthroid), but it seems to have only a minor effect on its bioavailability.[137]

LICORICE: Both licorice and grapefruit inhibit the enzyme 11β-hydroxysteroid dehydrogenase, which oxidizes cortisol to inactive cortisone. It was suggested that licorice and grapefruit, if taken together, may increase the risk of high blood pressure and other side effects.[121]

OPIATES: Theoretically, grapefruit may interact with metabolism of opioids by the liver and small intestine CYP3A4 enzyme. Grapefruit has been shown to increase the bioavailability of methadone[111,112] and alfentanil[31] in patients. Grapefruit juice was not associated with any change in the intensity of withdrawal symptoms by the patients.[111]

P-GLYCOPROTEIN SUBSTRATES: P-gp is a cell membrane–associated protein that transports a variety of drug substrates. Interaction with P-gp, including activation, inhibition, and induction, can lead to altered plasma or brain levels of P-gp substrates. Grapefruit has been shown to inhibit P-gp, which may explain its numerous drug interactions.[126,132]

PRAZIQUANTEL (BILTRICIDE): There is a documented interaction between grapefruit and the anthelmintic drug praziquantel in humans.[92] The biotransformation of praziquantel appeared to be mediated mainly by CYP3A4, which is inhibited by grapefruit; thus, concomitant administration of grapefruit and praziquantel resulted in significantly altered pharmacokinetics of the drug.

PROTEASE INHIBITORS: Based on clinical studies, grapefruit may increase bioavailability and adverse effects of protease inhibitors.[83,116-118,138,139] There is some clinical evidence that grapefruit juice may lead to small changes in pharmacokinetic parameters (C_{max} and t_{max}) of amprenavir.[116]

RED WINE: Red wine in combination with grapefruit juice appears to have an additive inhibitory effect on CYP3A4, which may theoretically increase the risk for interactions with other agents.[140] In contrast, white wine does not appreciably inhibit CYP3A4 activity.

SILDENAFIL (VIAGRA): Grapefruit modestly increases the absorption of sildenafil and plasma concentration in humans.[79,103]

THEOPHYLLINE (BRONKODYL, ELIXOPHYLLIN, SLO-BID): Grapefruit juice seems to modestly decrease theophylline levels when administered to subjects concurrently with sustained-release theophylline.[120] The mechanism of action is not understood. However, clinical studies show that the ingestion of grapefruit juice should not cause any pharmacokinetic or pharmacodynamic interaction when coadministered with another methylxanthine, caffeine.[141-143] There was no significant difference in ambulatory systolic and diastolic blood pressure or heart rate when grapefruit juice was coadministered with caffeine.[143]

TONIC WATER: Grapefruit's inhibitory effect on CYP450 isoenzymes may alter the metabolism of quinine in tonic water.[144] Grapefruit in combination with tonic water containing quinine should be avoided in people with cardiac rhythm disorders, such as long-QT syndrome, that may worsen with quinine.

Greater Celandine (Chelidonium majus)

Pharmacokinetics

After intraperitoneal administration, Ukrain (semisynthetic anticancer drug that contains alkaloids from the plant *Cheladonium majus* conjugated with thiophosphoric acid) was distributed rapidly throughout the body and into plasma, with a biological half-life of approximately 60 minutes. It is excreted primarily unchanged in urine.[1]

Adverse effects

There have been several reports of mild to severe hepatotoxicity associated with the use of *Chelidonium majus*. However, these reports did not specify the type of herb preparation used, manner the herb was administered, quantity of the herb taken, or duration of treatment. Patients appear to recover fully on discontinuation of the herb, and reports of liver failure have been lacking.[2-8] Studies investigating Ukrain state that it is generally well tolerated with minimal side effects.[9-12] "No untoward side effects" were observed when mice were treated intravenously, subcutaneously, or intraperitoneally with Ukrain.[13] Ukrain exhibits toxicity toward malignant cells; however, some experts have presented evidence that Ukrain is equally toxic to normal, transformed, and malignant cell lines.[14,15]

Interactions

ANTIBODY LEVELS: Ukrain has been shown to lower the antiovalbumin IgE antibody response and decrease antigen-induced histamine release from mast cells in ovalbumin-sensitized mice.[16]

BLOOD GLUCOSE: Greater celandine has traditionally been used for the treatment of diabetes. However, administration of dried leaves of celandine (6.25% of diet by weight) to streptozotocin-induced diabetic rats did not affect the development of hyperphagia, polydipsia, body weight loss, hyperglycemia, or hypoinsulinemia.[17]

BONE MARKERS: Ukrain may have antiosteoporotic effects because of its "anabolic effect" on bone in ovariectomized rats. The proposed mechanism of action is a stimulating effect on gonadal hormone production, especially estrogen. However, the animal data on Ukrain's effects on bone metabolism are conflicting.[18-21]

CYCLOPHOSPHAMIDE (CYTOXAN): In patients with advanced esophageal cancer, the combination of *C. majus* and cyclophosphamide appeared to mask the immunological response of the host without causing the degeneration of cancer tissue seen in patients who took *C. majus* alone.[22]

CYTOKINES AND INFLAMMATORY MARKERS: In vitro research showed that the combination of greater celandine and recombinant interferon gamma (rIFN-γ) resulted in a marked cooperative induction of nitrous oxide (NO) production and a significant increase in tumor necrosis factor alpha (TNF-α) in mouse peritoneal macrophages.[23] Based on laboratory tests, stylopine, a major constituent of *Chelidonium majus* leaf, suppresses NO and prostaglandin E_2 (PGE_2) production in macrophages by inhibiting iNOS and COX-2 expressions.[24] These biological activities of stylopine may contribute to the antiinflammatory activity of *C. majus*. It has also been proposed that quaternary benzophenanthridine alkaloids from *C. majus* may play a role in the antiinflammatory activity.[25]

DOPAMINERGIC AGENTS: Research with intraperitoneal administration of Ukrain in rats has shown that one of the primary actions of Ukrain involves stimulation of the dopaminergic system.[26] Concurrent use of Ukrain with dopaminergic agents may result in altered effects.

INDOMETHACIN (INDOCIN): Based on animal studies, *C. majus* extract alone and in a combination with extracts from the plants *Iberis amara, Melissa officinalis, Matricaria recutita, Carum carvi, Mentha x piperita, Glycyrrhiza glabra, Angelica archangelica,* and *Silybum marianum* (STW-5; Iberogast) produced a dose-dependent protective effect against indomethacin-induced gastric ulcers in rats.[27]

LIVER FUNCTION TESTS: There have been several reports of mild to severe liver damage associated with the use of *C. majus*. Concomitant use of greater celandine with other hepatotoxic agents may increase the risk of liver damage.[2]

MAO INHIBITORS: The major alkaloids from plants such as greater celandine and agents such as Ukrain (thiophosphoric acid derivative of a sum of the alkaloids isolated from greater celandine) have been shown to be irreversible inhibitors of the oxidative deamination reaction of serotonin and tyramine catalyzed by rat liver mitochondrial MAO.[28] Chelironine and the drug Ukrain were the strongest inhibitors of the reaction among the agents studied and may interact with MAO inhibitors.

SEDATIVES AND CENTRAL NERVOUS SYSTEM DEPRESSANTS: In rats and mice, intraperitoneal administration of Ukrain potentiated the action of hexobarbital. In rats, intraperitoneal administration of Ukrain potentiated the action of amphetamine and apomorphine, but did not affect the action of haloperidol (Apokyn, Haldol).[26]

SEROTONERGIC AGENTS: Research with intraperitoneal Ukrain in rats has shown that one of the primary actions of Ukrain involves inhibition of the serotonergic system.[26] Interactions with other serotonergic agents are possible.

TURMERIC: Several weeks after ingesting a combination herbal preparation containing greater celandine and curcuma root, a 42-year-old woman developed jaundice from acute hepatitis.[5] Her clinical recovery was rapid after withdrawal of the medication, and within 2 months her hepatic functions had returned to normal. This report raises the question of a possible interaction between greater celandine and curcuma root; however, causality remains unclear.

VIRAL LEVELS: A substance isolated from the freshly prepared crude extract of *C. majus* has been shown to have antiretroviral activity against HIV-1 in vitro.[29]

WHITE BLOOD CELL COUNTS: The immunomodulating effects of Ukrain include improvements in total T-cell, T-helper, and NK-cell counts, a decrease in T-suppressor cells, and a normalization of the helper/suppressor (H/S) ratio in cancer patients.[9,10] Treatment of peritoneal exudates from macrophages from tumor-bearing mice with Ukrain restored their defective cytolytic response against DA-3 tumor cells. These data suggest that the in vivo antitumor effects of Ukrain may be caused in part by Ukrain's ability to restore the cytolytic function of macrophages.[13]

Green Tea. See Tea *(Camellia sinensis)*

Guarana *(Paullinia cupana)*

Pharmacokinetics

The pharmacokinetics of guarana is unclear and largely related to its caffeine content.

Adverse effects

Note: Because caffeine is a constituent of guarana, theoretically, adverse reactions associated with caffeine may be seen with guarana ingestion (see Caffeine).

Guarana is generally well tolerated. The majority of information related to adverse effects of guarana is based in theory on the adverse effect profile of caffeine.

Interactions

Note: Interactions associated with guarana are predominantly theoretical and generally based on the adverse effect profile of caffeine (see Caffeine).

EPHEDRA: Use of concomitant ephedra and guarana has been associated with a case of cerebral infarction.[1]

Guggul *(Commifora mukul)*

Pharmacokinetics: Insufficient available evidence.

Adverse effects

Standardized guggulipid is generally regarded as being safe in healthy adults at recommended doses for up to 6 months.[1,2] Gastrointestinal upset is the predominant adverse effect that has been described in humans, most often involving loose stools or diarrhea. Headache and restlessness are also frequent complaints.

Hypersensitivity skin reactions were noted in a clinical trial and occurred in 5 of 34 patients (15%) receiving 50 mg of guggulsterones three times daily and in 1 of 33 (3%) patients receiving 25 mg of guggulsterones three times daily. In most cases, reactions occurred within 48 hours of starting therapy and resolved spontaneously within 1 week of therapy discontinuation, although one patient required oral steroids.[3]

Interactions

ANTICOAGULANTS/ANTIPLATELETS: Guggulipid administration has been associated with inhibition of platelet aggregation and increased fibrinolysis.[4-7] However, clinical reports of such drug interactions are lacking.

BETA-ADRENERGIC AGENTS: Coadministration of guggulipid to humans has been reported to decrease the bioavailability of the beta-blocker propranolol.[8]

BLOOD LIPIDS: Multiple small trials report that guggul lowers serum lipid levels with regular use of guggulipid (decreasing cholesterol, triglycerides, and LDLs and increasing HDLs).[5,9-18]

DILTIAZEM (CARDIZEM, DILACOR, TIAZAC): Coadministration of guggulipid to humans has been found to decrease the bioavailability of the calcium channel blocker diltiazem.[8] The chemical structure of other calcium channel blockers is sufficiently distinct that guggul may not affect other members of this class.

THYROID HORMONES: Guggul may stimulate thyroid function and may alter test results.[19-21]

Gymnema *(Gymnema sylvestre)*

Pharmacokinetics: Insufficient available evidence.

Adverse effects

Aside from hypoglycemia and potentiation of the effects of hypoglycemic agents after chronic use of gymnema, few clinically significant adverse effects have been associated with oral gymnema in the available literature, in studies up to 20 months in duration.[1-5] Gymnema has been reported to possess a sweet taste–suppressing effect, attributed to the peptide gurmarin.[6-10] This effect may result from interference with Na^+,K^+-ATPase activity of taste receptors[10] or from neural inhibition.[7]

Interactions

BLOOD GLUCOSE: Gymnema has been shown to lower blood glucose in diabetic patients.[1-5] Multiple animal studies have also reported hypoglycemic effects.[5,11-16]

BLOOD LIPIDS: Reductions in levels of serum triglycerides, total cholesterol, VLDL, and LDL have been observed in animals after administration of gymnema.[17,18]

Hawthorn (*Crataegus* spp.)

Pharmacokinetics: Insufficient available evidence.

Adverse effects

Limited clinical research has reported few side effects associated with hawthorne use,[1] however, other study has reported side effects associated with hawthorn. A 24-week multicenter observational trial of 1011 cardiac patients reported 14 total adverse events.[2] A large surveillance study of 3664 patients with class I or II cardiac insufficiency confirmed a causal link to side effects in 22 patients.[3] Reported adverse events have been infrequent, mild, and transient. They include abdominal discomfort, nausea, tachycardia, palpitations, hypotension, dyspnea, headache, dizziness, fatigue, sweating, mild macular skin eruptions, sleepiness, and agitation.[2-5]

Interactions

ANTICOAGULANTS/ANTIPLATELETS: Hawthorn should be used cautiously with antiplatelet agents; it has been shown to inhibit thromboxane A_2 (TXA_2) biosynthesis in vitro.[6] Clinical evidence of this interaction is lacking.

ANTIHYPERTENSIVE AGENTS: In a recent cross-sectional, point-of-care survey of 1818 patients, one case was identified as a potentially clinically significant interaction between hawthorn and antihypertensive agents.[7]

BLOOD PRESSURE: Animal and clinical studies[8,9] suggest that hawthorn may affect blood pressure.

DIGOXIN: A clinical study of healthy volunteers did not detect statistically significant effects of hawthorn on digoxin, suggesting possible safe coadministration.[8] Data on safe and efficacious dosing in this setting are still limited. Hawthorn has been noted to potentiate the inotropic effects (contraction stimulating or contraction decreasing) associated with cardiac glycoside agents without toxicity in study of isolated guinea pig hearts.[10] Hawthorn has been used concomitantly with cardiac glycosides to decrease glycoside dosage and potential toxicity.[11-13]

Hibiscus (*Hibiscus* spp.)

Pharmacokinetics: Insufficient available evidence.

Adverse effects

Reported safety data on hibiscus are limited, although it is popularly used as a tea. Hibiscus should be avoided in patients allergic or hypersensitive to hibiscus or its constituents.

Interactions

ACETAMINOPHEN (TYLENOL): A hibiscus drink has been shown to alter the half-life of acetaminophen in human volunteers.[1]

BLOOD PRESSURE: Hibiscus has been shown clinically to lower systolic and diastolic blood pressure.[2,3]

ESTROGENIC AGENTS: Hibiscus may have estrogenic activity, although the clinical significance is unclear.[4] Interactions with other estrogenic agents are possible.

HISTOLOGICAL TESTS: Hibiscus has shown anticancer effects in laboratory and animal studies[5-8] and theoretically may interact with antineoplastic agents.

KIDNEY FUNCTION TESTS: In healthy men, consumption of *Hibiscus sabdariffa* resulted in significant decreases in the urinary concentrations of creatinine, uric acid, citrate, tartrate, calcium, sodium, potassium, and phosphate, but not oxalate.[10]

QUININES: A hibiscus beverage has been shown to reduce the efficacy of quinine and chloroquine in human volunteers.[9]

VIRAL LEVELS: Antiviral effects of hibiscus have been observed in preliminary laboratory studies.[8]

Holy Basil (*Ocimum sanctum*)

Pharmacokinetics: Insufficient available evidence.

Adverse effects

Holy basil seems to be well tolerated in most people and has "generally recognized as safe" (GRAS) status in the United States. Based on animal studies, holy basil has demonstrated antispermatogenic and antifertility effects.[1-4]

Interactions

ANTICOAGULANTS/ANTIPLATELETS: Based on animal studies, holy basil may increase bleeding time.[5] However, clinical reports of such drug interactions are lacking.

BENZODIAZEPINES: In animals, holy basil has been shown to reduce the effects of diazepam (Valium).[6]

BLOOD GLUCOSE: Holy basil may have hypoglycemic properties, as demonstrated by clinical[7] and numerous animal studies. Proposed mechanisms of action include lowering corticosteroid levels, as demonstrated in vivo,[8] and stimulating insulin release, as shown in vitro.[9]

BLOOD LIPIDS: Based on animal research, holy basil may reduce serum lipid levels.[10]

CHOLINERGIC AGENTS: In animals, holy basil has been shown to reduce the effects of scopolamine.[6]

CYTOCHROME P450 SUBSTRATES: Based on animal studies, holy basil may inhibit CYP450 metabolism.[11] Caution is warranted when using holy basil with agents metabolized by this system.

SEDATIVES AND CENTRAL NERVOUS SYSTEM DEPRESSANTS: In animal studies, holy basil synergistically enhanced the sedative effects of pentobarbital, possibly through dopaminergic mechanisms.[5,6,12]

Hop (*Humulus lupulus*)

Pharmacokinetics: Insufficient available evidence.

Adverse effects

Based on traditional use and available clinical trials, no reported serious adverse effects have been associated with hop.[1,2] Hop may possess mild CNS depressant activities, particularly when used concomitantly with other CNS depressants.[3-5]

Phytoestrogens in hop may exert estrogenic agonist or antagonist properties, with unclear effects on hormone-sensitive conditions, such as breast, uterine, cervical, or prostate cancer or endometriosis.[6-9]

Interactions

BLOOD GLUCOSE: Animal studies show that hop both increases and decreases blood glucose levels.[10]

CYTOCHROME P450 SUBSTRATES: In vitro and in vivo studies have demonstrated induction of CYP3A and CYP2B by hop.[11-13] Hop may cause decreased plasma levels of agents metabolized by one or more of these enzymes.

ESTROGENIC AGENTS: Because the phytoestrogens in hop may exert estrogenic agonist or antagonist properties, hop should be used cautiously in patients receiving estrogen therapy. However, clinical evidence of interaction is lacking.

SEDATIVES AND CENTRAL NERVOUS SYSTEM DEPRESSANTS: Hop may cause drowsiness and theoretically may cause additive effects when used with other sedatives.

Horny Goat Weed (Epimedium grandiflorum)

Pharmacokinetics: Insufficient available evidence.

Adverse effects

In general, horny goat weed is well tolerated. Gastrointestinal side effects, including nausea, vomiting, and dry mouth, are the most common.[1] Based on anecdote, tachyarrhythmia may occur in individuals using products that contain horny goat weed,[2] which may dilate coronary vessels and lower blood pressure. Long-term use might cause aggressiveness or irritability. Large doses of Japanese *Epimedium* have been suggested to cause respiratory arrest.[3]

Interactions

ANTIBODY LEVELS: Based on research conducted in animals, the plant flavonoid baohuoside-1 (B-1), isolated from *Epimedium davidii*, may suppress antibody and delayed-type hypersensitivity responses.[4]

BLOOD LIPIDS: Horny goat weed may lower cholesterol.[1]

BLOOD PRESSURE: *Epimedium* may have hypotensive effects.[1]

CREATININE: In animals, *Epimedium sagittatum* decreased serum creatinine level.[5]

CYTOKINES AND INFLAMMATORY MARKERS: Horny goat weed may increase IL-2, IL-3, and IL-2 receptors. Based on human studies, horny goat weed may inhibit interleukin-6 (IL-6).[6] Theoretically, horny goat weed may interact with interleukin therapy.

ESTROGENIC AGENTS: Horny goat weed has been shown in vitro to have estrogenic activity.[7-11] Theoretically, it may interact with estrogen therapy and have additive effects.

HOMOCYSTEINE: Horny goat weed may increase or decrease homocysteine levels.[12]

KIDNEY FUNCTION TESTS: In animals, *E. sagittatum* decreased BUN level.[5]

MONAMINERGIC AGENTS: In animals, *Epimedium brevicorum* has been shown to inhibit MAO activity in the hypothalamus.[13] Horny goat weed should be avoided in patients using MAO inhibitors.

TESTOSTERONE: Horny goat weed may increase testosterone activity.[7-11]

THYROID HORMONES: Based on animal studies, prolonged use of excessive amounts of horny goat weed may be associated with decreased thyroid activity and T_3 and increased rT_3 and TRH.[14] Theoretically, horny goat weed may interact with thyroid hormones.

Horseradish (Armoracia rusticana, syn. Cochlearia armoracia)

Pharmacokinetics: Insufficient available evidence.

Adverse effects

There are few reported adverse effects associated with horseradish. Large oral doses can cause gastrointestinal upset, bloody vomiting, diarrhea, and irritation of mucous membranes and urinary tract. Topically, skin contact with fresh horseradish can cause irritation, blistering, or allergic reactions.

Interactions

ANTICOAGULANTS/ANTIPLATELETS: In animals, intravenous horseradish peroxidase has been shown to stimulate arachidonic acid metabolism and affect platelet aggregation.[1] However, clinical reports of drug interactions are lacking.

ANTIOXIDANTS: Based on in vitro study, horseradish root may have oxidative activity[2,3] and may counter the effects of antioxidants.

BACTERIAL LEVELS: Based on several early in vitro studies and one clinical trial, horseradish may have antimicrobial activity.[2,4-7]

BLOOD PRESSURE: In animals, horseradish in medicinal amounts has hypotensive activity.[1,8] Theoretically, concomitant use of horseradish and antihypertensive agents may result in additive blood pressure–lowering effects.

CYTOKINES AND INFLAMMATORY MARKERS: Horseradish has been demonstrated in vitro to inhibit COX-1 enzymes.[2,4]

ELECTROLYTES: Based on traditional use, horseradish may have strong diuretic effects.[14-16] Overuse may lead to electrolyte imbalance.

HISTOLOGICAL TESTS: Based on in vitro and animal studies, horseradish may have antineoplastic activity.[2,9-20] Theoretically, horseradish may interact with antineoplastic agents.

THYROID HORMONES: Based on in vitro evidence,[21] medicinal amounts of horseradish may alter thyroid hormone levels.

Horsetail (Equisetum spp.)

Pharmacokinetics: Insufficient available evidence.

Adverse effects

Horsetail has been associated with few reports of adverse effects. It is more often used in Germany and Canada, where it is regarded as generally safe when taken in therapeutic doses (300-mg capsule three times daily as needed to a maximum of 6 g daily). However, the silicon component of horsetail has the potential to break down thiamine and cause thiamine deficiency.[1] Horsetail contains small amounts of nicotine, which has numerous known adverse effects. Because of its diuretic activity, horsetail may increase potassium excretion, and very low potassium levels may cause arrhythmias.

Interactions

BLOOD GLUCOSE: *Equisetum myriochaetum* has reportedly caused low blood sugar levels in type 2 diabetic patients.[2] Effects of *Equisetum arvense* are not clear.

CORTICOSTEROIDS: Use of horsetail with corticosteroids that decrease potassium may theoretically cause hypokalemia. However, reports of this interaction have not been documented in the available literature.

ELECTROLYTES: Horsetail is believed to act as a weak diuretic because of equisetonin and flavone glycosides and has been demonstrated to act as a diuretic in humans.[3] Fluid loss and electrolyte imbalance may result with excessive use.

POTASSIUM: Horsetail possesses potassium-depleting properties and may alter electrolyte balance.

THIAMINE: The silicon component of horsetail can break down thiamine and may cause thiamine deficiency, as demonstrated only in animal observations.[1] Currently, clinical cases documenting this interaction are lacking.

Jackfruit (Artocarpus heterophyllus)

Pharmacokinetics: Insufficient available evidence.

Adverse effects

Jackfruit has few reported side effects. Patients with birch pollen–related allergies may be allergic to jackfruit as well.[1] According to animal research, jackfruit may cause decreased libido and altered sexual arousal, vigor, and performance.[2] However, jackfruit seeds do not appear to alter ejaculating competence and fertility. The lectins in jackfruit seeds have demonstrated hemagglutination activity and may affect blood clotting.[3,4]

Interactions

ANTIBODY LEVELS: Jackfruit and jackfruit seed lectins may selectively bind to IgA-1 in animals[5-7] and theoretically may alter test results.

ANTICOAGULANTS/ANTIPLATELETS: In vitro research has shown that jacalin extracted from jackfruit seeds was strongly erythroagglutinating but was nonspecific for A1-B0 erythrocytes.[4] This finding supports the effective hemagglutination produced by jacalin in Rhesus monkeys and humans. In another in vitro study, jackin also extracted from jackfruit seeds induced hemagglutination in human and rabbit erythrocytes.[3] Jackfruit seeds theoretically may antagonize the effects of anticoagulants/antiplatelets; however, clinical evidence is lacking.

BACTERIAL LEVELS: Various parts of the jackfruit plant have exhibited broad-spectrum antibacterial activity.[8]

BLOOD GLUCOSE: Based on clinical research, jackfruit leaves may improve glucose tolerance[9] and may affect blood glucose tests.

FUNGAL LEVELS: Jackfruit may inhibit the growth of various types of fungi (e.g., *Fusarium moniliforme*).[3]

VIRAL LEVELS: Based on in vitro research, jackfruit may inhibit the activity of various viruses, including herpes simplex virus type 2, varicella-zoster virus, and cytomegalovirus.[10]

WHITE BLOOD CELL COUNTS: Based on several in vitro studies, jackfruit and jackfruit seeds may have immunostimulative effects.[4,5,10-13] Theoretically, jackfruit may affect WBC counts.

Jiaogulan (Gynostemma pentaphyllum)

Pharmacokinetics: Insufficient available evidence.

Adverse effects: Insufficient available evidence.

Interactions

ANTICOAGULANTS/ANTIPLATELETS: Based on in vitro research, *Gynostemma pentaphyllum* may significantly inhibit platelet aggregation, accelerate disaggregation, and inhibit thrombosis. Conversely, *G. pentaphyllum* may contain a platelet aggregation factor.[1] Clinical reports of such drug interactions are lacking.

BLOOD GLUCOSE: Based on clinical research involving patients with nonalcoholic fatty liver disease, *G. pentaphyllum* may decrease insulin levels and insulin index scores.[2]

BLOOD LIPIDS: Based on clinical research involving patients with nonalcoholic fatty liver disease, *G. pentaphyllum* may decrease serum triglyceride levels.[2] In vitro research reports that *G. pentaphyllum* may activate liver X receptors, which play an important role in cholesterol homeostasis by serving as regulatory sensors of tissue cholesterol levels.[3]

CYTOKINES AND INFLAMMATORY MARKERS: Based on in vitro research, *G. pentaphyllum* may inhibit activation of nuclear factor kappa B (NF-κB), an important inflammatory factor.[4] Jiaogulan may interact with antiinflammatory agents. Clinical reports of such drug interactions are lacking.

HISTOLOGICAL TESTS: Based on in vitro studies, gypenosides extracted from *G. pentaphyllum* may have anticancer effects, such as decreasing cancer cell viability, arresting the cell cycle, and inducing apoptosis.[2,5-7] Jiaogulan may interact with antineoplastic agents.

LIVER FUNCTION TESTS: Based on clinical research involving patients with nonalcoholic fatty liver disease, *G. pentaphyllum* may decrease ALT, AST, or ALP levels.[2]

Jojoba (Simmondsia chinensis)

Pharmacokinetics: Insufficient available evidence.

Adverse effects

Topical jojoba oil may cause contact dermatitis.[1,2] Oral consumption of jojoba products intended for topical use should be avoided.

Interactions

BLOOD LIPIDS: The effects of jojoba oil on blood cholesterol levels have been demonstrated in animals.[3]

CYTOKINES AND INFLAMMATORY MARKERS: Jojoba has displayed antiinflammatory effects in animal and in vitro studies.[4]

GROWTH HORMONE: GH levels have been increased in animals fed 4% jojoba meal.[5]

THYROID HORMONES: Thyroxine levels increased and triiodothyronine levels decreased in animals fed 4% jojoba meal.[5]

WHITE BLOOD CELL COUNTS: In animals fed jojoba oil for 4 weeks (2.2%-9% of diet), there was a dose-related increase in WBC count.[6]

Kava (Piper methysticum)

Pharmacokinetics

The pharmacokinetic actions of kava are not well understood. Metabolites and unchanged lactones of kava are excreted in urine.[1]

Adverse effects

There is widespread concern regarding the potential hepatotoxicity of kava.[2-13] Many cases of liver damage have been reported in Europe, including hepatitis,[14-16] cirrhosis, fulminant liver failure,[17,18] and death.[19,20] These reports have been challenged, and researchers have maintained that kava is safe in most individuals at recommended doses.[21,22] Kava, when used for less than 1 to 2 months, has been generally regarded as safe and well tolerated.[23] The most common reported adverse effects are sedation, gastrointestinal complaints, and allergic rashes.[2,14-19,24-28] Chronic heavy use of kava has been associated with increased red blood corpuscle volume, reduced platelet size, and decreased lymphocyte counts.[29,30] Because kava may adversely affect the liver, it should be used with extreme caution in patients taking hepatotoxic agents because of an increased risk of liver damage.

Kava is still available in the United States, although the FDA has issued warnings to consumers and physicians.[6,7,31] It is unclear what dose or duration of use is correlated with the risk of liver damage, and whether the safety profile of kava is comparable to other agents used in the management of anxiety.

Interactions

ALBUMIN, TOTAL PROTEIN LEVELS: Chronic heavy use of kava has been associated with decreased albumin and total protein.[29] Causality is unclear and may involve poor nutrition in chronic kava users or hepatic damage.

ALCOHOL: Animal studies have demonstrated marked increases in the hypnosedative effects of alcohol when taken in combination with kava.[32] However, this effect has not been confirmed in healthy human volunteers.[33]

ANTICOAGULANTS/ANTIPLATELETS: Racemic kavain, present in kava preparations, has been shown to have antiplatelet effects from cyclooxygenase inhibition and inhibition of thromboxane synthesis.[34] Chronic heavy use of kava has been associated with increased red blood corpuscle volume and reduced platelet size.[29] However, clinical reports of such drug interactions are lacking.

CYTOCHROME P450 SUBSTRATES: Preliminary evidence suggests that kava may significantly inhibit multiple CYP450 enzymes, including 2C9, 2D6, and 3A(4,5,7).[35,36]

DOPAMINERGIC AGENTS: Kava has been reported to antagonize the effect of dopamine and elicit extrapyramidal effects in animals.[37-39] Therefore, kava may interfere with the effects of dopamine or dopamine agonists and may exacerbate the extrapyramidal effects of dopaminergic antagonists such as droperidol, haloperidol, risperidol, and metoclopramide. Kava (Piper methysticum) increases "off" periods in Parkinson's disease patients taking levodopa and can cause a semicomatose state when given concomitantly with alprazolam.[40]

ECHINACEA: Multiple reports detail hepatotoxicity associated with kava, most often with heavy or chronic use. Caution should be exercised with concomitant use of Echinacea, which some natural medicine practitioners have warned may cause liver toxicity as well. However, no clear evidence from basic science or clinical reports indicates that Echinacea causes significant liver toxicity. This potential interaction remains theoretical.

ELECTROLYTES: Because kava has purported diuretic properties, it should not be taken with diuretic agents.

HEMATOCRIT: Chronic heavy use of kava has been associated with increased red blood corpuscle volume and reduced platelet size.[29] It is not clear if poor nutrition or iron deficiency coincides with chronic kava use, thus confounding these findings.

LIVER FUNCTION TESTS: Because kava may adversely affect the liver, LFT may be altered. Kava should be used with extreme caution in patients taking hepatotoxic agents because of an increased risk of liver damage.

SEDATIVES AND CENTRAL NERVOUS SYSTEM DEPRESSANTS: Kava may potentiate CNS depressants, including barbiturates and benzodiazepines.[41] Lethargy and disorientation were reported in a 54-year-old man taking kava in combination with alprazolam.[42] Kavalactones have been shown to potentiate the effects of CNS depressants, such as ethanol, benzodiazepines, low-potency neuroleptics, beta blockers, and barbiturates in animals, with concurrent use being potentially toxic.[32,43] In a recent cross-sectional, point-of-care survey of 1818 patients, seven cases were identified as potentially clinically significant interactions between kava and sedatives.[44]

TYRAMINE-CONTAINING FOODS/BEVERAGES: Tyramine-containing foods may pose a risk of hypertensive crisis if eaten while taking kava, a result of the MAO inhibitory activity of kava found in vitro.[26,45] However, this interaction has not been reported in humans.

WHITE BLOOD CELL COUNTS: Chronic heavy use of kava has been associated with decreased lymphocyte counts.[29,30]

Kelp (Laminaria spp.). See Seaweed

Khat (Catha edulis)

Pharmacokinetics
When khat is chewed, absorption of cathinone is slow.[1] Cathinone is distributed in blood plasma; its plasma half-life is 90 minutes.[2] The primary metabolites are norpseudoephedrine, norephedrine, 3,6-dimethyl-2,5-diphenylpyrazine, and 1-phenyl-1,2-propanedione.[3-6] After oral administration, 22% to 52% of synthetic cathinone is excreted in 24-hour urine samples.[4] The half-life of khat was documented to be 260 ± 102 minutes.[1]

Adverse effects
Fresh khat leaves contain cathinone, a Schedule I drug under the Controlled Substances Act; however, the leaves typically begin to deteriorate after 48 hours, causing the chemical composition of the plant to break down.[2] Once this occurs, the leaves contain cathine, a controlled substance (Schedule IV).[7]

Based on historical use and available research, khat may increase blood pressure and heart rate[1,3-6,8-13] and cause insomnia, overalertness, constipation, dependency,[14] and psychosis.[15-20] Hemorrhoidal disease,[21] loss of appetite and anorexia,[16] gastritis, and malnutrition have also been associated with khat use.[15] There is a case report of fasciola hepatica (parasite) infection after chewing of khat leaves.[22] Khat chewing has also been associated with acute myocardial infarction[23] and oral carcinoma.[24]

Interactions
ALPHA-ADRENERGIC AGENTS: In one clinical study the effects of khat on urine flow rate were inhibited by indoramin (Baratol), an alpha blocker.[25]

ANTIBIOTICS: In a clinical study, khat chewing reduced urinary excretion of ampicillin and amoxicillin, possibly the result of formation of insoluble compounds between the tannins found in khat and the antibiotics.[26] These antibiotics should be administered 2 hours after khat chewing.

BLOOD PRESSURE: Khat has been reported to cause increases in systolic and diastolic blood pressure.[1,3-6,8-13]

CENTRAL NERVOUS SYSTEM STIMULANTS: Khat may cause CNS stimulation,[3] and use with other CNS stimulants may lead to additive effects.

DOPAMINERGIC AGENTS: Khat addiction has been successfully treated with the dopamine agonist bromocriptine.[27] A dose of 1.25 mg every 6 hours has been used, titrated downward over 4 weeks.[28]

HEART RATE: Khat has been reported to cause an increase in heart rate.[1,3-6,8-13]

Kiwi (Actinidia deliciosa, Actinidia chinensis)

Pharmacokinetics: Insufficient available evidence.

Adverse effects
No adverse effects were noted in athletes who consumed a kiwi-containing drink. Kiwi allergy is one of the more common allergies involving fruits, and caution is advised. There are numerous reports of allergy and cross-sensitization with kiwi and birch pollen, latex-containing plants, banana, avocado, chestnut figs, melons, nuts (hazelnuts), sesame seeds, poppy seeds, rye grain, flour, and grasses.[1-36]

Interactions
ANTICOAGULANTS/ANTIPLATELETS: Consuming two or three kiwi fruits daily for 28 days reduced platelet aggregation response in healthy human volunteers.[37] However, clinical reports of such drug interactions are lacking.

BLOOD LIPIDS: Kiwi fruit has reportedly lowered blood triglyceride levels by 15%.[37]

ELECTROLYTES: Kiwi contains potassium[38] and may alter electrolyte balance.

FUNGAL LEVELS: Based on preliminary laboratory data, kiwi may have antifungal activity[39] and may therefore alter or have an additive effect on other antifungal agents.

PHOSPHATASE TESTS: Kiwi fruit consumption caused false-positive results on a phosphate test, according to preliminary evidence.[40]

SEROTONERGIC AGENTS: Kiwi contains a high concentration of the neurotransmitter serotonin.[42] Concurrent use of kiwi with another agent that affects serotonin may increase the risk of serotonin syndrome, which is characterized by restlessness, loss of coordination, blood pressure changes, hallucinations, nausea, vomiting, increased body temperature, and overreactive reflexes.

URINE TESTS: Because of the serotonin content, kiwi may increase 5-hydroxyindoleacetic acid levels in the urine[36] and alter test results.

VITAMINS: Kiwi may increase the levels of vitamins in the body because of its high vitamin C[42,43] and vitamin E[38] content.

Kudzu (Pueraria lobata)

Pharmacokinetics

Puerarin is rapidly but incompletely absorbed from the gastrointestinal tract.[1,2] Based on animal research, crude extracts of diadzin from kudzu have approximately 10 times greater bioavailability than the pure compound, suggesting that other constituents in kudzu promote the update of diadzin.[3] When puerarin and daidzin were incubated for 24 hours with human intestinal bacteria, the metabolites daidzein and calycosin were produced.[4] At an early time, puerarin was converted to daidzin, then calycosin; the metabolic time course of daidzin was similar. Puerarin and daidzin were transformed to their aglycons (organic sugar compounds) by the bacteria producing β-glucuronidase, C-glycosidase, and β-glycosidase.[5] Puerarin is eliminated in the urine at a fairly rapid rate ($t_{1/2} \cong 4$ hours).[6]

Adverse effects

Currently, reports of side effects from oral kudzu are lacking. An allergic reaction has been reported after use of a combination herbal product containing kudzu. The patient developed a maculopapular eruption (bumpy skin rash) that started on the thighs and spread over the entire body and eventually led to hypothermia.[7]

Interactions

ALCOHOL: Kudzu extracts or individual isoflavones have been demonstrated to suppress alcohol intake in animal models of alcoholism.[8-12]

ANTICOAGULANTS/ANTIPLATELETS: Based on laboratory tests and animal studies, kudzu isoflavones possess antiplatelet activity.[5,13-20] Although documented interactions in humans are lacking, kudzu should be used cautiously to avoid bleeding risks.

BENZODIAZEPINES: In animals, kudzu has exhibited weak benzodiazepine agonism and reduced muscimol-stimulated chloride uptake by the benzodiazepine agonist flunitrazepam.[21]

BLOOD GLUCOSE: Based on animal studies, kudzu may lower blood glucose levels.[22]

BLOOD PRESSURE: Theoretically, kudzu may interact with hypotensive agents. Based on animal studies, kudzu possesses vasodilatory and hypotensive effects.[7,23-29]

BONE MARKERS: Based on in vitro research, puerarin may suppress bone resorption and promote bone formation in rats.[30]

CYTOCHROME P450 SUBSTRATES: Preliminary animal research suggests that kudzu inhibits and induces CYP450 isoenzymes. It is unclear which P450 isoenzymes are affected and to what degree.[31] Concurrent use of agents metabolized by the P450 liver enzyme system may result in altered therapeutic levels.

DOPAMINERGIC AGENTS: In animals the daidzin in kudzu has been shown to inhibit serotonin and dopamine metabolism.[32] Theoretically, concurrent use of kudzu with agents that affect the metabolism of serotonin and dopamine (e.g., MAO inhibitors) may lead to increased serotonin levels and increased risk of serotonin syndrome.

ESTROGENIC AGENTS: Laboratory tests and animal studies report that kudzu isoflavones have antiestrogenic activity.[27,33-39] Although clinical evidence of this interaction is lacking, kudzu should be used cautiously with agents that have estrogenic activity.

HEART RATE: In animal, the kudzu constituent daidzein has displayed antiarrhythmic properties.[40-43]

METHOTREXATE: Research conducted in rats has suggested that kudzu increases blood levels and decreases the body's elimination of methotrexate, an antineoplastic agent.[44]

NICOTINERGIC AGENTS: In animals, kudzu has been shown to weaken the effects of the nicotinic antagonist mecamylamine.[45]

PARATHYROID HORMONE: In animals, kudzu has been shown to decrease serum PTH levels.[46]

SEROTONERGIC AGENTS: In animals the daidzin in kudzu inhibits serotonin and dopamine metabolism.[36] Theoretically, concurrent use of kudzu with agents that affect the metabolism of serotonin and dopamine (e.g., MAO inhibitors) may lead to increased serotonin levels and increased risk of serotonin syndrome. The clinical relevance of this theoretical interaction is unclear.

THYROID HORMONE LEVELS: In animals, kudzu has been shown to increase TSH levels[47] and PTH levels.[46]

URINE TESTS: In animals, kudzu has been shown to increase urea nitrogen values.[47]

Lavender (Lavandula angustifolia)

Pharmacokinetics

Topically, lavender oil is quickly absorbed through the skin. The constituents linalool and linalyl acetate are detectable in the blood 5 minutes after topical application, reach peak levels at 19 minutes, and largely dissipate from the blood within 90 minutes of application.[1]

After oral administration, the constituents limonene and perillyl alcohol (POH) are metabolized into perillic acid (PA) and dihydroperillic acid (DHPA). In rats fed a diet containing POH or limonene, peak levels of PA were seen at 1 to 2.5 hours, peak levels of DHPA were noted at 2 to 3.5 hours, and half-life for each metabolite was 1 to 2 hours.[2] POH, PA, and DHPA are detectable in subjects' urine after high doses of POH ingestion. Approximately 9% of the total dose can be recovered in the first 24 hours. PA is the major metabolite found, with less than 1% of recovered POH.

Adverse effects

Common lavender use is 1 to 2 tsp of the herb taken as a tea (based on anecdote and expert opinion). The tea can be made by steeping 2 U.S. tsp (10 g) of leaves in 250 mL (1 cup) boiling water for 15 minutes. In recommended oral doses, lavender is generally considered to be well tolerated, with minimal adverse effects.[3-5]

Central nervous system depression has been noted with lavender aromatherapy,[6,7] including reports of significant deficits in working memory and impaired reaction times.[8] Additive narcotic effects have been noted in rats when oral lavender is taken concomitantly with barbiturates or chloral hydrate.[9,10] Headache has been observed in patients taking lavender tincture, which could be caused by the alcohol in the formulation (lavender 1:5 in 50% alcohol, 60 drops/day for 4 weeks).[11]

There have been case reports of mild dermatitis after use of topical lavender oil.[12] One individual developed an itchy dermatitis on his face after using lavender oil on his pillow;[13] patch testing subsequently confirmed a positive allergy to lavender. Photosensitization and changes in skin pigmentation have been reported after use of topical products containing lavender oil.[14,15]

Interactions

ANTICOAGULANTS/ANTIPLATELETS: Lavender contains varying amounts of coumarins[16] and therefore may theoretically increase the effects of blood-thinning agents. However, clinical evidence of this interation is lacking.

GABAERGIC AGENTS: Linalool, a monoterpene constituent of lavender, enhances GABAergic effects[17] and may intensify the sedative effects of gamma-aminobutyric acid (GABA)–specific antiepileptics and benzodiazepines.

IMIPRAMINE: Lavender may enhance the effects of antidepressant medications, as shown in a preliminary trial combining lavender with the TCA imipramine (Tofranil).[11]

SEDATIVES AND CENTRAL NERVOUS SYSTEM DEPRESSANTS: Lavender should be used cautiously in patients currently taking CNS depressants because concomitant use of lavender and pentobarbital or chloral hydrate significantly increased sleeping time and narcotic effects in animal studies.[9,10]

Lemon Balm *(Melissa officinalis)*

Pharmacokinetics: Insufficient available evidence.

Adverse effects

Lemon balm is included in the "generally recognized as safe" (GRAS) list of the U.S. Food and Drug Administration (FDA). Side effects are rare and generally mild, although research on long-term effects is limited. Mild side effects may include sleep disturbances and tiredness.[1]

Interactions

SEDATIVES AND CENTRAL NERVOUS SYSTEM DEPRESSANTS: Based on preclinical studies[2] and clinical research,[3] lemon balm may cause tiredness; thus, it should be used cautiously with other sedatives and alcohol. Clinical evidence of such an interaction is lacking.

SEROTONERGIC AGENTS: Lemon balm has been shown to inhibit brain concentrations of serotonin in vitro,[4] and therefore it may interact with agents whose primary action is to alter serotonin levels in vivo.

THYROID HORMONES: Lemon balm has been demonstrated to block binding of TSH to its receptor in human thyroid membranes.[5,6] These studies suggest that patients with thyroid problems, such as hypothyroidism, should use lemon balm cautiously because of the potential for thyroid hormone inhibition.

Lemongrass *(Cymbopogon* spp.*)*

Pharmacokinetics

The pharmacokinetics of lemongrass is not well understood. The metabolites of the citral component of lemongrass appear to be metabolized and eliminated rapidly in urine, with approximately 50% of the dose excreted in urine within 24 hours.[1] Beta-myrcene, an acyclic monoterpene in lemongrass oil, was found to induce cytochrome P450-2B1/2B2 isoenzymes in rats.[2,3]

Adverse effects

Lemongrass has "generally recognized as safe" (GRAS) status according to the U.S. Food and Drug Administration (FDA). Based on allergy tests, a common side effect of lemongrass oil is rash.[4-7]

Interactions

CYTOCHROME P450 SUBSTRATES: Beta-myrcene was found to induce CYP450-2B1/2B2 isoenzymes in rats.[2,3] Caution is warranted when considering concomitant use of lemongrass oil and other agents affected by these enzymes.

BLOOD GLUCOSE: Based on rat studies, lemongrass has shown hypoglycemic effects.[2,8] Caution should be used when administering lemongrass with blood sugar–lowering agents because of possible additive effects.

BLOOD LIPIDS: Lemongrass may have cholesterol-lowering effects.[9]

BLOOD PRESSURE: Based on in vitro and animal studies, lemongrass has shown blood pressure–lowering effects.[10-14] Caution should be used when taking lemongrass with antihypertensive agents because of possible additive effects.

LIVER FUNCTION TESTS: Based on clinical evidence, direct bilirubin and amylase levels were slightly elevated after a single dose or 2 weeks of daily oral administration of tea made from lemongrass.[15] However, the clinical significance of this finding is unclear.

Licorice *(Glycyrrhiza glabra)*

Pharmacokinetics

After oral administration, glycyrrhizin (active constituent of licorice) is metabolized to glycyrrhetinic acid by intestinal bacteria.[1] After intravenous administration of glycyrrhizin, both glycyrrhizin and glycyrrhetinic acid appear in the plasma. IV glycyrrhizin is metabolized in the liver by lysosomal beta-D-glucuronidase to 3-mono-glucuronide–glycyrrhetinic acid, which human liver is unable to metabolize to glycyrrhetinic acid; it is excreted with bile into the intestine, where bacteria metabolize it to glycyrrhetinic acid, which is reabsorbed.[2]

Adverse effects

Licorice contains glycyrrhizic acid, which is responsible for many of the reported side effects. Adverse effects from glycyrrhizin are primarily a result of hormonal and electrolyte disturbances. Possible effects include hypokalemia, hypernatremia, and metabolic alkalosis. Numerous cases of hypokalemia and hypertension have been associated with licorice use.[3,4] Metabolic abnormalities may also lead to irregular heartbeat, heart attack, kidney damage, muscle weakness, or muscle breakdown. Other side effects have included reduced body fat mass, decreased libido in men, and temporary vision problems. Serious, although rare, side effects reported with licorice use include acute pseudoaldosteronism syndrome, paralysis,[5] thyrotoxic periodic paralysis (TPP), metabolic alkalosis, seizure, and hypertensive encephalopathy with strokelike effects. Based on extensive in vivo and clinical evidence, a proposed acceptable daily intake is 0.015 to 0.229 mg glycyrrhizin/kg body weight.[6]

Deglycyrrhizinated licorice (DGL), used in many clinical trials, is free of glycyrrhizic acid and has had no significant reported adverse effects.

Interactions

BLOOD PRESSURE: Glycyrrhetinic acid derived from licorice has been demonstrated to inhibit renal 11β-hydroxysteroid dehydrogenase in vitro.[7] Licorice may increase blood pressure and theoretically may reduce the effects of antihypertensive agents.

CARDIAC GLYCOSIDES: Concurrent use of licorice with cardiac glycosides has been suggested to increase the risk of cardiac toxicity.[8]

CORTICOSTEROIDS: Numerous studies have shown that glycyrrhyzin inhibits 11β-hydroxysteroid dehydrogenase, the enzyme responsible for deactivating cortisol. Thus, long-term ingestion or overuse of licorice can produce hypermineralocorticoid-like effects in both animals and humans.[6] Licorice has also been shown in humans to potentiate the effects of topical hydrocortisone.[9]

CYTOCHROME P450 SUBSTRATES: There is conflicting evidence regarding the effect of licorice on CYP450 enzymes.[10,11] Licorice has been shown to induce and inhibit 2B6, 2C9, and 3A4.[11]

GRAPEFRUIT: Grapefruit may enhance the mineralocorticoid effect of licorice by blocking the conversion of cortisol to cortisone.[12]

HORMONE LEVELS: Licorice has been shown to alter the levels of numerous endogenous hormones[6] and may affect hormone therapy.

MILK: Hypercalcemia and renal failure were reported in a patient taking Caved-S (DGL product) and daily milk products.[13]

POTASSIUM: Licorice may deplete potassium, and overuse (or concurrent diuretic/laxative use) has been implicated in hypokalemia in numerous case reports.[6,14]

Lime (Citrus aurantifolia)

Pharmacokinetics: Insufficient available evidence.

Adverse effects

Lime juice, peel, and oil are generally considered safe to consume in food amounts. Rare reported side effects include photosensitivity, headaches, diarrhea, and dental effects (erosive effects on teeth).[1-5]

Interactions

ANTICOAGULANTS/ANTIPLATELETS: The furocoumarin content of lime juice may potentiate the action of anticoagulant/antiplatelet agents. However, clinical evidence of such an interaction is lacking.

CYTOCHROME P450 SUBSTRATES: Lime juice may inhibit CYP3A4,[3,6,7] causing increased drug levels and potentially increasing the risk of adverse effects.

DIGOXIN: As shown in vitro, fresh lime juice in concentrations greater than 5% may increase the transport of digoxin across cell membranes.[8]

FELODIPINE: In certain individuals, concomitant consumption of lime juice increased concentrations of the calcium channel blocker felodipine, presumably through CYP3A4 inhibition.[6]

GRAPEFRUIT: Bergamottin, a furocoumarin, is found in both grapefruit and lime juice,[6] and interactions may occur with concomitant use. Although bergamottin has not been studied extensively in lime, the concentrations found in lime juice are higher than those found in grapefruit juice. It has been proposed that bergamottin may interact with agents by competitive inhibition or mechanism-based inactivation.

IRON: Conflicting evidence exists as to whether ascorbic acid in limeade affects iron absorption. Although preliminary evidence suggests that lime may increase absorption of iron supplements, a randomized clinical trial (RCT) showed that ascorbic acid and limeade were unable to increase absorption of iron from food sources in nonpregnant women.[9]

MANNITOL: In vitro, 30% concentration of lime juice enhanced the absorption of ^{14}C-mannitol across cell lines by sixfold and eightfold.[10]

PHOTOSENSITIZING AGENTS: Because of the furocoumarin (psoralen) content of lemon oil,[2,11] lime oil may likewise increase the risk of phototoxicity.

Lingonberry (Vaccinium vitis-idaea)

Pharmacokinetics: Insufficient available evidence.

Adverse effects

Few adverse effects with lingonberry have been reported. However, animal research indicates that *Vaccinium vitis* leaf extract may adversely affect the male reproductive system.[1]

Interactions

ANDROGENIC AGENTS: *Vaccinium vitis* leaf extract has shown antigonadotropic effects in male frogs.[1]

CRANBERRY JUICE: A clinical trial reported that consumption of cranberry-lingonberry juice concentrate may significantly reduce the recurrence of urinary tract infections.[2]

CYTOKINES AND INFLAMMATORY MARKERS: Lingonberry has demonstrated antiinflammatory effects in vitro[3] and in animals[4] and may alter markers of inflammation such as C-reactive protein. Erythrocyte sedimentation rate, a nonspecific measure of inflammation, may be affected by lingonberry.

Maca (Lepidium meyenii)

Pharmacokinetics: Insufficient available evidence.

Adverse effects

It is recommended that fresh maca be consumed after boiling; otherwise it may cause stomach pain.[1] In clinical studies using up to 3 g daily for 12 weeks, no adverse effects were reported.[2,3] No side effects were noted in these trials, and maca was generally well tolerated. However, clinical studies have used only male subjects.

Interactions

ANTICOAGULANTS/ANTIPLATELETS: Plants in the Brassicaceae family are often rich in vitamin K, which may decrease the effects of warfarin; specific interactions with maca are unclear.

BLOOD PRESSURE: The maca constituent (1R,3S)-1-methyltetrahydro-β-carboline-3-carboxylic acid[4] is reportedly a CNS stimulant; thus, maca may affect blood pressure.

CENTRAL NERVOUS SYSTEM STIMULANTS: Because maca contains constituents that may act as CNS stimulants,[4] it may lead to additive or synergistic effects when used with other stimulants.

ESTROGENIC AGENTS: Both methanol and aqueous extracts of maca have shown estrogenic activity comparable with that of silymarin in a human breast cancer MCF-7 cell line.[5] However, clinical evidence of such an interaction is lacking.

Maitake Mushroom (Grifola frondosa)

Pharmacokinetics

The pharmacokinetics of maitake mushroom is not well understood. In animals, beta-glucans from maitake mushroom were distributed to the liver and spleen with a prolonged half-life.[1]

Adverse effects
The side effects of maitake mushroom are largely unknown because research is lacking. Safety in low doses is often assumed based on maitake's traditional use as a food.

Interactions
BLOOD GLUCOSE: Multiple animal studies have demonstrated hypoglycemic effects of maitake mushroom extracts. In insulin-resistant mice, a water-soluble maitake extract (Fraction X) has been associated with enhanced peripheral insulin sensitivity.[2] Decreased blood glucose levels and glucosuria and elevated serum insulin levels have been found with dietary maitake extract in experimental diabetic mice.[3,4] Maitake mushroom has also shown possible hypoglycemic effects in type 2 diabetes patients.[5]

BLOOD PRESSURE: Animal studies have shown reduced blood pressure with chronic oral use of maitake mushroom (8-10 weeks).[6,7] Theoretically, concomitant use of maitake mushroom and antihypertensive agents may cause additive blood pressure–lowering effects.

CYTOKINES AND INFLAMMATORY MARKERS: The D-fraction beta-glucan of maitake mushroom was shown in vitro to induce interferon gamma (IFN-γ), interleukin-12 (IL-12), p70, and IL-18, but suppress IL-4.[8] In mice, maitake beta-glucans enhanced NO synthesis by peritoneal macrophages through an IFN-γ–mediated mechanism.[9] In vitro, maitake was shown to synergize with IFN-α to inhibit hepatitis B virus (HBV) replication.[10]

HISTOLOGICAL TESTS: Animal studies have demonstrated that maitake extracts stimulate immune function and may prompt host-mediated antitumor activity.[11,12] Multiple antitumor mechanisms have been proposed based on results of in vitro and animal research.[9,13-23] Histological test results may be altered; however, systematic clinical evidence is lacking in this area.

VIRAL LEVELS: In vitro, maitake was shown to synergize with IFN-α to inhibit HBV replication.[10] A novel protein isolated from maitake was shown to inhibit herpes simplex virus 1 (HSV-1) replication in vitro and in mice.[24]

WHITE BLOOD CELL COUNTS: In vitro carcinoma models showed that the D-fraction beta-glucan of maitake mushroom shifted the balance between T-lymphocyte subsets from Th2 dominance to Th1 dominance.[8]

Mastic *(Pistacia lentiscus)*

Pharmacokinetics: Insufficient available evidence.

Adverse effects
Mastic was well tolerated in oral doses up to 2 g daily for up to 4 weeks to treat gastric or duodenal ulcer.[1,2] There were no reports of adverse effects in 44 patients participating in the available clinical trials at these doses.

Interactions
GENERAL: Available data are insufficient to identify any clinically important mastic/drug interactions.

BLOOD PRESSURE: In animals, extracts from *Pistacia lentiscus* have been shown to decrease diastolic, systolic, and mean arterial pressure with no change in heart rate in normotensive patients.[3,4]

Milk Thistle *(Silybum marianum)*

Pharmacokinetics
Bioavailability of orally administered silibinin, a constituent of milk thistle, ranges from 23% to 47% and appears to be higher when administered in a soft-gel capsule.[1] About 10% of silibinin was distributed in plasma.[2] The half-life of silibinin and silymarin is reported as less than 4 hours. Less than 3% of the free or conjugated form of silibinin is recovered in the urine.[1]

Adverse effects
In clinical trials and traditional use, oral milk thistle has generally been reported as well tolerated in recommended doses for up to 6 years. Several studies report mild gastrointestinal symptoms, including nausea, heartburn, diarrhea, epigastric pain, abdominal discomfort, dyspepsia, flatulence, and loss of appetite.[3-12] Urticaria, eczema, and headache have also been reported.[4,8,13,14] Hypersensitivity and anaphylactic reactions have been associated with milk thistle ingestion in case reports.[15-18]

Because many patients in available clinical trials have liver disease, it is unclear whether adverse effects are caused by milk thistle or by underlying liver disease; the rates of adverse effects are often similar to placebo.

Interactions
ALCOHOL: Milk thistle may reduce hepatotoxicity associated with ethanol ingestion.[19]

ANTINEOPLASTIC AGENTS: In cultured prostate carcinoma cells, silibinin has been shown to increase the efficacy of platinum compounds (cisplatin, carboplatin)[20] and doxorubicin.[21]

BLOOD GLUCOSE: Silymarin has been reported to decrease fasting plasma glucose, HbA_{1c}, and fasting insulin levels in patients with insulin-dependent diabetes associated with cirrhosis.[22] Concomitant use with other hypoglycemic agents may require dose adjustment.

BLOOD LIPIDS: Milk thistle may have cholesterol-lowering effects in humans.[23,24]

CYTOCHROME P450 SUBSTRATES: Data from in vivo and in vitro studies suggest inhibition of CYP450 3A4 and 2C9 to varying levels.[25,26] Caution is warranted because milk thistle may increase levels of agents metabolized by 3A4 and 2C9.

ESTROGENIC AGENTS: It has been suggested that silymarin may increase the clearance of estrogen by inhibiting β-glucuronidase activity.[27]

INDINAVIR: Although preclinical research suggests that milk thistle may inhibit CYP3A4 and potentially increase indinavir (Crixivan) levels,[26] milk thistle does not appear to affect the pharmacokinetics of indinavir in healthy volunteers.[28]

LIVER FUNCTION TESTS: Milk thistle may reduce hepatotoxicity associated with ethanol ingestion.[19]

URIDINE DIPHOSPHOGLUCURONOSYL TRANSFERASE SUBSTRATES: UGT is the primary phase II enzyme for the metabolism of several drugs. Silymarin has been shown to inhibit UGT in vitro[26] and may increase toxicity of drugs metabolized by this enzyme.

VITAMIN E: Silymarin and vitamin E have been reported to prevent amiodarone toxicity in animal studies.

Mistletoe *(Viscum album)*

Pharmacokinetics
The pharmacokinetics of mistletoe has not been thoroughly studied. However, a Phase I clinical trial in Germany revealed a

half-life of 13 minutes (and linear kinetics on doses ≥1600 ng/kg) for aviscumine.[1]

Adverse effects

Mistletoe is contraindicated in patients with protein hypersensitivity or chronic progressive infections (e.g., tuberculosis). It should also be avoided in patients with acute, highly febrile, inflammatory disease.[2] Most clinical trials were performed with unfractionated extracts, which contain numerous components, and were standardized primarily by the ML-1 lectin content.[3] This compound is believed to possess the properties of the active ingredient, although it is not necessarily the cause of adverse reactions. The minimal number of studies employing pure or purified ingredients makes it difficult to ascribe adverse effects to any one component of the mistletoe extracts.

Parenteral administrations of mistletoe may be accompanied by mild side effects, most of which are transient. The most common reactions were erythema and hyperemia.[2] Five patients in a Phase III clinical trial using Iscador-M discontinued the study because of World Health Organization (WHO) grade 3 to 4 toxicities (e.g., anorexia, general malaise, depressive moods, fever, and local skin inflammation at injection site).[4] In a Phase II trial with 23 patients, 34.8% had drug-related fever, 13.1% erythyema at injection site, and 17.4% pain at injection site. No drug-related discontinuation or toxic deaths occurred.[5]

Seizures have been reported anecdotally in poison control centers after ingestion of crude mistletoe plant material. Therefore, mistletoe may theoretically increase the risk of seizures.[6-12] Mydriasis and myosis/myalgia have been observed in patients using mistletoe.[7] Alleged adverse side effects and complications with mistletoe use also include dehydration.[2] Elevations of liver enzymes have been reported with high doses of mistletoe.[8]

Interactions

AGENTS THAT LOWER SEIZURE THRESHOLD: Anecdotal reports of seizures at poison control centers followed ingestion of crude mistletoe plant material.[6-12] Because mistletoe may theoretically increase the risk of seizures; concomitant use with other agents that lower seizure threshold should be avoided.

ANTICOAGULANTS/ANTIPLATELETS: A galactose-specific lectin has been shown to promote blood cell aggregation in vitro.[13] Mistletoe may thus interact with anticoagulants, athough clinical evidence is lacking.

BLOOD GLUCOSE: Chemicals in mistletoe contribute to insulin release, which lowers glucose levels.[14]

BLOOD PRESSURE: Mistletoe has been shown to cause hypertension and hypotension.[7,15] According to secondary sources, concomitant use of mistletoe with antihypertensive agents may result in enhanced hypotensive effects of antihypertensive drugs. One clinical trial reported both hypertension and hypotension as adverse effects.[7]

BUSULPHAN: Busulphan and mistletoe extract (Helixor) have been implicated in one case study involving organ fibrosis and death.[16] Although an interaction was possible, the mechanism remains unclear.

CHOLINERGIC AGENTS: According to secondary sources, concomitant use of mistletoe with agents used to treat glaucoma (cholinergics) may cause increased myosis from additive adverse effects.

CREATININE: Increased serum creatinine levels have been reported with mistletoe use.[17]

GARLIC: According to secondary sources, concomitant use of garlic and mistletoe may result in additive hypotensive action.

HAWTHORN (CRATAEGUS OXYACANTHA): According to secondary sources, concomitant use of hawthorn and mistletoe may result in additive hypotensive action.

IMMUNOMODULATORS: Mistletoe may stimulate the immune system and interfere with immunomodulating agents.[6,18,19]

KIDNEY FUNCTION TESTS: An increase in blood urea nitrogen (BUN) has been noted.[17]

LIME TREE (TILIA PLATYPHYLLOS): According to secondary sources, concomitant use of lime tree and mistletoe may result in additive hypotensive action.

LIVER FUNCTION TESTS: Elevated liver enzymes have been reported with high doses of mistletoe.[8] Caution is warranted with concomitant use of mistletoe and other hepatotoxic agents.

MONOAMINERGIC AGENTS MAO: Because of the tyramine content of mistletoe,[2] concomitant use of mistletoe and MAO inhibitors may increase the risks of hypertensive crisis.

SEDATIVES AND CENTRAL NERVOUS SYSTEM DEPRESSANTS: Concomitant use of mistletoe with CNS depressants has been suggested to enhance sedative effects.[6-12]

THYROID HORMONES: The manufacturer of Iscador noted that mistletoe may cause an inflammatory reaction when used during untreated hyperthyroidism.[20] Thyroid hormone levels may be altered. Caution is advised with mistletoe use in patients taking thyroid agents.

TOTAL SERUM PROTEIN: A slight decrease in total protein caused by a minor decrease in albumin concentration has been noted in clinical studies.[17]

TYRAMINE-CONTAINING FOODS: Mistletoe contains tyramine. Theoretically, mistletoe may interact with tyramine-containing foods, including red wine, cheeses, or aged foods, and may cause reactions that include hypertensive urgency.

WHITE BLOOD CELL COUNTS: An increase in CD3/25+ lymphocytes has been reported.[21] Increases in eosinophils have also been noted in patients using mistletoe.[12,17,22-25]

Modified Citrus Pectin

Pharmacokinetics

Although pectins are not digestible by humans,[1] modified citrus pectin (MCP) is altered to increase absorption. Pectin from citrus rinds is depolymerized through a treatment with sodium hydroxide and hydrochloric acid. The resultant smaller molecule comprises predominantly D-polygalacturonates, which may be more easily absorbed by the human digestive system.

Adverse effects

Few MCP-associated adverse effects have been reported. Like other dietary fibers, MCP may cause gastrointestinal adverse effects.

Interactions

BLOOD LIPIDS: Based on preliminary animal studies, pectin may lower cholesterol levels.[2-4]

HISTOLOGICAL TESTS: In animals, MCP has significantly inhibited carbohydrate-mediated tumor growth.[5-8]

ORAL AGENTS: As a form of dietary fiber, MCP may slow or reduce the absorption of oral agents; however, clinical evidence of such an interaction is lacking. Patients are recommended to take MCP 1 hour before or 2 hours after the intake of other oral agents.

PROSTATE-SPECIFIC ANTIGEN: In a Phase II pilot study, MCP significantly decreased PSA levels in patients with prostate cancer.[9]

URINE TESTS: Based on preliminary clinical evidence, MCP may significantly increase urinary excretion of metals.[10]

Muira Puama (Ptychopetalum olacoides)

Pharmacokinetics

The pharmacokinetics of muira puama is not well understood. Injections of muira puama (Ptychopetalum olacoides) extract appear to have a short duration of action.[1]

Adverse effects

Experts generally consider muira puama to be a safe herb, and reports of serious adverse effects are lacking in the available scientific literature. Muira puama may have the potential to increase blood pressure and cause CNS stimulation. Rarely, it may cause aggression, changes in appetite, changes in voice, or enlargement of genitalia.

Interactions

ANTICOAGULANTS/ANTIPLATELETS: Coumarin constituents of muira puama,[2-4] may potentiate actions of warfarin and other anticoagulant/antiplatelet agents. Clinical evidence of such interaction is lacking.

OPIATES: Interactions with opioids may result from similar analgesic mechanisms of action, shown in animals with the combination product Catuama (containing Ptychopetalum olacoides, Paullinia cupana, Zingiber officinalis, and Trichilia catigua).[5]

SEROTONERGIC AGENTS: Because of proposed serotonergic effects of muira puama,[6] actions of antidepressants may be altered.

YOHIMBE: Hydroalcoholic extract of muira puama has been suggested to potentiate yohimbine-induced toxicity.[6]

Myrcia (Myrcia spp.)

Pharmacokinetics: Insufficient available evidence.

Adverse effects

Reported side effects with myrcia currently are lacking in the available literature. Dizziness and drowsiness are possible, but not well documented.

Interactions

BLOOD GLUCOSE: Myrcia glucosides myrciacitrin I and myrciaphenone B have potent inhibitory activities on aldose reductase and α-glucosidase in vitro and may lower glucose levels.[1-4]

THYROID HORMONES: In vitro, Myrcia uniflora has been shown to inhibit thyroid peroxidase;[5] thus it may increase the effects of agents used for hyperthyroidism, leading to hypothyroidism. Because of potential effects on thyroid hormones, patients who begin taking M. uniflora may require dosage adjustments of their existing agents because of changes in metabolism.

Neem (Azadirachta indica)

Pharmacokinetics: Insufficient available evidence.

Adverse effects

Oral neem bark extract for up to 10 weeks has been tolerated well in adults.[1]

However, several cases of death from neem oil poisoning have occurred in children. Adverse effects have included vomiting, drowsiness, loose stools, metabolic acidosis, anemia, Reye-like syndrome, altered sensation and consciousness, seizures, decreased responsiveness, and liver enzyme increases with evidence of liver damage.[2-5]

Interactions

ACETAMINOPHEN (TYLENOL): Concomitant use of acetaminophen and aqueous leaf extract of Azadirachta indica has been reported to induce hepatotoxicity in rats.[6] Clinical reports of such drug interactions are lacking; however, because of multiple case reports that highlight the hepatotoxicity of neem,[2-5] concomitant use with acetaminophen should be avoided.

BLOOD PRESSURE: Because of possible hypotensive effects in rats, neem should be used cautiously with antihypertensive agents.[7]

COMPLETE BLOOD COUNT: In animals, oral administration of crude aqueous neem extract has significantly increased hemoglobin, lymphocytes, MCHC, RBCs, and WBCs.[8]

CYCLOPHOSPHAMIDE (CYTOXAN): Neem leaf extract has been shown to inhibit the clastogenic activity of cyclophosphamide in mice.[9]

CYTOCHROME P450 SUBSTRATES: Neem has been suggested to synergize with dillapiol, a CYP3A4 inhibitor in vivo.[10] Neem may enhance the effects of certain CYP450-metabolized agents.

ELECTROLYTES: Based on animal experiments, oral administration of crude aqueous neem extract resulted in significant decreases in potassium.[8]

GARLIC (ALLIUM SATIVUM): Administration of garlic and neem leaf extracts in rats significantly decreased the formation of lipid peroxides and enhanced the levels of antioxidants and detoxifying enzymes in the stomach, as well as in the liver and circulation.[11]

LIVER FUNCTION TESTS: In animals, oral administration of crude aqueous neem extract has significantly decreased bilirubin levels[8] and increased ammonia levels.[12] LFTs may be altered with neem use.

MITOMYCIN (MUTAMYCIN): Neem leaf extract has been shown to inhibit the clastogenic activity of mitomycin C in animals.[11]

OPIATES: The combination of a low dose of neem leaf extract (3.12 mg/kg) and a low dose of morphine (0.5 mg/kg) produced an increased loss of pain sensation in mice.[13]

QUININE: Concomitant use of neem extract and quinine hydrochloride has been reported to have positive synergistic effect on antimicrobial and spermicidal activity in vitro.[14]

TESTOSTERONE: Oral administration of crude aqueous neem extract resulted in significant decreases in testosterone in animals.[8]

THYROID HORMONES: High concentrations of neem leaf extract have been shown to inhibit thyroid function in rats, particularly conversion of T_3 and T_4.[15] High doses decreased T_3 and increased T_4 concentrations in rats after 100 mg/kg/day of neem leaf extract for 20 days. Thyroid hormone tests may be altered.

Nopal (Opuntia spp.)

Pharmacokinetics

The pharmacokinetics of nopal is not well understood. Insoluble fiber is not digested and passes through the gut unchanged.

Adverse effects

Nopal is generally well tolerated. Side effects include mild diarrhea, nausea, abdominal fullness, headache, and increase in stool volume and frequency.[1,2]

Interactions

ANTICOAGULANTS/ANTIPLATELETS: Based on clinical evidence, nopal may decrease fibrinogen levels.[3] Because fibrinogen plays a key role in blood clotting, reduced levels may result in interactions with anticoagulant and antiplatelet agents; however, clinical evidence of this potential interaction is lacking.

BLOOD GLUCOSE: Nopal has been demonstrated to lower blood glucose in numerous animal studies[4-7] and clinical studies.[8-15] It has traditionally been used as an antidiabetic remedy.

BLOOD PRESSURE: Based on animal evidence, nopal may lower blood pressure[16] and theoretically may have additive effects when used with antihypertensive agents.

LIVER FUNCTION TESTS: In animals, large doses of Opuntia extracts have shown adverse effects on the liver and spleen, though no mortality was observed even at high doses.[16]

ORAL AGENTS: When mixed with water or other fluids, nopal forms a sticky, slippery gel. Taking nopal by mouth could block the absorption of agents, other supplements, and nutrients from foods taken at the same time. Traditionally, patients are advised not to eat meals or take medication within 2 hours of oral consumption of nopal; however, this has not been evaluated clinically.

THYROID HORMONES: Based on animal research, consumption of nopal may decrease serum free thyroxin.[4] Caution is warranted when using nopal with thyroid hormones.

URIC ACID: There is some clinical evidence that nopal may decrease uric acid levels.[3]

Oleander (Nerium oleander, Thevetia peruviana)

Pharmacokinetics

The pharmacokinetics of oleander is not well understood. Oleandrin, the main cardiac glycoside found in oleander, is highly protein bound. The biological half-life of oleandrin was calculated at 16 to 44 hours.[1]

Administration of activated charcoal is thought to play a possible role in preventing oleander absorption after ingestion and enhancing elimination.[2-13]

Adverse effects

Clinical studies of oleander began in the 1930s but have largely been abandoned because of the significant gastrointestinal toxicity of oleander preparations. Any benefits of therapy may not outweigh the risk of toxicity. Generalized effects of oleander ingestion may include irritation of contacted membranes, buccal erythema, nausea, vomiting, diaphoresis, abdominal pain, diarrhea, headache, altered mental status, visual disturbances, mydriasis, cardiovascular toxicity, and risk of death.[14] Deaths have occurred after ingestion of all forms of oleander.[14-17]

Interactions

BLOOD PRESSURE: Because hypotension has been reported with oleander ingestion,[18] combined use with blood pressure–lowering agents may cause additive effects.

CREATININE: In reports of oleander toxicity and exposure, serum creatinine levels were elevated.[2]

HEART RATE: In humans, the cardiac glycoside content of oleander elicits significant atrioventricular nodal blocking effects and lowers the threshold for ventricular arrhythmia.[19,20] Any coadministered antiarrhythmic agent with similar properties may have additive and potentially adverse effects.

HISTOLOGICAL TESTS: Oleandrin and oleandrigenin, constituents of oleander, have been shown to possess cytotoxic properties[21,22] and theoretically may interact with antineoplastic agents.

IMMUNE PARAMETERS: An oleander preparations, Anvirzel, appears to contain polysaccharides that have immunostimulant effects[23] and may alter certain parameters of immunity.

KIDNEY FUNCTION TESTS: In four cases of oleander-induced renal toxicity, BUN was elevated.[2]

LIVER FUNCTION TESTS: In four cases of oleander-induced renal toxicity, bilirubin was elevated.[2]

SEDATIVES AND CENTRAL NERVOUS SYSTEM DEPRESSANTS: Four cardiac glycosides isolated from *Nerium oleander* (nerizoside, δ-dehydroadynerigen, neritaloside, and odoroside) have all demonstrated CNS depressant activity in mice.[2,24,25] Theoretically, use of oleander with other CNS depressants may cause additive effects.

Omega-3 Fatty Acids, Alpha-Linolenic Acid

Pharmacokinetics

Dietary omega-3 fatty acids are well absorbed[1] and are incorporated into fat tissues.[2] Alpha-linolenic acid (ALA), found mainly in green vegetables, canola oil, and soybeans, is the parent compound of all omega-3 fatty acids, including eicosapentaenoic acid (EPA) and docosahexaenoic acid (DHA). However, less than 10% of ALA is converted to EPA and DHA, making this an inefficient source of omega-3 fatty acids in the body. DHA is retroconverted to EPA.[3,4]

Adverse effects

The U.S. Food and Drug Administration (FDA) classifies intake of up to 3 g per day of omega-3 fatty acids from fish as "generally recognized as safe" (GRAS). Caution may be warranted in diabetic patients because of potential (but unlikely) increases in blood sugar levels, patients at risk of bleeding, or those with high LDL levels.[5-12]

Multiple clinical trials report small reductions in blood pressure with intake of omega-3 fatty acids.[13-19] Reductions of 2 to 5 mm Hg have been observed, and effects appear to be dose responsive (higher doses have greater effects).[14] DHA may have greater effects than EPA.[20] Caution is warranted in patients with low blood pressure.

Diets containing salmon oil, mackerel, or cod liver oil have been reported to prolong bleeding times significantly in healthy volunteers.[7,21-24] However, in other studies of omega-3 fatty acid supplementation, no adverse effects on bleeding time have been observed.[25,26]

Interactions

ANTICOAGULANTS/ANTIPLATELETS: Increased bleeding time is suggested to result from either less thromboxane (TXA_2) or higher prostacyclin I_3 levels. It is unclear if omega-3 fatty acids affect coagulation. Anecdotal evidence suggests that fish oil may increase INR.[27] However, clinical evidence suggests that fish oil does not affect coagulation, even when taken with anticoagulant therapy.[28,29] Nevertheless, caution is warranted when omega-3 fatty acids (from plant or fish) are taken with anticoagulant agents.

BLOOD GLUCOSE: Omega-3 fatty acids may lower blood sugar levels slightly.

BLOOD LIPIDS: Omega-3 fatty acids lower triglyceride levels but actually can slightly increase (worsen) LDL cholesterol levels.

BLOOD PRESSURE: Multiple clinical trials report small reductions in blood pressure with intake of omega-3 fatty acids.[13-19] Reductions of 2 to 5 mm Hg have been observed, and effects appear to be dose responsive.[14] DHA may have greater effects than EPA.[20] Caution is warranted in patients taking blood pressure–lowering agents because of potential additive effects.

VITAMINS: Any dietary oil increases the absorption of fat-soluble vitamins (A, D, E, K). Because certain vitamins (particularly A and D) can build up in the body and cause toxicity, patients taking multiple vitamins regularly or in high doses should discuss this risk with medical professionals.

Onion (Allium cepa)

Pharmacokinetics

The average absorption of quercetin after ingestion of onion has been reported to be 52%.[1] Absorbed quercetin was shown to be eliminated slowly from the blood.[2,3] Two major sites of metabolism are the liver and the colonic flora.[2] The urinary excretion of quercetin was 0.31%.[1] The elimination half-life ranges from 17 to 28 hours.[1]

Adverse effects

The primary adverse effects associated with onion are dermatological. Pemphigus (a rare skin disorder that causes blistering of skin and mucous membranes) and contact dermatitis have been reported. Gastrointestinal effects (heartburn, dyspepsia, gastric acidity, gastroesophageal reflux) have also been reported.[4-9]

Interactions

ANTICOAGULANTS/ANTIPLATELETS: Based on pharmacological and in vitro studies, onion and onion extract may inhibit platelet aggregation, reduce plasma viscosity, decrease hematocrit, and increase fibribolytic activity.[10-14] In theory, concurrent use of onion with anticoagulants/antiplatelets may increase the risk of bleeding; however, this interaction has not been evaluated clinically.

BLOOD GLUCOSE: Based on clinical studies, onion may reduce blood glucose levels.[15,16]

BLOOD LIPIDS: Based on clinical examination of alimentary hyperlipidemia, onion and onion essential oil may prevent fat-induced increases in serum cholesterol.[17,18]

BLOOD PRESSURE: According to clinical evidence, onion may decrease blood pressure.[11,19]

BONE MARKERS: Based on animal studies, onion may inhibit bone resorption[20-22] and theoretically may interact with osteoporosis agents.

HISTOLOGICAL TESTS: Based on in vitro, animal, and epidemiological studies, onion or onion extract may have anticancer effects.[23-32]

Papaya (Carica papaya)

Pharmacokinetics: Insufficient available evidence.

Adverse effects

Patients with known allergy or hypersensitivity to papain, papaya (Carica papaya), or other plants or foods that may contain papain[1] should avoid its use. Allergic sensitivity to papain may cause symptoms ranging from an itchy palate to abdominal cramps, diarrhea, and diaphoresis.[2] Other adverse effects of papain include gastric ulcer, esophageal perforation, and hypernatremia.[3]

Interactions

ANTICOAGULANTS/ANTIPLATELETS: An interaction between papain and warfarin has been proposed.[4] In one case report, a woman taking coumadin and Wobenzym (containing pancreatin, bromelain, papain, lipase, amylase, trypsin, α-chymotrypsin, and rutin) experienced coumadin overdose, possibly caused by coumadin contamination of the Wobenzym.[5]

ELECTROLYTES: Papain has been associated with hypernatremia, or elevated serum sodium levels.[3] Caution is warranted with sodium intake and papain use.

Passion Flower (Passiflora incarnata)

Pharmacokinetics: Insufficient available evidence.

Adverse effects

Experts generally consider passion flower to be a safe herb, with few adverse events reported. Adverse effects may result from adulterants in passion flower–containing products, rather than from passion flower itself.

Interactions

ANTICOAGULANTS/ANTIPLATELETS: Passion flower contains coumarin[1] and therefore may theoretically increase bleeding risk when used with blood-thinning agents. However, clinical evidence of this interaction is lacking.

ANXIOLYTICS: In animals, chrysin (a flavonoid in passion flower) displayed anxiolytic properties comparable to midazolam[2] and theoretically may cause additive effects when used with antianxiety agents.

BARBITURATES: Prolongation of barbiturate-induced sleep time in animals given passion flower has been demonstrated;[1,3,4] thus, passion flower may interact with barbiturates and other CNS depressants.

BLOOD ALCOHOL: Many tinctures contain high levels of alcohol and may affect blood alcohol levels. Adverse interactions may occur when taken with disulfiram (Antabuse) or metronidazole (Flagyl).

BLOOD PRESSURE: Passion flower was found to have hypotensive properties in animals.[5] Theoretically, concomitant use of other hypotensive agents and passion flower may result in additive blood pressure–lowering effects.

CYTOCHROME P450 SUBSTRATES: Theoretically, passion flower may interact with CYP450-metabolized agents.[6]

FLUMAZENIL (ROMAZICON): In animals the benzodiazepine antagonist flumazenil has been shown to suppress the anticonvulsant effects of Passiflora.[7]

FUNGAL TESTS: Antifungal activity has been observed in extracts of several species of passion flower[8,9] and theoretically may interact with antifungal agents.

GABAERGIC AGENTS: In animals, passion flower has been shown to affect GABAergic systems.[7] Interactions with other GABAergic agents are possible.

HISTOLOGICAL TESTS: A compound, 4-hydroxy-2-cyclopentanone, isolated from passion flower has been found to exert cytotoxic effects[8] and theoretically may interact with other agents with antineoplastic properties.

MONOAMINERGIC AGENTS: Harmala alkaloids of passion flower possess MAO-inhibiting activity.[1] Passion flower may therefore theoretically affect the activity of certain antidepressant agents.

NALOXONE (NARCAN): In animals the opioid receptor antagonist naloxone has been shown to suppress the anticonvulsant effects of Passiflora.[7]

Peony (Paeonia spp.)

Pharmacokinetics
The pharmacokinetics of peony is not well understood. Paeoniflorin, a bioactive monoterpene glucoside from peony root, is not well absorbed. However, its aglycon (nonsugar component of the glycoside), paeoniflorgenin, is absorbed and circulated in the bloodstream.

Adverse effects
Based on traditional use and available research, it appears that peony is well tolerated as part of Chinese herbal formulas when used for up to 3 months.[1-8] Based on secondary sources, peony may cause nausea and vomiting.

Interactions
ANTICOAGULANTS/ANTIPLATELETS: Theoretically, concomitant use of peony with anticoagulants/antiplatelets may increase risk of bleeding. This is suggested by a case of easy gum bleeding, epistaxis, and skin bruising with an international normalized ratio (INR) greater than 6.0 in a 61-year-old man previously stable on warfarin therapy.[9]

BACTERIAL TESTS: Peony has been used to treat *Campylobacter pyloridis* infection.[8] Microbiological assays may thus be altered by peony's purported antibacterial activity.

BLOOD LIPIDS: A combination product containing peony significantly increased apolipoprotein-A-I (APO-A) levels.[5]

BLOOD PRESSURE: A combination powder containing peony has been found to have blood pressure–lowering effects.[10] Based on in vitro research, PGG, a constituent of peony root, dilates vascular smooth muscle and suppresses the vascular inflammatory process via endothelium-dependent NO/cGMP signaling.[11] Blood pressure may be affected.

BODY TEMPERATURE: A combination product containing peony has been shown to improve low luteal-phase basal body temperature.[1]

CARBAMAZEPINE (TEGRETOL): According to animal research, concomitant use of peony and carbamazepine resulted in a decreased T_{max} of carbamazepine.[12] The clinical significance is not well understood.

CORTICOSTEROIDS: Based on clinical evidence, a combination product including peony may decrease the need for glucocorticoid medication in some patients with nephritis.[2]

CYTOKINES AND INFLAMMATORY MARKERS: In vitro, peony has been demonstrated to inhibit IL-8 expression through inactivation of NF-κB.[13] Antiinflammatory effects of peony have been observed in laboratory studies.[14-16] Theoretically, concomitant use of peony with antiinflammatory agents may have additive effects.

ESTROGENIC AGENTS: A combination product containing peony has been shown to significantly increase (estradiol) E_2 levels in postmenopausal women.[5]

FOLLICLE-STIMULATING HORMONE: A combination product containing peony has been shown to decrease FSH levels in postmenopausal women.[5]

HEMATOCRIT: In clinical research, both intravenous injection of 100% *Paeonia lactiflora* (5 mL daily) and a one-time pulmonary artery injection of 100% *P. lactiflora* (5 mL) have resulted in statistically significant improvements in hematocrit.[17]

HISTOLOGICAL TESTS: The peony constituent 1,2,3,4,6-penta-O-galloyl-β-D-glucose has exhibited antiangiogenic effects in vitro.[18] In humans, peony decreased tumor marker levels (CEA, CA-19-9, CA-125).[19] Scores tended to decrease with the decrease in size of myomas.[4,19]

LIGUSTICUM: Peony has significantly lowered the clinical bioavailability of ferulic acid derived from *Ligusticum wallichii*.[20]

PHENYTOIN (DILANTIN): In animals, peony root delayed the absorption and volume of distribution of the anticonvulsant phenytoin, reducing its therapeutic effectiveness.[21]

PROGESTOGENIC AGENTS: A combination product containing peony has been shown to improve low plasma progesterone levels in human subjects.[1] Hormonal therapy may be altered.

TAMOXIFEN: Tamoxifen has been shown to block the activation of the chimeric estrogen receptor by Bupleurum & Peony formula (Jia Wei Xiao Yao San) in vitro.[22] Theoretically, tamoxifen may interfere with the pharmacological effects of this formula if administered concomitantly.

VIRAL LEVELS: The methanol extract of *Paeonia suffruticosa* has demonstrated strong inhibition of HIV-1 integrase activity in vitro and may be a rich source of anti-HIV compounds.[23] Antiviral effects have also been observed in vitro.[23-25]

Peppermint (Mentha x piperita)

Pharmacokinetics
Peppermint oil is relatively rapidly absorbed after oral administration and is eliminated mainly through the bile.[1] The major biliary metabolite is menthol glucuronide, which undergoes enterohepatic circulation. Urinary metabolites are mono- and di-hydroxymenthols and carboxylic acids, with some excreted as glucuronic acid conjugates.

Adverse effects
Topical peppermint oil is generally well tolerated in quantities commonly consumed in food. Skin rash and irritation have been described from topical use of peppermint oil.[2,3]

When taken by mouth, peppermint oil can cause gastrointestinal effects such as heartburn, nausea, and vomiting. Allergic reactions resulting in flushing and headache have also occurred. Oral peppermint oil may cause oral ulcerations.[4]

Interactions
5-FLUOROURACIL: Peppermint oil may enhance skin absorption of topical 5-FU, based on animal research.[5]

ACIDITY: Some experts suggest agents that decrease stomach acid and increase gastric pH may cause premature dissolution of enteric-coated peppermint oil.

ANTIBIOTICS: In vitro, peppermint oil and menthol were shown to have synergistic effects with some antibiotics.[6]

BENZOIC ACID: Based on in vitro research, concomitant dermal exposure to low concentrations of peppermint oil may reduce the percutaneous penetration of benzoic acid.[7]

BLOOD PRESSURE: Calcium channel–blocking activity of peppermint oil has been observed in animal models,[8] and in theory, peppermint oil may add to the effects of agents that may also theoretically lower blood pressure.

CYTOCHROME P450 SUBSTRATES: Peppermint has been shown to inhibit CYP450 1A2, 2C9, 2C19, and 3A4[8-12] and may increase the levels or bioavailability of agents metabolized by these isoenzymes.

FUNGAL LEVELS: In vitro research has reported that peppermint oil showed antifungal activity against *Trichophyton mentagrophytes*.[13]

OXYTETRACYCLINE: Based on in vitro research, peppermint oil and menthol may have synergistic effects when combined with oxytetracycline.[6]

PARASITIC TESTS: In vitro studies have revealed that peppermint extracts may inhibit the growth and adherence of *Giardia lamblia* (parasite that causes giardiasis)[14] and theoretically may interact with antiparasitic agents.

Perilla (Perilla frutescens)

Pharmacokinetics: Insufficient available evidence.

Adverse effects

Perilla used in recommended doses is generally considered to be safe and well tolerated due to its history of use in food. Extensive safety data are lacking.

Interactions

BLOOD LIPIDS: In animals, perilla has been shown to lower HDL cholesterol levels.[1]

CYTOKINES AND INFLAMMATORY MARKERS: In vitro, perilla has been found to increase tumor necrosis factor production.[1,2]

INDOMETHACIN (INDOCIN): Perilla has been shown to suppress the effects of the nonsteroidal antiinflammatory drug indomethacin in rats, because of a change in fatty acid and eicosanoid status.[3] Similar interactions with other NSAIDs are possible.

SEDATIVES AND CENTRAL NERVOUS SYSTEM DEPRESSANTS: *Perilla frutescens* has been shown to prolong hexobarbital-induced sleep in animals because of the constituent dillapiol.[4]

Podophyllum (Podophyllum spp.)

Pharmacokinetics

The pharmacokinetics of podophyllum is not well understood. It appears to be well absorbed after ingestion.[1]

Adverse effects

Podophyllum applied topically for genital warts and oral hairy leukoplakia appears to be well-tolerated.[2-4] Generally, adverse effects are mild and include burning sensations, bad or altered taste, and mild pain in topical application. Adverse effects from oral ingestion may include gastrointestinal discomfort (diarrhea and abdominal pain).

Interactions

ANTIPSYCHOTIC AGENTS: According to animal research, podophyllum toxicity may cause a worsening of extrapyramidal symptoms that may occur with antipsychotic agents.[5]

ELECTROLYTES: Podophyllum has been historically used as a laxative. Overuse may cause dehydration and electrolyte disturbances.

HISTOLOGICAL TESTS: According to two case reports and clinical research, podophyllum is proposed to interrupt cellular mitosis at metaphase.[1,4,6] Podophyllum may interact with agents that have a similar mechanism. Additionally, antineoplastic agents may cause neutropenia.

LIVER FUNCTION TESTS: In animals, degenerative changes were observed in the liver after ingestion of podophyllum.[7] Podophyllum may alter liver function tests, and concurrent use with other hepatotoxic agents may increase the risk of liver damage.

WHITE BLOOD CELL COUNTS: Based on unsubstantiated reports, podophyllum may cause neutropenia; WBC counts should therefore be monitored.

Policosanol

Pharmacokinetics: Insufficient available evidence.

Adverse events

Policosanol appears to be safe and well tolerated, even in populations with high use of concomitant agents.[1] No drug-related clinical or biochemical adverse effects were reported in a number of clinical trials.[2-12] Frequency of mild, moderate, and severe adverse events and mortality has been shown to be lower in diabetic and nondiabetic individuals taking policosanol compared with placebo.[1,13,14]

Interactions

ANTICOAGULANTS/ANTIPLATELETS: Policosanol has been shown to inhibit platelet aggregation in vitro.[7,15-26] Theoretically, concomitant use of policosanol with anticoagulants/antiplatelets may increase the risk of bleeding. However, the addition of policosanol to warfarin therapy did not enhance the prolongation of the bleeding time induced by warfarin alone in humans.[24]

BETA-ADRENERGIC AGENTS: Several clinical studies have shown that policosanol decreased arterial pressure compared with placebo, and a pharmacological interaction with beta blockers was shown.[1,13,14] Pretreatment with high doses of policosanol significantly increased hypotensive effects induced by propranolol (Inderal) in animals.[27] Concurrent use of policosanol with antihypertensive agents was suggested to enhance hypotensive effects safely.

BLOOD LIPIDS: Policosanol may lower cholesterol,[5,8,16,28-30] and clinical studies have shown that its effects are comparable to those of statins.[16,28,29,31]

CREATINE PHOSPHOKINASE: Policosanol (10 mg) administered to elderly patients with hyperlipidemia significantly reduced CPK levels.[8]

CYTOKINES AND INFLAMMATORY MARKERS: Policosanol reduced malondialdehyde (MDA) serum levels in animals and humans.[22]

LEVODOPA: Increased dyskinesia has been reported in Parkinson's disease patients taking octacosanol with levodopa.[32] Caution is advised when taking policosanol with levodopa.

MARKERS OF INTERMITTENT CLAUDICATION: Policosanol (10-12 mg) significantly increased mean values of initial and absolute claudication distances.[7,15-17,33]

NITROPRUSSIDE (NITROPRESS): Because policosanol possesses an antioxidant effect and nitric oxide (NO) can be destroyed by oxygen-derived radicals, a scientific basis exists for an interaction between policosanol and nitroprusside. Pretreatment with policosanol significantly increased the nitroprusside-induced hypotensive effect in rats.[22]

OMEGA-3 FATTY ACIDS AND FISH OIL: In animals, concurrent therapy with policosanol and omega-3 fatty acids had additive cholesterol-lowering effect and reduced platelet aggregation in animals.[34]

Polypodium (Polypodium leucotomos)

Pharmacokinetics: Insufficient available evidence.

Adverse effects

Information is limited regarding the adverse effects of *Polypodium leucotomos*. Gastrointestinal discomfort has been reported.[1]

Interactions

BLOOD PRESSURE: A pharmacodynamic study of a different fern species, *Polypodium vulgare*, may cause hypotension.[2]

HEART RHYTHM: A pharmacodynamic study of a different fern species, *Polypodium vulgare*, reported positive inotropic and chronotropic effects.[2]

SEDATIVES AND CENTRAL NERVOUS SYSTEM DEPRESSANTS: A pharmacodynamic study of a different fern species, *Polypodium vulgare*, reported CNS depressant effects.[2] Concurrent use of *Polypodium leucotomos* with CNS depressants may have additive effects.

Pomegranate (Punica granatum)

Pharmacokinetics: Insufficient available evidence.

Adverse effects

Pomegranate has a long history of use as food and medicine in Asia and South America and is generally well tolerated. Several sources note that the fruit rind of pomegranate is actually contraindicated in diarrhea.[1-3]

Pomegranate root and stem contain pelletierine. Orally, overdoses can cause strychnine-like effects in the form of heightened reflex arousal that can escalate to paralysis. At amounts greater than 80 g, people experience vomiting, including bloody emesis, followed by dizziness, chills, vision disorders, collapse, and possibly death from respiratory failure. Ideally, the edible portion should contain no more than 0.25% tannin. The oral toxicity of plant tannins is low, as tannins are readily hydrolyzed in the gut to gallic acid and other metabolites; however, liver and kidney toxicity has occurred with high tannin doses used topically or intravenously.[4] Tannin consumption has been associated with certain cancers, such as esophageal cancer; however, it is unclear whether this is due to the tannins themselves or other compounds associated with tannins.[5]

Interactions

BLOOD PRESSURE: In hypertensive subjects, pomegranate juice has been shown to lower blood pressure through inhibition of angiotensin-converting enzyme (ACE).[6]

IRON: The fruit husk and root/stem bark of pomegranate contains up to 28% and 25% tannins, respectively, compared to 12.9% in black tea and 22.2% in green tea. The tannin content of various herbs may interact with iron, forming nonabsorbable complexes. Some experts have concluded that if herbs containing tannins are consumed at mealtime, nonabsorbable complexes will form with iron, zinc, and copper.[7,8] Concern has been raised that tannins may affect the administration of iron supplement products. However, limited evidence suggests only a negligible effect on iron administered by supplementation regimens.[9] The tannin complexes can dissolve in an acid environment such as the stomach. It is unclear to what extent the amount of tannin in pomegranate may affect iron absorption clinically. Until more is known, patients who need iron supplementation should be advised to separate administration times of these two compounds by 1 to 2 hours.

PSK (Coriolus versicolor)

Pharmacokinetics

According to animal research, radiolabeled PSK is absorbed within 24 hours after oral administration. It is partially decomposed in the digestive tract. PSK or its metabolites were detected in the digestive tract, bone marrow, salivary glands, brain, liver, spleen, pancreas, and tumor tissue in sarcoma-bearing mice. Approximately 70% of radiolabeled PSK is excreted in expired air, 20% in feces, 10% in urine, and 0.8% in bile.[1]

Adverse effects

PSK generally seems to have a low incidence of mild and tolerable side effects.[2-4] Cases of liver impairment and toxicity have been noted with PSK use.[5] Gastrointestinal upset, darkening of the fingernails, and coughing have been reported with extended use of PSK and with powdered supplemental forms.[7]

Low blood cell counts (leukopenia, thrombocytopenia, albuminuria) were observed in clinical trials.[3,8-10] Patients received chemotherapy in addition to PSK in these trials, which may have contributed to the low blood cell counts.

Interactions

ANTICOAGULANTS/ANTIPLATELETS: Thrombocytopenia (low blood platelet count) has been reported with PSK use.[8,10] Theoretically, concomitant use of PSK with anticoagulants/antiplatelets could increase risk of bleeding, although clinical evidence of this interaction is lacking.

CHEMOTHERAPY: Numerous animal and clinical studies have suggested that PSK may extend survival time in patients with lung cancer, gastric cancer, stomach cancer, colon cancer, or leukemia when used with chemotherapy.[5,7,11-16] Clinical studies have used PSK as an adjuvant to mitomycin C,[17] tegafur,[11,12,14] 5-fluorouracil,[12,14,15] and cisplatin.[21]

An antiangiogenic effect, in which inhibition of blood vessel growth theoretically slows tumor growth, has also been observed.[22]

LIVER FUNCTION TESTS: Liver impairment and toxicity have been reported in clinical trials.[8,10] Concomitant use of PSK with other hepatotoxic agents may increase the risk of liver damage.

URINE TESTS: Albuminuria (protein in urine) has been reported with PSK use.[8,10]

WHITE BLOOD CELL COUNTS: Leukopenia has been reported with PSK use.[8] These effects may be attributed to either PSK or concomitant chemotherapy.

Psyllium (Plantago spp.)

Pharmacokinetics

Psyllium remains predominantly in the gut as a "bulk" agent. It is somewhat resistant to fermentation and is passed largely unchanged through the gastrointestinal (GI) tract.[1,2] It has significant "water-holding" capacity because of its high hemicellulose content.[3] Onset of action is 12 to 24 hours; full effect may take 2 to 3 days.[4]

Adverse effects

Psyllium-containing laxatives, cereal, or other products are well tolerated and generally safe,[5-11] with the important exceptions of individuals with repeated psyllium exposure, known hypersensitivity, or preexisting bowel abnormalities, or when psyllium products are mixed with inadequate amounts of water.[12-21]

Anaphylaxis, wheezing or difficulty breathing, skin rash, and hives have been reported in patients who took psyllium or were exposed to psyllium laxatives in the workplace.[13,16-26] Cross-sensitivity may occur in people with allergy to English plantain pollen (*Plantago lanceolata*), grass pollen, or melon.[27]

Gastrointestinal side effects are generally mild and have not prompted discontinuation in clinical trials. Flatulence, bloating, diarrhea, indigestion, loose stool, abdominal pain, dyspepsia, and constipation have been reported.[28-33] Fecal obstruction of the GI tract has been noted in many case reports of patients taking psyllium-containing laxatives, and esophageal impaction and bezoars (indigestible mass) have also been reported after ingestion of psyllium products.[14,34-37]

Interactions

ANTICOAGULANTS/ANTIPLATELETS: Theoretically, psyllium may reduce the absorption of anticoagulant and antiplatelet agents. However, one study found no effect on warfarin levels by coadministered psyllium.[38]

ANTIDEPRESSANT AGENTS: Dietary fiber has been shown to lower the blood levels and effectiveness of tricyclic antidepressant (TCA) agents in three patients.[39] Reduced dietary fiber intake increased the blood levels and improved symptoms in these patients.

BLOOD GLUCOSE: Psyllium may delay the absorption of glucose from meals, leading to less postprandial hyperglycemia.[41]

BODY WEIGHT: Psyllium has been suggested as a possible weight loss aid, although studies have not produced conclusive results.[9,40]

CALCIUM: One clinical study demonstrated slightly (but not significantly) less absorption of calcium when administered with psyllium (Metamucil).[42]

CARBAMAZEPINE: Psyllium can decrease the absorption and concentration of carbamazepine.[43] Patients treated with carbamazepine and psyllium should have their administration times separated as much as possible and their plasma levels of carbamazepine monitored.

CHOLESTYRAMINE (QUESTRAN): Psyllium plus cholestyramine provided a modest but nonsignificant reduction in total and LDL cholesterol in human subjects. This combination significantly reduced constipation, abdominal discomfort, and heartburn compared with the group who continued taking cholestyramine alone.[44] Another study found no statistically significant lipid reduction after use of colestipol and psyllium.[45] One animal study showed greater LDL reduction with high-dose cholestyramine than with a lower dose plus psyllium. However, the study also found that the combination reversed cholestyramine-induced LDL receptor suppression and reduced hepatic cholesterol content.[46]

CYTOKINES AND INFLAMMATORY MARKERS: Acetoside and plantamajoside from *Plantago lanceolata* were found to inhibit arachidonic acid.[47]

DIGOXIN: Results are mixed regarding the effects of psyllium on digoxin levels. Limited study suggests that psyllium may lower digoxin levels.[48] However, another study found no effect.[49]

ELECTROLYTES: Excessive use of psyllium may lead to electrolyte loss.

HISTOLOGICAL TESTS: Some evidence suggests that psyllium might improve the chemoprotective effect of wheat bran.[50] Psyllium might help maintain normal cell proliferation in the colon.[51,52] Also, psyllium fiber is converted to butyrate, which appears to be important in protecting against colon cancer.[53]

HYDROPHILIC AGENTS: Psyllium may theoretically increase the effects of hydrophilic agents. Psyllium is hydrophilic because of its high content of hemicellulose.[3,13]

IRON: The long-term use of psyllium can reduce the absorption of iron.[54] Supplements should be taken 1 hour before or 4 hours after psyllium to avoid this interaction.

LITHIUM: Psyllium can decrease the plasma levels and effectiveness of lithium.[55,56] Psyllium should be separated from lithium by at least 2 hours to reduce the likelihood of this interaction. Lithium levels increased to therapeutic levels after stopping psyllium.[57]

ORAL AGENTS: Experts state that soluble fibers can decrease the absorption of oral agents.[58] Long-term use of psyllium with meals can reduce nutrient absorption, requiring vitamin or mineral supplementation. However, the use of blond psyllium husk for up to 6 months did not clinically alter vitamin or mineral status in a review of eight clinical trials.[30]

ORLISTAT (XENICAL, ALLI): One study of psyllium coadministered with orlistat versus orlistat alone found dramatically fewer GI events (e.g., diarrhea, oily discharge) in the combination-therapy group.[59]

SALICYLATES: Theoretically, salicylates may have decreased absorption when taken with psyllium. Administration times should be separated to minimize potential interactions.

STOOL TESTS: Psyllium and chitosan together may increase fat excretion in the stool.[54]

TETRACYCLINES: Theoretically, tetracyclines may have decreased absorption when taken with psyllium. Administration times should be separated to minimize potential interactions.

VITAMIN B_{12}: The long-term use of psyllium can reduce the absorption of vitamin B_{12}.[59] Supplements should be taken 1 hour before or 4 hours after psyllium to avoid this interaction.

Pycnogenol (*Pinus pinaster* subsp. *atlantica*)

Pharmacokinetics

Pycnogenol is rapidly absorbed after oral ingestion. Steady-state conditions have been reached after 5 days' ingestion of the pine bark extract. Pycnogenol metabolites include catechin, caffeic acid, ferulic acid, taxifolin, and the metabolite M1 (δ-(3,4-dihydroxy-phenyl)-γ-valerolactone).[1] Pycnogenol is excreted in the urine. Ferulic acid and taxifolin were excreted within 18 hours, with peak urinary excretion in 2 to 3 hours. Recovery of ferulic acid in urine was 36% to 43%, and recovery of taxifolin was 7% to 8%.[2]

Adverse effects

Pycnogenol is generally reported as being well tolerated. Low acute and chronic toxicity with mild unwanted effects may occur in a small percentage of patients after oral administration. Because of its astringent taste and occasional minor stomach discomfort, Pycnogenol is best taken with or after meals. To date, systematic safety data are insufficient. Possible side effects include mild and transient gastrointestinal complaints,[3] decreased blood glucose levels,[4] vertigo, headache, and nausea.[3]

Interactions

ANTICOAGULANTS/ANTIPLATELETS: Pycnogenol should be used cautiously with anticoagulants because of its potential to decrease coagulation.[5] Based on clinical research, Pycnogenol supplementation may significantly decrease serum thromboxane concentration.[6] In vitro, Pycnogenol was shown to improve the efficacy of acetylsalicylic acid (aspirin) in platelet inhibition.[5]

BACTERIAL LEVELS: In immunosuppressed mice, *Cryptosporidium parvum* infection was cleared more efficiently in animals given oral Pycnogenol.[7]

BETA-ADRENERGIC AGENTS: Based on a chick cardiomyocyte model, pretreatment with a beta-receptor antagonist may reduce the Pycnogenol-increased probability of contraction state.[8]

BLOOD GLUCOSE: Pycnogenol may reduce glucose levels[4,9] and should be used cautiously with hypoglycemic agents.

BLOOD LIPIDS: Pycnogenol may have cholesterol-lowering effects, as demonstrated in clinical research.[10]

BLOOD PRESSURE: Based on clinical trials, Pycnogenol may reduce blood pressure in hypertensive individuals.[3,6] Theoretically, Pycnogenol may cause additive effects when used with antihypertensives.

CYCLOPHOSPHAMIDE (CYTOXAN): Based on animal research, Pycnogenol may inhibit thymus DNA synthesis induced by cyclophosphamide.[11] Caution is warranted because Pycnogenol may interact with cyclophosphamide therapy.

CYTOKINES AND INFLAMMATORY MARKERS: Based on clinical studies[12,13] and in vitro studies,[14-16] Pycnogenol may have antiinflammatory effects and theoretically may interact with antiinflammatory agents. Based on clinical research, Pycnogenol treatment may significantly reduce serum leukotrienes.[17] In vitro, Pycnogenol was shown to increase TNF-α secretion[18] and IL-2 production[19] but to reduce elevated levels of IL-6.[19]

DOXORUBICIN (ADRIAMYCIN): Based on animal and in vitro studies, Pycnogenol may have a protective effect on the cardiotoxicity of doxorubicin (Adriamycin).[20] In combination with other antioxidants, Pycnogenol may elevate renal glutathione peroxidase, glutathione reductase, hepatic glutathione reductase activities, and glutathione disulfide or may reduce cardiac glutathione disulfide levels.[21] Hepatic GSH and cardiac glutathione peroxidase activity may also be elevated.

FLUORIDE: In animals, Pycnogenol was shown to prevent fluoride-induced kidney lysosomal damage.[22]

GROWTH HORMONE: In vitro, a combination of L-arginine, L-lysine, aged garlic extract (Kyolic), S-allyl cysteine, and Pycnogenol was shown to increase secretion of human GH.[23] The effects of Pycnogenol are not clear.

LOW-CARBOHYDRATE DIET: Based on research in diabetic rats, the combination of a low-carbohydrate diet with Pycnogenol treatment may increase retinal glutathione peroxidase and glutathione reductase activities.[24]

POLYPHENOL: An increase in plasma polyphenols has been noted in humans supplemented with Pycnogenol.[25]

TESTOSTERONE: Based on in vitro research, Pycnogenol may stimulate the synthesis of dihydrotestosterone.[26]

VITAMIN C: In vitro study has shown that Pycnogenol prolongs the life of the ascorbate radical.[27] However, there is limited clinical evidence to support these effects.

VITAMIN E: In vitro, Pycnogenol and vitamin E have been shown to have additive antioxidant effects. Pycnogenol may protect the α-tocopherol of endothelial cells and enhance the basal endogenous levels of α-tocopherol.[28]

WHITE BLOOD CELL COUNTS: In vitro, Pycnogenol was shown to increase natural killer (NK) cell cytotoxicity.[19]

Pygeum (*Prunus africanum*, syn. *Pygeum africanum*)

Pharmacokinetics: Insufficient available evidence.

Adverse effects

Pygeum has been well tolerated in most studies.[1-3] Individuals may experience abdominal discomfort, including diarrhea, constipation, stomach pain, or nausea. Stomach upset is usually mild and does not typically cause people to stop using pygeum.[3,4] The safety of pygeum has not been extensively or systematically studied; safety of use beyond 12 months has not been reliably studied.

Interactions

5α-REDUCTASE INHIBITORS: Pygeum extract appears to inhibit human prostatic 5α-reductase, but much less powerfully than finasteride.[5] 5α-Reductase inhibitors such as terazosin (Hytrin) or finasteride (Proscar) are used to treat symptoms of prostate enlargement and may increase the effects of pygeum, although this has not been clinically evaluated.

ESTROGENIC EFFECTS: Pygeum has demonstrated phytoestrogenic effects[6,7] and may interact with hormone therapies.

SAW PALMETTO AND STINGING NETTLE: If used with saw palmetto (*Serenoa repens*) or stinging nettle (*Urtica dioica*), pygeum may have additive effects on the prostate.[8] Combination products containing both stinging nettle and pygeum are available.

Quercetin

Pharmacokinetics

Pharmacokinetic studies with dietary quercetin glycosides showed marked differences in absorption rate and bioavailability. Flavonoids present in foods may be considered nonabsorbable because they are bound to sugars as beta-glycosides. Only free flavonoids without a sugar molecule, the so-called aglycones (aglycons), were thought to be able to pass through the gut wall. Quercetin is hydrolyzed in the small intestine and absorbed as aglycon, which is conjugated in the liver and secreted in bile into the intestinal lumen.[1] Quercetin does not appear to be well absorbed by the gut; quercetin chalcone (a modified version of quercetin) appears be better absorbed.[2] Quercetin glucoside is actively absorbed from the small intestine, whereas quercetin rutinoside is absorbed from the colon after deglycosylation.[3] In plasma, quercetin is extensively protein bound.[4-6] Carbon dioxide is the major metabolite of quercetin in humans[7] and is eliminated in the urine.[8] Plasma and urine levels reflect short-term intake.[9]

Adverse effects

Quercetin is a common food component and is found in various fruits, vegetables, and wines. It is generally safe and well tolerated at usual dietary intake. However, quercetin supplementation has been associated with headache, gastrointestinal effects, hematoma, and nephrotoxicity. Concern had been expressed about the possible tumorigenic effect of quercetin; however, it is not currently classified as a carcinogen.[10,11]

Interactions

GENERAL: There is anecdotal evidence that food may decrease or delay absorption of quercetin; therefore, it has been recommended to take quercetin on an empty stomach.

ANTICOAGULANTS/ANTIPLATELETS: Quercetin has been shown to inhibit platelet aggregation[12,13] and may increase risk of bleeding when used with anticoagulant/antiplatelet agents; however, clinical evidence is lacking on this interaction.

BROMELAIN: Use of bromelain in combination with quercetin may increase GI absorption of quercetin, as seen by increased improvement in symptoms of chronic pelvic pain syndrome in a controlled clinical trial.[14]

BUSULPHAN (BUSULFEX, MYLERAN): In cell culture, quercetin enhanced the antiproliferative activity of the chemotherapeutic agent busulphan in human leukemia cells.[15]

CAFFEINE: Quercetin has been reported to inhibit xanthine oxidase[16] and may affect caffeine and other methylxanthines, such as theophylline.

CISPLATIN (PLATINOL-AQ): In cell culture, quercetin inhibited the repair of cisplatin-induced DNA damage in hepatocytes,[17] and it inhibited cisplatin-induced damage to cultured renal tubular epithelial cells, possibly through free-radical scavenging.[18]

CYCLOSPORINE: Quercetin may affect the pharmacokinetics of oral cyclosporine. In animals it has been shown to reduce the bioavailability of cyclosporine; however, quercetin has also been shown to inhibit CYP450-3A4, which would lead to increased cyclosporine bioavailability.[19,20]

CYTOCHROME P450 SUBSTRATES: Given the antioxidant effect of quercetin, as well as that of other flavonoids, quercetin may be a significant environmental source of inhibitors of drug oxidation and may interact with agents metabolized by the CYP3A4 pathway, such as estradiol and nifedipine, anecdotally. Flavonoids such as quercetin interact with the metabolism of agents such as 17β-estradiol and other steroids that are extensively metabolized through the P450NF (P450-IIIA4) enzyme or closely related P450 systems.[21]

ESTROGENIC AGENTS: Inhibition of cytochrome P450 activity has been suggested as the mechanism by which quercetin alters the metabolism of 7β-estradiol.[22] In vitro, quercetin was found to act solely as an estrogen antagonist.[23]

NIFEDIPINE (ADALAT, PROCARDIA): Food rich in flavonoids, including quercetin, have been found to delay the first-pass metabolism of nifedipine in humans;[24] however, this effect has not been specifically attributed to quercetin.

QUINOLONE ANTIBIOTICS: Quercetin has been shown in vitro to bind to the DNA gyrase site on bacteria and competitively inhibit quinolone antibiotics.[25]

PAPAIN: Use of papain in combination with quercetin may increase GI absorption of quercetin, as suggested by increased improvement in symptoms of chronic pelvic pain syndrome in a controlled clinical trial.[14]

VITAMIN C: Vitamin C may enhance the antioxidant activity of quercetin, as represented in vitro as additive reductions in oxidative DNA damage.[10,26]

Red Clover *(Trifolium pratense)*

Pharmacokinetics

Red clover differs from the phytoestrogen soy in that the principal isoflavones in red clover are biochanin A and formononetin, whereas those in soy consist solely of genistein and daidzein. However, biochanin A and formononetin are metabolized extensively in vivo to genistein and daidzein, respectively.[1] Daidzein is further broken down to form the estrogenic metabolite equol and the less estrogenic *O*-desmethylangolensin (*O*-DMA). Metabolism and absorption (which may be influenced by food) are highly variable.[2] The half-life of the isoflavones daidzein and genistein is about 7 to 8 hours.[3]

Adverse effects

The few clinical studies using isoflavone extracts of red clover have reported good tolerance.[1,4,5] Because of estrogenic properties of red clover, weight gain, breast tenderness, and menstrual changes may theoretically occur.

Interactions

ANTICOAGULANTS/ANTIPLATELETS: Red clover contains coumarin and coumarin-like compounds, which theoretically may have additive effects when taken with anticoagulant or antiplatelet agents.[6] However, clinical evidence is insufficient regarding this interaction.

BLOOD GLUCOSE: Soy has been shown in clinical studies to have hypoglycemic effects.[7,8]

BLOOD LIPIDS: Red clover has been shown to reduce blood lipids in some clinical studies,[9] but not in others.[5,10]

CYTOCHROME P450 SUBSTRATES: In vitro evidence indicates that red clover may inhibit CYP450-3A4 enzyme. Theoretically, red clover may increase levels of CY3A4-metabolized agents.

ESTROGENIC AGENTS: Red clover isoflavones possess varying affinity for estradiol (estrogen) receptors (estradiol-α and estradiol-β) and are capable of acting as both agonists and antagonists.[11] Preliminary evidence suggests a preferential binding to ER-β, found in vasculature, brain, bone, and heart, versus ER-α, found in ovaries, breast, uterus, and adrenal glands. However, the clinical effects of isoflavone therapy on other therapy remain unclear. Isoflavones may affect levels of gonadotropin-releasing hormone (GrRH), follicle-stimulating hormone (FSH), and luteinizing hormone (LH) through hormonal feedback mechanisms.[12]

Red Yeast Rice *(Monascus purpureus)*

Pharmacokinetics: Insufficient available evidence.

Adverse effects

Note: Red yeast rice is the product of the yeast *Monascus purpureus* grown on rice and is a dietary staple in some Asian countries. It contains several compounds collectively known as monacolins, which are known to inhibit cholesterol synthesis. "Monacolin K" a potent inhibitor of HMG-CoA reductase, the liver enzyme responsible for producing cholesterol, is regulated and the target of pharmaceutical intervention. This active ingredient is also known as the prescription drug lovastatin (Mevacor), approved for marketing in the United States for high cholesterol. Of note, lovastatin can cause severe muscle, kidney, and liver damage. In 2007 the FDA issued a warning to consumers to avoid red yeast rice products promoted on the Internet because these products were found to contain lovastatin. Although red yeast rice is still available in the United States, it is fermented using a different process, and the active ingredient has been removed. Its ability to lower cholesterol is now questionable.

Limited data are available on adverse events associated with red yeast rice. Controlled trials report mild headache and gastrointestinal discomfort. In general, adverse effects, contraindications, and interactions for red yeast rice may be extrapolated from controlled trials with low-dose "statin" agents. In several case reports, patients using red yeast rice developed muscular dysfunction (myopathy) and muscle breakdown (rhabdomyolysis),[1-3] which have been described in numerous case reports of individuals taking statin agents.[4] Although the frequency of adverse effects appears to be low with moderate consumption of red yeast rice, standardization and data on the long-term safety of products containing red yeast rice are lacking. Red yeast rice should not be used in people with liver problems or in heavy alcohol users. Serious drug interactions have been reported.[4]

Interactions

Note: Because of the limited safety information for red yeast rice, many of these interactions are based on known interactions for statins. Whether these interactions are applicable to red yeast rice preparations will depend on the levels of monakolin K present.

ANTIBIOTICS: Certain antibiotics, in particular the macrolide antibiotics, are known to increase the risk of muscle breakdown (rhabdomyolysis) when taken with statins. A 2002 FDA report cited 42 cases (of 601 total cases of statin-associated rhabdomyolysis over 29 months) that also involved macrolide antibiotics,[4] which include azithromycin (Zithromax), clarithromycin (Biaxin), dirithromycin (Dynabac), erythromycin, and roxithromycin (Rulid). Because of the various types of statins and antibiotics involved in these cases, as well as the variable levels of statins in red yeast rice, these data should be interpreted carefully. Nonetheless, caution is warranted when taking red yeast rice and antibiotics concomitantly.

ANTICOAGULANTS/ANTIPLATELETS: The 2002 FDA report on statin-associated rhabdomyolysis cited 33 cases (of 601 total cases over 29 months) that also involved warfarin.[4] Because of the various types of statins, anticoagulants, and statin levels in red yeast rice, these data should be interpreted carefully. Nonetheless, caution is warranted when taking red yeast rice and anticoagulants or antiplatelets concomitantly.

AZOLE ANTIFUNGAL AGENTS: The 2002 FDA report on statin-associated rhabdomyolysis noted 12 cases (of 601 total cases) that also involved azole antifungals.[4] There are numerous types of azole antifungals, all with the suffix "-azole," such as clotrimazole (Lotrimin). Because of the various types of azoles and statins, as well as the variable levels of statins in red yeast rice, these data should be interpreted carefully. Nonetheless, caution is warranted when taking red yeast rice and antifungal medicines concomitantly.

BLOOD GLUCOSE: Based on clinical and animal studies, red yeast rice may decrease glucose.[5-7] Blood glucose tests may be affected.

BLOOD LIPIDS: Based on clinical trials, red yeast rice may lower cholesterol levels.[8-28] This effect may be caused by the monacolin K content.

BLOOD PRESSURE: In animals the aqueous extract of *Monascus purpureus* M9011 had antihypertensive and metabolic effects when used in fructose-induced hypertensive rats.[29,30] Theoretically, concurrent use of red yeast rice with antihypertensive agents may cause additive blood pressure–lowering effects.

CAROTENOIDS: In animals the combination of policosanol, red yeast rice extract, and astaxanthin has been shown to have additive antiatherosclerotic effects.[31]

COENZYME Q10 LEVELS: In animals, acute use of red yeast rice has been shown to deplete tissue CoQ10 levels.[32] Based on a case study of an elderly man, Chinese red rice may deplete muscle CoQ10 and maintain muscle damage after discontinuation of statin treatment.[33] Serum CoQ10 decreases by up to 30% with use of "statins."[34-36] The clinical implications of this reduction are unclear.

CYCLOSPORINE: The 2002 FDA report on statin-associated rhabdomyolysis noted 51 cases (of 601 total cases) that also involved the immunosuppressant cyclosporine.[4] Because of the various types of statins used in these cases, as well as the variable levels of statins in red yeast rice, these data should be interpreted carefully. Nonetheless, caution is warranted when taking red yeast rice and cyclosporine concomitantly.

CYTOCHROME P450 SUBSTRATES: Lovastatin is a substrate of CYP450-3A4 that is found in red yeast rice. Decreased lovastatin metabolism from CYP3A4 inhibition may increase the risk of myopathy and rhabdomyolysis.

DIGOXIN: The 2002 FDA report on statin-associated rhabdomyolysis noted 26 cases (of 601 total cases) that also involved the cardiac glycoside digoxin,[4] often used to treat heart conditions. Because of the various types of statins used in these cases, as well as the variable levels of statins in red yeast rice, these data should be interpreted carefully. Nonetheless, caution is warranted when taking red yeast rice and cardiac glycosides concomitantly.

FIBRIC ACID DERIVATES (FIBRATES): The 2002 FDA report on statin-associated rhabdomyolysis noted 80 cases (of 601 total cases) that also involved fibrates.[4] Fibrates are carboxylic acids often used with statins to treat hyperlipidemia; the various types include benzafibrate (Benzalip), ciprofibrate (Modalim), and fenofibrate (TriCor). Because of the various fibrates and statins, as well as the variable levels of statins in red yeast rice, these data should be interpreted carefully. Nonetheless, caution is warranted when taking red yeast rice and fibrates concomitantly.

FRUCTOSE: In animals, aqueous extract of *Monascus purpureus* M9011 has been shown to prevent and reverse fructose-induced hypertension.[29]

GABANERGIC AGENTS: Potentiation of side effects may occur when GABAnergic agonists are used in combination with red yeast rice.[7,37]

GRAPEFRUIT: Based on a documented clinical interaction between grapefruite juice and lovastatin,[38] grapefruit juice may elevate the bioavailability of red yeast rice.

HEMOGLOBIN LEVELS: In animals, red yeast rice has been shown to decrease hemoglobin.[39]

HMG-CoA REDUCTASE INHIBITORS: Taking red yeast rice with other HMG-CoA reductase inhibitors may increase the risk of adverse effects.[7,40,41]

INFLAMMATORY MARKER LEVELS: Based on results from clinical trials, use of red yeast may result in decreased C-reactive protein (CRP) levels.[42,43]

KIDNEY FUNCTION TESTS: In animals, decreased blood urea nitrogen (BUN) has been noted with use of red yeast rice.[39]

LACTATE: In animals, red yeast rice has been shown to decrease lactate levels.[39]

LEVOTHYROXINE: Two case reports have described interactions between simvastatin and levothyroxine (L-thyroxine).[44,45] It was postulated that the excess formation of CYP3A4 in the liver by simvastatin accelerated the metabolic breakdown of levothyroxine. Similar interactions are possible with lovastatin derived from red yeast rice.

LIVER FUNCTION TESTS: Based on clinical evidence, red yeast rice may increase aspartate transaminase (AST) and alanine transaminase (ALT).[7,40] Additionally, lovastatin found in red yeast rice may cause hepatotoxicity and may increase the risk of liver damage when used with hepatotoxic agents.

MIBEFRADIL (POSICOR): The 2002 FDA report on statin-associated rhabdomyolysis cited 99 cases (of 601 total cases) that involved mibefradil,[4] a calcium channel blocker used to treat hypertension and angina, before its withdrawal from the market because of serious side effects.[46] Although mibefradil is no longer available, caution is warranted when taking red yeast rice and calcium channel blockers concomitantly.

POLICOSANOL: Based on clinical research, a dietary supplement made of *Monascus purpureus*, octacosanols (policosanol), and niacin may decrease total cholesterol, LDL cholesterol, and triacylglycerols.[47]

PROTEASE INHIBITORS: Many common protease inhibitors are metabolized by CYP3A, which also metabolizes many statins, including lovastatin, simvastatin, atorvastatin, and cerivastatin.

Because of the known interactions between protease inhibitors, use of lovastatin is generally contraindicated in patients taking protease inhibitors.[48]

St. John's wort: Use of St. John's wort may reduce red yeast rice levels by inhibiting hepatic enzymes (CYP3A4).[43]

Vitamin A: Based on evidence of HMG-CoA reductase inhibitor use in individuals with high cholesterol level, use of red yeast may increase serum vitamin A levels.[49]

Zinc: Based on in vitro studies, red yeast rice may interact with zinc.[50]

Rehmannia (Rehmannia glutinosa)

Pharmacokinetics: Insufficient available evidence.

Adverse effects

Rehmannia has been well tolerated for 20 days to 1.2 years in clinical trials.[1-5]

Rehmannia is purported to cause dizziness, lack of energy, heart palpitations, edema, and gastrointestinal upset. Rehmannia can cause hypoglycemia.[6,7] In mice the antifertility effects of rehmannia were suggested by a decreased number of litters.[8,9] Liu Wei di huang t'ang, which is a decoction of rehmannia with six components, was tested on renally hypertensive rats and showed marked hypotensive effects.[10]

Interactions

Antibiotics: Animal evidence suggests that the concomitant use of aminoglycoside antibiotics and rehmannia may decrease the toxicity associated with aminoglycoside therapy.[11]

Antibody levels: In rats, rehmannia showed dose-dependent inhibition of systemic allergic reaction and anti-IgE antibody–induced cutaneous reaction.[12]

Anticoagulants/antiplatelets: In animals, Man-Shen-Ling (MSL), containing medicinal agents such as astragalus and rehmannia, exhibited anticoagulant effects.[13] Concomitant use of rehmannia with anticoagulants may result in additive effects, although clinical reports of such drug interactions are lacking.

Antineoplastic agents: Animal and clinical studies suggest that rehmannia may decrease toxicity associated with chemotherapy;[14,15] however, the evidence is unclear. Shi-Quan-Da-Bu-Tang (SQT), which contains *Rehmannia glutinosa, Paeonia lactiflora, Ligusticum wallichii, Angelica sinesis, Glycyrrhiza uralensis, Poria cocos, Atractyloides macrocephala, Panax ginseng, Astragalus membranaceus,* and *Cinnamomum cassia,* was found to potentiate therapeutic activity of chemotherapy and radiotherapy and to prevent or minimize associated adverse events in animal models of cancer.[15]

Blood glucose: Rehmannia may add to the effects of hypoglycemic agents and can cause hypoglycemia.[6] Seishin-kanro-to, composed of rehmannia radix, may reduce blood sugar levels in diabetic patients, according to a mouse study.[16]

Blood lipids: In a case-control study of patients with type 2 diabetes mellitus and hyperlipidemia, rehmannia resulted in reduced total and LDL cholesterol and triglycerides and incremental changes in HDL cholesterol.[17]

Blood pressure: Combination use of rehmannia and antihypertensives may result in additive effects. Liu Wei di huang t'ang, a decoction of rehmannia with six components, showed marked hypotensive effects in rats.[10]

Corticosteroids: Anecdotally, taking rehmannia concomitantly with corticosteroids has been reported to result in a synergistic effect and may reduce side effects.[1] Animal research showed that *Rehmannia glutinosa* used with dexamethasone maintained the therapeutic effect of the glucocorticoid and relieved side effects of both functional and morphological changes in pituitary and adrenal cortex caused by glucocorticoids.[17]

Kidney function tests: Rehmannia may have an additive effect when used with diuretics. In animals, Man-Shen-Ling (MSL), containing medicinal agents such as astragalus and rehmannia, caused an increase in renal blood flow and glomerular filtration, the excretion of urea-nitrogen, and a potassium/sodium-promoting function.[12] In rat study, *R. glutinosa* increased renal blood flow.[19]

Thyroid hormones: In a study of hyperthyroid rats, *R. glutinosa* lowered receptor affinity and the peripheral conversion of T_4 to T_3.[20] In another hyperthyroid rat study, rehmannia significantly reduced the binding capacity of the beta-adrenergic receptors in the kidney.[21] In a clinical study, *R. glutinsoa* may have improved clinical symptoms of Sheehan's syndrome and stimulated the hypothalamic-pituitary system.[4]

Reishi Mushroom (Ganoderma lucidum)

Pharmacokinetics: Insufficient available evidence.

Adverse effects

Acute and long-term studies have found *Ganoderma lucidum* to be generally well tolerated for up to 16 months.[1-11] The most common adverse events reported are skin rash, dizziness, and headaches. Reishi mushroom may be unsafe in patients with hemophilia because of its high adenosine content; however, in HIV-positive hemophilia patients, crude extracts of reishi mushroom did not exhibit antiplatelet effects.[12]

Interactions

Acyclovir: *G. lucidum* was shown in vitro to have synergistic antiherpetic effects when administered with acyclovir.[13]

Allografts: Reishi may have immunosuppressive effects, as demonstrated in an animal study in which reishi delayed allograft rejection.[14]

Anticoagulants/antiplatelets: Reishi may cause bleeding from prolongation of prothrombin time. In vitro and in vivo evidence shows that *Ganoderma lucidum* inhibits platelet aggregation.[15] However, in HIV-positive hemophilia patients, crude extracts of rehmannia did not exhibit antiplatelet effects.[12]

Blood glucose: Reishi has been shown to reduce blood sugar levels and increase insulin levels in mice.[16-21]

Blood lipids: Reishi may lower cholesterol by inhibiting cholesterol synthesis, as demonstrated in vitro.[22]

Blood pressure: *G. lucidum* has been demonstrated to lower blood pressure in animals.[23] In vitro, *G. lucidum* exhibited inhibitory effects on angiotensin-converting enzyme.[24]

HMG-CoA reductase inhibitors: Reishi has been shown to inhibit HMG-CoA reductase in cholesterol biosynthesis.[22] Because of the known adverse effects of HMG-CoA reductase inhibitors, concomitant use is discouraged, although clinical evidence of this interaction is lacking.

Viral levels: Reishi has demonstrated antiviral activities against HIV-1,[25,26] herpes simplex virus type 1 (HSV-1) and HSV-2,[27] and Epstein-Barr virus[28] in vitro.

Resveratrol

Pharmacokinetics

The absorption of a dietary relevant 25-mg oral dose of resveratrol was at least 70%, with peak plasma levels of resveratrol and metabolites of 491 ±90 ng/mL (~2 mcM) and a plasma half-life of 9.2 ±0.6 hours.[1] However, only trace amounts of unchanged resveratrol (<5 ng/mL) could be detected in plasma. A 25-mg dose per 70 kg was inadequate to permit circulating concentrations consistent with in vitro biological activity.[2] Urinary resveratrol and its metabolites were observed in human subjects receiving 600 and 1200 mL of grape juice. The cumulative amount of resveratrol excreted in the urine of mice receiving concentrated grape juice for 4 days was 2.3% of the ingested dose.[3] The glycoside form of resveratrol in grape juice may be absorbed to a lesser extent than the aglycon.[3] Resveratrol is also absorbed after oral wine ingestion, reaching peak plasma concentration of 1 mcM after 1 hour.[4] Total resveratrol concentrations in plasma, urine, heart, liver, and kidney were lower than that required for pharmacological activity after administration of red wine to rats.[5] In an isolated preparation of luminally and vascularly perfused rat small intestine, vascular uptake of administered resveratrol was 20.5%. The majority of the absorbed resveratrol was conjugated to yield resveratrol glucuronide (16.8%), which was also the main luminal metabolite (11.2%). Lesser amounts of resveratrol sulfate, 3.0% and 0.3%, were found on the luminal and vascular side, respectively, and small amounts of resveratrol and resveratrol conjugates (1.9%) were found in the intestinal tissue.[6]

Pharmacokinetic studies revealed that the target organs of resveratrol are the liver and kidneys, where it is concentrated after absorption and is mainly converted to a sulfated form and a glucuronide conjugate.[4,7] Tissue concentrations also show bioavailability in cardiac tissue.[4] In plasma, resveratrol was shown to interact with lipoproteins and could be largely delivered to body tissues in this way.[8]

In human liver, CYP1A2 likely plays a major role in the metabolism of trans-resveratrol into piceatannol and tetrahydroxystilbene M1.[9] Resveratrol also appears to be metabolized by CYP1B1, to form the antileukaemic agent, piceatannol.[10] In humans, resveratrol is metabolized into two resveratrol-3-O- and 4'-O-glucuronides.[11-13] Trans-resveratrol is rapidly converted in vivo primarily to trans-resveratrol-3-sulfate.[13,14] In serum, resveratrol is present mainly as glucuronide and sulfate conjugates.[2] Glucuronidation of resveratrol takes place in the human liver. After consumption by both humans and rats, total conjugates are greater than aglycon levels of resveratrol.[15] Compounds in the diet, such as quercetin and other flavonoids, may inhibit the sulfation and glucuronidation of resveratrol, improving its bioavailability.[16]

In vitro, trans-resveratrol inhibits a substrate oxidation reaction catalyzed by human recombinant CYP3A4 and 3A5.[17] Resveratrol inhibited the constitutive and induced expression and activity of CYP1A1, 1B1, and 3A4.[14,18-29] Resveratrol inhibited all CYP tested (1A1, 1A2, 1B1, 2A6, 2B6, 2E1, 3A4, 4A), except for 2E1.[30] Resveratrol is a marginal inhibitor of 3A4 and a weak inhibitor of CYP2C19.[14]

Most of the oral dose of resveratrol is excreted in urine as sulfate and glucuronic acid conjugates of the phenolic groups and hydrogenated derivatives of the aliphatic double bond.[1,2] Trans-resveratrol was influenced by the multidrug-related protein 2, an efflux pump present on the apical membrane.[31] In a second study, resveratrol was not a substrate for P-glycoprotein or the multidrug-resistance associated proteins.[32]

Adverse effects

There is limited long-term information regarding adverse effects associated with resveratrol supplements alone. Consumption of large quantities of red wine as a source of resveratrol is considered unsafe because of the alcohol content. The American Heart Association recommends up to two drinks daily for men and one drink daily for women; one drink is considered 4 oz of wine. Large amounts of alcohol consumption increase the risk of alcoholism, high blood pressure, obesity, stroke, breast cancer, psychiatric disordes, and accidents.[33]

Interactions

ANTIBIOTICS: Based on preliminary laboratory research, resveratrol may have additive effects when taken with actinomycin D and nystatin.[34,35] Trans-resveratrol may have a protective effect on gentamicin-induced kidney toxicity, as demonstrated in animals.[36]

ANTICOAGULANTS/ANTIPLATELETS: Laboratory study suggests that resveratrol has antiaggregating and antithrombin activity and may have additive effects when taken with other agents with the same actions.[5,37-47] Use of resveratrol with antiplatelets could cause increased risk of bleeding, although clinical reports of drug interactions are lacking.

ANTIVIRAL AGENTS: Resveratrol has been demonstrated in vitro to increase the effects of some antivirals, including antiretroviral HIV agents AZT, ddC, and ddI.[48]

BLOOD LIPIDS: Resveratrol has been shown to reduce cholesterol levels in rats.[49]

BLOOD PRESSURE: Theoretically, use of resveratrol with blood pressure–lowering agents may result in additive effects.[50,51]

CYCLOSPORINE: Based on preliminary in vitro data, resveratrol may enhance the immune suppression caused by cyclosporin A, as shown by its suppression of TNF-α, IL-2, and T-lymphocyte proliferation.[52]

CYTOCHROME P450 SUBSTRATES: Preliminary evidence suggests that resveratrol may weakly inhibit the way that the liver breaks down certain agents (inhibits multiple CYP450 enzymes).*

DIGOXIN: Resveratrol has been shown in vitro to antagonize the toxic effects of digoxin.[60,61]

ESTROGENIC AGENTS: Resveratrol has been demonstrated to both agonize[62,63] and antagonize[64-66] the effects of estrogenic agents. Resveratrol apparently has the potential to act as an estrogen agonist or antagonist, depending on such factors as cell type and estrogen receptor isoform (ER-α or ER-β).[67] Resveratrol has also been shown to inhibit vitamin D_3 receptor expression through estrogenic regulation.[68] Clinical evidence of estrogen interactions is lacking.

HISTOLOGICAL TESTS: Resveratrol has been shown in vitro to enhance radiation-induced cancer cell death.[69,70] Thus, it has been suggested as an adjunct to radiation therapy, although this has not been thoroughly studied. Histological findings may be altered.

LIVER FUNCTION TESTS: Drinking large quantities of red wine, which contains resveratrol, may have adverse effects on the liver.

MONOAMINERGIC AGENTS: Resveratrol competitively inhibits monoamine oxidase A.[71] Therefore, it may interact with other MAO inhibitors, such as phenelzine (Nardil) and tranylcypromine (Parnate), although this has not been studied extensively.

PACLITAXEL: Resveratrol has been suggested to have antineoplastic activity in several in vitro studies.[72-79] Some in vitro studies suggest that it may enhance the efficacy of paclitaxel;[76,77,79] other in vitro

---

*References 9, 10, 14, 19, 20, 23-26, 28, 29, 53-59.

studies suggest that resveratrol might interfere with paclitaxel.[74,75] In vitro, resveratrol has been shown synergistically to enhance the cytotoxic effects of ara-C (cytarabine) and tiazofurin.[80]

QUERCETIN AND RUTIN: Resveratrol has been shown to increase the growth-inhibitory effects of quercetin and rutin on cultured carcinoma cells.[81,82]

Rhodiola (Rhodiola rosea)

Pharmacokinetics
The pharmacokinetics of *Rhodiola* is not well understood. P-tyrosol, a constituent of *Rhodiola*, appears to be dose-dependently excreted in urine.[1]

Adverse effects
Anecdotal reports suggest that *R. rosea* might increase blood pressure, heart rate, and heart palpitations, as well as cause restlessness, irritability, and insomnia. However, reports of side effects from *Rhodiola rosea* (SHR-5) are currently lacking in the available literature.[2,3]

Interactions
ANTIBIOTICS: There is clinical evidence from a Phase III study that ADAPT-232 (combination product containing *R. rosea*, *S. chinensis*, and *E. senticosus*) may have additive effects with standard antibiotic therapy for pneumonia (cephazoline, with bromhexine and theophylline).[4]

ANTIBODY LEVELS: A combination product (Admax) containing *Leuzea carthamoides*, *Rhodiola rosea*, *Eleutherococcus senticosus*, and fruits of *Schisandra chinensis* was shown clinically to increase IgG and IgM.[4-5]

ANTIDEPRESSANTS: In animals, *R. rosea* extract significantly induced antidepressant-like and anxiolytic-like effects.[6] *Rhodiola* may interact with antidepressant or anxiolytic agents, although this has not been demonstrated.

ANTINEOPLASTIC AGENTS: In mice, *R. rosea* was found to inhibit tumor growth[7] and decrease the toxicity of doxorubicin (Adriamycin),[8] sarcolysin,[9] and cyclophosphamide.[10]

BACTERIAL LEVELS: In vitro, *R. rosea* has demonstrated antibacterial effects.[4]

BLOOD GLUCOSE: Animal and in vitro research suggest that *R. rosea* may decrease blood glucose.[11,12]

BLOOD PRESSURE: In vitro, ethanol and water extracts of *R. rosea* inhibited ACE activity[11] and may thus affect blood pressure.

CRANBERRY EXTRACT: A combination of water extracts of cranberry and *R. rosea* had additive effects on α-glucosidase, α-amylase, and ACE inhibition in vitro.[13]

CREATINE KINASE: In humans, *R. rosea* extract has been shown clinically to reduce CK levels after exhausting exercise.[14]

CYTOKINES AND INFLAMMATORY MARKERS: In humans, *R. rosea* extract has been shown to reduce levels of C-reactive protein after exhausting exercise.[14]

ESTROGENIC AGENTS: *R. rosea* has been suggested to interact with estrogen receptors, although this has not been clearly demonstrated.

HEMATOCRIT: In vitro, *R. rosea* did not modulate granulocytopoiesis[15] but did stimulate bone marrow erythropoiesis, followed by a decrease in bone marrow erythrokaryocytes.[16]

NEUROTRANSMITTER TESTING: Based on unsubstantiated reports, *R. rosea* may increase brain levels of dopamine, acetylcholine, and norepinephrine.[17]

OPIATES: In animal and in vitro research, *R. rosea* has been shown to activate opioid receptors.[18-22] Interactions with other opiates are possible, but not well understood.

SEDATIVES AND CENTRAL NERVOUS SYSTEM DEPRESSANTS: It has been suggested that *R. rosea* and neurological agents may have additive effects.[23] Based on unsubstantiated reports, *R. rosea* extract may potentiate the effect of pentobarbital.[24]

WHITE BLOOD CELL COUNTS: A combination product (Admax) containing *R. rosea* was shown clinically to increase CD3+, CD4+, CD5+, and CD8+ T-cell counts.[5] In another small clinical study, *R. rosea* extract improved parameters of leukocyte and T-cell immunity; however, the incidence of bladder cancer recurrence did not improve statististically.[25]

Rhubarb (Rheum spp.)

Pharmacokinetics
The pharmacokinetics of rhubarb is not well understood. Anthraquinone glycosides in rhubarb are hydrolyzed in the gut to aglycons, which are reduced by bacteria to anthranols and anthrones (the active compounds).[1] Only 2% to -5% of ingested oxalates have been shown to be absorbed in healthy human volunteers; oral oxalates given to animals have been excreted unchanged in the urine within 24 to 36 hours after ingestion.[2]

Adverse effects
Chronic use of rhubarb may cause electrolyte loss (especially potassium); other effects of overuse may include hyperaldosteronism, edema, inhibition of gastric motility, pseudomelanosis coli, intestinal griping, colic, atonic colon,[3-10] nephropathies, albuminuria, hematuria, bone deterioration and muscular weakness, arrhythmias, and cardiac toxicity (especially if cardiac glycosides, diuretics, or corticosteroids are used concomitantly).[11-13] Rhubarb root contains tannins; while the oral toxicity of plant tannins is low (as it is readily hydrolyzed in the gut to gallic acid and other metabolites), liver and kidney toxicity has occurred with high tannin doses used topically or intravenously.[14] Tannin consumption has been associated with certain cancers, such as esophageal cancer; however, it is unclear whether this is due to the tannins themselves or other compounds associated with tannins.[15]

Short-term use of raw rhubarb may cause gastrointestinal complaints, including abdominal pain, diarrhea, nausea, and vomiting.[4,5,16] Handling rhubarb leaves may cause contact dermatitis.[8,13]

Oxalic acid in rhubarb may form insoluble calcium oxalate crystals in the blood that may be deposited in the kidneys and may lead to renal stones. Bright-yellow or red, discolored urine may occur with rhubarb ingestion. Hyperkalemia has been reported in one person taking rhubarb (amount unspecified).[17] Abuse of rhubarb may cause dependence with need for increased doses.

Interactions
ALISMATIS ORIENTALIS: In a clinical trial, rhubarb showed hypolipidemic properties when used with *Alismatis orientalis*.[18]

ANGIOTENSIN-CONVERTING ENZYME INHIBITORS: Rhubarb root contains tannins shown in vitro to inhibit angiotensin converting enzyme (ACE).[19] In clinical trials, rhubarb has shown a synergistic effect with captopril, an ACE inhibitor, to reduce serum creatinine levels.[17,20-23] Hyperkalemia, corrected with furosemide, occurred in one person taking rhubarb and captopril.[17]

ANTIPSYCHOTIC AGENTS: Rhubarb reduced the need for higher doses of antipsychotic agents in schizophrenic patients.[24]

BLOOD LIPIDS: Rhubarb may have cholesterol-lowering effects, as demonstrated in human subjects.[25-27]

BLOOD PRESSURE: Rhubarb may lower blood pressure.[28,29] Theoretically, concomitant use with antihypertensive agents may enhance blood pressure–lowering effects.

CALCIUM: In theory, concurrent use of rhubarb and sorrel may decrease mineral absorption, although animal research involving rhubarb stalk fiber did not reveal altered bioavailability of calcium.[30]

CHLORHEXIDINE: In a clinical trial, rhubarb reduced gingivitis when used with chlorhexidine.[31]

CISPLATIN: In mice treated with cisplatin, cotherapy with rhubarb significantly reduced the lethal toxicity and renal toxicity of this common chemotherapeutic agent; the combination did not interfere with the chemotherapeutic effect of cisplatin.[32]

CORTICOSTEROIDS: Rhubarb along with dexamethasone (Decadron) reduced the lung edema in rats because of endotoxin-induced lung injury.[33]

CREATININE: In clinical trials, rhubarb has shown a synergistic effect with captopril, an ACE inhibitor, to reduce serum creatinine levels.[17,20-22]

ELECTROLYTES: Overuse of rhubarb may compound diuretic-induced potassium loss.[17] Rhubarb also possesses laxative effects,[34] which may contribute to fluid and/or electrolyte loss.

ESTROGENIC AGENTS: Uterus segments taken from estrogen-pretreated rats decreased in spontaneous contractility after the addition of rhein.[35]

GINSENG: In a clinical trial, rhubarb and sanchi powder *(Panax notoginseng)* were used together for hemorrhagic fever from nephritic syndrome.[36]Fu 2005

GLAUBER'S SALT (MIRABILITE): In a clinical trial, rhubarb enhanced the laxative effects of Glauber's salt.[37]

IRON: Herbal texts and anecdotal reports suggest that rhubarb impairs absorption of iron because of oxalate content.[38] However, based on laboratory research, rhubarb *(Rheum rhaponticum)* may have a moderately enhancing effect on iron absorption.[39]

KIDNEY FUNCTION TESTS: Rhubarb has been shown to induce nephrotoxicity in animal studies.[40] However, rhubarb tannins have been shown to improve BUN, creatinine, GFR, renal plasma flow, and renal blood flow.[41] Caution is warranted.

LIVER FUNCTION TESTS: The high tannin level of rhubarb root may increase the chance of hepatic necrosis.[15] In large amounts, ingestion of sorrel may lead to liver damage and should be avoided with hepatotoxic agents.

MILK: Anecdotally, the effectiveness of rhubarb may be decreased when taken concurrently with milk or other dairy products.

MINERALS: Absorption of minerals from food may be decreased with concomitant rhubarb ingestion.[42,43] Rhubarb's oxalate content may bind multivalent metal ions in the GI tract and decrease their absorption.

NIFEDIPINE (PROCARDIA): In a clinical trial, rhubarb enhanced the effects of the calcium channel blocker nifedipine.[44]

ORAL AGENTS: Rhubarb's laxative effects may reduce the absorption of other oral agents because of reduced GI transit time. Clinical evidence of such an interaction is lacking.

SAGE: In a clinical trial, rhubarb and sage cream reduced the symptoms of herpes labialis.[45]

URINE TESTS: Rhubarb may discolor urine bright yellow to red and may interfere with certain diagnostic tests. Rhubarb use has been associated with hematuria.[12]

ZINC: In humans, use of rhubarb has been shown to decrease the absorption of zinc.[38]

Rose Hip (*Rosa* spp.)

Pharmacokinetics: Insufficient available evidence.

Adverse effects

Based on historical use and available research, rose hip preparations appear to be well tolerated in recommended doses for up to 3 months.[1-3] Some adverse effects may be related to the amount of vitamin C present in rose hips. However, individuals who work in rose cultivation or manufacturing of rose products are susceptible to developing IgE-mediated hypersensitivity to rose.[4-7]

Interactions

Note: Secondary sources report several interactions between vitamin C and such agents as aspirin, estrogens, fluphenazine, salicylates, and warfarin. It is not clear how much vitamin C remains in dried and stored rose hips, or whether the remaining vitamin C may cause similar interactions.

ALUMINUM: The vitamin C found in rose hips may interact with aluminum-containing antacids and increase aluminum absorption.

ANTIBODY LEVELS: Rose plant workers have significantly higher serum IgE levels than control subjects.[5] In other studies, IgE has been detected in rose workers and villagers living in rose-cultivating areas (statistical significance not stated).[6,7]

ANTICOAGULANTS/ANTIPLATELETS: Rugosin E, a constituent of *Rosa rugosa*, was the most potent platelet-aggregating agent among nine ellagitannins tested in rabbit and human platelets.[8] Interactions with anticoagulants/antiplatelets are possible, but clinical evidence is lacking.

BACTERIAL LEVELS: In vitro evidence indicates that the essential oil of *Rosa damascena* petals, an extract of *Rosa canina* seeds, an extract of petals of *Rosa canina*, and compounds isolated from *R. canina* extract (tellimagrandin I and rugosin B) all have antibacterial activity.[9-11]

BLOOD LIPIDS: A clinical trial with a standardized rose hips powder extract (Hyben Vital) reported an unexpected 8.5% decrease in total cholesterol.[1]

CYTOKINES AND INFLAMMATORY MARKERS: Hyben Vital has been shown to reduce serum C-reactive protein (CRP) levels in humans.[2] This rose hips preparation has also reduced the rate of migration of polymorphonuclear leukocytes in vitro.[1,2] Extracts or fractions obtained from *Rosa canina* roots have demonstrated inhibitory activity in vitro against one of the following models of inflammation: interleukin-1 (IL-1α, IL-1β) and tumor necrosis factor (TNF-α) biosynthesis.[12]

ELECTROLYTES: Theoretically, rose hips may have additive effects when taken concomitantly with laxatives.

ESTROGENIC AGENTS: With a documented interaction between ethinyl estradiol and vitamin C in humans,[13] similar interactions are likely with rose hips.

HISTOLOGICAL TESTS: The juice of *Rosa rugosa* has strongly inhibited the proliferation of all cancer cell lines examined in vitro and strongly induced differentiation of HL-60 cells.[14,15] Equiguard (containing *Rosa laevigatae* fruit extract and eight other Chinese herbs) has demonstrated anti–prostate cancer effects in vitro.[16]

IRON: Vitamin C promotes iron absorption in the small intestine and may increase the absorption of dietary iron.[17]

PROSTATE-SPECIFIC ANTIGEN: Equiguard (containing *Rosa laevigatae* fruit extract and eight other Chinese herbs) has been shown to lower intracellular and secreted PSA in vitro.[16]

SALICYLATES: Administration of 900 mg of aspirin was found to block GI absorption of a single oral dose of 500 mg vitamin C in humans.[18] Concomitant use of rose hips and salicylates may increase urinary excretion of ascorbic acid and decrease excretion of salicylates.

SKIN PRICK TESTS: Workers in a rose-processing plant showed 53.84% positive responses to a specifically prepared skin prick test using a rose allergen (*Rosa domescena*).[5]

VIRAL TESTS: Extracts from the root of *Rosa rugosa* have been shown to have effects against HIV-1 protease in vitro.[19]

WHITE BLOOD CELL COUNTS: In a randomized controlled trial (RCT), natural killer (NK) cell activity increased significantly in the group supplemented with Long-Life CiLi.[20] Rose plant workers have significantly higher eosinophil counts than control subjects.[5]

Rosemary *(Rosmarinus officinalis)*

Pharmacokinetics
Rosmarinic acid is well absorbed in the GI tract. One-half hour after IV administration in rat, rosmarinic acid was detected and measured in the brain, heart, liver, lung, muscle, spleen, and bone tissue, showing the highest concentration in lung tissue, which was 13 times the blood concentration, followed by the spleen, heart, and liver tissue.[1] In 16 human samples, a correlation between coumarin 7-hydroxylation and (–)-verbenone 10-hydroxylation in the liver was observed, indicating that cytochrome P450-2A6 is the principal enzyme in verbenone (constituent of rosemary) metabolism in the liver.[2,3]

Adverse effects
Based on historical use and available research, rosemary seems well tolerated, with few documented cases of adverse events. Ingestion of rosemary oil can be toxic, and the maximum safe dose is not currently available. Although rare, seizures associated with rosemary have been reported.[4]

Interactions
ANTICOAGULANTS/ANTIPLATELETS: Rosemary has shown significant antithrombotic activity in animals.[5] Caution is advised when using rosemary with blood-thinning agents.

ANTINEOPLASTIC AGENTS: Rosemary has been shown in vitro to enhance the sensitivity of cancer cells to doxorubicin and vinblastine.[6]

ANXIOLYTICS: Theoretically, rosemary should be used cautiously in combination with anxiolytic agents because of possible additive effects.

BACTERIAL LEVELS: Based on multiple in vitro studies, rosemary and rosemary extracts may have antibacterial activity.[7-10]

BLOOD PRESSURE: Based on in vitro evidence, the water extracts of rosemary may inhibit ACE.[11] Blood pressure may be affected.

BLOOD GLUCOSE: Rosemary has been shown to increase as well as decrease glucose levels.[11-13]

BLOOD LIPIDS: As demonstrated in vitro, constituents in rosemary extract may inhibit cholesterol oxidation product formation from nucleus and lateral chain of the cholesterol molecule.[14,15] Blood lipid levels may be affected.

BONE MARKERS: In animals, rosemary, rosemary essential oil, and their monoterpene components have been shown to inhibit bone resorption.[16]

CYTOCHROME P450 SUBSTRATES: Results from in vitro and rat studies suggest that rosemary may selectively induce CYP450 enzymes in the liver, particularly 2A6, 2B, 1A1, 2B1/2B2, and 2E1.[17-19]

ELECTROLYTES: In animals, aqueous extracts of rosemary significantly increased urinary excretion of sodium, potassium, and chloride and decreased creatinine clearance.[20] Electrolyte balance may thus be altered with rosemary ingestion.

ESTROGENIC AGENTS: In animals, rosemary was shown to enhance deactivation of estrogen by the liver.[21] Clinical interactions are possible, although evidence is lacking.

FUROSEMIDE: Rosemary has been shown to increase the effects of the diuretic furosemide in vitro.[22] Caution is advised when using rosemary with all diuretic agents.

IRON: Rosemary extract has been shown to decrease the absorption of nonheme iron in humans.[23]

LITHIUM: As an herbal diuretic, rosemary has been suggested to exacerbate lithium toxicity.[24]

SEDATIVES AND CENTRAL NERVOUS SYSTEM DEPRESSANTS: Theoretically, rosemary should be used cautiously in combination with CNS depressants because of possible additive effects.

Rutin ($C_{27}H_{30}O_{16}$)

Pharmacokinetics
The pharmacokinetics of rutin has been studied in healthy volunteers. Absorption of an oral dose of hydroxyethylrutosides was less than 10%.[1] Rutosides are distributed in the blood, lungs, spleen, and muscles.[2] Rutosides are metabolized by intestinal flora and liver[1,2] and are primarily eliminated in the bile. A small amount is excreted in the urine.[2]

Adverse effects
Rutins, oxerutins, and troxerutins have been used effectively and safely in several clinical and equivalence trials. Numerous studies have reported no adverse side effects with rutin treatment.[3-20] Gastrointestinal disturbances have included diarrhea, dry mouth, constipation, and vomiting.[21-27]

Interactions
ANTICOAGULANTS/ANTIPLATELETS: Rutin is often used in combination with warfarin (Coumadin).[28-30] Clinical studies have confirmed the anti–erythrocyte aggregation effect of troxerutin,[31] a constituent of rutin, and suggest a favorable effect on blood fibrinolytic activity.[32]

DOCETAXEL: Rutin (300 mg hydroxyethylrutoside) has been given to breast cancer patients to counteract docetaxel-fluid retention.[33]

HORSE CHESTNUT EXTRACT: Oxerutins may have an additive effect when used concomitantly with horse chestnut extract, although the mechanism for this interaction is not well understood.[24]

NITRATES: Theoretically, rutin may convert compounds to nitroso derivatives and may form potentially mutagenic substances with nitrates found in some processed meat products.[34]

WHITE BLOOD CELL COUNTS: Rutin was shown to reduce lymphedema in patients after breast cancer surgery.[35] Altered WBC counts were rare events in a clinical trial involving elderly patients.[21]

Rye *(Secale cereale)*

Pharmacokinetics: Insufficient available evidence.

Adverse effects
Side effects occur rarely with rye grass use.[1] Rye grass pollen extract has been reported to cause gastrointestinal side effects, including dyspepsia, nausea, and abdominal distention.[2]

Interactions: Insufficient available evidence.

Safflower (Carthamus tinctorius)

Pharmacokinetics
Safflower oil pharmacokinetics has been studied extensively. In cystic fibrosis patients, safflower oil (triglyceride) consumed in the absence of pancreatic enzymes did not raise in mean plasma linoleic acid levels over the next four hours.[1] When linoleic acid monoglyceride (LAM) was consumed, the increase in plasma linoleic acid levels was significantly greater than for safflower oil. When free fatty acid (hydrolyzed safflower oil) was ingested, there was almost no increase in plasma linoleic acid levels in cystic fibrosis or control children. The absorption of linoleic acid from triglyceride, but not from linoleic acid monoglyceride, was greater when the cystic fibrosis children also took pancreatic enzymes. Three children with cystic fibrosis had greater increases in plasma linoleic acid levels following ingestion of safflower oil when they took antacid and cimetidine with their pancreatic capsules, compared to when they only took the pancreatic capsules. In a clinical trial, plasma samples obtained 0, 2, 4, 6, and 8 hours after a meal with a high safflower oil content showed that the cystic fibrosis patients absorbed all safflower preparations when administered with their regular dose of pancreatic enzyme supplement.[2] Many calculated parameters useful as indices of essential fatty acid status indicated that essential fatty acid deficiency exists in cystic fibrosis.[3] Treatment of 11 cystic fibrosis patients with safflower oil (1g/kg daily) failed to correct the aberrations in fatty acid pattern. The biochemical data suggest that there may be impairment in the conversion of linoleate to arachidonate as well as an impairment of absorption. However, malabsorption alone cannot account for the inadequate or marginal essential fatty acid status of cystic fibrosis patients.[4] One absorption study with safflower oil demonstrated normal enteral absorption of essential fatty acids and the ability to cross the blood-cerebrospinal fluid barrier.[5] Restricted linoleic acid availability in cystic fibrosis patients causes a change in red blood cell shape either directly by decreasing the linoleoylphosphatidylcholine content of the membrane or indirectly by affecting enzyme activity.[6]

Administration of 0.1g of fat per kilogram body weight as 10% or 20% safflower oil emulsion (Liposyn) to healthy volunteers did not show a significant difference in the clearance rate between the two emulsions.[7] It was concluded that 20% fat emulsion is as safe as 10% fat emulsion for use in intravenous nutritional support. Another study found that small neonates may have a relative deficit in clearance of free fatty acids.[8]

Safflower yellow B is metabolized by human intestinal bacteria.[9]

There is a rapid transfer of dietary fatty acids from plasma chylomicrons, specifically linoleic acid, into human milk.[10] Maximum increase occurred 10 hours after safflower oil ingestion and remained significantly elevated in milk for 10 to 24 hours (p < 0.05).

Plasma concentrations of 18:2 n-6 fatty acids increased for two hours when 609 ± 37 mcM/L was ingested during a continuous low-dose heparin infusion in 80 healthy volunteers.[11]

Metabolism in theonin 54 (T54) carriers: Postprandial lipemia in obese and T54 carriers is significant for the areas under the chylomicron cholesterol and chylomicron triacylglycerol curves (higher values for safflower 0.635 ± 0.053 and 2.48 ± 0.30mmol. hour/L, respectively) than olive oil (0.592 ± 0.052 and 2.48 ± 0.32mmol. hour/L, respectively) or (0.425 ± 0.043 and 1.69 ± 0.20mmol. hour/L, respectively; p<0.05).[12] The stability of 1:1-soybean/safflower intravenous lipid emulsions in three different all-in-one admixtures intended for neonatal and infant patients was investigated.[13] The stability of soybean/safflower-based admixtures significantly and rapidly deteriorated in one of the three all-in-one compositions studied. This significant and rapid deterioration of stability was likewise observed in an earlier study.[14]

Adverse effects
Safflower is a member of the daisy family (Asteraceae/Compositae) and may cause allergic reactions in patients sensitive to daisies. Other members of this family include ragweed, chrysanthemums, marigolds, and many other plants. Rarely, safflower may cause diarrhea, low blood pressure, tachycardia, loss of appetite, nausea, bad aftertaste, stomach cramps, and a feeling of fullness.[15-17]

Interactions
ACIDITY: In a case series, children with cystic fibrosis had greater increases in plasma linoleic acid after ingestion of safflower oil when they took antacids and the H_2 receptor blocker cimetidine with their pancreatic capsules, than when they took the pancreatic capsules alone.[1]

ALBUMIN LEVELS: An increase in serum albumin was noted in pediatric patients receiving 20% safflower oil emulsion for 2 weeks.[18]

ANTICOAGULANTS/ANTIPLATELETS: Based on clinical and laboratory studies, safflower (taken orally) may have antiplatelet aggregation activity[19-23] and may increase the effects of blood-thinning agents. However, clinical evidence indicates that safflower infusion may develop hypercoagulability of blood. Small doses of heparin added to large doses of Liposyn 10% (emulsion of safflower oil) in total parenteral nutrition (TPN) reversed hypercoagulation caused by safflower oil.[20]

BLOOD GLUCOSE: Based on clinical research, safflower oil may adversely affect glycemic control in type 2 diabetic patients.[24] This is supported by animal evidence that a high-fat safflower oil diet produced insulin resistance.[25]

BLOOD LIPIDS: According to clinical trials and laboratory study, ingestion of safflower oil may decrease serum total cholesterol, HDL, LDL, apolipoprotein B, and malondialdehyde-LDL.[21,26-31] However, some clinical trials found that safflower may increase some serum lipids, including cell cholesterol in the plasma, and may increase triglyceride-rich lipoproteins.[32-35] Several other clinical trials found that safflower oil did not significantly change any measured lipid/lipoprotein values.[31,36-43]

BLOOD PRESSURE: Safflower may cause a modest fall in blood pressure.[44]

CYTOKINES AND INFLAMMATORY MARKERS: Based on clinical research involving hormone replacement therapy (HRT), safflower oil may cause additive effects with fish oil to reduce CRP and IL-6.[45] In the peritoneal macrophages of animals fed safflower, hemorrhage increased PGE_2 release but decreased antigen presentation capacity; IL-1 and IL-2 were enhanced.[46] In vitro, safflower activated NF-κB and increased cytokine production by macrophages.[47] However, in a clinical study, safflower did not alter cytokine and eicosanoid production during human immunodeficiency virus (HIV) infection.[48]

LITHIUM: Based on a case series, safflower oil may reverse the symptoms of low-dose lithium neurotoxicity caused by inhibited synthesis of prostaglandin E_1 (PGE_1).[49]

PENTOBARBITAL: In animals, safflower oil has been shown to decrease pentobarbital-associated mortalities.[50]

RICE BRAN OIL: Blending rice bran oil with safflower oil, at a definite proportion (7:3 wt/wt), may magnify the hypocholesterolemic efficacy, compared with the effect of each oil alone.[51-53]

WHITE BLOOD CELL COUNT: In humans, safflower supplementation resulted in enhanced NK-cell activity.[54] However, safflower emulsion was not shown to alter parameters of cellular immunity in some in vitro studies.[48,55-57]

Sage (Salvia officinalis)

Pharmacokinetics

The pharmacokinetics of sage is not well understood. The rosmaric acid constituent of sage apparently is poorly absorbed.[1] Some constituents of sage are metabolized in the liver.[2]

Adverse effects

Sage is approved for food use as a spice or seasoning in the United States and appears in the FDA's "generally recognized as safe" (GRAS) list. Sage appears to be a safe product in most patients; however, doses of 12 drops or more have been documented to induce seizures.[3,4] Large amounts or prolonged use of sage leaf or ingestion of sage oil may cause restlessness, vomiting, vertigo, tachycardia, tremors, seizures, and kidney damage.[5]

Interactions

AGENTS THAT MAY LOWER SEIZURE THRESHOLD: Some species of sage may cause convulsions[6-8] and should be used with caution when combined with agents that lower the seizure threshold.

ALFALFA: Sage has been used in combination with alfalfa (Medicago sativa) to treat menopausal symptoms.[9]

BACTERIAL LEVELS: In vitro studies have demonstrated the antimicrobial effects of sage.[10-12] Clinical effects are not clear.

BENZODIAZEPINES: Based on in vitro research, some flavones in sage may competitively inhibit benzodiazepine receptor binding[13,14] and theoretically may interact with benzodiazepine agents.

BLOOD GLUCOSE: Based on in vitro studies, sage may have blood sugar–lowering activity.[15,16]

CHOLINERGIC AGENTS: Sage has displayed anticholinergic properties.[16-18] Certain cholinergic agents may interact with sage.

CYTOCHROME P450 SUBSTRATES: Sage has been found to inhibit CYP3A4 and should be used cautiously in patients taking CYP3A4 substrates.

CYTOKINES AND INFLAMMATORY MARKERS: Based on in vitro studies, sage may have antiinflammatory activity.[19,20]

ESTROGENIC AGENTS: Sage essential oil has displayed estrogenic activity[19] and may cause additive effects when used with estrogen therapy. Sage has been used in combination with alfalfa (Medicago sativa) to treat menopausal symptoms.[9] Clinical reports of such drug interactions are lacking.

RHUBARB: In a clinical trial, rhubarb and sage cream reduced the symptoms of herpes labialis.[21]

SEDATIVES AND CENTRAL NERVOUS SYSTEM DEPRESSANTS: Sage may have sedative properties[5] and may cause additive effects when used with CNS depressants.

THYROID HORMONES: Sage may induce a significant increase in thyroid-stimulating hormone (TSH)[9] and theoretically may affect test results.

Sandalwood (Santalum album)

Pharmacokinetics: Insufficient available evidence.

Adverse effects

In a case study, sandalwood incense appeared to cause itchy lesions.[1]

Interactions

ANXIOLYTIC AND HYPNOTIC AGENTS: Because it may have relaxation properties,[2] sandalwood aromatherapy should be used cautiously with other anxiolytic and hypnotic agents. The interactions between oral sandalwood and other agents are not well understood.

Sanicle (Sanicula europaea)

Pharmacokinetics

Sanicle has been found to contain saponins,[1-4] which are reported to be poorly absorbed by the body. However, the pharmacokinetics of sanicle is currently unclear.

Adverse effects

Reports of adverse effects associated with *Sanicula* species are currently lacking in the scientific literature. Phytodermatosis has been reported.[5] Gastrointestinal irritation may result from saponin content.

Interactions

BLOOD PRESSURE: According to secondary sources, sanicle has caused edema reduction in animal research.

FUNGAL LEVELS: Based on laboratory research, *Sanicula* saponins may have antimycotic effects.[6]

VIRAL LEVELS: In vitro, a *Sanicula europaea* leaf extract has shown activity against influenza virus[7,8] and HIV.[1]

Saw Palmetto (Serenoa repens)

Pharmacokinetics: Insufficient available evidence.

Adverse effects

Overall, there appear to be few safety concerns with short-term use of saw palmetto, although large-scale and longer-term safety studies are lacking.[1] Saw palmetto appears to be well tolerated by most patients for 3 to 5 years. The most common complaints are gastrointestinal and include abdominal discomfort or pain, nausea, vomiting, and diarrhea (anecdotally, lipidosterolic extract of *Serenoa repens* [LSESR] may be a better-tolerated formulation).[2-6] Taking saw palmetto extract with food may decrease these GI side effects. Clinically significant bleeding has been associated with saw palmetto products in case reports.[7,8] Erectile dysfunction and decreased libido have also been reported.[9] Saw palmetto contains tannins. The oral toxicity of plant tannins is low, as it is readily hydrolyzed in the gut to gallic acid and other metabolites; however, liver and kidney toxicity has occurred with high tannin doses used topically or intravenously.[10] Tannin consumption has been associated with certain cancers, such as esophageal cancer; however, it is unclear whether this is due to the tannins themselves or other compounds associated with tannins.[11]

Interactions

AGENTS THAT MAY LOWER SEIZURE THRESHOLD: Theoretically, saw palmetto may have additive effects with agents that lower the seizure threshold. However, clinical reports of this drug interaction are lacking.

ANTIBIOTICS: Saw palmetto, in combination with antibiotics (ciprofloxacin, azithromycin), has been clinically effective in treating chronic bacterial prostatitis.[12]

ANTICOAGULANTS/ANTIPLATELETS: Based on case studies of severe hemorrhage,[7,8] saw palmetto should be used cautiously with other agents that increase the risk of bleeding. However, clinical reports of such drug interactions are lacking.

BLOOD ALCOHOL: Many saw palmetto tinctures contain high amounts of alcohol and may affect blood alcohol levels. Adverse interactions may occur when taken with disulfiram (Antabuse) or metronidazole (Flagyl).

BLOOD PRESSURE: Occasional cases of hypertension with use of saw palmetto have been reported in controlled trials.[7,9,13]

CAT'S CLAW: Because cat's claw and saw palmetto have been shown to stimulate macrophage phagocytosis in vitro; additive effects may occur when taken concomitantly.[14]

CYTOKINES AND INFLAMMATORY MARKERS: Based on its ability to inhibit lipoxygenase and cyclooxygenase, saw palmetto has antiinflammatory properties in vitro.[15-17] Interactions with antiinflammatory agents are possible, although clinical evidence is lacking.

ECHINACEA: Because echinacea and saw palmetto were shown to stimulate macrophage phagocytosis and NK-cell synthesis of interferon-γ in vitro, additive effects may occur when taken concomitantly.[14]

HISTOLOGICAL TESTS: Antiproliferative and proapoptotic properties have been attributed to saw palmetto based on other in vitro studies.[18-22] Theoretically, saw palmetto may interact with antineoplastic agents.

HORMONAL AGENTS: Based on in vitro observations that saw palmetto may be antiandrogenic and may exert activity on estrogen receptors,[23-25] saw palmetto therapy may interact with oral contraceptive (OC) use and hormone replacement therapy (HRT). However, clinical evidence of such an interaction is lacking.

IRON: The tannins that may be present in saw palmetto may prevent the absorption of iron in the body.

WHITE BLOOD CELL COUNTS: Saw palmetto may have additive effects when taken with immunostimulants because saw palmetto has been shown to stimulate macrophage phagocytosis and NK-cell synthesis of IFN-γ in vitro.[14]

Sea Buckthorn *(Hippophae rhamnoides)*

Pharmacokinetics: Insufficient available evidence.

Adverse effects: Insufficient available evidence.

Interactions

ANTICOAGULANTS/ANTIPLATELETS: Sea buckthorn has been shown to decrease platelet aggregation in vitro.[1-3] Theoretically, concomitant use of anticoagulants/antiplatelets with sea buckthorn may increase the risk of bleeding; however, clinical evidence is lacking.

BACTERIAL LEVELS: Sea buckthorn has displayed antibacterial properties in vitro.[4]

BLOOD GLUCOSE: In animals, flavonoids from sea buckthorn have been shown to reduce serum glucose levels.[5]

BLOOD LIPIDS: Sea buckthorn oil may increase high-density lipoprotein (HDL) levels.[1,2,5-8]

BLOOD PRESSURE: Based on in vitro research, the total flavones of sea buckthorn may have an inhibitory effect on angiotensin-converting enzyme (ACE) activity and on angiotensin II formation.[9] In animals, sea buckthorn has been shown to lower blood pressure.[10]

CISPLATIN: In mice, sea buckthorn juice has been shown to decrease the genotoxic effects of cisplatin on bone marrow and sperm cells.[11]

CYCLOPHOSPHAMIDE: Sea buckthorn oil has been demonstrated to decrease the cytogenetic action of cyclophosphamide in vitro.[12]

FARMORUBICIN AND EPIRUBICIN: Sea buckthorn oil has been shown in vitro to decrease the cytogenetic action of farmorubicin (equivalent to the FDA-approved drug epirubicin [Ellence]) in vitro.[12]

HISTOLOGICAL TESTS: Sea buckthorn may have anticancer effects.[7,13-16] However, it has been demonstrated to reduce the efficacy of some anticancer agents.

WHITE BLOOD CELL COUNTS: Based on animal and in vitro studies, sea buckthorn may inhibit lymphocyte proliferation.[17,18] WBC counts may be affected.

Seaweed

Pharmacokinetics: Insufficient available evidence.

Adverse effects

Bladderwrack *(Fucus vesiculosus)* contains varying amounts of iodine, up to 600 mcg/g, and regular use may elicit hyperthyroidism, hypothyroidism, goiter, or myxedema (normal human iodine intake, 100-200 mcg/day).[1-4] Bladderwrack also concentrates heavy metals found in the ocean, including arsenic, cadmium, and lead; thus, ingestion carries the risk of heavy metal poisoning.[5] Also, high doses of iodine from seaweed may cause a brassy taste, increased salivation, gastric irritation, and acneiform skin lesions.[3] For these reasons, prolonged therapy may be inadvisable.

In addition, bladderwrack should be avoided in patients with heart failure or renal insufficiency, because of its potentially high sodium content, and in hyperthyroid patients because of its iodine content.[2] Furthermore, a case report illustrates adverse effects from bladderwrack's anticoagulant properties.[6] A 54-year-old woman taking kelp *(Laminaria)* tablets presented to her physician with abnormal bleeding and petechiae. She was diagnosed with autoimmune thrombocytopenic purpura with dyserythropoiesis, attributed to contaminants in the kelp preparation. Three months after discontinuation of the kelp supplement and treatment with immunoglobulin, prednisolone, and azathioprine, her dyserythropoiesis was reversed.[6]

Interactions

ANTICOAGULANTS/ANTIPLATELETS: Bladderwrack may increase the risk of bleeding if taken concomitantly with anticoagulants/antiplatelets because of its in vitro exhibition of anticoagulant properties.[7,8] Clinical reports of such drug interactions are lacking.

BLOOD GLUCOSE: Extracts of bladderwrack have been found to cause significant hypoglycemia in laboratory animals, and may also have hypoglycemic effects in humans.[9]

ELECTROLYTES: Bladderwrack may contain vitamins and minerals (calcium, magnesium, potassium, sodium) and therefore may increase serum levels. Because of its high sodium content, seaweed may alter electrolyte balance and water levels. Electrolyte levels may also be altered by the laxative properties of seaweed. Mechanistically, this may be caused by the component alginic acid, a hydrophilic colloidal polysaccharide present in bladderwrack.

KIDNEY FUNCTION TESTS: The presence of heavy metal contaminants in bladderwrack preparations, including arsenic, cadmium, chromium, and lead, may potentiate renal damage if taken with known nephrotoxic agents.

LITHIUM CARBONATE: Concomitant use of iodine-containing agents, such as bladderwrack or kelp, may alter thyroid function when used with lithium.

ORAL AGENTS: Seaweed could theoretically slow down or decrease the absorption of other oral agents because of its hydrophilic colloidal polysaccharides, although reports of actual interactions are lacking.

STIMULANTS: Stimulants may act synergistically with bladderwrack because of its purported hypermetabolic, thyroid-stimulating properties.

THYROID HORMONES: In case reports, transient hyperthyroidism has been associated with kelp products taken alone.[1-4] In theory, the high iodine content of bladderwrack may interfere with the function of agents that act on the thyroid.

Shiitake Mushroom (Lentinus edodes)

Pharmacokinetics: Insufficient available evidence.

Adverse effects

Overall, side effects associated with shiitake are rare and thought to be caused by lentinan. Side effects attributed to shiitake include dermatological effects (shiitake dermatitis or contact dermatitis),[1-7] fever and chills,[8-12] hematological changes,[13] and abdominal discomfort.[13]

Interactions

ALBUMIN: In a clinical trial, serum albumin level increased in 58% of gastric cancer patients treated with lentinan plus tegafur.[14] It is unclear if this is caused by lentinan use.

ANTIBODY LEVELS: In cultured sheep red blood cells (RBCs), shiitake was shown to stimulate humoral immune responses.[15] Cultured murine macrophages were also activated by shiitake in an antibody-dependent manner.[16] Lentinan may also directly stimulate antibody production, as shown by enhanced immunoglobulin production by peripheral mononuclear cells in vitro and in vivo.[17]

ANTICOAGULANTS/ANTIPLATELETS: Shiitake has been shown in vitro to inhibit platelet aggregation.[18] Theoretically, concomitant use of shiitake and anticoagulant/antiplatelets may increase the risk of bleeding.

ANTIFUNGAL AGENTS: In vitro, lentin isolated from *L. edodes* was shown to inhibit mycelial growth in a variety of fungal species, including *Physalospora piricola*, *Botrytis cinerea*, and *Mycosphaerella arachidicola*.[19]

ANTINEOPLASTIC AGENTS: In clinical trials, lentinan has been demonstrated to interact with cancer therapies TS-1 (tegafur-gimeracil-oteracil potassium),[20] tegafur,[14] tegafur and cisplatin,[21] 5-fluorouracil (5-FU),[22,23] levamisole,[24] uracil, mitomycin C, and other chemotherapeutic agents.[25-45] It has also shown benefit in survival rates of cancer patients.[20,21,46-50] Based on in vitro research, lentin may inhibit proliferation of leukemia cells.[19] Shiitake has been proposed as an adjunct to standard antineoplastic therapy.

AZIDOTHYMIDINE: In vitro, lentinan was shown to enhance the effect of AZT in terms of HIV replication blockage.[51]

BACTERIAL LEVELS: Based on in vitro studies, the juice of shiitake mushroom and the culture fluid of *Lentinus (Lentinula) edodes* mycelium may inhibit bacterial growth.[52] Theoretically, shiitake mushroom may interfere with or cause additive effects with antibacterial agents.

BLOOD LIPIDS: In animals, shiitake has been shown to reduce plasma levels of free cholesterol, triglycerides, and phospholipids.[53]

CRANBERRY: In vitro, β-glucosidase from shiitake was shown to release phenolic aglycons from cranberry.[54]

CYTOCHROME P450 SUBSTRATES: Based on in vitro evidence, lentinan may suppress hepatic constitutive and inducible CYP1A expression through the production of TNF-α and DNA-binding activity of NF-κB.[55]

CYTOKINES AND INFLAMMATORY MARKERS: Several in vitro and clinical studies have shown shiitake to modulate cytokine production in cell-mediated immunity.[9,55-59] Based on in vitro evidence, *L. edodes* may also inhibit 12-(S)-HHTrE production, a marker of COX activity.[51]

DIDANOSINE (2′,3′-DI, VIDEX): Concomitant use of the antiretroviral drug didanosine (ddI, Videx) with lentinan was shown to augment drug-induced increases in CD4+ levels in HIV-positive patients.[60]

IMMUNOSUPPRESIVE ACIDIC PROTEIN LEVELS: Based on clinical research involving gastric cancer patients, lentinan plus tegafur may decrease serum IAP.[14] It is unclear if this is caused by lentinan use.[61,62]

PHOTOSENSITIZING AGENTS: Based on a case report, lentinan may cause photosensitivity.[1] Thus, combination with photosensitizing agents (e.g., doxycycline) may increase side effects.

PROLACTIN LEVELS: Based on clinical research involving cancer patients, a combination of lentinan and surgical therapy may result in a decrease in blood levels of prolactin.[63]

WHITE BLOOD CELL COUNTS: Numerous in vitro and clinical studies have demonstrated shiitake to enhance cell-mediated immunity.[9-11,16,24,56-59,64-80] Based on clinical research involving normal humans, shiitake (4 g powder daily for 10 weeks) may induce eosinophilia when taken orally.[13] Shiitake may also induce granulocytopenia in cancer patients,[8] and the lentinan component may cause grade 2 leukopenia.[20] Furthermore, studies in HIV and cancer patients have shown that lentinan may significantly increase T cells, B cells, and macrophages.[57,60,63,68,81] Concomitant use of the antiretroviral drug didanosine and lentinan was suggested to augment drug-induced increases in CD4+ levels in HIV-positive patients.[60]

Skullcap (Scutellaria spp.)

Pharmacokinetics

The pharmacokinetics of skullcap are not well understood. Five metabolites have been isolated from barbat skullcap (*Scutellaria barbata*), including scutellarin, 6-methyl-scutellarin, 6-methyl-scutellarein, and conjugates of scutellarin with two sulfate groups.[1]

Adverse effects

Few adverse effects reports are in the available literature. According to a Phase I trial of BZL101, an aqueous extract from *S. barbata*, the most frequently reported adverse effects included nausea, diarrhea, headache, flatulence, vomiting, constipation, and fatigue.[2]

Interactions

ANTINEOPLASTIC AGENTS: Based on animal studies, Baikal skullcap (*Scutellaria baicalensis*) extract may potentiate the antimetastatic effect of cyclophosphamide.[3,4] Based on further research conducted in animals, *Scutellaria baicalensis* extract may ameliorate cyclophosphamide-induced myelotoxicity.[5]

BACTERIAL LEVELS: In laboratory research, apigenin and luteolin isolated from *S. barbata* showed antibacterial activity against methicillin-resistant *Staphylococcus aureus* (MRSA).[6,7]

CYTOCHROME P450 SUBSTRATES: Based on mutagenesis studies, Baikal skullcap may inhibit CYP450 and alter levels and effects of agents metabolized by this enzyme system.[8,9]

CYTOKINES AND INFLAMMATORY MARKERS: Baikal skullcap has been used historically for its antiinflammatory activity[10,11] and may alter or cause additive effects with antiinflammatory agents.

ELECTROLYTES: Baikal skullcap has been used historically for diuretic effects.[10] Excessive use may lead to fluid loss and electrolyte imbalance.

5-FLUOROURACIL: In animals, baikal skullcap has been shown to ameliorate 5-FU–induced myelotoxicity.[5]

FUNGAL CULTURE: Based on laboratory research, baikal skullcap may have antifungal effects against *Candida* spp.[6,12]

HEMATOCRIT: *S. baicalensis* dry extract and baicalin (found in blue skullcap) stimulate erythropoiesis[13] and may alter the outcomes of RBC and WBC counts.

HISTOLOGICAL TESTS: Although clinical evidence is lacking, numerous in vitro and animal studies have demonstrated *S. barbata* to have anticancer properties;[3,8,10,14-36] thus, it theoretically may alter or cause additive effects if used with antineoplastic agents.

SEDATIVES AND CENTRAL NERVOUS SYSTEM DEPRESSANTS: Baikal skullcap is suggested to cause drowsiness[11] and may have additive effects with sedative agents.

VIRAL LEVELS: Baikal skullcap has been suggested to have antiviral activity[11] and may interact with antiviral agents.

WHITE BLOOD CELL COUNTS: *S. baicalensis* dry extract and baicalin (found in blue skullcap) stimulate erythropoiesis[13] and may alter the outcomes of RBC and WBC counts.

Slippery Elm (*Ulmus rubra*, syn. *Ulmus fulva*)

Pharmacokinetics: Insufficient available evidence.

Adverse effects

Contact dermatitis and urticaria have been reported after exposure to slippery elm or an oleoresin contained in the slippery elm bark. Slippery elm contains plant tannins. The oral toxicity of plant tannins is low, as tannins are readily hydrolyzed in the gut to gallic acid and other metabolites; however, liver and kidney toxicity has occurred with high tannin doses used topically or intravenously.[1] Tannin consumption has been associated with certain cancers, such as esophageal cancer; however, it is unclear whether this is due to the tannins themselves or other compounds associated with tannins.[2]

Interactions

ORAL AGENTS: Slippery elm could theoretically slow down or decrease the absorption of other oral agents because of hydrocolloidal fibers, although reports of interactions are lacking. Slippery elm contains tannins, which could theoretically decrease absorption of nitrogen-containing substances such as alkaloids, although reports of actual interactions are lacking.

Sorrel (*Rumex acetosa, Rumex* spp.)

Pharmacokinetics

There is limited reliable information on the pharmacokinetics of sorrel. Approximately 2% to 5% of ingested oxalates are absorbed in healthy human volunteers. Oral oxalates administered to animals are excreted unchanged in the urine 24 to 36 hours after ingestion.[1]

Adverse effects

Scientific evidence on the use of sorrel alone is limited. Sorrel is likely safe when used in very small amounts in foods. However, toxicity may occur when taken in larger amounts and may include damage to the kidneys, liver, and GI tract. These outcomes are likely related to oxalate (oxalic acid) content in sorrel. Sorrel leaves contain 0.3% oxalate.[1] In a case-report, a 53-year-old man died after ingestion of 500 g of sorrel in soup (6-8 g oxalic acid).[2] The mean lethal dose of oxalic acid for adults is estimated at 15 to 30 g, although doses as low as 5 g have been shown to be fatal.[1,2] Sorrel may be unsafe in children because of its oxalic acid content (ingestion of rhubarb leaves, another source of oxalic acid, is reported to have caused death in a 4-year-old child).[1] The combination formula Sinupret anecdotally is well tolerated and includes sorrel in combination with gentian root, European elderflower, verbena, and cowslip flower (infrequent GI upset has been reported).

Interactions

ALKALOIDS: In theory, precipitation of some agents (especially alkaloid agents) may occur when taken concomitantly with sorrel. Therefore, separate administration is recommended.

ANTIBIOTICS: Concurrent use of doxycycline with Quanterra Sinus Defense or Sinupret was reported in a clinical trial synergistically to improve outcomes in patients with acute bacterial sinusitis.[3] There is limited additional evidence supporting this observation.

ANTICOAGULANTS/ANTIPLATELETS: Oxalate constituents have been reported to decrease coagulation time.[2] However, clinical reports of drug interactions are lacking.

CALCIUM: Oxalate constituents have been reported to alter calcium concentrations.[2] However, clinical reports of drug or supplement interactions are lacking.

COPPER: The oxalate content may bind multivalent metal ions and decrease their absorption.[2] In humans, use of sorrel has been shown to decrease the absorption of copper.[4]

ELECTROLYTES: Polyuria has been reported anecdotally with the use of sorrel and may add to the effects of diuretics.

IRON: The oxalate content may bind multivalent metal ions and decrease their absorption.[2] Anecdotal reports suggest impaired absorption of iron because of oxalate content.[4,5]

KIDNEY FUNCTION TESTS: In large amounts, ingestion of sorrel may lead to kidney stones or kidney damage, likely caused by its oxalate content; sorrell should be avoided with renotoxic agents.

LIVER FUNCTION TESTS: In large amounts, ingestion of sorrel may lead to liver damage and should be avoided with agents that are hepatotoxic.

ZINC: The oxalate content may bind multivalent metal ions and decrease their absorption.[2] In humans, use of sorrel has been shown to decrease the absorption of copper and zinc.[4]

Soy (*Glycine max*)

Pharmacokinetics

On ingestion, soy isoflavones are metabolized by intestinal bacteria, absorbed from the intestinal tract, transported by the portal vein, and then metabolically processed by the liver. About 10% to 22% of soy isoflavones are excreted in urine.[1,2] The half-life of soy isoflavones, daidzein and genistein, is about 7 to 8 hours.[3]

Adverse effects

Soy is "generally regarded as safe" according to the United States Food and Drug Administration (FDA), and has long been a staple of Asian diets. The most frequent adverse effects related to soy are allergic reactions and stomach and intestinal difficulties such as bloating, nausea, and constipation. Soy allergy is a common food allergy; individuals with soy allergy may also cross-react to certain foods, including peanuts, legumes, wheat, rye, and barley. The use of soy is often discouraged in patients with hormone-sensitive malignancies such as breast, ovarian, or uterine cancer, because of concerns about possible estrogen-like effects (which theoretically may stimulate tumor growth). Other hormone-sensitive conditions (e.g., endometriosis) may also theoretically be worsened. In laboratory studies it is unclear whether isoflavones stimulate or block the effects of estrogen, or both (acting as a receptor agonist/antagonist). Until additional research is available, patients with these conditions should be cautious and seek medical advice before starting use.[4,5]

Interactions

BLOOD GLUCOSE: Soy has been shown in clinical studies to lower blood glucose levels.[6,7]

BLOOD PRESSURE: Soy may lower blood pressure.[8] Theoretically, concomitant use with antihypertensive agents may enhance blood pressure–lowering effects.

ESTROGENIC AGENTS: Despite a large body of research on soy phytoestrogens, it is not clear if isoflavones stimulate and/or block the effects of estrogen. It is not known whether taking soy or soy isoflavone supplements increases or decreases the risk of adverse effects of estrogen on the body (e.g., blood clots).[4,5]

GINSENG (PANAX SPP.): Some experts believe that there may be a potential interaction between soy extract and *Panax ginseng*, although this potential interaction is not well described.

IRON: The effects of soy protein or soy flour on iron absorption are not clear. Studies have reported decreases in iron absorption, although other research has noted no effects or increased iron absorption in people taking soy. People using iron supplements as well as soy products should consult their qualified health care practitioner to monitor blood iron levels.

THYROID HORMONES: Based on human case reports and animal research, decreased thyroid hormone and increased TSH levels may occur with use of soy and should therefore be used cautiously in combination with thyroid agents.[4,5]

Spirulina (*Arthrospira* spp.)

Pharmacokinetics: Insufficient available evidence.

Adverse effects

Spirulina appears to be well tolerated.[1-4] Rare reports of reported adverse effects include headache, muscle pain, facial flushing, and sweating.[3,4] Contamination of blue-green algae with heavy metals is possible, especially in species that are often harvested in uncontrolled settings.[5] The phenylalanine content of blue-green algae may exacerbate the condition phenylketonuria.[6]

Interactions

ANTICOAGULANTS/ANTIPLATELETS: C-phycocyanin is an in vitro inhibitor of platelet aggregation, which may involve inhibition of thromboxane A_2 formation, intracellular calcium mobilization, and platelet surface glycoprotein IIb/IIIa expression, accompanied by increasing cyclic AMP formation and platelet membrane fluidity.[7] Interactions with other anticoagulants or antiplatelets are possible, despite the lack of clinical evidence.

BLOOD GLUCOSE: In humans, spirulina may have hypoglycemic effects.[4,8]

BLOOD LIPIDS: Based on animal and clinical studies, spirulina may decrease total and LDL cholesterol and triglycerides.[1,2,9-11]

BLOOD PRESSURE: Biochemical screens have identified potential ACE inhibitors.[12] Spirulina may thus alter blood pressure, although these effects are not well documented.

BONE MARKERS: Spirulina decreased bone mineral density in the trabecular bone of rodents under estrogen-deficient conditions; however, the exact mechanism is unclear.[13]

CALCIUM: A weight loss study of 15 volunteers receiving 200-mg spirulina tablets for 4 weeks detected small, statistically significant increases in serum calcium.[4]

CYTOKINES AND INFLAMMATORY MARKERS: C-phycocyanin has been shown in vitro to inhibit TXA_2 formation.[7] In vitro the ethanolic extracts of *Spirulina maxima* inhibited COX-dependent inflammatory marker production.[14] Purported immune-enhancing effects were shown in rats, in which spirulin supplementation induced IL-4 and IFN-γ.[15]

DOXORUBICIN: In animals, spirulina served as a cardioprotective agent during doxorubicin treatment; additionally, spirulina did not compromise the antitumor activity of doxorubicin and was suggested to improve its therapeutic index.[16]

HISTAMINE: Spirulina has been shown to inhibit IgE-mediated histamine release from activated mast cells in rats, preventing anaphylactic reactions after exposure with a known allergen.[17]

VIRAL LEVELS: Polysaccharides found in *Arthrospiria platensis* (formerly known as *Spirulina platensis*) have been shown to inhibit both herpes simplex virus type 1 (HSV-1) and human immunodeficiency virus type 1 (HIV-1) in vitro and in animals.[18,19]

WHITE BLOOD CELL COUNTS: Purported immune-enhancing effects were shown in rats, in which spirulin supplementation enhanced cell-mediated immunity.[15]

Squill (*Urginea maritima*, syn. *Scilla maritima*)

Pharmacokinetics: Insufficient available evidence.

Adverse effects

Because of its cardiac glycoside constituents, squill may have similar adverse effects as digitalis, including arrhythmia and atrioventricular (AV) block. Other common adverse effects include abdominal pain, vomiting, nausea, and seizures.

In one case report a 55-year-old woman presented with nausea, vomiting, seizures, hyperkalemia, AV block, and ventricular arrhythmias similar to digitalis toxicity after ingesting two bulbs of *Urginea maritima*. Her serum digoxin level was 1.59 ng/mL (normal, 0.5-2 ng/mL), and she later died of ventricular arrhythmias.[1]

Interactions

CORTICOSTEROIDS: Theoretically, concomitant use of squill with long-term corticosteroids may increase effects and cause adverse effects.

DIGOXIN: *Urginea maritima* contains cardiokinetic 3β-ramnoside-14β-hydroxy-δ-4,20,22-bufatrienolide (proscillaridine A).[2] Squill has shown similar toxic effects to cardiac glycoside toxicity, resulting in increased serum digoxin, arrhythmia, and death.[1] In theory, squill may have additive toxic effects when used with digoxin or other cardiac glycosides.

ELECTROLYTES: Historical texts document squill's diuretic effects.[3,4] Decreased potassium levels may lead to hypokalemia. Concurrent use with potassium-depleting agents (e.g., licorice), laxatives, or diuretics may further alter electrolyte balance and increase the toxicity of cardiac agents.

QUINIDINE: Concomitant use of squill and quinidine theoretically may increase the risk of cardiac and adverse effects.

St. John's Wort (Hypericum perforatum)

Pharmacokinetics

In 18 healthy male volunteers who received 612 mg of dry extract of St. John's wort (STW-3, Laif 600), either as a single oral dose or as a multiple once-daily dose over 14 days, concentration-time curves were determined for hypericin, pseudohypericin, hyperforin, the flavonoid aglycon quercetin, and its methylated form isorhamnetin, for 48 hours after single dosing and for 24 hours on day 14 at the end of the 2 weeks of continuous daily dosing regimen. After single-dose intake, results were, for hypericin, area under the curve (AUC[0-infinity]) = 75.96 hours × ng/mL, maximum plasma concentration (C_{max}) = 3.14 ng/mL, time to reach C_{max} (t_{max}) = 8.1 hours, and elimination half-life ($t_{1/2}$) = 23.76 hours; for pseudohypericin, AUC(0-infinity) = 93.03 hours × ng/mL, C_{max} = 8.50 ng/mL, t_{max} = 3.0 hours, $t_{1/2}$ = 25.39 hours; and for hyperforin, AUC(0-max) = 1009.0 hours × ng/mL, C_{max} = 83.5 ng/mL, t_{max} = 4.4 hours, $t_{1/2}$ = 19.64 hours. Under steady-state conditions achieved through administration of the multidose regimen, similar results were obtained.[1]

St. John's wort (SJW) may have multiple effects on various enzymes (inhibition and induction) of the liver cytochrome P450 system.[2] Clinical studies have reported that SJW is able to induce CYP450-3A4.[2-5] SJW (hyperforin) has also been shown to activate a regulator (pregnane X receptor) of 3A4 transcription and thereby induce the expression of 3A4 in human liver cells.[6] There are mixed results regarding SJW on other CYP450 isoenzymes.[4] However, SJW has been shown to induce 1A2, 2C9, 2D6, 2C19, and 2E1.[7-11]

Various SJW constituents (including hypericin, xanthon, and flavonols) have been shown in vitro to inhibit monoamine oxidase (MAO) A and B by hypericin and other components, such as xanthon and flavonols of SJW; however, it is widely agreed that the magnitude of MAO inhibition is inadequate for its purported antidepressant activity.[12-15] Even at concentrations up to 10 mcM, hypericin lacked significant MAO inhibition.[16] Based on these data and other pharmacokinetic findings,[17] the MAO inhibition may not be clinically relevant.

Adverse effects

Multiple reports of headache have been documented with SJW use.[18-25] Several cases of reversible photosensitivity to SJW have also been reported.[26]

In rare cases, SJW may cause serotonin syndrome, characterized by rigidity, hyperthermia, delirium, confusion, autonomic instability, and coma. In a case report of possible serotonin syndrome associated with SJW, a 40-year-old man manifested transient flushing, diaphoresis, hypertension, disorientation, dyspnea, and tremors. The patient, who had a history of depression and SSRI-induced mania, was not taking other agents.[27] Another report described a 33-year-old woman with mild anxiety who experienced multiple anxiety episodes with autonomic arousal (blood pressure maximum, 195/110 mm Hg) after three doses of SJW.[28] In a telephone survey, a woman reported nausea, diaphoresis, muscle cramping, weakness, and elevated pulse and blood pressure after a single dose of a combination product containing SJW, kava, and valerian.[29]

Anorgasmia, decreased libido, orgasmic delay, and erectile dysfunction are among the sexual side effects reported with SJW use.[30-34] Inhibition of sperm motility has been observed in vitro from SJW.[34] Frequent urination has been noted, albeit rarely.[30]

Interactions

ANESTHETIC AGENTS: It has been hypothesized that SJW may interact with anesthetic agents.[35] In a case report, cardiovascular collapse during anesthesia was reported in a healthy 23-year-old woman who had been taking SJW daily for 6 months before surgery; the patient had undergone uneventful general anesthesia 2 years earlier when she was not taking SJW.[36]

ANTICOAGULANTS/ANTIPLATELETS: There have been several cases of reduced international normalized ratio (INR) in patients using warfarin and SJW concomitantly.[37] This was confirmed in a trial of healthy men given 25 mg of warfarin.[38] In most cases the patients had been stabilized on warfarin for some time before ingesting SJW. None of these patients developed thromboembolic events; however, the decrease in INR was thought to be clinically significant. Increases in warfarin dose or discontinuation of SJW resulted in the INR returning to target values.

ANTIDEPRESSANTS: It has been widely suggested that SJW may potentiate the effects of selective serotonin reuptake inhibitors (SSRIs) and MAO inhibitors, theoretically leading to clinical toxicity such as serotonin syndrome or hypertensive crisis.[39-42] There have been multiple case reports of interactions between SJW and SSRIs, including sertraline[39] and paroxetine.[40,41,43] However, given the unclear MAO inhibitory activity of hypericin,[12-16,44] the interaction with other MAO inhibitors may not be clinically significant. Nonetheless, caution is warranted with concomitant use. Possible interactions between SJW and the serotonergic antidepressant nefazodone have been noted,[39] as well as interactions with tricyclic antidepressants (TCAs); two 14-day studies of depressed patients found a significant reduction in amitriptyline concentration with concurrent ingestion of SJW.[45,46] A number of CYP enzymes, including 1A2, 2C19, 3A4, and 2D6, are involved in the metabolism of TCAs.[47] In a recent cross-sectional, point-of-care survey of 1818 patients, eight cases were identified as potentially clinically significant interactions between SJW and antidepressants.[48]

BENZODIAZEPINES: SJW has been reported to induce the metabolism of benzodiazepine agents. In humans, SJW has been reported to reduce midazolam concentrations, presumably from CYP3A4 induction.[3,4,49,50]

CYCLOSPORINE: There are numerous clinical reports of significant reductions in cyclosporine drug levels and possible organ rejections with concomitant use of SJW.[49,51-63] The mechanism for this interaction is likely caused by induction of CYP3A4 and induction of intestinal P-gp drug transporter.

CYTOCHROME P450 SUBSTRATES: Concurrent use of agents metabolized via the CYP450 liver enzyme system may result in altered therapeutic levels of pharmacological agents, because of induction or inhibition of enzymes by SJW.[64] Human studies have reported SJW to induce CYP3A4.[2-5] SJW (hyperforin) has been shown to activate a regulator (pregnane X receptor) of 3A4 transcription and thereby induce expression of 3A4 in human liver cells.[6] Results are mixed regarding SJW on other CYP450 isoenzymes.[4] However, SJW has been shown to induce 1A2, 2C9, 2D6, 2C19, and 2E1.[7-11,65] Many agents, such as chemotherapeutic drugs (irinotecan, etoposide, vinblastine, vincristine, vindesine), protease inhibitors (ritonavir, amprenavir), and antifungals (ketoconazole, itraconazole), should be avoided with SJW.

DIGOXIN: In humans, *Hypericum* extract was demonstrated to decrease digoxin levels by 25%;[66,67] this effect was likely caused by induction of the P-glycoprotein drug transporter.[46,66-72] Bigemeny was reported in an 80-year-old man taking both digoxin and SJW.[73]

The interaction of SJW and digoxin varies within SJW preparations and seems to depend on the dose of hyperforin.[74,75]

ESTROGENIC AGENTS: SJW causes an induction of ethinyl estradiol–norethindrone metabolism, consistent with increased CYP3A activity.[76] In 16 healthy women treated with a low-dose OC (Loestrin 1/20), treatment with SJW (300 mg three times daily) resulted in increased metabolism of norethindrone and ethinyl estradiol, breakthrough bleeding, follicle growth, and ovulation.[77] There are multiple reports of reduced serum level/half-life of OCs in association with SJW use; alterations in hormone levels, and altered menstrual bleeding (including breakthrough bleeding).[37,67,78-81] It was suggested that bleeding irregularities may adversely affect compliance to OCs; furthermore, together with SJW-induced decreases in serum 3-ketodesogestrel concentrations, concomitant use may enhance the risk of unintended pregnancies.[79] In early 2002, warnings emerged after several reports, in Sweden and the United Kingdom, of unwanted pregnancies in women taking OCs and SJW.

HMG-CoA REDUCTASE INHIBITORS: In healthy subjects, SJW was shown to reduce the serum concentrations for simvastatin (but not pravastatin), likely from the induction of CYP3A4 by SJW and induction of P-gp.[82]

IMATINIB (GLEEVEC): SJW has been shown to increase the clearance of the anticancer drug imatinib in humans,[83,84] thus possibly reducing its effectiveness. The mechanism for this interaction is likely caused by the induction of CYP3A4 metabolism of imatinib by SJW.

IRINOTECAN (CAMPTOSAR): SJW has been shown to reduce irinotecan's effectiveness in humans, leading to treatment failure.[85,86] The mechanism for this interaction likely results from induction of CYP3A4 by SJW.

LINEZOLID (ZYVOX): There have been case reports of serotonin syndrome resulting from the interaction of linezolid and SSRIs.[87,88] Theoretically, concomitant use with SJW may increase the risk of serotonergic side effects and serotonin syndrome–like symptoms.

METHADONE: Long-term use of SJW has been shown to reduce methadone levels and increase the risk of withdrawal in humans, attributed to CYP3A4 induction by SJW.[89]

NONNUCLEOSIDE REVERSE-TRANSCRIPTASE INHIBITORS: SJW has been shown to decrease plasma concentrations of the antiretroviral NNRTIs, possibly from CYP450 induction. The oral clearance of the NNRTI nevirapine was significantly increased in five HIV-positive patients treated with nevirapine and concomitant SJW.[90] Effects on these medications may also be caused by P-gp induction.[72] The FDA issued an advisory discouraging the concomitant use of SJW and certain antiretroviral medications.

OPIATES: In a recent cross-sectional, point-of-care survey of 1818 patients, one case was identified as a potentially clinically significant interaction between St. John's wort and the opiate tramadol.[48]

P-GLYCOPROTEIN SUBSTRATES: P-glycoprotein is a cell membrane–associated protein that transports a variety of drug substrates. Interaction with P-gp, including activation, inhibition, and induction, can lead to altered plasma or brain levels of P-gp substrates. SJW increases P-gp expression, suggesting that the herb may interact with agents that act as P-gp substrates.[91-94]

PHOTOSENSITIZING AGENTS: The most widely reported adverse effect of SJW is photosensitivity.[95] Concurrent use of SJW with other photosensitizing agents may increase the risk of photosensitivity.

PROTEASE INHIBITORS: SJW has been shown to decrease plasma concentrations of protease inhibitors (PIs), possibly from CYP450 induction. An open-label study demonstrated a significant reduction in concentrations of the PI indinavir when taken concurrently with SJW by healthy volunteers.[96] Effects on these medications may also be caused by an induction of the drug pump P-gp.[72] The FDA issued an advisory discouraging the concomitant use of SJW and certain antiretroviral medications.

SEROTONERGIC AGENTS: Concomitant use of SJW with 5-HT1 agonists (triptans) may result in additive serotonergic adverse effects and possibly serotonin syndrome. However, clinical evidence of such an interaction is unclear.

TACROLIMUS (PROGRAF): Several reports indicate that SJW may decrease the levels of the immunosuppressant tacrolimus, likely from induction of CYP3A4 and P-gp.[97-99]

THEOPHYLLINE (BRONKODYL, ELIXOPHYLLIN, SLO-BID): It has been suggested that SJW may affect serum levels of theophylline or its metabolites; however, this remains unclear.[72] In one case report, serum theophylline levels decreased with concomitant SJW (300 mg daily); theophylline levels increased after discontinuation of SJW.[100] However, controlled studies found that SJW likely is insufficient to cause a change in plasma theophylline concentrations.[101]

TYRAMINE-CONTAINING FOODS/BEVERAGES: Weak MAO inhibitory activity of SJW has been observed in vitro.[12-17,102] Similar to warnings accompanying the use of MAO inhibitor antidepressants, consumption of tyramine-containing foods with SJW may pose an increased risk of hypertensive crisis. In a telephone survey of 43 subjects who had taken SJW, 39 persons reported ingesting tyramine-rich foods or products. Two persons taking 600 to 900 mg daily reported associated flushing and pounding headaches.[103] However, given the unclear MAO inhibitory activity of hypericin,[12-16,44] the potential interaction with tyramine-containing foods may not be clinically significant.

VERAPAMIL (ISOPTIN): Repeated administration of SJW significantly decreased the bioavailability of R- and S-verapamil in humans, attributed to induction of first-pass CYP3A4 metabolism, most likely in the gut.[104]

Stevia (Stevia rebaudiana)

Pharmacokinetics

Based on rat studies, stevia appears to be metabolized in the intestinal wall and liver.[1,2] Stevia remained constant after a 2-hour perfusion into isolated rat livers.[2]

Adverse effects

Long-term stevia therapy (up to 2 years) has not been associated with significant adverse effects.[3,4] Occasionally, stevia has been reported to cause nausea, abdominal fullness, myalgia, muscle weakness, and dizziness.[4,5] Stevia should be avoided in patients with impaired kidney function or other kidney diseases because animal studies have shown stevia to affect renal activity, sodium excretion, and urinary flow.[6-8]

Interactions

BLOOD GLUCOSE: Stevia may lower blood sugar and increase the risk of hypoglycemia.[9,10]

BLOOD PRESSURE: Stevia has been shown to act as a vasodilator in vitro[7] and may affect blood pressure.

CALCIUM: Stevia may act as a calcium antagonist[7,11] and may interact with calcium supplements. Stevia may alter calcium levels, as well as agents that affect calcium channels; however, this interaction has not been well documented.

ELECTROLYTES: Stevioside is secreted by renal tubular epithelium and induces diuresis and natriuresis[12] in animals. Electrolyte balance may be altered, and stevia should be used cautiously with other diuretics.

Stinging Nettle (Urtica dioica)

Pharmacokinetics
The pharmacokinetics of stinging nettle is not well understood. After oral administration of 20 mg of *Urtica dioica* agglutinin (UDA) to healthy volunteers, 30% to 50% of the dose was excreted in the feces.[1] The total amount of UDA in the urine was less than 1%.

Adverse effects
Nettle therapy was generally well tolerated for up to 2 years in available clinical trials.[2-13] Gastrointestinal irritation is the most frequently reported adverse effect.[9,11,14,15]

Interactions
ANDROGENIC AGENTS: Stinging nettle has been shown in vitro to inhibit 5α-reductase, the enzyme that converts testosterone to the more potent form dihydrotestosterone.[1,16-18] Although interactions with androgenic agents are possible, stinging nettle has not been shown to inhibit 5α-reductase in clinical studies.[19]

ANTICOAGULANTS/ANTIPLATELETS: Nettle root contains a coumarin constituent;[1,20,21] administration of nettle root may theoretically interact with anticoagulants/antiplatelets and may increase risk of bleeding. Because nettle leaves contain vitamin K,[20] high doses may theoretically alter response to anticoagulants. However, clinical reports of drug interactions are lacking.

BLOOD PRESSURE: Nettle has been associated with acute hypotensive action.[22] Theoretically, concurrent use of nettle with antihypertensive agents may cause additional lowering of blood pressure.

CYTOKINES AND INFLAMMATORY MARKERS: Stinging nettle has displayed antiinflammatory properties[23,24] and theoretically may interact with similar agents.

ELECTROLYTES: An aqueous extract of aerial parts administered to male rats demonstrated diuretic and natriuretic effects.[22] Overuse (or concomitant use with other diuretics) may result in dehydration and hypokalemia.

Strawberry (Fragaria spp.)

Pharmacokinetics
Based on clinical evidence, strawberry anthocyanins are recovered in urine as glucuroconjugates and sulfoconjugates; four hours after strawberry consumption, more than two thirds of anthocyanin metabolites were excreted.[1]

Adverse effects
Other than allergic responses, there are relatively few reports of adverse effects caused by strawberries. In sensitive subjects, strawberry has caused contact urticaria[2] and pruritic dermatoses (eczema and neurodermite).[3]

Fresh strawberries and cut strawberry salads have been found to be contaminated with pesticides,[4] fungi,[5] bacteria,[6,7] and other microorganisms.[8] Strawberry jam has been contaminated by pyrethroid insecticide residues[9] and possibly the norovirus, although the norovirus contamination was most likely caused by postmarket food handlers.[10] Part of the problem may be the difficulty in removing contamination either before or after strawberries go to the market.

Interactions
ANTICOAGULANTS/ANTIPLATELETS: Based on in vitro studies, strawberry may have antiplatelet properties.[11,12] Concomitant use of strawberry and anticoagulants/antiplatelets may increase risk of bleeding, although clinical evidence is lacking.

BACTERIAL LEVELS: Based on in vitro studies, strawberries may have antibacterial properties.[13,14]

HISTOLOGICAL TESTS: Based on in vitro studies, individual compounds in strawberries have demonstrated anticancer activity in several different studies, by blocking initiation of carcinogenesis dose-dependently, inducing apoptosis, and suppressing progression and proliferation of tumors.[15-19] Based on in vitro research, strawberry extracts may be cytotoxic against leukemia cells.[20]

IRON: Based on clinical research involving parous women, strawberry (*Fragaria* spp.) may have a mild to moderate enhancing effect on iron absorption.[21]

NONSTEROIDAL ANTIINFLAMMATORY DRUGS: Based on in vitro research, strawberry extracts may inhibit COX enzymes and theoretically may interfere or cause additive effects with NSAIDs.[15] However, clinical evidence of such an interaction is lacking.

ORAL AGENTS: Based on in vitro studies, strawberry extracts may inhibit intestinal P-glycoprotein–related functionality[22,23] and may interfere with gastrointestinal absorption of agents.

SALICYLATES: Based on tests performed in allergic patients, there may be a connection between acetylsalicylic acid (aspirin) intolerance and strawberry sensitivity.[24]

Sweet Almond (Prunus amygdalus dulcis)

Pharmacokinetics: Insufficient available evidence.

Adverse effects
In most reports, sweet almond is generally considered to be safe when taken orally. Few nonallergic adverse reactions have been reported in the literature. However, hypersensitivities to almonds are common and may lead to severe reactions.

Interactions
BLOOD GLUCOSE: According to research in rats, almonds may have a significant hypoglycemic effect.[1]

BLOOD LIPIDS: Almonds have been reported to lower cholesterol levels.[2-6]

ESTROGENIC AGENTS: Because almonds have exerted estrogenic activity in rats, sweet almonds may theoretically have additive effects when taken with estrogen. Subsequent samples of different varieties of almonds have not confirmed this finding.[7]

Sweet Annie (Artemisia annua)

Pharmacokinetics
In a pharmacokinetic study, artemisinin (active constituent in sweet Annie) was absorbed faster from herbal tea preparations than from oral solid-dosage forms, but bioavailability was similar. One liter of an aqueous preparation of 9 g of *Artemisia annua* contained 94.5 mg of artemisinin. The elimination half-life of *A. annua* is 2 to 4 hours.[1,2] Its main metabolite, dihydroartemisin, has a half-life of approximately 40 minutes.[1]

Adverse effects
Sweet Annie appears to be generally well tolerated.[1,3] A related species *(Artemisia composita)* may have potential CNS and cardiovascular toxicities.[4]

Interactions
ANTIMALARIAL AGENTS: Constituents of sweet Annie, including artemisin, arteether, artemether, artemotil, artenimol, artesunate, and dihydroartemisinin, are currently being used to treat drug-resistant and non–drug-resistant malaria.[5-12] Because these antimalarial compounds are found in sweet Annie, interactions with antimalarial treatments are likely; however, they have not been thoroughly evaluated.

BACTERIAL LEVELS: The essential oil of *Artemisia annua* aerial parts was shown to inhibit bacterial growth in vitro.[13]

FUNGAL LEVELS: The essential oil of *A. annua* aerial parts has been shown to inhibit fungal growth in vitro.[13]

HISTOLOGICAL TESTS: Based on several in vitro studies, *A. annua* constituents, including artesunate, artemisinin, dihydroartemisinin, and quercetagetin 6,7,3′,4′-tetramethyl ether, may have antineoplastic activity.[14-19] Furthermore, artesunate (semisynthetic derivative of artemisinin) has been shown to inhibit angiogenesis in vivo and in vitro.[20] Histological tests may be altered. Interactions with antineoplastic agents are possible but not yet clinically evaluated.

QUINOLINES: Based on review conclusions, artesunate may be chemically incompatible with quinolines;[21] however, clinical evidence is lacking. Quinolines are aromatic organic bases synthesized or obtained from coal tar and used as food preservatives and in making antiseptics. These should not be confused with *quinolones*, a family of broad-spectrum antibiotics.

SODIUM BUTYRATE: Based on in vitro studies, extracts from *Artemisia annua* and analogs of *A. annua* constituents have been found to have anticancer properties, especially when combined with sodium butyrate.[16]

WHITE BLOOD CELL COUNTS: A water soluble derivative of artemisinin was shown to inhibit peripheral lymphocytes and thymocytes in vitro, in contrast to reports of immunostimulatory activity in vivo.[22] The mechanisms of inhibition and discrepancy with in vivo results were unclear. Immunological tests, such as lymphocyte count, may be affected by sweet Annie.

Tea *(Camellia sinensis)*

Pharmacokinetics
The pharmacokinetic parameters of black tea are related to its caffeine content (see Caffeine). Green tea is metabolized in the body to epigallocatechin gallate (EGCG), epigallocatechin (EGC), and epicatechin (EC). Catechins from green tea are rapidly absorbed.[1-3] An increase in catechins in the blood has been found to be rapid, with an average maximum change of 13% approximately 2 hours after ingestion.[4] Blood levels rapidly decline, with an elimination half-life of 4.8 hours for green tea.[5]

Adverse effects
Studies of the specific side effects of black and green tea are limited. However, black tea and green tea are sources of caffeine, for which multiple reactions are reported (see Caffeine).

Caffeine is a CNS stimulant and may cause insomnia in adults, children, and infants (including nursing infants of mothers taking caffeine). Caffeine acts on the kidneys as a diuretic, increasing urine and urinary sodium/potassium levels and potentially decreasing blood sodium/potassium levels, and may worsen incontinence. Caffeine-containing beverages may increase the production of stomach acid and may worsen ulcer symptoms. Caffeine in certain doses can increase heart rate and blood pressure, although people who consume caffeine regularly do not seem to experience these effects long term. Tannin in tea can cause constipation. The oral toxicity of plant tannins is low, as it is readily hydrolyzed in the gut to gallic acid and other metabolites; however, liver and kidney toxicity has occurred with high tannin doses used topically or intravenously.[6] Tannin consumption has been associated with certain cancers, such as esophageal cancer; however, it is unclear whether this is due to the tannins themselves or other compounds associated with tannins.[7]

An increase in blood sugar levels may occur after drinking black tea containing high levels of caffeine. Caffeine-containing beverages such as black tea should be used cautiously in patients with diabetes. People with severe liver disease should use caffeine cautiously because levels of caffeine in the blood may build up and last longer. Skin rashes have been associated with caffeine ingestion. In laboratory and animal studies, caffeine has been found to affect blood clotting, although effects in humans are unclear.

Interactions
GENERAL: Interactions associated with black and green tea are predominantly theoretical and largely based on the adverse effect profile of caffeine.

ANTICOAGULANTS/ANTIPLATELETS: Both catechins in green tea and caffeine in tea may have antiplatelet activity. Theoretically, black and green tea might increase the risk of bleeding when used with anticoagulants/antiplatelets. In one case report, large amounts (½-1 gallon) of green tea antagonized the effects of warfarin, possibly from the small amounts of vitamin K in green tea.[8,9] Dry green tea leaves contain significantly more vitamin K than black tea leaves; green tea may contain 1428 mcg vitamin K/100 g leaf, whereas black tea may contain only 262 mcg vitamin K/100 g leaf.[10]

CYTOCHROME P450 SUBSTRATES: Green tea and black tea have been reported to induce CYP450 enzymes 1A1, 1A2, and 2B1. In theory, clinically significant alterations of the metabolism of concomitant agents may occur.

MILK: Black tea polyphenols significantly reduced hamster buccal pouch carcinogenesis alone and acted synergistically with concomitant milk ingestion.[11,12]

SALICYLATES: The concomitant administration of tannin-containing agents may result in a malabsorption of salicylic acid.[13] Salicylates such as aspirin may be affected when taken with tea.

Tea Tree *(Melaleuca alternifolia)*

Pharmacokinetics: Insufficient available evidence.

Adverse effects
Tea tree oil is generally believed to be well tolerated when applied topically.[1-7] The most common adverse effects associated with topical tea tree oil are contact dermatitis and mucous membrane irritation. Oral ingestion has been associated with numerous case reports of toxicity.

Interactions
TOPICAL DRYING AGENTS/ASTRINGENTS: Topical tea tree oil preparations may result in drying of the skin and may act additively with other agents, such as tretinoin (Retin-A, Renova).

Thyme (Thymus vulgaris)

Pharmacokinetics
In one study of thymol and carvacrol in rats, urinary excretion of metabolites occurred rapidly; only small amounts were excreted after 24 hours.[1]

Adverse effects
Based on historical use and clinical anecdote, thyme flower and leaves appear to be safe in culinary and limited medicinal use. However, caution is warranted with the use of thyme oil, which should not be taken orally and should be diluted for topical administration because of potential toxic effects.

Thyme should be avoided in persons with known allergy/hypersensitivity to members of the Lamiaceae (mint) family or to any component of thyme. Thyme is not recommended during pregnancy or lactation because data are insufficient. A 1975 review of plants as possible new antifertility agents classified thyme as an "emmenagogue" and abortifacient.[2]

Interactions
ESTROGENIC AGENTS: Thyme has demonstrated estradiol receptor–binding activity in vivo,[3] although this has not been systematically studied or demonstrated in humans.

5-FLUOROURACIL: Topical thymol significantly enhanced percutaneous absorption of 5-FU through porcine epidermis compared with control.[4]

PROGESTOGENIC AGENTS: Thyme has demonstrated progesterone receptor-binding activity in vivo,[4] although this has not been systematically studied or demonstrated in humans.

PROLACTIN: Based on preclinical data, prolactin levels theoretically may be decreased at high thyme doses.[5]

THYROID HORMONES: An extract of *Thymus serpyllum*, a species related to *Thymus vulgaris*, has been shown to exert antithyrotropic effects in rats, causing a decline in TSH and prolactin.[5] Therefore, thyme may theoretically decrease levels of thyroid hormone, although this has not been systematically studied or demonstrated in humans.

Tribulus (Tribulus terrestris)

Pharmacokinetics: Insufficient available evidence.

Adverse effects
Tribulus terrestris appears to be generally safe. Few adverse events have been reported and include insomnia and menorrhagia.[1] A case of pneumothorax on digestion of tribulus fruit has been reported.[2]

Interactions
BETA-ADRENERGIC ANTAGONISTS: Tribulus may add to beta-blocker effects because of its negative chronotropic activity in cardiac muscle.[3]

BLOOD GLUCOSE: In animals, tribulus has been shown to lower blood glucose levels.[4]

BLOOD PRESSURE: Tribulus has been found to have a hypotensive action and may cause additive effects when used with agents that lower blood pressure.[5]

CARDIAC GLYCOSIDES: A water-soluble extract of tribulus was found to have a positive inotropic activity, thus possibly exacerbating the effects of cardiac glycosides.[6]

KIDNEY FUNCTION TESTS: A water extract of tribulus was found to exhibit diuretic effects.[7] In dogs an ether extract of tribulus fruit produced diuresis and increased renal creatinine clearance, suggesting an increase in glomerular filtration rate (GFR).[5]

STEROIDS: Preliminary evidence suggests that tribulus may increase serum testosterone and reduce the estrogenic effects of androstenedione.[8] However, clinical evidence is unclear. Studies suggest that herbal preparations (300 mg androstenedione, 150 mg DHEA, 750 mg *Tribulus terrestris*, 625 mg chrysin, 300 mg indole-3-carbinol, and 540 mg saw palmetto) may increase serum testosterone concentrations,[9,10] but do not appear to reduce the estrogenic effects of androstenedione.[9-11] Thus, it remains unclear whether tribulus affects steroid hormone levels, but it does not appear to affect androstenedione conversion to estradiol and dihydrotestosterone.

Turmeric (Curcuma longa)

Pharmacokinetics
Animal research found that the absorption of curcumin after oral administration varies from 25% to 60%, with most of the absorbed flavonoid being metabolized in the intestinal mucosa and liver.[1] The remainder is excreted in the feces.[2]

Adverse effects
The most common side effect with turmeric reported in humans is gastrointestinal upset, including epigastric burning, dyspepsia, nausea, and diarrhea.[3,4] High doses of turmeric are thought to be safe based on toxicology studies.[5] Increased bleeding risk is a concern with high doses of curcumin.[6]

Interactions
ANTIBIOTICS: An ethyl acetate extract of *Curcuma longa* greatly lowered the minimum inhibitor concentration (MIC) of ampicillin and oxacillin in vitro.[7] Clinical evidence of such an interaction is lacking.

ANTICOAGULANTS/ANTIPLATELETS: In vitro and animal studies report that turmeric inhibited platelet aggregation,[8-11] possibly from effects on eicosanoids.[8,12-15] Therefore, turmeric may potentiate the effects of other agents that increase the risk of bleeding; however, clinical evidence is lacking. In a recent cross-sectional, point-of-care survey of 1818 patients, two cases were identified as potentially clinically significant interactions between turmeric and anticoagulant/antiplatelet agents.[16]

ANTINEOPLASTIC AGENTS: Multiple preclinical studies have explored potential anticancer and chemoprotective mechanisms of turmeric and its constituent curcumin.[17-40] Theoretically, it may interact with antineoplastic agents, although clinical evidence is lacking.

BLOOD GLUCOSE: In animal research, turmeric extracts exhibited hypoglycemic effects on blood glucose levels.[41]

BLOOD LIPIDS: Turmeric has been found to decrease low-density lipoprotein, increase high-density lipoprotein, and decrease serum lipid peroxides; rat studies suggest that turmeric may produce changes in cholesterol metabolism by stimulating cholesterol-7α-hydroxylase activity.[42,43]

BLOOD PRESSURE: Transient hypotension has been noted in dogs after administration of curcumin.[44] Administering turmeric oil daily for 3 months to healthy volunteers, however, did not affect pulse or blood pressure.[17]

CYTOCHROME P450 SUBSTRATES: There is evidence that turmeric may interfere with cytochrome P450 (CYP450) enzymes, which are responsible for breaking down various agents in the liver. As a result, turmeric may cause high levels of agents in the body, leading to serious side effects. In rats, curcumin is reported to be a potent inhibitor of CYP450-1A1/1A2, a less potent inhibitor of 2B1/2B2, and a weak inhibitor of 2E1.[45] Inhibition of CYP450 has also been demonstrated in vitro and in other animal studies.[22,36,46,47] Clinical data are lacking.

CYTOKINES AND INFLAMMATORY MARKERS: In animal and in vitro research, turmeric and its constituent curcumin have shown various antiinflammatory effects.* Drug interactions are possible, although clinical evidence is lacking.

DOXORUBICIN (ADRIAMYCIN, DOXIL): Curcumin (200 mg/kg) protects against acute doxorubicin-induced myocardial toxicity in rats.[58] However, clinical evidence of such an interaction is lacking.

GREATER CELANDINE: Several weeks after ingesting a combination herbal preparation containing greater celandine and curcuma root, a 42-year-old woman developed jaundice from acute hepatitis.[59] Her clinical recovery was rapid after withdrawal of the medication, and within 2 months her hepatic functions had returned to normal. This report raises the question of a possible interaction between greater celandine and curcuma root; however, causality remains unclear.

HORMONAL THERAPY: Theoretically, turmeric may interact with hormonal agents, although clinical evidence is lacking. In mice, turmeric was associated with enlargement of sexual organs and increased sperm motility.[60]

LIVER FUNCTION TESTS: The turmeric constituent curcumin has been reported to induce LFT abnormalities in rats and may be mildly hepatotoxic in high doses.[6] Caution is warranted when using turmeric with hepatotoxic agents.

RESERPINE: Turmeric root solid alcoholic extract significantly reduced the frequency of reserpine-induced gastric and duodenal ulcers in rats. In high doses, however, turmeric may be ulcerogenic.[61] Clinical evidence is lacking.

Tylophora (Tylophora indica)

Pharmacokinetics: Insufficient available evidence.

Adverse effects

Tylophora is generally well tolerated but occasionally may cause gastrointestinal complaints. It has been reported to cause nausea, vomiting, altered taste perception, and mouth soreness.[1-5] Drowsiness has also been reported.[2]

Interactions

ACIDITY: Tylophora may inhibit gastric acid.[6] Clinical evidence is lacking, but Tylophora may interact with antacids, H$_2$ antagonists, or proton pump inhibitors (PPIs) if used concomitantly.

CORTICOSTEROIDS: According to animal research, Tylophora antagonized dexamethasone/hypophysectomy-induced suppression of the pituitary.[7] Clinical interactions are possible, although evidence is lacking.

SEDATIVES AND CENTRAL NERVOUS SYSTEM DEPRESSANTS: In animals, tylophorine, the major alkaloid of Tylophora, potentiated pentobarbital sleep time.[8] Similar interactions are possible in humans, despite the lack of clinical evidence.

---

*References 8, 9, 12, 13, 15, 48-57.

Uva Ursi (Arctostaphylos uva-ursi)

Pharmacokinetics

Arbutin, a constituent of uva ursi, is rapidly absorbed after oral administration.[1] Uva ursi is primarily excreted in urine.[2,3] Arbutin, a constituent of uva ursi and other herbs (including sweet marjoram and damiana), may result in increased serum and urinary levels of hydroquinone and its metabolites.[4]

Adverse effects

Uva ursi is generally well tolerated in short-term, traditional doses, but there is limited clinical safety evidence. The herb may cause skin irritations, greenish brown urine color, irritation and inflammation of the urinary tract mucous membranes, insomnia, irritability, motor restlessness, and headaches. Because of the tannin content, uva ursi may cause nausea, vomiting, diarrhea, stomach upset, and hepatotoxicity. The oral toxicity of plant tannins is low, as it is readily hydrolyzed in the gut to gallic acid and other metabolites; however, liver and kidney toxicity has occurred with high tannin doses used topically or intravenously.[5] Tannin consumption has been associated with certain cancers, such as esophageal cancer; however, it is unclear whether this is due to the tannins themselves or other compounds associated with tannins.[6]

Interactions

ACIDITY: Concomitant use of uva ursi and urine acidifiers may reduce the effects of uva ursi.

ALOESIN: When combined, uva ursi and aloesin inhibited tyrosinase activity in a synergistic manner in vitro by noncompetitive and competitive inhibition.[7]

BACTERIAL LEVELS: Uva ursi has been used traditionally as an antiseptic and treatment for urinary tract infections and may decrease bacterial levels in certain infections.

CORTICOSTEROIDS: In an animal model of contact dermatitis, arbutin synergistically enhanced the antiinflammatory properties of prednisolone in mice, whereas arbutin alone required a dose of 100 mg/kg or higher to produce significant therapeutic effects.[8]

In mice, arbutin inhibited delayed-type hypersensitivity caused by picryl chloride or sheep RBCs 24 hours after induction (but not before or 16 hours after). Further, arbutin enhanced the effects of prednisolone or dexamethazone when administered concurrently.[9]

ELECTROLYTES: Uva ursi has been shown to increase urine flow in rats.[10] Electrolyte balance may be altered.

NONSTEROIDAL ANTIINFLAMMATORY DRUGS: In rats the arbutin in uva ursi was shown to enhance the antiinflammatory activity of indomethacin on contact dermatitis, hypersensitivity, and arthritis.[11]

URINE TESTS: Uva ursi has been reported to turn urine greenish brown and may interfere with colormetric urine tests. Uva ursi has been shown to increase urine flow in rats;[10] further, arbutin may increase urinary levels of hydroquinone and its metabolites.[4]

Valerian (Valeriana officinalis)

Pharmacokinetics

Valerian appears to be metabolized in the liver;[1] its route of excretion is unclear. Valepotriates are poorly absorbed and subject to a significant first-pass effect when administered orally. Degradation may occur in the presence of heat or alkaline conditions. Valepotriates and their metabolites have been found in the stomach lining, intestines, blood, liver, kidneys, heart, lungs, and brain.

Adverse effects

Short-term mild impairments in vigilance, concentration, and processing time for complex thoughts, as well as mild fatigue, have been reported in trials (lasting for several hours), although residual sedative effects appear to be less pronounced than those associated with benzodiazepines.[2-5] Preliminary evidence suggests that valerian does not have sedative effects in recommended doses.[2,3,6] In one trial, use of a combination product containing valerian and lemon balm *(Melissa officinalis)* did not impair performance on psychometric tests that correlate with the ability to drive or operate machinery.[7] A drug "hangover" effect has been reported in patients taking high doses of valerian extracts.[8] A "valerian withdrawal" effect has been reported with chronic high-dose use; delirium, ameliorated by benzodiazepines, was reported in a single patient undergoing withdrawal from high doses of valerian.[9] Dizziness and headache have been reported in clinical studies, although they are rare.[10,11] Anecdotally, some patients may develop a "paradoxical reaction" leading to nervousness or excitability, and use for longer than 2 to 4 months may result in insomnia.

It remains unclear if valerian is hepatotoxic. Hepatotoxicity has been associated with some multiherb preparations that include valerian;[12] however, the contribution of valerian itself cannot be determined from these reports, because of the potential hepatotoxicity of other ingredients (e.g., skullcap), as well as the possibility of adulteration with unlisted herbs (e.g., known hepatotoxic herb germander, which is often mistakenly harvested as skullcap).

Valerian is not recommended for use in pregnant and lactating women because of theoretical concerns over the teratogenic effects of valepotriates, and theoretical properties as a uterine stimulant, abortifacient, and "emmenagogue." Valepotriates and baldrinals have been shown to be cytotoxic and mutagenic in vitro.[13,14] However, these substances are unstable and generally not found in commercial valerian products.

Interactions

ANTICONVULSANTS: Anecdotal reports suggest that valerian products may interact with antiseizure agents, although published scientific evidence is lacking.

BETA-ADRENERGIC ANTAGONISTS: In a randomized trial, a combination of 100 mg valerian extract and 20 mg propranolol was found to impair performance on a written concentration test more than valerian alone (reported to slightly improve performance).[4] However, there was no comparison to propranolol alone, so it is unclear whether the effects resulted from the beta blocker only or from the combination with valerian.

BLOOD ALCOHOL: Valerian tinctures often contain high alcohol content (15%-90%), and may affect blood alcohol levels. Adverse interactions may occur when taken with disulfiram (Antabuse) or metronidazole (Flagyl).

LOPERAMIDE (IMODIUM): A brief episode of acute delirium was reported in one patient during concomitant use of loperamide and valerian.[15] However, causality could not be established because the patient was also taking St. John's wort. The condition resolved rapidly with discontinuation of treatment.

SEDATIVES AND CENTRAL NERVOUS SYSTEM DEPRESSANTS: Valerian may theoretically potentiate the effects of CNS depressants, although studies in patients taking CNS-active agents concurrently with valerian report no increase in adverse effects.[2,3,16] In a recent cross-sectional, point-of-care survey of 1818 patients, 15 cases were identified as potentially clinically significant interactions between valerian and sedatives.[17]

SEROTONERGIC AGENTS: A patient taking the SSRI fluoxetine (Prozac) for a mood disorder (in the setting of alcohol use) reported that approximately 12 hours after taking valerian tablets, he experienced mental status changes and lost control of his left arm.[18] Other reported symptoms included agitation and obsession that led him to self-inflict cuts to his hand. After another 12 hours, his symptoms resolved. The specific role of valerian in this isolated case is not clear.

Wheatgrass *(Triticum aestivum)*

Pharmacokinetics: Insufficient available evidence.

Adverse effects

Wheatgrass is generally considered safe. No serious side effects have been reported using 100 mL of wheatgrass juice daily for up to 1 month.[1] Reported adverse effects are lacking in the literature.[1,2] Because it is grown in soils or water and consumed raw, wheatgrass may be contaminated with bacteria, molds, or other substances.

Interactions: Insufficient available evidence.

White Horehound *(Marrubium vulgare)*

Pharmacokinetics

The pharmacokinetics of white horehound is not well understood. White horehound administered to mice for analgesia had a maximum duration of action for analgesia of 4 hours.[1]

Adverse effects

White horehound is generally considered safe. Large doses of white horehound have caused arrhythmias in animal studies.[2] Hypotension has been reported in animals, perhaps mediated by the vascular relaxant activity of *Marrubium*.[3] Theoretically, aldosterone-enhancing properties of white horehound may cause hypernatremia and edema based on the proposed mechanism of action, including loss of potassium and distal sodium reabsorption in the kidneys. Decreases in blood glucose have been reported in hyperglycemic rabbits compared with a control (water ingestion).[4] White horehound has been used traditionally as an emetic and cathartic; in large doses it may cause diarrhea resulting from its purported mechanism of action on the GI tract.

Interactions

BLOOD GLUCOSE: White horehound may lower blood glucose.[4]

DIGOXIN: White horehound contains glycosides that theoretically could potentiate the activity of similar agents such as digoxin.[5]

DIURETICS: Because white horehound may enhance aldosterone action, it may interact with aldosterone-blocking diuretic agents.[5] However, clinical evidence of this interaction is lacking.

ESTROGENIC AGENTS: White horehound may possess phytoestrogenic chemicals that antagonize or agonize estrogen receptors and thus may interact with estrogen therapies.[5] However, clinical evidence of such an interaction is lacking.

HEART RATE: Large amounts of white horehound may cause arrhythmias, and should be avoided with agents that affect cardiac rhythm.[2]

HORMONE LEVELS: Because of proposed hypothalamic-pituitary-adrenal axis (HPA) effects of white horehound constituents, it may alter hormone levels.[5]

SEROTONERGIC AGENTS: Preclinical studies with aqueous extracts of white horehound suggest that it may antagonize the effects of serotonin.[2] Theoretically, this antagonism may interact with antidepressants, certain antiemetics, and certain antimigraine agents ("triptans"); however, clinical evidence is lacking.

Wild Indigo (Baptisia australis, Baptisia tinctoria)

Pharmacokinetics: Insufficient available evidence.

Adverse effects

Scant information is available on the adverse effects of wild indigo. However, the plant is listed on the FDA's list of toxic plants. When used in a combination of *Baptisiae tinctoriae* root, *Echinaceae pallidae/purpureae* root, and *Thujae occidentalis*, two clinical studies found no adverse effects.[1,2]

Interactions

VIRAL LEVELS: Based on a review, the herbal combination of echinacea, wild indigo, and white cedar has antiviral characteristics.[2] Viral counts may be affected.

WHITE BLOOD CELL COUNTS: Based on preliminary in vitro studies and clinical studies using combination products, wild indigo may have nonspecific immunostimulative or immunomodulating effects, probably by activating macrophages.[3-8]

Wild Yam (Dioscorea villosa)

Pharmacokinetics

Diosgenin, the active component of wild yam, is poorly absorbed. It is distributed into the liver, adrenals, and walls of the GI tract and undergoes extensive biotransformation. Diosgenin is eliminated through the bile and excreted in feces.[1,2]

Adverse effects

Topical application of wild yam has been well tolerated.[3] Contact dermatitis has been reported after rubbing the skin with *Dioscorea batatas*, a related yam species.[4]

Interactions

BLOOD ALCOHOL: Some wild yam tinctures contain high concentrations of alcohol and may affect blood alcohol levels. Adverse interactions may occur when taken with disulfiram (Antabuse) or metronidazole (Flagyl).

BLOOD LIPIDS: Diosgenin has been shown to reduce total and LDL cholesterol levels as well as triglycerides in animal and clinical studies.[1,2,5-13] HDL levels have been shown to be increased.[5,6,12-14]

ESTROGENIC AGENTS: Based on in vitro research, wild yam root may possess antiestrogenic activity and theoretically may antagonize the effects of estrogen/phytoestrogen therapy.[15] However, clinical evidence is lacking.

INDOMETHACIN: Wild yam has been found to lower serum levels of the antiinflammatory drug indomethacin, as well as attenuate indomethacin-induced intestinal inflammation, in rats.[16] Clinical data are lacking.

PROGESTOGENIC AGENTS: Wild yam was found to suppress progesterone synthesis.[17] Wild yam may interact with progesterone, although clinical evidence is lacking.

VITAMIN C: Vitamin C has been shown to enhance the cholesterol-lowering effects of diosgenin and clofibrate.[12]

Willow (Salix spp.)

Pharmacokinetics

Willow bark extract is absorbed into the bloodstream.[1] More than 80% of the salicin in willow bark is absorbed after oral administration.[2] Salicin and its derivatives are absorbed through the gut, and small amounts are absorbed in the small intestine. Salicylic acid was the major metabolite of salicin detected in the serum (86% of total salicylates), followed by salicyluric acid (10%) and gentisic acid (4%). Peak levels were reached less than 2 hours after oral administration. Renal elimination occurred predominantly in the form of salicyluric acid.[3] Willow bark extract is primarily excreted renally in the form of salicyluric acid.[1,4]

Adverse effects

Although current U.S. regulations do not require manufacturers of willow bark products to include any cautions on the label, the dietary supplement contains salicylates that may present a safety risk to some people. The same precautions taken with aspirin should be taken with willow bark.

Willow bark extract has been reported to cause various gastrointestinal problems, headaches, and allergic reactions.[5] Plants containing salicylates have a very bitter taste, so willow bark tea may be unpalatable for most patients, particularly children. Willow bark may cause GI side effects, including diarrhea, heartburn, and dyspepsia.[6,7] It may also cause blood pressure instability.[6] Willow bark should be avoided in patients with kidney disorders because it may reduce renal blood flow and may contribute to renal failure in patients predisposed to such diseases.[8,9] Based on a meta-analysis, the combination of salicin and alcohol may increase the risk of GI bleeding and gastritis.[10]

Interactions

ACETAZOLAMIDE: In vitro research and two case reports suggest a toxic interaction between salicylates and the carbonic anhydrase inhibitor acetazolamide. Pharmacokinetic studies in human subjects showed that salicylate reduced the plasma protein binding and renal clearance of acetazolamide; further, in two case reports of elderly patients chronically receiving aspirin, concomitant use of acetazolamide resulted in lethargy, incontinence, and confusion, likely from elevated unbound plasma acetazolamide concentrations and reduced plasma protein binding.[8] Salicylic acid toxicity may also be increased. Because of the salicylic acid content of willow bark, caution is advised when using it concomitantly with acetazolamide or related compounds.

ALCOHOL: A meta-analysis found that the combination of salicin and alcohol may increase the risk of GI bleeding and gastritis.[10]

ANTICOAGULANTS/ANTIPLATELETS: Willow bark increases bleeding by decreasing platelet aggregation[11,12] and should be avoided in patients taking anticoagulant/antiplatelet agents. However, willow bark extract containing 240 mg salicin had lesser inhibitory effects on platelet aggregation than aspirin in human subjects.[11,12] Concomitant willow bark and warfarin use was suggested as a risk factor for increased bleeding;[13] however, clinical data are lacking.

BLOOD LIPIDS: Based on clinical evidence, willow bark extract may induce hypertriglyceridemia.[7]

BLOOD PRESSURE: Willow bark may cause blood pressure instability[6] and should be used cautiously with hypotensive agents.

CYTOKINES AND INFLAMMATORY MARKERS: Based on laboratory studies, willow bark may have antiinflammatory effects[14-16] and theoretically may interact with other anti-inflammatory agents.

KIDNEY FUNCTION TESTS: Willow bark has been suggested to reduce renal blood flow and may contribute to renal failure in patients predisposed to such diseases.[8,9]

METHOTREXATE: Theoretically, white willow may decrease the renal excretion of methotrexate, resulting in toxic levels because of its salicin content.

PHENYTOIN (DILANTIN): Theoretically, the concomitant use of phenytoin and willow bark's salicylates may cause plasma protein–binding displacement, thereby increasing phenytoin levels in the blood and potentially causing toxicity.

PROBENECID: Theoretically, the concomitant use of probenecid with willow bark may impair the effectiveness of probenecid because of willow bark's proposed aspirin-like pharmacological actions.

PROTEIN-BOUND AGENTS: White willow bark's plasma protein–binding salicylate component may displace some other plasma protein–bound agents and may alter drug levels in the body.

SPIRONOLACTONE: Theoretically, the concomitant use of spironolactone with willow bark may result in antagonistic or additive effects.

SULFONYLUREAS: Theoretically, the concomitant use of sulfonylureas with willow bark may increase the effect of sulfonylureas and may increase side effects and risk for toxicity.

TANNINS: The concomitant administration of tannin-containing agents may result in a malabsorption of salicylic acid.[17]

VALPROIC ACID: Theoretically, the concomitant use of valproic acid with willow bark may impair the effectiveness of valproic acid.

WHITE BLOOD CELL COUNTS: Willow bark extract may have antileukemic activity and alter WBC test results.[18]

Yohimbe (Pausinystalia yohimbe)

Pharmacokinetics

Yohimbine, the major alkaloid of the yohimbe plant, seems to be poorly absorbed after oral administration. Bioavailability is highly variable (7%-87%).[1] Yohimbine is distributed in liver, RBCs, brain, and intestinal wall.[2,3] Yohimbine appears to be eliminated through metabolism because urinary excretion is minimal.[2] Yohimbine has an elimination half-life of less than 1 hour, whereas an active metabolite, 11-hydroxy-yohimbine, has a half-life of about 6 hours.[4]

Adverse effects

Because of the potential for serious side effects and interactions, the FDA has determined yohimbine to be unsafe for over-the-counter sale. Because yohimbe bark may contain clinically significant amounts of yohimbine alkaloid, similar risks may apply. However, a 1995 chemical analysis of 26 commercial yohimbe products reported that most contained virtually no yohimbine.[5]

Yohimbine is likely to be safe when taken by adults in recommended oral doses under the direction and supervision of a qualified health care professional. In large doses, yohimbine may cause severe hypotension and cardiac conduction disorders.[6-11] Yohimbine should be avoided in pregnancy because it may act as a uterine relaxant and fetal toxin. It should also be avoided during lactation and in children (deaths have been reported in children).

Interactions

Note: Yohimbe bark extract contains approximately 6% indole alkaloids, of which 10% to 15% is yohimbine. A 1995 chemical analysis of 26 commercial yohimbe products reported that most contained virtually no yohimbine.[5] The pharmacological activity of yohimbine has been well characterized in studies, although these effects may or may not apply to yohimbe, depending on the concentration of yohimbine present.

ALPHA-ADRENERGIC AGENTS: Yohimbine is an alpha-adrenergic blocker and has been reported to antagonize the effects of alpha-adrenergic agents such as clonidine.[12-14] In theory, this interaction may also apply to yohimbe bark extract, which contains variable (but low) concentrations of yohimbine alkaloid. Concomitant use of yohimbe and phenothiazines is contraindicated because of an increased risk of alpha-2-adrenergic antagonism.

AMPHETAMINES: Use of yohimbine with amphetamines has been cautioned anecdotally, although reliable scientific evidence is limited in this area.

ANTIDEPRESSANTS: TCAs and concomitant yohimbine should be used cautiously because of potential increases or decreases in blood pressure.

BETA-ADRENERGIC AGENTS: Beta blockers may have a protective role against yohimbine toxicity.

BLOOD GLUCOSE: Anecdotally, yohimbine increases the effects of hypoglycemic agents, including insulin, but reliable scientific evidence is limited in this area. It is unclear whether these potential effects extend to hypoglycemic agents.

BLOOD PRESSURE: Yohimbine may interfere with blood pressure control and should be used cautiously with other hypotensive agents. In theory, this interaction may also apply to yohimbe bark extract, which contains variable (but low) concentrations of yohimbine alkaloid.

CAFFEINE: Caffeine-containing agents such as coffee, tea, cola, guarana, and mate may theoretically increase the risk of hypertensive crisis when taken with yohimbine. In theory, this interaction may also apply to yohimbe bark extract, which contains variable (but low) concentrations of yohimbine alkaloid.

CENTRAL NERVOUS SYSTEM STIMULANTS: Over-the-counter products containing stimulants, including caffeine, phenylephrine, and phenylpropanolamine (removed from the U.S. market), may lead to additive effects when used in combination with yohimbe bark extract. However, evidence for this interaction is largely anecdotal.

CHOLINERGIC AGENTS: Concomitant cholinergic agents should be used with caution.

CYTOCHROME P450 SUBSTRATES: Agents that inhibit CYP450 3A3 or 3A4 may elicit increases in serum levels of yohimbine. Likewise, agents that induce these enzymes may result in decreases in serum levels.

EPHEDRA: Anecdotal reports cite a risk of hypertensive crisis when yohimbine is used concomitantly with ephedra.

ETHANOL: Concomitant use of ethanol with yohimbine produces an additive effect of increasing the severity of acute intoxication.[15] In theory, this interaction may also apply to yohimbe bark extract, which contains variable (but low) concentrations of yohimbine alkaloid.

GOLDENSEAL AND BERBERINE: Berberine, an alkaloid present in goldenseal, competitively inhibits the binding of yohimbine to cell surface receptors in vitro, which may or may not affect pharmacological actions when the two agents are administered concurrently.[16] In theory, this interaction may also apply to yohimbe bark extract, which contains variable (but low) concentrations of yohimbine alkaloid.

HISTAMINE: Use of yohimbine with antihistamine has been cautioned anecdotally, although reliable scientific evidence in this area is limited.

LINEZOLID: As a weak MAO inhibitor, linezolid should not be used with yohimbine because of the potential additive effects and toxicity.

MONOAMINERGIC AGENTS: Because of yohimbine's MAO inhibitory activity, concomitant use may produce additive effects and is contraindicated because of an increased risk of hypertensive crisis. In theory, this interaction may also apply to yohimbe bark extract, which contains variable (but low) concentrations of yohimbine alkaloid.

MUSCARINIC AGENTS: Concomitant yohimbine use with antimuscarinic agents may increase risk of toxicity; however, the evidence for this interaction is largely anecdotal.

OPIATES: Although yohimbine by itself does not appear to possess analgesic effects, yohimbine may enhance morphine analgesia, based on the results of a controlled trial.[17,18] In theory, this interaction may also apply to yohimbe bark extract, which contains variable (but low) concentrations of yohimbine alkaloid. Yohimbine may increase or decrease naloxone-precipitated opiate withdrawal symptoms.[19-21] Again, in theory, this interaction may also apply to yohimbe bark extract.

PHYSOSTIGMINE: In preliminary clinical research, concomitant use of yohimbine and physostigmine in patients with Alzheimer's disease has been associated with anxiety, agitation, restlessness, and chest pain.[22] In theory, this interaction may also apply to yohimbe bark extract.

TYRAMINE-CONTAINING FOODS: Because of the MAO inhibitor activity of yohimbine, tyramine-containing foods, including red wines, fermented meats, and aged cheeses, theoretically may increase the risk of hypertensive crisis when taken concomitantly with yohimbine. In theory, this interaction may also apply to yohimbe bark extract, which contains variable (but low) concentrations of yohimbine alkaloid.

Yucca (*Yucca schidigera*)

Pharmacokinetics: Insufficient available evidence.

Adverse effects

The few reports on yucca and its adverse effects cite urticaria and allergic rhinitis.[1]

Interactions

BLOOD LIPIDS: A blend of *Yucca schidigera* and *Quillaja saponaria* extract filtrates has been shown to decrease total and LDL cholesterol levels in hypercholesterolemic patients.[2]

CYTOKINES AND INFLAMMATORY MARKERS: Based on in vitro research,[3] yuccaols and resveratrol from yucca may reduce inflammation and theoretically may interact with antiinflammatory agents.

FUNGAL LEVELS: Based on in vitro research, alexin extracted from *Yucca gloriosa* flowers may have a broad spectrum of antifungal activity.[4]

HISTOLOGICAL TESTS: Based on in vitro research, yuccaols and resveratrol from yucca may reduce cell proliferation[3] and may interact with antineoplastic agents.

QUILLAJA SAPONARIA: Based on clinical research, ingestion of a blend of *Yucca schidigera* and *Quillaja saponaria* extract filtrates may decrease total and LDL cholesterol levels in hypercholesterolemic patients.[2]

VIRAL LEVELS: In vitro research reports that yucca leaf protein isolated from the leaves of *Yucca recurvifolia* Salisb. inhibited herpes simplex virus type 1 (HSV-1), HSV-2, and human cytomegalovirus.[5] Theoretically, yucca may interact with antiviral agents.

B Pregnancy and Lactation

This appendix contains herb safety information for pregnant or lactating women. This is not an all-inclusive or comprehensive list of known or potential safety considerations. A qualified health care practitioner should be consulted with specific questions or concerns regarding the safety of herb use during pregnancy or lactation. The U.S. Food and Drug Administration (FDA) currently classifies pharmaceuticals into pregnancy categories (A, B, C, D, or X) based on potential fetal risks weighed against benefit (Table B-1). Although the FDA does not regulate dietary supplements, including herbal supplements, it has classified some herbs (e.g., belladonna, foxglove) based on their pharmacologically active constituents using the current five-letter classification system. Other organizations may also use available evidence to assess herbal safety based on these guidelines.

Abuta (Cissampelos pareira)
There is insufficient information regarding the safety of abuta during pregnancy or lactation. Abuta may have abortifacient properties, based on anecdotal reports, although abuta has traditionally been used to prevent abortion.[2,3] Scientific evidence is limited in this area.

Acacia (Acacia senegal)
According to the Central Drug Research Institute in Lucknow, India, in collaboration with the U.S. National Institutes of Health (NIH) and World Health Organization (WHO), acacia displays antiimplantation effects and may hold potential as an herbal contraceptive.[4] However, there is insufficient evidence regarding the safety of acacia during pregnancy or lactation.

Acai (Euterpe oleracea)
Insufficient available evidence.

Acerola (Malpighia glabra, Malpighia punicifolia)
Insufficient available evidence.

Ackee (Blighia sapida)
Insufficient available evidence.

Aconite (Aconitum napellus)
Because there are numerous reports of toxicity and adverse effects during oral and topical aconite treatment,[5-11] it is not recommended during pregnancy or lactation.

African Wild Potato (Hypoxis hemerocallidea)
Insufficient available evidence.

Agaric (Amanita muscaria)
Agaric should be avoided in pregnant or lactating women because of its known toxicity; potential adverse effects include hallucinations, confusion, and dizziness.[12]

TABLE B-1 Current Categories for Drug Use in Pregnancy.*

CATEGORY	DESCRIPTION
A	Adequate, well-controlled studies in pregnant women have not shown an increased risk of fetal abnormalities.
B	Animal studies have revealed no evidence of harm to the fetus, however, there are no adequate and well-controlled studies in pregnant women.
	or
	Animal studies have shown an adverse effect, but adequate and well-controlled studies in pregnant women have failed to demonstrate a risk to the fetus.
C	Animal studies have shown an adverse effect and there are no adequate and well-controlled studies in pregnant women.
	or
	No animal studies have been conducted and there are no adequate and well-controlled studies in pregnant women.
D	Studies, adequate well-controlled or observational, in pregnant women have demonstrated a risk to the fetus. However, the benefits of therapy may outweigh the potential risk.
X	Studies, adequate well-controlled or observational, in animals or pregnant women have demonstrated positive evidence of fetal abnormalities. The use of the product is contraindicated in women who are or may become pregnant.

*The FDA has recently proposed to replace these classifications with a new labeling system. Under the proposed rule, drug labeling will contain pregnancy and lactation subsections that each contains 1) a risk summary, 2) clinical considerations, and 3) a data section. (From U.S. Food and Drug Administration, Center for Drug Evaluation and Research, Summary of Proposed Rule on Pregnancy and Lactation Labeling, May 28, 2008. http://www.fda.gov.

Agave (*Agave* spp.)
Women from rural areas of the central plateau of Mexico drink a mild alcoholic beverage called *pulque* to increase breast milk production. Pulque is believed to stimulate milk production in lactating women. Although alcohol is contraindicated in pregnancy and lactation (see Alcohol), the relatively small amounts excreted in breast milk after pulque consumption is unlikely to have harmful effects on breastfed infants.[13] However, pulque intake during lactation has been suggested to adversely affect postnatal growth in some Mexican populations.[14]

Anordin and dinordin, prepared with steroids derived from the sisal plants *Agave sisilana* and *Agave americana*, have antifertility properties, as shown by Swedish and U.S. scientists. This new family of contraceptives has the advantage of administration only once or twice a month versus the 20 times necessary with typical oral contraceptives.[15]

Agrimony (*Agrimonia* spp.)
There is insufficient information regarding the safety of agrimony during pregnancy or lactation. Agrimony has been used traditionally to treat heavy menstrual bleeding.[16] Oral use of agrimony during pregnancy may be unsafe because of possible effects on the menstrual cycle.

Alcohol, Ethanol
Alcohol is a component of some herbal preparations, such as tinctures.[2,3] The American Academy of Pediatrics (AAP) states that "prenatal exposure to alcohol is one of the leading preventable causes of birth defects, mental retardation, and neurodevelopmental disorders" and recommends that pregnant women (or those attempting to conceive) abstain from alcohol.[17] According to the AAP, alcohol is "usually compatible" with lactation; however, large amounts (>1 g/kg daily) may result in decreased milk ejection reflex in the mother and drowsiness, diaphoresis, or growth abnormalities in the infant.[18]

Alder Buckthorn (*Frangula alnus*)
Alder buckthorn should not be taken orally during pregnancy and lactation because of safety concerns.[19]

Alfalfa (*Medicago sativa*)
The potential uterine stimulant stachydrine is found in the variety *Medicago sativa* var. *italica*.[20] Alfalfa seeds are traditionally reputed to be lactogenic and to affect the menstrual cycle (i.e., promote menstruation).[20] The coumestrol present in alfalfa may possess estrogenic properties,[21] with unclear effects on pregnancy or lactation. Alfalfa should be avoided during pregnancy or lactation because of insufficient available data.

Alkanna (*Alkanna* spp.)
Insufficient available evidence.

Allspice (*Pimenta dioica*)
Insufficient available evidence.

Aloe (*Aloe vera*)
Although topical application is unlikely to be harmful during pregnancy or lactation,[22] internal use of aloe is not recommended because its anthroquinones purportedly may stimulate uterine contraction. It is not known whether anthroquinones or other pharmacologically active constituents of aloe may be excreted with breast milk. Consumption of the dried juice from the pericyclic region of aloe leaves is contraindicated during lactation by many herbal texts because of a lack of safety data.

Alpinia (*Alpinia galanga*)
Insufficient available evidence.

Amaranth (*Amaranthus hypochondriacus*)
Insufficient available evidence.

Ambrette (*Abelmoschus moschatus*)
There is insufficient information regarding the safety of ambrette during pregnancy or lactation. Lactating women should avoid oral and topical ambrette formulations because it is excreted in breast milk.[23]

American Hellebore (*Veratrum viride*)
See False Hellebore (*Veratrum* spp.).

American Pawpaw (*Asimina triloba*)
Because of the cytotoxic effects of pawpaw extracts,[24-36] use during pregnancy and lactation is contraindicated.

American Pennyroyal (*Hedeoma pulegioides*)
See False Pennyroyal (*Hedeoma* spp.).

American Skullcap (*Scutellaria barbata*)
See Skullcap (*Scutellaria* spp.).

Andiroba (*Carapa* spp.)
Insufficient available evidence.

Andrographis (*Andrographis paniculata*)
Andrographis should be avoided during pregnancy because of possible contraceptive effects observed in animal studies.[2,3] There is insufficient information regarding the safety of andrographis during lactation.

Angel's Trumpet (*Brugmansia* and *Datura* spp.)
Based on case reports and epidemiological research, the entire angel's trumpet plant is considered to be poisonous and is unsafe when used orally during pregnancy and lactation.[37,38]

Angostura (*Galipea officinalis*, syn. *Angostura trifoliata*)
Insufficient available evidence.

Anise (*Pimpinella anisum*)
Anise should be avoided during pregnancy because it has been traditionally used to induce abortions. In Mexico, Turkey, and China, anise is used as a galactagogue (substance that enhances milk production). Many anise-containing beverages contain alcohol, which should be avoided by pregnant and lactating patients (see Alcohol).

Annatto (*Bixa orellana*)
The use of annatto during pregnancy and lactation has not been thoroughly studied in humans. However, annatto is considered likely safe when used orally in amounts found in foods because of its long history of use as a food additive. Annatto seeds are used to make a brightly colored paste that is added to numerous foods to impart color. In animals, doses up to 500 mg/kg of annatto given by gavage (forced feeding) for 7 days had no adverse effects on mother or fetus.[39]

Apple (*Malus sylvestris*)
Maternal food consumption of apples is likely safe during pregnancy and lactation and has been suggested to protect children from developing asthma later in life.[40]

Apricot (Prunus armeniaca)
Apricot fruit is generally recognized as safe during pregnancy and lactation. Medicinal amounts have not been studied. Apricot pit contains amygdalin, a cyanide-like plant compound. Adverse reactions similar to cyanide poisoning, such as vomiting, diarrhea, lethargy, tachypnea, and cyanosis, have been reported with apricot pit consumption.[41]

Aristolochia (Aristolochia spp.)
Aristolochic acid A, a constituent of *Aristolochia mollissima*, has been associated with abortifacient effects and toxicity.[42] Aristolochia is not recommended during pregnancy or lactation because of insufficient safety data.

Arnica (Arnica spp.)
Internal use of arnica is contraindicated during pregnancy because of known toxicity and the potential for uterine stimulation (based on animal and in vitro data).[2,3] Signs of arnica poisoning are characterized by severe mucous membrane irritation (vomiting, diarrhea, mucous membrane hemorrhage) and brief stimulation of cardiac activity, followed by cardiac muscle palsy. With insufficient safety information, use should be avoided during lactation.

Arrowroot (Maranta arundinacea)
Insufficient available evidence.

Arum (Arum maculatum)
Because of toxicity and adverse effects,[43] arum should be avoided during pregnancy and lactation.

Asafoetida (Ferula assafoetida)
Asafoetida has traditionally been used as an abortifacient and may be unsafe during pregnancy and breastfeeding. Alcohol extracts of asafoetida should be avoided because of alcohol content (see Alcohol). Alcohol extracts of asafoetida have also demonstrated cytotoxic and antiproliferative effects in vitro[44] and could harm developing embryos.

Asarum (Asarum spp.)
Insufficient available evidence.

Ash (Fraxinus spp.)
Insufficient available evidence.

Ashwagandha (Withania somnifera)
Although evidence of safety during pregnancy is lacking, ashwagandha is not recommended based on anecdotal reports of abortifacient properties. It is also not recommended during lactation because of insufficient safety data.

Asparagus (Asparagus officinalis)
Asparagus is likely safe during pregnancy or lactation when consumed in reasonable dietary quantities by nonallergic women. There is insufficient safety evidence for supplemental doses.

Astragalus (Astragalus membranaceus)
Insufficient available evidence.

Autumn Crocus (Colchicum autumnale spp.)
Colchicine, an alkaloid derived from autumn crocus, should be avoided in pregnant women, as well as in men and women planning to conceive, because of teratogenic effects. Using colchicine during the first 2 weeks of gestation has been linked to numerous birth defects, including congenital deformities such as agnathia (missing lower jaw), cleft palate, exencephaly (brain outside skull), and polydactyly (abnormal number of digits).[45,46] Colchicine is excreted in breast milk; therefore, autumn crocus should also be avoided in lactating women.[47,48]

Avocado (Persea americana)
Modest food consumption of avocado is likely safe during pregnancy and lactation. There is a lack of safety information regarding the medicinal use of avocado during pregnancy. Some varieties of avocado may be unsafe during lactation. In animals the Guatemalan variety of avocado resulted in mammary gland damage and reduced milk production at doses greater than 20 g/kg.[49]

Ayurveda
Ayurvedic herbs are potent, and some contain compounds that may be toxic if taken in large amounts or over an extended period. In addition, some herbs imported from India have been reported to contain high levels of toxic metals. Certain Ayurvedic herbs or herbal combinations may be contraindicated during pregnancy and lactation. For example, *Terminalia hebula* (harda), a powerful purgative used to stimulate gastrointestinal motility, should be avoided during pregnancy.[2,3] Supervision of a trained practitioner is recommended.

Ba Ji Tian (Morinda officinalis)
Insufficient available evidence.

Babassu (Orbignya phalerata)
Insufficient available evidence.

Bach Flower Remedies
Bach flower remedies are usually consumed as alcohol-based preparations, and alcohol intake should be avoided in pregnant or breastfeeding women (see Alcohol). However, according to the Dr. Edward Bach Centre, the amount of alcohol is so small in Bach flower remedies that it can usually be disregarded.[50] Nonetheless, because of the lack of safety data, use is not recommended in pregnant or lactating women.

Bacopa (Bacopa monnieri)
Insufficient available evidence.

Bael (Aegle marmelos)
Bael is not recommended for use during pregnancy, as Indian bael leaves have been traditionally used to induce abortion and to sterilize women. It is not recommended during lactation because of insufficient safety data.

Baikal Skullcap (Scutellaria baicalensis)
See Skullcap (*Scutellaria* spp.).

Bamboo (Arundinaria japonica)
Insufficient available evidence.

Banaba (Lagerstroemia speciosa)
Insufficient available evidence.

Barbat Skullcap (Scutellaria barbata)
See Skullcap (*Scutellaria* spp.).

Barberry (Berberis spp.)
Based on unsubstantiated reports, barberry has exhibited uterine stimulant properties, and berberine (found in barberry) has been shown to have antifertility activity (see Berberine). It is not recommended during lactation because of insufficient safety data.

Barley (Hordeum vulgare)
Barley is likely safe when ingested in reasonable dietary quantities by nonsensitive women.[2,3] However, excessive consumption of barley sprouts is not advised during pregnancy based on traditional use. Barley may not be safe during breastfeeding, according to anecdotal reports.

Bay Leaf (Laurus nobilis)
Insufficient available evidence.

Bean (Phaseolus vulgaris)
Beans, particularly red kidney beans, contain the toxin phytohemagglutinin (PHA). Many cases of red kidney bean poisoning are attributable to insufficient soaking or cooking of the beans.[51] However, properly prepared beans are likely safe when consumed in reasonable dietary quantities by nonallergic women. There is insufficient safety information for supplemental doses in pregnant or lactating women.

Bear's Garlic (Allium ursinum)
Insufficient available evidence.

Beet (Beta vulgaris)
Beet is likely safe in amounts found in food during pregnancy. The use of medicinal amounts of beet during pregnancy should be avoided because of a lack of safety data. Beets contain nitrates; however, according to AAP, breastfed infants of mothers who ingest beets and other foods high in nitrates are not believed to be at risk of nitrate poisoning because nitrate concentration does not increase significantly in breast milk.[52]

Belladonna (Atropa spp.)
Belladonna is not recommended during pregnancy because of the potential for toxicity and adverse outcomes. Belladonna is listed under FDA Category C, meaning that adverse effects have been observed in animal reproduction studies. One small case-control study of neonatal death and congenital malformations showed no increase in these outcomes in mothers ingesting belladonna alkaloids.[53] In another study, there was an increase in birth defects in the offspring of mothers who had taken belladonna, although no relationship between first-trimester use of atropine and birth defects was found.[54] In anecdotal reports, use of belladonna during pregnancy may increase the risk of respiratory abnormalities, hypospadias (penile urethral anomalies in males), and eye/ear malformations.

Belladonna alkaloids are excreted in breast milk, thereby exposing infants to potential toxicity. However, AAP has identified atropine (a constituent of belladonna) as "usually compatible with breast feeding."[18]

Berberine
Berberine, the active component of goldenseal (Hydrastis canadensis) and plants of the genus Berberis, has been reported to have antifertility activity.[55] Berberine has been reported to increase the risks of kernicterus, a type of brain damage caused by jaundice, because of its ability to displace bilirubin from albumin in vitro and in vivo.[56] Berberine-containing herbs have been suggested historically as abortifacients and uterine stimulants; however, scientific evidence is lacking. There is insufficient information regarding the safety of berberine during lactation.

Bergamot Oil (Citrus bergamia)
There is insufficient evidence regarding the safety of bergamot oil during pregnancy or lactation.[23] However, a maternal cohort study correlated high citrus intake during pregnancy with increased incidence of food allergies in children.[57]

Beta-Glucan (β-Glucan)
As a naturally occurring component of plant products, beta-glucan is likely safe when consumed in reasonable dietary quantities by pregnant or lactating women. However, there is insufficient evidence regarding the safety of supplemental doses.

Beta-Sitosterol (β-Sitosterol), Sitosterol (22,23-Dihydrostigmasterol, 24-Ethylcholesterol)
As a naturally occurring component of plant products, beta-sitosterol is likely safe when consumed in reasonable quantities in the diet by pregnant or lactating women. However, there is insufficient evidence regarding the safety of supplemental doses.

Betel Nut (Areca catechu)
Pregnant or lactating women should not use betel nut because of potential carcinogenic or fetotoxic effects. Betel nut also has central nervous system (CNS) stimulant and cholinergic effects that may adversely affect fetuses or breastfed babies. In mouse reproduction studies, betel nut ingestion resulted in fetal death, reduced fetal weight, and delayed skeletal maturity.[58] In addition, parental betel quid chewing has been associated with early manifestation of metabolic syndrome in children.[59] The clinical adverse effects of betel nut in pregnant women were found to be 2.8-fold greater than in women who did not use betel.[60] In an earlier study, however, no adverse fetal effects were found when betel nut was administered to pregnant women.[61] There has also been a case report of withdrawal in an infant whose mother was a chronic betel nut user.[62]

Betony (Stachys spp.)
Betony has traditionally been used to stimulate the uterus and cause amenorrhea, which suggests a possibility of premature birth or miscarriage. Thus, betony should not be used during pregnancy. There is insufficient information regarding the safety of betony during lactation.

Bilberry (Vaccinium myrtillus)
The safety of bilberry during pregnancy or lactation has not been established or studied systematically. However, one study used bilberry extract to treat pregnancy-induced lower-extremity edema, and no adverse effects were reported.[63] Bilberry fruit is presumed to be safe on the basis of its use as a food product.

Birch (Betula spp.)
There is insufficient safety information for the use of birch during pregnancy or lactation. Maternal birch pollen allergy seems to have a stronger influence on the development of rhinoconjunctivitis in children with atopy (genetic tendencies to develop atopic dermatitis, allergic rhinitis, and asthma) than on the degree of allergen exposure during pregnancy.[64]

Bishop's Weed (Ammi majus)
Insufficient available evidence.

Bitter Almond (Prunus amygdalus)
Bitter almond or laetrile, an FDA-banned drug made from bitter almond, is not recommended in pregnant women because it may lead to birth defects. When administered to pregnant hamsters, oral laetrile resulted in skeletal malformations in offspring. However, intravenous (IV) laetrile did not result in malformations. Oral laetrile reportedly increased in situ cyanide concentration significantly, whereas IV laetrile in these animals did not.[65] Bitter almond is not recommended during lactation because of insufficient safety information.

Bitter Apple (Citrullus colocynthis)
Oral use of *Citrullus colocynthis* is not recommended during pregnancy. The fruit pulp has been used as an abortifacient in Europe and India.[66,67] There is insufficient information regarding the safety of bitter apple during lactation.

Bitter Melon (Momordica charantia)
Bitter melon is not recommended during pregnancy. Two proteins (alpha- and beta-momocharin) isolated from the raw fruit possess properties that may cause abortions in animals; lowered fertility rates are also possible.[2,3] There is insufficient safety information available on bitter melon during lactation.

Bitter Orange (Citrus aurantium)
Insufficient available evidence.

Black Bryony (Tamus communis, syn. Dioscorea communis)
According to plant and herbal textbooks, all parts of the black bryony plant may be poisonous, presumably because of saponin content. Based on these secondary sources, ingestion should be avoided during pregnancy and lactation.

Black Cohosh (Actaea racemosa, formerly Cimicifuga racemosa)
According to a systematic review by researchers in the Motherisk Program at the Hospital for Sick Children in Toronto, black cohosh should be used cautiously during pregnancy because of labor-inducing effects.[68] In a survey of 500 nurse-midwives in the United States, 33% of the 172 respondents indicated that they use black cohosh to stimulate labor.[69] There is one report of severe multiorgan hypoxic injury in a child delivered with the aid of both black cohosh and blue cohosh *(Caulophyllum thalictroides)*.[70] The child survived with permanent CNS damage. Notably, blue cohosh possesses a vasoconstrictive glycoside, which may have been responsible for the adverse effects. Based on in vitro evidence, black cohosh could have labor-inducing effects, hormonal effects, emmenagogic (menstrual-stimulant) properties, and anovulatory effects. Therefore, black cohosh should be avoided during pregnancy. Furthermore, black cohosh tinctures may be inadvisable during pregnancy because of their high alcohol content (see Alcohol), although the absolute quantity of alcohol ingested from tinctures at recommended doses is likely to be relatively small.

According to a systematic review, black cohosh should be avoided during lactation because of possible hormonelike effects.[68]

Black Currant (Ribes nigrum)
Insufficient available evidence.

Black Haw (Viburnum prunifolium)
There is insufficient information regarding the safety of black haw during pregnancy or lactation. According to secondary sources, black haw has traditionally been used to relax the uterus, reduce uterine contractility, and prevent miscarriages. Black haw has been studied for its potential effects on uterine activity,[71] although safety information is limited.

Black Horehound (Ballota nigra)
Insufficient available evidence.

Black Mulberry (Morus nigra)
Based on its historical use as food, black mulberry is likely safe when consumed by nonallergic pregnant women as part of the diet in reasonable quantities. There is insufficient safety information for supplemental doses.

Black Mustard (Brassica nigra)
Because of possible abortifacient and menstrual-stimulant effects,[48] black mustard oil should be avoided in medicinal amounts during pregnancy. Because of a lack of sufficient safety data, the use of black mustard (orally or topically) should also be avoided during pregnancy and lactation.

Black Pepper (Piper nigrum)
Insufficient available evidence.

Black Seed (Nigella sativa)
Black seed should be avoided during pregnancy when taken orally in doses exceeding food amounts. Black seed may decrease or block uterine contractions,[72] and it may also have contraceptive effects.[73] Use should be avoided during breastfeeding because of insufficient safety data.

Blackberry (Rubus fructicosus)
Based on traditional use of the fruit as a food, blackberry is likely safe when consumed in reasonable amounts by pregnant or breastfeeding patients. Medicinal uses are not recommended because of a lack of safety information.

Bladderwrack (Fucus vesiculosus)
See Seaweed.

Blessed Thistle (Cnicus benedictus)
Blessed thistle has been used traditionally to stimulate menstruation or induce abortion and therefore should be avoided during pregnancy. Although blessed thistle has been used traditionally to stimulate lactation, it is not recommended because of insufficient safety information.

Bloodroot (Sanguinaria canadensis)
There is insufficient safety information regarding the safety of bloodroot during pregnancy or lactation. Traditionally, bloodroot was used to stimulate menstruation and therefore should not be used during pregnancy.

Blueberry (Vaccinium angustifolium)
Based on traditional use of the fruit as a food, blueberry is likely safe when consumed in reasonable amounts by pregnant or breastfeeding patients.[74] It should be avoided for medicinal purposes during pregnancy and lactation because of insufficient safety data.

Blue Cohosh (Caulophyllum thalictroides)
According to a systematic review by researchers in the Motherisk Program at the Hospital for Sick Children in Toronto, blue cohosh should be used only with extreme caution and vigilant medical supervision during pregnancy because of potential teratogenic, embryotoxic, and oxytoxic effects.[75] The roots of *Caulophyllum thalictroides* contain teratogenic alkaloids, together with saponins, which are considered to be responsible for the uterine-stimulant effects.[76] Based on rat studies, the constituent tapsine may be embryotoxic, and *N*-methylcytisine may be teratogenic.[77] The use of blue cohosh to induce abortion is frequently associated with adverse effects in the mother or fetus.[78] There have been case reports of cardiotoxicity in newborns of mothers who ingested blue cohosh; the resulting adverse effects included congestive heart failure (CHF), myocardial infarction (MI) or toxicity, stroke, and shock.[79-82] Adverse effects noted in perinatal infants with maternal blue cohosh use include MI with CHF and shock,[79] seizures,[80] and breathing difficulties with subsequent CNS ischemic damage.[70] Nicotinic toxicity was also observed in a pregnant women attempting to induce abortion with blue cohosh; the symptoms of tachycardia, muscle weakness and twitching, sweating, vomiting, and abdominal pain were believed to be caused by the blue cohosh constituent methylcytisine.[78]

There is insufficient safety information regarding blue cohosh during lactation.

Blue Flag (Iris versicolor)
Insufficient available evidence.

Boldo (Peumus boldus)
There is insufficient information regarding the safety of boldo during pregnancy or lactation. When administered to rats, boldo demonstrated anatomical alterations in the fetus.[2,3] However, the German Commission E reports no contraindications during pregnancy or lactation with the ascaridole-free boldo preparations.

Boneset (Eupatorium spp.)
There is currently a lack of reliable data on the clinical uses of boneset, and the following information is based on traditional use and expert opinion.

Boneset may be toxic and should be avoided by pregnant or breastfeeding women. Boneset is used in large doses to induce vomiting and evacuation of the bowels. According to secondary sources, hepatotoxic unsaturated pyrrolizidine alkaloids are common in the *Eupatorium* genus and might exist in boneset as well. Fresh boneset contains tremerol, a toxic chemical that can cause nausea, vomiting, weakness, muscle tremors, and increased respiration. Higher doses can cause coma and death. Dried boneset apparently does not contain tremerol.

Borage (Borago officinalis)
According to the conclusions of a review, borage oil may be contraindicated during pregnancy because of the teratogenic and labor-inducing effects of prostaglandin E agonists, such as the gamma-linolenic acid (GLA) in borage oil.[83] However, in a survey of 150 pregnant women (45 of whom used dietary supplements during pregnancy), adverse effects were mild, with one woman who used borage seed oil complaining of mild intestinal gas.[84] Borage oil is not recommended during lactation. In a study of GLA supplementation on arachidonic acid content in the breast milk of atopic mothers, supplementation with either high or low doses of GLA increased GLA and dihomo-GLA in the breast milk but did not increase arachidonic acid content.[85]

Boswellia (Boswellia serrata)
Reports suggest that resin from boswellia is a menstrual-flow stimulant (an emmenagogue) and may induce abortion.[86] Safety of boswellia during pregnancy has not been systematically studied, and therefore it cannot be recommended. Boswellia should be avoided during lactation because of a lack of sufficient safety data.

Boxwood (Buxus sempervirens)
Insufficient available evidence.

Brewer's Yeast (Saccharomyces cerevisiae)
Insufficient available evidence.

Bromelain (Bromeliaceae)
Insufficient available evidence.

Broom Corn (Sorghum bicolor)
Insufficient available evidence.

Bryonia (Bryonia spp.)
Bryonia is a poisonous plant that is *not* safe during pregnancy or lactation. In its pure form, bryonia may cause adverse gastrointestinal effects that may result in death. Consumption of either the berries or the roots of bryonia is not considered safe during pregnancy because of the risk of abortion.[45,89]

Buchu (Agathosma betulina)
There is insufficient information regarding the safety of buchu during pregnancy or lactation. According to traditional use, buchu may be an abortifacient and may stimulate uterine contractions.

Buckhorn Plantain (Plantago lanceolata)
Buckhorn plantain may stimulate contraction of the uterus,[88] and thus it should be avoided during pregnancy. There is insufficient data regarding the safety of buckhorn plantain use during lactation.

Buckwheat (Fagopyrum esculentum)
Small human studies have reported no toxic adverse effects to the embryo from buckwheat.[89,90] However, there is insufficient available evidence regarding the safety of buckwheat during pregnancy or lactation.

Bugleweed (Lycopus spp.)
Based on secondary sources and herbal tradition, bugleweed may not be safe during pregnancy because it may have hormonelike and antihormone-like actions,[91,92] such as antigonadotropic and antithyrotropic activity. Bugleweed should be avoided during lactation because of purported antiprolactin activity.

Bulbous Buttercup (Ranunculus bulbosus)
Insufficient available evidence.

Bupleurum (Bupleurum spp.)
Insufficient available evidence.

Burdock (Arctium lappa)
Traditionally, burdock has been avoided during pregnancy and lactation, especially during the first trimester, because of the presence of anthraquinone glycosides in burdock root and uterine-contracting (oxytocic) and uterine-stimulating activities observed in

animals.[20] Many burdock tinctures contain high levels of alcohol and should be avoided during pregnancy (see Alcohol). Burdock should also be avoided during lactation because of insufficient safety data.

Butcher's Broom (Ruscus aculeatus)
Insufficient available evidence.

Butterbur (Petasites hybridus)
Insufficient available evidence.

Cabbage (Brassica oleracea. Capitata)
Cabbage and other cultivar groups of *B. oleracea*, such as broccoli (Italica Group), Brussels sprouts (Gemmifera Group), cauliflower (Botrytis Group), and kale (Acephala Group), are likely safe when consumed in amounts found in food. Medicinal use of cabbage during pregnancy should be avoided. Animal studies demonstrated toxicity to the embryo, but no teratogenic effects were observed.[93] Topical use of cabbage leaves during lactation is safe and often recommended to reduce breast swelling and engorgement.[94-97] However, when consumed by lactating women, cabbage may increase the risk of infantile colic (excessive crying) for unknown reasons.[98]

Caffeine
Caffeine is a constituent in many herbs, including coffee (*Coffea* spp.), kola nut (*Cola acuminata*), guarana (*Paullinia cupana*), and tea (*Camellia sinensis*). According to a prospective cohort study, pregnant women who consume 200 mg or more of caffeine had double the risk of miscarriage as those who had no caffeine.[99] Large amounts of green tea should be used cautiously in pregnant women, because caffeine crosses the placenta and has been associated with spontaneous abortion, intrauterine growth retardation, and low birth weight. Heavy caffeine intake during pregnancy may increase the risk of later developing SIDS (sudden infant death syndrome). Very high doses of caffeine have been associated with birth defects, including limb and palate malformations.

Caffeine is readily transferred into breast milk. Infants nursing from mothers consuming high levels of caffeine daily have been reported to experience tremors and heart rhythm abnormalities. Components present in breast milk may reduce the infant's ability to metabolize caffeine, resulting in higher-than-expected blood levels. Caffeine ingestion by infants can lead to sleep disturbances and insomnia and has been associated with anemia, reduced iron metabolism, and irritability. Belladonna alkaloids are excreted in breast milk, thereby exposing infants to potential toxicity. However, AAP has identified moderate intake of caffeinated beverages (up to 2-3 cups daily) as "usually compatible with breast feeding."[18]

Cajeput (Melaleuca quinquenervia)
Insufficient available evidence.

Calamus (Acorus calamus)
Sterility occurred in male houseflies that were exposed to vapors of calamus oil.[100] Reproductive effects on female houseflies or humans are unclear.

Calendula (Calendula officinalis)
In vitro, calendula has exhibited moderate "uterotonic" effects in isolated rabbit and guinea pig uterine tissues.[88] Anecdotal reports indicate that calendula may possess spermicidal and abortifacient effects.[48] The effects of calendula use during pregnancy and lactation are not clear.

California Poppy (Eschscholzia californica)
Insufficient available evidence.

Camphor (Cinnamomum camphora)
Oral and topical camphor should be avoided during pregnancy and lactation.[101,102] Oral camphor crosses the placenta and has been associated with fetal and neonatal death.[103-105] It is not clear whether the same effects may occur with topical use.

Canadian Hemp (Apocynum cannabinum)
Because it contains digitalis-like glycosides that may have toxic effects on the heart,[43] Canadian hemp should be avoided during pregnancy and lactation.

Caper (Capparis spinosa)
Insufficient available evidence.

Capsicum (Capsicum spp.)
Capsicum is likely safe during pregnancy and lactation when used appropriately as a topical agent.[106] Capsicum should be avoided orally for medicinal uses during pregnancy because of insufficient available evidence. Because oral capsicum has been associated with dermatitis in breastfed infants,[107] it should be avoided during lactation.

Caraway (Carum carvi)
Caraway oil has been used to stimulate menstruation,[108] and should be avoided during pregnancy and lactation in medicinal amounts.

Cardamom (Elettaria cardamomum)
Although cardamom is widely used as a spice, there is insufficient evidence on its safety (particularly in quantities greater than those normally found in foods) during pregnancy or lactation.

Carob (Ceratonia siliqua)
Insufficient available evidence.

Carqueja (Baccharis spp.)
Insufficient available evidence.

Carrot (Daucus carota)
Carrot is likely safe during pregnancy and lactation when consumed in reasonable dietary amounts. In humans, carrot juice was found to alter the flavor of breast milk 2 to 3 hours after carrot juice ingestion.[109] In addition, babies whose mothers had consumed carrot juice for a few weeks consumed less carrot-flavored cereal and spent less time eating than babies whose mothers had consumed water. In another clinical trial, ingestion of 100 g of grated carrots daily for 60 days significantly improved the serum vitamin A and iron levels of lactating mothers at risk of deficiency.[110]

Cascara (Rhamnus purshiana)
There is insufficient data regarding the safety of cascara in pregnant women. Cascara is thought to be excreted into breast milk; however, the AAP has deemed it compatible with breastfeeding.[18]

Cashew (Anacardium occidentale)
Tree nuts are common causes of food allergies in children, and a recent study suggests that cashew allergies can be more severe than peanut allergies in children.[111] However, moderate consumption of cashew

nuts during pregnancy is likely safe. Cashew for medicinal purposes is not recommended because of insufficient available evidence.

Castor (*Ricinus* spp.)
Castor oil is used historically to induce labor in full-term pregnant women. Traditionally, oral castor oil is not recommended earlier in pregnancy because of the risk of premature labor and miscarriage.[19,112] Castor oil should be avoided in lactating women because of insufficient safety data.

Cat's Claw (*Uncaria* spp.)
Historically, cat's claw was used as a contraceptive and as an abortifacient. Although the data are insufficient, its use should be avoided in women who are pregnant or attempting to conceive.

Catnip (*Nepeta cataria*)
Insufficient available evidence.

Catuaba (*Erythroxylum catuaba*)
Insufficient available evidence.

Cedar (*Cedrus* spp.)
Insufficient available evidence.

Cedar Leaf (*Thuja occidentalis*)
Cedar leaf (also known as eastern arborvitae or northern whitecedar) is unrelated to cedars of the genus *Cedrus*. Because of possible abortifacient effects,[19,113] cedar leaf oil should be avoided orally during pregnancy. Oral and topical use is not recommended during lactation because of potential toxic adverse effects.[114]

Celery (*Apium graveolens*)
Celery is likely safe when consumed by pregnant women as part of the diet in reasonable quantities. However, a maternal cohort study correlated high celery intake during pregnancy with increased incidence of food allergies in children.[57]

Chamomile (*Matricaria recutita*, syn. *Matricaria suaveolens*, *Matricaria chamomilla*, *Anthemis nobilis*, *Chamaemelum nobile*, *Chamomilla chamomilla*, *Chamomilla recutita*)
There is currently a lack of formal studies on the effects of chamomile on pregnant women. However, because of its theoretical properties as a uterine stimulant, abortifacient, and menstrual-flow stimulant (emmenagogue), most experts agree that excessive ingestion of chamomile should be avoided during pregnancy. Roman chamomile has a Class 2b safety rating from the American Herbal Products Association, advising against its use during pregnancy because of potential abortifacient effects when taken at high doses.

Chamomile is generally not recommended during lactation because of the lack of safety data. Based on secondary sources, chamomile may cause changes in lactation, particularly in nutritional quality and flavor.

A life-threatening anaphylactic reaction was reported in a woman given a glycerol and Kamillosan (a combination of chamomile, corn oil, lanolin, beeswax, yellow soft paraffin, and emulsifying wax) enema during labor, resulting in the infant also becoming asphyxiated.[115]

Chaparral (*Larrea tridentata*, *Larrea divaricata*)
Chaparral and its constituent nordihydroguaiaretic acid (NDGA) are potentially toxic or fatal and are not recommended for general use. Anecdotally, chaparral has induced uterine contractions in animals. NDGA was shown to inhibit prolactin effects on RNA, lipid, and casein biosynthesis in cultured mouse mammary gland explants.[116] The clinical significance of this finding is unclear.

Chasteberry (*Vitex agnus-castus*)
Some clinicians have used chasteberry in progesterone-deficient women during their first trimester to prevent miscarriage,[117] but it is not known if chasteberry is safe or effective for this indication. According to a systematic review by researchers in the Motherisk Program at the Hospital for Sick Children in Toronto, there is unclear evidence (based on theory, expert opinion, and in vitro studies) that chasteberry may have estrogenic and progesteronic effects, uterine-stimulant activity, or emmenagogic activity. Its effects on miscarriage and lactation are also unclear.[118]

The use of chasteberry during lactation is controversial. Chasteberry competitively binds to dopamine receptors and has been shown to affect prolactin secretion,[119,120] possibly resulting in decreased breast milk production. However, based on its traditional use as a galactagogue, some clinicians actually use low doses to stimulate milk production, with some reported benefits.[121] A study involving 20 healthy men noted increased prolactin levels in those receiving low doses of chasteberry (120 mg/day), but a decrease of prolactin secretion was reported with higher doses (480 mg/day).[122]

Cherry (*Prunus avium*, *Prunus cerasus*, and various *Prunus* spp.)
Insufficient available evidence.

Chia (*Salvia hispanica*)
Insufficient available evidence.

Chickweed (*Stellaria* spp.)
Insufficient available evidence.

Chicory (*Cichorium intybus*)
When used orally during pregnancy, chicory has been suggested to induce menstruation or miscarriage.[48] There is insufficient available evidence regarding chicory use during lactation.

Chinese Angelica
See Dong Quai (*Angelica sinensis*).

Chirata (*Swertia chirayita*)
Insufficient available evidence.

Chocolate (*Theobroma cacao*)
Moderate maternal intake of chocolate has not adversely affected the fetus.[123-127] In breastfeeding women who consume moderate amounts of chocolate, the amount of theobromine passed to the infant is likely insignificant.[23] Excessive chocolate consumption (>16 oz daily) is not recommended during lactation because it has been suggested to cause irritability and increased bowel activity in the nursing infant.[18] Chocolate contains 2 to 35 mg of caffeine per serving.[123,128] Pregnant women should not consume more than 200 mg daily of caffeine (see Caffeine).

Chrysanthemum (*Chrysanthemum* spp.)
There is insufficient information regarding the safety of chrysanthemum during pregnancy or lactation. Pyrethrins found in the seed

casings of *Chrysanthemum cinerariifolium* and *C. coccineum* are used as insecticides and insect repellents and may have adverse effects, such as neurotoxicity and allergic reactions, if ingested.[129,130]

Cinchona (*Cinchona officinalis*)
Oral cinchona is not recommended during pregnancy because of safety concerns such as labor induction.[19] Use of cinchona during lactation should be avoided because of insufficient safety information.

Cleavers (*Galium odoratum*)
Insufficient available evidence.

Clove (*Syzygium aromaticum*, syn. *Eugenia aromaticum*)
There is insufficient evidence regarding the safety of clove use during pregnancy or lactation. In mice, clove essential oil supplementation appeared to have a negative impact on embryonic development.[131]

Club Moss (*Lycopodium clavatum*)
Insufficient available evidence.

Cnidium (*Cnidium monnieri*)
Insufficient available evidence.

Coca (*Erythroxylum coca, Erythroxylum novogranatense*)
Coca contains cocaine and is contraindicated during pregnancy and lactation because of known adverse effects.[18] Use of coca may increase risk of miscarriage and preterm labor.

Coccinia indica (*Coccinia grandis*)
Insufficient available evidence.

Coconut (*Cocos nucifera*)
Evidence suggests that coconut oil is safe during pregnancy and lactation when used in reasonable dietary quantities.[108] There is insufficient evidence regarding the safety of supplemental doses during pregnancy or lactation.

Codonopsis (*Codonopsis pilosula*)
There is insufficient information regarding the safety of codonopsis during pregnancy or lactation. Because codonopsis has demonstrated antifertility activity in rats,[132] it should be avoided in women attempting to conceive.

Coffee (*Coffea* spp.)
Most of the risks associated with coffee are attributed to its caffeine content (see Caffeine). Coffee contains about 100 to 200 mg of caffeine per 8 oz.[123,128]

Coleus (*Coleus forskohlii*)
There is insufficient information regarding the safety of coleus during pregnancy or lactation.

In animals, treatment with 880 mg/kg/day of the extract of the related *Coleus barbatus* before embryo implantation caused delayed fetal development and had an antiimplantation effect.[133]

Coltsfoot (*Tussilago farfara*)
Insufficient available evidence.

Comfrey (*Symphytum* spp.)
Comfrey should be avoided during pregnancy and lactation because it contains pyrrolizidine alkaloids; maternal consumption of these constituents has been implicated in vascular occlusive disease and neonatal death.[134] Toxins from comfrey can be found in the milk from grazing animals that have consumed comfrey.[135] Thus, it is likely that comfrey toxins would also be excreted in human milk. Comfrey is also potentially hepatotoxic.[136-143]

Condurango (*Marsdenia cundurango*)
Insufficient available evidence.

Copaiba Balsam (*Copaifera* spp.)
Insufficient available evidence.

Cordyceps (*Cordyceps sinensis*)
Cordyceps may be unsafe in pregnant women because it may affect steroid hormone levels, based on laboratory and human data.[144-146] An in vitro study showed that cordyceps increases 17β-estradiol production in a dose- and time-dependent manner.[145] The influence of 17β-estradiol directly influences the quality of maturing oocytes and thus potentially the outcome of assisted-reproduction treatment. There is insufficient information regarding the safety of cordyceps during lactation.

Coriolus Mushroom (*Coriolus versicolor*)
Insufficient available evidence.

Corn Poppy (*Papaver rhoeas*)
Insufficient available evidence.

Corn Silk (*Zea mays*)
Oral corn silk should be avoided in excessive quantities during pregnancy because it has been shown to stimulate uterine contractions in animals.[147] There is insufficient information regarding the safety of corn silk during lactation.

Cornflower (*Centaurea cyanus*)
Insufficient available evidence.

Corydalis (*Corydalis* spp.)
Because it may induce uterine contractions,[19,148] oral corydalis may be unsafe during pregnancy. It should also be avoided during lactation because of insufficient available evidence.

Couch Grass (*Agropyron repens, Elymus repens*)
Insufficient available evidence.

Cow Parsnip (*Heracleum maximum*)
Insufficient available evidence.

Cowhage (*Mucuna pruriens*)
There is insufficient information regarding the safety of cowhage during pregnancy or lactation. However, cowhage has been suggested to inhibit prolactin secretion in men with hyperprolactinaemia;[149,150] thus it may also affect prolactin secretion in lactating women.

Cowslip (*Primula veris*)
Insufficient available evidence.

Cramp Bark *(Viburnum opulus)*
Insufficient available evidence.

Cranberry *(Vaccinium macrocarpon)*
Cranberry or cranberry juice is likely to be safe when consumed in reasonable dietary quantities. According to a systematic review by researchers in the Motherisk Program at the Hospital for Sick Children in Toronto, cranberry may pose little risk when used during pregnancy or lactation.[151] Pharmacologists from the same group ranked a number of herbs according to the FDA guidelines and placed cranberry in Pregnancy Category A.[152]

Cranesbill *(Geranium spp.)*
Insufficient available evidence.

Cypress *(Cupressus sempervirens)*
Insufficient available evidence.

Daisy *(Bellis perennis)*
Daisy should be avoided during pregnancy and lactation because of the possibility of growth retardation in the fetus and infant. A homeopathic preparation containing *Bellis perennis* and arnica was tested clinically for its effects on postpartum bleeding; however, its effects were uncertain.[153]

Damiana *(Turnera diffusa)*
Traditionally, damiana has been used as an abortifacient and is contraindicated during pregnancy.[2,3] There is insufficient information regarding the safety of damiana during lactation.

Dandelion *(Taraxacum officinale)*
Dandelion has traditionally been used safely as a food; however, there is insufficient information regarding the safety of dandelion in supplemental doses during pregnancy or lactation. Many dandelion tinctures contain high levels of alcohol and thus should be avoided during pregnancy (see Alcohol).

Danshen *(Salvia miltiorrhiza)*
Danshen should be avoided during pregnancy, particularly in the third trimester, because it may increase the risk of bleeding. In theory, the blood-thinning properties of danshen may increase the risk of miscarriage or bleeding; effects on the fetus or nursing infants are not known.[2,3]

Date Palm *(Phoenix dactylifera)*
Insufficient available evidence.

Desert Parsley *(Lomatium dissectum)*
Insufficient available evidence.

Devil's Claw *(Harpagophytum procumbens)*
There is insufficient information regarding the safety of devil's claw during pregnancy or lactation. Devil's claw has exhibited oxytocin-like effects ex vivo,[154] and use in pregnancy is generally not recommended.

Devil's Club *(Oplopanax horridus)*
There is insufficient information regarding the safety of devil's club during pregnancy or lactation. Devil's club has been reported anecdotally to expel afterbirth and to start postpartum menstrual flow.[2,3]

Dogwood *(Cornus spp.)*
There is insufficient information regarding the safety of dogwood during pregnancy or lactation. In a case report, a woman with premature ovarian failure and secondary amenorrhea used a traditional Chinese combination herbal remedy containing dogwood to enhance fertility; she conceived after 1 month of use.[155] However, the effects of dogwood are difficult to discern from this report.

Dong Quai *(Angelica sinensis)*
Dong quai may be unsafe during pregnancy because of possible hormonal and anticoagulant/antiplatelet properties. Animal research has noted conflicting effects on the uterus, with reports of both stimulation and relaxation. There is a published report of miscarriage in a woman taking dong quai, although it is not clear that dong quai was the cause.[156] Dong quai is traditionally viewed as increasing the risk of abortion. There is insufficient evidence regarding the safety of dong quai during breastfeeding.

Drosera *(Drosera intermedia, Drosera anglica)*
Insufficient available evidence.

Eastern Hemlock *(Tsuga canadensis)*
Insufficient available evidence.

Echinacea *(Echinacea spp.)*
In preliminary studies, oral echinacea has not appeared to pose a teratogenic risk. Results of a controlled, prospective study of 206 pregnant women suggested no effect on the incidence of birth defects, gestational age, maternal weight gain, birth weight, pregnancy outcome, or fetal distress from echinacea use.[157,158] In this study, pregnant women used different formulations; 58% used capsule/tablet (250-1000 mg/day) and 38% used tinctures (5-30 drops/day) that varied in alcoholic content from 25% to 45%. Duration of use was typically continuous for 5 to 7 days. The statistical power of this study was limited, however, leaving the possibility of undetected adverse gestational effects.

The German Commission E considers oral *Echinacea* in recommended doses safe for use in pregnancy and lactation. However, some experts do not recommended parenteral administration during pregnancy. Tinctures may be inadvisable because of 15% to 90% alcohol content (see Alcohol), although the absolute quantity of alcohol ingested from tinctures at recommended doses is likely to be relatively small. Nonetheless, according to a systematic review by researchers in the Motherisk Program at the Hospital for Sick Children in Toronto, there is sufficient evidence to suggest the safety and low teratogenic potential of echinacea use during pregnancy, even during the first trimester.[159] Pharmacologists from the same group ranked a number of herbs according to the FDA guidelines and placed echinacea in Pregnancy Category A.[152] However, safety information for lactation is insufficient.

Elder *(Sambucus nigra)*
Elder may be unsafe during pregnancy and lactation because of a possible risk of toxicity; however, safety evidence is currently lacking. One study reports gastrointestinal discomfort in pregnant women taking elderberry.[84]

Elecampane *(Inula helenium)*
Insufficient available evidence.

English Ivy (Hedera helix)
Insufficient available evidence.

English Walnut (Juglans regia)
English walnut is likely safe during pregnancy and lactation when the fruit, leaf, or hull is consumed appropriately in food amounts.[108] However, there is insufficient evidence regarding the safety of supplemental doses.

Ephedra (Ephedra sinica)
Ephedra is generally considered unsafe during pregnancy. Ephedrine, a metabolite of ephedra, crosses the placenta and has been found to increase fetal heart rate.[160,161] Ephedra may induce uterine contractions. Ephedra is unsafe during breastfeeding. Ephedrine crosses into breast milk and has been associated with irritability, crying, and insomnia in infants.[162]

Essiac Herbal Combination Tea
In general, there is a lack of safety and efficacy data for Essiac herbal combination tea. However, Essiac may be unsafe during pregnancy or lactation because of toxicities of various components. Oxalic acid, which may be found in components of Essiac, is considered unsafe in pregnancy and lactation because it may potetially induce uterine contractions.[20,163,164] Traditionally, burdock found in Essiac has been avoided during pregnancy and lactation, especially during the first trimester, because of the anthraquinone glycosides in burdock root and the oxytocic and uterine-stimulant activities.[20] The inner bark of slippery elm, another ingredient in Essiac, has historically been used for abortions, although well-documented reports are lacking. Rhubarb, found in Essiac, also contains anthraquinones, which are potentially mutagenic and genotoxic,[165] although there is a lack of evidence in this area.

Although studies exploring excretion of rhubarb's active principle in breast milk are lacking, small amounts of active metabolites from other anthroids are excreted in the milk.[166]

Eucalyptus (Eucalyptus spp.)
All forms of eucalyptus oil are considered unsafe during pregnancy or lactation because of its known toxicity, which may lead to CNS depression, coma, seizure, aspiration of stomach contents, and death.[167] It is not clear if eucalyptus oil is passed to babies through breast milk, but there have been cases of infant deaths from taking eucalyptus oil by mouth.

Euphorbia (Euphorbia spp.)
Insufficient available evidence.

European Buckthorn (Rhamnus cathartica)
Insufficient available evidence.

European Pennyroyal (Mentha pulegium)
See False Pennyroyal (Hedeoma spp.).

Evening Primrose (Oenothera biennis)
Evening primrose oil is used traditionally to stimulate labor;[69] however, clinical evidence suggests that it is ineffective for this purpose.[168] It is unclear whether evening primrose oil is safe to use during pregnancy or lactation.

Eyebright (Euphrasia officinalis)
Insufficient available evidence.

False Hellebore (Veratrum spp.)
Known for its potent toxic and teratogenic effects,[169] false hellebore (also known as skunk cabbage or cornlily) should not be used during pregnancy and lactation. In a clinical study involving pregnant women, bradycardia, nausea, and vomiting were all encountered regularly after administration of Veratrone, a pharmaceutical product containing jervine alkaloids found in false hellebore.[170] The common species Veratrum californicum contains teratogenic alkaloids that inhibit important developmental pathways[171] and have been associated with multiple severe birth defects when ingested by pregnant animals.[172-176] False hellebore is not related to another species also commonly known as skunk cabbage (Symplocarpus foetidus).

False Pennyroyal (Hedeoma spp.)
The volatile oil of pennyroyal is traditionally considered to be an abortifacient;[20] based on several case reports, it may increase the risk of uterine contractions and stimulate menstruation.[177-180] Therefore, pennyroyal is not recommended in pregnant women. There is a case report of pennyroyal oil association with an aborted fetus 4 days after ingestion,[180] although pennyroyal leaf combined with other herbs in a tea had no effect on pregnancy outcome in a different case report.[181] Pennyroyal is not recommended for nursing women because its harmful constituents (pulegones) may be transferred through breast milk.

Fennel (Foeniculum vulgare)
Fennel is likely unsafe when used orally by pregnant women.[19] Based on secondary sources, fennel preparations (other than fennel seed infusions and fennel honey) are contraindicated during pregnancy because of possible uterine-stimulating effects; however, there are no known restrictions for fennel during lactation.[50] Fennel has been traditionally used to stimulate milk production; however, the safety and efficacy of this use is unclear.

Fenugreek (Trigonella foenum-graecum)
Both water and alcoholic extracts of fenugreek have been shown to exert a stimulating effect on the isolated guinea pig uterus, especially during late pregnancy.[182] Fenugreek may possess abortifacient effects and is usually not recommended for use in doses higher than found in foods (when used as a spice) during pregnancy.[20] Traditionally, fenugreek has been used as a galactogogue to stimulate milk production. Fenugreek may lower blood glucose levels[183] and should thus be used with caution in women with diabetes (including gestational diabetes). Because of the coumarin content,[183] fenugreek may increase the risk of bleeding and should be used only with extreme caution around the time of childbirth.

Feverfew (Tanacetum parthenium)
There is insufficient information regarding the safety of feverfew during pregnancy or lactation. Historical use suggests possible emmenagogic and abortifacient effects; however, scientific evidence is lacking.

Fig (Ficus carica)
Fresh or dried fruit is likely safe during pregnancy and lactation when used as part of the diet in reasonable quantities. There is insufficient evidence about the safety of fig leaf or fruit used in medicinal amounts during pregnancy and lactation.

Fireweed (Epilobium angustifolium)
Insufficient available evidence.

Flax (Linum usitatissimum)
The use of flaxseed or flaxseed oil during pregnancy and lactation may be unsafe. Animal studies show possible harmful effects, and human data are insufficient. Flaxseed may stimulate menstruation or exert other hormonal effects and could be detrimental in pregnancy. Male offspring of female rats fed 20% to 40% flaxseed or 13% to 26% flaxmeal during pregnancy and lactation had increased levels of luteinizing hormone and testosterone, increased cauda epididymal weight and sperm number, and decreased prostatic weight.[184] However, they experienced no effects on testis structure or spermatogenesis.[185] Female rats exposed to 5% flaxseed during gestation and lactation had altered mammary gland development, delayed onset of puberty, and reduced number of estrous cycles, whereas female rats exposed to 10% flaxseed experienced earlier puberty onset and lengthened estrous cycles.[186]

Fo-Ti (Polygonum multiflorum)
There is insufficient information regarding the safety of fo-ti during pregnancy. It is known to enter the breast milk and may be unsafe during breastfeeding because it may cause diarrhea in breastfed infants.[112]

Foxglove (Digitalis purpurea, Digitalis lanata)
Data are lacking to associate foxglove or the various digitalis glycosides with congenital defects. Animal studies have failed to show teratogenic effects. Digoxin has been used for both maternal and fetal indications (e.g., supraventricular tachycardia) during all stages of gestation without reports of fetal harm. Digoxin is excreted into breast milk, although reports of adverse effects in nursing infants are lacking. The AAP considers digoxin to be compatible with breastfeeding.[18]

Fuzheng Jiedu Tang
Insufficient available evidence.

Galium (Galium aparine)
Insufficient available evidence.

Garcinia (Garcinia cambogia)
Insufficient available evidence.

Garlic (Allium sativum)
Garlic is likely safe during pregnancy in amounts usually ingested in food, based on historical use. Pharmacologists at the Hospital for Sick Children in Toronto, Canada ranked a number of herbs according to the FDA guidelines and placed garlic in Pregnancy Category A.[158] Garlic supplementation should be avoided around the time of labor because of a theoretical increased risk of bleeding. In addition, uterine-stimulant activity was reported in early animal research.[187] In a controlled study of 10 pregnant women, the odor of amniotic fluid samples was reported to smell more like garlic in women who had ingested capsules containing the essential oil of garlic 45 minutes before amniocentesis than in women who had not ingested garlic.[188]

Garlic is also likely to be safe during lactation in amounts usually ingested in food, based on historical use. Maternal consumption of garlic supplements has been associated with increases in nursing time, milk odor,[189] and infant milk consumption.[190]

Gentian (Gentiana lutea; Gentiana acaulis)
Insufficient available evidence.

Germander (Teucrium chamaedrys)
Germander is hepatotoxic[191-194] and may be unsafe during pregnancy and lactation.

Giant Knotweed (Polygonum cuspidatum)
Insufficient available evidence.

Ginger (Zingiber officinale)
Consumption of ginger in amounts greater than those typically found in food (<1 g dry weight/day) is not advised by some authors during pregnancy because of purported emmenagogic effects, as well as abortifacient, mutagenic, or antiplatelet effects.[19] However, others report a lack of scientific or medical evidence for a pregnancy contraindication.[19,195] This matter is further confused because traditional Chinese medicine (TCM) cautions against ginger use in pregnancy, although much higher doses are generally used in TCM. Ginger may effectively treat nausea and vomiting during pregnancy[196] and is widely believed to be safe to use during pregnancy. Pharmacologists at the Hospital for Sick Children in Toronto, Canada ranked a number of herbs according to the FDA guidelines and placed ginger in Pregnancy Category A.[158]

Ginkgo (Ginkgo biloba)
According to a systematic review by researchers in the Motherisk Program at the Hospital for Sick Children in Toronto, ginkgo should be used cautiously during pregnancy, especially around the time of labor when its antiplatelet activity may increase the risk of bleeding.[197] Furthermore, gingko preparations have been contaminated with colchicine, a known teratogen associated with numerous birth defects. In one study, increased levels of colchicine in placental blood (49-763 mcg/L) was found in patients taking *Ginkgo biloba* herbal pregnancy supplements.[198] However, experts argue that many pregnant women have used ginkgo without experiencing harmful effects. Nonetheless, the safety of ginkgo use during pregnancy remains inconclusive. Colchicine has been identified by the AAP as "usually compatible with breastfeeding."[18]

Ginseng (Panax spp.)
According to WHO, ginseng is not teratogenic in vivo and has been used traditionally in pregnant and lactating women. However, the safety of ginseng in women during pregnancy and lactation has not been systematically evaluated. In cultured rat embryos, ginsenoside Rb1 induced teratogenicity.[199] TCM suggests that *Panax ginseng* should not be used by pregnant or nursing mothers. Safety in young children or people with severe liver or kidney disease has not been established. An intoxication-like syndrome has been reported in a few newborns given *P. ginseng* or whose mothers took it while pregnant or breastfeeding. One documented case of an infant death has been attributed to *P. ginseng* intoxication.[200] According to a systematic review by researchers in the Motherisk Program at the Hospital for Sick Children in Toronto, ginseng should be used cautiously during pregnancy (particularly during the first trimester) and lactation.[101]

Globe Artichoke (Cynara scolymus)
Insufficient available evidence.

Goji (Lycium spp.)
There is insufficient information regarding the safety of goji during pregnancy or lactation. According to anecdotal reports, *Lycium* may have uterine-stimulant properties. Chinese physicians have traditionally used goji berries to treat infertility.[202]

Goldenrod (Solidago virgaurea)
There is insufficient information regarding the safety of Phytodolor (which contains goldenrod plus aspen and ash) during pregnancy.[203] A species from the same family as goldenrod (Haplopappus heterophyllus) called rayless goldenrod may contain the toxic substance tremetol or tremetone and has been responsible for intoxication of cows and their calves, as well as for human poisonings after consumption of milk from intoxicated cows.[140,204] The toxin is excreted in the milk of lactating animals; thus goldenrod may be best avoided during lactation.

Goldenseal (Hydrastis canadensis)
Berberine-containing herbs, such as goldenseal, have been suggested historically as abortifacients and uterine stimulants; however, scientific evidence is lacking (see Berberine). Hydrastine, a different active constituent of goldenseal, may induce labor and should not be used by pregnant women.[205] There is insufficient information regarding the safety of berberine or hydrastine during lactation.

Goose Grass (Galium aparine)
Insufficient available evidence.

Gotu Kola (Centella asiatica)
Insufficient available evidence.

Grape (Vitis vinifera)
Modest consumption of grapes as part of a healthy diet is likely safe during pregnancy and lactation. There is insufficient available evidence regarding the medicinal use of grapes or their constituents.

Grape Seed (Vitis spp.)
Insufficient available evidence.

Grapefruit (Citrus x paradisi)
A maternal cohort study correlated high citrus intake during pregnancy with increased incidence of food allergies in children.[62]

Grass Pea (Lathyrus savitus)
Insufficient available evidence.

Graviola (Annona muricata)
Graviola has been associated with parkinsonism and myeloneuropathies,[206,207] and it thus may be unsafe to use during pregnancy or lactation.

Greater Celandine (Chelidonium majus)
There is insufficient information regarding the safety of greater celandine during pregnancy or lactation. In rat reproduction studies the product Ukrain (containing thiophosphoric acid alkaloid derivatives from the plant Chelidonium majus) did not induce signs of toxicity or teratogenic effects.[208] However, slight embryotoxic effects (increased postimplantation losses) and small litter sizes were noted in hamsters exposed to Ukrain at doses not embryotoxic to rats.

Ground Ivy (Glechoma hederacea)
Insufficient available evidence.

Guarana (Paullinia cupana)
Guarana is a source of caffeine, which is implicated in most adverse effects associated with guarana use (see Caffeine).

Guayule (Parthenium argentatum)
Insufficient available evidence.

Guggul (Commiphora mukul)
Insufficient available evidence.

Gumweed (Grindelia camporum)
There is insufficient information regarding the safety of gumweed during pregnancy or lactation. However, oral preparations of gumweed may contain alcohol, which is unsafe to use during pregnancy (see Alcohol).

Gymnema (Gymnema sylvestre)
Insufficient available evidence.

Haritaki (Terminalia arjuna)
Insufficient available evidence.

Hawthorn (Crataegus spp.)
Hawthorn is a component of Menoprogen, a combination herbal remedy for menopausal symptoms that displayed estrogenic effects in animals.[209] The contribution of hawthorn to the observed effects is unclear. There is insufficient information regarding the safety of hawthorn use during lactation.

Hazelnut (Corylus avellana, Corylus heterophylla)
Tree nuts are common causes of food allergies in children and may also increase the risk of asthma in children. However, moderate consumption of hazelnuts during pregnancy is likely safe. There is insufficient evidence regarding the safety of medicinal doses.[2,3]

Heartsease (Viola tricolor)
Insufficient available evidence.

Hemlock (Conium maculatum)
Hemlock is contraindicated during pregnancy and lactation. It is a poisonous herb that has been associated with congenital defects in animals.[210,211]

Hemp (Cannabis sativa)
Although hemp seed oil is composed primarily of essential fatty acids, which are beneficial during pregnancy, it also contains small amounts of cannabidiol from Cannabis plants. Cannabinols in marijuana may pass through the placenta, and maternal use may result in low birth weight and developmental problems.[212-215] Hemp seed oil also appears to be excreted in breast milk,[216-218] and thus the AAP does not recommend it during lactation.[18]

Hibiscus (Hibiscus spp.)
Hibiscus tiliaceus has been used traditionally to speed childbirth.[212] In animals, excessive doses of hibiscus for relatively long periods could have a deleterious effect on the testes of rats.[220] Hibiscus rosa-sinensis has exhibited antifertility activity, and the benzene extract of the flower petals may suppress implantation.[4] There is insufficient information regarding the safety of hibiscus during lactation.

Holy Basil (Ocimum sanctum)
Based on traditional use as a uterine stimulant, holy basil may be unsafe to use during pregnancy.[2,3]

Honeysuckle (*Lonicera* spp.)
According to the Central Drug Research Institute in Lucknow, India, in collaboration with NIH and WHO, honeysuckle displays antiimplantation effects and may hold potential as an herbal contraceptive.[4]

Hoodia (*Hoodia gordonii*)
Insufficient available evidence.

Hop (*Humulus lupulus*)
Caution is warranted during pregnancy and lactation because of possible hormonal (estrogenic) and sedative effects of hop or other ingredients found in combination products.[221-225] There is insufficient evidence regarding safety in these areas. Some hop preparations contain high levels of alcohol and should be avoided during pregnancy (see Alcohol).

Horny Goat Weed (*Epimedium grandiflorum*)
Insufficient available evidence.

Horse Chestnut (*Aesculus hippocastanum*)
There is insufficient information regarding the safety of horse chestnut or horse chestnut seed extract (HCSE) during pregnancy or lactation. In a randomized controlled trial, 52 women with pregnancy-induced venous insufficiency used Venostasin retard (240-290 mg HCSE, standardized to 50 mg escin) and showed no serious adverse effects after 2 weeks.[226]

Horseradish (*Armoracia rusticana*, syn. *Cochlearia armoracia*)
Horseradish is likely safe when consumed in moderate amounts, based on its historical use as a spice. However, based on herbal textbooks and folkloric precedent, medicinal use of horseradish has been used to induce abortion. Published reports are lacking. Glucosinolates from horseradish are considered toxins that can be excreted through breast milk and may pose a hazard.[135] Because horseradish contains mustard oil constituents, which may be toxic and irritating, it may be unsafe to use in large quantities during pregnancy or lactation.

Horsetail (*Equisetum* spp.)
There is insufficient information regarding the safety of horsetail during pregnancy or lactation. Caution should be taken during pregnancy and breastfeeding because of theoretical effects of thiamine depletion, hypokalemia, and nicotine toxicity.[2,3]

Hoxsey Formula
Insufficient available evidence.

Hydrangea (*Hydrangea arborescens*)
Insufficient available evidence.

Hyssop (*Hyssopus officinalis*)
Insufficient available evidence.

Indian Snakeroot (*Rauwolfia serpentina*)
Reserpine alkaloids found in Indian snakeroot may cross the placenta and have teratogenic effects.[43,50,102] Indian snakeroot should be avoided during lactation because reserpine alkaloids are excreted in breast milk.[102]

Indian Tobacco (*Lobelia inflata*)
Indian tobacco should be avoided during pregnancy because of evidence suggesting emetic effects.[19,147,227] There is insufficient information regarding the safety of Indian tobacco during lactation.

Isatis indigotica (*Isatis tinctoria*)
Insufficient available evidence.

Jackfruit (*Artocarpus heterophyllus*)
Insufficient available evidence.

Jasmine (*Jasminum grandiflorum*)
Insufficient available evidence.

Jequirity (*Abrus precatorius*)
Although *Abrus precatorius* seeds have been used historically to stimulate labor or abortion, oral use is not recommended because of known toxicity. Abrin, a constituent of *A. precatorius*, is toxic at 5 mg, and ingestion of one bean by a child may be fatal.[228]

Jewelweed (*Impatiens biflora*, *Impatiens pallida*)
There is insufficient information regarding the safety of jewelweed during pregnancy or lactation. Because of purportedly high mineral content, particularly calcium oxalate, which is a common constituent of kidney stones, large quantities of jewelweed should be avoided.

Jiaogulan (*Gynostemma pentaphyllum*)
Insufficient available evidence.

Jimson Weed (*Datura* spp.)
There is insufficient evidence regarding the safety of jimson weed in pregnant or lactating women. Jimson weed has been associated with poisoning, and the constituent hyoscyamine is known to be excreted into breast milk.[229] Atropine and scopolamine found in California jimson weed may decrease milk production, based on anecdotal reports. However, atropine and scopolamine have been identified by the AAP as "usually compatible with breast feeding."[18]

Jointed Flatsedge (*Cyperus articulatus*)
Insufficient available evidence.

Jojoba (*Simmondsia chinensis*)
There is insufficient information regarding the safety of jojoba during pregnancy or lactation. In broiler breeding females fed jojoba meal, the size of the eggs laid were smaller and the overall production rate lower than in birds not fed jojoba.[230] Ovary and oviduct weights were also reduced. In female rats fed defatted jojoba meal or pure simmondsin, the number of corpora lutea on gestation day 16 was reduced, thought to be caused by decreased food intake in this group.[231] Fetal and placental weights were also reduced in these groups.

Juniper (*Juniperus communis*)
Based on expert opinion, juniper may increase uterine tone and interfere with fertility or implantation; thus it may be unsafe during pregnancy because of the potential for abortions and the induction of labor contractions. Abortifacient activity of juniper has been observed in rats after oral administration of a 50% ethanolic extract at 300 mg/kg.[232] There is insufficient information regarding the safety of juniper during lactation.

Katuka (*Picrorhiza kurroa*)
Insufficient available evidence.

Kava (*Piper methysticum*)
The safety of kava has not been thoroughly studied during pregnancy or lactation; however, it is known to be hepatotoxic (see Appendix A). Use is discouraged during pregnancy because of possible decreases in uterine tone and during lactation because of possible kava pyrone transport into milk (with unknown effects).[233] There is insufficient information regarding the safety of kava during lactation.

Kelp (*Laminaria* spp.)
See Seaweed.

Khat (*Catha edulis*)
Unsubstantiated sources have reported reduced birth weight, birth defects, and lactation inhibition caused by maternal khat use. Therefore, khat should be avoided in pregnancy and lactation.[2,3]

Khella (*Ammi visnaga*)
The active constituent of khella (khellin) has uterine stimulant activity; therefore, khella is contraindicated during pregnancy.[54] There is insufficient information regarding the safety of khella during lactation.

Kiwi (*Actinidia deliciosa, Actinidia chinensis*)
Because of its historical use as a food, kiwi is likely safe to consume in reasonable quantities by nonallergic pregnant or lactating women. However, there is insufficient information regarding the safety of kiwi during pregnancy or lactation.

Kola Nut (*Cola acuminata*)
Caffeine is found in kola (cola) nut and is associated with most of the risks of kola nut use (see Caffeine).

Kudzu (*Pueraria lobata*)
Insufficient available evidence.

Labrador Tea (*Ledum groenlandicum*)
Insufficient available evidence.

Ladies Mantle (*Alchemilla vulgaris*)
Traditionally, ladies mantle has been used as a conception aid and for excessive menstruation.[2,3] However, evidence of safety during pregnancy or lactation is lacking.

Lady's Slipper (*Cypripedium acaule, Cypripedium calceolus*)
Insufficient available evidence.

Laetrile
See Bitter Almond (*Prunus amygdalus*).

Lavender (*Lavandula angustifolia*)
Because of its purported properties as an emmenagogue, excessive internal use of lavender may be unsafe during pregnancy. However, definitive evidence is lacking in this area. There is also insufficient information regarding the safety of lavender during lactation.

Ledum (*Rhododendron groenlandicum*)
Because of possible abortifacient properties,[43] ledum should be avoided during pregnancy. There is insufficient information regarding the safety of ledum during lactation.

Lemon Balm (*Melissa officinalis*)
There is insufficient information regarding the safety of lemon balm during pregnancy or breastfeeding. Anecdotally, lemon balm may elicit emmenagogic, antithyrotropic, and antigonadotropic effects.[234]

Lemongrass (*Cymbopogon* spp.)
Lemongrass infusions (or <0.5 g/kg of its terpene constituent, beta-myrcene) resulted in no significant adverse effects in the rats or their offspring when given before mating, during pregnancy, or during lactation.[235-237] However, greater than 0.5 g/kg of beta-myrcene prenatally resulted in increased resorption rate, decreased birth weight, increased perinatal mortality, delayed postnatal development, and skeletal anomalies.[236,237] Anecdotal evidence suggests avoiding lemongrass during pregnancy because of its effects on the uterus and menstruation, although primary clinical evidence is lacking. There is insufficient information regarding the safety of lemongrass during lactation.

Lesser Celandine (*Ranunculus ficaria*)
Insufficient available evidence.

Licorice (*Glycyrrhiza glabra*)
Because heavy licorice consumption (>500 mg glycyrrhizin weekly) has been associated with preterm delivery,[238] large amounts of licorice may be unsafe during pregnancy. Glycyrrhizin has been detected in human breast milk;[239] however, breastfeeding safety is unclear.

Ligustrum (*Ligustrum lucidum*)
Insufficient available evidence.

Lime (*Citrus aurantifolia*)
Insufficient available evidence. However, a maternal cohort study correlated high citrus intake during pregnancy with increased incidence of food allergies in children.[59]

Lime Flower (*Tilia europaea*)
Insufficient available evidence.

Lingonberry (*Vaccinium vitis-idaea*)
Lingonberry is likely safe to consume during pregnancy by nonallergic women in reasonable quantities. There is insufficient safety information regarding supplemental doses. *Vaccinium vitis* leaf extract has shown antigonadotropic effects in male frogs;[240] effects on female reproduction are unclear.

Liverwort (*Hepatica* spp.)
Insufficient available evidence.

Lotus (*Nelumbo nucifera*)
There is insufficient information regarding the safety of lotus during pregnancy or lactation. Limited evidence suggests that *Nelumbo nucifera* seed has antifertility activity in animals.[241]

Lousewort (*Delphinium staphisagria*)
Insufficient available evidence.

Lovage (Levisticum officinale)
There is insufficient information regarding the safety of lovage during pregnancy or lactation. Spanish New Mexicans have reportedly used lovage as an abortifacient.[242]

Ma Huang
See Ephedra (Ephedra sinica).

Maca (Lepidium meyenii)
Insufficient available evidence.

Magnolia (Magnolia spp.)
Magnolia flower bud may be unsafe during pregnancy because of possible uterine-stimulant effects.[243] It is unclear if magnolia bark is safe during pregnancy or lactation.

Maitake Mushroom (Grifola frondosa)
Insufficient available evidence.

Mangosteen (Garcinia mangostana)
Insufficient available evidence.

Marijuana (Cannabis sativa)
See Hemp (Cannabis sativa).

Marshmallow (Althaea officinalis)
Insufficient available evidence.

Mastic (Pistacia lentiscus)
In animals, mastic has demonstrated angiotensin-converting enzyme (ACE) inhibition activity.[244] Because pharmacological ACE inhibitors have known adverse effects in fetuses,[245] mastic may be unsafe to use during pregnancy. However, safety information in pregnancy or lactation is lacking.

Meadowsweet (Filipendula ulmaria)
Meadowsweet may be unsafe during pregnancy because it may increase uterine tone and stimulate uterine activity.[2,3] Meadowsweet contains salicylates, which are associated with fetal abnormalities.[246] Drugs in this class are listed by the FDA in Pregnancy Category D (positive evidence of human fetal risk). There is insufficient information regarding the safety of meadowsweet during lactation. Salicylate should be given to nursing mothers with caution because it has been associated with metabolic acidosis in infants.[18]

Mexican Scammony Root (Ipomoea orizabensis)
Insufficient available evidence.

Mezereon (Daphne mezereum)
Insufficient available evidence.

Milk Thistle (Silybum marianum)
There is some evidence to support the safety of milk thistle during pregnancy or lactation. The constituent silymarin has been used safely to treat mothers with intrahepatic cholestasis[247] and minor liver disorders.[248] There has been historical use of milk thistle during lactation, and herbalists recommend it to improve lactation in nursing mothers. This traditional use may be a result of the white veins on the plant's spiked green leaves, which are fabled to carry the milk of the Virgin Mary. However, systematic safety data are lacking.

Mistletoe (Viscum album)
Mistletoe has been shown to have uterine-stimulant activities in animals[20] and therefore should be avoided in pregnancy. There is insufficient information regarding the safety of mistletoe during lactation.

Momordica grosvenori (Momordica charantia)
Momordica grosvenori may be unsafe during pregnancy because of evidence that suggests that it may stimulate menstruation and has caused abortion in animals.[48,249,250] There is insufficient information regarding the safety of Momordica grosvenori during lactation.

Morinda (Morinda citrifolia)
Morinda should be avoided during pregnancy because evidence suggests that it has abortifacient effects.[251] There is insufficient information regarding the safety of morinda during lactation.

Motherwort (Leonurus artemisia, Leonurus cardiaca)
Motherwort should be avoided during pregnancy because evidence suggests it may have uterine-stimulating effects.[19,48,152] There is insufficient information regarding the safety of motherwort during lactation.

Moutan (Paeonia lactiflora)
Moutan should be avoided during pregnancy because evidence suggests it may cause uterine contractions.[252] There is insufficient information regarding the safety of moutan during lactation.

Mugwort (Artemisia vulgaris)
There is insufficient information regarding the safety of mugwort during pregnancy or lactation. Traditionally, mugwort has been used as an abortifacient. The German Commission E lists mugwort as an unapproved herb with insufficient evidence of safety or effectiveness.

Muira Puama (Ptychopetalum olacoides)
Muira puama may be unsafe during pregnancy because of reported idiosyncratic motor/sacral stimulant properties. There is insufficient information regarding the safety of muira puama during lactation.[50]

Mulberry (Morus nigra)
Insufficient available evidence.

Mullein (Verbascum thapsus)
Insufficient available evidence.

Myrcia (Myrcia spp.)
There is insufficient information regarding the safety of myrcia during pregnancy or lactation. Also, uncontrolled diabetes or thyroid dysfunction during pregnancy can lead to abnormal fetal development.[2,3] Because of the theoretical potential to affect blood glucose and thyroid function, myrcia should not be used during pregnancy or lactation.

Myrrh (Commiphora myrrha)
The oral use of myrrh may be unsafe during pregnancy because it may stimulate uterine tone and blood flow and may have abortifacient effects.[19,50,152] It is unclear if topical use of myrrh is safe during pregnancy because of lack of sufficient evidence. There is insufficient information regarding the safety of myrrh during lactation.

Neem (Azadirachta indica)
Neem is not considered to be safe for use during pregnancy because of abortifacient and antiimplantation effects noted in animal

studies.253-258 Teratogenic effects have not been reported in the subsequent offspring of animals treated with neem.253,255,256,259-261 safety during lactation has not been established.

Noni (Morinda citrifolia)
Insufficient available evidence.

Nopal (Opuntia spp.)
Insufficient available evidence.

Northern Prickly Ash (Zanthoxylum americanum)
Northern prickly ash is not recommended during pregnancy or lactation because of a lack of sufficient evidence.

Nutmeg (Myristica fragrans)
Because nutmeg may have abortifacient effects,19,262 it may be unsafe during pregnancy when taken for medicinal purposes. Ingestion of 1 tablespoon of nutmeg at 30 weeks' gestation resulted in signs of anticholinergic intoxication; fetal heartbeat increased for 12 hours, but mother and fetus completely recovered within 24 hours.263 There is insufficient information regarding the safety of nutmeg during lactation.

Nux Vomica (Strychnos nux-vomica)
Nux vomica should not be taken during pregnancy or lactation because of the risk of ingesting toxic levels of strychnine, which can cause muscular convulsions and death. The safety of homeopathic nux vomica during pregnancy or lactation has not been clinically established.

Oak Moss (Evernia prunastri)
Oak moss should be avoided during pregnancy because of possible uterine-stimulating effects.48 There is insufficient information regarding the safety of oak moss during lactation.

Oats (Avena sativa)
Oats are generally considered safe when consumed in reasonable dietary quantities during pregnancy and lactation.19,264,265

Oleander (Nerium oleander, Thevetia peruviana)
Oleander is toxic and should be avoided during pregnancy and lactation. Human use of oleander in its unprocessed or medicinal forms is not recommended because of known toxicity. Folkloric use of oleander as an abortifacient is not supported by scientific research. There is a case report of a mother who consumed two yellow oleander seed kernels 12 hours before giving birth.266 The intention of this ingestion is unclear. The fetus, while still in utero, developed evidence of cardiac glycoside toxicity, with a moderate decrease in fetal heart rate immediately prepartum and postpartum. At 40 hours postpartum the baby suffered left-sided seizures, followed by generalized seizures at 70 hours. Laboratory studies were normal, and the child eventually recovered uneventfully and was doing well 3 years later. It was hypothesized that maternal-fetal transmission of lipid-soluble thevetin, the chief cardiac glycoside in yellow oleander, may have occurred.

Olive (Olea europaea)
Olive oil is likely safe to consume in reasonable quantities during pregnancy and lactation, because of its historical use in foods. There is insufficient safety information regarding other parts of the olive plant (such as the leaf) or supplemental doses of olive products.

Omega-3 Fatty Acids, Alpha-Linolenic Acid
It is not known conclusively whether omega-3 fatty acid supplementation in women during pregnancy or breastfeeding is beneficial to infants. It has been suggested that high intake of omega-3 fatty acids during pregnancy, particularly docosahexaenoic acid (DHA) found in fish, may increase birth weight and gestational length.267 However, higher doses may not be advisable because of the potential risk of bleeding.

Reported as integral in the growth and functional development of the brain in infants, DHA appears to be taken up by the brain in preference to other fatty acids.268-270 DHA and arachidonic acid are often included in infant formulas. DHA in the diet has also been associated with visual (retinal) development in infants271-274 and with retinal pathology during aging.275 In a case of severe deficiency, supplementation was reported to alleviate severe growth retardation.276 In contrast, it has been reported that high doses of eicosapentaenoic acid (EPA, found naturally in algae and fish that consume algae) in addition to DHA may be harmful in preterm infants,277 who frequently appear to be DHA deficient.272 The consequences of deficiency in alpha-linolenic acid (ALA, a precursor of DHA derived from plant sources) include anomalies in the composition of nervous membranes, perturbation of electrophysiological parameters, and greater sensitivity to neurotoxins.278

Onion (Allium cepa)
Insufficient available evidence.

Oregano (Origanum vulgare)
There is insufficient evidence regarding the safety of supplemental sage use during pregnancy or lactation. In mice, oregano essential oil supplementation appeared to have a negative impact on embryonic development.131 An over-the-counter product (Carachipita) containing oregano, in addition to pennyroyal (Mentha pulegium), yerba de la perdiz (Magiricarpus pinnaus), and guaycuru (Statice brasiliensis), has been linked with case reports of induced abortion.279

Pagoda Tree (Styphnolobium japonicum)
Insufficient available evidence.

Palm (Elaeis guineensis)
Palm oil may be used during pregnancy and lactation when used appropriately and in moderation by healthy individuals. It is likely safe when used during pregnancy for up to 6 months.280-282

Parsley (Petroselinum crispum)
Parsley is likely safe when consumed by nonallergic women in amounts generally found in foods. However, supplemental doses of parsley may not be safe during pregnancy when taken for medicinal purposes because of evidence that it may have abortifacient effects and stimulate menstrual flow.19,147,283 There is insufficient information regarding the safety of parsley supplementation during lactation.

Parsnip (Pastinaca sativa)
Insufficient available evidence.

Passion Flower (Passiflora incarnata)
Constituents found in some species of Passiflora, such as harman and harmaline, were reported to stimulate the uterus in several animal studies during the early 1930s.20 These effects have not been investigated in recent available studies. Whether passion flower contains the cyanogenic glycoside gynocardin remains controversial.284

Passion flower should thus be avoided in pregnancy until additional data are available. Many tinctures contain high levels of alcohol and should be avoided during pregnancy (see Alcohol). There is insufficient information regarding the safety of passion flower during lactation.

Pau d'Arco (Tabebuia impetiginosa)
Oral pau d'arco is contraindicated during pregnancy in high doses because of known toxicities (liver and kidney damage).[23,283] Topical use should be avoided during pregnancy because of insufficient available evidence. Information is also insufficient on the safety of pau d'arco during lactation.

PC-SPES
PC-SPES, a product based on a TCM formulation, contains saw palmetto (Serenoa repens), chrysanthemum (Chrysanthemum morifolium), reishi mushroom (Ganoderma lucidum), licorice (Glycyrrhiza glabra), dyer's woad (Isatis indigotica), san qi (Panax pseudoginseng), rubescens (Rabdosia rubescens), and baikal skullcap (Scutellaria baicalensis). Because of undeclared prescription drugs present in PC-SPES, it has been banned by the FDA and is not considered safe for use.

Peanut (Arachis hypogaea)
Peanut oil is likely safe when consumed as part of the diet, in reasonable quantities, by nonallergic pregnant or lactating women. There is insufficient safety information regarding supplemental doses.

Pear (Pyrus communis)
Pear is safe when consumed as part of the diet in reasonable quantities by nonallergic pregnant women. There is insufficient safety information regarding supplemental doses.[43]

Pellitory-of-the-Wall (Parietaria officinalis)
Insufficient available evidence.

Peony (Paeonia spp.)
Peony should be avoided in pregnancy because evidence suggests it may cause uterine contractions.[252] There is insufficient information regarding the safety of peony during lactation.

Peppermint (Mentha x piperita)
Peppermint oil and menthol may be unsafe in pregnancy and lactation because of insufficient information and the potential for toxicity. Excessive use is contraindicated in early pregnancy because of possible emmenagogic effects.[45]

Perilla (Perilla frutescens)
Insufficient available evidence.

Peyote (Lophophora williamsii)
The use of hallucinogens, as with peyote, is not recommended during pregnancy. Studies in mice and monkeys indicate that mescaline, a constituent of peyote, may cross the placenta[285-287] and has been linked to congenital malformations.[288,289]

Phyllanthus (Phyllanthus emblica)
Insufficient available evidence.

Pine Bark Extract (Pinus pinaster)
Insufficient available evidence.

Pleurisy (Asclepias tuberosa)
Insufficient available evidence.

Podophyllum (Podophyllum spp.)
Podophyllum may be unsafe to use during pregnancy or lactation because of teratogenic effects associated with topical use in pregnancy.[290,291]

Poison Ivy (Toxicodendron radicans)
Poison ivy may be found in topical preparations and used for disorders such as arthritis. It may also be found in homeopathic medicine. Available evidence is insufficient on the safety of oral and topical use of poison ivy during pregnancy or lactation.[23]

Pokeweed (Phytolacca americana)
Because of purported uterine-stimulant and abortifacient effects, pokeweed may be unsafe during pregnancy and lactation.[48,147]

Policosanol
There is insufficient information regarding the safety of policosanol during pregnancy or lactation. According to animal studies, policosanol does not affect the reproductive performance or fetal/neonatal development or lactation at levels of up to 500 mg/kg daily over three successive generations.[292-294]

Polygonum cuspidatum (Polygonum cuspidatum)
Insufficient available evidence.

Polypodium (Polypodium leucotomos)
Insufficient available evidence.

Pomegranate (Punica granatum)
Pomegranate is likely safe when consumed as part of the diet in reasonable quantities by nonallergic women. Pomegranate is a source of folic acid, which may be beneficial for fetal development. In animals, supplementation with pomegranate juice had neuroprotective effects in neonates.[295,296] However, according to anecdotal reports, the bark, root, and fruit rind of pomegranate may stimulate menstruation or uterine contractions.

Populus (Populus spp.)
Insufficient available evidence.

Psyllium (Plantago spp.)
Psyllium-containing laxatives appear to be safe in all three trimesters, but reproductive safety studies in humans and animals are lacking. Psyllium may lower blood sugar levels, which lead to interactions or other complications during pregnancy (especially in cases of gestational diabetes). Psyllium-containing products are considered "apparently safe" during lactation.[147]

Pulsatilla (Anemone pulsatilla)
Oral and topical use of pulsatilla is not recommended during pregnancy because of abortifacient and teratogenic effects.[45,297] There is insufficient information regarding the safety of pulsatilla during lactation.

Pumpkin (Cucurbita spp.)
Pumpkin is likely safe when consumed as part of the diet in reasonable quantities by nonallergic women. There is insufficient safety information regarding supplemental doses.

Pycnogenol (Pinus pinaster subsp. atlantica)
Insufficient available evidence.

Pygeum (Prunus africanum, syn. Pygeum africanum)
Insufficient available evidence.

Quassia (Picraena excelsa, Quassia undalata, Quassia amara)
Quassia is considered unsafe during pregnancy and lactation. Quassia may have cytotoxic and emetic properties.[43,47,114]

Quercetin
Insufficient available evidence.

Quinoa (Chenopodium quinoa)
Insufficient available evidence.

Rabdosia (Rabdosia rubescens)
Insufficient available evidence.

Raspberry (Rubus idaeus)
Raspberry is likely safe when consumed as part of the diet in reasonable quantities by nonallergic women. According to anecdotal reports, raspberry leaf may induce labor if taken in large amounts during the first or second trimester; however, a clinical trial using raspberry leaf tablets in pregnant women (32 weeks of gestation) reported no adverse effects.[298] The safety of raspberry supplementation has not been established in pregnancy or lactation.

Red Clover (Trifolium pratense)
Red clover should be avoided during pregnancy and lactation because of its estrogenic activity.[221] In rats, maternal exposure to subcutaneous genistein (an isoflavone) was shown to increase the incidence of mammary tumors in offspring, mimicking the effects of in utero estrogenic exposures.[299] Red clover has been implicated as a cause of infertility and abortion in grazing livestock.

Red Yeast Rice (Monascus purpureus)
Red yeast rice should be avoided during pregnancy and lactation. Traditional red yeast rice contains small amounts of lovastatin, an HMG-CoA reductase inhibitor, a drug listed as FDA Pregnancy Category X. This indicates demonstrated fetal abnormalities, or evidence of fetal risk based on human experience, and the risk of the drug's use in pregnant women clearly outweighs any possible benefit. Lovastatin is contraindicated in women who are pregnant or attempting to conceive.

In vitro, pigments purified from the mycelium of *Monascus purpureus* (rubropunctatin, monascorubrin, monascin, and ankaflavin) were found to be toxic toward chicken embryos.[300]

The presence of the mycotoxin *citrinin*, a secondary metabolite of *Monascus* species, in fermentation products is potentially hazardous to health.[301] High doses are teratogenic in rats and embryonically lethal in mice. There is no established tolerance limit for humans; therefore, caution should be used when consuming products containing citrinin.[302]

Rehmannia (Rehmannia glutinosa)
Insufficient available evidence.

Reishi Mushroom (Ganoderma lucidum)
Insufficient available evidence.

Resveratrol
There is insufficient available evidence regarding the use of resveratrol-containing supplements during pregnancy and lactation. Resveratrol is a natural component of red wine; the American College of Obstetricians and Gynecologists does not recommend alcohol consumption in pregnant women[303] because it can lead to serious fetal damage (see Alcohol).

Rhodiola (Rhodiola rosea)
Insufficient available evidence.

Rhubarb (Rheum spp.)
Because of its putative effect as a uterine stimulant, rhubarb root may be unsafe during pregnancy. Because of anthraquinone alkaloids, which are potentially mutagenic and genotoxic, rhubarb should not be used during lactation.[20] Although studies exploring excretion of rhubarb's active principle in breast milk are lacking, small amounts of active metabolites from other anthroids are known to be excreted in milk.[157] Rhubarb should be avoided during lactation because it contains potentially genotoxic emodin and aloe-emodin, which may have cathartic effects in infants. In case reports, rhubarb has caused neonatal jaundice.[304]

Rooibos (Aspalathus linearis)
Insufficient available evidence.

Rose Hip (Rosa spp.)
Rose hip is likely safe when consumed as part of the diet in reasonable quantities by nonallergic women. There is insufficient available evidence on supplemental doses. Based on secondary sources, some experts recommend rose hips herbal tea for nursing women because of its vitamin C content.

Rosemary (Rosmarinus officinalis)
Rosemary is likely safe when consumed in reasonable amounts (as a spice) in foods. Available evidence on medicinal doses is insufficient. Rosemary was traditionally used for abortion, and there is a risk of embryo toxicity and abnormalities caused by altered hormone levels.[305,306] There is insufficient information regarding the safety of rosemary supplementation during lactation.

Rue (Ruta graveolens)
Ruta graveolens should be avoided during pregnancy because of possible uterine-stimulant and abortifacient effects.[19,307] Deaths have been reported in women using *R. graveolens* as an abortifacient.[42] Use of *R. graveolens* during lactation should be avoided because of insufficient safety information.

Rutin ($C_{27}H_{30}O_{16}$)
Rutin supplements have been safely used during pregnancy to treat venous insufficiency,[308,309] hemorrhoids,[310] and varicose veins.[311] Administration of O-(β-hydroxyethyl)-rutoside for 8 weeks showed minimal side-effects, and healthy babies were delivered with good Apgar scores.[312] Another trial confirmed no drug-related problems in the pregnancies, delivery, or the babies.[313]

Rye (Secale cereale)
Insufficient available evidence.

Safflower (Carthamus tinctorius)
Safflower oil is likely safe when used in the diet in reasonable quantities by healthy patients. In 32 case reports of soybean oil–based or soybean/safflower oil–based emulsions used in total parenteral nutrition programs for pregnant patients, no relationship was found between onset of labor or harmful maternal/fetal effects and administration of lipid emulsion.[314] The flower of safflower may be unsafe because it has shown a stimulating action on the uterus in vitro.[315] According to clinical evidence, there is a rapid transfer of dietary fatty acids from plasma chylomicrons into human milk, with maximum increase occurring 10 hours after safflower oil ingestion.[309,316]

Sage (Salvia officinalis)
There is insufficient evidence regarding the safety of sage use during pregnancy or lactation. In mice, sage essential oil supplementation appeared to have a negative impact on embryonic development.[131] Theoretically, the sage constituent thujone may have menstrual-stimulant and abortifacient effects. In a study of menopausal women, extracts of the leaves of *Salvia officinalis* (sage) and *Medicago sativa* (alfalfa), when used together, induced a significant increase in prolactin in some women.[317] Because sage is a potential phytoestrogen and has a historical use as an antihidrotic (antiperspirant), it may be useful as a treatment during weaning to decrease lactation, according to secondary sources. However, because of lack of available evidence, women should use sage cautiously during normal lactation.

Saiko-Keishi-To
Insufficient available evidence.

Salvia (Salvia divinorum)
Insufficient available evidence.

Sandalwood (Santalum album)
Insufficient available evidence.

Sanicle (Sanicula europaea)
Insufficient available evidence.

Sarsaparilla (Smilax spp.)
Insufficient available evidence.

Sassafras (Sassafras spp.)
Sassafras tea and oil should be avoided during pregnancy and lactation; these preparations contain the known carcinogen safrole.[318-320]

Saw Palmetto (Serenoa repens)
Because of potential antiandrogenic activity and effects on estrogen receptors, saw palmetto extract is contraindicated in women who are pregnant or lactating.[321-323] Use has been discouraged during pregnancy and lactation because of saw palmetto's proposed ability to inhibit the conversion of testosterone to dihydrotestosterone (DHT), which may cause abnormalities in the genitalia of a male fetus/infant. One study of sperm motility suggests that saw palmetto adversely affects sperm metabolism, whereas other reports from the same authors found no adverse effects on sperm, oocytes, or fertilization.[324]

Schisandra (Schisandra chinensis)
Schisandra berry should be avoided during pregnancy because of possible uterine-stimulating effects.[119,325] There is insufficient information regarding the safety of schisandra berry during lactation.

Scotch Broom (Cytisus scoparius)
Scotch broom should be avoided during pregnancy because it contains the alkaloid sparteine, which is known to cause uterine contractions and carries a theoretical risk of inducing abortion (abortifacient properties).[2,3] Scotch broom should be avoided during breastfeeding because of insufficient evidence and a hypothetical risk of serious toxicity.[2,3]

Sea Buckthorn (Hippophae rhamnoides)
There is insufficient information regarding the safety of sea buckthorn during pregnancy or lactation. Pregnant and lactating patients should not consume more than food amounts of sea buckthorn because of insufficient safety data.

Seaweed
Seaweeds, such as bladderwrack, are often not recommended during pregnancy and lactation because of high variability of iodine concentrations, frequent contamination with heavy metals, and potential for teratogenic effects.[326]

Senna (Senna alexandrina)
There is insufficient evidence regarding the use of senna when used appropriately for a short duration. Senna has not been found to be teratogenic in animals. High doses and long-term use should be avoided, however, because senna has been associated with laxative dependence and hepatotoxicity.[327,328] Senna appears to be safe during lactation when used appropriately for a short time; it has been identified by the AAP as "usually compatible with breast feeding."[18] Sennosides A and B do not appear to be excreted into breast milk; however, the active metabolite, rhein, is excreted into the milk in small amounts. Reports of adverse effects in infants are lacking.[96,329-331]

Shakuyaku-Kanzo-To
Insufficient available evidence.

Shepherd's Purse (Capsella bursa-pastoris)
Shepherd's purse may be unsafe during pregnancy or lactation because it has traditionally been used as an abortifacient and emmenagogue and was shown to enhance uterine tone in uterine horn samples from rabbits and guinea pigs.[88]

Shiitake Mushroom (Lentinus edodes)
Insufficient available evidence.

Skullcap (Scutellaria spp.)
Insufficient available evidence.

Skunk Cabbage (Symplocarpus foetidus)
Based on unsubstantiated reports, *Symplocarpus foetidus* may alter the menstrual cycle; uterine contractions may result from irritant properties.[2,3] Unrelated plants in the genus *Veratrum*, also commonly known as skunk cabbage and corn lily, contain alkaloids that have known toxic and teratogenic effects and should not be taken during pregnancy or lactation (see False Hellebore).

Slippery Elm (*Ulmus rubra*, syn. *Ulmus fulva*)
Use should be avoided during pregnancy because of the risk of contamination with slippery elm whole bark, which may have abortifacient properties. There is insufficient information regarding the safety of slippery elm during lactation.

Sophora (*Styphnolobium japonicum*)
Insufficient available evidence.

Sorrel (*Rumex acetosa*, *Rumex* spp.)
Sorrel may cause oxalate toxicity, although insufficient evidence exists on the safety of sorrel during pregnancy and lactation. A surveillance study of Sinupret (herbal preparation containing sorrel) in pregnant women reported no excess teratogenicity compared to controls not using Sinupret.[332]

Soy (*Glycine max*)
Soy as a part of the regular diet is generally considered safe during pregnancy and breastfeeding. It is not clear whether large doses of soy or soy isoflavones, which may have estrogen-like properties, adversely affect fetal or neonatal development. Female mice given genistein during pregnancy more frequently gave birth to male pups with hypospadias.[333] Similar effects have not been observed in humans.

Soy isoflavones have been detected in human breast milk;[334] however, it is not clear whether soy affects infant development. Compared to breast milk, soy-based formula has been associated with slight alterations in breast tissue development in infants,[335] although the clinical significance of this finding is unclear. Soy formula, substituted for milk-based formulas or breast milk, has been associated with significantly lower bone mineral density in infants.[336,337] However, soy formulas with improved mineral suspension resulted in comparable bone mineral metabolism to human milk or cow's milk,[338] suggesting that the mineral content of the formula, rather than the soy content, contributes to any observable differences in infant bone mineral density.

Soybean oil is likely safe when consumed as part of the diet in reasonable quantities by nonallergic women. Limited data suggest that parenteral use of lipids with soybean oil may be safe because it has been used to treat severe morning sickness without adverse effects.[102] There is insufficient information regarding the safety of soybean oil during lactation.

Spinach (*Spinacia oleracea*)
Spinach is likely safe when consumed as part of the diet in reasonable quantities by nonallergic women. There is insufficient safety information on medicinal doses.

Spirulina (*Arthrospira* spp.)
There is insufficient information regarding the safety of spirulina during pregnancy or lactation in humans. When fed to pregnant mice through week 19 of gestation, diets of up to 30% spirulina did not cause toxic effects to mother or fetus.[339]

Squill (*Urginea maritima*, syn. *Scilla maritima*)
Squill should be avoided by pregnant patients because of purported abortifacient effects. There is insufficient information regarding the safety of squill during lactation.

St. Ignatius Bean (*Strychnos ignatii*)
Insufficient available evidence.

St. John's Wort (*Hypericum perforatum*)
According to a systematic review by researchers in the Motherisk Program at the Hospital for Sick Children in Toronto, St. John's wort (SJW) should be used cautiously or avoided by pregnant women until further safety data are acquired.[340] In one case, a woman who took SJW from gestation week 24 until delivery had no complications, and her child was normal.[341] Currently, it is unclear if SJW is safe during pregnancy or breastfeeding.[342] Use in breastfeeding women appears to have little risk; however, side effects are possible.[340] In animals, SJW reportedly increased uterine muscle tone,[93] which may potentially cause uterine contractions. No adverse effects have been noted in infants from mothers taking SJW postnatally for depression.[343-345]

Star Anise (*Illicium verum*)
Insufficient available evidence.

Stevia (*Stevia rebaudiana*)
There is limited available information regarding the use of stevia during pregnancy and lactation. In hamsters, stevioside (in daily doses as high as 2.5 g/kg) affected neither growth nor reproduction.[346]

Stinging Nettle (*Urtica dioica*)
Stinging nettle may be unsafe during pregnancy and lactation because it may induce uterine stimulation.[347]

Strawberry (*Fragaria* spp.)
Strawberry is likely safe when consumed as part of the diet in reasonable quantities by nonallergic women. There is insufficient safety information regarding medicinal doses during pregnancy or lactation.

Suma (*Hebanthe eriantha*)
Insufficient available evidence.

Sunflower (*Helianthus annuus*)
Sunflower is likely safe when consumed as part of the diet in reasonable quantities by nonallergic women. There is insufficient safety information regarding medicinal doses.

Sweet Almond (*Prunus amygdalus dulcis*)
Tree nuts are common causes of food allergies in children, and consumption of nuts during pregnancy may increase the risk of asthma in the infant. However, moderate consumption of almonds is likely safe in nonallergic pregnant women. There is insufficient safety information regarding medicinal doses. In animals, almond extracts may increase sperm count and sperm motility.[348] The clinical significance, especially pertaining to pregnancy or lactation, is unclear.

Sweet Annie (*Artemisia annua*)
Insufficient available evidence.

Sweet Basil (*Ocimum basilicum*)
Sweet basil is likely safe in nonallergic women when consumed in amounts generally found in foods. There is insufficient safety information regarding medicinal doses. Based on in vitro study, sweet basil may be a potent spermicide in humans,[349] although the clinical significance (especially pertaining to pregnancy or lactation) is unclear.

Sweet Woodruff (Galium odoratum)
It has been suggested that sweet woodruff should be avoided during pregnancy.[350] There is insufficient information regarding the safety of sweet woodruff during lactation.

Tamanu (Calophyllum inophyllum)
Insufficient available evidence.

Tangerine (Citrus reticulata)
Tangerine is likely safe to use during pregnancy or lactation, when consumed as part of the diet in reasonable quantities by nonallergic women. However, a maternal cohort study correlated high citrus intake during pregnancy with increased incidence of food allergies in children.[59]

Tamarind (Tamarindus indica)
Tamarind is likely safe when consumed as part of the diet in reasonable quantities by nonallergic women. There is insufficient safety information regarding medicinal doses.

Tansy (Tanacetum vulgare)
Tansy may be unsafe during pregnancy and lactation. Herbal texts and ethnobotanical studies have documented that tansy may induce abortion, and thus it is considered unsafe for internal use in pregnant women.[242,351] The thujone constituent is potentially toxic.[23]

Tea (Camellia sinensis)
The adverse effects associated with tea (e.g., green tea, black tea, jasmine tea) are largely attributed to its caffeine content (see Caffeine).

Tea Tree (Melaleuca alternifolia)
Topical tea tree oil may be safe when used appropriately.[352] Oral tea tree oil is unsafe during pregnancy and lactation because of known toxicity. Animal studies suggest that tea tree oil should be used cautiously during childbirth because it has been anecdotally reported to decrease the force of spontaneous contractions.

Terminalia (Terminalia arjuna)
Insufficient available evidence.

Thunder God Vine (Tripterygium wilfordii)
Thunder god vine is likely unsafe during pregnancy because of possible teratogenic effects.[353] There is insufficient information regarding the safety of thunder god vine during lactation.

Thyme (Thymus vulgaris)
Thyme is likely safe when consumed in reasonable quantities or as a spice by nonallergic women. There is insufficient evidence regarding the safety of thyme supplementation during pregnancy or lactation. In mice, sage essential oil supplementation appeared to have a negative impact on embryonic development.[131] A 1975 review of plants as possible new antifertility agents classified thyme as an emmenagogue and abortifacient.[20]

Tree Tobacco (Nicotiana glauca)
Tree tobacco may be unsafe to use during pregnancy or lactation. Animals that eat tree tobacco may give birth to offspring with developmental abnormalities, especially bone and joint abnormalities and cleft palate.[354-367] Fetal malformations may likewise occur in humans.

Tribulus (Tribulus terrestris)
Tribulus may be unsafe during pregnancy or lactation; it has been traditionally used as an abortifacient. There is insufficient information regarding the safety of tribulus during lactation.

Turmeric (Curcuma longa)
Based on historical use, turmeric is generally considered to be safe when used as a spice in foods during pregnancy and lactation. However, turmeric may be unsafe when ingested in high doses from foods or when used medicinally, because of potential emmenagogic or uterine-stimulant effects. Oral turmeric has not been found to be teratogenic in mice or rats.[368-370] In mice, turmeric has been associated with weight gain of sexual organs and increased sperm motility, without spermatotoxic effects.[371]

Turpentine (Pinus palustris)
Turpentine oil should be avoided during pregnancy because it may have abortifacient effects.[48,372] There is insufficient information regarding the safety of turpentine oil during lactation.

Tylophora (Tylophora indica)
Tylophora may be unsafe during pregnancy and lactation because of reported abortifacient properties.[20]

Usnea (Usnea spp.)
Insufficient available evidence.

Uva Ursi (Arctostaphylos uva-ursi)
Uva ursi may be unsafe during pregnancy or lactation, because of reported potential to induce labor.[88]

Valerian (Valeriana officinalis)
Valerian may be unsafe during pregnancy or lactation, based on theoretical concerns over the teratogenic effects of valepotriates. Valerian constituents (valepotriates and baldrinals) have been shown to be cytotoxic and mutagenic in vitro.[373,374] However, these substances are unstable and generally not found in commercial valerian products. In rats, 30-day administration of a mixture of valepotriates failed to demonstrate any changes in fertility, estrous phases, or development of offspring.[375] No teratogenic actions have been reported in the few known cases of valerian intoxication during pregnancy.[376] Because of the lack of human safety data, however, it is prudent to discontinue valerian use during pregnancy and lactation.

Vanilla (Vanilla planifolia)
Because of historical use as a food flavoring, vanilla is likely safe when consumed by nonallergic women in amounts generally found in foods. There is insufficient safety information regarding medicinal doses. Some aromatic compounds, such as vanilla, mint, garlic, and alcohol, can flavor a woman's milk, thereby altering the chemosensory experience of the nursing infant.[377] The infant's response to a particular flavor may depend on recent prior exposure and duration of exposure to that flavor. One study of 133 adults who had been breastfed or bottle-fed as infants showed that neonatal experience with vanilla influenced food preferences later in life.[378] Because commercial vanilla extracts contain high amounts of alcohol, they should be used cautiously by pregnant or lactating women (see Alcohol).

Verbena (*Verbena officinalis*)
There is a lack of available systematic studies evaluating safety and efficacy in pregnant or lactating women. Contraceptive effects of *Verbena hybrida* and *Verbena bonariensis* were observed after administration of oral doses of 100 to 200 mg/kg in animals,[379] and these plants have been used traditionally in Ayurvedic medicine as contraceptives.

Vetiver (*Chrysopogon* spp.)
Insufficient available evidence.

Wasabi (*Wasabia japonica*)
Insufficient available evidence.

Water Hemlock (*Cicuta* spp.)
Insufficient available evidence.

Watercress (*Nasturtium officinale*)
Watercress is likely safe when consumed as part of the diet in reasonable quantities by nonallergic women. There is insufficient safety information on supplemental doses. Based on secondary sources, watercress may be unsafe when used during pregnancy because of its purported abortifacient effects.[48] There is insufficient information regarding the safety of watercress during lactation.

Wheatgrass (*Triticum aestivum*)
Because it is grown in soils or water and consumed raw, wheatgrass may be contaminated with bacteria, molds, or other substances. Theoretically, women who are pregnant or breastfeeding should use wheatgrass cautiously.

White Horehound (*Marrubium vulgare*)
White horehound may be unsafe during pregnancy because of emmenagogic and abortifacient effects demonstrated in animals.[20] In addition, anecdotal reports have noted that white horehound may stimulate uterine contractions. There is insufficient information regarding the safety of white horehound during lactation.

White Oak (*Quercus alba*)
Insufficient available evidence.

White Water Lily (*Nymphaea odorata*)
Insufficient available evidence.

Wild Arrach (*Chenopodium vulvaria*)
Insufficient available evidence.

Wild Cherry (*Prunus africana, Prunus emarginata, Prunus serotina*)
Insufficient available evidence.

Wild Indigo (*Baptisia australis, Baptisia tinctoria*)
Insufficient available evidence.

Wild Yam (*Dioscorea villosa*)
Wild yam may be unsafe during pregnancy and lactation because it is believed to induce uterine contractions.[380] Wild yam is purported to possess progestogenic or estrogenic effects, and there are anecdotal reports of contamination with synthetic progesterone.

Willow (*Salix* spp.)
There is insufficient information regarding the safety of willow bark during pregnancy or lactation. However, salicylates (which are found in willow bark) are associated with fetal abnormalities,[246] and drugs in this class are listed in FDA Pregnancy Category D (positive evidence of human fetal risk). There is anecdotal evidence that salicylates in breast milk may cause rash in breastfed infants.[2] Salicylates should be given to nursing mothers with caution because it has been associated with metabolic acidosis in infants.[18]

Witch Hazel (*Hamamelis virginiana*)
Insufficient available evidence.

Wormwood (*Artemisia absinthium*)
Wormwood may be unsafe during pregnancy and lactation.[381,382] The CNS stimulant thujone can be found in wormwood, which may have uterine and menstrual-stimulant effects.[2,3] There is insufficient information regarding the safety of wormwood during lactation.

Yarrow (*Achillea millefolium*)
Yarrow has traditionally been used as an abortifacient, emmenagogue, contraceptive, and stimulant for uterine contractions. In rats, a dose 56 times the daily human dose of yarrow reduced fetal weight and increased placental weight; it was concluded that the dose used was not maternotoxic, and there was no increase in preimplantation or postimplantation losses, suggesting that yarrow was neither an abortifacient nor a contraceptive.[383] There is insufficient information regarding the safety of yarrow during lactation.

Yellow Dock (*Rumex crispus*)
Based on expert opinion, pregnant women should not ingest harsh laxatives. Yellow dock is thought to fall into this category, perhaps because of the anthraquinone content.[384] However, some herbal experts have recommended yellow dock in pregnancy because of its iron content,[385] although this use has not been shown to be safe in clinical trials. There is insufficient information regarding the safety of yellow dock during lactation.

Yerba Santa (*Eriodictyon californicum*)
The safety of yerba santa has not been established in pregnancy or lactation. Tinctures of yerba santa may contain high levels of alcohol, which is not recommended for use in pregnant women (see Alcohol). However, 1 mL of yerba santa ethanol extract has been used traditionally in pregnant women.

Yew (*Taxus* spp.)
Yew may be unsafe during pregnancy or lactation because of its historical use as an abortifacient.[66] There is insufficient information regarding the safety of yew during lactation.

Yohimbe (*Pausinystalia yohimbe*)
Yohimbe is contraindicated during pregnancy and lactation because it may act as a uterine relaxant and fetal toxin. Adverse effects have been reported in breastfed babies whose mothers consumed yohimbe.[386]

Yucca (*Yucca schidigera*)
Insufficient available evidence.

Answers to Chapter Review Questions

CHAPTER 3
Psychiatric Disorders

1. d. seizures
Several case reports cite seizures associated with use of evening primrose oil (EPO) in patients with/without known seizure disorders, and possibly with the combination of EPO and anesthetics.

2. a. Arecoline
Extrapyramidal symptoms (EPS) such as tremor and stiffness have been reported in patients who chewed betel while receiving antipsychotic drugs; these effects have been attributed to the active alkaloid ingredient in betel nut, arecoline, which possesses cholinergic properties.

3. False
Betel nut–chewing schizophrenic patients scored significantly lower on both positive and negative subscales of the Positive and Negative Syndrome Scale (PANSS).

4. c. 3 g daily for up to 1 year
EPO has been well tolerated in doses up to 3 g daily for 1 year, according to available studies. Although other doses may also be well tolerated, there is a lack of systematic safety or efficacy data for other doses.

5. All true *except*: b. Based on studies demonstrating abnormal membrane phospholipid metabolism in patients with schizophrenia, it has been theorized that betel nut may play a role in the treatment of schizophrenia.
Unlike evening primrose oil, which contains essential fatty acids that are thought to play a role in membrane phospholipid metabolism, betel nut's principal active constituent is the cholinergic component arecoline.

CHAPTER 4
Anxiety and Insomnia

1. All options *except*: c. Bitter orange
Bitter orange contains synephrine, an alkaloid with similar properties to the CNS stimulant ephedrine.

2. b. Liver damage
There is concern regarding kava's potential toxicity, based on multiple reports of liver damage in Europe and a number of cases in the United States, including hepatitis, cirrhosis, and liver failure.

3. b. Hop
Phytoestrogens in hop may exert estrogenic agonist or antagonist properties, with unknown effects on hormone-sensitive conditions, such as breast, uterine, cervical, or prostate cancer, or endometriosis.

4. False
Although the name is similar to kola ("cola") nut, gotu kola is not the same and does not contain caffeine.

5. d. All the above
Rosemary extract is frequently used in aromatherapy to treat anxiety as well as enhance mood, alter pain perception, and increase alertness.

6. d. 30 mL bacopa syrup daily (representing 12 g dry crude extract) for one month
In published studies, patients with anxiety have used 30 mL of bacopa syrup daily (representing 12 g dry crude extract) for 1 month.

7. False
The most common current application of St. John's wort is the treatment of depressive disorders. Though it has also been associated with depression, anxiety has not been a major focus of St. John's wort research.

8. c. Limbic system
Kavapyrones may inhibit the limbic system, which may cause suppression of mood and emotions. Its effects on other parts of the brain are not well understood.

CHAPTER 5
Depressive Disorders

1. d. All of the above
St. John's wort appears to inhibit serotonin, norepinephrine, and dopamine synaptic reuptake.

2. False
Preliminary research suggests that lavender tincture may be helpful as an adjunct to prescription antidepressant medications; as a monotherapy, the beneficial effects of lavender in depression are not as clear.

3. d. All the above

St. John's wort may cause sexual side effects, headache, and photosensitivity.

4. c. Ginkgo

Monoamine oxidase (MAO) inhibition by Ginkgo has been demonstrated in animals. To date, the effects of ginger, elder, and lavender on MAO inhibition have not been clearly demonstrated.

5. d. 300 to 600 mg daily

The recommended dose of Ginkgo for maintenance therapy is 300 to 600 mg daily. For starting doses, 300 to 600 mg three times daily are usually recommended; safety and/or efficacy of high doses (3 to 6 g daily) or low doses (30 to 60 mg) are unclear.

6. False

Preliminary evidence suggests that ginkgo (Ginkgo biloba) is not effective in preventing seasonal affective disorder (SAD).

7. All true except: a. Short-term studies suggest that St. John's wort is more effective than TCAs for severe depression.

Though the efficacy of St. John's wort may be comparable to tricyclic antidepressants (TCAs) for treating mild to moderate major depression, studies thus far have not shown it to be consistently superior to TCAs or other standard antidepressant medications.

8. d. All the above

Adverse effects associated with ginkgo use include increased risk of bleeding, increased risk of hypertensive crisis when ingested with tyramine-containing foods, and increased plasma insulin levels.

9. True

There is some clinical evidence suggesting that chasteberry may be comparable to fluoxetine in relieving symptoms of PMDD.

10. a. Anxiety

There is some clinical evidence suggesting that sage may decrease anxiety, improve alertness, and have a calming effect. Its effects in treating bloating, backache, and uncontrollable crying (colic) have not been thoroughly demonstrated to date.

CHAPTER 6
Physical and Cognitive Enhancement

1. a. Evening primrose oil

There is some clinical evidence suggesting symptomatic improvements in patients with postviral fatigue syndrome who took evening primrose oil and fish oil. Though other treatments may have also been used, their efficacy may not be as clear.

2. c. Borage has been hypothesized as being effective for narcotic concealment.

In available research, narcotic concealment has not been a major indication for borage seed oil or its constituent GLA; however, borage has been hypothesized as a remedy for preventing and treating alcohol hangover.

3. b. Tribulus

Tribulus has been promoted for athletic performance, muscle mass enhancement, and as a testosterone booster; however, its efficacy has not clearly been demonstrated in available studies, and its proposed mechanism of action remains unclear.

4. a. Warfarin

A clinical interaction between warfarin and a papain-containing combination product has been proposed; however, this interaction was possibly caused by contamination of the combination product with warfarin. Though additional interactions may be possible, clinical reports of interactions with other agents are lacking.

5. True

Kudzu extracts or individual isoflavones have been demonstrated to suppress alcohol intake in animal models of alcoholism (see Appendix A). Kudzu is used as a remedy for alcoholism; however, supportive evidence is lacking.

6. a. Pycnogenol

A randomized controlled study found that Pycnogenol improved attention and various rating scales in children with ADHD. Though bitter orange contains alkaloids that exert stimulant effects, its use in ADHD has not been rigorously examined.

7. True

Rhodiola has been used traditionally to enhance physical and mental performance, and several Russian studies have examined its efficacy.

CHAPTER 7
Parkinson's Disease

1. b. Catechin polyphenols (including theaflavin and ECGC)

The major antioxidants found in green tea are the catechin polyphenols. Studies suggest that green tea catechin polyphenols possess potent antioxidant activity and may invoke neuroprotective effects.

2. b. Psychosis

Cowhage has also caused acute toxic psychosis, likely due to its levodopa content.

3. d. All the above

Ashwagandha may interact with anticoagulants (warfarin), antidiabetic agents (repaglinide), and cholinesterase inhibitors (rivastigmine).

4. c. Kava

Based on reports of extrapyramidal effects associated with kava use, it should be avoided in patients with Parkinson's disease or in patients with a history of medication-induced extrapyramidal effects.

5. False

A multiherb preparation (a concoction in cow's milk of powdered Mucuna pruriens and Hyoscyamus reticulatus seeds and Withania somnifera and Sida cordifolia roots) reduced improved symptoms of Parkinson's disease. The direct effects of ashwagandha is not clear.

6. a. L-dopa
Cowhage (Mucuna pruriens) seeds have been used in traditional Ayurvedic medicine to treat Parkinson's disease. This traditional use is supported by laboratory analysis that show cowhage contains 3.6% to 4.2% levodopa (L-dopa; 3,4-dihydroxy-L-phenylalanine), the same chemical used in several Parkinson's disease drugs that is a precursor to dopamine.

7. b. 22.5 to 67.5 grams
Specific cowhage extracts standardized to 3.3% L-dopa (HP-200) have been used. Dosages have ranged from 22.5 to 67.5 grams divided into two to five daily doses.

CHAPTER 8
Seizure Disorders

1. False
Bacopa, not lavender, was found to reverse the expression of N-methyl-D-aspartate receptor 1 (NMDA R1)– and glutamate receptor–binding alterations to near-control levels in epileptic rats. The effects of lavender on NDMA and glutamate receptor binding are unclear.

2. d. All of these agents may interact with bacopa.
Because of its sedative effects, bacopa may interact with central nervous system (CNS) depressants (chloral hydrate). Because animal research has suggested that bacopa affects thyroid hormone levels, it may potentially interact with thyroid medications (methimazole). It may also interact with anticonvulsants (phenytoin) and other agents metabolized by CYP450.

3. True
Although false hellebore was prescribed for epilepsy and convulsions in the eighteenth and nineteenth centuries, its potentially toxic and irritating constituents now preclude its use.

4. a. Euphorbia fisheriana
The active alkaloid in Euphorbia fisheriana reportedly has anticonvulsant effects.

5. d. All the above
Atkins Diet, vitamin E, and chiropractic medicine may be useful adjunct therapies for epilepsy.

CHAPTER 9
Pain

1. True
Bromelain has proteolytic activity, and is thought to lower kininogen and bradykinin in serum and tissues, thereby altering prostaglandin synthesis.

2. b. Eugenol
The clove component eugenol is popular in dentistry for its mild anesthetic and analgesic effects, but its mechanism of action is not well understood.

3. d. Both a and c
Dong quai and feverfew should be used cautiously with photosensitizing agents.

4. a. Menstrual pain
Dong quai has historically been used for various types of pain associated with menstruation.

5. d. All the above
White horehound may interact with drugs that affect serotonin because of evidence suggesting it may antagonize the effects of serotonin. Because of proposed hypothalamic-pituitary-adrenal (HPA) axis effects of white horehound constituents, it may alter hormone levels. Because white horehound may enhance aldosterone action, it may interact with aldosterone-blocking diuretic agents. However, clinical evidence of this interaction is lacking.

6. c. Sesquiterpene lactones
Sesquiterpene lactones are thought to be the principal antiinflammatory components of dandelion.

7. c. Aspirin
Because willow contains salicin, which is chemically related to aspirin and other salicylates, it may present a risk of anaphylactic reaction in patients with a history of allergy to salicylates, such as aspirin.

8. True
Soy's potential to relieve breast pain may be due to its isoflavones (phytoestrogens).

CHAPTER 10
Alzheimer's Disease and Related Disorders

1. False
Cathinone, an alkaloid structurally related to amphetamine, is thought to be the main constituent of khat. The main active components of ginseng are the ginsenosides.

2. d. All the above
Flavonoids in ginkgo have been shown to reduce oxidative cellular damage in Alzheimer's disease; monoamine oxidase (MAO) inhibition by ginkgo has been reported in animals; and ginkgo has also been found to increase serotonin levels and norepinephrine levels.

3. d. All the above
Based on clinical reports, ginkgo may potentially interact with antiplatelet medications such as clopidogrel, as well as drugs that lower the seizure threshold such as carbamazepine and the calcium channel blocker nifedipine.

4. c. 300 mg daily for 12 weeks
For cognitive function, 300 mg daily of Keenmind Bacopa monnieri extract has been used for 12 weeks.

5. True
Ginseng appears to exert acute effects on cognitive performance, according to clinical evidence.

6. a. Soy isoflavones (daidzein and genistein) act as weak agonists at estrogen receptors in the brain.
Soy isoflavones (daidzein and genistein) are widely believed to be the pharmacologically active constituents of soy. Studies have suggested that soy isoflavones act as weak agonists at estrogen receptors in the brain.

7. a. Lavender
Lavender aromatherapy has been shown to improve emotion and aggressive behavior in patients with Alzheimer's dementia.

CHAPTER 11
Hypertension

1. b. Captopril
In one study, hibiscus standardized extract worked as well as captopril (Capoten) in lowering blood pressure.

2. a. Has exhibited antifertility activity.
Hibiscus has displayed antifertility activity and should be avoided in women attempting to conceive.

3. d. All the above
Based on pharmacological effects suggested in basic science studies, as well as clinical observations, hibiscus should be used cautiously in patients taking drugs that may affect blood pressure (propranolol), as well as acetaminophen, quinine, and chloroquine.

4. False
In one randomized controlled trial, Pycnogenol reduced systolic blood pressure significantly, but diastolic blood pressure was not significantly lowered compared with placebo.

5. d. Both a and b
Because it has been shown to lower blood glucose, Pycnogenol may interact with hypoglycemic agents such as metformin. Pycnogenol has also been shown clinically to reduce thromboxane levels and thus may interact with anticoagulants such as warfarin. Grape seed extract and Pycnogenol are not the same, even though they both contain oligomeric proanthocyanidins (OPCs).

6. False
Stevioside therapy (up to 2 years) has not been associated with significant adverse effects; thus it is not likely that short-term use will carry a significant risk of adverse effects.

7. a. 600 to 900 mg daily in three divided doses
Multiple clinical trials have used 600 to 900 mg daily of non-enteric-coated, dehydrated garlic powder in three divided doses for hypertension.

8. c. Oxalic acid
Rhubarb leaves contain poisonous oxalic acid.

9. d. Both a and b
Ancient Chinese monks used reishi to calm their minds for meditation. Reishi has also displayed ACE inhibitory activity. However, the active ingredients in Ganoderma lucidum have not been fully determined or standardized.

10. All true *except:* d. Pycnogenol is best taken on an empty stomach.
It may be best to take Pycnogenol with or after meals.

CHAPTER 12
Congestive Heart Failure and Diuresis

1. False
Numerous well-conducted human clinical trials have demonstrated safety and efficacy of hawthorn leaf and flower in NYHA Class I-II heart failure, characterized by slight or no limitation of physical activity. Its safety and efficacy for Class IV heart failure remain uncertain.

2. d. All the above
Adverse effects of hawthorn include hypotension, dyspnea, and fatigue, and therefore it should be used cautiously in patients with low blood pressure, asthma, or chronic fatigue syndrome.

3. a. 160 to 900 mg daily
Doses of 160 to 900 mg of hawthorn daily have been effective in the treatment of mild to moderate CHF, improving exercise capacity and alleviating symptoms of cardiac insufficiency.

4. True
Deaths have resulted from ingestion of all forms of oleander, a poisonous plant.

5. d. All the above
Goldenseal and/or berberine may interact with anticoagulants, beta blockers, and tetracyclines due to similar mechanisms of action.

6. b. Equisetonin and flavonoids
Diuretic properties of horsetail may be attributed to equisetonin and flavonoids.

7. b. Oligomeric proanthocyanidins
The active components of grape seed extract (GSE) are the oligomeric proanthocyanidins (OPCs).

8. True

9. d. All the above
Dandelion may interact with potassium-sparing diuretics (triamterene), anticoagulants (warfarin), and antidiabetic agents (insulin) due to known pharmacological effects and its constituents.

10. c. Scoparin and scoparoside
Diuretic effects of scotch broom may be attributed to the constituents scoparin and scoparoside.

CHAPTER 13
Angina

1. All *except:* c. Kava
Kava has not been shown to benefit symptoms of angina.

2. True

3. **d.** All the above
Danshen may alter lipid panel, prolong prothrombin time/INR, and falsely elevate digoxin level.

4. **All true** *except:* **c.** Injection of safflower oil has been shown to reduce symptoms of angina pectoris in patients with coronary artery disease.
Injection of safflower, not safflower oil, has been shown reduce symptoms of angina pectoris in CAD patients.

5. **All true** *except:* **a.** Ginseng, as a monotherapy, may reduce symptoms of coronary artery disease, such as anginal chest pain.
Ginseng in combination with other herbs such as Radix ophiopogonis and Schisandra chinensis may reduce CAD symptoms such as anginal chest pain. The effects of ginseng monotherapy are unclear.

6. **d.** Because of in vitro evidence of thromboxane A_2 inhibition, hawthorn should be used cautiously with anticoagulants/antiplatelets such as warfarin and aspirin.
Hawthorn has been associated with mild adverse effects; however, safety has not been systematically evaluated in humans. The evidence to date does not unequivocally support the use of hawthorn for angina.

7. True

CHAPTER 14
Ischemic Disease and Heart Rhythm Disorders

1. **c.** Aspirin
Salicylic acid is the chemical precursor to aspirin (acetylsalicylic acid).

2. **d.** Flaxseed oil contains omega-3 fatty acids, but not omega-6 fatty acids.
This statement is false because flaxseed oil contains both omega-3 and omega-6 fatty acids.

3. **d.** All the above
Studies have suggested that arnica may inhibit platelet aggregation, reduce serum lipids, and reduce inflammation.

4. **a.** Fiber
The proposed lipid-lowering effects of flaxseed (not flaxseed oil) have been attributed to the fiber component. The fatty acids in flaxseed and flaxseed oil (omega-3 and omega-6) may also offer some benefit. Flaxseed does not contain statins.

5. **b.** Meadowsweet *(Filipendula ulmaria)*
Meadowsweet, but not chia, contains significant amounts of salicylic acid.

6. **d.** All the above
Both golden chia and danshen are Salvia species, and their roots have been traditionally used to treat stroke.

7. **d.** All the above
Constituents of betel nut have cholinergic activity and are potentially carcinogenic. Long-term use has been associated with oral submucous fibrosis (OSF), cervical dysplasia, precancerous oral lesions, and squamous cell carcinoma.

8. True
The toxic effects associated with the administration of aconite, including dizziness and flushing of the face, limit its ability to be used clinically as an agent to treat bradycardia (slow heart rate).

9. **All** *except:* **d.** Echinacea
Echinacea has not been found to have antiarrhythmic properties; however, bloodroot, devil's claw, and mistletoe may be used in the management of arrhythmias.

10. False.
In most people, arrhythmias are minor and are not dangerous; they may occur as normal responses to physiological and psychological stimuli.

CHAPTER 15
Coagulation Disorders

1. **d.** It has been reported to cause hyperthyroidism.
Garlic has both fibrinolytic and antiplatelet activity. It has been reported to cause both intraoperative bleeding and decreased serum level of the protease inhibitor saquinavir. Anecdotal reports cite hypothyroidism, not hyperthyroidism, with garlic ingestion.

2. **b.** Serum glucose
Animal studies have shown garlic to reduce serum glucose concentration and increase insulin secretion. This has not been recorded in human studies but is theoretically possible.

3. **d.** Both a and b
Ginger might interact with a variety of different drug classes, including antiarrhythmics (procainamide), cardiac glycosides (digoxin), and antihypertensives. Ginger has not been shown to interact with the acne medication isotretinoin (Retin-A).

4. **All** *except:* **c.** Increased O_2 production
In vitro, grape seed extract enhances NO release and reduces superoxide production, O_2 production, and platelet aggregation.

5. False
Policosanol is generally well tolerated and has been shown to decrease the rate of adverse events in diabetic patients compared to placebo.

6. **c.** Pycnogenol treatment may be effective in preventing deep vein thrombosis and superficial vein thrombosis.
Pycnogenol has been shown to increase the effect of salicylates in vitro and decrease platelet aggregation. Studies have suggested that Pycnogenol treatment may be effective in preventing thrombotic events, particularly during airplane flights.

7. True

8. a. It binds to the α_2-adrenoreceptor on platelets.

Yohimbe decreases epinephrine-induced platelet aggregation and binds to the α_2-adrenoreceptor on platelets. It is poorly absorbed after oral administration. Yohimbe has a half-life of 1 hour, and its active metabolite has a half-life of 6 hours. It should be avoided in pregnancy because of potential fetal toxicity and uterine-relaxing effects.

9. False

The FDA has determined yohimbine to be unsafe for over-the-counter sale because of potential adverse effects and interactions. Most commercial yohimbe bark products do not contain appreciable amounts of yohimbine.

10. c. Cimetidine

Grape seed extract is not known or suspected to interact with H_2 blockers. It may theoretically interact with allopurinol, methotrexate, and enalapril based on in vitro evidence of angiotensin-converting enzyme (ACE) and xanthine oxidase inhibition.

CHAPTER 16
Lipid Disorders

1. True

2. c. 500 to 1000 mg

Current recommended doses of guggul for hyperlipidemia are 500 to 1000 mg of the constituent guggulipid.

3. a. Psyllium should not be taken within 1 hour after taking medications or other oral agents.

Because it may interfere with the absorption of oral agents, psyllium should not be taken within 1 hour of taking medications and other oral agents. Psyllium is not absorbed, is considered safe during all three trimesters of pregnancy, and has strong scientific evidence supporting its use in reducing cholesterol levels.

4. True

5. c. Triterpenes

Triterpenes, found in reishi, appear to be responsible for the inhibition of cholesterol absorption and inhibition of cholesterol synthesis.

6. b. Allergy or hypersensitivity to grass or wheat

Multiple cases of allergy have been reported with barley, and cross-reactivity may occur with allergy to grass or wheat.

7. d. Monacolins

Several compounds collectively known as monacolins (found in red yeast rice) are statins known to inhibit cholesterol synthesis.

8. True

The FDA has approved health claims that soy products (containing at least 6.25 g soy protein per serving, one-fourth the effective level of 25 g/day) may reduce the risk of coronary heart disease (CHD) by lowering blood cholesterol levels.

9. d. Oleanolic acid and ursolic acid

In vitro and in vivo studies have demonstrated that both oleanolic acid and ursolic acid constituents of hyssop have antihyperlipidemic properties.

10. False

Hawthorn contains monomeric catechins and oligomeric procyanidins, which are thought to contribute to hypocholesterolemic effects. Hawthorn is not noted to contain oleoresin; however, it is a constituent of cayenne and other Capsicum species.

11. d. Both a and c

Specific components of soybean, such as the isoflavones genistein and daidzein, may be responsible for the cholesterol-lowering properties of soy.

12. c. 3.4 to 45 g daily in two or three divided doses for 8 to 12 weeks

To lower cholesterol, 3.4 to 45 g daily of psyllium, in two or three divided doses for 8 to 12 weeks, may be recommended.

13. False

Fenugreek has been shown to reduce total and LDL cholesterol levels, but not HDL-C levels.

CHAPTER 17
Respiratory Disorders

1. b. Inhibiting the release of leukotrienes.

Animal studies have demonstrated that boswellia inhibits the release of leukotriene B_4 (LTB_4), a potent inducer of bronchoconstriction and asthma.

2. a. 200 to 1200 mg three times daily

To treat asthma, 200 to 1200 mg boswellia three times daily has been used.

3. a. Safflower

Patients with cystic fibrosis usually have decreased linoleic acid from reduced absorption of nutrients. Safflower, which is a good source of linolenic acid, has been used to supplement CF patients; however, its efficacy remains unclear.

4. False

These effects of forskolin have been compared to fenoterol, a beta-2-adrenergic receptor agonist, but fenoterol appears to have a stronger effect.

5. d. All of the above

Goji may decrease triglycerides, elevate INR, and increase leukocyte counts.

6. b. Potential antiinflammatory properties of butterbur have been attributed to ephedrine content.

Potential anti-inflammatory properties of butterbur extracts have been attributed to the petasin content. Butterbur is not known to contain ephedrine.

7. **True**

8. **c.** 150 mg in three divided daily doses for 2 to 4 months

To treat asthma, 150 mg of standardized butterbur (Petadolex) has been taken in three divided daily doses for 2 to 4 months.

9. **a.** 10 to 20 g daily for 4 weeks

For asthma, perilla seed oil at 10 to 20 g daily for 4 weeks has been used.

10. **b.** Kiwi contains a high concentration of the neurotransmitter serotonin.

Kiwi may decrease (rather than increase) platelet aggregation. Furthermore, cross-sensitization with banana has been reported and may not be safe for those with banana allergies; thus, those with banana allergies should use kiwi only with caution.

CHAPTER 18
Diabetes Mellitus

1. **d.** Both a and c

Although several constituents of bitter melon have been found to possess hypoglycemic properties, most interest has focused on a polypeptide isolated from the seeds called polypeptide p and a mixture of two steroid glycosides referred to as charantin.

2. **False**

Multiple human trials have failed to demonstrate significant effects of oral garlic preparation on measures of glycemic control in diabetic or non-diabetic patients.

3. **a.** Stevia

Stevia rebaudiana standardized extracts are used as natural sweeteners or dietary supplements in different countries for their content of stevioside or rebaudioside A.

4. **d.** All the above

The total triterpenic (hydrocarbons) fraction of gotu kola contains three main components: asiatic acid, madecassic acid, and asiaticoside.

5. **c.** Alfalfa

Alfalfa should also be avoided in patients with systemic lupus erythematosus (SLE) because of a possible risk of disease exacerbation.

6. **b.** Inulin

Inulin, a constituent in dandelion, may act as a glucose modulator.

7. **d.** Weight gain

Chronic ingestion of a devil's club infusion can cause weight gain.

8. **True**

Numerous studies have demonstrated that nopal may reduce blood glucose levels in patients with diabetes.

9. **d.** All the above

Bladderwrack may interact with propylthiouracil (high iodine content of bladderwrack may interfere with function of drugs that act on thyroid), lithium (altered thyroid function), and warfarin (increased bleeding risk).

10. **b.** Kudzu

Puerarin is an isoflavone derived from kudzu. Puerarin injections may reduce blood viscosity, improve microcirculation, and play a positive therapeutic role in diabetic retinopathy.

CHAPTER 19
Pituitary and Thyroid Disorders

1. **c.** It is a phytoestrogen.

In vitro, constituents in chasteberry bind selectively to estrogen receptor beta, and the flavonoid apigenin has been identified as an active phytoestrogen in chasteberry.

2. **a.** It may be standardized to agnuside, aucubin, or casticin content.

There is good scientific evidence supporting the efficacy of chasteberry in treating hyperprolactinemia.

3. **b.** Urticaria

Adverse effects reported with maca include stomach pain, bloating, flatulence, leukocytosis, and increased PT/INR. Urticaria has not been reported as a significant side effect associated with maca use.

4. **a.** It has been used in traditional medicine to enhance fertility and libido.

In one clinical study, maca had no effect on reproductive hormone levels, including luteinizing hormone, follicle-stimulating hormone, prolactin, 17α-hydroxyprogesterone, testosterone, and 17β-estradiol.

5. **c.** 1%

A preparation of rehmannia, standardized to contain 1% glutannic acid per dose, has been used.

6. **False**

Rehmannia has been found to decrease aminoglycoside toxicity in animals.

7. **c.** Both a and b

Bladderwrack may have very high levels of arsenic, cadmium, and lead. It has also been reported to have anticoagulant effects.

8. **c.** Goiter

The high iodine content of bladderwrack may be effective in preventing hypothyroidism and goiter, although trace amounts are generally sufficient for this purpose.

9. **d.** Rehmannia (Rehmannia glutinosa)

In a study evaluating the effects of Rehmannia glutinosa in the treatment of Sheehan's syndrome (postpartum hypopituitarism), subjects showed marked improvement in clinical symptoms after 2 to 5 months of treatment.

CHAPTER 20
Obesity

1. True
Persons with a BMI of 30 and above are obese.

2. All true except: c. Hoodia acts as a stimulant, similar to ephedra, to aid in weight loss.
Unlike ephedra, hoodia does not work as a stimulant; it acts as an appetite suppressant.

3. b. Methylxanthines
Methylxanthines (which include the stimulant caffeine) appear to elevate free fatty acid mobilization and enhance weight loss.

4. All true except: d. There is strong evidence to support the use of spirulina as an appetite suppressant.
Spirulina is marketed as an appetite suppressant; however, limited research thus far shows no benefit of spirulina over placebo.

5. a. 4.7 g daily
There is clinical evidence that HCA in garcinia, given three times daily 30 to 60 minutes before meals (for a total of 4.7 g daily), may reduce body weight and BMI.

6. True
According to clinical trials, consuming soy milk appears to be as effective in reducing weight, fat, and abdominal circumference as consuming skim milk.

CHAPTER 21
Menopause

1. All true except: c. Clinical research shows that black cohosh combined with kava improves climacteric complaints as well as psychological disorders.
A combination of black cohosh and St. John's wort appears to be beneficial for climacteric complaints, including the related psychological components. It is unclear if combination of black cohosh and kava has a similar effect.

2. b. 20 to 40 mg twice daily
For perimenopausal symptoms, studies have used 20-mg to 40-mg Remifemin tablets (corresponding to 1-2 mg 27-deoxyactein) twice daily.

3. True

4. a. 20 to 60 g of soy protein providing 40 to 80 mg of isoflavones
Doses of 20 to 60 g of soy protein providing 40 to 80 mg of isoflavones have been used in research.

5. False
Manufacturers of a vaginal cream containing wild yam (Dioscorea villosa) have claimed that the cream possesses progesterone-like effects and is a source of "natural hormones," although this is not supported by animal or human studies.

6. b. The brand of soy isoflavone extract used in most trials and most available commercially is Promensil.
Promensil contains red clover isoflavones, not soy isoflavones.

7. b. Alfalfa
Sage in combination with alfalfa reduced menopausal symptoms, including hot flushes and night sweating, in one available clinical trial.

8. d. All the above
Black cohosh may interact with agents that alter serotonin (fluoxetine), antihypertensive agents (enalapril), and cytochrome P450 substrates (ketoconazole).

9. b. 1200 mg calcium and 800 IU vitamin D daily
Daily elemental calcium and vitamin D intake for postmenopausal women should be about 1200 mg and 800 IU, respectively.

10. True
St. John's wort may help treat psychological and psychosomatic symptoms associated with perimenopause or menopause, including depression, as measured by self-rating and physician rating in clinical studies.

CHAPTER 22
Osteoporosis

1. d. Silicon
Animal and in vitro studies suggest that silicon plays a role in bone development, may increase the rate of bone mineralization, and may enhance calcium deposition in bone.

2. False
If the T-score is −2.5 or lower, the individual is considered to have osteoporosis and therefore at high risk for fracture.

3. d. Both a and c
Doses of 57.7 mg and 85.5 mg of red clover isoflavones daily (Rimostil containing genistein daidzein, formonetin, and biochanin) for 6 months increased BMD in postmenopausal women.

4. All true except: b. Soy isoflavones act only on osteoblasts, not osteoclasts.
Soy isoflavones act on both osteoblasts and osteoclasts.

5. True
Soy isoflavones appear to have beneficial effects on BMD, bone turnover markers, and bone mechanical strength in postmenopausal women in some (but not all) available studies.

CHAPTER 23
Arthritis

1. a. Gamma-linolenic acid (GLA)
GLA is thought to exert borage seed oil's antiinflammatory effects.

2. b. Aucubin
Aucubin has been shown in vitro to prevent the release of the inflammatory mediator leukotriene C_4. Curcumin is the active

antiinflammatory component of turmeric. Procumben is not a known constituent of any herbal therapy. Rhynchophylline is a component of cat's claw that may inhibit platelet aggregation.

3. **c.** Both a and b

Extracts of devil's claw have been reported to inhibit leukotriene B_4 and decrease COX-2 expression.

4. **b.** Soybean

The effects of avocado/soybean unsaponifiables (ASU) on osteoarthritis have been studied clinically, with some promising (but still inconclusive) evidence.

5. **b.** Salicylate

The active constituents of willow bark are the salicylates, which are chemical precursors to aspirin (acetylsalicylate).

6. **c.** Both a and b

Bromelain may inhibit the biosynthesis of proinflammatory prostaglandins by lowering the levels of kininogen and bradykinin in serum and tissues.

7. **All true** *except:* **c.** The medicinal uses of *Rosa* spp. are confined to the fruits.

The fruits, seeds, husks, and roots of Rosa species have all been used medicinally.

8. **a.** Two purified semisynthetic lignan glycosides

One study evaluated the use of 300 mg of CPH 82, which is composed of two purified semisynthetic lignan glycosides of Podophyllum emodi.

9. **a.** Reducing plasma urate

Cherry consumption has been shown to lower plasma urate concentrations and increase urate elimination in the urine; this may explain the purported antigout effects of cherry.

10. **c.** Ginger may suppress leukotriene biosynthesis by inhibiting 5-lipoxygenase.

Ginger shares pharmacological properties with nonsteroidal antiinflammatory drugs (NSAIDs) because it suppresses prostaglandin synthesis through inhibition of COX-1 and COX-2. However, ginger can be distinguished from NSAIDs based on its ability to suppress leukotriene biosynthesis by inhibiting 5-lipoxygenase.

CHAPTER 24
Gastrointestinal Disorders

1. **b.** Soluble fiber

The constituent responsible for psyllium's laxative effects is soluble fiber.

2. **d.** Anthraquinone glycosides

Aloe latex contains anthraquinone glycosides (aloin, aloe-emodin, and barbaloin) that act as potent colonic-specific stimulant laxatives.

3. **False**

Arrowroot has been primarily studied for its effect on diarrhea. Asparagus, not arrowroot, has been shown to be equivalent to metoclopramide in reducing gastric emptying time.

4. **d.** All the above

Peppermint has been used and studied for postoperative nausea (as inhalation), irritable bowel syndrome, and abdominal distention.

5. **a.** Warfarin

Artichoke may increase the risk of bleeding, based on a case report of significantly reduced platelet aggregation in patients taking artichoke extract; thus, interactions with warfarin are possible.

6. **True**

7. **d.** All the above

Psyllium has been used for constipation, diarrhea, and irritable bowel syndrome.

8. **b.** Cipro

Fennel contains high amounts of minerals, and formation of a ciprofloxacin-cation complex results. This formation may reduce ciprofloxacin absorption, as shown in rodents; however, clinical evidence of this interaction is lacking.

9. **All true** *except:* **c.** Flaxseed oil produces laxative effects.

Though oils may produce laxative effects, flaxseed (not flaxseed oil) is noted for its laxative effects because of its soluble fiber content.

10. **True**

Numerous studies report that infants and young children (2-36 months old) with diarrhea who are fed soy formulas experience fewer daily bowel movements and fewer days of diarrhea than those fed milk-based formulas. Soy has also been shown to improve weight gain.

CHAPTER 25
Liver Disorders

1. **All true** *except:* **b.** There is strong evidence supporting the use of milk thistle for all liver disorders.

Systematic reviews and meta-analyses concluded that the clinical efficacy of milk thistle for liver disease (e.g., hepatitis) has not been clearly established.

2. **False**

Neo-Minophagen C (SNMC) contains glycyrrhizin.

3. **d.** All the above

Kava kava (Piper methysticum), comfrey (Symphytum officinale), and germander (Teucrium chamaedrys) are all herbs with potential hepatotoxic effects.

4. **All true** *except:* **c.** Mistletoe is a key herb in *sho-saiko-to* for hepatitis C.

Bupleurum, not mistletoe, is a key herb in sho-saiko-to. The commercial preparation Iscador, containing mistletoe, has been used for hepatitis C.

5. True

6. b. 420 mg silymarin daily in three divided doses
Silymarin (Legalon) at 420 mg daily in three divided doses has been used for chronic hepatitis.

7. d. Both a and b
Cordyceps appears to inhibit hepatic fibrogenesis from liver injury and inhibition of transforming growth factor beta.

8. d. All the above
Varying mechanisms may lead to inflammation of the liver, including mitochondrial abnormalities, enhanced delivery of fatty acids to the liver, and defects in the uptake, metabolism, and secretion of lipids in liver.

9. False
Compound K is a metabolite of ginseng. p-Methoxybenzoic acid is the constituent of capers that appears to have hepatoprotective effects.

10. a. ELISA
Hepatitis C is usually diagnosed through an ELISA (enzyme-linked immunosorbent assay) that detects the presence of antibody to two regions of the hepatitis C genome.

CHAPTER 26
Genitourinary Disorders

1. b. Yohimbe is an active indole alkaloid constituent found in the bark of the yohimbine tree.
Because of the potential for serious side effects and interactions, the FDA has determined yohimbine to be unsafe for over-the-counter sale. Moreover, a 1995 chemical analysis of 26 commercial yohimbe products reported that most contained virtually no yohimbine. The pharmacological activity of yohimbine has been well characterized in studies, although these effects may or may not apply to yohimbe, depending on the concentration of yohimbine present.

2. False
The most popular use of Cernilton, prepared from rye grass pollen, is for treating benign prostatic hyperplasia (BPH).

3. d. Both a and c
Numerous human studies report that pygeum significantly reduced the number of nighttime urinary episodes, urinary hesitancy, urinary frequency, and pain with urination (dysuria) in men who experience mild to moderate symptoms.

4. All true except: b. Nettle does not appear to be well tolerated.
Nettle oral therapy was generally well tolerated for up to 2 years in available clinical trials.

5. d. Both a and b
Nopal and stinging nettle both appear to inhibit aromatase, a key enzyme in steroid hormone metabolism.

6. True
Panax ginseng has been shown to be superior to placebo and trazodone in the treatment of erectile dysfunction. However, it remains equivocal whether ginseng can be considered a standard therapy for erectile disorders.

7. a. Inhibition of nitric oxide
Ginkgo may be efficacious in the treatment of erectile dysfunction based on vasodilatory effects, possibly related to inhibition of nitric oxide.

8. c. 320 mg daily in one or two divided doses
For BPH, saw palmetto at 320 mg daily in one dose or two divided doses (80%-90% liposterolic content) has been used in multiple clinical trials and is recommended by the German Commission E.

9. All true except: a. Maca is rich in isoflavones.
Maca is not noted to contain significant amounts of isoflavones; however, maca is rich in plant sterols such as beta-sitosterol.

10. False
Numerous controlled trials have reported saw palmetto to be superior to placebo and possibly equivalent (but not superior) to the antiandrogenic agent finasteride (Proscar).

CHAPTER 27
Bacterial Infections

1. *False:* b. All bacteria are pathogenic to humans.
Not all bacteria are pathogenic to humans. Some bacteria, such as those that reside in the colon, are beneficial to humans.

2. True
Arbutin in uva ursi is reported to be active against Staphylococcus aureus (gram positive) and Escherichia coli (gram negative).

3. *False:* c. Cranberry hinders bacterial proliferation in the urinary tract by acidifying urine.
Cranberry was originally thought to prevent UTI by acidifying urine, but it is now widely believed to prevent bacteria from adhering to the cells that line the bladder.

4. d. All the above
Calendula, chiropractic manipulation, and belladonna have been suggested and used as adjunctive therapies for children with recurrent/chronic otitis media; however, not all have been proven to be effective.

5. d. All the above
Sanguinarine has demonstrated antibacterial activity against gram-positive and gram-negative bacteria. Sanguinarine may also kill animal cells by blocking the action of Na^+, K^+-ATPase transmembrane proteins. The reduction in bacterial growth may be caused by inhibition of bacterial adherence and plaque formation.

6. **False**

The standardized extract Kan Jang contains andrographis, not ginseng as its main active ingredient.

7. **d.** All the above

Angostura, garlic, and lavender have each demonstrated activity against mycobacteria.

8. **d.** Both a and b

Human studies have reported favorable effects of berberine ophthalmic preparations on trachoma. Berberine has also been used to treat cholera. Trachoma may also cause vaginal infections; however, the use of berberine for vaginitis has not been studied extensively.

9. **a.** The active ingredients are chlorhexidine and rhubarb.

The active ingredients of Pyralvex are rhubarb extract and salicylic acid.

10. **d.** Both a and c

Listerine is a broad-spectrum antibacterial mouthrinse that contains a combination of essential oils and other plant constituents (eucalyptol, menthol, thymol, methyl salicylate).

CHAPTER 28
Parasitic and Fungal Infections

1. **a.** Estrogen

Thyme has demonstrated estradiol and progesterone receptor-binding activity in vivo, although this has not been systematically studied or demonstrated in humans.

2. **c.** Tea tree oil is toxic when ingested.

Tea tree oil (derived from Melaleuca alternifolia) should not be used orally because of multiple reports of CNS toxicity and cutaneous allergic responses. Terpinen-4-ol is the component most likely responsible for tea tree's antimicrobial properties.

3. **False: d.** Sweet Annie should be avoided in patients taking antiplatelet or anticoagulant medications because of potential thrombotic effects.

Sweet Annie has not been reported to have effects on coagulation.

4. **c.** Lectinlike mucopolysaccharide

A lectinlike mucopolysaccharide isolated from Fucus vesiculosus has been found to cause agglutination of the yeast Candida guilliermondii and also inhibits its growth.

5. **False.**

Pomegranate extract may be effective in the treatment of oral candidiasis, but studies involving vaginal infections are lacking.

6. **c.** Both a and b

Berberine is an active constituent in both goldenseal and barberry.

7. **All except: c.** Plasmodium

Berberine has displayed activity against various types of parasites and fungi, including Alternaria spp., Candida albicans, Curvularia spp., Drechslera spp., Fusarium spp., Mucor spp., Rhizopus oryzae, Aspergillus flavus, Aspergillus fumigatus, Entamoeba histolytica, Giardia lamblia, Trichomonas vaginalis, and Leishmania donovani. However, in vitro research has reported no activity of berberine against Plasmodium in malaria.

8. **Incorrect: b.** It has been suggested that antimicrobial activity of garlic powder is more potent than garlic oil on a unit-weight basis.

Conversely, it has been suggested that garlic oil's antimicrobial activity is more potent than garlic powder on a unit-weight basis.

9. **d.** All the above.

Synephrine alkaloids and p-octopamine are usually cited as "active ingredients" on product labels; however, bitter orange also contains the furocoumarins bergapten and oxypeucedanin, which have well-established photosensitizing and photoreactive properties.

10. **False**

The potential for increased melanoma risk warrants caution when using any psoralens to accelerate skin pigmentation.

CHAPTER 29
Viral Infections

1. **b.** CD4+ T cells

HIV primarily infects and destroys immune cells with the CD4 receptor protein on their cell surfaces (CD4+ T cells).

2. **d.** All the above

Reactivation of latent herpesvirus infections may be triggered by menstruation, sun exposure, illness with fever, stress, immune system imbalances, and other unknown causes.

3. **False**

A sage and rhubarb cream decreased skin swelling and reduced pain, appeared to be as effective as acyclovir (Zovirax) cream, and was more effective than sage alone.

4. **d.** All the above

The antiviral effects of aloe may be caused by interference with DNA synthesis, inhibition of the replication of human immunodeficiency virus type 1 (HIV-1) and herpes simplex virus type 1 (HSV-1), and modification of the glycosylation of viral glycoproteins.

5. **True**

According to a clinical study, administration of lentinan with didanosine significantly increased CD4+ levels for up to 38 weeks.

6. **True**

Immunostimulatory properties of echinacea appear to target both nonspecific and specific immune function. Nonspecific effects include increases in macrophage proliferation and phagocytosis, as well as secretion of interferon (IFN), tumor necrosis factor (TNF), and interleukin-1 (IL-1), in vitro and in vivo. Specific immune responses include the activation of alternate complement pathway components and elevated levels/activity of T lymphocytes and natural killer (NK) cells.

7. **c.** Significant adverse effects and interactions with protease inhibitors (PIs) and nonnucleoside reverse transcriptase inhibitors (NNRTIs) have been reported with concurrent use of St. John's wort.

Multiple reports of significant adverse effects and interactions with PIs and NNRTIs may preclude any use in patients with HIV/AIDS.

8. **d.** All the above

Research suggests that elder may reduce mucus production. Oral elderberry has been reported to improve flulike symptoms, and rescue medication was required less in those receiving elderberry.

9. **c.** Both a and b

Glycyrrhizin, a glycoside of licorice, has been reported to inhibit HIV replication and may be beneficial as an alternative or adjunct to antiviral therapy in patients with herpes zoster.

10. **True**

Mistletoe has been shown to increase production of IFN-α, TNF, and IL-1 and activity and number of NK cells.

CHAPTER 30
Cancer

1. **All true except: b.** The half-life of aloe-emodin is 4 to 6 hours.

The half-life of aloe-emodin is 48 to 50 hours.

2. **True**

3. **d.** All these are true.

NDGA has been theorized to block cellular respiration and inhibit cell metabolism. It has also been demonstrated to release stored calcium from the endoplasmic reticulum. However, NDGA has been demonstrated to have mutagenic potential as well; stimulation of tumor growth was reported in an early study using NDGA to treat cancer.

4. **False**

Cranberry should be used cautiously to treat cancer because there is some evidence that cranberry pills are strongly associated with bladder cancer.

5. **d.** All the above

Panax quinquefolius synergistically inhibited cancer cell growth when used in combination with the breast cancer therapeutic agents cyclophosphamide (Cytoxan), doxorubicin, fluorouracil, and methotrexate.

6. **c.** *Coriolus versicolor* mushroom

PSK, or polysaccharide K, is obtained from cultured mycelia of the mushroom *Coriolus versicolor*.

7. **All true except: b.** Shiitake lentinan has not been shown to benefit mean survival time in cancer patients.

When combined with standard chemotherapeutic agents, lentinan resulted in reduced tumor size, improvement of symptoms, and improved survival time in various clinical trials and case studies.

8. **a.** Mistletoe is a widely used cancer treatment in Europe.

Mistletoe is one of the most widely used alternative cancer treatments in Europe. However, efficacy has not been conclusively demonstrated for any one condition. Mistletoe plants and berries are toxic to humans, and their extracts are not sold in the United States.

9. **a.** Antiproliferative and/or proapoptotic effects in numerous cell lines

In vitro, curcumin derivatives demonstrated antiproliferative and/or proapoptotic effects in numerous cell lines, including multidrug-resistant cell lines, rat aortic smooth muscle cells, leukemic cells, human breast cancer cells, and human epidermoid carcinoma cells. Turmeric has been shown to be nonmutagenic by the Ames test and may reduce protein kinase C activity and oxidative damage.

10. **c.** Silymarin

Silymarin, composed of silydianin, silychristine, and silibinin, is considered the active constituent of milk thistle. Silica, salicylic acid, and aviscumine are major constituents of horsetail, willow bark, and mistletoe, respectively.

Index

A

AAMI *See* Age-associated memory impairment (AAMI)
Abana
  for angina, 131b
  for hypertension, 109b
Abdomen
  massage of for constipation, 339
  peppermint for distention of, 330
Abdominal obesity, 253
Abdominal pain in irritable bowel syndrome, 319-320
Absence seizure, 62, 62t
Abuse, substance, 40
Abuta *(Cissampelos pareira)*, 570
Acacia *(Acacia senegal)*
  adverse effects, interactions, and pharmacokinetics of, 486
  for dental plaque, 389
  for lipid disorders, 189
  pregnancy and lactation and, 570
ACE inhibitors. *See* Angiotensin-converting enzyme (ACE) inhibitors, cough associated with
Acetaminophen, hepatic toxicity of, 345, 356
Acetylcholinesterase inhibitors, ginkgo *versus*, 91
Acetyl coenzyme A, 171
Acid-fast bacilli, 383
Acid reflux disease, 316
Aconite *(Aconitum napellus)*
  adverse effects, interactions, and pharmacokinetics of, 486-487
  for arrhythmias, 141
  for congestive heart failure, 117
  for pain, 72
  pregnancy and lactation and, 570
  for thyroid disease, 247
Acquired immunodeficiency syndrome (AIDS), 427. *See Also* Human immunodeficiency virus (HIV)
Acromegaly, 242
ACS *See* Acute coronary syndrome (ACS)
ACTH *See* Adrenocorticotropic hormone (ACTH)
Activated partial thromboplastin time (aPTT), 159

Acupressure
  auricular, for smoking cessation, 210, 213
  for nausea and vomiting and irritable bowel syndrome, 339
  for pain, 82
Acupuncture
  for angina, 132
  for arthritis, 309
  for cholesterol levels and heart health, 191
  for genitourinary disorders, 376
  for irritable bowel syndrome, 339
  for nausea and vomiting, 339
    chemotherapy-induced, 480
  for weight loss, 262
Acute coronary syndrome (ACS), 135, 136f
Acute pain, 70-71
Acute respiratory distress syndrome (ARDS), 201-209
Adenoma, pituitary, 242
ADH *See* Antidiuretic hormone (ADH)
Adjustment disorders, 30-31
Adolescent, depression in, 29
Adrenocorticotropic hormone (ACTH), 241
  disorders of, 243
Adult-onset asthma, 197
Adverse effects, 486-568
Aerobes, 383
African eye worm infection, 411
African wild potato *(Hypoxis hemerocallidea)*
  for arthritis, 306
  for benign prostatic hyperplasia, 364
  for diabetes mellitus, 234
Agaric *(Amanita muscaria)*
  pregnancy and lactation and, 570
  for psychiatric disorders, 13
Agave *(Agave* spp.), 571
Age-associated memory impairment (AAMI), 91-92
Agitation in dementia
  aromatherapy and music therapy for, 99
  bitter orange for, 97
  grape seed for, 92-93
  lemon balm for, 94

Agrimony *(Agrimonia* spp.)
  adverse effects, interactions, and pharmacokinetics of, 487
  for diabetes mellitus, 234
  for gastrointestinal disorders, 320-322
  pregnancy and lactation and, 571
  for tuberculosis, 398-399
AIDS. *See* Acquired immunodeficiency syndrome (AIDS)
Airway obstruction, asthmatic, 197
  belladonna for prevention of, 200
ALA. *See* Alpha-linolenic acid (ALA)
Alcohol
  acacia interaction with, 486
  cancer and, 483
  diabetes mellitus and, 237
  gout and, 310
  irritable bowel syndrome and, 341
  liver disease due to, 343-344
    case study, 356-357
    milk thistle for, 350
  osteoporosis and, 288-289
  pregnancy and lactation and, 571
Alcoholism, chronic, 345
Alder buckthorn *(Frangula alnus)*, 571
Alertness, sandalwood for, 48
Alfalfa *(Medicago sativa)*
  adverse effects, interactions, and pharmacokinetics of, 487-488
  for diabetes mellitus, 220
  for fungal infections, 419
  for lipid disorders, 173
  for menopausal symptoms, 268
  pregnancy and lactation and, 571
Allergy
  asthma due to, 197
  food, asthma and, 212
  onion for, 206
  rhinitis due to, 198-199
    butterbur for, 202
    ephedra for, 204-205
    stinging nettle for, 208
Aloe *(Aloe vera)*
  adverse effects, interactions, and pharmacokinetics of, 488
  for cancer prevention, 450
  for diabetes mellitus, 220
  for gastrointestinal disorders, 320-323

Aloe *(Aloe vera) (Continued)*
   pregnancy and lactation and, 571
   for viral infection, 431, 442
Alpha-granule deficiency, 157
Alpha-herpesvirinae, 429
Alpha-linolenic acid (ALA)
   adverse effects, interactions, and pharmacokinetics of, 540-541
   for cardiovascular health, 177
   for hypertension, 105
   for lipid disorders, 182
   pregnancy and lactation and, 586
Alport syndrome, 157
Alternative medical systems, 1
Alzheimer's disease, 86-101
   adjunct therapies for, 97-99
   case studies for, 99-100
   depression and, 35
   diagnosis of, 88-89, 88b
   herbal therapies for, 89-97, 97t-98t
      with negative evidence, 97
   integrative therapy plan for, 99-100
   overview of, 86-89
   signs and symptoms of, 87-88, 87b
Amanita phalloides mushroom poisoning, 349
Ambrette *(Abelmoschus moschatus)*, 571
American ginseng. *See* Ginseng *(Panax* spp.)
American hellebore *(Veratrum viride)*. *See* False hellebore *(Veratrum* spp.)
American pawpaw *(Asimina triloba)*
   adverse effects, interactions, and pharmacokinetics of, 488
   for cancer treatment, 450, 483
   pregnancy and lactation and, 571
American pennyroyal *(Hedeoma pulegioides)*. *See* False pennyroyal *(Hedeoma* spp.)
Amoxicillin, acacia interaction with, 486
Anaerobes, 383
Anal fissure, 331-332
Analgesia, 79t *See Also* Pain
   arnica for, 72
Anapsos. *See* Polypodium *(Polypodium leucotomos)*
Ancylostoma duodenale, 410
Andrographis *(Andrographis paniculata)*
   adverse effects, interactions, and pharmacokinetics of, 488-489
   for diabetes mellitus, 234
   pregnancy and lactation and, 571
   for upper respiratory tract infection, 389
   for viral infections, 431, 442
Anemia, radiotherapy-induced, 479
Aneurysm, 138
Angel's trumpet *(Brugmansia* and *Datura* spp.)
   pregnancy and lactation and, 571
   for psychiatric disorders, 13

Angina, 127
   adjunct therapies for, 132, 150
   associated with myocardial infarction, 135
   case studies for, 132-133
   diagnosis of, 128-129
   herbal therapies for, 129-131, 131t
      with limited evidence, 131-132
   integrative therapy plan for, 132-133
   overview of, 127-129
   signs and symptoms of, 128
Angiography, computed tomographic, 128-129, 138
Angioplasty, 128
Angiotensin-converting enzyme (ACE) inhibitors
   for angina, 128
   cough associated with, 124
Angostura *(Galipea officinalis*, syn. *Angostura trifoliata)*, 399
Anise *(Pimpinella anisum)*
   pregnancy and lactation and, 571
   for respiratory disorders, 209
Annatto *(Bixa orellana)*, 571
Antibiotics, 381-383
   for leprosy, 385
   resistance to, 404
Antibodies, asthma and, 197
Antibody titer in viral diagnosis, 430-431
Antidiuretic hormone (ADH), 242
   disorders of, 243
Antigen detection in viral diagnosis, 431
Antigenic shift in influenza, 428
Antimicrobials, 381-383
Antineoplastic agents
   acacia interaction with, 486
   in cancer treatment, 481
Antioxidants
   in cancer treatment, 482, 484
      interference of, 449
   for congestive heart failure, 124
Antivirals, 428
Anxiety
   in heart disease patients, panchakarma for, 131b
   during menopause, 277
   seizure disorders and, 66-67
Anxiety disorders, 17-28
   adjunct therapies for, 25-26
   case studies associated with, 26
   herbal therapies for, 20-24, 25t
      with limited evidence, 24-25
      with negative evidence, 24
   integrative therapies for, 26-27
   overview of, 17-19
   signs and symptoms of, 18
Aphasia in Alzheimer's disease, 88
Apoptosis, 445
Apple *(Malus sylvestris)*, 571
Apraxia in Alzheimer's disease, 88

Apricot *(Prunus armeniaca)*
   adverse effects, interactions, and pharmacokinetics of, 489
   for cancer, 474-475
   pregnancy and lactation and, 572
aPTT. *See* Activated partial thromboplastin time (aPTT)
Arabinoxylan in cancer treatment, 481
Arbutin, 398
Arcus senilis, 171
ARDS. *See* Acute respiratory distress syndrome (ARDS)
Arecoline, 12
Arginine for growth hormone deficiency, 248
Aristolochia *(Aristolochia* spp.), 572
Arjuna *(Terminalia arjuna)*, 131b
Arnica *(Arnica* spp.)
   for acute diarrhea in children, 321
   adverse effects, interactions, and pharmacokinetics of, 489
   for osteoarthritis, 296
   for pain, 72
   pregnancy and lactation and, 572
   propranolol and, 153
   for stroke, 141
Aromatase inhibition by stinging nettle, 373
Aromatherapy
   for Alzheimer's disease, 99-100
   in cancer treatment, 480
Arrhythmia, 30, 134-154
   aconite for, 141
   case study for, 152
   diagnosis of, 140
   foxglove for, 149
   herbal therapies for, 148t-149t
   herbs causing, 150
   integrative therapy plan for, 151-154
   signs and symptoms of, 140
   Traditional Chinese medicine for, 147b
   types of, 139
Arrowroot *(Maranta arundinacea)*
   adverse effects, interactions, and pharmacokinetics of, 489-490
   for gastrointestinal disorders, 321, 341
Artemisinin. *See* Sweet Annie *(Artemisia annua)*
Arteriography, 128, 138
Arteriovenous malformation (AVM), rupture of, 137-138
Arthritis, 291-314
   adjunct therapies for, 309-310
   case studies associated with, 311-313
   gouty, 296
   herbal therapies for, 296-306, 307t-308t
      with limited evidence, 306-309
      with negative evidence, 306

Arthritis *(Continued)*
　infectious, 295
　integrative therapy plan for, 310-313
　osteoarthritis, 292
　overview of, 291-296
　periarthritis, 294-295
　reactive, 295-296
　rheumatoid, 293-294
　　juvenile, 295
Art therapy
　in cancer treatment, 480
　for elderly patients, 99-100
Arum *(Arum maculatam)*, 572
Asafoetida *(Ferula assafoetida)*, 572
Ascariasis, 410
　elecampane for, 419
　noni for, 420
Ash *(Fraxinus* spp.)
　adverse effects, interactions, and pharmacokinetics of, 490
　for gouty arthritis, 296-297
Ashwagandha *(Withania somnifera)*
　adverse effects, interactions, and pharmacokinetics of, 490
　for congestive heart failure, 117
　for depressive disorders, 34
　for diabetes mellitus, 221
　for lipid disorders, 173
　for osteoarthritis, 297
　for Parkinson's disease, 55-57, 59
　pregnancy and lactation and, 572
Asian ginseng. *See* Ginseng *(Panax* spp.)
Asparagus *(Asparagus officinalis)*
　adverse effects, interactions, and pharmacokinetics of, 490
　for dyspepsia, 321
　pregnancy and lactation and, 572
Aspirin, 3
　bleeding stomach ulcer due to, 328
Asthma, 197-198, 211t-212t
　ayurveda for, 209
　belladonna for, 200
　borage for, 200
　boswellia for, 201
　butterbur for, 201-202
　case study, 213-214
　choline for, 210
　danshen for, 203
　English ivy for, 204
　ephedra for, 204
　eucalyptus for, 205
　evening primrose for, 209
　forskolin for, 203
　integrative therapy plan for, 212-214
　magnesium for, 210
　peppermint for, 206
　perilla for, 207
　pycnogenol for, 207
　St. John's wort for, 210

Asthma *(Continued)*
　tea for, 208
　tylophora for, 208-209
Astragalus *(Astragalus membranaceus)*
　adverse effects, interactions, and pharmacokinetics of, 490-491
　for Alzheimer's disease and related disorders, 89
　for cancer treatment, 450-451, 476
　for chemotherapy-induced nausea and vomiting, 476, 483-484
　for cognitive and physical enhancement, 44
　for congestive heart failure, 118
　for coronary artery disease, 141-142, 152
　for diabetes mellitus, 221
　for lipid disorders, 173
　for liver disorders, 346, 356
　for smoking cessation, 210
　for tuberculosis, 174
　for viral infections, 432, 442
ASU. *See* Avacado/soybean unsaponifiables (ASU)
Ataxia in Parkinson's disease, 58-59
Atherosclerosis, 137
　alfalfa for, 173
　chia for, 176
　flax for, 143, 177
　garlic for, 143-144, 178
　horny goat weed for, 144-145
　lemon grass for, 181
　pomegranate for, 145
　safflower for, 146, 186
Athlete's foot, 413
　garlic for, 416
　tea tree for, 417
Athletic performance, 44, 51
　adjunct therapies, 51
　astragalus for, 44
　cordyceps for, 45
　evening primrose for, 45
　garcinia for, 45
　ginseng for, 46
　kiwi for, 47
　papaya for, 47
　rhodiola for, 47
　tribulus for, 48, 51
Atkins Diet
　in epilepsy treatment, 66
　for weight loss, 261
Atonic seizure, 63
Atrial fibrillation, 137, 139-140
Atrial flutter, 139
Attachment of virus, 428
Attention disorders, 41-42, 42b
　adjunct therapies for, 49-51
　evening primrose for, 45
　pycnogenol for, 47, 51
Atypical depression, 30
Aura before seizure, 61

Auricular acupressure for smoking cessation, 210, 213
Autoantibodies in thyroid disorders, 246
Automatisms in complex partial seizures, 62
Autumn crocus *(Colchicum autumnale* spp.), 572
Avacado/soybean unsaponifiables (ASU)
　for osteoarthritis, 297, 311-312
AVM. *See* Arteriovenous malformation (AVM), rupture of
Avocado *(Persea americana)*
　adverse effects, interactions, and pharmacokinetics of, 491
　for lipid disorders, 174
　for osteoarthritis, 297-298
　pregnancy and lactation and, 572
Ayurveda, 56b
　for Alzheimer's disease, 97b
　for angina, 131b
　for asthma, 209b
　for depression, 34b
　for hypertension, 109b
　for osteoarthritis, 306b
　pregnancy and lactation and, 572
　for viral hepatitis, 353b

B

Bach flower remedies, 48b
　for attention disorders, 48b
　for depression, 34b
　pregnancy and lactation and, 572
Back pain, lower, 69
　devil's claw for, 75, 84
　willow for, 78-79
Bacopa *(Bacopa monnieri)*
　adverse effects, interactions, and pharmacokinetics of, 491
　for Alzheimer's disease and related disorders, 89-90, 100
　for anxiety and insomnia, 20-23
　diazepam and, 341
　for irritable bowel syndrome, 321
　for psychiatric disorders, 13
　for seizure disorders, 64, 67
Bacterial infection, 380-407, 382t
　adjunct therapies for, 400-403
　case studies associated with, 404-406
　cholera, 384-385
　conjunctivitis, 383-384
　in diarrhea, 318
　in foodborne illness, 385
　gram-negative, 383
　gram-positive, 383
　herbal therapies for, 389, 401t-403t
　　with limited evidence, 398-400
　　with negative evidence, 398
　in infectious arthritis, 295
　integrative therapy plan for, 403-406
　in leprosy, 385-386

Bacterial infection *(Continued)*
   in meningitis, 384
   methicillin-resistant *Staphylococcus aureus*, 386
   mycobacterial, 383
   Mycobacterium avium complex, 386
   in otitis media, 386-387
   overview of, 380-389, 381f
   oxygen dependence and, 383
   periodontal, 387
   in prostatitis, 362-363, 363t
   in Reiter's syndrome, 295
   in trachoma, 387
   in tuberculosis, 388
   types of, 383-389
   upper respiratory tract, 388
   urinary tract, 388-389
Bael *(Aegle marmelos)*
   for irritable bowel syndrome, 321
   pregnancy and lactation and, 572
Baikal skullcap *(Scutellaria baicalensis)*. See Skullcap *(Scutellaria* spp.)
Baker cyst, 292
Balloon angioplasty, 128
Balneotherapy for arthritis, 309-310
Bamboo *(Arundinaria japonica)*, 399
Banaba *(Lagerstroemia speciosa)*
   adverse effects, interactions, and pharmacokinetics of, 491
   for diabetes mellitus, 221
Barbat skullcap *(Scutellaria barbata)*. See Skullcap *(Scutellaria* spp.)
Barberry *(Berberis* spp.) See Berberine
Barley *(Hordeum vulgare)*
   adverse effects, interactions, and pharmacokinetics of, 491-492
   for diabetes mellitus, 221
   for gastrointestinal disorders, 322-328
   for lipid disorders, 174
   pregnancy and lactation and, 573
   for weight loss, 259
Basophils, 197
Bean *(Phaseolus vulgaris)*, 573
Beaver fever, 409-410
Bedwetting, 361
Beef tapeworm, 410
Bee pollen in cancer treatment, 481
Beet *(Beta vulgaris)*
   adverse effects, interactions, and pharmacokinetics of, 492
   for diabetes mellitus, 222
   for lipid disorders, 174
   pregnancy and lactation and, 573
Belladonna *(Atropa* spp.)
   adverse effects, interactions, and pharmacokinetics of, 492
   for headache, 73
   for irritable bowel syndrome, 322b

Belladonna *(Atropa* spp.) *(Continued)*
   for menopausal symptoms, 268-269
   for Parkinson's disease, 57
   pregnancy and lactation and, 573
   for radiodermatitis, 479
   for respiratory disorders, 200
Bellergal for menopausal symptoms, 269
Benign prostatic hyperplasia (BPH), 360
   African wild potato for, 364
   beta-sitosterol for, 365
   case study for, 376
   integrative therapy plan for, 376
   nopal for, 370
   pygeum for, 370
   red clover for, 371
   rye for, 371
   saw palmetto for, 372
   stinging nettle for, 373
Benign tumor, 445
Berberine
   adverse effects, interactions, and pharmacokinetics of, 493
   for bacterial infection, 404-406
   for cholera, 403
   for diabetes mellitus, 222
   for gastrointestinal disorders, 327
   for infectious diarrhea, 394
   for parasitic and fungal infection, 416, 419, 424
   pregnancy and lactation and, 573
   for trachoma, 394
Bergamot oil *(Citrus bergamia)*, 573
Bernard-Soulier syndrome, 157
Beta blockers for angina, 128
Beta-glucan (β-glucan)
   adverse effects, interactions, and pharmacokinetics of, 493-494
   for diabetes mellitus, 222
   for HIV, 432
   for lipid disorders, 175
   pregnancy and lactation and, 573
   for weight loss, 259
Beta-herpesvirinae, 429
Beta-sitosterol (β-sitosterol)
   adverse effects, interactions, and pharmacokinetics of, 494-495
   for benign prostatic hyperplasia, 365
   for lipid disorders, 175, 192
   pregnancy and lactation and, 573
   for tuberculosis, 399
Betel nut *(Areca catechu)*
   adverse effects, interactions, and pharmacokinetics of, 153, 495
   for cognitive and physical enhancement, 44
   for dental caries, 390-391
   for inflammatory bowel disease, 335
   pregnancy and lactation and, 573
   for psychiatric disorders, 12

Betel nut *(Areca catechu) (Continued)*
   for stroke, 142
   for xerostomia, 476-479
Betony *(Stachys* spp.)
   pregnancy and lactation and, 573
   for seizure disorders, 64-65
Bifidobacterium as probiotic, 400
Bilberry *(Vaccinium myrtillus)*
   adverse effects, interactions, and pharmacokinetics of, 496
   for coronary artery disease, 148-150
   for diabetes mellitus, 234
   for peptic ulcer disease, 335
   pregnancy and lactation and, 573
Bile flow stimulant, white horehound as, 334
Biologically based therapies
Bipolar disorder, 15, 31
   omega-3 fatty acids for, 98
Birch *(Betula* spp.), 573
Bisabolol, 399
Bishop's weed *(Ammi majus)*
   adverse effects, interactions, and pharmacokinetics of, 496
   for tinea versicolor, 414-415
Bitter almond *(Prunus amygdalus)*
   adverse effects, interactions, and pharmacokinetics of, 496
   for cancer, 474
   pregnancy and lactation and, 574
Bitter apple *(Citrullus colocynthis)*, 574
Bitter melon *(Momordica charantia)*
   adverse effects, interactions, and pharmacokinetics of, 496-497
   for cancer, 475
   for diabetes mellitus, 223
   for HIV, 432-433, 442
   for parasitic infection, 419
   pregnancy and lactation and, 574
Bitter orange *(Citrus aurantium)*
   adverse effects, interactions, and pharmacokinetics of, 497
   for Alzheimer's disease and related disorders, 97
   for cognitive and physical enhancement, 49
   for fungal infections, 415
   for weight loss, 51, 253, 264
Blackberry *(Rubus fructicosus)*, 574
Black bryony *(Tamus communis,* syn. *Dioscorea communis)*, 574
Black cohosh *(Actaea racemosa,* formerly *Cimicifuga racemosa)*
   adverse effects, interactions, and pharmacokinetics of, 497-498
   for arthritis, 298
   in breast cancer treatment, 451, 484
   for menopausal symptoms, 269, 277-279

Black cohosh *(Actaea racemosa,* formerly
    Cimicifuga racemosa) (Continued)
    for osteoporosis, 285
    pregnancy and lactation and, 574
Black currant *(Ribes nigrum)*
    adverse effects, interactions, and pharmacokinetics of, 498-499
    for hypertension, 103
    for rheumatoid arthritis, 298
Black haw *(Viburnum prunifolium),* 574
Black mulberry *(Morus nigra),* 574
Black mustard *(Brassica nigra),* 574
Black pepper *(Piper nigrum),* 499
    adverse effects, interactions, and pharmacokinetics of, 499
    for masking withdrawal symptoms from stimulants, 51
    in stoke recovery therapy, 151
Black seed *(Nigella sativa),* 574
Black tea. *See* Tea *(Camellia sinensis)*
Bladder. *See Also* Genitourinary disorders
    anatomy of, 360f
    cancer of
        rhodiola for, 465-466
        signs and symptoms of, 446
    infection of, 388
    neurogenic, 362
        saw palmetto for, 372
Bladderwrack *(Fucus vesiculosus). See*
    Seaweed
Bleeding
    gastric ulcer due to aspirin use, licorice for, 328
    herbs that may increase risk of, 165t-166t
    increased in coagulation disorders, 158
    diagnosis of, 158-159
    perioperative considerations, cancer and, 449
    postpartum, daisy for, 160
    upper gastrointestinal, rhubarb for, 162, 332
Blessed thistle *(Cnicus benedictus)*
    adverse effects, interactions, and pharmacokinetics of, 499-500
    for bacterial infection, 399, 405-406
    for gastrointestinal disorders, 322-330
    pregnancy and lactation and, 574
    for viral infection, 433, 442
Blindness, river, 411
Blood
    coagulation disorders of (*See* Coagulation disorders)
    coagulopathy and, 157-158
    hemostasis and, 155-156
Blood clot. *See Also* Embolus; Thrombosis
    in coagulation, 155
    dissolution of, 156
    turmeric for prevention of, 163

Blood glucose testing in diabetes mellitus
    for diagnosis, 219
    for monitoring, 220
Blood pressure, 102
    high (*See* Hypertension)
    low (*See* Hypotension)
Bloodroot *(Sanguinaria canadensis)*
    adverse effects, interactions, and pharmacokinetics of, 500
    for dental plaque, gingivitis and periodontal disease, 391, 404
    pregnancy and lactation and, 574
Blood vessel wall, hemostasis and, 155-156
Blueberry *(Vaccinium angustifolium),* 574
Blue cohosh *(Caulophyllum thalictroides)*
    pregnancy and lactation and, 575
    for seizure disorders, 64
BMD. *See* Bone mineral density (BMD) in osteoporosis
BMI. *See* Body mass index (BMI)
Body mass index (BMI), 253, 262
Boldo *(Peumus boldus),* 575
Bone
    cancer of, 447
    osteoporosis and, 281-283
    remodeling of, 281-282
        in osteoarthritis, 292
    resorption of, 245, 281
Bone mineral density (BMD) in osteoporosis, 283, 283t, 286
    tea and, 285
Boneset *(Eupatorium* spp.)
    adverse effects, interactions, and pharmacokinetics of, 500
    for common cold and influenza, 433
    pregnancy and lactation and, 575
Borage *(Borago officinalis)*
    adverse effects, interactions, and pharmacokinetics of, 500-501
    for anxiety and insomnia, 20
    for lipid disorders, 175
    pregnancy and lactation and, 575
    for respiratory disorders, 200-201
    for rheumatoid arthritis, 298-299, 311
    seizures due to, 65
Boswellia *(Boswellia serrata)*
    adverse effects, interactions, and pharmacokinetics of, 501
    for arthritis, 299
    for brain cancer, 451-452
    for inflammatory bowel disease, 323-330
    pregnancy and lactation and, 575
    for respiratory disorders, 201, 209, 212
Bowel cleansing, cascara for, 324
Boxwood *(Buxus sempervirens)*
    adverse effects, interactions, and pharmacokinetics of, 501
    for HIV/AIDS, 433-434, 442

BPH. *See* Benign prostatic hyperplasia (BPH)
Bradycardia, 138-140. *See Also* Arrhythmia
Bradykinesia in Parkinson's disease, 55
Brain
    Alzheimer's disease and, 87-88
    anatomy of, 12f
    cancer of
        boswellia for, 451-452
        signs and symptoms of, 447
    cerebrovascular accident in, 137-138
    injury of
        bupleurum for, 90
        peppermint for, 94
    normal, 54f
    pain and, 69
    Parkinson's disease and, 54f
    psychiatric disorders and, 12f
    seizures and, 61
    stimulants and, 39
Brain scan in Alzheimer's disease diagnosis, 89
Breakthrough pain, 71, 83
Breast cancer
    bromelain for, 452-454
    case study associated with, 484
    evening primrose for, 455
    flax for, 455
    milk thistle for, 460
    prevention of
        black cohosh for, 451
        soy for, 469-470
    PSK for, 464, 475
    screening for, 447-448
    signs and symptoms of, 447
    tea for, 473
Breast pain, soy for, 77-78
Breast self-examination (BSE), 447-448
Breviscapine *(Erigeron breviscapus),* 164
Bromelain (Bromeliaceae)
    adverse effects, interactions, and pharmacokinetics of, 502
    for cancer, 452
    for pain and inflammation, 73, 83-84
    for respiratory disorders, 201
    for rheumatoid arthritis, 299
    for urinary tract infection, 391-392
Bronchitis, 198
Bronchoconstriction, asthmatic, 204
Bronchospasm, asthmatic, 197
Brugia malayi, 411
Bryonia *(Bryonia* spp.), 575
BSE. *See* Breast self-examination (BSE)
Buchu *(Agathosma betulina),* 575
Buckhorn plantain *(Plantago lanceolata),* 575
Buckwheat *(Fagopyrum esculentum),* 575
Bugleweed *(Lycopus* spp.), 575

Bupleurum (*Bupleurum* spp.)
    adverse effects, interactions, and pharmacokinetics of, 502
    for brain injury, 90
    for hepatitis, 346-347
    for hepatocellular carcinoma prevention, 453
Burdock (*Arctium lappa*)
    adverse effects, interactions, and pharmacokinetics of, 502-503
    for diabetes mellitus, 223
    pregnancy and lactation and, 575-576
Butterbur (*Petasites hybridus*)
    adverse effects, interactions, and pharmacokinetics of, 503
    for migraine prophylaxis, 73-74
    for respiratory disorders, 201-202
Bypass graft, coronary artery, 128

C

Cabbage (*Brassica oleracea* var. Capitata), 576
CABG *See* Coronary artery bypass graft (CABG)
CAD *See* Coronary artery disease (CAD)
Caffeine, 46
    adverse effects, interactions, and pharmacokinetics of, 503-504
    for asthma, 208
    for fatigue and low energy, 43-44
    in guarana, 46
    Parkinson's disease and, 56
    pregnancy and lactation and, 576
Calamus (*Acorus calamus*)
    pregnancy and lactation and, 576
    for psychiatric disorders, 13
Calcitonin, 244
Calcium
    daily requirements, 282t
    elevated blood levels of, 245
    for hypertension, 110
    low blood levels of, 245
    for menopausal symptoms, 276, 278
    for osteoporosis, 285-286, 288
    for thyroid disorders, 248
    for weight loss, 261
Calcium channel blockers for angina, 128
Calculi, renal, 363-364
    cornflower for, 374
    cranberry for, 366-371, 377
    grapefruit for, 368
Calendula (*Calendula officinalis*), 576
Calorie intake during menopause, 274-276
CAM. *See* Complementary and alternative medicine (CAM)
Camphor (*Cinnamomum camphora*)
    for pain, 79
    pregnancy and lactation and, 576
Canadian hemp (*Apocynum cannabinum*), 576

Cancer, 444-485. *See Also* specific types
    adjunct therapy for, 479-482
    case studies associated with, 483-484
    diagnosis of, 447-449
        diagnostic testing in, 448
        screening in, 447-448
        staging in, 449
    herbal therapies for, 450-452, 477t-479t
        with limited evidence, 475-476
        with negative evidence, 474-475
    integrative therapy plan for, 482-484
    management of toxicity and side effects due to treatment of, 476-479
    new cases of and deaths associated with, 445t
    overview of, 445-450, 445t
    remission of, 449-450
    safety concerns in, 449
    signs and symptoms of, 446-447
    thyroid, 245
Candidemia, 414
Candidiasis, 413-414
    case study associated with, 424
    cinnamon for, 415
    eucalyptus for, 393
    kiwi for, 420
    pomegranate for, 417
    probiotics for, 423-424
    propolis for, 420-423
    tea tree for, 417
Caper (*Capparis spinosa*)
    adverse effects, interactions, and pharmacokinetics of, 504-505
    for cirrhosis, 347-350
Capsaicin for pain, 83
Capsicum (*Capsicum* spp.)
    for lipid disorders, 190
    pregnancy and lactation and, 576
    for weight loss, 254
Caraway (*Carum carvi*), 576
Cardamom (*Elettaria cardamomum*), 576
Cardiac cycle, 140
Cardiac remodeling, 124
Cardiac stress test, 128
Cardiomyopathy, 118, 151
Cardiopulmonary bypass (CPB), 74
Cardiovascular disorders
    angina, 127-133
    chia for prevention of, 176
    congestive heart failure, 114-126
    hypertension, 102-113
    ischemic, 134-154
    lipid disorders and, 170-195
    menopause and, 276
    rhythm, 134-154
Caries, dental
    betel nut for, 390-391
    tea for, 397

Carnitine for thyroid disorders, 248
Carob (*Ceratonia siliqua*)
    adverse effects, interactions, and pharmacokinetics of, 505
    for gastrointestinal disorders, 323
    for lipid disorders, 176
Carotid ultrasonography, 128, 138
Carrot (*Daucus carota*), 576
Cartilage, osteoarthritis and, 292
Cascara (*Rhamnus purshiana*)
    adverse effects, interactions, and pharmacokinetics of, 505
    for bowel cleansing, 324
    pregnancy and lactation and, 576
Cashew (*Anacardium occidentale*), 576
Cassia (*Cortex cinnamomi*), 247
Castor (*Ricinus* spp.), 577
Cataplexy in narcolepsy, 42
Catecholamines in asthma, 197
Categorical pain scale, 71
Cat's claw (*Uncaria* spp.)
    adverse effects, interactions, and pharmacokinetics of, 505-506
    for arthritis, 299-300, 312
    in cancer treatment, 453, 484
    for pain, 79
    pregnancy and lactation and, 577
    for respiratory disorders, 202
Cayenne pepper (*Capsicum annum*). *See* Capsicum (*Capsicum* spp.)
CD4+ cell count in human immunodeficiency virus, 429
Cedar leaf (*Thuja occidentalis*), 577
Celery (*Apium graveolens*), 577
Central nervous system. *See Also* Brain
    normal, 54f
    Parkinson's disease and, 54f
    psychiatric disorders and, 12f
    stimulants and, 39
Cerebral insufficiency, 45, 90-92, 151
Cerebrovascular accident (CVA), 137-138, 158
    arnica for, 141
    betel nut for, 142
    danshen for, 142-143
    diagnosis of, 138
    embolic, 158
    ginkgo for, 144
    high blood pressure and, 102-103
    signs and symptoms of, 138
    tea for, 147
    thrombotic, 137, 158
Cernilton, 371
Cervical cancer
    milk thistle for, 460
    screening for, 448
CF. *See* Cystic fibrosis (CF)
CFS. *See* Chronic fatigue syndrome (CFS)

Coronary artery disease (CAD) *(Continued)*
   myocardial infarction as first sign of, 137
   policosanol for, 145
   red yeast rice for, 185
   reishi mushroom for, 130, 186
   safflower for, 131, 146
   soy for, 187
   squill for, 147
   Traditional Chinese medicine for, 147b-148b
Corticotropin-releasing hormone (CRH) disorders, 243
Corydalis *(Corydalis* spp.)
   pregnancy and lactation and, 578
   for tapeworm, 419
Cough associated with angiotensin-converting enzyme (ACE) inhibitors, 124
Cough-variant asthma, 197
Counseling, 7 *See Also* Psychotherapy
   in erectile dysfunction, 375
Cowhage *(Mucuna pruriens)*
   adverse effects, interactions, and pharmacokinetics of, 511-512
   for Parkinson's disease, 26, 56, 59
   case study for, 59
   pregnancy and lactation and, 578
COX. *See* Cyclooxygenase (COX)
CPB. *See* Cardiopulmonary bypass (CPB)
CPH 82 for rheumatoid arthritis, 303
Crack cocaine, 41
Cranberry *(Vaccinium macrocarpon)*
   adverse effects, interactions, and pharmacokinetics of, 512
   for Alzheimer's disease and related disorders, 90
   for cancer, 475, 483
   for dental plaque, 392
   for fungal infections, 419
   for gastrointestinal disorders, 335
   for kidney stones, 366, 377
   pregnancy and lactation and, 579
   for urinary tract infection, 375-376, 392, 398, 404-405
   for viral infections, 438
C-reactive protein (CRP), omega-3 fatty acids for lowering of, 183
Creutzfeldt-Jakob disease, 87
CRH. *See* Corticotropin-releasing hormone (CRH) disorders
Crohn's disease, 319 *See Also* Inflammatory bowel disease (IBD)
   boswellia for, 323
Crown chakra, 21
CRP. *See* C-reactive protein (CRP), omega-3 fatty acids for lowering of
CRPS. *See* Complex regional pain syndrome (CRPS)
Cryptococcus neoformans, 419
CT. *See* Computed tomography (CT)

CTA. *See* Computed tomographic angiography (CTA)
CTZ. *See* Chemoreceptor trigger zone (CTZ)
Culture, viral, 431
Curcumin *See* Turmeric *(Curcuma longa)*
Cushing's disease, 243
Cushing's syndrome, 243
Cutaneous leishmaniasis, 409
   zinc for, 420
CVA. *See* Cerebrovascular accident (CVA)
Cyanosis in chronic obstructive pulmonary disease, 198
Cyclooxygenase (COX), garlic for inhibition of, 160
CYP450 system, drug interactions in cancer treatment and, 449
Cyst, Baker, 292
Cystic fibrosis (CF), 199
   borage for, 201-202
   safflower for, 208
   turmeric for, 210
Cystine kidney stone, 363
Cystitis, 388
   case study for, 405
   interstitial, 361-362
     chamomile for, 365-369
Cytochrome P450 system, drug interactions in cancer treatment and, 449
Cytokines
   in asthma, 197
   in bacterial infection, 381
Cytomegalovirus (CMV), 430

D

Daisy *(Bellis perennis)*
   adverse effects, interactions, and pharmacokinetics of, 512
   for coagulation disorders, 160
   pregnancy and lactation and, 579
Damiana *(Turnera diffusa)*
   adverse effects, interactions, and pharmacokinetics of, 512
   for depressive disorders, 34
   pregnancy and lactation and, 579
   for psychiatric disorders, 13
   for sexual dysfunction, 366
   for weight loss, 255
Dandelion *(Taraxacum officinale)*
   adverse effects, interactions, and pharmacokinetics of, 512-513
   for arthritis, 306
   for cancer, 475
   for congestive heart failure, 118-119
   for diabetes mellitus, 224
   fertility and, 249
   for gastrointestinal disorders, 325
   for hepatitis B, 348
   for pain, 79
   pregnancy and lactation and, 579

Dandruff, 417
Danshen *(Salvia miltiorrhiza)*
   adverse effects, interactions, and pharmacokinetics of, 513-514
   for cardiovascular disease and angina, 129
   for chemotherapy toxicity, 476
   for hepatitis B, 348
   for ischemic stroke, 142-143
   for kidney disease, 366-367
   for lipid disorders, 176
   pregnancy and lactation and, 579
   propranolol and, 153
   for respiratory disorders, 203
Data analysis for research, 9
Decoction, 3
Deep vein thrombosis (DVT), 158
   integrative therapy plan for, 167
   mesoglycan for, 166
   pycnogenol for prevention of, 162
Defibrillator, 139-140
Degenerative joint disease (DJD), 292. *See Also* Osteoarthritis (OA)
Deglycyrrhizinated licorice (DGL). *See* Licorice *(Glycyrrhiza glabra)*
Dehydroepiandrosterone (DHEA)
   for gout, 300
   for psychiatric disorders, 14
   for weight loss, 261
Delusions, 12
Dementia, 86-87. *See Also* Alzheimer's disease
   agitation in
     aromatherapy and music therapy for, 99
     bitter orange for, 97
     grape seed for, 92-93
     lemon balm for, 94
   coenzyme Q for, 98
   ginkgo for, 45, 90, 92
   jojoba for, 93
   lavender for, 94
   omega-3 fatty acids for, 98
   polypodium for, 94-95
   rhodiola for, 95
   Traditional Chinese medicine for, 97
   vitamin E for, 98
Dental caries
   betel nut for, 390-391
   tea for, 397
Dental pain, 74
Dental plaque
   acacia for, 389
   bloodroot for, 391, 404
   cranberry for, 392
   eucalyptus for, 393
   mastic for, 396
   neem for, 396
   pycnogenol for, 396-397

Dental plaque *(Continued)*
　tea tree for, 397-398
　thyme for, 398
Depressive disorders, 29-38
　adjunct therapies for, 35
　anxiety with, 25-26
　in cancer, 446
　case studies associated with, 36
　in children and elderly, 31-32
　diagnosis of, 32
　herbal therapies for, 14, 32-34, 36t
　　with limited evidence, 34-35
　　with monoamine oxidase inhibitor properties, 35b
　　with selective serotonin reuptake inhibitor properties, 35b
　insomnia and, 26
　integrative therapy plan for, 35-38
　during menopause, 277-278
　omega-3 fatty acids for, 98
　overview of, 29-32
　in Parkinson's disease, 58
　psychiatric disorders accompanied by, 14
　signs and symptoms of, 31-32
　types of, 30-31
De Quervain's thyroiditis, 244
Dermatophytes, 412
Devil's claw *(Harpagophytum procumbens)*
　adverse effects, interactions, and pharmacokinetics of, 514
　for arthritis, 300-301, 311
　for pain and inflammation, 75, 83
　for physical symptoms associated with depression, 35
　pregnancy and lactation and, 579
Devil's club *(Oplopanax horridus)*
　adverse effects, interactions, and pharmacokinetics of, 514
　for diabetes mellitus, 224
　pregnancy and lactation and, 579
DEXA. *See* Dual-energy x-ray absorptiometry (DEXA) in osteoporosis diagnosis
DHA. *See* Docosahexaenoic acid (DHA) for cardiovascular health
DHEA. *See* Dehydroepiandrosterone (DHEA)
Diabetes insipidus, 243
Diabetes mellitus, 216-240
　adjunct therapies for, 235-237
　case studies associated with, 237
　diagnosis of, 219-220
　herbal therapies for, 220-227, 235t-236t
　　with limited evidence, 234-235
　　with negative evidence, 234
　hyperglycemia in, 217-218
　hypoglycemia in, 218

Diabetes mellitus *(Continued)*
　integrative care plan for, 237-239
　overview of, 217-220
　types of, 218-219
　weight management and, 263
Diabetic nephropathy, 235-236
Diabetic peripheral neuropathy
　adjunct therapies for, 235-236
　evening primrose for, 224
　ginseng for, 226
　kudzu for, 228
Diagnostic and Statistical Manual of Mental Disorders (DSM), 19
Diarrhea, 318
　arnica for, 321
　arrowroot for, 321
　carob for, 323
　chamomile for, 324
　false hellebore for, 335
　goldenseal for, 327, 394
　in inflammatory bowel disease, 319
　in irritable bowel syndrome, 319-320
　psyllium for, 331-332
　rhubarb for, 332
　seizures and, 66
　slippery elm for, 333
　soy for, 333
　traveler's, 318
　vitamin and mineral deficiencies due to, 339
Diastolic pressure, 103
DIC. *See* Disseminated intravascular coagulation (DIC)
Diet
　Atkins, 66, 261
　in cancer treatment, 483
　epilepsy and, 66
　for gout, 310
　in HIV treatment, 440
　hypertension and, 109-111
　for liver disease, 353-355
　macrobiotic, 261-262
　during menopause, 274-276
　metabolism and, 252
　myocardial infarction and stroke, 151
　therapeutic lifestyle changes, 172-173, 190
　vitamin K in, 166
Dietary Supplement Health and Education Act of 1994 (DSHEA), 2
Dietary Supplement Ingredient Database (DSID), 3
Dietary supplements, 2-5
　active ingredients in, 4
　adverse effects, interactions, and pharmacokinetics of, 486-569
　combination products, 4
　dosages of, 6
　evidence-based integrative care and, 5-6
　herbs, 3

Dietary supplements *(Continued)*
　interactions with, 4-5
　for menopausal symptoms, 276
　patient counseling and, 7
　pregnancy and lactation and, 570-592
　prevalence of, 2
　regulations of, 5-6
　safety and purity of, 4
　standardization of, 6
　supplements, 4
Digestion, 315-316
Digitalis. *See* Foxglove *(Digitalis purpurea, Digitalis lanata)*
Diphyllobothrium latum, 410
Disseminated intravascular coagulation (DIC), 158
Diuresis
　ashwagandha for, 117
　dandelion for, 118-119
　horsetail for, 120-121
　rutin for, 122
Diuretics for congestive heart failure, 114-115
DJD. *See* Degenerative joint disease (DJD)
DNA abnormalities in cancer, 446
Docosahexaenoic acid (DHA) for cardiovascular health, 177-178, 181, 193
Dogwood *(Cornus* spp.), 579
Dong quai *(Angelica sinensis)*
　adverse effects, interactions, and pharmacokinetics of, 514
　for arthritis, 296
　for cardiovascular disease and angina, 129
　for cognitive and physical enhancement, 49
　for menopausal symptoms, 269-270
　for pain, 79
　pregnancy and lactation and, 579
　for respiratory disorders, 203-204
Dopamine loss in Parkinson's disease, 53
Dosage, 6
Double depression, 30
Dracunculiasis, 410-411
Drugs
　abuse of, 40-41
　categories of for use in pregnancy, 570t
　goldenseal for masking of illicit drugs from urinalysis, 51
　insomnia due to, 20
　interaction in cancer treatment, 449
　liver disorders due to, 345
　milk thistle for, 349
DSHEA. *See* Dietary Supplement Health and Education Act of 1994 (DSHEA)
DSID. *See* Dietary Supplement Ingredient Database (DSID)

DSM. *See* Diagnostic and Statistical
    Manual of Mental Disorders (DSM)
Dual-energy x-ray absorptiometry
    (DEXA) in osteoporosis diagnosis,
    283
Duodenal ulcer. *See* Peptic ulcer disease
DVT. *See* Deep vein thrombosis (DVT)
Dwarf tapeworm, 410
Dyslipidemia. *See* Lipid disorders
Dyspepsia, 316
    asparagus for, 321
    blessed thistle for, 322-323
    globe artichoke for, 327
    lemon balm for, 328
    licorice for, 328
    peppermint for, 330
    turmeric for, 333
    white horehound for, 334
Dyspnea
    in emphysema, 198
    in interstitial lung disease, 200
Dysrhythmia. *See* Arrhythmia

E

EBV. *See* Epstein-Barr virus (EBV)
Echinacea *(Echinacea* spp.)
    adverse effects, interactions, and pharmacokinetics of, 514-515
    bacopa and, 100
    for cancer, 454-455
    for genital herpes, 438
    pregnancy and lactation and, 579
    for radiation-induced leukopenia, 479
    for upper respiratory tract infection,
        399, 405-406, 434,
        438, 441
Echocardiogram, 140
Eclampsia, tonic-clonic seizure during,
    62
Ectoparasite, 408-409
Ectopic adrenocorticotropic hormone
    syndrome, 243
ED. *See* Erectile dysfunction (ED)
Eicosapentaenoic acid (EPA) for cardiovascular health, 177-178, 181, 193
Ejaculation, premature
    clove for, 374
    ginseng for, 368
Elderly
    Alzheimer's disease in, 86-101
    depression in, 31-32
Elder *(Sambucus nigra)*
    adverse effects, interactions, and pharmacokinetics of, 515
    for influenza, 435
    for lipid disorders, 177
    pregnancy and lactation and, 579
Elecampane *(Inula helenium)*, 419
Electrocardiography in arrhythmias, 140
Elephantiasis, 411

Embolus, 135, 155, 156f, 158
    pulmonary, 158
    stroke due to, 137, 158
Emphysema, 198
Endometrial cancer, 469-470
Endoparasite, 408-409
Endotracheal intubation, coleus
    administration before, 203
End-stage renal disease (ESRD), 245
Energy, low, herbal stimulants for,
    43-44
Energy drinks, 51
Energy therapies
    in cancer treatment, 480
English ivy *(Hedera helix)*
    adverse effects, interactions, and pharmacokinetics of, 515
    for respiratory disorders, 204
English walnut *(Juglans regia)*, 580
Enterotoxin, 384
Enuresis, nocturnal, 361
Eosinophils in asthma, 197
EPA. *See* Eicosapentaenoic acid (EPA) for cardiovascular health
Ephedra *(Ephedra sinica)*
    adverse effects, interactions, and pharmacokinetics of, 516-517
    arrhythmia due to, 150
    for cognitive and physical enhancement, 49
    pregnancy and lactation and, 580
    for respiratory disorders, 204, 212
    for sexual arousal, 367
    for weight loss, 51, 255, 263
Epilepsy, 61. *See Also* Seizure disorders
    Jacksonian, 62
Epstein-Barr virus (EBV), 430
Erectile dysfunction (ED), 360-361
    case study for, 377
    coleus for, 366
    ginkgo for, 367
    ginseng for, 368
    grapefruit for, 377-378
    integrative therapy plan for, 376
    muira puama for, 369
    psychological counseling for, 375
    pycnogenol, 370
    yohimbe for, 373
ERr 731, 272
Esberitox N, 438
Escherichia coli, 380-381
    bromelain for, 391
    cranberry for, 392
    eucalyptus for, 393
    seaweed for, 400
    uva ursi for, 398
Esophagus
    cancer of
        greater celandine for, 458-459
        PSK for, 464

Esophagus *(Continued)*
    candidal infection of, 414
    peptic ulcer of, 317
    spasm of, 330
ESRD. *See* End-stage renal disease (ESRD)
Essences, 4
Essential oils, 4
Essiac herbal combination tea
    adverse effects, interactions, and pharmacokinetics of, 517
    for cancer, 474b
    pregnancy and lactation and, 580
Estrogenic activity, herbs with, 275t-276t
Estrogen therapy for osteoporosis, 286
Ethanol, 571. *See Also* Alcohol
Ethereal oils, 4
Eucalyptus *(Eucalyptus* spp.)
    adverse effects, interactions, and pharmacokinetics of, 517
    for dental plaque and gingivitis, 393
    for headache, 75
    pregnancy and lactation and, 580
    for respiratory disorders, 205
Eugenol. *See* Clove *(Syzygium aromaticum,* syn. *Eugenia aromatica)*
Euphorbia *(Euphorbia* spp.)
    adverse effects, interactions, and pharmacokinetics of, 517-518
    for bacterial infection, 399
    for pain, 79
    for seizure disorders, 64, 67
European barberry *(Berberis vulgaris)*. *See* Berberine
Evening primrose *(Oenothera biennis)*
    adverse effects, interactions, and pharmacokinetics of, 518
    for breast cancer, 455
    for cardiovascular health, 148
    for cognitive and physical enhancement, 45
    for diabetes mellitus, 224
    for hypertension, 104
    for menopausal symptoms, 274
    pregnancy and lactation and, 580
    for psychiatric disorders, 13
    for respiratory disorders, 209
    for rheumatoid arthritis, 301
    seizures or lower seizure threshold
        due to, 65
    for weight loss, 256
Evidence-based integrative care, 7f, 8-10,
    10b
Exercise
    for arthritis, 309, 311
    asthma induced by, 197
    cholesterol levels and, 190
    for gastrointestinal disorders, 340
    for hypertension, 110-111
    Kegel, 278, 375
    during menopause, 276-277

Exercise (Continued)
    for osteoporosis prevention, 286, 288
    for pain, 83
    for weight loss, 262-263
Exercise performance. See Athletic performance
Extract, 3-4
Extrinsic asthma, 197
Eyebright (Euphrasia officinalis)
    adverse effects, interactions, and pharmacokinetics of, 518
    for bacterial conjunctivitis, 393-394
    for liver disorders, 353
    for pain, 79
Eye infection
    African worm, 411
    bacterial conjunctivitis, 383-384
    Chlamydia, 387
        goldenseal for, 394

F

Faces pain scale, 71, 71f
Facial pain, 69
Factor X, 156
Fainting. See Syncope
Fall prevention in osteoporosis, 288
False hellebore (Veratrum spp.)
    adverse effects, interactions, and pharmacokinetics of, 518
    for diarrhea, 335
    for hypertension, 104
    pregnancy and lactation and, 580
    for seizure disorders, 64
False pennyroyal (Hedeoma spp.)
    pregnancy and lactation and, 580
    for psychiatric disorders, 13
Familial hyperlipidemia
    garlic for, 178
    safflower for, 186
Fasting blood glucose test, 219
Fatigue
    in cancer, 446
    in depression, 31
    ginseng for, 46
    herbal stimulants for, 43-44
Fat intake, cancer and, 483
Fatty liver, 343-344
    rhubarb for, 352
FDA. See Food and Drug Administration (FDA)
FDAMA. See Food and Drug Administration Modernization Act (FDAMA)
Fecal incontinence, 318
Female reproductive system, 268f
Fennel (Foeniculum vulgare)
    adverse effects, interactions, and pharmacokinetics of, 518
    for gastrointestinal disorders, 325, 339
    pregnancy and lactation and, 580

Fenugreek (Trigonella foenum-graecum)
    adverse effects, interactions, and pharmacokinetics of, 519
    for coagulation disorders, 164
    for diabetes mellitus, 225
    for lipid disorders, 177
    pregnancy and lactation and, 580
Festinating gait, 55
Fever
    in cancer, 446
    in common cold, 428
Fever blister. See Oral herpes
Feverfew (Tanacetum parthenium)
    adverse effects, interactions, and pharmacokinetics of, 519
    for migraine headache, 75-76, 83-84
    pregnancy and lactation and, 580
    for rheumatoid arthritis, 301
Fibrillation
    atrial, 137, 139-140
    ventricular, 135, 139-140
Fibrin, 156
Fibrinogen, 156
Fibrinolysis, 156
    garlic for increase of, 160-162
Fibrosis
    liver, 344
    pulmonary, 199-200
        ginkgo for, 205
Fig (Ficus carica)
    adverse effects, interactions, and pharmacokinetics of, 519
    for diabetes mellitus, 225
    pregnancy and lactation and, 580
Filariasis, lymphatic, 411
Fingernail, fungal infection of, 413
    tea tree for, 418
    thyme for, 418-419
Fish oil. See Omega-3 fatty acids
Fish tapeworm, 410
Fissure, anal, 331-332
Flatulence, 322-331
Flax (Linum usitatissimum)
    adverse effects, interactions, and pharmacokinetics of, 519-520
    for arthritis, 306
    for atherosclerosis and coronary artery disease, 143
    for cancer
        breast, 455
        prostate, 474-475
    for constipation, 325, 340
    for diabetes mellitus, 226
    for hypertension, 105
    for lipid disorders, 177
    for lupus nephritis, 367
    for menopausal symptoms, 270
    pregnancy and lactation and, 581
Flower diagnosis, 48

Flower remedies. See Bach flower remedies
Flu. See Influenza
Fluid extract, 3-4
Flutter, atrial, 139
Focal seizure, 61
Focusing in cancer treatment, 480
Follicle-stimulating hormone (FSH), 241
    disorders of, 243-244
    menopause and, 266
Food allergy, asthma and, 212
Food and Drug Administration (FDA)
    on dietary supplements, 2
    on health claims, 5-6
    pharmaceutical pregnancy categories of, 570t
Food and Drug Administration Modernization Act (FDAMA), 5
Foodborne bacterial illness, 385
    kudzu for, 399
Forskolin. See Also Coleus (Coleus forskohlii), 12
    for asthma, 203
    for cardiomyopathy, 118
    for hypertension, 109
    for increasing lean body mass, 254
Fo-ti (Polygonum multiflorum), 581
Foxglove (Digitalis purpurea, Digitalis lanata)
    for arrhythmia, 149
    for congestive heart failure, 122
    pregnancy and lactation and, 581
Fracture due to osteoporosis, 283
Freebasing, 41
Freezing in Parkinson's disease, 53-55
French lilac. See Galega (Galega officinalis)
Frozen shoulder, 294
Fruits and vegetables for cancer prevention, 483
FSH. See Follicle-stimulating hormone (FSH)
Fungal infection, 408-426, 412-414
    adjunct therapies for, 420-423
    case studies associated with, 424
    herbal therapies for, 414-416, 421t-423t
    with limited evidence, 419-420
    integrative therapy plan for, 423-425
Fusarium, 419
Fusobacterium nucleatum, 390

G

GABA. See Gamma-aminobutyric (GABA)
GAD. See Generalized anxiety disorder (GAD)
Gait
    festinating, 55
    Parkinsonian, 53-54

Galectin-3, 462
Galega (Galega officinalis)
　for diabetes mellitus, 226b
　for weight loss, 259
Gamma-aminobutyric (GABA), 17-18, 44
Gamma-herpesvirinae, 429
Gamma-linolenic acid (GLA). See Also Borage (Borago officinalis); Evening primrose (Oenothera biennis)
　for arthritis, 298, 301
　for asthma, 200
　for diabetic peripheral neuropathy, 224-225, 236
　for hypertension, 104
Gamma oryzanol for hypothyroidism, 248
Garcinia (Garcinia cambogia)
　adverse effects, interactions, and pharmacokinetics of, 520
　for cognitive and physical enhancement, 45
　for weight loss, 256
Garlic (Allium sativum)
　adverse effects, interactions, and pharmacokinetics of, 520-521
　for atherosclerosis, 143-144, 152
　for bacterial infection, 399, 405-406
　for cancer prevention, 456
　for cardiovascular health, 151
　for coagulation disorders, 160
　for diabetes mellitus, 234
　for fungal infections, 415-416
　for *Helicobacter pylori* infection, 335
　for hypertension, 105, 111
　for lipid disorders, 178
　pregnancy and lactation and, 581
　for upper respiratory tract infection, 435
Gastric cancer, 330
　ginkgo for, 456
　ginseng for, 457-458
　PSK for, 464
　signs and symptoms of, 447
　soy for, 469-470
Gastric spasm, 330
Gastric ulcer. See Peptic ulcer disease
Gastroesophageal reflux disease (GERD), 316
　carob for, 323
Gastrointestinal disorders, 315-342
　accessory organs of, 317f
　adjunct therapies for, 335
　associated with depression, 35
　case studies associated with, 340
　chemotherapy-induced, 482
　herbal therapies for, 320-323, 336t-338t
　　with limited evidence, 335
　　with negative evidence, 335
　integrative therapy plan for, 339
　lower, 318-320

Gastrointestinal disorders (Continued)
　overview of, 315-320, 316-317f
　upper, 316-318
GBF. See Germinated barley foodstuff (GBF)
GDS. See Global Deterioration Scale (GDS)
Generalized anxiety disorder (GAD), 18-19
Generalized seizure, 62-63
Genetics
　in Alzheimer's disease diagnosis, 89
　in cancer, 446, 448, 482
Genital herpes, 429-430
　aloe for, 431
　case studies associated with, 442
　echinacea for, 438
　licorice for, 438
Genital warts, 437
Genitourinary disorders, 359-379
　adjunct therapies for, 375
　benign prostatic hyperplasia, 360
　case studies associated with, 376
　erectile dysfunction, 360-361
　herbal therapies for, 364-365, 375t
　　with limited evidence, 374
　integrative therapy plans for, 376
　interstitial cystitis, 361-362
　kidney stones, 363-364
　lupus nephritis, 364
　neurogenic bladder, 362
　overview of, 360
　pelvic inflammatory disease, 364
　prolapsed uterus, 362
　prostatitis, 362-363, 363t
　urinary incontinence, 361
Genotyping, 383
GERD. See Gastroesophageal reflux disease (GERD)
German measles, 430
Germinated barley foodstuff (GBF), 322
Gerson therapy, 481
Gestational diabetes, 219
　diagnosis of, 220
GH. See Growth hormone (GH)
Ghrelin, 252-253
Giardiasis, 409-410
Gigantism, 242
Ginger (Zingiber officinale)
　adverse effects, interactions, and pharmacokinetics of, 521-522
　for arthritis, 301-302
　for cancer, 456
　for coagulation disorders, 161
　for nausea and vomiting, 326, 341
　pregnancy and lactation and, 581
　for weight loss, 256
Gingivitis, 387
　bloodroot for, 391
　eucalyptus for, 393

Gingivitis (Continued)
　rhubarb for, 397
　tea tree for, 397-398
Ginkgo (Ginkgo biloba)
　adverse effects, interactions, and pharmacokinetics of, 522-523
　for Alzheimer's disease and related disorders, 35, 90-91, 100
　for anxiety and insomnia, 24
　for cognitive and physical enhancement, 45
　for depressive disorders, 32, 35
　for erectile dysfunction, 367, 378
　for ischemic stroke, 144
　for memory impairment, 14
　pregnancy and lactation and, 581
　for psychiatric disorders, 14
　for respiratory disorders, 205
　warfarin and, 99-100
Ginseng (Panax spp.)
　adverse effects, interactions, and pharmacokinetics of, 523-524
　for Alzheimer's disease and related disorders, 92
　arrhythmia due to, 150, 152
　in cancer treatment, 457-458, 482, 484
　coagulation disorders and, 167
　for cognitive and physical enhancement, 46
　for congestive heart failure, 119
　for coronary artery disease, 129-130
　for diabetes mellitus, 226
　for erectile dysfunction, 378
　for hypertension, 106
　for lipid disorders, 179
　for liver disorders, 348
　for menopausal symptoms, 270
　for methicillin-resistant *Staphylococcus aureus*, 405, 394
　for Parkinson's disease, 57
　pregnancy and lactation and, 581
　for respiratory disorders, 205
　for sexual function, 368, 378
　for weight loss, 259
GLA. See Gamma-linolenic acid (GLA)
Global Deterioration Scale (GDS), 87b
Globe artichoke (Cynara scolymus)
　adverse effects, interactions, and pharmacokinetics of, 524-525
　for gastrointestinal disorders, 327, 339
　for lipid disorders, 179
Glucagon, 217
Gluconeogenesis, 217
Glucosamine, 309, 311
Glucose
　diabetes mellitus and, 217
　impaired fasting, 219
　impaired tolerance, 218-219
　　jackfruit for, 228

Glucose *(Continued)*
   metabolism of, 217
      safflower and, 234
   self-monitoring of, 220
   St. John's wort and, 483
   testing of
      for diagnosis, 219
      for monitoring, 220
Glutamate, 17-18
Glycogen, 217
Glycosylation, 220
Glycyrrhizin. *See* Licorice *(Glycyrrhiza glabra)*
Goat's rue. *See* Galega *(Galega officinalis)*
Goiter, 244
   seaweed for, 247
Goji *(Lycium* spp.)
   adverse effects, interactions, and pharmacokinetics of, 525
   for cancer, 458
   pregnancy and lactation and, 581-582
Goldenrod *(Solidago virgaurea)*, 582
Goldenseal *(Hydrastis canadensis)*. *See Also* Berberine
   for congestive heart failure, 119-120, 125
   for lipid disorders, 180
   for masking of illicit drugs from urinalysis, 51
   pregnancy and lactation and, 582
Goldenthread *(Coptis chinensis)*. *See* Berberine
Gonadotropins, 243
Gotu kola *(Centella asiatica)*
   adverse effects, interactions, and pharmacokinetics of, 525-526
   for anxiety and insomnia, 21
   for diabetes mellitus, 227
Gout, 296
   alcohol intake and, 310
   ash for, 296-297
   cherry for, 300
   diet for, 310
   willow for, 306
Grading scale, *Natural Standards*, 9-10, 9t
Gram-negative bacteria, 383
Gram-positive bacteria, 383
Gram staining, 383
Grand mal seizure, 62, 62t
Grapefruit *(Citrus* x *paradisi)*
   adverse effects, interactions, and pharmacokinetics of, 526-528
   for erectile dysfunction, 377-378
   for kidney stones, 368
   for lipid disorders, 180
   pregnancy and lactation and, 582
Grape Seed extract. *See* Pycnogenol *(Pinus pinaster* subsp. *atlantica)*

Grape seed *(Vitis* spp.)
   adverse effects, interactions, and pharmacokinetics of, 526
   for Alzheimer's disease and related disorders, 92-93
   for cancer, 475
   for coagulation disorders, 161
   for lipid disorders, 180
   pregnancy and lactation and, 582
Graves' disease, 242-243, 246
Graviola *(Annona muricata)*, 582
Gray platelet syndrome, 157
Greater celandine *(Chelidonium majus)*
   adverse effects, interactions, and pharmacokinetics of, 528-529
   for cancer, 458-459
   for fungal infections, 419
   pregnancy and lactation and, 582
Green tea. *See* Tea *(Camellia sinensis)*
Growth hormone (GH), 241
   disorders of, 242
      arginine for, 248
Guarana *(Paullinia cupana)*
   adverse effects, interactions, and pharmacokinetics of, 529
   for Alzheimer's disease and related disorders, 93
   arrhythmia due to, 150, 152
   for cognitive and physical enhancement, 46
   for depressive disorders, 33
   pregnancy and lactation and, 582
   for psychiatric disorders, 13
   for weight loss, 257
Guar *(Cyamopsis tetragonoloba)*, 335
Guggul *(Commiphora mukul)*
   adverse effects, interactions, and pharmacokinetics of, 529
   for arthritis, 302
   for lipid disorders, 180, 192
   for weight loss, 257
Guinea worm disease, 410-411
Gumweed *(Grindelia camporum)*, 582
Gymnema *(Gymnema sylvestre)*
   adverse effects, interactions, and pharmacokinetics of, 529-530
   for diabetes mellitus, 227, 238
   for lipid disorders, 181
   for weight loss, 259

H

Hallucinogen herbs for psychiatric disorders, 13-14
Hansen's disease, 385-386
Hashimoto's thyroiditis, 244
Hawthorn *(Crataegus* spp.)
   adverse effects, interactions, and pharmacokinetics of, 530
   for angina, 130, 132

Hawthorn *(Crataegus* spp.) *(Continued)*
   for congestive heart failure, 120, 124-125
   for hypertension, 109
   for lipid disorders, 190
   pregnancy and lactation and, 582
Hay fever, 198
Hazelnut *(Corylus avellana, Corylus heterophylla)*, 582
HBV. *See* Hepatitis B virus (HBV)
HDLs. *See* High-density lipoproteins (HDLs)
Headache, 69
   belladonna for, 73
   eucalyptus for, 75
   migraine, 69
      butterbur for, 73-74
      feverfew for, 75-76
      willow bark for, 84
Healing touch (HT), 480
Health claims
Heart. *See Also* Cardiovascular disorders
   anatomy of, 115f
   conduction system of, 135f
   remodeling of in congestive heart failure, 124
Heart attack. *See* Myocardial infarction (MI)
Heart beat, abnormal. *See* Arrhythmia
Heartburn, 316
Helicobacter pylori infection
   cinnamon for, 325
   cranberry for, 335
   garlic for, 335
   goldenseal for, 327
Helminthic infection, 410-412
Hemlock *(Conium maculatum)*, 582
Hemoglobin A monitoring in diabetes mellitus, 220, 237
Hemophilia, 157
Hemorrhagic cystitis, 365-366
Hemorrhagic stroke, 137-138
Hemorrhoids, 331-332
Hemostasis, 155-156
Hemp *(Cannabis sativa)*, 582
Hepatic disorders, 343-358
   adjunct therapies for, 353
   cancer
      bupleurum for, 453
      PSK for, 464
   case studies associated with, 356
   diagnosis of, 345-346
   drug-induced, 345
   herbal therapies for, 346, 354t-355t
      with limited evidence, 353
      with negative evidence, 353
   integrative therapy plan for, 355
   overview of, 343-346
   stages of, 343-344
   Wilson's disease, 345

Hepatic failure, 344
Hepatitis, 344-345
   bupleurum for, 346-347
   chicory for, 347
   milk thistle for, 349
   mistletoe for, 351
   peony for, 351
   rhubarb for, 352
   schisandra for, 353
   spirulina for, 353
Hepatitis A, 344
Hepatitis B virus (HBV), 344
   cordyceps for, 347-348
   dandelion for, 348
   danshen for, 348
   reishi mushroom for, 351
Hepatitis C, 345
   case study for, 357
   licorice for, 349
   safflower for, 352
   St. John's wort for, 353
Hepatitis D virus, 345
Hepatitis E, 345
Hepatocellular carcinoma, 453
Herbs, 3
   active ingredients in, 4
   adverse effects, interactions, and pharmacokinetics of, 486-569
   dosages of, 6
   evidence-based integrative care and, 6-7
   forms of, 3-4
   interactions with, 4-5
   patient counseling and, 7
   pregnancy and lactation and, 570-592
   prevalence of, 2
   safety and purity of, 4
   standardization of, 6
Hernearin, 399
Herpesviruses, 429-430
   adjunct therapies for, 440
   aloe for, 431
   case studies associated with, 442
   echinacea for, 438
   lemon balm for, 435
   licorice for, 435-436, 438
   Reishi mushroom for pain following, 77
   rhubarb for, 436
   sage for, 436
   shiitake mushroom for, 437
   tea tree for, 437
Hibiscus (*Hibiscus* spp.)
   adverse effects, interactions, and pharmacokinetics of, 530
   for hypertension, 106, 111-112
   pregnancy and lactation and, 582
High blood pressure. *See* Hypertension
High blood sugar. *See* Hyperglycemia
High-density lipoproteins (HDLs), 171-172

High-protein diet in epilepsy treatment, 66
Histamine in asthma, 197
Histoplasmosis, 414
HIV. *See* Human immunodeficiency virus (HIV)
HLE. *See* Human leukocyte elastase (HLE)
Holy basil (*Ocimum sanctum*)
   adverse effects, interactions, and pharmacokinetics of, 530
   for diabetes mellitus, 228
   for parasitic infection, 419
   pregnancy and lactation and, 583
Homeopathy, 3
Honeysuckle (*Lonicera* spp.), 583
Hoodia (*Hoodia gordonii*), 259
Hookworm infection, 410
Hop (*Humulus lupulus*)
   adverse effects, interactions, and pharmacokinetics of, 530-531
   for anxiety and insomnia, 21
   for arthritis, 302-303
   for menopausal symptoms, 270-271
   pregnancy and lactation and, 583
Hormone replacement therapy (HRT), 268, 277
Horny goat weed (*Epimedium grandiflorum*)
   adverse effects, interactions, and pharmacokinetics of, 531
   arrhythmia due to, 152
   for atherosclerosis, 144-145
   for osteoporosis prevention, 283-284
   for sexual dysfunction in renal failure patients, 369
Horse chestnut (*Aesculus hippocastanum*)
   for congestive heart failure, 122
   pregnancy and lactation and, 583
Horseradish (*Armoracia rusticana*, syn. *Cochlearia armoracia*)
   adverse effects, interactions, and pharmacokinetics of, 531
   pregnancy and lactation and, 583
   for urinary tract infection, 395
Horsetail (*Equisetum* spp.)
   adverse effects, interactions, and pharmacokinetics of, 531
   for congestive heart failure, 120-121, 125
   for osteoporosis, 284
   pregnancy and lactation and, 583
Host
   parasitic, 408
   viral, 427
Hot flashes during menopause, 267, 277
   soy for, 272
Hoxsey formula for cancer, 476
HPV. *See* Human papillomavirus (HPV)

HRT. *See* Hormone replacement therapy (HRT)
HT. *See* Healing touch (HT)
Human immunodeficiency virus (HIV), 429
   adjunct therapies for, 440
   aloe for, 431
   andrographis for, 431
   beta-glucan for, 432
   bitter melon for, 432-433
   blessed thistle for, 433
   boxwood for, 433-434
   case studies associated with, 442
   integrative therapy plan for, 441
   licorice for, 435-436
   mistletoe for, 436
   St. John's wort for, 438
   Syzygium claviflorum for, 438b
   tea tree for oral thrush in, 418
   turmeric for, 437
Human leukocyte elastase (HLE), 304
Human papillomavirus (HPV), 464
Human skeleton, 282f
Huperzine, 98-99
Hydrastine, 119
Hydrazine in cancer treatment, 481
Hydrotherapy for arthritis, 309-310
Hydroxycitric acid. *See* Garcinia (*Garcinia cambogia*)
Hydroxymethylglutaryl-coenzyme A for Alzheimer's disease, 87
5-Hydroxytryptophan
   for Parkinson's disease ataxia, 58-59
   for weight loss, 261
Hymenolepis nana, 410
Hyperactive-impulsive behavior in attention disorders, 41, 42b
Hypercalcemia, 245
Hypercholesterolemia. *See Also* Lipid disorders
   acacia for, 190
   ashwagandha for, 173
   avocado for, 174
   beta-sitosterol for, 175
   carob for, 176
   elder for, 177
   goldenseal for, 180
   grape. Seed for, 180
   omega-3 fatty acids for, 181-182
   policosanol for, 183
   psyllium for, 182
   pycnogenol for, 184
   red clover for, 185
   red yeast rice for, 185
   rhubarb for, 186
   safflower for, 186
   soy for, 187
   spirulina for, 187
   sweet almond for, 188
   tea for, 188

Hypercholesterolemia *(Continued)*
   turmeric for, 188
   white horehound for, 189
   wild yam for, 189
   yucca for, 189
Hyperemesis gravidarum, 318
   ginger for, 326
Hyperglycemia, 217-218. *See Also* Diabetes mellitus
   barley for, 221
   beet for, 222
   flax for, 226
   garlic for, 234
   ginseng for, 226
   jackfruit for, 228
   psyllium for, 230
   seaweed for, 232
   stevia for, 233
Hyperlipidemia, 150, 171. *See Also* Lipid disorders
   alfalfa for, 173
   barley for, 174
   beet for, 174
   beta-glucan, 175
   borage for, 175
   cordyceps for, 176
   danshen for, 176
   fenugreek for, 177
   flax for, 177
   garlic for, 178
   ginseng for, 179
   globe artichoke for, 179
   guggul for, 180
   gymnema for, 181
   lemon grass for, 181
   milk thistle, 181
   niacin for, 191
   nopal for, 182
   safflower for, 186
Hyperparathyroidism, 245, 248
Hyperprolactinemia, 246
Hypertension, 102-113
   adjunct therapies for, 109-111
   case studies for, 111
   diagnosis of, 103
   herbal therapies for, 103-109, 110t
      with limited evidence, 109
   herbs associated with, 111t
   integrative therapy plan for, 111-112
   malignant, 103
   overview of, 102-103
   pulmonary, 200
   signs and symptoms of, 103
Hyperthyroidism, 242-244
Hypertriglyceridemia
   omega-3 fatty acids for, 182
   tea for, 188
Hypnotherapy
   in HIV treatment, 440
   for irritable bowel syndrome,

Hypnotherapy *(Continued)*
   for pain, 82
   for weight loss, 262
Hypocalcemia, 245
Hypoglycemia, 218
Hypogonadism, erectile dysfunction due to, 361
Hypoparathyroidism, 245, 248
Hypophonia in Parkinson's disease, 55
Hypophysis, 241
Hypopituitarism, 246
Hypotension, 103
Hypothyroidism, 242-245, 248-249
Hypsarrhythmia in West syndrome, 63
Hyssop *(Hyssopus officinalis)*
   for lipid disorders, 190
   seizures or lower seizure threshold due to, 66
Hysterectomy, 267

I

IBD. *See* Inflammatory bowel disease (IBD)
Iberogast, 324, 328, 329
IBS. *See* Irritable bowel syndrome (IBS)
Ictus, 61
IdB 1027 for bilberry, 335
Idiopathic pain, 70
IFG. *See* Impaired fasting glucose (IFG)
IgE. *See* Immunoglobulin E (IgE)
IGT. *See* Impaired glucose tolerance (IGT)
ILD. *See* Interstitial lung disease (ILD)
Immune system
   cancer and, 446
   enhancement of
      aloe for, 431
      astragalus for, 432, 442, 451
      echinacea for, 434
   response of
      in asthma, 197
      in bacterial infection, 381
      to virus, 428
Immunization, 428
   influenza, 441
   measles, mumps, rubella, 430
Immunoglobulin E (IgE) in asthma, 197
Immunomodulators, 428
Impaired fasting glucose (IFG), 219
Impaired glucose tolerance (IGT), 218-219
Impotence, 360. *See Also* Erectile dysfunction (ED)
Impulsive behavior in attention disorders, 41, 42b
Inattention in attention disorders, 41, 42b
Incontinence
   fecal, 318
   urinary, 361

Incontinence *(Continued)*
   adjunct therapies for, 375
   during menopause, 276
Indeterminate colitis, 319
Indian belladonna *(Atropa acuminata)*. *See* Belladonna *(Atropa* spp.)
Indian snakeroot *(Rauwolfia serpentina)*
   for hypertension, 109
   pregnancy and lactation and, 583
Indian tobacco *(Lobelia inflata)*, 583
Indigestion, 316
Infant. *See Also* Child
   acute diarrhea in, soy for, 333
   colic in
      chamomile for, 324
      fennel for, 325
   postoperative pain in, aconite for, 72
Infarction, myocardial, 127, 135-137
   diagnosis of, 137
   high blood pressure and, 103
   integrative therapy plan for, 151-154
   signs and symptoms of, 137
   types of, 135-137
Infection
   bacterial (*See* Bacterial infection)
   fungal (*See* Fungal infection)
   in irritable bowel syndrome, 319-320
   opportunistic, in human immunodeficiency virus, 429
   parasitic (*See* Parasitic infection)
   upper respiratory tract (*See* Upper respiratory tract infection [URI])
   urinary tract (*See* Urinary tract infection [UTI])
Infectious arthritis, 295
Infectious diarrhea, 318
   goldenseal for, 394
Infertility, 249
Inflammation. *See Also* Pain
   in Alzheimer's disease, 97
   in asthma, 79t-82t, 197
   bromelain for, 73, 83-84
   comfrey for, 74-75
   devil's claw for, 83
   turmeric for, 78
Inflammatory bowel disease (IBD), 319
   aloe for, 320-321
   barley for, 322
   betel nut for, 335
   boswellia for, 323
   psyllium for, 331-332
   wheatgrass for, 334
Influenza, 428-429
   adjunct therapies for, 440
   andrographis for, 431
   boneset for, 433
   cranberry for, 438
   elder for, 435
   vaccination, 441

Infusion, 3
Inhibin B, 267
INR. See International normalized ratio (INR)
Insomnia
　adjunct therapies for, 26
　case studies associated with, 26
　herbal therapies for, 20-24, 25t
　　with limited evidence, 24-25
　　with negative evidence, 24
　integrative therapies for, 26-27
　overview of, 19-20
　signs and symptoms of, 20
Insulin
　diabetes mellitus and, 217
　in glucose metabolism, 217
　resistance to, 217-219
　　kudzu for, 228
Integrative care, 7f, 8-10, 10b
Integrative medicine, 2
Interactions, 486-569
International Classification of Epileptic Seizure, 61, 62t
International normalized ratio (INR), 159
Interstitial cystitis, 361-362
Interstitial lung disease (ILD), 199-200
Intracerebral hemorrhage, 138
Intrinsic asthma, 197
Intubation, coleus administration before, 203-204
Iodine in thyroid function, 244
　deficiency of, 249
　supplementation of, 248
Irritable bowel syndrome (IBS), 319-320
　acupressure and acupuncture for, 339
　arrowroot for, 321
　bacopa for, 321
　belladonna for, 322b
　case study for, 340
　globe artichoke for, 327
　hypnotherapy for, 339
　peppermint for, 330
　psyllium for, 331-332
　turmeric for, 333
Iscador. See Mistletoe (Viscum album)
Ischemia, cardiac, 127, 135
Ischemic heart disease, 134-154
　adjunct therapies for, 150-151
　case study for, 152
　cerebrovascular accident, 137-138
　herbal therapies for, 141-147, 148t-149t
　　with limited evidence, 148
　　with negative evidence, 148
　integrative therapy plan for, 151-154
　myocardial infarction, 135-137
Ischemic stroke, 137
　danshen for, 142-143
　ginkgo for, 144

Islets of Langerhans, 217
Isoflavones
　for menopausal symptoms, 271, 273f, 277
　for osteoporosis, 284, 288

J

Jackfruit (Artocarpus heterophyllus)
　adverse effects, interactions, and pharmacokinetics of, 531-532
　for diabetes mellitus, 228
Jacksonian epilepsy, 62
Jequirity (Abrus precatorius), 583
Jewelweed (Impatiens biflora, Impatiens pallida), 583
Jiaogulan (Gynostemma pentaphyllum)
　adverse effects, interactions, and pharmacokinetics of, 532
　for cancer, 459
Jimson weed (Datura spp.), 583
Jock itch, 413
Joint
　gout and, 296
　infectious arthritis and, 295
　osteoarthritis and, 292
　Reiter's syndrome and, 295
　rheumatoid arthritis and, 293, 294f
　　juvenile, 295
　synovial, 292f
Jointed flatsedge (Cyperus articulatus), 64
Jojoba (Simmondsia chinensis)
　adverse effects, interactions, and pharmacokinetics of, 532
　for Alzheimer's disease and related disorders, 93
　pregnancy and lactation and, 583
JRA. See Juvenile rheumatoid arthritis (JRA)
Juniper (Juniperus communis)
　for diabetes mellitus, 234
　pregnancy and lactation and, 583
Juvenile osteoporosis, 282-283
Juvenile rheumatoid arthritis (JRA), 295

K

Kamalahar for viral hepatitis, 353b
Katuka for viral hepatitis, 353b
Kava (Piper methysticum)
　adverse effects, interactions, and pharmacokinetics of, 425, 532-533
　for anxiety, 21, 26-27
　　during menopause, 277
　for depressive disorders, 34
　for Parkinson's disease, 57, 59
　pregnancy and lactation and, 584
　for psychiatric disorders, 14
　for seizure disorders, 65
Kegel exercises, 375
Kelp (Laminaria spp.). See Seaweed

Ketoacidosis, 217-218
Khat (Catha edulis)
　adverse effects, interactions, and pharmacokinetics of, 533
　for Alzheimer's disease and related disorders, 93-94
　for cognitive and physical enhancement, 49
　pregnancy and lactation and, 584
Khella (Ammi visnaga), 584
Kidney
　anatomy of, 360f
　congestive heart failure and, 114-115, 116f
　high blood pressure and, 102-103
Kidney disease. See Also Genitourinary disorders
　cancer, 447
　danshen for, 366-367
　end-stage, 245
　lupus nephritis, 364
　　flax for, 367
　renal calculi, 363-364
　　cornflower for, 374
　　cranberry for, 366, 377
　　grapefruit for, 368
　soy for, 372
Kiwi (Actinidia deliciosa, Actinidia chinensis)
　adverse effects, interactions, and pharmacokinetics of, 533-534
　for cognitive and physical enhancement, 47
　for fungal infections, 420
　pregnancy and lactation and, 584
　for respiratory disorders, 206
Kola nut (Cola acuminata)
　for cognitive and physical enhancement, 49
　for depressive disorders, 34
　pregnancy and lactation and, 584
Korean Red Ginseng. See Ginseng (Panax spp.)
Kudzu (Pueraria lobata)
　adverse effects, interactions, and pharmacokinetics of, 534
　for angina, 130, 132
　for bacterial infection, 399
　for diabetes mellitus, 228
　for menopausal symptoms, 271
Kundalini yoga for angina, 132
Kwai, 105, 144

L

Labeling, 5, 5f
Lactation, 570-592
Lactobacillus as probiotic, 400
Ladies mantle (Alchemilla vulgaris), 584
Laetrile. See Also Bitter almond (Prunus amygdalus), 474

Lavender (*Lavandula angustifolia*)
  adverse effects, interactions, and pharmacokinetics of, 534-535
  for Alzheimer's disease and related disorders, 94, 100
  for anxiety, 22, 26
  for bacterial infection, 399-400
  for cancer, 459-460
  for depressive disorders, 33
  for methicillin-resistant *Staphylococcus aureus*, 405
  for perineal pain after childbirth, 76, 84
  pregnancy and lactation and, 584
LDLs. *See* Low-density lipoproteins (LDLs)
Lean body mass increase
  cinnamon for, 254
  coleus for, 254
Ledum (*Rhododendron groenlandicum*), 584
Leishmaniasis, 409
  barberry for, 419
  goldenseal for, 416
  zinc for, 420
Lemon balm (*Melissa officinalis*)
  adverse effects, interactions, and pharmacokinetics of, 535
  for Alzheimer's disease and related disorders, 94
  for anxiety and insomnia, 22
  for gastrointestinal disorders, 328
  for herpesvirus, 435
  pregnancy and lactation and, 584
Lemongrass (*Cymbopogon* spp.)
  adverse effects, interactions, and pharmacokinetics of, 535
  pregnancy and lactation and, 584
Lennox-Gastaut syndrome, 63
Lentinan
  in cancer treatment, 479
  in HIV treatment, 441
Lepromatous leprosy, 385
Leprosy, 385-386
  bamboo for, 399
Leukemia
  PSK for, 464
  signs and symptoms of, 447
Leukopenia, radiotherapy-induced, 479
Leukotrienes in asthma, 197
LFTs. *See* Liver function tests (LFTs)
LH. *See* Luteinizing hormone (LH)
Libido. *See* Sexual function
Licorice (*Glycyrrhiza glabra*)
  adverse effects, interactions, and pharmacokinetics of, 357, 535-536
  for depressive disorders, 34
  for gastrointestinal disorders, 328, 340
  for genital herpes, 438
  infertility and, 249

Licorice (*Glycyrrhiza glabra*) (Continued)
  for liver disease, 349, 356
  pregnancy and lactation and, 584
  for reduction in body fat mass, 257
  for viral infection, 435-436
Lime (*Citrus aurantifolia*)
  adverse effects, interactions, and pharmacokinetics of, 536
  for cholera prevention, 395
  pregnancy and lactation and, 584
Lingonberry (*Vaccinium vitis-idaea*)
  adverse effects, interactions, and pharmacokinetics of, 536
  for parasitic infection, 420
  pregnancy and lactation and, 584
  for urinary tract infection prevention, 395-396
Lipid disorders, 170-195
  adjunct therapies for, 190
  case studies associated with, 192
  in diabetes mellitus, 236-237
  diagnosis of, 171-173
  herbal therapies for, 173, 191t
    with limited evidence, 190
    with negative evidence, 189
  integrative therapy plan for, 192
  overview of, 171-173
  signs and symptoms of, 171
Lipoproteins, 171
  diet for lowering, 172-173, 190
  levels of, 172
Listerine, 393
Liv-52, 347
Liver disorders, 343-358
  adjunct therapies for, 353
  cancer
    bupleurum for, 453
    PSK for, 464
  case studies associated with, 356
  diagnosis of, 345-346
  drug-induced, 345
  hepatitis, 344-345. (*See Also* Hepatitis)
  herbal therapies for, 346, 354t-355t
    with limited evidence, 353
    with negative evidence, 353
  integrative therapy plan for, 355
  overview of, 343-346
  stages of, 343-344
  Wilson's disease, 345
Liver failure, 344
Liver function tests (LFTs), 345-346
Loa loa, 411
Lobelia (*Lobelia inflata*), 209
Loiasis, 411
Long-QT syndrome, 140
Lotus (*Nelumbo nucifera*), 584
Lovage (*Levisticum officinale*), 585
Low back pain, 69
  devil's claw for, 75, 84
  willow for, 78-79

Low blood sugar. *See* Hypoglycemia
Low-density lipoproteins (LDLs), 171. *See Also* Lipid disorders
  diet for lowering, 172-173, 190
  levels of, 172
Lung. *See Also* Respiratory disorders
  cancer of
    case study associated with, 483-484
    greater celandine for, 458-459
    peony for, 463
    PSK for, 464
    sage for prevention of, 466-467
    screening for, 448
    signs and symptoms of, 447
  chronic obstructive pulmonary disease, 198
  function tests of in, 198, 212
  embolism of, 158
  fibrosis of, 199-200
    ginkgo for, 205
  histoplasmosis of, 414
  pulmonary hypertension and, 200
Lupus nephritis, 364
  flax for, 367
Luteinizing hormone (LH), 241
  disorders of, 243-244
Lycopene for reduced cancer risk, 481
Lymphatic filariasis, 411
Lymphoma, non-Hodgkin's, 447

M

MAC. *See Mycobacterium avium* complex (MAC)
Maca (*Lepidium meyenii*)
  adverse effects, interactions, and pharmacokinetics of, 536
  for cognitive and physical enhancement, 49
  effects of on male reproductive hormone levels, 247
  for fertility problems, 249
  for menopausal symptoms, 274
  for sexual function, 369
Macrobiotic diet, 261-262
Magnesium
  for asthma, 210
  for cardiovascular health, 150-151
Magnetic resonance imaging (MRI)
  in Alzheimer's disease, 89
  in angina, 129
  in stroke, 138
Magnet therapy for arthritis, 309
Magnolia (*Magnolia* spp.), 585
Ma huang. *See* Ephedra (*Ephedra sinica*)
Maitake mushroom (*Grifola frondosa*)
  adverse effects, interactions, and pharmacokinetics of, 536-537
  for cancer, 460
  for diabetes mellitus, 229
  for genitourinary disorders, 374

Major depression, 30
Malaria, 409
　case study associated with, 424
　chloroquine-resistant, goldenseal for, 416
　integrative therapy plan for, 424
　sweet Annie for, 417
　vitamin A for, 423
　yerba santa for, 420
Malignant cell, 445
Malignant hypertension, 103
Manic-depressive disorder, 31
Manipulative and body-based therapies, 1-2
MAP. See *Mycobacterium avium* subsp. *paratuberculosis* (MAP)
Marijuana *(Cannabis sativa)*, 306
Marjoram *(Origanum majorana)*, 164
Masking in Parkinson's disease, 55
Massage, abdominal, for constipation, 339
Massage therapy in cancer treatment, 480
Mast cells in asthma, 197
Mastic *(Pistacia lentiscus)*
　adverse effects, interactions, and pharmacokinetics of, 537
　for dental plaque, 396
　for gastric and duodenal ulcers, 329
　pregnancy and lactation and, 585
Maturity-onset diabetes of the young (MODY), 219-220
May-Hegglin anomaly, 157
MCP. See Modified citrus pectin (MCP)
Meadowsweet *(Filipendula ulmaria)*
　aspirin *versus*, 149
　pregnancy and lactation and, 585
Measles, 430
Meditation
　in HIV treatment, 440
　in seizure disorders treatment, 66
Mefloquine, 424
Melanocyte-stimulating hormone (MSH), 242
Melanoma, 447
Melatonin
　in cancer treatment, 480
　for sleep disorders, 26
　for smoking cessation, 210
Memory impairment, 14
　bacopa for, 89-90
　cranberry for, 90
　ginkgo for, 45, 90-92
　rhubarb for, 95
　tea for, 96
Meningitis, bacterial, 384
Menopause, 266-280
　adjunct therapies for, 274-277
　case studies associated with, 278
　diagnosis of, 268
　herbal therapies for, 268-274, 275t-276t

Menopause *(Continued)*
　　with limited evidence, 274
　　with negative evidence, 274
　hormone replacement therapy for, 268
　integrative therapy plan for, 277-279
　overview of, 266-268
　perimenopause, 267
　postmenopause, 267
　signs and symptoms of, 267-268
　sleep disturbances due to, 26
　surgical, 267
Mental status evaluation (MSE), 89
Menthol, 206-207
Mescaline, 14
Mesoglycan, 166
Metabolic syndrome, 219
　case study associated with, 238
　diagnosis of, 220
　obesity in, 253
Metabolism, glucose, 217
　diabetes mellitus and, 217
　safflower and, 234
Metastasis, 445
Metformin, 3
　for diabetes mellitus, 226b
　for weight reduction, 259
Methamphetamine abuse, 41
Methicillin-resistant *Staphylococcus aureus* (MRSA), 386
　case study associated with, 404-405
　ginseng for, 394
　lavender for, 399-400
　tea for, 397
8-Methoxypsoralen (8-MOP), 415
Mexican horsetail. See Horsetail *(Equisetum* spp.)
MF101 for menopausal symptoms, 274
MI. See Myocardial infarction (MI)
Microangiopathy, diabetic, 236
　gotu kola for, 227
　pycnogenol for, 230
Micrographia in Parkinson's disease, 55
Migraine headache, 69
　butterbur for, 73-74
　feverfew for, 75-76, 83-84
　willow bark for, 84
Milk thistle *(Silybum marianum)*
　adverse effects, interactions, and pharmacokinetics of, 537
　for cancer prevention, 460-461
　for diabetes mellitus, 229
　for lipid disorders, 181
　for liver disorders, 349, 356
　pregnancy and lactation and, 585
　for prostate cancer, 374
　for respiratory disorders, 209-210
Mind-body interventions, 1-2
　for arthritis, 310
　in cancer treatment, 480
　in HIV, 440

Minerals
　deficiencies of due to diarrhea, 339
　in HIV treatment, 440
Minor motor seizure, 63
Mistletoe *(Viscum album)*
　adverse effects, interactions, and pharmacokinetics of, 357, 537-538
　for arthritis, 303
　for cancer, 461, 482
　for hepatitis, 351, 357
　for HIV, 436, 442
　for hypertension, 109
　pregnancy and lactation and, 585
　for respiratory disorders, 206
　for seizure disorders, 65
Mixed dementia, 86-87
Mixing study in coagulation disorder, 159
Modified citrus pectin (MCP)
　adverse effects, interactions, and pharmacokinetics of, 538-539
　for prostate cancer, 462
MODY. See Maturity-onset diabetes of the young (MODY)
Momordica grosvenori (Momordica charantia), 585
Monoamine oxidase inhibitor (MAOI), herbal therapies with properties of, 35b
Mood
　changes in due to depression, 31
　enhancement of
　　caffeine for, 46
　　guarana for, 33, 46
　　sage for, 33
Morbid obesity, 252, 264
Morinda *(Morinda citrifolia)*, 585
Morning sickness, 318
　ginger for, 326
Motherwort *(Leonurus artemisia, Leonurus cardiaca)*, 585
Motion sickness
　case study for, 341
　ginger for, 326
Moutan *(Paeonia lactiflora)*, 585
Mouth, candidiasis infection of. See Oral thrush
Moxibustion
　in cancer treatment, 480
　for weight loss, 262
MRI. See Magnetic resonance imaging (MRI)
MRSA. See Methicillin-resistant *Staphylococcus aureus* (MRSA)
MSE. See Mental status evaluation (MSE)
MSH. See Melanocyte-stimulating hormone (MSH)
Mucositis, radiotherapy-induced, 479
Mucoviscidosis, 199

Mugwort *(Artemisia vulgaris)*
    pregnancy and lactation and, 585
    for seizure disorders, 65
Muira puama *(Ptychopetalum olacoides)*
    adverse effects, interactions, and pharmacokinetics of, 539
    pregnancy and lactation and, 585
    for sexual dysfunction, 369
Mullein *(Verbascum thapsus)*, 210
Multiple sleep latency test, 43
Mumps, 430
Mushrooms
    maitake
        adverse effects, interactions, and pharmacokinetics of, 536-537
        for cancer, 460
        for diabetes mellitus, 229
        for genitourinary disorders, 374
    reishi
        adverse effects, interactions, and pharmacokinetics of, 549
        for cancer, 465
        for cardiovascular disease and angina, 130
        for diabetes mellitus, 232
        for hepatitis B, 351
        for hypertension, 107, 112
        for lipid disorders, 186
        for postherpetic pain, 77
    shiitake
        adverse effects, interactions, and pharmacokinetics of, 557
        as chemotherapy adjuvant, 467-468, 479
        for fungal infection, 420
        for genitourinary disorders, 374
        for herpesvirus, 437
Music therapy
    for Alzheimer's disease, 99-100
    for pain, 83
Mycobacteria, 383
    nontuberculous, 386
Mycobacterium avium complex (MAC), 386
Mycobacterium avium subsp. *paratuberculosis* (MAP), 319
Mycobacterium leprae, 385
Mycobacterium tuberculosis, 388
Myocardial infarction (MI), 127, 135-137
    diagnosis of, 137
    high blood pressure and, 103
    integrative therapy plan for, 151-154
    signs and symptoms of, 137
    types of, 135-137
Myoclonic seizure, 62-63
Myrcia (Myrcia spp.)
    adverse effects, interactions, and pharmacokinetics of, 539
    for diabetes mellitus, 229
    pregnancy and lactation and, 585
Myrrh *(Commiphora myrrha)*, 585

N

Nails, fungal infection of, 413
    tea tree for, 418
    thyme for, 418-419
NASH. *See* Nonalcoholic steatohepatitis (NASH)
Nasopharyngeal cancer
    PSK for, 464
    rhubarb for, 466
Nasopharyngitis, acute viral, 428
National Cancer Institute (NCI), 2
National Center for Complementary and Alternative Medicine (NCCAM), 2
Native extract, 4
Natural Standards
    grading scale of, 9-10, 9t
    research collaboration and
Nausea, 317-318
    acupressure and acupuncture for, 339
    chemotherapy-induced, management of, 327, 476
    ginger for, 326
    peppermint for, 330
NCCAM. *See* National Center for Complementary and Alternative Medicine (NCCAM)
Necator americanus, 410
Neck pain, 69
Neem *(Azadirachta indica)*
    adverse effects, interactions, and pharmacokinetics of, 539
    for dental plaque, 396
    for gastric and duodenal ulcer, 329
    pregnancy and lactation and, 585-586
Neisseria meningitidis, 400
Nephritic syndrome, rhubarb for bleeding associated with, 162-163
Nephritis, lupus, 364
    flax for, 367
Nephrolithiasis, 363-364
    cornflower for, 374
    cranberry for, 366-371, 377
    grapefruit for, 368
Nephropathy, diabetic, 235-236
Nerve pain, 70
Nervous system
    central (*See* Brain; Central nervous system)
    sympathetic, activation of in anxiety disorders, 17-18, 18f
Neuralgia, postherpetic, 430
    Reishi mushroom for, 77
Neurogenic bladder, 362
    saw palmetto for, 372
Neurogenic pain, 70
Neuroleptics, 11
Neuromuscular symptoms in cancer, 446
Neurons, 17-18, 18f
    Alzheimer's disease and, 88

Neuropathy, diabetic peripheral
    adjunct therapies for, 235-236
    evening primrose for, 224
    ginseng for, 226
    kudzu for, 228
Neurotransmitters
    activation of in anxiety disorders, 17-18, 18f
    depression and, 30, 30f
New breviscapine. *See* Breviscapine *(Erigeron breviscapus)*
Niacin for hyperlipidemia, 191
NIC. *See* National Cancer Institute (NCI)
Nicotine addiction, 40-41
Nicotine replacement therapy (NRT), 210
Nitrates for angina, 127-128, 132
Nitric oxide in hemostasis, 155-156
NLEA. *See* Nutrition Labeling and Education Act (NLEA)
Nociceptive pain, 70
Nocturnal enuresis in children, 361
Nodules
    rheumatoid, 294
    thyroid, 245
Nonalcoholic steatohepatitis (NASH), 343-344
    rhubarb for, 352
Nonallergic asthma, 197
Non-Hodgkin's lymphoma, 447
Noni *(Morinda citrifolia)*
    for parasitic infection, 420
    for weight loss, 260
Non-ST-segment elevation myocardial infarction (NSTEMI), 136
Nontuberculous mycobacteria (NTM), 386
Nopal *(Opuntia* spp.)
    adverse effects, interactions, and pharmacokinetics of, 539-540
    for benign prostatic hyperplasia, 370
    for diabetes mellitus, 229
    for lipid disorders, 182
    for weight loss, 260
Nordihydroguaiaretic aced (NDGA). *See* Chaparral *(Larrea tridentata, Larrea divaricata)*
North American skullcap *(Scutellaria lateriflora)*. *See* Skullcap *(Scutellaria* spp.)
Northern prickly ash *(Zanthoxylum americanum)*, 586
NRT. *See* Nicotine replacement therapy (NRT)
NSTEMI. *See* Non-ST-segment elevation myocardial infarction (NSTEMI)
NTM. *See* Nontuberculous mycobacteria (NTM)
Numerical pain scale, 71
Nutmeg *(Myristica fragrans)*, 586
Nutrient content claims, 5

Nutrition Labeling and Education Act (NLEA), 5
Nux vomica *(Strychnos nux-vomica)*, 586

O

OA. *See* Osteoarthritis (OA)
Oak moss *(Evernia prunastri)*, 586
Oats *(Avena sativa)*, 586
Obesity, 252-265
   abdominal, 253
   adjunct therapies for, 261-262
   asthma and, 197
   case studies associated with, 263
   diagnosis of, 253, 253t
   herbal therapies for, 253-258, 260t
     with limited evidence, 259-261
     with negative evidence, 259
   integrative therapy plan for, 262-265
   morbid, 252, 264
   overview of, 252-253
   signs and symptoms of, 253
Obsessive-compulsive disorder (OCD), 19
Obstruction, airway, due to asthma, 197
Occlusion, coronary, 127
Occupational asthma, 197
OCD. *See* Obsessive-compulsive disorder (OCD)
ODS. *See* Office of Dietary Supplements (ODS)
Office of Dietary Supplements (ODS), 3
Oleander *(Nerium oleander, Thevetia peruviana)*
   adverse effects, interactions, and pharmacokinetics of, 540
   for cancer, 462-463
   for congestive heart failure, 121
   pregnancy and lactation and, 586
   for psychiatric disorders, 13
Olive *(Olea europaea)*
   for hypertension, 109
   pregnancy and lactation and, 586
Omega-3 fatty acids
   adverse effects, interactions, and pharmacokinetics of, 540-541
   for arthritis, 309
   for cancer, 481
   for congestive heart failure, 124
   for dementia, 98
   for hypertension, 109-110
   for lipid disorders, 182, 192-193
   pregnancy and lactation and, 586
Onchocerciasis, 411
Onion *(Allium cepa)*
   adverse effects, interactions, and pharmacokinetics of, 541
   for diabetes mellitus, 230
   for hypertension, 106
   for osteoporosis, 285
   for respiratory disorders, 206

Onycholysis, 413
Onychomycosis, 413
   case study associated with, 425
   tea tree for, 417
Opportunistic infection in human immunodeficiency virus, 429
Oral cancer
   signs and symptoms of, 447
   spirulina for, 470-471
Oral glucose tolerance test, 219
Oral herpes, 429-430
   tea tree for, 437
Oral thrush, 413-414
   case study associated with, 424
   cinnamon for, 415
   tea tree for, 417
Oregano *(Origanum vulgare)*
   for fungal infection, 420
   pregnancy and lactation and, 586
Oregon grape *(Berberis aquifolium)*. *See* Berberine
Osteoarthritis (OA), 292, 293f
   adjunct therapies for, 309-310
   arnica for, 296
   ashwagandha for, 297
   avocado for, 297-298, 311
   black cohosh for, 298
   boswellia for, 299
   case study associated with, 312
   cat's claw for, 299-300
   devil's claw for, 300-301, 311
   ginger for, 301-302
   glucosamine and chondroitin for, 309, 311
   guggul for, 302
   integrative therapy plan for, 310-313
   magnet therapy for, 309
   pathologic changes in, 293f
   rose hip for, 304, 311
   turmeric for, 304-305
   willow for, 305, 311
Osteoblasts, 281
Osteoclasts, 245, 281
Osteocytes, 281
Osteopathy for otitis media, 403
Osteopenia, 281-282
Osteophyte, 292
Osteoporosis, 281-290
   adjunct therapies for, 285-286
   case studies associated with, 288
   diagnosis of, 283
   herbal therapies for, 283-285, 286t
     with limited evidence, 285
   integrative therapy plan for, 286-289, 287f
   during menopause, 274, 278
   overview of, 281-283, 282f
   prevention of, 282f
   signs and symptoms of, 283
   treatment algorithm for, 287f

Otitis media (OM), 386-387
   chiropractic for, 403
   osteopathy for, 403
   sanicle for, 400
Ovaries
   cancer of
     ginkgo for, 456
     ginseng for, 457
     signs and symptoms of, 447
   premature failure of, 266
Oxygen dependence, bacterial, 383

P

Pacemaker cells, 138-139
Pain, 69-85
   abdominal, in irritable bowel syndrome, 319-320
   adjunct therapies for, 82-83
   case studies associated with, 84
   chest (*See* Angina)
   defined, 69
   diagnosing causes of, 71
   due to cancer, 446
   herbal therapies for, 72-82, 79t-82t
     with limited evidence, 79
   integrative therapy plan for, 83-84
   in myocardial infarction, 137
   in osteoarthritis, 292
   overview of, 69-71
   in periodontal disease, 387
   scales, 71
   signs and symptoms of, 71
   types of, 70
Palm *(Elaeis guineensis)*, 586
Panax ginseng. *See* Ginseng *(Panax* spp.)
Panchakarma for anxiety in heart disease patients, 131b
Pancreas
   anatomy of, 317f
   cancer of
     ginkgo for, 456
     greater celandine for, 458-459
     signs and symptoms of, 447
   in glucose metabolism, 217
Panic disorder, 19
Papain. *See* Papaya *(Carica papaya)*
Papanicolaou smear, 448
Papaya *(Carica papaya)*
   adverse effects, interactions, and pharmacokinetics of, 541
   for arthritis, 303
   for cognitive and physical enhancement, 47
   for gastrointestinal disorders, 329
Paralysis
   sleep, 42-43
   Todd's, 62
Parasitic infection, 408-426
   adjunct therapies for, 420-423
   case studies associated with, 424

Parasitic infection *(Continued)*
   helminthic, 410-412
      herbal therapies for, 414-416, 421t-423t
         with limited evidence, 419-420
      integrative therapy plan for, 423-425
      overview of, 408-414
   protozoal, 409-410
Parathyroid hormone (PTH), 244
   disorders of (*See* Thyroid and parathyroid disorders)
   osteoporosis and, 282
Parkinsonian gait, 53-54
Parkinsonism, 53
Parkinson's disease (PD), 53-60
   adjunct therapies for, 58
   anxiety in, 26
   case studies for, 59
   diagnosis of, 55
   herbal therapies for, 55-57, 57t-58t
      with limited evidence, 57-58
      with negative evidence, 57
   integrative therapy plan for, 59
   overview of, 53-55
   signs and symptoms of, 53-55
Paronychia, fungal, 413
   thyme for, 418-419
Parsley *(Petroselinum crispum)*, 586
Partial seizure, 61-62
Passion flower *(Passiflora incarnata)*
   adverse effects, interactions, and pharmacokinetics of, 541
   for anxiety and insomnia, 23-24
   for congestive heart failure, 121-122
   pregnancy and lactation and, 586-587
   for seizure disorders, 65
Patient counseling, 7
Pau d'arco *(Tabebuia impetiginosa)*, 587
PC-SPES
   for cancer, 475-476
   pregnancy and lactation and, 587
PCTA. *See* Percutaneous transluminal coronary angioplasty (PCTA)
PD. *See* Parkinson's disease (PD)
Peanut *(Arachis hypogaea)*, 587
Pear *(Pyrus communis)*, 587
Pelvic examination in menopause diagnosis, 268, 268f
Pelvic floor exercise, 375
Pelvic inflammatory disease (PID), 364
Pelvic pain syndrome, 77, 372
Penetration of virus, 428
Penicillin, 381-383
Peony *(Paeonia* spp.)
   adverse effects, interactions, and pharmacokinetics of, 542
   for liver disorders, 351
   for lung cancer, 463
   pregnancy and lactation and, 587
Pepper. *See* Black pepper *(Piper nigrum)*; Capsicum *(Capsicum* spp.)

Peppermint *(Mentha x piperita)*
   adverse effects, interactions, and pharmacokinetics of, 542-543
   for Alzheimer's disease and related disorders, 94
   for bacterial infection, 400
   for gastrointestinal disorders, 330
   for headache, 75-76
   pregnancy and lactation and, 587
   for respiratory disorders, 206-207
   in stoke recovery therapy, 151
Peptic ulcer disease, 317
   bilberry for, 335
   licorice for, 328
   mastic for, 329
   neem for, 329
   sea buckthorn for, 332
   turmeric for, 333
Peptidoglycan
   on gram-negative bacteria, 383
   on gram-positive bacteria, 383
Percutaneous transluminal coronary angioplasty (PCTA), 128
Periarthritis, 294-295
Perilla *(Perilla frutescens)*
   adverse effects, interactions, and pharmacokinetics of, 543
   for respiratory disorders, 207
Perillyl alcohol (POH) for cancer, 459-460
Perimenopause, 267
   black cohosh for, 269
   St. John's wort for, 273
Perineal pain after childbirth, 76, 84
Periodontal bacterial disease, 387
   acacia for, 389
   bloodroot for, 391
   eucalyptus for, 393
   rhubarb for, 397
   tea tree for, 397-398
Peristalsis, 316
Petit mal seizure, 62, 62t
Peyote *(Lophophora williamsii)*
   pregnancy and lactation and, 587
   for psychiatric disorders, 14
Peyronie disease, 361
PFTs. *See* Pulmonary function tests (PFTs)
Phagocytosis, 381
Phantom pain, 70
Pharmacokinetics, 486-569
Pharmacotherapy, 1-7
Pharyngitis, 436
Phobias, 19
Phosphatidylserine for Alzheimer's disease, 99
Physical activity. *See* Exercise
Physical enhancement. *See* Cognitive and physical enhancement
Physical therapy for pain, 83

Phytobezoar, papaya for, 329
Phytoestrogens, 270, 279, 284, 288
PID. *See* Pelvic inflammatory disease (PID)
Pineapple *(Ananas comosus)*. *See* Bromelain *(Bromeliaceae)*
Pituitary disorders
   adenoma, 242
   adjunct therapies for, 248
   of adrenocorticotropic hormone and corticotropin-releasing hormone, 243
   of antidiuretic hormone, 243
   case studies associated with, 249
   diagnosis of, 244
   of growth hormone, 242
   herbal therapies for, 246-247, 247t
      with limited evidence, 247-248
   integrative therapy plan for, 248-250
   of luteinizing hormone and follicle-stimulating hormone, 243-244
   overview of, 241-246
   of prolactin, 243
   of thyroid-stimulating hormone, 242-243
Pituitary gland, 241, 242f
Pityriasis capitis, 417
Pityriasis versicolor, 413
   bishop's weed for, 414-415
   selenium for, 423
   zinc for, 420
Plaque
   arterial, 171
   dental (*See* Dental plaque)
Plasmin, 156
Plasminogen, 156
Plasmodium. *See* Malaria
Platelets, 156
   disorders of, 157
Platelet count, 158-159
Platelet inhibitors
   for angina, 128
   garlic, 160
   ginger, 161
   grape seed, 161
   policosanol, 161, 167
   pycnogenal, 161
   yohimbe, 163
Pleural effusion, 446
Plummer's disease, 244
PMDD. *See* Premenstrual dysphoric disorder (PMDD)
Podophyllum *(Podophyllum* spp.)
   as adjunct cancer therapy, 480
   adverse effects, interactions, and pharmacokinetics of, 543
   for gastrointestinal disorders, 335
   pregnancy and lactation and, 587
   for rheumatoid arthritis, 303-304, 312
   for uterine cancer, 463-464

POH. *See* Perillyl alcohol (POH) for cancer
Poison ivy *(Toxicodendron radicans)*, 587
Pokeweed *(Phytolacca americana)*, 587
Policosanol
   adverse effects, interactions, and pharmacokinetics of, 543
   for coagulation disorders, 161, 167
   for coronary heart disease, 145
   for lipid disorders, 182
   pregnancy and lactation and, 587
Polydipsia in diabetes mellitus, 217
Polyphagia in diabetes mellitus, 217
Polypodium *(Polypodium leucotomos)*
   adverse effects, interactions, and pharmacokinetics of, 543-544
   for Alzheimer's disease and related disorders, 94-95
Polysomnography, 43
Polyuria in diabetes mellitus, 217
Pomegranate *(Punica granatum)*
   adverse effects, interactions, and pharmacokinetics of, 544
   for atherosclerosis, 145
   for fungal infection, 417
   pregnancy and lactation and, 587
Pork tapeworm, 410
Porphyromonas gingivalis, 398
Positron emission tomography (PET), 89
Postherpetic neuralgia, 430
Postictal state of seizure, 61
Postmenopause, 267, 277-278
Postoperative nausea and vomiting, 327
Postoperative pain
   aconite for, 72
   arnica for, 72
Postpartum bleeding, 160
Postpartum depression, 31
Postpartum psychosis, 31
Postpericardiotomy syndrome, 128
Posttraumatic stress disorder (PTSD), 19
Postural instability in Parkinson's disease, 55
Postvoid residual (PVR) measurement, 361
Potassium sensitivity test, 362
Poultice, 4
Powdered extract, 4
Prana, 97
Prayer in cancer treatment, 480
Prebiotics, 403
Prediabetes, 218
Preeclampsia, 62-63, 103
   evening primrose for, 104
   false hellebore for, 104
   rhubarb for, 108
Pregnancy, 570-592
   caffeine consumption during, 46-47
   gestational diabetes during, 219
      diagnosis of, 220

Pregnancy *(Continued)*
   ginger for morning sickness during, 326
   hypertension during (*See* Preeclampsia)
   lavender for perineal pain after childbirth, 76
   morning sickness during, 318
      ginger for, 326
Premature ejaculation
   clove for, 374
   ginseng for, 368
Premature heartbeat, 140
Premature ovarian failure, 266
Premenstrual dysphoric disorder (PMDD), 31
   chasteberry for, 32, 36-37
Prions, 86-87
Probiotics, 400
   for chemotherapy-induced gastrointestinal symptoms, 482
   for gastrointestinal problems, 339
   for liver disease, 355
   for vaginal candidiasis, 423-424
Prodromal symptoms, 430
Progestogenic activity, herbs with, 275t-276t
Prolactin, 241
   disorders of, 243
      case study associated with, 249
      chasteberry for, 246
Prolapsed uterus, 362
Propolis for candidiasis, 420-423
Propranolol
   arnica and, 153
   danshen and, 153
Prostacyclin, 155-156
Prostaglandins in asthma, 197
Prostate disorders
   benign hyperplasia, 360
      African wild potato for, 364
      beta-sitosterol for, 365
      integrative therapy plan for, 376
      nopal for, 370
      pygeum for, 370
      red clover for, 371
      rye for, 371
      saw palmetto for, 77, 372
      stinging nettle for, 373
   cancer
      case study associated with, 483
      chaparral for, 454
      flax for, 474-475
      milk thistle for, 374, 460
      modified citrus pectin for, 462
      saw palmetto for, 467
      screening for, 448
      signs and symptoms of, 447
      soy for prevention of, 469-470
      tea for, 473
      maitake and shiitake mushroom for, 374

Prostate-specific antigen (PSA) testing, 360, 376
Prostatitis, 362-363, 363t
   danshen for, 366-367
   quercetin for, 374
   rye for, 371
   saw palmetto for, 372
   types of, 363, 363t
Protein intake in epilepsy treatment, 66
Proteinuria, soy for, 372
Prothrombin, 156
Prothrombin time (PT), 159
Protozoal infection, 409-410
Pseudoephedrine, 255
PSK *(Coriolus versicolor)*
   adverse effects, interactions, and pharmacokinetics of, 544
   for cancer, 464, 475
   as adjunct therapy, 479
Psoralens, 415
Psychiatric disorders, 11-16
   adjunct therapies for, 14
   anxiety and insomnia, 17-28
   case studies associated with, 15
   depressive disorders, 29-38
   diagnosis of, 12
   herbal therapies for, 12, 14t
      hallucinogenic, 13-14
      with limited evidence, 13
   integrative therapy plan for, 15
   overview of, 11-12
   psychotic disorders and, 11-12
   signs and symptoms of, 12
Psychoeducation, 11
Psychogenic pain, 70
Psychotherapy
   in cancer treatment, 480
   for depression during menopause, 277
   for diabetes mellitus, 236
   for weight loss, 262
Psychotic disorders, 11-12
   postpartum, 31
Psyllium *(Plantago* spp.)
   adverse effects, interactions, and pharmacokinetics of, 544-545
   for colon cancer, 464-465
   for constipation
      in epilepsy, 66-67
      in Parkinson's disease, 58
   for diabetes mellitus, 230
   for gastrointestinal disorders, 331, 339
   for lipid disorders, 184
   for obesity, 257, 263
   pregnancy and lactation and, 587
PT. *See* Prothrombin time (PT)
PTH. *See* Parathyroid hormone (PTH)
PTSD. *See* Posttraumatic stress disorder (PTSD)
Pulmonary embolism, 158

Pulmonary fibrosis, 199-200
  ginkgo for, 205
Pulmonary function tests (PFTs), 198, 212
Pulmonary hypertension, 200
Pulsatilla (*Anemone pulsatilla*), 587
Pumpkin (*Cucurbita* spp.), 587
Purity, 4
PVR. *See* Postvoid residual (PVR) measurement
P wave, 140
Pycnogenol (*Pinus pinaster* subsp. *atlantica*)
  adverse effects, interactions, and pharmacokinetics of, 545-546
  for arthritis, 306
  for attention disorders, 47, 51
  for coagulation disorders, 162
  for dental bleeding and plaque, 396-397
  for diabetes mellitus, 230
  for erectile dysfunction, 370
  for hypertension, 107, 111
  for lipid disorders, 182
  for pain, 76-77
  for respiratory disorders, 207
Pyelonephritis, 388
Pygeum (*Prunus africanum*, syn. *Pygeum africanum*)
  adverse effects, interactions, and pharmacokinetics of, 546
  for benign prostatic hyperplasia, 370, 376-377
Pyralvex, 397
Pyrosis, 316

Q

QRS wave, 140
QT interval, weight loss and, 263
Quassia (*Picraena excelsa, Quassia undalata, Quassia amara*), 588
Quercetin
  adverse effects, interactions, and pharmacokinetics of, 546-547
  for cardiovascular disease, 145-146
  for hypertension, 106, 110
  for prostatitis, 374
  for respiratory disorders, 210

R

RA. *See* Rheumatoid arthritis (RA)
Radioallergosorbent test (RAST), 198-199
Radiotherapy, management of toxicity and side effects of, 476-479
Radix aconiti. *See* Aconite (*Aconitum napellus*)
Raspberry (*Rubus idaeus*), 588
RAST. *See* Radioallergosorbent test (RAST)

Reactive arthritis, 295-296, 310
Receptor, viral, 428
Rectal cancer. *See* Colorectal cancer
Red clover (*Trifolium pratense*)
  adverse effects, interactions, and pharmacokinetics of, 547
  for benign prostatic hyperplasia, 371
  for cardiovascular disorders, 149
  for diabetes mellitus, 231
  for lipid disorders, 185
  for menopausal symptoms, 271-272, 277
  for osteoporosis, 284, 288
  pregnancy and lactation and, 588
  for prostate cancer, 465
Red yeast rice (*Monascus purpureus*)
  adverse effects, interactions, and pharmacokinetics of, 547-549
  for diabetes mellitus, 231
  for lipid disorders, 185, 192
  pregnancy and lactation and, 588
Rehmannia (*Rehmannia glutinosa*)
  as adjunct cancer therapy, 480
  adverse effects, interactions, and pharmacokinetics of, 549
  for pituitary disorders, 246
Reishi mushroom (*Ganoderma lucidum*)
  adverse effects, interactions, and pharmacokinetics of, 549
  for cancer, 465
  for cardiovascular disease and angina, 130
  for diabetes mellitus, 232
  for hepatitis B, 351
  for hypertension, 107, 112
  for lipid disorders, 186
  for postherpetic pain, 77
Reiter's syndrome, 295-296, 310
Relaxation response, 262
Relaxation therapy
  for angina, 132
  in HIV treatment, 440
Release of virus, 428
Remission, cancer, 449-450
Remodeling
  bone, 281
    osteoarthritis and, 292
    osteoporosis and, 282
  cardiac, 124
Renal calculi, 363-364
  cornflower for, 374
  cranberry for, 366, 377
  grapefruit for, 368
Renal system. *See* Genitourinary disorders; Kidney
Replication, viral, 428
Reproductive system, female, 268f
Research, *Natural Standard*, 8-9
Reserpine for hypertension, 109
Resistance, antibiotics, 404

Resorption, bone, 245, 281
Respiratory disorders, 196-215
  adjunct therapies for, 210
  allergic rhinitis, 198-199
  asthma, 197-198
  case studies for, 213-214
  chronic obstructive pulmonary disease, 198
  cystic fibrosis, 199
  due to cancer, 446
  herbal therapies for, 200-209, 211t-212t
    with limited evidence, 209-210
    with negative evidence, 200
  integrative therapy plan for, 212-214
  overview of, 197-200
  pulmonary fibrosis, 199-200
  pulmonary histoplasmosis, 414
  pulmonary hypertension, 200
  upper respiratory tract infection, 388
    andrographis for, 389
    case study associated with, 405-406
    echinacea for, 399, 434, 438
    garlic for, 435
    wild indigo for, 437-438
    yerba santa for, 400
Resting tremor in Parkinson's disease, 55
Resveratrol
  adverse effects, interactions, and pharmacokinetics of, 550-551
  for cardiovascular disease, 146
  for lipid disorders, 190
  pregnancy and lactation and, 588
Retinal vein occlusion, 163-164
Review of systematic reviews, 9
RF. *See* Rheumatoid factor (RF)
Rheumatoid arthritis (RA), 293-294, 294f
  adjunct therapies for, 309-310
  black cohosh for, 298
  black currant for, 298
  borage for, 298-299, 311
  boswellia for, 299
  bromelain for, 299
  case study associated with, 311-312
  cat's claw for, 299-300
  evening primrose, 301
  feverfew for, 301
  ginger for, 301-302
  guggul for, 302
  integrative therapy plan for, 310-313
  joint destruction in, 293, 294f
  juvenile, 295
  medications for, 311
  mistletoe for, 303
  papaya for, 303
  podophyllum for, 303-304
  turmeric for, 304-305
  willow for, 305

Rheumatoid factor (RF), 292, 294
Rhinitis, allergic, 198-199
   butterbur for, 202
   ephedra for, 204-205
   stinging nettle for, 208
Rhinovirus in common cold, 428
Rhodiola (*Rhodiola rosea*)
   adverse effects, interactions, and pharmacokinetics of, 551
   for Alzheimer's disease and related disorders, 95
   for bladder cancer, 465-466
   for cognitive and physical enhancement, 47
   for respiratory disorders, 207
Rhubarb (*Rheum* spp.)
   adverse effects, interactions, and pharmacokinetics of, 551-552
   for Alzheimer's disease and related disorders, 95
   for coagulation disorders, 162
   for gastrointestinal disorders, 162, 332, 340
   for gingivitis, 397
   for herpes, 436
   for lipid disorders, 186
   for liver disorders, 352
   for menopausal symptoms, 272
   for nasopharyngeal carcinoma, 466
   for obesity, 258
   for parasitic infection, 420
   for preeclampsia, 108
   pregnancy and lactation and, 588
Rhythmic heart disorders. *See* Arrhythmia
Riboflavin for malaria, 423
Rigidity
   herbs for, 97t-98t
   in Parkinson's disease, 55
Ringworm, 412-413
River blindness, 411
Rose hip (*Rosa* spp.)
   adverse effects, interactions, and pharmacokinetics of, 552-553
   for osteoarthritis, 304, 311
   pregnancy and lactation and, 588
Rosemary (*Rosmarinus officinalis*)
   adverse effects, interactions, and pharmacokinetics of, 553
   for anxiety and insomnia, 23-24
   for coagulation disorders, 164
   for parasitic infection, 420
   pregnancy and lactation and, 588
Roundworm infections
   ascariasis, 410
   dracunculiasis, 410
   trichinosis, 412
Rubella, 430
Rue (*Ruta graveolens*), 588

Rupture of arteriovenous malformation, 137-138
Rutin ($C_{27}H_{30}O_{16}$)
   adverse effects, interactions, and pharmacokinetics of, 553
   for cirrhosis, 347
   for coagulation disorders, 163
   for congestive heart failure, 122
   for hypertension, 110
   pregnancy and lactation and, 588
Rye (*Secale cereale*)
   adverse effects, interactions, and pharmacokinetics of, 553-554
   for benign prostatic hyperplasia and prostatitis, 371

S

Saccharomyces boulardii probiotic, 339
SAD. *See* Seasonal affective disorder (SAD); Social anxiety disorder (SAD)
Safety, 4, 486-569
Safflower (*Carthamus tinctorius*)
   adverse effects, interactions, and pharmacokinetics of, 554-555
   for angina, 131
   for atherosclerosis and coronary artery disease, 146
   for diabetes mellitus, 234
   for hepatitis C, 352
   for hypertension, 108
   for lipid disorders, 186
   for Parkinson's disease, 57
   pregnancy and lactation and, 589
   for respiratory disorders, 208
Sage (*Salvia officinalis*)
   for acute pharyngitis, 403, 436
   adverse effects, interactions, and pharmacokinetics of, 555
   for Alzheimer's disease and related disorders, 95
   for depressive disorders, 33
   for diabetes mellitus, 234
   for herpesvirus, 436
   for lung cancer prevention, 466-467
   for menopausal symptoms, 272
   for osteoporosis, 285
   pregnancy and lactation and, 589
   seizures or lower seizure threshold due to, 66
Sahaja yoga in seizure disorders treatment, 66
Salvia (*Salvia divinorum*), 14
Sandalwood (*Santalum album*)
   adverse effects, interactions, and pharmacokinetics of, 555
   for anxiety and insomnia, 24
   for cognitive and physical enhancement, 48

Sanicle (*Sanicula europaea*)
   adverse effects, interactions, and pharmacokinetics of, 555
   for otitis media, 400
   for respiratory disorders
SA node. *See* Sinoatrial (SA) node
Sassafras (*Sassafras* spp.), 589
Savory (*Satureja* spp.), 164
Saw palmetto (*Serenoa repens*)
   adverse effects, interactions, and pharmacokinetics of, 555-556
   for benign prostatic hyperplasia, 372, 376-377
   for cancer prevention and prostate cancer treatment/prevention, 467, 483
   for genitourinary disorders, 372
   pregnancy and lactation and, 589
   for prostatitis and pelvic pain syndrome, 77
Scales, pain, 71, 71f
Schisandra (*Schisandra chinensis*)
   for cognitive and physical enhancement, 49
   for liver disorders, 353
   pregnancy and lactation and, 589
Schistosoma mansoni, 420
Schizoaffective disorder, 12
Schizophrenia, 11-12
   adjunct therapies for, 14
   betel nut for, 12
   case study for, 15
   coleus for, 12-13
   evening primrose for, 13
Schizophreniform disorder, 12
Scopolamine, 341
Scotch broom (*Cytisus scoparius*)
   for cardiovascular disorders, 149
   for congestive heart failure, 122
   pregnancy and lactation and, 589
Screening, cancer, 447-448
Sea buckthorn (*Hippophae rhamnoides*)
   adverse effects, interactions, and pharmacokinetics of, 556
   for cardiovascular disease, 146-147
   for cirrhosis, 352
   for gastric ulcer, 332, 340
   for hypertension, 108
   pregnancy and lactation and, 589
Seasonal affective disorder (SAD), 31
   ginkgo for, 32
Seaweed
   adverse effects, interactions, and pharmacokinetics of, 556-557
   for bacterial infection, 400
   for cancer, 476
   for coagulation disorders, 164
   for diabetes mellitus, 232

Seaweed *(Continued)*
   for fungal infection, 420
   pregnancy and lactation and, 589
   for thyroid disorders, 247, 249
   for weight loss, 260
Secondary adrenal insufficiency, 243
Seizure disorders, 61-68
   adjunct therapies for, 66
   case studies for, 67
   classification of, 61, 62t
   diagnosis of, 63
   herbal therapies for, 63-64, 65t
     with limited evidence, 64-66
   herbs associated with, 65
   integrative therapy plan for, 66-67
   overview of, 61-63
   signs and symptoms of, 63
   types of, 61-63, 62t
Selective serotonin reuptake inhibitor (SSRI)
   herbal therapies with properties of, 35b
   yohimbe for sexual side effects of, 373
Selenium
   for bacterial infection, 403
   in cancer treatment, 481
   for thyroid disorders, 248
   for tinea versicolor, 423
Selenomonas artemidis, 398
Self-examination, breast, 447-448
Self-monitoring of blood glucose (SMBG), 220
Senescence, 445
Senility
   ginseng for, 92-94
   rhubarb for, 95
   Traditional Chinese medicine for, 97
Senna *(Senna alexandrina)*, 589
Sepsis, 381
Septic arthritis, 295
Septic shock, 381
Serum cholesterol, 172
Sexual function
   damiana for, 366
   depression and, 35
   ephedra for, 367
   erectile, 360-361. (*See Also* Erectile dysfunction (ED))
   ginkgo for, 367
   ginseng for, 368
   horny goat weed for, 369
   maca for, 369
   during menopause, 267
   muira puama for, 369
   yohimbe for, 373
Shark cartilage in cancer treatment, 481
Sheehan's syndrome, 246
Sheep's sorrel *(Rumex acetosella)*. *See* Sorrel *(Rumex acetosa, Rumex* spp.)

Shepherd's purse *(Capsella bursa-pastoris)*, 589
Shiitake mushroom *(Lentinus edodes)*
   adverse effects, interactions, and pharmacokinetics of, 557
   as chemotherapy adjuvant, 467-468, 479
   for fungal infection, 420
   for genitourinary disorders, 374
   for herpesvirus, 437
Shingles, 430
Shock, septic, 381
Shortness of breath. *See* Dyspnea
Sho-saiko-to, 346, 453
Shoulder, periarthritis of, 294
SIADH. *See* Syndrome of inappropriate antidiuretic hormone secretion (SIADH)
Sick sinus, 140
Silymarin. *See* Milk thistle *(Silybum marianum)*
Simple partial seizure, 62, 62t
Sinoatrial (SA) node, 138-139
Sitosterol (22,23-Dihydrostigmasterol, 24-Ethylcholesterol). *See* Beta-sitosterol (β-Sitosterol)
Skeleton, human, 282f
Skin
   cancer of
     melanoma as, 447
     screening for, 448
   changes in due to cancer, 446
   fungal infection of, 412
     fungal paronychia, 413
     tinea capitis and tinea corporis, 412-413
     tinea cruris, 413
     tinea pedis, 413
     tinea unguium, 413
     tinea versicolor, 413
   Parkinson's disease and, 55
   radiotherapy-induced dermatitis of, 479
Skullcap *(Scutellaria* spp.)
   adverse effects, interactions, and pharmacokinetics of, 557-558
   for anxiety and insomnia, 25
   for cancer, 468-469
   for chemotherapy toxicity, 476
   for seizure disorders, 65
Skunk cabbage *(Symplocarpus foetidus)*, 589
SLE. *See* Systemic lupus erythematosus (SLE), kidney disease due to
Sleep disturbances. *See Also* Insomnia
   in depression, 31, 35
   during menopause, 277
   narcolepsy, 42-43
   in Parkinson's disease, 58
Sleep paralysis in narcolepsy, 42-43

Slippery elm *(Ulmus rubra,* syn. *Ulmus fulva)*
   adverse effects, interactions, and pharmacokinetics of, 558
   for cancer, 469
   for gastrointestinal disorders, 333
   pregnancy and lactation and, 590
SMBG. *See* Self-monitoring of blood glucose (SMBG)
Smoking
   cancer and, 483
   cessation of, 210, 212-213, 237
   chronic obstructive pulmonary disease and, 198
   diabetes mellitus and, 237
   green tea and, 472
   irritable bowel syndrome and, 341
   osteoporosis and, 288-289
   upper respiratory tract infection and, 405
Social anxiety disorder (SAD), 19
Sodium intake in hypertension, 111
Solid extract, 4
Somatic pain, 70
Somatic symptoms in menopause, 268
Somatostatin, 217
Sorrel *(Rumex acetosa, Rumex* spp.)
   adverse effects, interactions, and pharmacokinetics of, 558
   for bacterial infection, 400
   for cancer, 469
   pregnancy and lactation and, 590
   for viral infections1120, 438, 441
Soy *(Glycine max)*
   adverse effects, interactions, and pharmacokinetics of, 558-559
   for Alzheimer's disease and related disorders, 96
   for breast pain, 77-78
   for cancer, 469-470
   for diabetes mellitus, 232
   for diarrhea, 333
   for hypertension, 108
   for kidney disease, 372
   for lipid disorders, 187, 192-193
   for menopausal symptoms, 272, 273f, 277
   for osteoporosis, 284, 288
   pregnancy and lactation and, 590
   for weight loss, 258, 263
Spasm
   colonic, gastric, and esophageal peppermint for, 330
   infantile in West syndrome, 63
Spastic colon, 319
Spinach *(Spinacia oleracea)*, 590
Spinal cord, 12f
Spinal manipulative therapy, 82. *See Also* Chiropractic

Spirometry in asthma diagnosis, 197-198
Spirulina *(Arthrospira* spp.)
   adverse effects, interactions, and pharmacokinetics of, 559
   for diabetes mellitus, 233
   for lipid disorders, 187
   for oral cancer, 470-471
   pregnancy and lactation and, 590
   for viral hepatitis, 353
   for weight loss, 258
Squill *(Urginea maritima,* syn. *Scilla maritima)*
   adverse effects, interactions, and pharmacokinetics of, 559
   for coronary artery disease, 147
   pregnancy and lactation and, 590
SSRI. *See* Selective serotonin reuptake inhibitor (SSRI)
St. John's wort *(Hypericum perforatum)*
   adverse effects, interactions, and pharmacokinetics of, 560-561
   in Alzheimer's disease treatment, 100
   for anxiety and insomnia, 23
   for asthma, 210
   for depressive disorders, 14, 33, 35-37
      during menopause, 273, 277
   glucose control and, 483
   for hepatitis C, 353
   for HIV, 438, 442
   infertility and, 249
   for inflammation, 84
   interaction in cancer treatment, 449
   pregnancy and lactation and, 590
Stable angina, 127
Staging of cancers, 449
Staphylococcus, 383
Staphylococcus aureus, 380-381, 383
   betel nut for, 390
   eucalyptus for, 393
   methicillin-resistant, 386
      case study associated with, 404-405
      ginseng for, 394
      lavender for, 399-400
      tea for, 397
      uva ursi for, 398
Staphylococcus epidermidis, 383
Statins for Alzheimer's disease, 87
Status epilepticus, 63
Steatohepatitis, 343-344
STEMI. *See* ST-segment elevation myocardial infarction (STEMI)
Stenosis
   cardiac, 127
   due to plaque, 171
Stevia *(Stevia rebaudiana)*
   adverse effects, interactions, and pharmacokinetics of, 561-562
   for diabetes mellitus, 233
   for hypertension, 109, 111
   pregnancy and lactation and, 590

Stimulants, 39
   abuse of, 40-41, 49
   Controlled Substance Act classification of, 40
   herbal, 44-48, 50t
      adjunct therapies, 49-51
      for athletic performance, 44
      for attention disorders, 41
      case studies associated with, 51
      for chronic fatigue syndrome, 43
      for fatigue and low energy, 43-44
      with limited evidence, 49
      for narcolepsy, 42-43
      overview of, 39-44
      for weight loss, 44
Stinging nettle *(Urtica dioica)*
   adverse effects, interactions, and pharmacokinetics of, 562
   for arthritis, 304
   for benign prostatic hyperplasia, 373
   for congestive heart failure, 122
   for pain, 79
   pregnancy and lactation and, 590
   for respiratory disorders, 208
Stomach, 330
   cancer of
      ginkgo for, 456
      ginseng for, 457-458
      PSK for, 464
      signs and symptoms of, 447
      soy for, 469-470
   spasm of, peppermint for, 330
   ulcer of(*See* Peptic ulcer disease)
Stomatitis, radiotherapy-induced, 479
Strawberry *(Fragaria* spp.)
   adverse effects, interactions, and pharmacokinetics of, 562
   for colorectal cancer prevention, 471
   pregnancy and lactation and, 590
Streptococcus, 383
Streptococcus faecalis, 389
Streptococcus mutans
   andrographis, 389
   thyme for, 398
Streptococcus pyogenes, 394
Streptococcus salivarius, 390
Streptococcus sobrinus, 398
Stress, seizure disorders and, 66
Stress incontinence, 361
   during menopause, 276
Stress test, cardiac, 128
Stroke. *See* Cerebrovascular accident (CVA)
Strongyloidiasis, 411
Structure and function claims, 5
ST-segment elevation myocardial infarction (STEMI), 136-137
Subarachnoid hemorrhage, 138
Substance abuse, 40
Succussion, 104

Sugar cane wax *(Saccharum officinarum).* *See* Policosanol
Suicidal thoughts in depression, 31, 35
Summer savory *(Satureja hortensis). See* Savory *(Satureja* spp.)
Sunflower *(Helianthus annuus)*, 590
Superinfection, 388
Supplement facts, 5, 5f
Supplements. *See* Dietary supplements
Supraventricular tachycardia (SVT), 139
Surgery
   nausea and vomiting following
      ginger for, 327
      peppermint for, 330
   pain following
      aconite for, 72
      arnica for, 72
Sweat test in cystic fibrosis, 199
Sweet almond *(Prunus amygdalus dulcis)*
   adverse effects, interactions, and pharmacokinetics of, 562
   for lipid disorders, 188
   pregnancy and lactation and, 590
Sweet Annie *(Artemisia annua)*
   adverse effects, interactions, and pharmacokinetics of, 562-563
   for cancer, 471
   for malaria, 417, 424
Sweet basil *(Ocimum basilicum)*, 590
Sweet woodruff *(Galium odoratum)*, 591
Sympathetic nervous system activation in anxiety disorders, 17-18, 18f
Synbiotic, 403
Syncope, 140
Syndrome of inappropriate antidiuretic hormone secretion (SIADH), 243
Syndrome X, 219, 253
Synovial joint, 292f
Systemic lupus erythematosus (SLE), kidney disease due to, 364
   flax for, 367
Systolic pressure, 103
Syzygium claviflorum for HIV infection, 438b

T

T_3. *See* Triiodothyronine (T_3)
T_4. *See* Thyroxine (T_4)
Tachycardia, 138-140, *See Also* Arrhythmic
   supraventricular, 139
   ventricular, 139
Taenia saginata, 410
Taenia solium, 410
Tamanu *(Calophyllum inophyllum)*, 420
Tamarind *(Tamarindus indica)*, 591
Tangerine *(Citrus reticulata)*, 591
Tannin, adverse effects of, 486

Tansy *(Tanacetum vulgare)*, 591
Tapeworm infection, 410
   corydalis for, 419
Tarragon *(Artemisia dracunculus)*, 164
Taurine for weight loss, 261
TB. *See* Tuberculosis (TB)
TCM. *See* Traditional Chinese medicine (TCM)
Tea *(Camellia sinensis)*, 3
   adverse effects, interactions, and pharmacokinetics of, 563
   for Alzheimer's disease and related disorders, 96
   for anxiety and insomnia, 24
   for arthritis, 306-307
   for cancer prevention and treatment, 471-472
   for cognitive and physical enhancement, 49
   for congestive heart failure, 122
   for dental caries, 397
   for diabetes mellitus, 233
   for heart attack prevention, 147
   for lipid disorders, 188
   for menopausal symptoms, 274
   for Methicillin-resistant *Staphylococcus aureus*, 405, 397
   for osteoporosis prevention, 285
   for Parkinson's disease, 56, 59
   pregnancy and lactation and, 591
   for respiratory disorders, 208
   for weight loss, 258, 263
Tea tree *(Melaleuca alternifolia)*
   adverse effects, interactions, and pharmacokinetics of, 563
   for dental plaque and gingivitis, 397-398
   for fungal infection, 417, 425
   for methicillin-resistant *Staphylococcus aureus*, 397-398
   for oral herpes, 437
   pregnancy and lactation and, 591
TENS. *See* Transcutaneous electrical nerve stimulation (TENS)
Tension headache, 76
Terbinafine, 425
Testing, third-party, 6
TGs. *See* Triglycerides (TGs)
TGV. *See* Thunder god vine *(Tripterygium wilfordii)*
Theophylline for asthma, 208
Therapeutic lifestyle changes (TLC) diet, 172-173, 190
Therapeutic touch for pain, 83
Thiamin in cancer treatment, 482
Third-party testing, 6
Threadworm infection, 411-412
Thrombin, 156
Thrombocytopenia, 158-159
Thromboembolus, 158

Thrombosis, 155, 158
   coronary, 127, 135
   deep vein, 158
      integrative therapy plan for, 167
      pycnogenol for prevention of, 162
   integrative therapy plan for, 167
   rutin for, 163
   stroke due to, 137, 158
Thrush, oral, 413-414
   case study associated with, 424
   cinnamon for, 415
   tea tree for, 417
Thunder god vine *(Tripterygium wilfordii)*
   for arthritis, 307
   pregnancy and lactation and, 591
Thyme *(Thymus vulgaris)*
   adverse effects, interactions, and pharmacokinetics of, 564
   for coagulation disorders, 164
   for dental plaque, 398, 404
   for fungal infections, 418-419, 425
   pregnancy and lactation and, 591
Thymol. *See* Thyme *(Thymus vulgaris)*
Thyroid and parathyroid disorders, 244-246
   adjunct therapies for, 248-250
   case studies associated with, 249
   diagnosis of, 245-246
   herbal therapies for, 246-247, 247t
      with limited evidence, 247-248
   hyperparathyroidism, 245
   hyperthyroidism, 244
   hypoparathyroidism, 245
   hypothyroidism, 244-245
   nodules, 245
   tumors and cancer, 245
Thyroid-stimulating hormone (TSH), 241
   disorders of, 242-243
Thyrotropin, 241
Thyrotropin receptor-stimulating antibody (TRS-Ab), 246
Thyroxine (T_4), 241, 244
TIA. *See* Transient ischemic attack (TIA)
Tincture, 4
Tinea, 412
Tinea capitis, 412-413
Tinea corporis, 412-413
   garlic for, 416
Tinea cruris, 413
   garlic for, 416
Tinea pedis, 413
   garlic for, 416
   tea tree for, 417
Tinea unguium, 413
Tinea versicolor, 413
   bishop's weed for, 414-415
   selenium for, 423
   zinc for, 420
TLC diet. *See* Therapeutic lifestyle changes (TLC) diet

TNM staging of cancer, 449
Todd's paralysis, 62
Toenail, fungal infection of, 413
   tea tree for, 418
   thyme for, 418-419
Tonic-clonic seizure, 62, 62t
Total cholesterol levels, 172
Toxicity of cancer treatment, 476-479
Toxins, hepatic, 349, 355b, 356
Trachoma, 387
   goldenseal for, 394
Traditional Chinese medicine (TCM)
   for angina, 131b
   in cancer treatment, 482
   for congestive heart failure, 122b
   for dementia and senility, 97
   for ischemic heart disease and arrhythmias, 147b-148b
   for menopausal symptoms, 274
   for respiratory disorders, 209
   for thyroid disorders, 246
Transcutaneous electrical nerve stimulation (TENS), 481-482
Transient ischemic attack (TIA), 138
TRAUMEEL S, 479
Travel, malaria and, 424
Traveler's diarrhea, 318
Tree tobacco *(Nicotiana glauca)*, 591
Tree turmeric *(Berberis aristata)*. *See* Berberine
Tremor in Parkinson's disease, 55
Tribulus *(Tribulus terrestris)*
   adverse effects, interactions, and pharmacokinetics of, 564
   for angina, 131
   for cognitive and physical enhancement, 48, 51
   pregnancy and lactation and, 591
Trichinosis, 412
Trichomonas vaginalis, rhubarb for, 420
Trichuriasis, 412
Triglycerides (TGs), 171-172
   lowering of
      omega-3 fatty acids for, 181
      tea for, 188
Triiodothyronine (T_3), 241, 244
TRS-Ab. *See* Thyrotropin receptor-stimulating antibody (TRS-Ab)
Trypanosomes, 409
Tryptophan for weight loss, 261
T-score in osteoporosis diagnosis, 283
TSH. *See* Thyroid-stimulating hormone (TSH)
Tuberculoid leprosy, 385
Tuberculosis (TB), 388
   agrimony for, 398-399
   angostura for, 399
   astragalus for, 390
   bamboo for, 399
   beta-sitosterol for, 399

Tumor. *See Also* Cancer
  benign, 445
  thyroid, 245
Tumor markers, 448
Turmeric *(Curcuma longa)*
  adverse effects, interactions, and pharmacokinetics of, 564-565
  for Alzheimer's disease and related disorders, 96
  for arthritis, 304-305, 312
  for cancer prevention and treatment, 473
  for coagulation disorders, 163
  for gastrointestinal disorders, 333
  for HIV/AIDS, 437, 442
  for inflammation, 78
  for lipid disorders, 188
  for liver disorders, 353
  pregnancy and lactation and, 591
  for respiratory disorders, 210
Turpentine *(Pinus palustris)*, 591
T wave, 140
Tylophora *(Tylophora indica)*
  adverse effects, interactions, and pharmacokinetics of, 565
  pregnancy and lactation and, 591
  for respiratory disorders, 208-209
Type 1 diabetes, 218. *See Also* Diabetes mellitus
  fenugreek for, 225
  fig for, 225
Type 2 diabetes, 218. *See Also* Diabetes mellitus
  ashwagandha for, 221
  beet for, 222
  berberine for, 222
  cinnamon for, 224
  fenugreek for, 225
  ginseng for, 226
  myrcia for, 229
  pycnogenol, 230
  reishi mushroom for, 232
  soy for, 232
  weight management and, 263

U

Ukrain, 458-459
Ulcer. *See* Peptic ulcer disease
Ulcerative colitis, 319. *See Also* Inflammatory bowel disease (IBD)
  aloe for, 320-321
  barley for, 322
Ultrasonography, carotid, 128, 138
Uncoating of virus, 428
United States Department of Agriculture (USDA), 3
Unstable angina, 127, 135
Upper gastrointestinal disorders, 162, 316-318

Upper respiratory tract infection (URI), 388
  andrographis for, 389
  case study associated with, 405-406
  echinacea for, 399, 434, 441
  garlic for, 435
Urethritis, 388
Urge incontinence, 361
  during menopause, 276
URI. *See* Upper respiratory tract infection (URI)
Uric acid kidney stone, 363
Uric acid levels in gout, 296
Urinalysis, 389
Urinary incontinence, 361
  adjunct therapies for, 375
  during menopause, 276
Urinary system, 360f. *See Also* Genitourinary disorders
Urinary tract infection (UTI), 388-389
  bromelain for, 391-392
  case study for, 405
  cranberry for, 375-376, 392, 398, 404
  horseradish for, 395
  lingonberry for, 395-396
  uva ursi for, 398
  vitamin C for, 403
  zinc for, 403
Urolithiasis, 363-364
  cornflower for, 374
  cranberry for, 366, 377
  grapefruit for, 368
Urosepsis, 388
USDA. *See* United States Department of Agriculture (USDA)
Uterus
  cancer of
    podophyllum for, 463-464
    signs and symptoms of, 447
  prolapsed, 362
Uva ursi *(Arctostaphylos uva-ursi)*
  adverse effects, interactions, and pharmacokinetics of, 565
  for congestive heart failure, 124
  pregnancy and lactation and, 591
  for urinary tract infection, 398, 405
U wave, 140

V

Vaccination, 428
  influenza, 441
  measles, mumps, rubella, 430
Vagina
  candidiasis infection of, 414
  probiotics for, 423-424
  tea tree for, 417
  changes in during menopause, 267
Vaginal cones and balls for urinary incontinence treatment, 375

Vaginitis
  case study for, 377
  chamomile for, 365-366
  tea tree for, 417
Valerian *(Valeriana officinalis)*
  adverse effects, interactions, and pharmacokinetics of, 565-566
  for anxiety and insomnia, 24, 26-27
  in Parkinson's disease, 58
  pregnancy and lactation and, 591
  for seizure disorders, 65
Vanilla *(Vanilla planifolia)*, 591
Varicella-zoster virus, 429-430
  licorice for, 435-436
Vascular dementia, 86-87
Vasomotor symptoms in menopause, 267
Vasopressin. *See* Antidiuretic hormone (ADH)
Venoruton for diuresis, 122
Ventricular fibrillation, 135, 139-140
Ventricular tachycardia (VT), 139
Verbena *(Verbena officinalis)*, 592
Very-low-density lipoproteins (VLDLs), 171
Vessel wall, hemostasis and, 155-156
Vibrio cholerae, 384, 395
Viral infection, 427-443
  adjunct therapies for, 440
  case studies associated with, 441
  in diarrhea, 318
  in hepatitis, 344
    astragalus for, 346-350
    ayurveda for, 353b
    milk thistle for, 349
    spirulina for, 353
  herbal therapies for, 431, 439t-430t
    with limited evidence, 438-440
    with negative evidence, 438
  in infectious arthritis, 295
  integrative therapy plan for, 440-442
  life cycle of virus in, 428
  overview of, 427-431
  types of, 428-430
Visceral pain, 70
Visual analog pain scale, 71
Vitamins
  deficiencies due to diarrhea, 339
  in HIV treatment, 440
Vitamin A in cancer treatment, 480-481
Vitamin B_6
  in epilepsy treatment, 66
  versus ginger for morning sickness, 326
Vitamin B_2 for malaria, 423
Vitamin C
  in cancer treatment, 482
  for urinary tract infection, 403
Vitamin D
  in epilepsy treatment, 66
  for hyperparathyroidism, 248

Vitamin D *(Continued)*
    for menopausal symptoms, 276
    for osteoporosis, 285-286, 288
Vitamin E
    for dementia, 98
    in epilepsy treatment, 66
Vitamin K
    in coagulation cascade, 156
    intake of in healthy diet, 166
    for reversal of effects of warfarin, 166
VLDLs. *See* Very-low-density lipoproteins (VLDLs)
Volatile oils, 4
Vomiting, 317-318
    acupressure and acupuncture for, 339
    carob for, 323
    chemotherapy-induced, 327, 476
    ginger for, 326
    during pregnancy, 318
        ginger for, 326
Von Willebrand disease, 157, 159

W

Waist circumference, abdominal obesity and, 253
Waist-to-hip ratio (WHR), 262
Walking. *See* Gait
Warfarin
    astragalus and, 152
    bacopa and, 100
    chia and, 152
    garlic and, 152
    ginkgo and, 99-100
    vitamin K for reversal of effects of, 166
Warts, genital, 437
Watercress *(Nasturtium officinale)*, 592
Water hemlock *(Cicuta* spp.), 66
Weight loss, 44, 253-258, 260t. *See Also* Obesity
    for arthritis, 310
    bitter orange for, 49, 51
    capsicum for, 254
    due to cancer, 446
    guarana for, 46
    in HIV, 440
West syndrome, 63

Wheatgrass *(Triticum aestivum)*
    adverse effects, interactions, and pharmacokinetics of, 566
    for inflammatory bowel disease, 334
    pregnancy and lactation and, 592
Whipworm infection, 412
White hellebore *(Veratrum album)*. *See* False hellebore *(Veratrum* spp.)
White horehound *(Marrubium vulgare)*
    adverse effects, interactions, and pharmacokinetics of, 566
    for diabetes mellitus, 234
    for gastrointestinal disorders, 334
    for lipid disorders, 189
    for pain, 78
    pregnancy and lactation and, 592
WHR. *See* Waist-to-hip ratio (WHR)
Wild indigo *(Baptisia australis, Baptisia tinctoria)*
    adverse effects, interactions, and pharmacokinetics of, 567
    for respiratory tract infection, 437-438
Wild yam *(Dioscorea villosa)*
    adverse effects, interactions, and pharmacokinetics of, 567
    for lipid disorders, 189
    for menopausal symptoms, 273-274
    pregnancy and lactation and, 592
Willow *(Salix* spp.)
    adverse effects, interactions, and pharmacokinetics of, 567-568
    for arthritis, 305-306, 311
    for cardiovascular health, 147b-148b, 150
    for coagulation disorders, 164
    for pain, 78-79, 83
    pregnancy and lactation and, 592
Wilson's disease, 345
Wiskott-Aldrich syndrome, 157
Withdrawal, black pepper for masking symptoms of, 51
Wolff-Parkinson-White syndrome, 139
Wong-Baker Faces Pain Rating Scale, 71f
Worms, parasitic, 410-412
Wormwood *(Artemisia absinthium)*, 592
Wound healing
    arnica for, 72
    cat's claw for, 79
Wuchereria bancrofti, 411

X

Xanthelasma, 171
Xanthoma, 171
Xerostomia, radiotherapy-induced, 476-479

Y

Yarrow *(Achillea millefolium)*
    for bacterial infection, 400
    pregnancy and lactation and, 592
Yeast infection, 413-414
Yellow dock *(Rumex crispus)*
    for liver disorders, 353
    pregnancy and lactation and, 592
Yerba santa *(Eriodictyon californicum)*
    for malaria and trypanosomes, 420
    pregnancy and lactation and, 592
    for respiratory infection, 400
Yew *(Taxus* spp.), 592
YGD for weight loss, 255
Yoga
    for angina, 132
    in cancer treatment, 480
    for hypertension, 110-111
    in seizure disorders treatment, 66
    for smoking cessation, 210
    for weight loss, 262
Yohimbe *(Pausinystalia yohimbe)*
    adverse effects, interactions, and pharmacokinetics of, 568-569
    for coagulation disorders, 163
    for Parkinson's disease, 57
    pregnancy and lactation and, 592
    for psychiatric disorders, 14
    seizures or lower seizure threshold due to, 66
    for sexual function, 373, 376, 378
Yucca *(Yucca schidigera)*
    adverse effects, interactions, and pharmacokinetics of, 569
    for lipid disorders, 189

Z

Zinc
    for cutaneous leishmaniasis, 420
    for urinary tract infection, 403